Nanoparticle-Based Drug Delivery in Cancer Treatment

Nanotechnology for Drugs, Vaccines and Smart Delivery Systems

Series Editors:
Ram K. Gupta, Tuan Anh Nguyen

This book series aims to provide an overview of the recent development in vaccine and drug design, smart delivery systems, and characterizations. Many topics related to the applications of nanotechnology in the advancement of drugs, vaccines, and delivery systems will be discussed. Each book in this series will be authored or contributed by experts and global research teams will participate. The level of presentation is intended for students, scientists, researchers, and industries dealing with nanotechnology for advanced drugs, vaccines, and targeted delivery systems.

RNA Delivery Function for Anticancer Therapeutics
Loutfy H. Madkour

Nanoparticle-Based Drug Delivery in Cancer Treatment
Loutfy H. Madkour

For more information on this book series, please visit https://www.routledge.com/Nanotechnology-for-Drugs-Vaccines-and-Smart-Delivery-Systems/book-series/CRCNANDRUVAC

Nanoparticle-Based Drug Delivery in Cancer Treatment

Loutfy H. Madkour

CRC Press
Taylor & Francis Group
Boca Raton London New York

CRC Press is an imprint of the
Taylor & Francis Group, an **informa** business

First edition published 2022
by CRC Press
6000 Broken Sound Parkway NW, Suite 300, Boca Raton, FL 33487-2742

and by CRC Press
2 Park Square, Milton Park, Abingdon, Oxon, OX14 4RN

Library of Congress Cataloging-in-Publication Data
Names: Madkour, Loutfy H. (Loutfy Hamid), author.
Title: Nanoparticle-based drug delivery in cancer treatment / Loutfy H. Madkour.
Description: First edition. | Boca Raton : CRC Press, 2022. | Series:
Nanotechnology for drugs, vaccines and smart delivery systems |
Includes bibliographical references and index.
Identifiers: LCCN 2021039307 (print) | LCCN 2021039308 (ebook) |
ISBN 9781032135205 (hardback) | ISBN 9781032135212 (paperback) |
ISBN 9781003229674 (ebook)
Subjects: LCSH: Nanoparticles—Therapeutic use. | Cancer—Treatment. |
Drug delivery systems. | Nanomedicine.
Classification: LCC RC271.N36 M33 2022 (print) | LCC RC271.N36 (ebook) |
DDC 616.99/4061—dc23/eng/20211201
LC record available at https://lccn.loc.gov/2021039307
LC ebook record available at https://lccn.loc.gov/2021039308

ISBN: 9781032135205 (hbk)
ISBN: 9781032135212 (pbk)
ISBN: 9781003229674 (ebk)

DOI: 10.1201/9781003229674

Typeset in Times
by codeMantra

Contents

Preface

Cancer has become one of the most complex diseases due to numerous genetic disorders and cellular abnormalities. Cancer disease continues to be a major health concern worldwide being the second leading cause of death in the world. According to the World Health Organization (WHO), nearly ten million people are estimated to die of cancer by the year 2020. Cancer is caused by various mutations in hundreds of genes including both proto-oncogenes and tumor suppressor genes. Nanotechnology offers a variety of conjugate and particle-packaging methods that utilize the special characteristics of nucleic acids and could mediate the delivery of oligonucleotides directly into blood cancer cells. While most of these developments were able to silence genes in various blood cancer cell lines *in vitro*, only few of them demonstrated *in vivo* gene silencing, in disperse mouse models of leukemia/lymphoma, or *ex vivo*, in patients' primary cells and in clinical trials. For many years, studies of siRNA have progressively advanced toward novel treatment strategies against cancer. Recently, the clinical success rate of RNAi therapeutics is increasing and now some are on the right track to gain Food and Drug Administration (FDA) approval in the next year or two.

Emerging therapeutics that utilize RNA interference (RNAi) have the potential to treat broad classes of diseases due to their ability to reversibly silence target genes. In August 2018, the FDA approved the first siRNA therapeutic, called ONPATTRO™ (Patisiran), for the treatment of transthyretin-mediated amyloidosis. This was an important milestone for the field of siRNA delivery that opened the door for additional siRNA drugs. Currently, more than 20 small interfering RNA (siRNA)-based therapies are in clinical trials for a wide variety of diseases including cancers, genetic disorders, and viral infections. To maximize therapeutic benefits of siRNA-based drugs, a number of chemical strategies have been applied to address issues associated with efficacy, specificity, and safety. This book focuses on the chemical perspectives behind nonviral siRNA delivery systems, including siRNA synthesis, siRNA conjugates, and nanoparticle (NP) delivery using nucleotides, lipids, and polymers. Tracing and understanding the chemical development of strategies to make siRNAs into drugs is important to guide development of additional clinical candidates and enable prolonged success of siRNA therapeutics.

siRNA is a promising drug candidate, expected to have broad therapeutic potentials toward various diseases including viral infections and cancer. With recent advances in bioconjugate chemistry and carrier technology, several siRNA-based drugs have advanced to clinical trials. However, most cases address local applications or diseases in the filtering organs, reflecting the remaining challenges in systemic delivery of siRNA. The difficulty in siRNA delivery is in large part due to poor circulation stability and unfavorable pharmacokinetics and biodistribution profiles of siRNA. siRNA has gained attention as a potential therapeutic reagent due to its ability to inhibit specific genes in many genetic diseases. In order to develop siRNAs as therapeutic agents for cancer treatment, delivery strategies for siRNA must be carefully designed and potential gene targets carefully selected for optimal anticancer effects.

The use of nanotechnology applications to develop nanodelivery systems has allowed researchers to overcome limitations of antineoplastic drugs by increasing the solubility of the drug and decreasing the toxicity to healthy tissues. Great efforts have been made over the past decades in biology with the aim of searching novel and more efficient tools in therapy. However, RNA drugs, typically siRNAs, are rapidly degraded by RNases and filtrated in the kidney, thereby requiring a delivery vehicle for efficient transport to the target cells. To date, various delivery formulations have been developed from cationic lipids, polymers, and/or inorganic NPs for systemic delivery of siRNA to solid tumors.

In recent years, application of NPs in diagnosis and treatment of cancer has been the object of extensive research. Among these studies, some have focused on the dose enhancement effect of gold nanoparticles (GNPs) in radiation therapy of cancer. It is clear from the introduced work that functional-molecule-coated MSNs are stable and biocompatible. Moreover, such nanocomposites display much potential applications in the biomedical field, such as photodynamic therapy, cell imaging, and selective recognition. These strategies may be universal methods for constructing hybrid organic–inorganic nanomaterials that can be widely applied in the biomedical field.

Nanomaterials such as carbon nanotubes (CNTs), quantum dots, and dendrimers have unique properties that can be exploited for diagnostic purposes, thermal ablation, and drug delivery in cancer.

Cancer occurs as a result of a series of gene mutations in a cell. The activation of anti-apoptotic pathways is a defense mechanism that rescues cells from cell death. Cancer is one of the most complex diseases that have resulted in multiple genetic disorders and cellular abnormalities. Cancer is a generic term that encompasses a group of diseases characterized by an uncontrolled proliferation of cells. There are more than 200 different types of cancer, each of which gains its nomenclature according to the type of tissue the cell originates in. Many patients who succumb to cancer do not die as a result of the primary tumor, but because of the systemic effects of metastases on other regions away from the original site. One of the aims of cancer therapy is to prevent the metastatic process as early as possible. There are currently many therapies in clinical use, and recent advances in biotechnology lend credence to the potential of nanotechnology in the fight against cancer.

Key challenges to siRNA usage in clinic lay both in selecting the best of this vast selection of possible targets and in optimizing delivery of the siRNA agents to individual tumors. Choice of target and delivery route are very important for enhancing therapeutic efficacy in cancer and should be done in a manner designed to minimize side effects in normal tissue. Since delivery and target selection are perhaps the ultimate limitations for siRNA-based therapy, we will conclude with a few thoughts on these final challenges.

In this book, various modifications and delivery strategies for siRNA delivery are discussed. In addition, we present current thinking on target gene selection in major tumor types. The progress of siRNA therapy as well as its medical application via NP-mediated delivery for cancer treatment has been discussed. In addition, siRNAs have been studied for the treatment of various human diseases such as genetic disorders, ocular conditions, cardiovascular diseases, viral infections, and cancers. siRNA has received much attention due to its sequence-specific gene-silencing efficacy and universality in therapeutic target. Despite its promising potentials as gene therapeutics, a lot of limitations to clinical applications of siRNA remain to be overcome; not only the inherent properties of siRNA but also delivery barriers have been considered as serious challenges in clinical translation of siRNA drugs. There are many efforts to develop safe and efficient gene carriers, but recently, the improvement of physicochemical properties of siRNA itself has been accompanied through chemical and structural modifications. The chemically or structurally modified siRNA could exhibit enhanced stability, reduced off-target effects, and minimized immunogenicity. Furthermore, the development of siRNA conjugates, the increase in siRNA size, and the construction of nucleic acid nanostructures could achieve the advancements in siRNA delivery properties. Thus, rational design of the modified siRNA and integrating it with an efficient delivery carrier can overcome hurdles to clinical translation of siRNA therapeutics.

Better elucidation of the mechanism of action, the impact of chemical modifications that stabilize and reduce nonspecific effects of siRNA molecules, and the key design considerations for effective delivery systems has spurred progress toward developing clinically successful siRNA therapies.

In this book, we discuss recent advances in NP-mediated siRNA delivery systems and the application of these systems in clinical trials for cancer therapy. Furthermore, we offer perspectives on future applications of siRNA therapeutics.

Cancer tissue is usually characterized by rapid and abrupt angiogenesis processes, resulting in leaky and defective blood vessels with large fenestrations, due to extensive endothelial cell disorganization. Also, the smooth-muscle layer is frequently absent or abnormal in the vascular wall, leading to passive dilatation of vessels. The consequence is the enhanced extravasation of macromolecules in the tumor tissue, in contrast to low-molecular-weight molecules that undergo rapid renal clearance.

In the last decades, there have been tremendous research efforts to develop efficient and powerful cancer therapies. Cancer nanotechnology is a rapidly emerging field that holds great promise for revolutionizing cancer detection, diagnosis, treatment, and cure. Most cancer nanotechnology advances are primarily focused on developing nanoengineered materials that can significantly impact noninvasive molecular-scale imaging techniques and targeted delivery of drugs. Further, multifunctional nanostructures are being developed that can simultaneously serve as contrast agents for enhanced imaging and nanovectors for targeted drug delivery or therapies. However, it is critical to identify/synthesize specific biomarkers, which, when conjugated to nanostructures, will target them only to specific tumor sites. The achievement of the goals of nanotechnology-mediated early cancer detection and more efficacious therapies requires synergistic integration and convergence of a variety of disciplines. These include cancer biology, materials science and engineering, biomedical engineering, toxicology, computer science and engineering, chemistry, physics, and mathematics. Engineered properties of NPs are opening the door to new, noninvasive strategies for cancer therapy, not previously possible. This would include photothermal therapy, NP-enhanced radiotherapy, targeted combinatorial cancer therapy, and NP-enhanced radiofrequency cancer therapy. With more synthetic approaches for the preparation of carrier-free nanodrugs than ever, we expect a range of new carrier-free formulations to be developed and employed in cancer therapy in the future. With more knowledge about immunosuppressive and activating cells and pathways, the combinational use of immunotherapy with anticancer agents will promote the success of carrier-free nanodrugs. Eventually, these nanodrugs should be tuned to optimize their key properties such as size, shape, surface chemistry, and long-term stability. Furthermore, cancer nanotechnology holds the potential to ultimately improve access to cancer care worldwide.

To date, enormous investigations have been conducted to enhance medicines' target-oriented delivery to improve their therapeutic index. In this regard, lipid-based carrier systems might have been regarded as prime delivery systems that are very close to the natural cell-derived vesicles used for biomolecular communication among cells from occasionally remote tissues. Upon examination of the literature, we found a chasm between groups of investigations in drug pharmaceutics and thought that maybe holistic research could provide better information with respect to drug delivery inside the body, especially when they are going to be injected directly into the bloodstream for systemic distribution.

Recent promising clinical results of RNA therapeutics have drawn significant attention of academia and industries to RNA therapeutics and their carrier systems. To improve their feasibility in clinics, systemic evaluations of currently available carrier systems under clinical trials and preclinical studies are needed. In this book, we focus on recent noticeable preclinical studies and clinical results regarding siRNA-based conjugates for clinical translations. Advantages and drawbacks of siRNA-based conjugates are discussed, compared to particle-based delivery systems. Then, representative siRNA-based conjugates with aptamers, peptides, carbohydrates, lipids, polymers, and nanostructured materials are introduced. To improve the feasibility of siRNA conjugates in preclinical studies, several considerations for the rational design of siRNA conjugates in terms of cleavability, immune responses, multivalent conjugations, and mechanism of action are also presented. Lastly, we discuss lessons from previous preclinical and clinical studies related to siRNA conjugates and perspectives of their clinical applications.

The direct conjugation of siRNA and carriers or the use of polymerized siRNA can improve the loading efficiency of siRNA into gene carriers. Finally, recent advances in nucleic acid NP systems for efficient siRNA delivery are highlighted.

Cancer immunotherapy aimed at boosting cancer-specific immunoresponses to eradicate tumor cells has evolved as a new treatment modality. NPs incorporating antigens and immunomodulatory agents can activate immune cells and modulate the tumor microenvironment to enhance antitumor immunity. The nanotechnology approach has been demonstrated to be superior to standard formulations in *in vivo* settings. NP-based cancer immunotherapy, including peptide- and nucleic acid-based nanovaccines, nanomedicines containing an immunoadjuvant to activate antitumor immunity, NP delivery of immune checkpoint inhibitors, and the combination of the above approaches. In addition, combination of the compound nanoparticles with molecules of immune checkpoint inhibitors or photodynamic therapy could complement each other and more efficiently suppress tumor proliferation at the primary and metastatic sites. Nanoparticles with specific features could also control the release of payloads in response to typical conditions in the tumor microenvironment including hypoxia, specific protease and decreased pH condition, and further alter the immunosuppressive microenvironment into immune-supportive features. Thus, the redox-sensitive-based delivery strategy was often utilized as an effective way for controlled release of drugs into the tumor microenvironment. Encouraging results and new emerging nanotechnologies in drug delivery promise the continuous growth of this field and ultimately clinical translation of enhanced immunotherapy of cancer.

Clinical applications of many anticancer drugs are restricted due to their hydrophobic nature, requiring the use of harmful organic solvents for administration, and poor selectivity and pharmacokinetics resulting in off-target toxicity and inefficient therapies. A wide variety of carrier-based NPs have been developed to tackle these issues, but such strategies often fail to encapsulate drug efficiently and require significant amounts of inorganic and/or organic nanocarriers, which may cause toxicity problems in the long term. Preparation of nanoformulations for the delivery of water-insoluble drugs without using carriers is thus desired, requiring elegantly designed strategies for products with high quality, stability, and performance. These strategies include simple self-assembly or involving chemical modifications via coupling drugs together or conjugating them with various functional molecules such as lipids, carbohydrates, and photosensitizers. During nanodrug synthesis, insertion of redox-responsive linkers and tumor-targeting ligands endows them with additional characteristics such as on-target delivery, and conjugation with immunotherapeutic reagents enhances immune response alongside therapeutic efficacy.

Cancer immunotherapy, which could utilize the host's immune system to kill tumor cells, has great potential in long-term inhibition of tumor growth and recurrence compared to chemotherapy and radiotherapy. Tumors exhibit powerful adaption to escape the destruction of immune system at the late stage of diseases due to overactivation of immune checkpoint pathways that function as natural "brakes" for immune responses. The newly emerging immune checkpoint inhibitors are regarded as the breakthrough for cancer immunotherapy as they can re-boost the host's immune system by restoring T-cell function and promoting cytotoxic T lymphocyte (CTL) responses.

Although NPs incorporating small immunomodulatory compounds have shown efficiency in preclinical models, their clinical application is limited due to the lack of potency. To induce potent immunoresponse for effective anticancer therapy, these immunomodulatory small molecules may need to combine with other agents. Additionally, their delivery needs to be targeted or localized to minimize the side effects and improve the efficacy.

The objective of this book was to develop a topical siRNA delivery system that can permeate through the stratum corneum and viable epidermis and efficiently deposit therapeutic levels of siRNA to the basal epidermis/upper dermis where melanoma cells reside. To achieve this objective, a series of liposome compositions that contained various concentrations of edge activator in their structures were prepared and then complexed with siRNA at different ratios to generate a small library of liposome–siRNA complexes (lipoplexes) with different physicochemical properties. In this book, we used melanoma as a disease model. Through the use of quantitative imaging analysis, we identified the necessary design parameters for effective permeation of lipoplexes through the skin layers and deposition at the upper dermis. The ability of the formulated lipoplexes to internalize into melanoma cells, knock down the expression of the BRAF protein, and induce cell death in melanoma cells was studied by fluorescent microscopy, in-cell immunofluorescence assay, and WST-1 cell proliferation assay. By providing direct quantitative and qualitative microscopy evidence, the results of this study demonstrate for the first time that the passive delivery of an edge-activated liposomal formulation can effectively carry siRNA through the stratum corneum and deposit it at the lower epidermis/upper dermis.

Despite significant advances, anticancer therapy strategies still suffer from severe drawbacks. One of the main limitations of most treatments is the lack of selectivity for the tumor tissues resulting in severe side effects for patients that limit their compliance.

This book presents relevant published data related to microRNA (miRNA) and RNAi delivery using NPs in cancer therapy. Due to the high incidence of death among cancer patients, there is an urgent demand for the development of novel and innovative delivery systems for therapeutic agents. For most cases, a single targeted therapeutic agent may not be sufficient [1], and therefore, NPs are designed to assure an efficient delivery. The book summarizes the most recent data in the field of NP design and functionalization in the context of targeted and efficient therapy. The book presents in a well-structured manner the newest developments in the field of nanotechnology, one of the most rising research niches from our times. Besides the basic strategies, we also discuss the latest forms of therapy involving nucleic acid delivery at targeted sites in the form of miRNA and siRNA. The present book is also complemented by the comprehensive presentation of the chimeric antigen receptor (CAR) T-cell therapy, a novel domain with high-ranking chances of success in the clinical scenario. Therefore, we hope that this book will feed the need of both researchers and clinicians in the attempt to develop and implement superior forms of therapies for the benefit of patients. Moreover, the comprehensive presentation of the current achievements will stimulate the idea of hybrid nanostrategies that will combine their advantages of different therapies, minimizing at the same time the downsides associated with each type of therapy.

SUMMARY

Recent progress in RNA biology has broadened the scope of therapeutic targets of RNA drugs for cancer therapy. This book describes the current status of clinical trials related to siRNA-based cancer therapy, as well as the remaining issues that need to be overcome to establish a successful therapy. It, then, introduces various promising design strategies of delivery vehicles for stable and targeted siRNA delivery, including the prospects for future design.

This book describes the pharmacokinetics and biodistribution of siRNA nanomedicines, focusing on those reported in the past 3 years, and their pharmacological effects in selected disease models such as hepatocellular carcinoma, liver infections, and respiratory diseases. The examples discussed here will provide an insight into the current state of the art and unmet needs in siRNA delivery.

There are several general concepts that are important in NP drug delivery. These include the enhanced permeability and retention (EPR) effect, NP clearance by the mononuclear phagocyte system (MPS), and desirable NP characteristics for cancer applications. To fully take advantage of the EPR effect, NPs must remain in circulation long enough for tumor accumulation. However, NPs are prone to clearance by the MPS, previously called the reticuloendothelial system. The MPS is part of the immune system that is mainly responsible for clearing macromolecules from circulation [2]. The MPS comprises bone marrow progenitors, blood monocytes, and tissue macrophages. It also includes the Kupffer cells of the liver and macrophages of the spleen, which are responsible for clearance of macromolecules from circulation. NPs can interact with MPS cells and lead to their opsonization. Since premature elimination from circulation will prevent NPs from accumulating in tumors, much effort has been devoted to creating "stealth" NPs. The most common strategy has been grafting polyethylene glycol (PEG) or other macromolecules such as polysaccharides onto the NP surface [3]. The presence of PEG or other molecules enables steric stabilization, preventing protein adsorption, interactions among particles, and interactions with immune cells.

The development of technologies for detecting cancer at an early stage, before metastasis, presents a major challenge.

Although nanotechnology has not yet been deployed clinically for cancer diagnosis, it is already on the market in a variety of medical tests and screens, such as the use of GNPs in home pregnancy tests [4]. For cancer diagnosis, NPs are being applied to capture cancer biomarkers, such as cancer-associated proteins, circulating tumor DNA, circulating tumor cells, and exosomes [5]. An essential advantage of applying NPs for cancer detection lies in their large surface area-to-volume ratio relative to bulk materials [6]. Due to this property, NP surfaces can be densely covered with antibodies, small molecules, peptides, aptamers, and other moieties. These moieties can bind and recognize specific cancer molecules (Figure 1).

By presenting various binding ligands to cancer cells, multivalent effects can be achieved, which can improve the specificity and sensitivity of an assay [8].

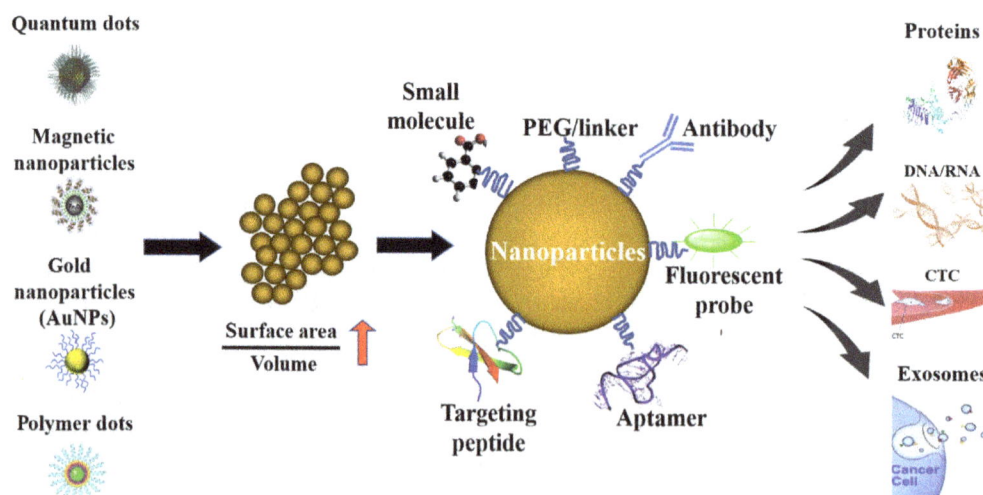

FIGURE 1 Nanotechnology improves cancer detection and diagnosis [7].

Nanotechnology-based diagnostic methods are being developed as promising tools for real-time, convenient, and cost-effective cancer diagnosis and detection [9]. This book summarizes recent progress in the development of nanotechnology and addresses the application of nanotechnology in cancer diagnosis. We also provide our perspective on challenges in the use of nanotechnology for cancer diagnosis.

MYC, an oncoprotein deregulated in over half of all human malignancies, has thus far been considered "undruggable" with conventional approaches. RNAi, a therapeutic approach that can be used to silence the *MYC* oncogene, has been shown to inhibit cancer growth in animal models. Synthetic DsiRNA with specificity for *MYC* has demonstrated highly potent activity *in vitro* (picomolar IC_{50}), and anti-MYC DsiRNA formulated in EnCore lipid NPs (DCR-MYC) has demonstrated activity *in vivo* across various tumor models. DCR-MYC is the first MYC-targeting siRNA to enter clinical trials.

RNAi can be considered a promising alternative for cancer therapy as it is less toxic than classical chemotherapy.

In the last 10 years, there has been an intense focus on miRNA research including miRNA targets and their impact on the up- or downregulation of various genes and on pathological processes. The high incidence of cancers has triggered a pressing need to develop new cancer therapeutics. miRNAs are associated with cell proliferation, metastasis, tumor progression, invasion, sustained angiogenesis, apoptosis, and drug resistance and radioresistance. Furthermore, many miRNAs are remarkably changed in almost all human cancers. As miRNAs exert their effect by targeting protein-coding messenger RNAs (mRNAs), verifying targets of dysregulated miRNAs is of utmost importance.

siRNA promises high efficacy and excellent specificity to silence the target gene expression, which shows potential for cancer treatment. However, systemic delivery of siRNA with selectivity to the tumor site and into the cytosol of tumor cells remains a major limitation. To achieve this, we generated oligoaminoamide-based sequence-defined polycationic oligomers by solid-phase-assisted synthesis, which can form polyplexes with anionic siRNA by electrostatic interaction to serve as siRNA carrier. Delivery of macromolecules such as siRNA into cells that reside in the basal epidermis of the skin is a major challenge due to the transport barriers that need to be overcome. siRNAs have potential therapeutic applications in various dermatological diseases such as psoriasis, atopic dermatitis, and cancer. Unfortunately, a low permeability of siRNA through the stratum corneum and epidermis has significantly limited its use for topical application.

A logical aim for initial siRNA translation is local therapies, as delivering siRNA directly to its site of action helps to ensure that a sufficient dose reaches the target tissue, lessens the potential for off-target side effects, and circumvents the substantial systemic delivery barriers. While locally injected or topically applied siRNA has progressed into numerous clinical trials, an enormous opportunity exists to develop sustained-release, local delivery systems that enable both spatial and temporal control of gene silencing. siRNA has the ability to disrupt cellular pathways by knocking down genes, opening the door to new treatments of diseases caused by aberrant gene expression. The use of nanocarriers prevents both renal clearance and RNase degradation by protecting siRNA chains and increasing their half-life in blood. siRNAs have been considered one of the most noteworthy developments that are able to regulate gene expression following a process known as RNAi. RNAi is a posttranscriptional mechanism that involves the inhibition of gene expression through promoting cleavage on a specific area of a target mRNA. This technology has shown promising therapeutic results for a good number of diseases, especially in cancer. However, siRNA therapeutics have to face important drawbacks in therapy including stability and successful siRNA delivery *in vivo*. In this regard, the development of effective siRNA delivery systems has helped addressing these issues by opening novel therapeutic windows that have allowed building up important advances in nanomedicine.

Thanks to a multitude of large-scale sequencing efforts, numerous genetic alterations have been identified in tumors, opening the way for the generation of siRNA therapeutics targeting both the mutant genes and in lesions in cancer signaling pathways arising from these genetic defects. Small-molecule or antibody drugs have proven quite effective for targeting certain cell surface and intracellular protein targets.

As already mentioned, the dysregulation of a given miRNA may alter the expression of hundreds of genes in cancer affecting the entire network in which targets are involved. By considering all experimental validation studies in cancer, genes targeted by miR-193a-3p are involved in several biological processes, including proliferation, apoptosis, migration, and metastasis. To acquire major advancements in knowledge and comprehension of the canonical and noncanonical mRNA targets, more studies involving the use of proteomics profiling and RNA pull-down with biotinylated miRNA mimics are needed.

The book focuses on material platforms that establish both localized and controlled gene silencing, with an emphasis on the systems that show most promise for clinical translation. In this book, we will survey the latest progress in the field of oligonucleotide-based nanomedicine in the heterogeneous group of hematological malignancies. We will describe the most advanced nonviral nanocarriers for oligonucleotide delivery to malignant blood cells, and a special emphasis will be made on the *ex vivo*, *in vivo*, and clinical trials, which are currently under development. However, a multi-sensitization individualized therapy designed specifically for each type of cancer cell may be more likely to prove viable to overcome cancer cell resistance. In the long term, future work should focus on identifying effective concentrations, dosage regimens, and combination with chemotherapy and radiotherapy, apart from the vectors. Once in use, the long-term results following miRNA therapy will need to be assessed.

Recently, small molecules and antibodies for cancer immunotherapy have been shown to have strong antitumor effects [10,11]. However, transcription factors and certain key oncoproteins such as Ras have proven difficult to access and block with conventional drug-based or antibody-mediated approaches. In terms of "undruggable" disease targets, siRNA therapeutics has the potential to specifically target and silence almost any gene target [12]. In addition, their process of identifying and optimizing a siRNA for a target is relatively rapid and siRNAs are easy to synthesize [13,14]. These characteristics strongly support the need to develop siRNA therapeutics for cancer treatment.

In this book, we introduce the basic mechanisms of the immune checkpoint pathways and outline the recent successes of immune checkpoint blockade (ICB) therapy in combination with NP delivery system. Furthermore, the underexplored potential in application of nanotechnology to enhance the efficacy of immune checkpoint therapy and overcome the limits of immune checkpoint inhibitors is also discussed.

These strategies necessitate the interaction of hematologists with fundamental cell biologists, immunologists, and materials scientists to focus on better understanding current pathology and potential opportunities to develop novel therapies based on receptor expression and biology.

Though these novel strategies increase the complexity of the delivery systems and will need approval for therapeutic use in humans, they may pave the way for improved RNA therapy in hematological malignancies, cancer, and other leukocyte-related diseases.

The recent progress in nanotechnology-based applications in cancer diagnosis is summarized in Figure 2.

Nanoparticle-Based Drug Delivery in Cancer Treatment, is a compilation of 15 chapters written by Loutfy H. Madkour.

These chapters will cover the fundamentals of technical advances in the nanotechnological developments of interfering RNA-based NPs and delivery vehicles and validated therapeutic RNAi–molecular target interactions. The book explains the results of clinical and preclinical trials including NP interfering RNA applications. NPs conjugated to the targeting ligand for effective siRNA delivery increase the chance of binding the tumor surface receptor; however, the process also increases the overall size of the NP. The book gives strategies that might be universal methods for constructing hybrid organic–inorganic nanomaterials and can be widely applied in the biomedical field. The applications of SiNPs in *in vitro* and *in vivo* tumor imaging demonstrated the potential for further developing the SiNPs

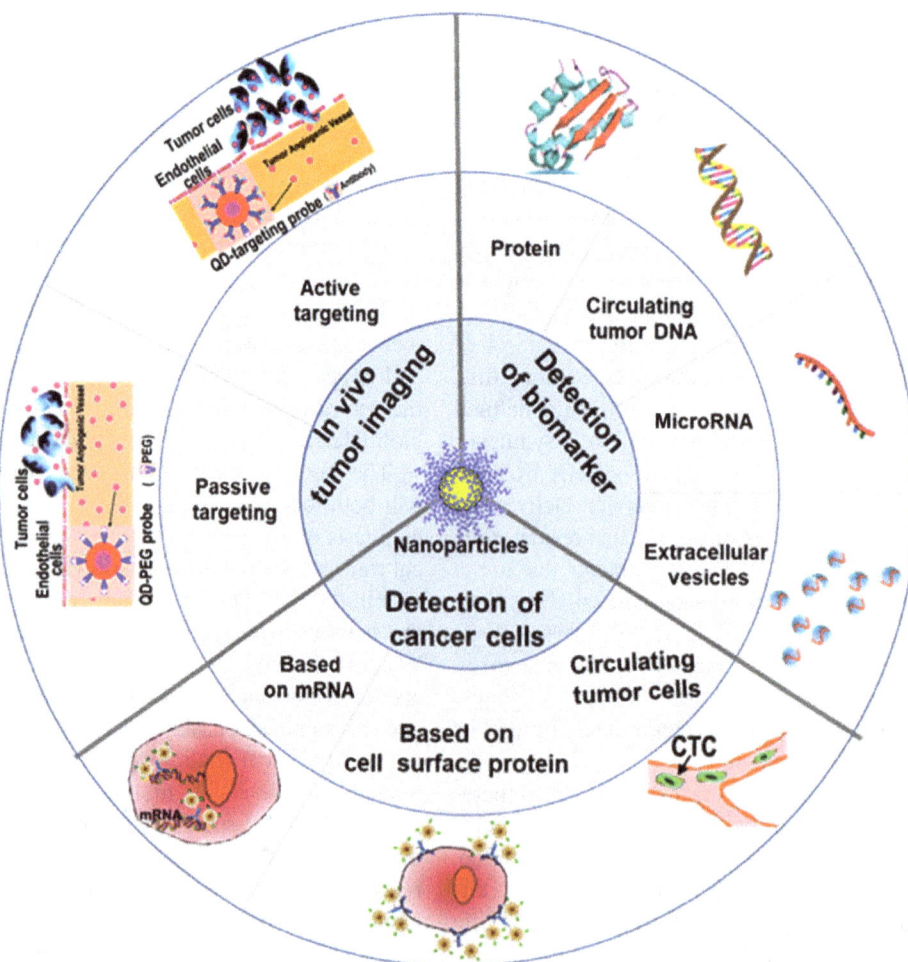

FIGURE 2   Schematic illustration of nanotechnology applications in cancer diagnosis [7].

into clinically useful reagents. Fluorescence imaging and MRI are currently the main strategies for the applications of SiNPs in cancer imaging. X-ray/CT may also be used along with SiNPs as imaging agents. Thus, the selection of appropriate cell-specific targeting moieties and careful design of stable and potent NP delivery systems are required for future development. A list of references at the end of each chapter is provided for the readers to learn more about a particular topic. Typically, these references include basic research, research papers, review articles, and articles from the popular literature. This book will be useful for students, teachers, and researchers in the various disciplines of life sciences, agricultural sciences, medicine, and biotechnology in universities, research institutions, and biotech companies.

REFERENCES

1. Y. Ma, X. Fan, L. Li, pH-sensitive polymeric micelles formed by doxorubicin conjugated prodrugs for co-delivery of doxorubicin and paclitaxel, *Carbohydr. Polym.* 137 (2016) 19–29.
2. I. Pastan, R. Hassan, D.J. Fitzgerald, et al. Immunotoxin therapy of cancer, *Nat. Rev. Cancer* 6 (2006) 559–565.
3. D. Peer, P. Zhu, C.V. Carman, et al. Selective gene silencing in activated leukocytes by targeting siRNAs to the integrin lymphocyte function-associated antigen-1, *Proc. Natl. Acad Sci. U. S. A.* 104 (2007) 4095–4100.
4. W. Zhou, X. Gao, D. Liu, X. Chen, Gold nanoparticles for in vitro diagnostics, *Chem. Rev.* 115 (2015) 10575. doi: 10.1021/acs.chemrev.5b00100.
5. S. Jia, R. Zhang, Z. Li, J. Li, Clinical and biological significance of circulating tumor cells, circulating tumor DNA, and exosomes as biomarkers in colorectal cancer, *Oncotarget* 8 (2017) 55632. doi: 10.18632/oncotarget.17184.
6. S. Song, Y. Qin, Y. He, Q. Huang, C. Fan, H.Y. Chen, *Chem. Soc. Rev.* 39 (2010) 4234.
7. Y. Zhang, M. Li, X. Gao, Y. Chen, T. Liu, Nanotechnology in cancer diagnosis: progress, challenges and opportunities, *J. Hematol. Oncol.* 12 (2019) 137, 1–13. doi: 10.1186/s13045-019-0833-3.
8. B. Kumar, R. Kumar; I.I. Skvortsova, V. Kumar, Mechanisms of tubulin binding ligands to target cancer cells: Updates on their therapeutic potential and clinical trials, *Curr. Cancer Drug Targets* 17 (2016) 357–375. doi: 10.2174/1568009616666160928110818.
9. X.J. Chen, X.Q. Zhang, Q. Liu, J. Zhang, G. Zhou, Nanotechnology: A promising method for oral cancer detection and diagnosis, *J. Nanobiotechnol.* 16 (2018) 52. doi: 10.1186/s12951-018-0378-6.
10. D.M. Pardoll, The blockade of immune checkpoints in cancer immunotherapy, *Nat. Rev. Cancer* 12 (2012) 252–264.
11. M.M. Gubin, X. Zhang, H. Schuster, E. Caron, J.P. Ward, T. Noguchi, Y. Ivanova, J. Hundal, C.D. Arthur, W.J. Krebber, G.E. Mulder, M. Toebes, M.D. Vesely, S.S. Lam, A.J. Korman, J.P. Allison, G.J. Freeman, A.H. Sharpe, E.L. Pearce, T.N. Schumacher, R. Aebersold, H.G. Rammensee, C.J. Melief, E.R. Mardis, W.E. Gillanders, M.N. Artyomov, R.D. Schreiber, Checkpoint blockade cancer immunotherapy targets tumour-specific mutant antigens, *Nature* 515 (2014) 577–581.
12. M. Toyoshima, H.L. Howie, M. Imakura, R.M.Walsh, J.E. Annis, A.N. Chang, J. Frazier, B.N. Chau, A. Loboda, P.S. Linsley, M.A. Cleary, J.R. Park, C. Grandori, Functional genomics identifies therapeutic targets for MYC-driven cancer, *Proc. Natl. Acad. Sci. U. S. A.* 109 (2012) 9545–9550.
13. O. Milhavet, D.S. Gary, M.P. Mattson, RNA interference in biology and medicine, *Pharmacol. Rev.* 55 (2003) 629–648.
14. S.J. Lee, M.J. Kim, I.C. Kwon, T.M. Roberts, Delivery strategies and potential targets for siRNA inmajor cancer types, *Adv. Drug Delivery Rev.* 104 (2016) 2–15

Author

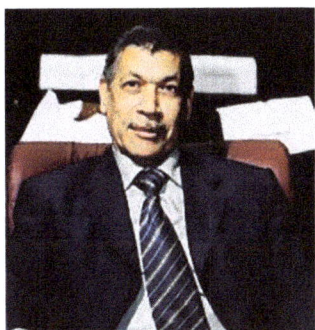

Prof. Loutfy H. Madkour is a professor of physical chemistry and nanoscience at Tanta University (Egypt). He earned his BSc, MSc, and PhD in physical chemistry from the Cairo, Minia, and Tanta universities in Egypt, respectively. He has published 200 peer-reviewed original research articles, 20 review articles, and 8 books. He is an editorial board member of several international journals, including *International Journal of Industrial Chemistry* (*IJIC*—Springer); *International Journal of Ground Sediment & Water; Global Drugs and Therapeutics; Chronicles of Pharmaceutical Science; Journal of Targeted Drug Delivery; UPI Journal of Pharmaceutical, Medical and Health Sciences; Global Journal of Nanomedicine; Clinical Pharmacology and Toxicology Research; Journal of Pharmacology & Pharmaceutical Research; LOJ Pharmacology & Clinical Research; CPQ Medicine; Pharmaceutical Sciences & Analytical Research Journal; Japan Journal of Research; Organic & Medicinal Chemistry International Journal; Nanotechnology & Applications; Materials Science Journal; Journal of Chemical Science and Chemical Engineering (JCSCE); United Journal of Nanotechnology and Medicine; Clinical Practice (Therapy)* journal; *Journal of Materials New Horizons; Journal of Radiology and Medical Imaging*; MedDocs Publishers; *World Journal of Pharmacy and Pharmaceutical Sciences (WJPPS); Journal of Material Science and Technology Research—RBM; Ecronicon: EC Clinical & Medical Case Reports (ECCMC); Medical Research and Health Sciences an Open Access Publication ISSN: 2589-9023 2589-9031; Acta Scientific Women's Health Journal as Women's Health Journal ; PHARMACOGNOSY Journal; and Journal of Community Medicine and Health Care Management.*

1 The Advantages and Versatility of Carrier-Free Nanodrug and Nanoparticle Systems for Cancer Therapy

1.1 NANOPARTICLES' (NPs) FABRICATION AND THEIR APPLICATIONS IN CANCER TREATMENT

Current cancer treatments include surgical intervention, radiation, and chemotherapeutic drugs, which often also kill healthy cells and cause toxicity to the patient. Conventional chemotherapeutic agents also do not show targeted action and are distributed nonspecifically in the body where they affect both cancerous and normal cells, thereby limiting the dose achievable within the tumor cells and also resulting in suboptimal treatment due to excessive toxicities.

Nanotechnology is the science of nanoscale, which is the scale of nanometers or one-billionth of a meter. Nanotechnology encompasses a broad range of technologies, materials, and manufacturing processes that are used to design and/or enhance many products, including medicinal products.

Green synthesis of nanoparticles (NPs) [1] is a global eco-friendly method to develop and produce nanomaterials with unique biological, physical, and chemical properties. This technology has achieved considerable progress in the oncology field in recent years. Recently, attention has shifted toward biological synthesis, owing to the disadvantages of physical and chemical synthesis, which include toxic yields, time and energy consumption, and high cost. Many natural sources are used in green fabrication processes, including yeasts, plants, fungi, actinomycetes, algae, and cyanobacteria. Cyanobacteria are among the most beneficial natural candidates used in the biosynthesis of NPs, due to their ability to accumulate heavy metals from their environment. They also contain a variety of bioactive compounds, such as pigments and enzymes, which may act as reducing and stabilizing agents. Cyanobacteria-mediated NPs have potential antibacterial, antifungal, antialgal, anticancer, and photocatalytic activities.

Most chemotherapeutic agents are not specific to the cancer cells they are intended to treat, and they can harm healthy cells, leading to numerous adverse effects. Due to this nonspecific targeting, it is not feasible to administer high doses that may harm healthy cells. Moreover, low doses can cause cancer cells to acquire resistance, thus making them hard to kill. A solution that could potentially enhance drug targeting and delivery lies in understanding the complexity of nanotechnology. Engineering pharmaceutical and natural products into nanoproducts can enhance the diagnosis and treatment of cancer. Novel nanoformulations such as liposomes, polymeric micelles, dendrimers, quantum dots (QDs), nanosuspensions, and gold nanoparticles (Au-NPs) have been shown to enhance the delivery of drugs. Improved delivery of chemotherapeutic agents targets cancer cells rather than healthy cells, thereby preventing undesirable side effects and decreasing chemotherapeutic drug resistance. Nanotechnology has also revolutionized cancer diagnosis by using nanotechnology-based imaging contrast agents that can specifically target and therefore enhance tumor detection. In addition to the delivery of drugs, nanotechnology can be used to deliver nutraceuticals like phytochemicals that have multiple properties, such as antioxidant activity, that protect cells from oxidative damage and reduce the risk of cancer. There have been multiple advancements and implications for the use of nanotechnology to enhance the delivery of both pharmaceutical and nutraceutical products in cancer prevention, diagnosis, and treatment [1].

Nanotechnology is an emerging field that includes synthesis, characterization, and development of various nanomaterials [2,3] that have significant roles in daily life, providing valuable products that improve industrial production, agriculture, communication, and medicine [4]. Currently, around 1000 commercial nanoproducts are available in world markets [5,6]. The term "nano" denotes any particles or materials with at least one nanosized (1–100 nm) dimension. NPs differ significantly from their bulk materials in terms of physical, chemical, and biological properties [7]. These differences are mainly due to their high surface area-to-volume ratio, which results in considerable differences in catalytic and thermal activities, melting point, conductivity, mechanical properties, and optical absorption. These properties make NPs applicable in almost all fields [8].

NPs have significant roles in bio-diagnostic and optical biosensing, nanophotonics, and imaging and treatment of many diseases affecting human health [9]. Silver nanoparticles (Ag-NPs) can interact effectively with microbe surfaces due to their small size and large surface area and are thus used as antimicrobial agents [10]. Ag-NPs synthesized using *Fusarium keratoplasticum* and embedded in cotton fiber showed significant antibacterial activity against pathogenic bacteria [11]. Carbon nanotubes (CNTs) have a key role in drug delivery, because of their capacity to carry drugs and control their release into target cells [12]. QD NPs have been used to detect the location of malignant cells inside the body [13]. Iron oxide NPs are used in resonance imaging and diagnosis of tumors [14]. Au-NPs are in high demand for various applications in multiple fields owing to their low toxicity [15]. In addition, Au-NPs have high photothermal and photoacoustic activity, making them suitable for use in photothermal therapy (PTT) for cancer. Other biogenic NPs such as copper oxide NPs [16], zinc oxide NPs [17], selenium NPs [18] acted as potent anticancer agents. The variation in NP shapes, including spherical, cubic, needles, triangular, and rod, enables them to be used in diverse areas such as device manufacture, electronics, optics, and biofuel cells (Figure 1.1) [19].

The physicochemical routes used to produce NPs are often unwieldy and expensive and result in liberation of toxic byproducts that threaten ecological systems [20]. To avoid these drawbacks, green synthesis of NPs using biogenic agents has become an alternative to chemical and physical synthesis [21]. Diatoms, mushrooms, algae, plants, fungi, bacteria, actinomycetes, lichen, cyanobacteria, and microalgae have been shown to successfully reduce metal precursors to their corresponding NPs [22]. Intra- and extracellular green synthesis techniques have been developed to reduce bulk materials to nanoforms using biological extracts [23]. These nanomaterials can be synthesized in the presence of biocompounds such as flavanones, amides, enzymes, proteins, pigments, polysaccharides, phenolics, terpenoids, or alkaloids, to aid the reduction and stabilization of NPs [22]. A high surface area-to-volume ratio is the target physical feature of NPs, as it confers their versatile applicability and ability to withstand harsh conditions [24]. The shape and size of NPs synthesized by microorganisms can be controlled by various abiotic and biotic factors, including pH, temperature, the nature of the microorganisms, their biochemical activity, and interactions with heavy metals [25–27].

In the past few years, the synthesis of NPs using cyanobacteria has become an active research field [25,28]. Cyanobacteria are a diverse group of photoautotrophic prokaryotes that exist in a wide range of ecosystems [29]. They are distinguished by their ability to fix atmospheric nitrogen (N_2) by reducing nitrogen gas to ammonia using nitrogen reductase enzymes. This is a significant advantage in their role in biotransformation of metals to NPs [20], as they possess the ability to eliminate heavy metal ions from their surrounding environment. Furthermore, they contain various biomolecules including secondary metabolites, proteins, enzymes, and pigments that confer important biological properties such as antimicrobial and anticancer activity [28,30,31]. In addition to these features, cyanobacteria have a high growth rate that facilitates high biomass production. Thus, they represent important nanotechnology-mediated microorganisms that can act as nanobiofactories for NPs [32,33]. Although there have been several detailed reviews of biological synthesis using microorganisms, few studies have focused on synthesis of NPs using cyanobacteria.

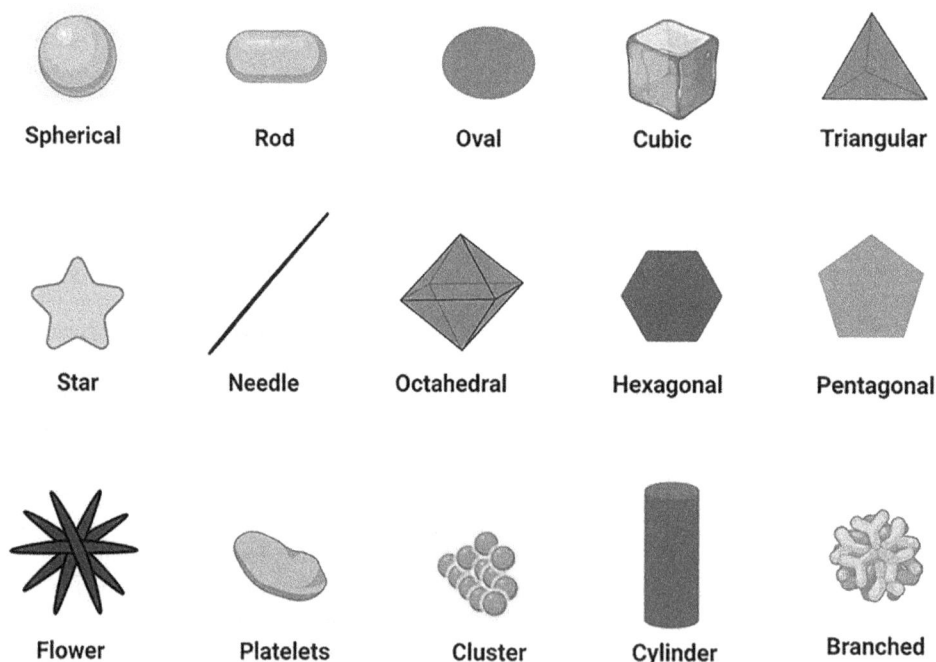

FIGURE 1.1   Various shapes of nanoparticles.

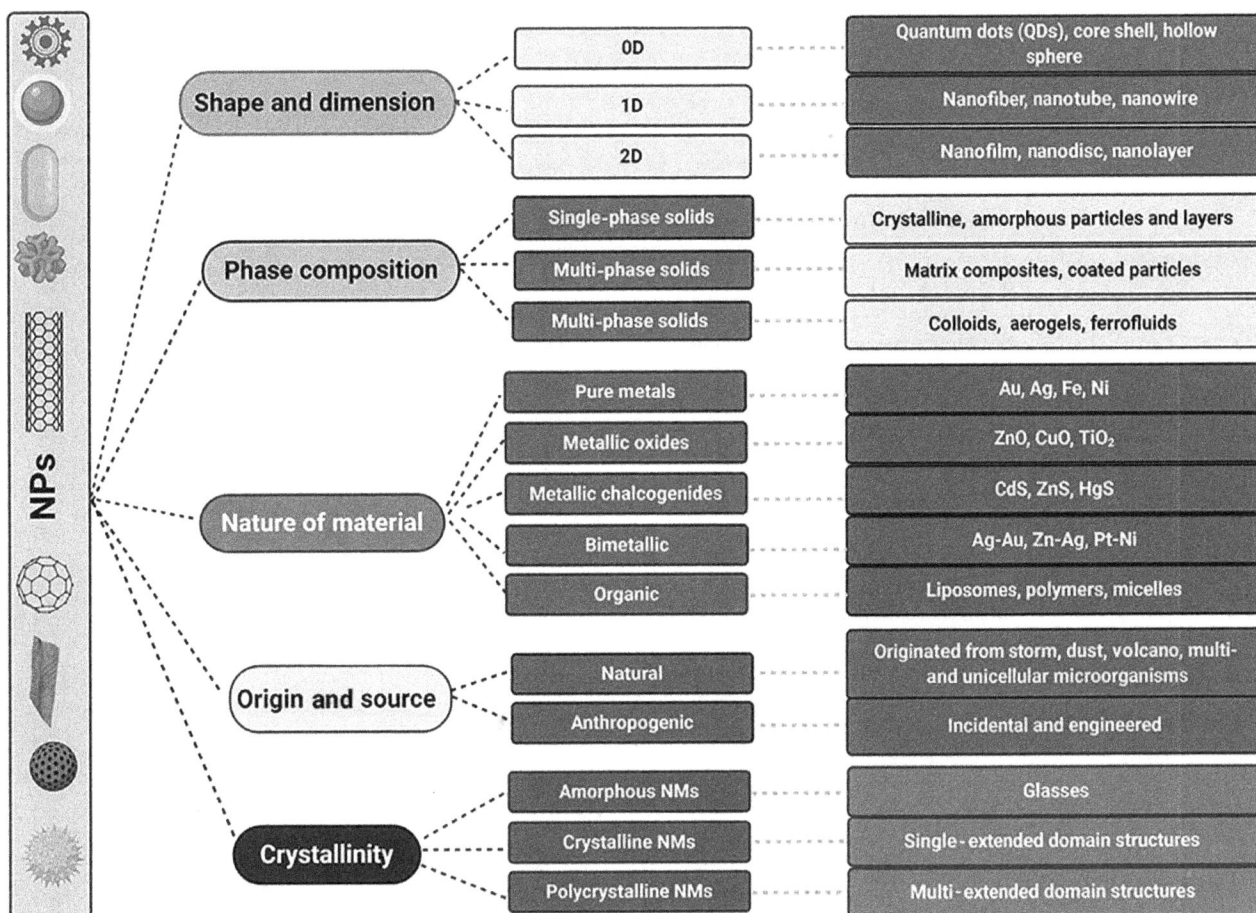

FIGURE 1.2 Nanoparticles' classifications. (©2019. Dove Medical Press. Adapted from Refs. [34] and [20] with permission from Elsevier.)

1.2 CLASSIFICATION OF NPs

NPs can be classified according to various factors, such as shape and dimension, phase compositions, nature, and origin (Figure 1.2) [34]. For instance, natural NPs include those that exist in the biosphere as a result of fabrication from heavy metals by living organisms, as well as those generated incidentally by forest fires, volcanic eruptions, weathering of rocks, and explosion of clay minerals, soil erosions, and sandstorms [35]. By contrast, engineered NPs are produced using chemical and physical routes. NPs can also be classified according to their chemical nature. Inorganic NPs include metal and metal oxide NPs such as silver, gold, platinum, titanium oxide, iron oxide, copper oxide, and zinc oxide NPs. Organic NPs include carbon NPs, N-halamine compounds, and chitosan (CS) NPs [22].

1.3 SYNTHESIS AND CHARACTERIZATION OF NPs

There are several methodologies for NP synthesis, including conventional methods such as chemical and physical approaches as well as modern methods such as biological synthesis using natural living organisms [26], enzymes [36], vitamins [37], etc. [7]. The chemical routes are a type of bottom-up fabrication method, in which the atom is assembled to nuclei and then grown to NPs [38]. In chemical methods, the main components are the precursor metals and the stabilizing and reducing agents. Reducing agents include sodium citrate, ascorbate, and sodium borohydride [39]; stabilizing agents include polyvinylpyrrolidone, starch, and sodium carboxyl methylcellulose [40]. Physical synthesis strategies belong to top-down route, in which the metals are converted to their nanoforms using physical approaches such as laser ablation [41], mechanical milling [42], and sputtering [38,43].

The drawbacks of the physicochemical approaches include power consumption, high cost, and a slow production rate, and most importantly, these processes are not more eco-friendly due to their toxic yields that threaten ecological systems [7,19]. Thus, there are global efforts toward development and usage of eco-friendly methods to synthesize NPs.

Green chemistry represents an advanced version of bottom-up nanotechnology approaches used to fabricate NPs [20]. But still now, biological synthesis process fights many obstacles to compete physicochemical synthesis such as obtaining uniform shape and size of NPs [44]. The aim of the biological synthesis methodology is to utilize natural sources to convert bulk material into nanoscaled particles

TABLE 1.1

Techniques Performed to Characterize Nanoparticles

Type of Analysis	Characterization Analyses	Function	References
Spectroscopic techniques	Ultraviolet (UV)–visible spectroscopy	Confirm the formation of NPs and detect their wavelength ranges	[28]
	Fourier transform infrared spectroscopy (FTIR)	Determine the chemical composition of biocoats surrounding biogenic NPs	[32]
	Zeta potential	Characterize NPs' charge	[54]
	Dynamic light scattering (DLS)	Estimate hydrodynamic diameter	[54]
	Nuclear magnetic resonance (NMR) spectroscopy	Determine the content and purity of NPs	[55]
X-ray-based analyses	X-ray diffraction (XRD)	Evaluate composition, structure, and crystal phase of NPs	[50]
	X-ray photoelectron spectroscopy (XPS)	Evaluate the structure of NPs	[24]
	Energy-dispersive spectroscopy (EDAX or EDS)	Evaluate the atomic structure of NPs	[50]
Microscopic techniques	Scanning electron microscopy (SEM)	Determine the size and morphological appearance of NPs	[44]
	Transmission electron microscopy (TEM) and high-resolution TEM	Determine the size and morphological appearance of NPs	[44]
	Atomic force microscopy (AFM)	Determine the geometries, size, morphology, and surface roughness of NPs	[51,56]
Magnetic techniques	Superconducting quantum interference device (SQUID), vibrating sample magnetometer (VSM), and ferromagnetic resonance (FMR)	Estimate magnetization saturation, magnetization remanence, magnetic anisotropic constant, and demagnetization field	[52,53,57]

with unique properties [33]. The natural sources used in biofabrication of NPs vary from unicellular to multicellular organisms; moreover, this process can be carried out in the presence of single proteins, enzymes, pigments, etc. [22]. The unicellular organisms include bacteria [45], cyanobacteria [32], and diatoms [46], while multicellular organisms include algae and plant [47,48]. The variety of potential natural sources and biomolecules facilitates the production of NPs with different unique properties. NPs are also subjected to various characterization analyses to assess their physical and chemical properties, including size, distribution, dispersion, stability, charge, and surface morphology [49,50]. These analyses use spectroscopic techniques such as ultraviolet (UV)–visible spectroscopy, Fourier transform infrared spectroscopy (FTIR), zeta potential, dynamic light scattering, and nuclear magnetic resonance (NMR) spectroscopy to determine wavelength ranges [28] and the chemical composition of biocoats surrounding biogenic NPs [32] and to confirm the formation of NPs, as well as characterizing their charge and hydrodynamic diameter. X-ray-based analyses such as X-ray diffraction (XRD) [50], X-ray photoelectron spectroscopy (XPS) [24], and energy-dispersive spectroscopy (EDAX or EDS) are employed to evaluate composition, structure, and crystal phase [50]. Microscopic techniques such as scanning electron microscopy (SEM), transmission electron microscopy (TEM), high-resolution TEM (HR-TEM), and atomic force microscopy (AFM) are used to determine the size and morphological appearance of NPs [44,51]. Also, there are several techniques to estimate the magnetic properties of NPs, such

as ferromagnetic resonance (FMR) and vibrating sample magnetometer (VSM) (Table 1.1) [52,53].

1.4 BIOFABRICATION SYNTHESIS METHODS OF NPs

The method of biofabrication of NPs differs from organism to another [58]. Moreover, differences are found among different strains of the same species [59,60]. Naturally, NPs are synthesized when microorganisms are exposed to toxic substances, in response to which they secrete extracellular substances to capture the material, or mediated through electrostatic interactions [58,61]. Mukherjee et al. showed that attraction electrostatic forces were among the factors aiding the reduction process of NPs in fungal cells [61]. The biotransformation of NPs follows a general pattern wherein metal ions are trapped in the microbial cells or on the microbial surface in the presence of enzymes and then reduced to form NPs [58]. Furthermore, the reduction of NPs by microorganisms can be classified into intracellular and extracellular synthesis (Figure 1.3).

1.4.1 INTRACELLULAR SYNTHESIS OF NPs

Intracellular formation of NPs refers to cases where the reduction of bulk material into NPs is performed inside host cells under the control of various biological factors [21]. Methods for *in vivo* synthesis of NPs in the laboratory involve three general steps: (i) culturing the target microorganisms; (ii) the interaction between the precursor solution and living cells;

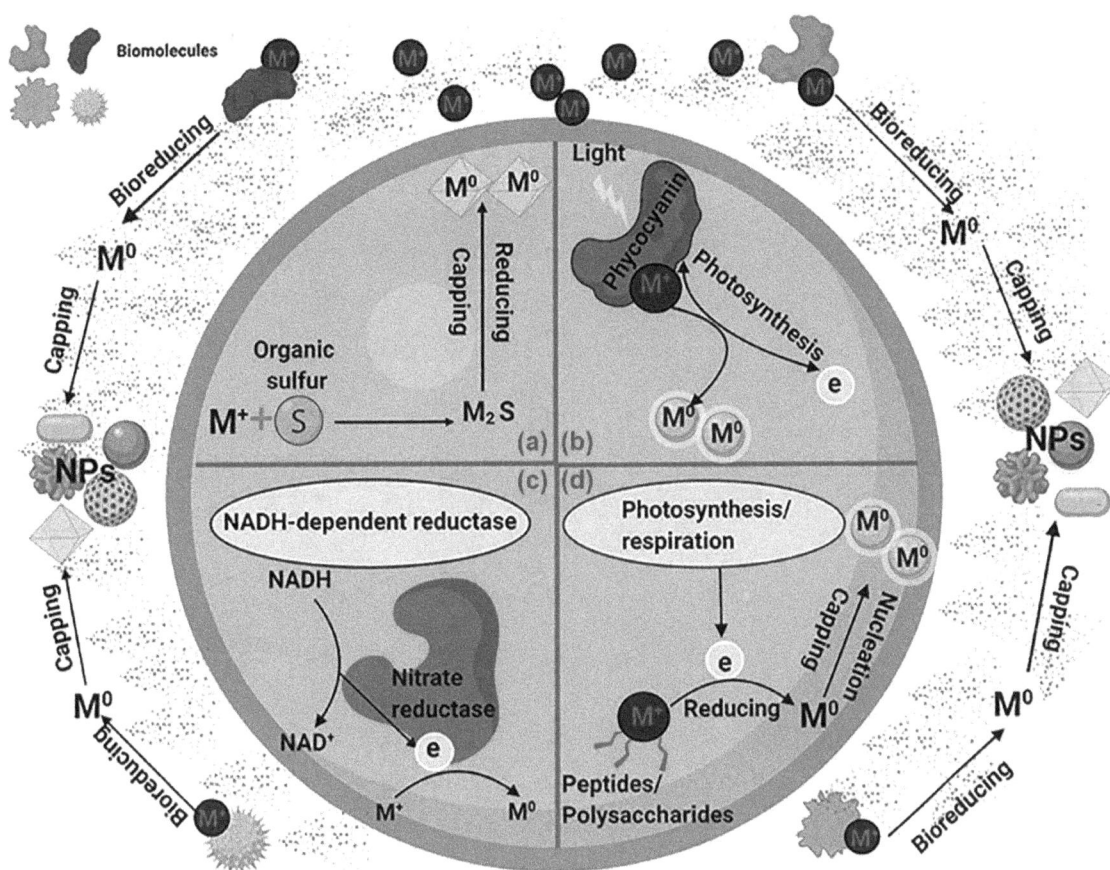

FIGURE 1.3 Potential mechanisms of green synthesis methods. (a–d) Different intracellular synthesis methods. (a) Organic sulfur-mediated synthesis of NPs. (b) Pigment-mediated synthesis of NPs. (c) Enzyme-mediated synthesis of NPs. (d) Biomolecule-mediated synthesis of NPs. M^+, metal; M^0, reduced NPs; e, electron; S, sulfur, M_2S, metal sulfide.

and (iii) the separation and purification of NPs from cells for characterization using physicochemical techniques [25]. In the latter step, the mixture of living microorganisms and precipitated NPs is centrifuged at 12,000 g. The pellets are then washed multiple times with distilled water for direct examination, and/or the cells are lysed using methods such as sonication to extract NPs for analysis (Figure 1.4) [62].

Intracellular interactions between bulk materials and microorganisms can be achieved by two different protocols. The first involves collecting cellular biomass of target microorganisms in the logarithmic phase by centrifugation and then washing this biomass to remove any traces of salts from the medium [63]. The cleaned biomass is dissolved in water and mixed with a suitable concentration of precursor material solution. In the second method, microorganisms are individually cultured along with the bulk material solution and kept under culture conditions for 2 weeks [64].

In cyanobacteria, ions are intracellularly reduced by electrons produced via the electron transport system, including energy-generating reactions in photosynthesis and, to some extent, in the respiratory electron transport system as a result of the existence of enzymes such as NADH-dependent reductases and redox reactions occur in the cytoplasm, thylakoid membranes, and cell membranes [23,65,66].

Lengke et al. showed that after reaction between *Plectonema boryanum* UTEX 485 system and silver nitrate, spherical, octahedral, and anhedral Ag-NPs were precipitated inside cells and in the culture solution [25]. They suggested that the silver ions were reduced by an intracellular electron donor or exported by a membrane transporter system. This indicates that the metabolic status (e.g., respiration or photosynthesis) and the growth phase of an organism determine its ability to synthesize NPs. Remarkably, *P. boryanum* was shown to reduce gold(III) chloride solutions to Au-NPs intracellularly [67]. The authors attributed the biorecovery mechanism of *P. boryanum* strains to either the gold(III) chloride solution or the acidic medium, which killed cyanobacteria and liberated more organic sulfur, leading to further precipitation of gold particles. The interactions of cyanobacteria or organic material released through the cyanobacterial membrane with gold(III) chloride enhanced the growth of metallic Au-NPs.

Kalishwaralal et al. suggested that nitrate reductase enzymes may help to induce the enzyme responsible for synthesis of Ag-NPs in *Bacillus licheniformis* [68]. Another study showed that nitrogenases (nitrogen-fixing enzymes) may be potent reducing agents for fabrication of gold ions into Au-NPs [69]. Shabnam and Pardha-Saradhi reported that thylakoids extracted from *Potamogeton nodosus* (an

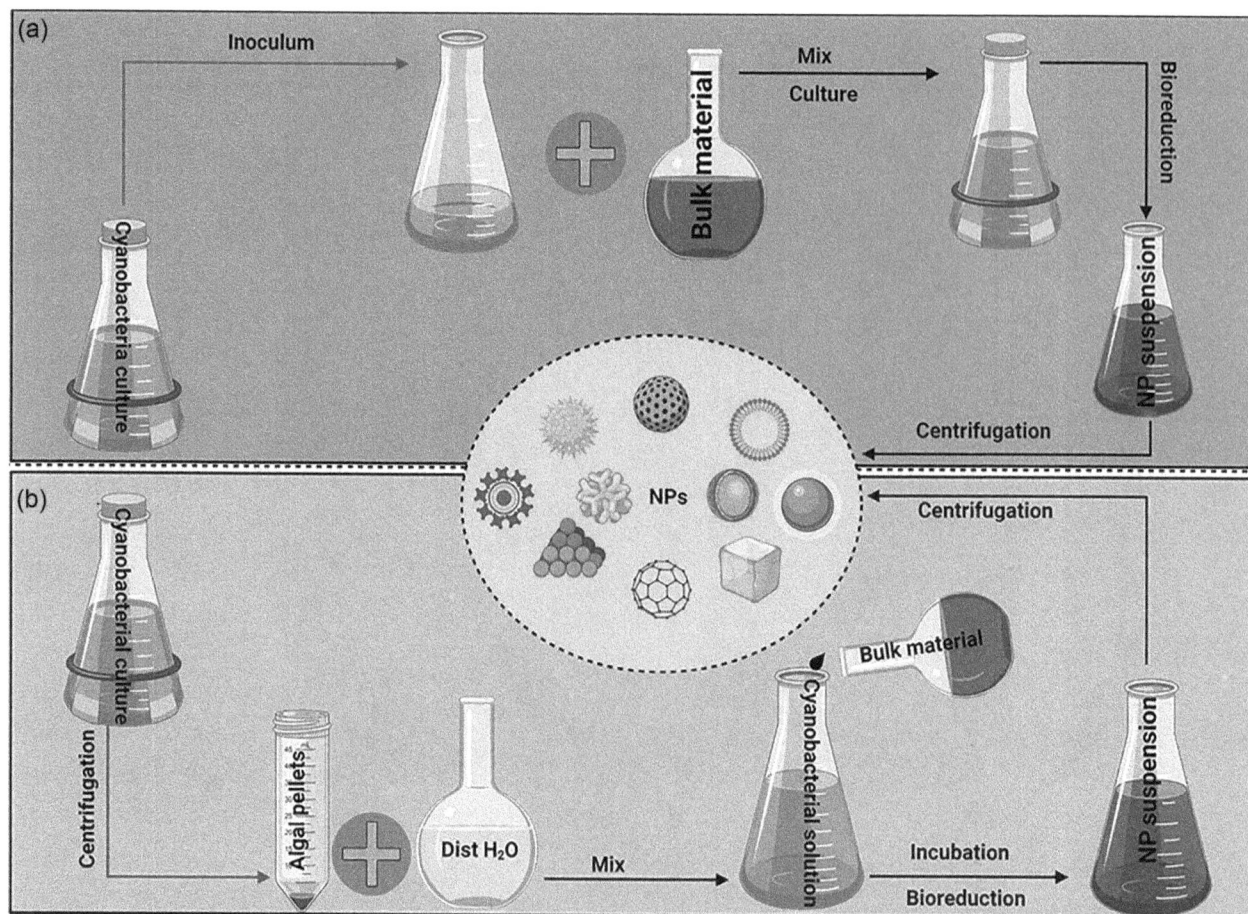

FIGURE 1.4 Potential protocols of intracellular synthesis methods. (a) Microorganisms are individually cultured along with the bulk material solution and kept under culture conditions. (b) Synthesis of NPs utilizing algal biomass in the logarithmic phase.

aquatic plant) and *Spinacia oleracea* (a terrestrial plant) may have been responsible for the fabrication of gold ions into Au-NPs during photochemical reactions [70]. Dahoumane et al. suggested that polysaccharides and other macromolecules may be responsible for internal reduction and stabilization of NPs [71]. Other reports have suggested that cyanobacterial pigments act as potent bioreductant molecules that intracellularly reduce bulk material into NPs [72,73].

1.4.2 EXTRACELLULAR SYNTHESIS OF NPs

Extracellular synthesis takes place outside the cell, with exuded biological molecules such as pigments, ions, proteins, enzymes, hormones, and antioxidants having a significant role in the reduction process of NPs [74,75]. These biomolecules act as reducing and capping agents during the biofabrication process. Various methods exist for extracellular synthesis of NPs, including use of cell-free culture media, cell biomass extracts, and biomolecules (Figure 1.5).

1.4.3 CELL-FREE MEDIA

NPs can be synthesized using the culture media of microorganisms after removal of biomass by centrifugation. The filtrated extracellular culture media are mixed with metal

precursor solutions under certain conditions to synthesize NPs. Keskin et al. tested five cyanobacterial strains and showed that cell-free culture media of *Synechococcus* sp. were able to synthesize Ag-NPs under light conditions [76]. Ag-NPs were also extracellularly synthesized using the supernatant of *Pseudomonas* sp. THG-LS1.4 strain [77]. Many studies have demonstrated the vital role of biocontents such as enzymes, antioxidants, and phenolic and alkaloid compounds present in the cell-free culture in controlling the bioreduction process of NPs. Shivaji et al. suggested that biomolecules such as NADH-reductases and sulfur-containing proteins in the cell-free supernatant are involved in the biofabrication of metallic NPs [78].

1.4.4 CELL BIOMASS FILTRATE

Several reports describe the cell biomass filtrate synthesis approach, in which microorganism cultures are centrifuged and the pellets washed at least three times with distilled water to eliminate any excess metal from the medium [32,33,79]. Then, the cleaned pellets are freeze-dried using a lyophilizer or dried in an oven almost at 40°C, and then crushed using a mortar and pestle. The resulting fine powder is mixed with distilled water and then filtrated using Whatman filter paper. Finally, the filtrate is mixed with a

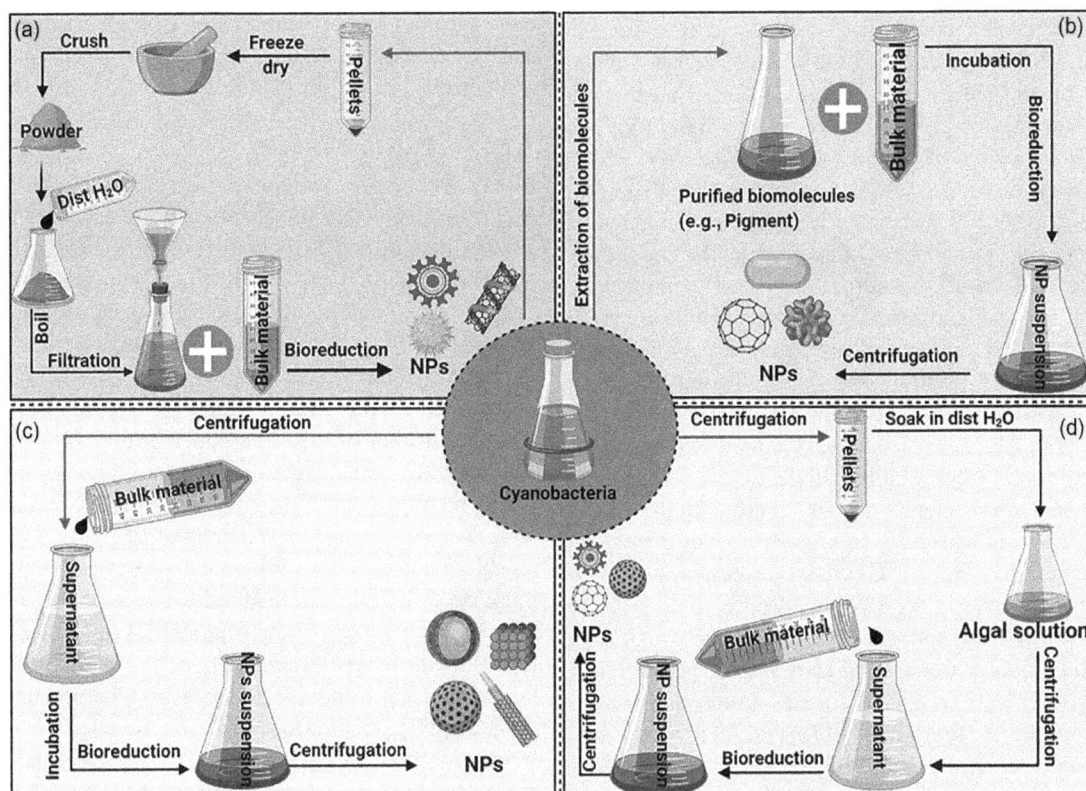

FIGURE 1.5 Potential protocols of extracellular synthesis methods. (a–d) Different protocols of extracellular synthesis of NPs. (a) Cell biomass-mediated synthesis of NPs. (b) Biomolecule-mediated synthesis of NPs. (c) Cell-free medium-mediated synthesis of NPs. (d) Cell filtrate-mediated synthesis of NPs.

metal precursor solution and incubated under suitable conditions. In this method, active biomoieties such as proteins and enzymes in the cell filtrate have significant roles in the biofabrication and stabilization of NPs [32]. Other route mentioned by Hassan et al. in which cell biomass collected at mid-exponential phase and wash several times to exclude any trace elements then soaked in distilled water for specific time. Afterward, the mixture is centrifuged, and the supernatant is used for NP synthesis [16].

1.4.5 BIOMOLECULE-BASED NP SYNTHESIS

1.4.5.1 Pigments

Cyanobacteria, microalgae, actinomycete, algae, etc., are distinguished by the predominance of pigments in their cells, such as carotenoid [80], C-phycocyanin [73], and R-phycoerythrin [81], that are able to synthesize NPs. C-phycocyanin is a blue photosynthetic accessory pigment that forms part of phycobilisomes, structures attached to thylakoids involved in light harvesting and transferring electrons toward photosystem II reaction centers [82,83]. It has been shown that C-phycocyanin controls electron transfer and has the ability to bind to heavy metals [84,85]. Recent studies have demonstrated the role of C-phycocyanin in the fabrication of NPs; Patel et al. showed that utilizing C-phycocyanin extracted from two different cyanobacterial

species (*Spirulina* and *Limnothrix* species) resulted in production of Ag-NPs with different shapes and sizes [59]. The authors attributed these differences in morphological features to the fact that the two C-phycocyanin preparations differed in purity and molecular weight. Also, they showed that there was a relationship between the ability of C-phycocyanin to synthesize NPs and the presence of light, as the pigment failed to reduce silver nitrate into Ag-NPs under dark conditions. Wei et al. demonstrated the importance of C-phycocyanin extracted from Spirulina as a protective (capping) agent during the reduction process of silver nitrate into Ag-NPs [86]. El-Naggar et al. reported that a proteinaceous pigment, phycocyanin, isolated from *Nostoc linckia* reduced silver nitrate into Ag-NPs under direct illumination (2400–2600 lux) for 24 h at room temperature [73]. In another study, phycoerythrin was extracted from *Nostoc carneum* and used as a reducing agent to synthesize Ag-NPs [87]. Mubarak Ali et al. successfully synthesized cadmium sulfide (CdS) NPs using C-phycoerythrin (CPE) extracted from cyanobacterial species *Phormidium tenue* NTDM05 [28]. The mechanism by which C-phycocyanin mediates Ag-NP synthesis is not clear; however, Patel et al. suggest that it is similar to the mechanism of the red pigment R-phycoerythrin extracted from red algae, which can synthesize Ag-NPs without the addition of any reductant materials [59].

1.4.5.2 Proteins

Many studies have considered the role of proteins in the stabilization and reduction of NPs [21,32,73]. Bharde et al. showed that cationic proteins secreted by *Verticillium* sp. and *Fusarium oxysporum* had hydrolytic activity, which enabled them to reduce and/or cap magnetite NPs [88]. Reddy et al. found that a bacterial protein of molecular weight between 25 and 66 kDa contributed to the reduction process of Au-NPs, whereas a protein of molecular weight between 66 and 116 kDa was responsible for SNP fabrication [89]. Khalifa et al. suggested that amino acids and proteins acted as stabilizing and reducing agents in the biofabrication process of metal nanoparticles (MNPs) [90]. Mubarak Ali et al. showed that the presence of groups such as amino, carboxyl, and sulfate in the amino acid sequence of cyanobacterial proteins facilitates the bioreduction process of extremely small NPs with uniform particle size distribution [91]. Govindaraju et al. performed extracellular synthesis of silver–gold core shell NPs, in addition to Ag-NPs and Au-NPs, using the single-cell protein *Spirulina platensis* [9]. They identified the FTIR bands at 1653, 1541, and 1242 cm^{-1} as amide I–III bands of polypeptides/proteins and suggested that algal proteins played a crucial part in the stabilization process of these NPs. Rahman et al. reported that under metal stress, new or modified proteins were expressed to perform dual functions, fabricating precursor materials into CuO NPs and acting as stabilizing agents [92]. They showed that a 22-kDa protein of *Phormidium* was responsible for the reduction of copper sulfate into copper oxide NPs. Rosken et al. first detected Au-NPs in the extracellular polymeric material of vegetative cells and the heterocyst polysaccharide layer of *Anabaena cylindrica* [93].

1.4.5.3 Enzymes

Many studies have investigated the roles of various enzymes, including nitrate reductases and NADH-dependent enzymes in the bioreduction process of NPs [69]. Furthermore, Yin et al. reported that superoxide dismutase has a vital role in the extracellular production of Ag-NPs using *F. oxysporum* [58]. Mostly, the assimilatory type of nitrate reductases is metalloproteins having molybdenum ions as cofactor and catalyzes several reactions in nitrogen, carbon, and sulfur cycle. Many studies have demonstrated the importance of these enzymes as a potent reducing agent in the biofabrication process of MNPs [94].

Oza et al. suggested that nitrate reductase aided the NADH-dependent extracellular synthesis of Au-NPs by *Chlorella pyrenoidosa* [69]. Brayner et al. synthesized Au-NPs, Ag-NPs, Pt NPs, and Pd NPs in the presence of cyanobacteria using nitrogenases as reducing agents [95]. They chose three strains, *Calothrix pulvinata*, *Anabaena flos-aquae*, and *Leptolyngbya foveolarum*, to form the NPs. C. pulvinata synthesized Pd and Pt NPs after 30 min and 15 days, respectively; Au-NPs after a few hours; and Ag-NPs after 24 h. By contrast, when the same precursor materials and strains were incubated with nitrogenases, Pd and Pt, Au, and Ag NPs formed after 2 h, 72 h, and 10 min, respectively.

1.4.5.4 Polysaccharides

Morsy et al. used extracellular polysaccharides (EPSs) from *Nostoc commune* to reduce silver nitrate to Ag-NPs [96]. Briefly, they mixed 10 g of dried cyanobacteria with water, suspended the mixture in 100 mL of potassium phosphate buffer (pH 7), and homogenized it in a blender at medium velocity for 10 s, followed by stirring overnight at ambient temperature. The suspension was then homogenized again at least three times for 10 s and left to stand at ambient temperature for 10 min. The upper layer (polysaccharides) was removed using a spatula, and the lower aqueous layer was centrifuged at 6000× g for 10 min at 20°C. The pellets were discarded, and the supernatant containing the water-soluble fraction of the EPSs was dialyzed overnight against distilled water and freeze-dried using a lyophilizer. Then, 50 mL of the aqueous EPS solution (10 mg/mL) was added to 30 mM of silver nitrate solution. The reaction was auto-claved at 15 psi and 121°C for 5 min. To precipitate biogenic Ag-NPs, the mixture was centrifuged at 15,000× g for 30 min at 20°C. They reported that the EPSs functioned as potent reducing and capping agents, and showed that coating Ag-NPs with EPSs prevented the particles from coming into contacting with oxygen and increased their stability.

1.5 FACTORS INFLUENCING THE BIOFABRICATION OF NPs USING MICROORGANISMS

Many factors should be considered during biological synthesis, including illumination, time of exposure, pH, temperature, and concentration. Control of these factors can facilitate the production of NPs with suitable physicochemical properties [23,71].

1.5.1 Illumination

The presence or absence of light has an important role in the biosynthesis of NPs. Some researchers report that light is needed at least to accelerate the bioreduction process for synthesis of NPs [97]. Patel et al. suggested that illumination conditions are significant factors controlling the intracellular and extracellular synthesis of Ag-NPs using phototrophic cyanobacteria [59]. They found that some cyanobacteria could not produce NPs under dark conditions. However, under the same conditions but after exposure to light, the same strains were able to fabricate Ag-NPs from silver nitrate. On the other hand, other strains including *Anabaena* sp., *Limnothrix* sp., and *Synechocystis* sp. were able to produce NPs under both light and dark conditions. This can be explained by the fact that different strains produce different compounds capable of NP synthesis, only some of which require light activation [59]. Another important point related to illumination is the light intensity. Mankad et al. reported complete extracellular reduction of silver ions to Ag-NPs after exposure of a mixture of *Azadirachta indica* leaf extract and silver nitrate solution to sunlight for only 5 min [97].

1.5.2 TIME OF EXPOSURE

The time of reaction varies among different microorganisms, with some able to synthesize NPs within minutes whereas others require weeks. Lengke et al. reported that *P. boryanum* UTEX 485 took 28 days to synthesize Ag-NPs, whereas Zada et al. showed that *Leptolyngbya* sp. JSC-1 fabricated Ag-NPs extracellularly from silver nitrate after 20 min [98,99]. A recent study showed that the dispersivity and stability of Ag-NPs synthesized using *Oscillatoria limnetica* changed with increasing time. After 48 h of synthesis, the UV spectrum wavelength value was constant, and after 9 months of incubation, the optical intensity had shifted from 0.71 to 0.599 nm, indicating the stability of Ag-NPs with low agglomeration [27]. The stability of Anabaena-mediated Ag-NPs was evaluated after 6 months of storage by Singh et al. [100]. The results showed that the Ag-NPs were stable with no change in spectral absorbance, at least in the first 3 months.

1.5.3 pH

El-Naggar et al. reported that pH significantly affected the size and distribution of Ag-NPs [87]. They reported that Ag-NPs' extracellular synthesis using phycoerythrin was inhibited in acidic media (pH), whereas the reaction was enhanced under alkaline conditions (pH 10). In addition, smaller and more highly dispersed NPs were observed at pH 10, whereas larger and more aggregated NPs were observed at pH 12.

1.5.4 TEMPERATURE

Lengke et al. reported the first successful alternative to abiotic chemical approaches for fabricating NPs [98]. They screened the ability of *P. boryanum* UTEX 485 to form extra- and intracellular platinum NPs. The results demonstrated the effects of a variable range of temperatures on NP formation, showing that crystallization and recrystallization of NPs depend on temperature. Decreasing temperature resulted in amorphous distribution, while a crystalline structure was dominant at higher temperatures.

1.5.5 CONCENTRATION OF PRECURSORS AND NATURAL REDUCING AGENTS

The concentration of bioreductant materials has an important influence on the features of NPs, including shape and size [27]. The synthesis of NPs is dose-dependent and is also related to the type of algae used [69,71]. Hamouda et al.

showed that increasing the concentration of the cyanobacteria *Oscillatoria limnetica* increased the absorbance of the resulting peaks [27]. Moreover, they reported that peaks shifted in position from 420 to 430 nm, accompanied by broadening of peaks, indicating an increase in the size of particles. They also found that the extracellular biofabrication reaction of Ag-NPs was dependent on the dose of silver nitrate. Overall, increasing the concentration of precursor materials resulted in an increased optical intensity recorded by UV spectrophotometry.

1.5.6 NATURE OF MICROORGANISMS

The nature of microorganisms is related to their biomolecular contents and the types of these molecules, such as polysaccharides, peptides, and pigments [22,91]. Thus, different microorganisms vary in their ability to form NPs. Brayner et al. screened the reduction activity of three cyanobacterial cultures and observed that the size and shape of NPs varied according to the genus of cyanobacteria used [95]. Moreover, different strains from the same species were found to produce NPs with different physicochemical and biological characteristics. Recent studies used different strains from the same *Nostoc* species, including *Nostoc* sp. Bahar M [33], *Nostoc* HKAR-2 [102], and *Nostoc muscorum* NCCU-442 [60], resulting in different nanosize ranges (8.5–26.44, 51–100, and 42 nm, respectively) of the resulting Ag-NPs.

Other factors may control NP features, including the microorganisms' habitats and their ability to eliminate metals from their environment [22]. Blue-green algae are distinguished by their ability to accumulate heavy metals from the surrounding environment and degrade these metals into NPs [21]. Husain et al. showed that 30 cyanobacterial strains isolated from a marine habitat had significant potential to extracellularly reduce silver nitrate to Ag-NPs [60]. By contrast, other eubacteria known to be resistant to heavy metals such as *Aphanizomenon* sp. could not fabricate Ag-NPs from silver metal under laboratory conditions [59].

1.6 CYANOBACTERIA AS BIOMACHINERY FOR NP SYNTHESIS

The blue-green algae (cyanobacteria) are the only known oxygen-producing prokaryotes. All cyanobacteria are microscopic and widespread in aquatic environments, with some terrestrial species. The aquatic forms mostly occur in freshwater, and few are marine [103]. Cyanobacteria contain non-membrane-bound organelles including chloroplasts, unstacked thylakoids, phycobiliprotein pigments, and cyanophycean starch and peptidoglycan matrices or walls. In addition, they are a rich source of biomolecules such as proteins, enzymes, antioxidants, vitamins, and polysaccharides [28]. Although there have been many reports of biological synthesis with different micro- or

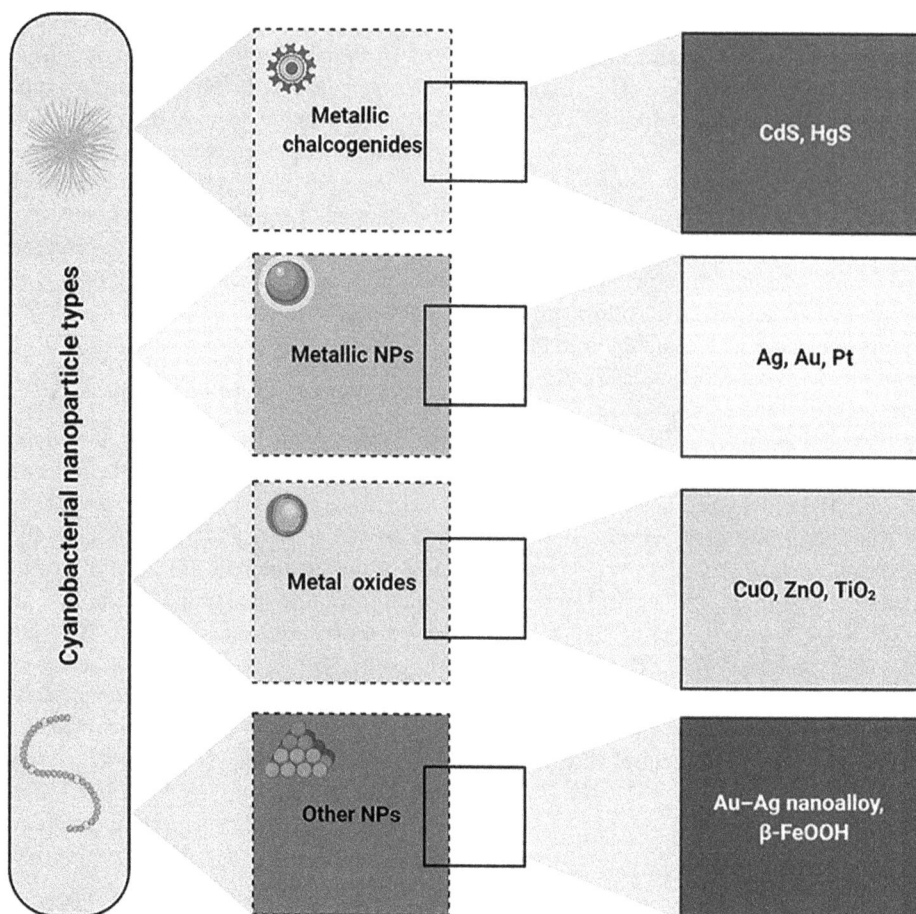

FIGURE 1.6   Type of metallic NPs synthesized by cyanobacteria. CdS, cadmium sulfide; HgS, mercury sulfide; Au, gold; Ag, silver; Pt, platinum; CuO, copper oxide; ZnO, zinc oxide; β-FeOOH, akaganéite.

macroorganisms, using plants, algae, bacteria, and fungi to obtain NPs of various sizes and shapes, few studies have used cyanobacteria as the biological machinery for NP fabrication [13]. Cyanobacteria are considered to be important biofactories that can be used to synthesize NPs by either extracellular or intracellular methods, owing to their ease of culture at ambient temperature and under atmospheric pressure, their high growth rate, the variable biocompounds inside their cells, their capacity to take up heavy metal ions, and the environmental safety of their products [21]. Different studies have demonstrated the capacity of different cyanobacterial strains to form different types of NPs, including metallic NPs such as Ag-NPs and Au-NPs, and metal oxide NPs such as ZnO NPs and CuO NPs, as well as other nanomaterials such as Ag–Au nanoalloys and semiconductor NPs such as CdS NPs (Figure 1.6) [3,67,103,104].

1.6.1 Silver Nanoparticles (Ag-NPs)

Ag-NPs are the most commonly used MNPs in various fields and can be found in many industrial and medical products including dressings, surgical instruments and masks, detergents, and care products [105,106]. Conventionally, Ag-NPs have been fabricated by chemical and physical approaches.

Due to the drawbacks of these routes including their high cost, high energy requirements, and toxic byproducts, green synthesis methods have been developed to produce clean NPs and avoid the harmful effects of physicochemical techniques [7,13]. For instances, Kim et al. mentioned that the injection rate and reaction temperature are crucial factors to synthesize Ag-NPs using polyol process and a modified precursor injection approach [107]. They generated spherical Ag-NPs with nanosize of 17 nm at 100°C. In contrast, many studies using neutral organisms could synthesize Ag-NPs with smallest size ranging from 10, 10–15, to 14.9 nm at room temperature [33,95,108]. Also, Jin et al. synthesized Ag-NPs utilizing photoinduced route [109]. They found that Ag-NPs have triangular shape with size range between 30 and 120 nm. The scholars used chemically stabilizing agents such as citrate and poly(styrene sulfonate) to obtain stable Ag-NPs, while *Arthrospira maxima SAE* and *Arthrospira platensis* were able to generate triangular Ag-NPs (61 and 46 nm, respectively) at 30°C for 24 h without needing to any stabilizing agents [60].

Eco-friendly synthesis research has expanded rapidly to discover new microbes with hydrolytic capacity to synthesize NPs. Among these biological entities, blue-green algae provide a straightforward route for producing the desired

Ag-NPs. *Desertifilum* IPPAS B-1220 was explored for the fabrication of Ag-NPs for the first time by Hamida et al. [32], who extracellularly synthesized Ag-NPs using a cell biomass extract under direct illumination for 24 h at room temperature. The formation of D-SNPs was confirmed by UV absorption peak at 421 nm. XRD diffraction pattern exhibited five 2θ degree at 29.7, 38.4, 44.6, 64.7, and 77.7 indicates the nanocrystallinity of D-SNPs. FTIR data demonstrated different IR peaks at 601.81, 1042.35, 1626.05, 2353.23, and 3453.72 cm^{-1} for D-SNPs. According to dominant FTIR spectra, the scholars reported that the main biomolecules responsible for the bioreduction and stabilization processes were proteins and polysaccharides. Also, they found that *Desertifilum* IPPAS B-1220 sp. could produce spherical Ag-NPs with sizes ranging from 4.5 to 26 nm.

Lengke et al. used *P. boryanum UTEX 485* for the first time for both intracellular and extracellular synthesis of Ag-NPs [110]. They found that Ag-NPs have octahedral and spherical shapes with nanosize ranging from 1 to 200 and 10 nm, respectively. EDS and XPS indicated the association of trace of iron, phosphorus, and sulfur with Ag-NPs. They reported that the biofabrication process of silver nitrate could be linked with metabolic process using nitrate by reducing nitrate to nitrite and ammonium which is fixed as glutamine before cyanobacterial death. However, liberation of organic materials after bacterial death resulted in precipitation of Ag-NPs in solution. A recent study investigated the hydrolytic activity of a new strain of cyanobacteria, *Nostoc* sp. Bahar M, to extracellularly fabricate Ag-NPs from silver nitrate [33]. The authors mentioned that the plasmon resonance of *Nostoc*-mediated Ag-NPs was at 403 nm, indicating the smaller size of these NPs. Also, XRD pattern confirmed the face-centered cubic crystalline structure of Ag-NPs. TEM and SEM showed that Ag-NP produced by *Nostoc* sp. Bahar M was uniformly distributed and spherical in shape, with average nanosize of 14.9 nm. Also, FTIR data exhibited that protein molecules play an important role in the biofabrication process of Ag-NPs. Recently, an aqueous extract of *Oscillatoria limnetica* biomass was also used to synthesize Ag-NPs at room temperature for 18 h [27]. The Ag-NPs were spherical in shape and have diverse sizes ranging between 3.30 and 17.97 nm. Also, the authors studied variable abiotic factors such as pH, time, and concentration of natural reducing materials and silver nitrate to determine the optimal conditions for Ag-NP synthesis. They found that the most suitable conditions to produce Ag-NPs from *Oscillatoria limnetica* are at pH of 6.7 and for 18 h as well as the synthesis process is dose-dependent manner for both silver nitrate and cyanobacterial extract concentrations.

Thirty cyanobacterial species were screened for extracellular synthesis of Ag-NPs [60]. The results showed that all 30 cyanobacteria were able to form Ag-NPs from their precursor materials, with variable size ranges. *Cylindrospermum stagnale* performed the best, producing the smallest Ag-NPs with nanosizes of 38–40 nm. Similarly, Sudha et al. screened the Ag-NP fabrication ability of several cyanobacterial species isolated from Muthupet mangroves, including *Aphanothece, Oscillatoria, Microcoleus, Aphanocapsa, Phormidium, Lyngbya, Gloeocapsa, Spirulina,* and *Synechococcus* [72]. Of all the tested microorganisms, only *Microcoleus* sp. could reduce silver nitrate and form spherical Ag-NPs, with an average diameter of 55 nm.

Patel et al. performed both extracellular and intracellular syntheses of Ag-NPs with light and dark incubation using different cyanobacterial isolates, including *Anabaena* sp., *Aphanizomenon* sp., *Cylindrospermopsis* sp. 121–1, *Cylindrospermopsis* sp. USC CRB3, *Lyngbya* sp., *Limnothrix* sp., *Synechocystis* sp., and *Synechococcus* sp. With the exception of *Aphanizomenon* sp., all tested cyanobacteria reduced silver nitrate to Ag-NPs under direct light exposure using either cell-free culture liquids or cell biomass extracts. In addition, only the cell biomass extracts of *Anabaena* sp., *Limnothrix* sp., and *Synechocystis* sp. were able to synthesize Ag-NPs under dark incubation. Only *Aphanizomenon* sp. failed to tailor the bulk material into its nanoform [59].

1.6.2 Gold Nanoparticles

Au-NPs are known to be good heat conductors and low-toxicity NPs against normal cells that are suitable for use in PTT to treat cancer [111]. As well as physiochemical methods, biological synthesis can be used to synthesize Au-NPs in an eco-friendly manner. The first investigation of the ability of *Anabaena laxa* to catalyze the conversion of hydrogen tetrachloroaurate(III) into Au-NPs was performed by Lenartowicz et al. [112]. They reported that *A. laxa* were able to intracellularly fabricate Au-NPs with diverse morphologies and sizes using three different concentrations of auric chloride (HAuCl$_4$; 0.1, 0.5, and 1 mM). The authors reported that the maximum UV spectra peak was formed at 545 and 560 nm for 0.5 and 1 mM of HAuCl$_4$. Three 2θ degrees (38.2°, 44.3°, and 64.6°) were detected by X-ray diffraction analysis indicating the crystallinity of Au-NPs. Also, TEM micrographs showed that the Au-NPs appearing at 0.5 mM were spherical; however, few NPs with other shapes (triangular, hexagonal, and irregular) were observed. The size of these NPs ranged from 0 to 30 nm; however, the largest particles have a size range from 30 to 100 nm. At a higher concentration (1 mM of HAuCl$_4$), triangular, hexagonal, and irregular shapes of Au-NPs appeared with a nanosize range from 20 to 50 nm. In addition, living cyanobacterial cultures were able to form Au-NPs more efficiently than dead ones, indicating a role of metabolic activity in the bioreduction process of Au-NPs.

Similarly, Dahoumane et al. and Brayner et al. demonstrated the bioreduction ability of *A. flos-aquae* to intracellularly synthesize Au-NPs [23,95]. Rosken et al. showed that *A. cylindrica* and other *Anabaena* sp. reduced gold ions to Au-NPs without releasing toxic anatoxin-a [93,113]. They mentioned that *A. cylindrica* were able to intracellularly produce Au-NPs after 4 h under direct illumination incubation. XRD pattern of Au-NPs showed that these NPs have ellipsoidal shape with an aspect ratio of 1.15. The biosynthesized Au-NPs were spherical, and their average size was 10 nm. Moreover, TEM micrographs showed that the Au-NPs were mainly distributed in vegetative cells (50%) in comparison with heterocysts and found to be located along the thylakoid membranes. The scholars suggested that heterocysts are not as important for NP fabrication, because their results showed that more than ten vegetative cells contained Au-NPs while only one heterocyst contained NPs. The bioreduction activities of three species of cyanobacteria, *Phormidium valderianum, P. tenue,* and *Microcoleus chthonoplastes,* were screened against HAuCl$_4$ solution at different pH values by Parial et al. [15]. They reported that all three tested cyanobacterial strains were able to synthesize Au-NPs; however, only *P. valderianum* was able to produce Au-NPs of different shapes and sizes, including nanospheres (15 nm) and triangular (24 nm) and hexagonal (25 nm) NPs, in response to variations in pH. *Gloeocapsa* sp. were exploited for intracellular synthesis of Au-NPs using cleaned whole cells [114]; 90 mL of 10^{-3} HAuCl$_4$ solution was mixed with 10 mL of *Gloeocapsa* culture and incubated with stirring at ambient temperature. After a few hours, Au-NPs had formed, and their UV absorbance was 547 nm. Moreover, FTIR results showed that algal proteins were responsible for the bioreduction process that formed these NPs, as strong peaks were observed at 3424.96 cm^{-1}, corresponding to N-H stretching, and at 1640.16 cm^{-1}, corresponding to amide I. In addition, SEM and TEM micrographs showed that the Au-NPs had spherical shape and diameters of <100 nm.

1.6.3 COLLOIDAL AU-NPS

Au-NPs are good contrast agents because of their small size, good biocompatibility, and high atomic number. Research shows that Au-NPs work by both active and passive ways to target cells. The principle of passive targeting is governed by a gathering of the Au-NPs to enhance imaging because of the permeability tension effect (EPR) in tumor tissues [115]. Active targeting, on the other hand, is mediated by the coupling of Au-NPs with tumor-specific targeted drugs, such as EGFR monoclonal antibodies (mAbs), to achieve Au-NP active targeting of tumor cells (Figure 1.7) [116]. When the energy exceeds 80 keV, the mass attenuation rate of gold becomes higher than that of alternative elements such as iodine, indicating a greater prospect of Au-NPs [117]. Rand et al. mixed Au-NPs with liver cancer cells and found, using X-ray imaging, that the clusters of liver cancer cells in the gold nanocomposite group were significantly stronger than those in the liver cancer cells alone. These findings have important implications for early diagnosis, with the technique allowing tumors as small as a few millimeters in diameter to be detected in the body [118].

1.6.4 OTHER NANOMATERIALS

The ability of cyanobacteria to reduce metallic NPs is not limited to Ag-NPs and Au-NPs, but extends to other metals including platinum, palladium, and cadmium, as well as metal oxides including copper oxide and zinc oxide. Lengke et al. screened the ability of *P. boryanum UTEX 485* to form platinum and palladium NPs under variable temperatures [100,119]. The scholars mentioned that Pd NPs formed after incubation with *P. boryanum* for 28 days at 25°C–100°C. TEM micrographs of Pd NPs showed that these particles have spherical and elongated shapes, but at 100°C, only spherical palladium hydride appeared. XRD analysis of Pd NPs synthesized at 100°C and 60°C showed different peaks at a Bragg angle (2θ) of 46.9, 54.5, and 81.2, indicating the nanocrystalline of Pd NPs; however, at 25°C no diffraction peaks were detected. Similarly, different physicochemical analyses of Pt NPs synthesized by *P. boryanum UTEX 485* at 25°C–100°C for 28 days and at 180°C for 1 day were performed by Lengke et al. XPS results showed the association of sulfur, phosphorus, and nitrogen with platinum(II), and

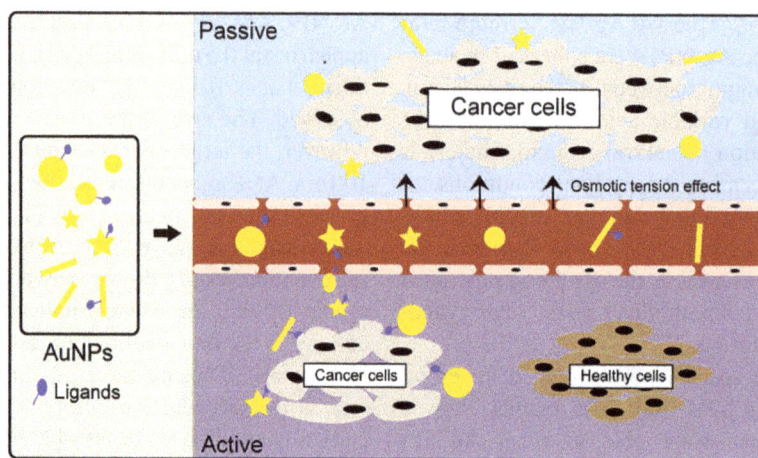

FIGURE 1.7 Various types of gold nanoparticles (different sizes, morphologies, and ligands) accumulate in tumor tissues by the action of osmotic tension effect (termed passive targeting) or localize to specific cancer cells in a ligand–receptor binding way (termed active targeting).

EDX analysis indicated the presence of sulfur with platinum. So, the authors speculated that these organic elements play a significant role in the reduction process of platinum ions into Pt NPs. Brayner et al. intracellularly synthesized Au-NPs, Ag-NPs, Pt NPs, and Pd NPs utilizing the biomass of *C. pulvinata*, *A. flos-aquae*, and *L. foveolarum* [95]. They suggested that polysaccharides were responsible for NP stabilization. CdS NPs are well-known and widely studied semiconductors. They have been synthesized using various microorganisms, including yeasts, algae, and fungi [120–122]. CPE pigment extracted from *P. tenue* was also used to synthesize 5-nm CdS NPs from their precursors, using an aqueous mixture of CdCl2 and Na2S [28]. The CdS NPs formed after incubation with CPE pigment for 24 h at 37°C. The formation of CdS NPs was confirmed by the absorption peak at 470 nm. FTIR analysis demonstrated that new bands at 1543, 1364, and 1223 cm^{-1} appeared only in CPE-coated CdS NPs, which indicates a new vibration due to C/S band. Other bands seen at 1364 and 1034 cm^{-1} were related to the C-N stretching vibrations of the aromatic amino amines. Furthermore, EDAX analysis confirmed the existence of both Cd and S in biosynthesized CdS NPs.

1.6.5 METAL OXIDES AND AKAGANÉITE NPS

Nostoc sp. [103] and *Anabaena* sp. [99] have been used to generate ZnO NPs, whereas copper oxide (CuO) NPs were produced by *Phormidium cyanobacterium* and *S. platensis*, respectively [92,104]. Brayner et al. synthesized beta-iron oxyhydroxide (β-FeOOH) NPs using *A. flos-aquae*, *C. pulvinata*, and *Klebsormidium* sp. [123]. They found that there were two basic mechanisms by which iron had acquired higher plants, denoted strategy I and strategy II. Strategy I involves soil acidification and formation of lateral roots and specific transfer cells in the rhizodermis, as well as induction of an Fe^{3+}-chelate reductase and of Fe^{2+} transporters. This strategy was used in all plants except grasses. Grasses followed strategy II, in which iron is taken up as a Fe^{3+}-siderophore complex. Based on these observations, the authors proposed that the mechanism of iron oxide fabrication by cyanobacteria followed strategy II (siderophore-based iron acquisition). Owing to the limited availability of iron, the cells released organic Fe^{3+} metal-chelating molecules (siderophores) that could solubilize and scavenge iron ions from the environment and internalize them into the cells. Similarly, Dahoumane et al. biologically generated akaganéite NPs using *A. flos-aquae* [124]. They showed that XRD analysis of freeze-dried cyanobacteria after reaction with iron salts exhibited the existence of tetragonal akaganéite NPs with some amorphous phase related to the cyanobacteria biomass. TEM ultrathin sections of cyanobacteria treated with iron precursors showed distribution of dark β-FeOOH akaganéite nanorods inside the bacterial cells. However, HR-TEM provided more information about the distribution pattern of akaganéite NPs inside the cells, in which the nanorods appeared as a complex arrangement of pores forming a spongelike structure.

1.6.6 BIMETALLIC NPS

Bimetallic NPs include a combination of two different metals, the ratio of which can be varied to provide novel physicochemical features derived from the constituting metals [9,13]. These NPs are attractive for various applications due to the extra degree of freedom they afford. Govindaraju et al. used extracellular synthesis to produce silver–gold core shell NPs, in addition to Ag-NPs and Au-NPs, using the single-cell protein *S. platensis* [9]. The spectral wavelength of silver–gold bimetallic NPs was 509 nm, and their size was 17–25 nm. Roychoudhury et al. exposed *Lyngbya majuscula* to an equimolar solution of gold and silver (1 mM, pH 4) for 72 h to produce an Au-Ag nanoalloy [125]. They reported that *Lyngbya* sp. acted as environmentally friendly factories for Au–Ag nanoalloy fabrication. The UV absorbance of the nanoalloy was 481 nm, with a nanosize ranging from 5 to 25 nm.

1.7 PASSIVE AND ACTIVE OF NP TARGETING DELIVERY IN CANCER TREATMENT

Ideally, for the effectiveness of anticancer drugs in cancer treatment, they should first, after administration, be able to penetrate through the barriers in the body and reach the desired tumor tissues with minimal loss of their volume or activity in the blood circulation. Second, after reaching the desired site, drugs should have the ability to selectively kill tumor cells without affecting normal cells. These two basic approaches are also associated with improvements in patient survival and quality of life by increasing the intracellular concentration of drugs and reducing dose-limiting toxicities simultaneously.

Increasingly, NPs seem to have the potential to satisfy both of these requirements for effective drug carrier systems.

Cancer nanotechnology has the potential to dramatically improve current approaches to cancer detection, diagnosis, imaging, and therapy while reducing toxicity associated with traditional cancer therapy. Cancer nanotechnology has tremendous potential to safely revolutionize current approaches to imaging, early diagnosis, treatment, and prevention of cancer [126].

A wide variety of nanomaterials are currently under investigation and development for application relative to cancer nanotechnology. These include polymers, dendrimers, lipids, organometallic materials, and carbon-based materials (reviewed extensively in Refs. [127,128]). Considerations on the selection of specific nanomaterials for cancer nanotechnology applications necessarily include biocompatibility, toxicity, size, surface chemistry, and their properties in biologic systems.

As described by Heath and Davis [129], NPs have four unique properties that distinguish them from other cancer therapeutics: (i) the NP, which can itself have therapeutic or diagnostic properties, can be designed to carry a large therapeutic "payload"; (ii) NPs can be attached to multivalent targeting ligands that yield high affinity and specificity for target cells; (iii) NPs can be made to accommodate multiple drug molecules that simultaneously allow combinatorial cancer therapy; and (iv) NPs can bypass traditional drug resistance mechanisms.

NPs and nanoparticulate formulations of established therapeutics have been integrated into cancer therapeutics and ongoing clinical trials [130]. These formulations offer improved efficacy and reduced toxicity compared to conventional therapeutics.

Consideration must be given to the toxicological impacts of nanomaterials intended for human administration [131]. Material, structure, size, size dispersion, agglomeration, shape, surface charge, surface chemistry, and adsorbed species are important and need to be considered as each of these characteristics ultimately affects not only biodistribution but also patterns of clearance and ultimately toxicological effects on end organs [132]. Consideration also needs to be given to the ability of nanomaterials administered *in vivo* to suppress or stimulate the immune system as these factors can have a significant impact on the well-being of the host [133].

There are no harmonized standards for assessing the toxicology of nanomaterials, and this remains a major challenge in the development of nanomaterials for human use. There is a need for reliable predictive assays that are much needed to accelerate the safe transition of nanomaterials toward human cancer applications [134].

In order to achieve many imaging and therapeutic applications in cancer nanotechnology *in vivo*, nanomaterials must be delivered to sites of cancer [135]. For many imaging and therapeutic applications, selective or preferential delivery of nanomaterials to sites of cancer would be optimal. Two general approaches have been utilized to accomplish this: passive targeting and active targeting [128].

Passive targeting of NPs relies on abnormal gap junctions (100–600 nm) in the endothelium of tumor blood vessels for accumulation of NPs in tumors [136]. In order to achieve passive targeting of NPs, engineering of particles with long circulation half-lives [such as coating particles with hydrophilic polymer such as polyethylene glycol (PEG)] is most desirable and this type of construct favors passive accumulation of particles inside tumors [128,135]. Altered lymph drainage is a characteristic of tumors which favors retention of NPs inside tumors. In general, small particle size is thought to favor intratumoral extravasation [137,138]. Particle composition and shape are also determinants of particle uptake, although these relationships have not been well characterized [139].

Active targeting of NPs relies on conjugation of a tumor-specific ligand(s) to NPs for their specific delivery to tumor sites [140,141]. Targeting moieties that have been investigated include antibodies, peptides, cell surface ligands, and aptamers [135,142]. Targets in tumors have included tumor antigens, cell surface receptors that are internalized (e.g., folate receptors [143] and transferrin receptors [144]), and tumor vasculature [145]. Active targeting has

been extensively studied in preclinical models but has not been effectively translated into current clinical applications [135]. In preclinical models, targeting has inconsistently led to increased accumulation in tumors [146,147]. In many instances, cancer cell uptake has been increased with targeting without an increase in overall tumor accumulation of NPs [146,147]. Development of novel, specific targeting strategies for NPs to cancer remains an important area of active investigation.

"Controlled release" occurs when a natural or synthetic polymer combines with a drug in such a way that the drug is encapsulated within the polymer system for subsequent release in a predetermined manner (Figure 1.8) [148].

Polymeric drug delivery vehicles can be designed as NPs that release the encapsulated drugs through surface or bulk erosion, diffusion, or swelling, followed by diffusion in a time- or condition-dependent manner. The release of the active agent may be constant over a long period or cyclic over a long period, or it may be triggered by environmental or other external events [149] such as changes in pH [149–152] or temperature [153], or the presence of an analyte such as glucose [154]. In general, controlled-release polymer systems can provide drug levels in an optimum range over a longer period of time compared to other drug delivery methods. Thus, they increase the efficacy of the drug and maximize patient compliance, while enhancing the ability to use highly toxic, poorly soluble, or relatively unstable drugs. The primary consideration of drug delivery is to achieve more effective therapies while eliminating the potential for both under- and overdosing. Other advantages of using controlled-release delivery systems include the maintenance of drug levels within a desired range, the need for fewer administrations, optimal use of the drug in question, and increased patient compliance. This is particularly relevant to cancer therapy in which the effectiveness of the treatment is directly related to the ability to kill cancer cells while affecting as few healthy cells as possible. By administering bolus doses of cytotoxic chemotherapeutic drugs, adverse effects are commonly observed and these may be sufficiently intense to limit continuation of the chemotherapy course.

Molecular targeting therapy has emerged as one approach to overcome the lack of specificity of conventional chemotherapeutic agents [155]. However, the resistance development in cancer cells can dodge the cytotoxicity not only of conventional chemotherapeutics but also of newer molecular targeting therapeutics [156]. By using both passive and active targeting strategies, intracellular concentration of drugs in cancer cells can be improved by NPs while avoiding toxicity in normal cells (Figure 1.9) [157,158].

Passive targeting feats the characteristic features of tumor biology that allows nanocarriers to accumulate in a tumor by the enhanced permeability and retention (EPR) [160]. Active approaches achieve this by conjugating nanocarriers containing chemotherapeutics with molecules that bind to overexpressed antigens or receptors on the target

(a)

Passive targeting

(b)

Active targeting

Endothelium

NP

Targeted NP

Cancer cells

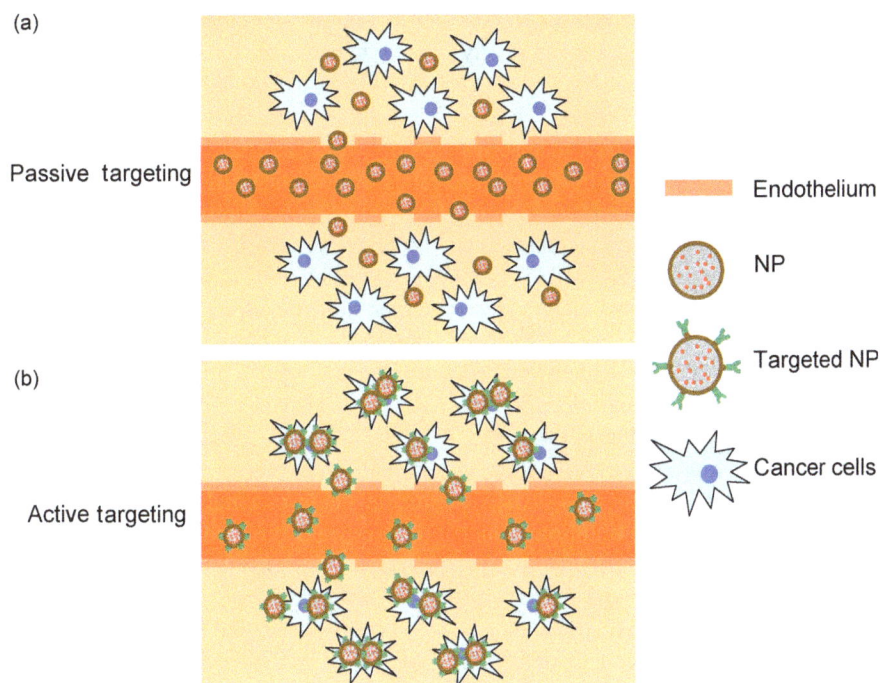

FIGURE 1.8 Schematic representation of nanoparticle targeting. (a) Nanoparticles are concentrated in the tumor interstitium via passive extravasation through the leaky microvasculature shown as gaps in the endothelial layer (light orange). This process has been named the EPR effect. In this case, the efficacy of nanoparticles is largely mediated through the local release of the drug near the cancer cells. (b) Targeted nanoparticles similarly concentrate in the tumor interstitium through the EPR effect, but once there, nanoparticles are actively taken up by cancer cells after binding to their target antigens on the surface of the cancer cells. In this case, the drugs are released largely inside the cancer cells, resulting in enhanced efficacy.

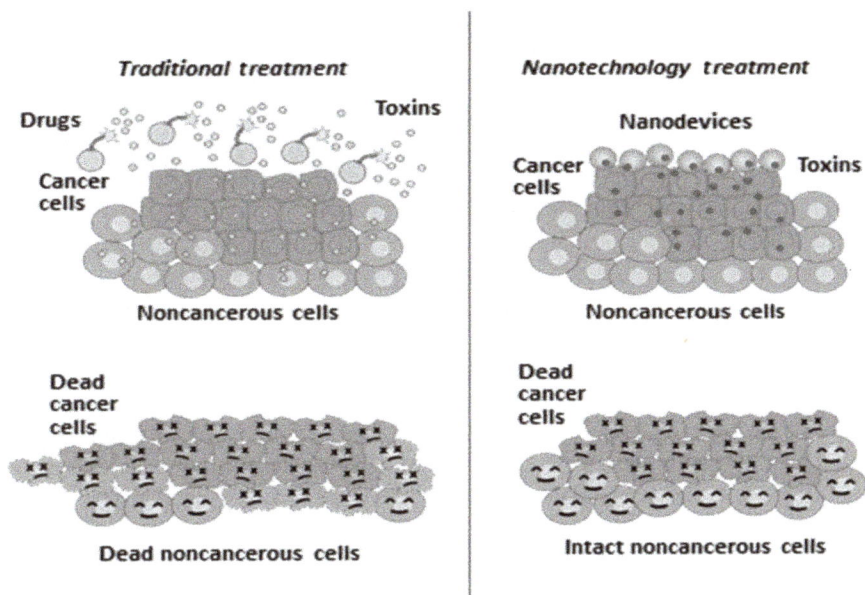

Traditional treatment

Drugs   Toxins

Cancer
cells

Noncancerous cells

Dead
cancer
cells

Dead noncancerous cells

Nanotechnology treatment

Nanodevices

Cancer
cells   Toxins

Noncancerous cells

Dead
cancer
cells

Intact noncancerous cells

FIGURE 1.9 Improving cancer treatment [159].

cells. However, although NPs offer many advantages as drug carrier systems, there are still many limitations to be solved, such as poor oral bioavailability, instability in circulation, inadequate tissue distribution, and toxicity. Reviews provide a perspective on the use of nanotechnology as a fundamental tool in cancer research and nanomedicine [161,162]. Here, we focus on the types and characteristics of NPs, how NPs are being used as drug delivery systems to kill cancer cells more effectively and also to reduce or overcome drug resistance, and how NPs will be developed to improve their therapeutic efficacy and functionality in future cancer treatments.

The precise relationship between physicochemical properties of NPs and their biodistribution continues to be poorly understood [132,163]. This is largely due to the complexity and variety of biological interactions between NPs and the host as well as the widely varying properties of NPs themselves [164] and the dynamic status of the biologic host. Particle characteristics change in different environments and should be measured in conditions as close to the point of application (e.g., in serum or in cell culture medium) as possible [132]. As the relationship of the material properties of NPs to intratumoral accumulation is poorly understood, studies that do not thoroughly characterize material properties likely will not reproduce consistent results [132]. This remains an important area of ongoing investigation. An understanding of these principles will be essential to safe and reproducible utilization of nanomaterials for human cancer applications.

NPs have tremendous potential for traditional and emerging cancer imaging modalities. The ability to specifically engineer nanomaterials has the potential to improve contrast agent specificity, sensitivity, and functionality, leading to new paradigms in early cancer detection and image-guided cancer therapy [165]. In addition, new nanoscale contrast agents are expected to exhibit reduced toxicity compared to traditional imaging contrast agents.

A variety of nanoscale magnetic resonance imaging (MRI) contrast agents have been developed [166]. These particles have received significant attention, given the widespread use of MR in clinical practice currently [167]. These contrast agents have been designed to improve detection sensitivity and may be biologically targeted to sites of cancer to offer imaging specificity [168]. Further, nanoscale MR contrast agents have also been used to mediate noninvasive cancer therapy (e.g., neutron capture therapy and radiofrequency ablation) and for targeted drug delivery [169].

Malignant cells are resistant to the anticancer action [170] of chemotherapeutic agents and cell division inhibitors, which reflects their ability to change at molecular level and develop tumor survival strategies that activate the angiogenic mechanism, in order to prevent hypoxic conditions and to support nutrient intake. Therefore, the main therapeutic approaches are targeting the hallmarks of cancer, particularly aiming to inhibit tumor angiogenesis. Multiple cellular processes related to apoptosis or cell proliferation lead to alterations in signaling pathways that are responsible for resistance to chemotherapy and drug tolerance in a cancer cell [171–173].

The progress of nanotechnology-based screening techniques has led to target-based drug development regimens that increase the survival rate of cancer patients [174]. Therapeutic agents are becoming highly specific and have a high affinity for various molecular targets, depending on the malignancy's genotype and phenotype [175]. Cancer treatment strategies include a wide range of combination chemotherapy drugs, in addition to radiotherapy and adjuvant/neoadjuvant surgery. The main drawbacks related to chemotherapy are the unwanted side effects. Therefore, intensive research is carried out to develop novel therapeutic formulation using specific NPs for targeted delivery in order to avoid the cytotoxic effects on healthy cells [176].

NP-based drug delivery systems show remarkable progress due to their ability to have a "controlled-release reservoir," which can safely deliver therapeutic agents to injury sites or specific cells [177,178]. For safe use in medicine, NPs must be biocompatible, that is, able to integrate within a biological system without causing immune response or negative side effects when the construct is directly released either into the tumor or into the bloodstream [179]. NPs must also provide controlled drug release, increasing the therapeutic agent's protection and circulation time and thus decreasing toxicity to healthy cells [178,180]. This can lead to an EPR effect [181].

Nanotechnology is a rapidly growing research area in the fields of catalysts, biosensors, bioimaging, energy devices, and targeted drug delivery [182–185]. The large surface-to-volume ratio of NPs and their size, ability to carry other compounds, binding ability, and their adsorption properties make them suitable for biomedical applications. NPs can also improve bioavailability, protect drugs from degradation, and control release rates, i.e., provide sustained drug release. These unique characteristics of NPs offer a viable platform for their use as an effective drug delivery system [186]. Biodegradable carboxymethyl cellulose/graphene oxide (CMC/GO) nanohybrid hydrogel beads physically crosslinked with $FeCl_3.6H_2O$ have been used for the controlled release of an anticancer drug (doxorubicin, DOX) [187]. The π–π stacking interaction between GO and DOX caused higher drug loading efficiency. The release profile from hydrogels was highly pH-dependent, based on hydrogen-bonded interactions, and exhibited a faster release at pH ~ 6.8 than in slightly basic media (pH ~ 7.4). Furthermore, greater amounts of filler/GO reduced the release rate because of enhanced interactions between the components. Halloysite nanotube-embedded hybrid hydrogels of poly(hydroxyethyl methacrylate) with sodium hyaluronate were very effective for colon cancer drug delivery [188]. Anticancer drugs, such as 5-fluorouracil (5-FU), have been encapsulated not only in hydrogel networks but also in halloysite nanotubes using an equilibrium swelling method, followed by pulling and breaking the vacuum. *In vitro* release of 5-FU from nanohybrid hydrogels exhibited pH-dependent controlled release following diffusion-controlled non-Fickian transport behavior. 5-FU was also intercalated within the gallery of natural montmorillonite (Mt) clay, which could be compounded using alginate (Alg), followed by a coating with CS, to prepare a complex drug release system with controlled-release behavior [189]. The release rate of 5-FU was found to be retarded when using an Alg–CS/5-FU/Mt nanohybrid system in gastric and intestinal environments. Hybrids of nanoclay and CS–polylactide blends also released paclitaxel (PTX) in a pronounced manner in basic conditions compared to their release in acidic environments [190]. Biodegradable poly(ϵ-caprolactone) (PCL) nanohybrid scaffolds with organically modified nanoclay, which were prepared through an electrospinning technique, exhibited sustained delivery of an anticancer drug (dexamethasone) vis-à-vis pure polymer by creating a maze or "tortuous path" that retarded the diffusion of the drug from the matrix in the presence of a two-dimensional (2D) filler [191]. Biocompatible polyurethane nanohybrids using an aliphatic diisocyanate and aliphatic chain extender with varying chain lengths and 2D nanoclay were designed for sustained drug delivery of an anticancer drug in which the tortuous path was created through larger crystallites from self-assembly of a hard segmented zone [192]. Graphene-based polyurethane nanohybrids have been prepared by grafting long-chain polyurethane onto the surface of functionalized GO for sustained drug delivery of an anticancer drug (dexamethasone) [193]. Chemically tagged amine- and sulfonate-functionalized graphene within long-chain polyurethane molecules has been developed for the sustained release of dexamethasone [194,195]. A hard segment in pure polyurethane was responsible for delayed drug release, whereas the self-assembled structure and graphene moieties acted as a barrier for the diffusion of loaded drugs in nanohybrids. Several other polymer NP hybrid systems have been reported as sustained-release systems for cancer therapy using different drugs, such as DOX, 5-FU, and MTX [196–200]. The dual administration of DOX with MTX had higher cytotoxicity toward T47D breast cancer cells than free dual drug forms. Dual anticancer drug-loaded antibacterial smart polymer nanohybrids have the potential to be used for combination cancer therapy.

1.8 SIZE AND SURFACE CHARACTERISTICS OF NPs

NPs must have the ability to remain in the bloodstream for a considerable time without being eliminated for effective delivery of drug to the targeted tumor tissue. Conventional surface particles and non-modified NPs are usually caught in the circulation by the reticuloendothelial system (RES), such as the liver and the spleen, depending on their size and surface characteristics [201]. The fate of injected NPs can be controlled by adjusting their size and surface characteristics.

Surface characteristics: Surface characteristics of NPs are an important factor for determining their lifespan and destiny during circulation relating to their capture by macrophages. Ideally, NPs should have hydrophilic surface so that they can escape macrophage capture [202]. This can be achieved by two methods: first, coating the surface of NPs with a hydrophilic polymer, such as PEG, and second, protecting them from opsonization by repelling plasma proteins; alternatively, NPs can be formed from block copolymers with hydrophilic and hydrophobic domains [203].

Size: In addition to their surface characteristics, there is one more advantage of NPs: their size can be adjusted. The size of NPs used in a drug delivery system should be small enough to escape capture by fixed macrophages that are lodged in the RES, such as the liver and spleen, but should be large enough to prevent their rapid leakage into

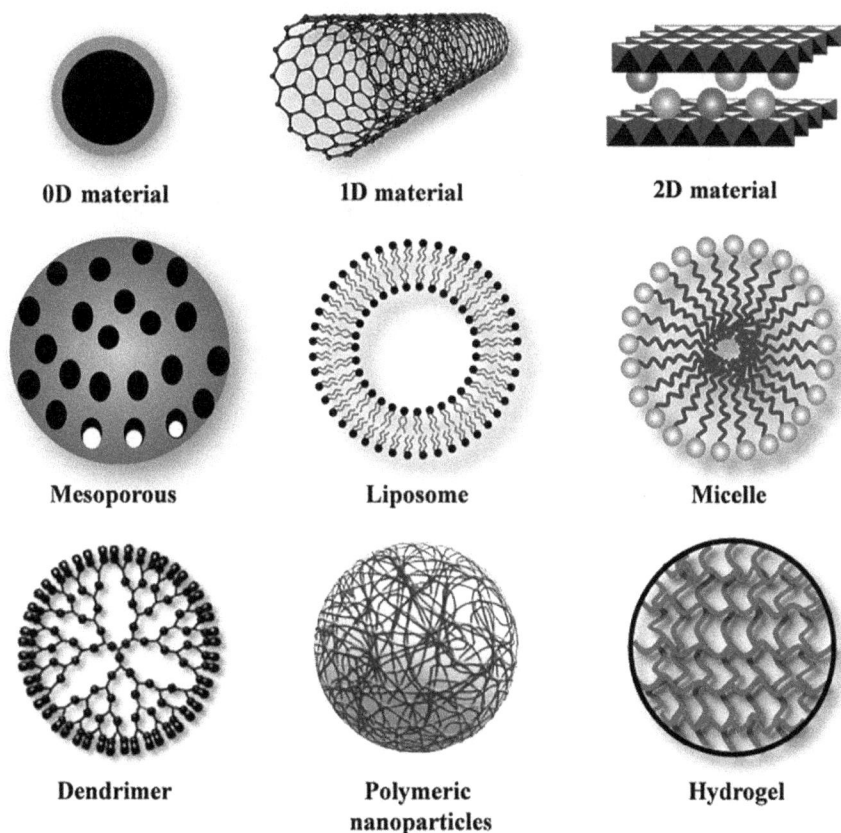

0D material   **1D material**   **2D material**

Mesoporous   **Liposome**   **Micelle**

Dendrimer   **Polymeric nanoparticles**   **Hydrogel**

SCHEME 1.1 Different types of nanocarriers used as controlled-delivery vehicles for cancer treatment.

blood capillaries. The size of the sinusoid in the spleen and fenestra of the Kupffer cells in the liver varies from 150 to 200 nm [204], and the size of gap junction between endothelial cells of the leaky tumor vasculature may vary from 100 to 600 nm [205]. Thus, the size of NPs should be up to 100 nm to reach tumor tissues by passing through these two particular vascular structures.

1.9 TYPES OF NANOCARRIERS USED AS CONTROLLED DELIVERY VEHICLES FOR CANCER TREATMENT

Several innovative methods of drug delivery are being used in cancer treatment. A wide range of nanoscale compounds based on synthetic polymers, proteins, lipids, and organic and inorganic particles have been employed for the development of cancer therapeutics. Compared with the direct administration of bare chemo-drugs, drug encapsulation in a carrier offers a number of advantages, such as protection from degradation in the bloodstream, better drug solubility, enhanced drug stability, targeted drug delivery, decreased toxic side effects, and improved pharmacokinetic and pharmacodynamic drug properties. To date, an impressive library of various drug delivery vehicles has been developed with varying sizes, architectures, and surface physicochemical properties with targeting strategies (Scheme 1.1).

NPs are used in medicine to improve bioavailability [206,207], to enhance the delivery of therapeutic agents [208], or to develop novel imaging techniques [209–211], in order to assure the control of biological systems for single molecules or groups of molecules [212]. A wide range of nanostructures such as liposomes, nanodiamonds, QDs, peptides, cyclodextrin (CD), CNTs, and graphene and metal-based NPs are used for diagnostic or therapeutic purposes (Figure 1.10) [207].

NPs are able to enhance the accumulation and release of pharmacologically active agents at the tumor site, improve therapeutic efficacy, and decrease the intensity of side effects on the healthy tissues. Due to the intrinsic features of NPs, it is possible to integrate both diagnostic and therapeutic agents into a single NP. These features allow monitoring the biodistribution and accumulation of agents at the target site, and thus, the release of drugs can be visualized and quantified, which may lead to proper assessment of their therapeutic efficiency [213,214].

The low size of NPs allows them to cross cellular membranes and avoid detection by the RES, thus preventing their degradation. Their high surface area enhances the loading of therapeutic agents, making them ideal for medical purposes [215]. A wide range of anticancer drugs such as rituximab, lestaurtinib, carboplatin, PTX, DOX, and tyrosine kinase inhibitors have been loaded onto NPs with

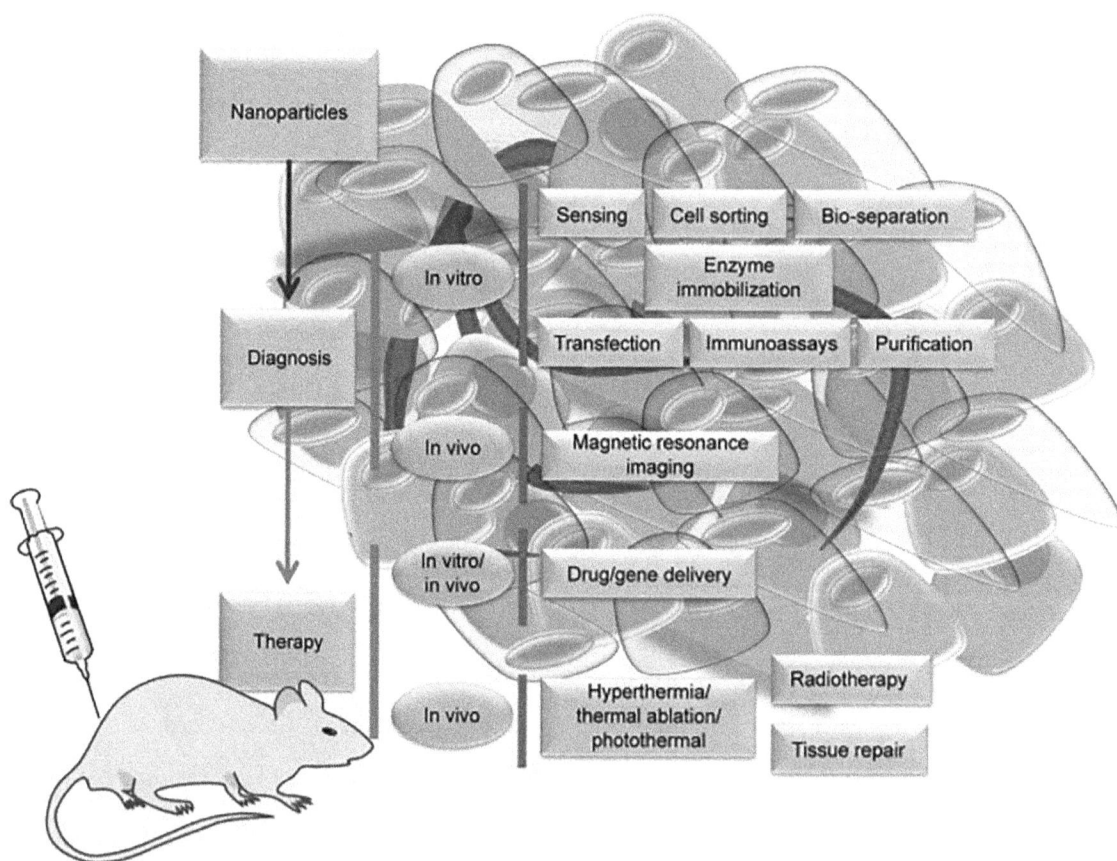

FIGURE 1.10   Different applications of nanoparticles involved in therapy and diagnosis.

a potential effect against various cancers, and a superior therapeutic efficacy than free chemotherapeutics [216–220].

1.10 KINETICS AND BIODISTRIBUTION OF NPs

The kinetics, biodistribution, and release profile of the active compounds are modified by the nanodrug formulation, thus improving cancer treatment while enhancing EPR. To be more effective, the nanodrugs must be accumulated at the target tissues, for which the NPs must be smaller than the mean pore size of the vasculature of the target tissues.

Nanodrugs are complex, and scientists must understand their structure and physical and chemical characteristics, as well as the biological principles employed to attach or encapsulate the therapeutic agents [221]. Drugs could be selectively targeted to tumors through "active targeting" by using a peptide or an antibody that specifically binds to a molecule that is selectively expressed on targeted cancer cells. Drugs should "passively target" cell-specific functions or local environments in order to facilitate the uptake and accumulation in tumor tissues and inflammatory sites (Figure 1.11) [222]. In addition, there are some NP properties that determine their *in vivo* distribution, such as particle size, charge, core, surface properties, shape, flexibility, multivalence, and controlled synthesis.

Key areas of investigation in NP research are the pharmacokinetics and biodistribution, related to the NP size and its behavior. It was shown that the optimal size for the drug delivery systems is between 1 and 100 nm. Small NPs increasingly accumulate and penetrate into tumor tissues through the EPR effect, with elimination in the spleen being avoided. Multivalence is characterized by a high surface area-to-volume ratio, which offers high loading capacity for different imaging agents, targeting ligands, and therapeutic agents. The shape of NPs influences their internalization into cells, determining the *in vivo* behavior and biological function (Figure 1.12). To improve or reduce

circulation time, the surface and charge of the NPs can be changed; positive charge is correlated with a higher rate of nonspecific internalization and a shorter blood circulation time, when compared to negative and neutral charges [213].

An important mechanism by which therapeutic agents are taken up by the cells is the endocytic pathway. After passing through the cellular membrane, these agents are entrapped in endosomes and are degraded in lysosomes by specific enzymes. The main advantage of this mechanism is that it facilitates the endosomal escape and ensures cytosolic delivery of the agents, which helps achieving an effective biological-based therapy.

There are various mechanisms for endosomal escape that facilitate the release of the therapeutic agents into the cytosol. Pore formation occurs through the interactions between the membrane tension that extends the pores and the line tension that closes the pores. This causes the forming of pores in the lipid bilayer mediated by aggregates of peptides that enter into the membrane in a perpendicular orientation, thus leading to an inward curving of the membrane. The proton sponge effect (pH-buffering effect) is a mechanism caused by the ability of agents to inflate when protonated. Through this step, called "protonation," the entrapped components are released due to the inflow of ions and water into the endosomal environment, leading to endosomal membrane ruptures. Another mechanism is represented by the fusogenic peptides that have the ability to destabilize the endosomal membrane, which plays an important role in cellular trafficking and endocytosis. Endosomal membrane can be destroyed photochemically, by exposure to light. This method induces the formation of reactive singlet oxygen with a short lifetime which destroys the endosomal membrane, allowing the therapeutic agent to be delivered to the cytosol [223].

A NP's intracellular fate is based on the selected endocytic pathway. However, many researches showed that the transport pathway can be affected by the physicochemical characteristics of NPs, such as size, charge, shape, different

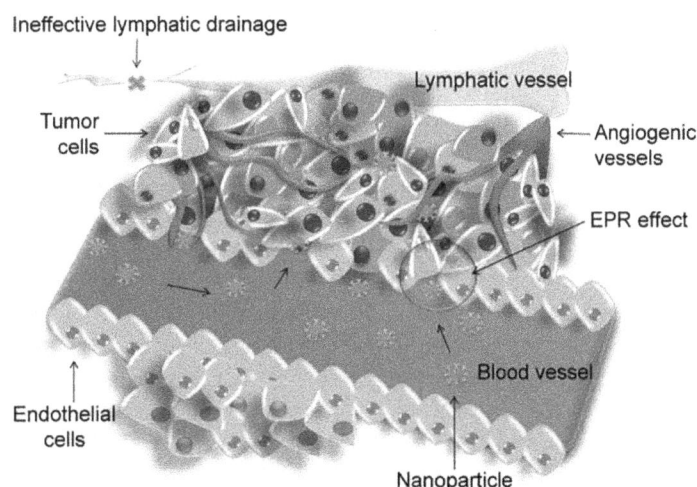

FIGURE 1.11 Passive targeting relies on cell-specific functions or local environments specific to the target tissue to facilitate uptake and accumulation in tumor tissues and inflammatory sites. EPR, enhanced permeability and retention.

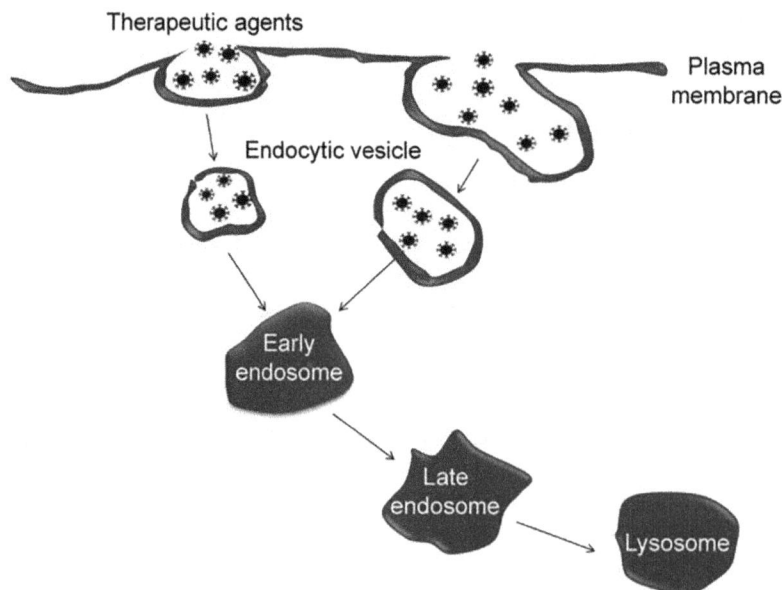

FIGURE 1.12 Nanoparticle internalization. Nanoparticles enter the cell via endocytosis, which is the main pathway for crossing the cellular membrane. Also, nanoparticles are internalized into the cells, and the cargo is released inside. Nanoparticles administered are cleared in the liver and spleen, which remain in these organs for a long time and are then taken up by macrophages. Then, the nanoparticles exit the cell via exocytosis.

endocytic machineries in various cell types [224], aggregation state, and surface chemistry [225]. Peñaloza et al. showed that NPs can be taken by recycling endosomes back to the extracellular environment, or may be degraded in lysosomes or trapped in an organelle, without releasing their content at the desired site [207,226].

1.11 MECHANISMS OF NANOCARRIERS FOR DRUG DELIVERY

Nanocarriers come across numerous barriers in their route to the target, such as mucosal barriers and nonspecific uptake [227,228]. To report the challenges in targeting tumors with nanotechnology, it is essential to combine the rational design of nanocarriers with the fundamental understanding of tumor biology. General features of tumors include poor lymphatic drainage and leaky blood vessels. Whereas free drugs may diffuse nonspecifically, a nanocarrier can escape into the tumor tissues via the leaky vessels by the EPR effect [229] (Figure 1.13).

There is rapid and defective angiogenesis (formation of new blood vessels from existing ones), because of which there is increased permeability of blood vessels in tumor cells. Furthermore, the dysfunctional lymphatic drainage in tumors also helps in retaining the accumulated nanocarriers and allows them to release drugs into the locality of the tumor cells. Experiments using liposomes of different mean size suggest that the threshold vesicle size for extravasation into tumors is ~400 nm [205], but other studies have shown that particles having diameters <200 nm are more effective [230,231]. Based on clinical therapy, passive targeting approaches suffer from several limitations. Some drugs cannot diffuse efficiently so targeting cells within tumor is

not always possible and the random nature of the approach makes it difficult to control the process because of this lack of control multiple-drug resistance (MDR) may induce— a situation where chemotherapy treatments fail patients shows resistance of cancer cells toward one or more drugs MDR occurs because of the overexpression of transporter proteins that expel drugs from cells on the surface of cancer cells [156,232,233]. Expelling drugs inevitably lowers the therapeutic effect, and cancer cells soon develop resistance to a variety of drugs. The passive strategy is further limited because certain tumors do not exhibit the EPR effect, and the permeability of vessels may not be the same throughout a single tumor [234]. One way to overcome these limitations is to modify the nanocarriers in such a way that they actively bind to specific cells after extravasation. This can be achieved by attaching targeting agents such as ligands— molecules that can bind to specific receptors on the cell surface—to the surface of the nanocarrier by a variety of conjugation chemistries. Nanocarriers will recognize the receptor and bind to target cells through ligand–receptor interactions, and drug will be released inside the cell (Figure 1.13). In general, targeting agent which is used to deliver nanocarriers to cancer cells, it is imperative that the agent should bind with high selectivity to molecules that are uniquely expressed on the cell surface. Other important consideration is that to maximize specificity, a surface marker, which can be an antigen or receptor, should be overexpressed on target cells than in the normal cells. For example, to efficiently deliver liposomes to B-cell receptors using the anti-CD19 mAb, the density of receptors should be in the range of 104–105 copies per cell. Those with lower density are less effectively targeted [235]. In a breast cancer model, a receptor density of 105 copies of ErbB2

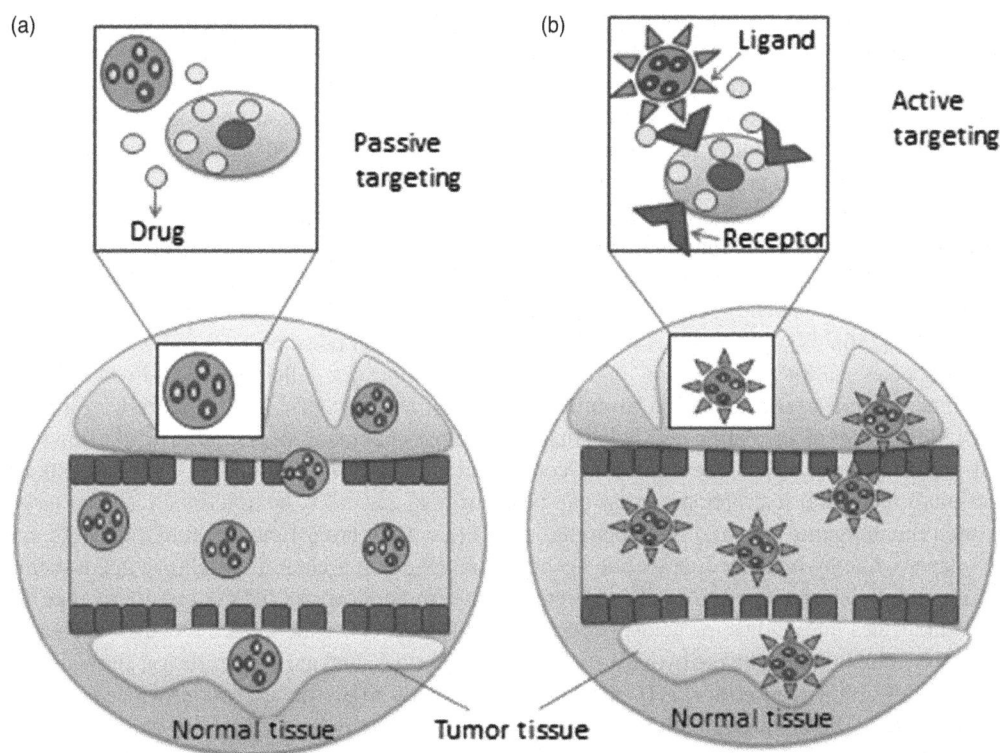

FIGURE 1.13 Schematic representation of different mechanisms by which nanocarriers can deliver drugs to tumors. (a) Passive tissue targeting and (b) active cellular targeting.

receptors per cell was necessary to improve the therapeutic efficacy of an anti-ErbB2-targeted liposomal DOX relative to its non-targeted counterpart [236]. The binding of certain ligands to their receptors may cause receptor-mediated internalization, which is often necessary if nanocarriers are to release drugs inside the cells [158,237,238]. For example, when immunoliposomes targeted to human blood cancer (B-cell lymphoma) were labeled with an internalizing anti-CD19 ligand, a more significant therapeutic outcome was achieved rather than a non-internalizing anti-CD20 ligand [239]. In contrast, owing to the bystander effect, targeting nanocarriers to non-internalizing receptors may sometimes be advantageous in solid tumors, where cells lacking the target receptor can be killed through drug release at the surface of the neighboring cells, where carriers can bind [240]. It is generally known that higher binding affinity increases targeting efficacy. However, for solid tumors due to a "binding-site barrier," high binding affinity can decrease penetration of nanocarriers, where the nanocarrier binds to its target so strongly that penetration into the tissue is prevented. In addition to enhanced affinity, multivalent binding effects may be used to improve targeting. The collective binding in a multivalent interaction is much stronger than monovalent binding. For example, dendrimer nanocarriers conjugated to 3–15 folate molecules showed a 2500- to 170,000-fold enhancement in dissociation constants (KD) over free folate when attaching to folate-binding proteins immobilized on a surface. This was attributed to the avidity of the multiple folic acid (FA) groups on the periphery of the dendrimers [241].

Nanomedicine is a rapidly developing area that is revolutionizing cancer diagnosis and therapy. NPs have unique biological properties given their small size (diameter within 1–100 nm) and large surface area-to-volume ratio, which allows them to bind, absorb, and carry anticancer agents, such as drugs, deoxyribonucleic acid (DNA), ribonucleic acid (RNA), and proteins, along with imaging agents with high efficiency. Nanocarriers used in chemotherapy can be classified into two major types designed for targeted or non-targeted drug delivery: vehicles that use organic molecules as a major building block material and those that use inorganic elements (usually metals) as a core. Organic nanocarriers are comprised of liposomes, lipids, dendrimers, CNTs, emulsions, and synthetic polymers.

1.11.1 Inorganic Nanocarriers

Inorganic nanocarrier platforms have been intensively investigated for therapeutic and imaging treatments in recent years due to their great advantages, such as large surface area, better drug loading capacity, better bioavailability, lower toxic side effects and controlled drug release, and their tolerance toward most organic solvents, unlike polymer-based NPs. QDs, CNTs, layered double hydroxides (LDHs), mesoporous silica, and magnetic NPs are commonly used in cancer treatment in various ways. QDs have already been proven to be powerful imaging probes, especially for long-term, multiplexed, and quantitative imaging and diagnostics [242–244]. Zero-dimensional (0D) fluorescent NPs, such as QDs within the size of 1–10 nm, have emerged as one of the most promising NPs for targeted and traceable drug delivery systems, real-time monitoring of intracellular processes, and *in vivo* molecular imaging due to their unique physicochemical properties, such as uniform size, large surface-to-volume ratio, biocompatibility, highly tunable photoluminescence property, improved signal brightness, resistance against photobleaching, and multicolor fluorescence imaging and detection [245]. However, the main challenge with QDs in biological applications is their hydrophobic nature, high tendency of aggregation, and nonspecific adsorption [246,247]. QD surfaces are usually coated with polar species and/or monolayer or multilayer ligand shells to make them water-soluble and to enhance their bioactivity [248]. This type of coating also helps in the development of multifunctional QDs, where imaging contrast agents and small molecular hydrophobic drugs can be embedded between the inorganic core and the amphiphilic polymer coating layer while hydrophilic therapeutic agents (hydrophilic drug, small interfering RNA (siRNA), etc.) and targeting biomolecules (antibodies, proteins, peptides, and aptamers) can be immobilized onto the hydrophilic side of the amphiphiles [249,250]. Gao et al. [251] developed polymer-encapsulated and bioconjugated QD probes for cancer targeting and *in vivo* imaging. d-α-Tocopheryl polyethylene glycol 1000 succinate monoester (TPGS)-coated multifunctional (theranostic) liposomes have been developed in the form of docetaxel and QD for cancer imaging and targeted therapy [252]. Recently, multifunctional QDs have been synthesized, making them a promising targeted drug delivery vehicle for the diagnosis and image-guided chemotherapy of various cancers [253,254].

Carbon nanotubes (CNTs): CNTs are synthetic one-dimensional (1D) nanomaterials made from carbon, and they structurally contain rolled sheets of graphene rings built from sp^2 hybridized carbon atoms into hollow tubes. CNTs are well known for ideal near-infrared (NIR) photothermal ablation therapy because they increase the temperature within tumors as a function of light intensity and CNT dose [255,256]. Functionalized water-soluble CNTs are being investigated for their use in gene and drug delivery because they can readily cross biological barriers and can effectively transport molecules into the cytoplasm without producing a toxic effect [257,258]. Chemotherapeutic drug molecules have been conjugated to functional groups on the CNT surface or through polymer coatings of CNTs, which are usually formed via cleavable bonds. CNTs for antitumor immunotherapy can act as antigen-presenting carriers to improve weakly immunogenic tumor-based peptides/antigens to trigger a humoral immune response within the tumor [259,260]. Among the inorganic nanocarriers, 2D LDHs, also known as hydrotalcite-like compounds, have recently attracted a great deal of interest for their potential as delivery carriers mainly because of their excellent biocompatibility, anion exchange capability, high drug loading efficacy, full protection for loaded drugs, pH-responsive drug release, ease of preparation, low cost, easy and efficient penetration into the cell membrane and considerable

drug delivery, biodegradation in the cellular cytoplasm (pH between 4 and 6), and good endosomal escape; moreover, the drug release rate can be tuned by changing the interlayer anion. LDHs consist of layers of a divalent metal ion, such as Mg^{2+}, Ca^{2+}, Ni^{2+}, and Zn^{2+}, with a trivalent metal ion isomorphically substituted to give the layers a net positive charge [261]. This charge is balanced by interlayer hydrated anions, resulting in a multilayer of alternating host layers with exchangeable gallery anions, such as Cl^-, NO_3^-, and CO_3^{2-}. Anionic drugs and biofunctional molecules (genetic materials, peptides, proteins, etc.) can easily be intercalated in the interlayer gallery through direct synthesis, coprecipitation, anion exchange, etc., thereby conferring protection against enzymatic degradation while flowing in biological fluids [262–264]. In addition, their internal and/or external surfaces can easily be functionalized and modified to incorporate a targeting function, and their high specific surface area and better chemical stability make them attractive for diverse applications. LDHs can intercalate various important anionic biofunctional molecules, such as DNA, siRNA, nucleotides, and anticancer drugs, showing sustained delivery with high therapeutic efficiency and bioactivity. A unique strategy for the delivery of non-ionic insoluble drugs using LDH as carrier can also be made through micellization [265]. The intercalation of an anticancer drug, raloxifene hydrochloride (RH), into a series of magnesium–aluminum LDHs with varying interlayer exchangeable anions (NO_3^-, CO_3^{2-}, PO_4^{3-}) through an ion exchange technique has been reported and was found to release the drug in a controlled manner [261]. Figure 1.14a illustrates the rapid release rate using phosphate-bound LDH-drug (LP-R) while sustained delivery is obtained using nitrate-based LDH (LN-R). Spectroscopic (XPS, UV–Vis) and thermal (DSC) studies confirm the strong interactions between drug molecules and LDH host layers, which lead to sluggish delivery in LN-R against LP-R. *In vitro* anticancer studies demonstrate better efficacy of cell death using drug-intercalated LDHs instead of a pure drug arising from sustained release of the intercalated drug (Figure 1.14b).

Among the drug-intercalated LDHs, LP-R/pure drug exhibits better tumor suppression efficiency, whereas the body weight loss index suggests organ damage. In contrast, LN-R shows slight, slow tumor healing but exhibits minimum body weight loss, indicating a better drug delivery vehicle (Figure 1.14c). Histograms of different organs and analyses of biochemical parameters suggest damaged liver cells of mice treated with a fast-release vehicle (pure drug and LP-R), whereas no damage occurs in mouse liver cells treated with LN-R or a slow-release vehicle (Figure 1.14d). Further, positively charged LDH NPs can easily penetrate into negatively charged cell membranes through the clathrin-mediated endocytosis pathway. Li et al. [266] employed a combined strategy using LDH to simultaneously deliver CD-siRNA and a chemotherapeutic drug (5-FU) to cancer cells, leading to significantly higher cytotoxicity than single treatments with either CD-siRNA or 5-FU.

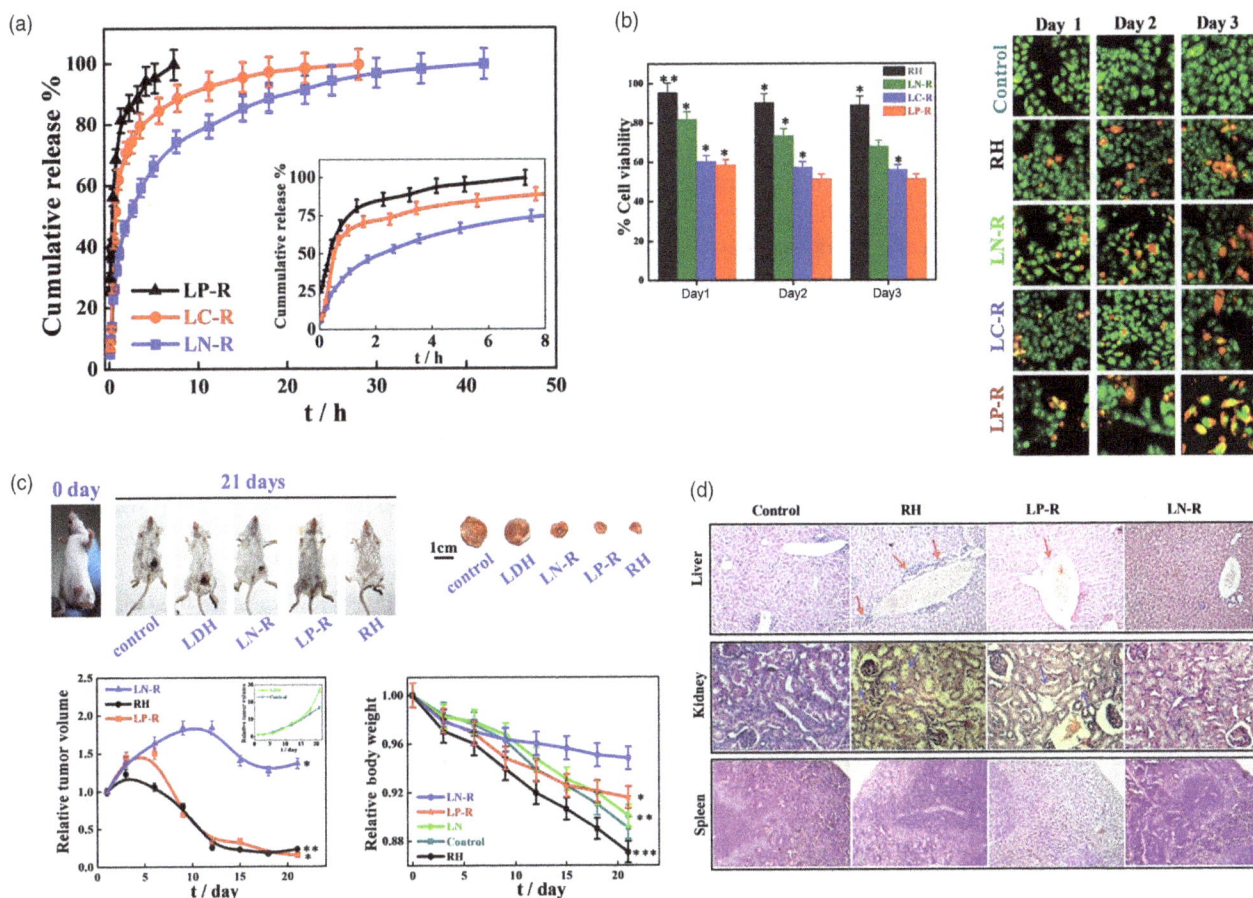

FIGURE 1.14 *In vitro* and *in vivo* controlled release of drug using layered double hydroxides and its effects. (a) *In vitro* drug release profiles for drug-intercalated nitrate, carbonate, and phosphate LDHs (LN-R, LC-R, and LP-R, respectively); the inset figure describes the release pattern of the above-mentioned systems in a time frame of 0–8 h. (b) *In vitro* cytotoxicity of free drug and drug-intercalated LDHs against HeLa cells at different time intervals. (c) *In vivo* antitumor effect and systematic toxicity of pure RH and drug-intercalated LDHs in comparison with control. (d) Histological analysis of the liver, kidney, and spleen of tumor-bearing mice treated with control (saline), pure RH, LN-R, and LP-R [261].

Based on the structure and the diameter, CNTs can be categorized into two kinds: the single-walled CNTs (SWNTs) and the multiwalled CNTs (MWNTs) [267]. The SWNTs are composed of monolithic cylindrical graphene, and the MWNTs are composed of concentric graphene [267]. Because of the physical and chemical properties of CNTs, including surface area, mechanical strength, metal properties, and electrical and thermal conductivity, it is a candidate well suited for large-scale biomedical applications [268]. CNTs also possess a property that allows them to absorb light from the NIR region, causing the nanotubes to be heated up by the thermal effect, thus targeting tumor cells [269–271]. The natural forms of CNTs promote noninvasive penetration of biofilms and are regarded as highly competent carriers for the transport of various drug molecules into living cells [272]. Due to the suitability of CNTs, drugs such as PTX are assembled with them and administered both *in vitro* and *in vivo* for cancer treatment [273].

Fullerenes: Fullerenes are carbon allotropes with a large spheroidal molecule consisting of a hollow cage of 60 or more atoms. They behave like electron-deficient alkenes and react readily with electron-rich species [274]. The photodynamic effect of two new decacationic fullerene and red light-harvesting antenna–fullerene conjugated monoadduct derivatives generated reactive oxygen species (ROS) for anticancer therapy. Mesoporous silica nanoparticles (MSNs) are extensively used as drug delivery vehicles due to their unique properties, such as their large specific surface area and pore volume, controllable particle size, ease of functionalizing good biocompatibility, and ability to provide a physical casing to protect and house drugs from degeneration or denaturation. MSNs with tunable pore sizes offer great potential for controlling drug loading percentages and release kinetics and can deliver antitumor drugs in a targeted fashion, releasing them on demand to increase their cellular uptake without any premature release prior to reaching the target site [275]. Another advantage of MSNs is their ability to deliver membrane-impermeable hydrophobic drugs, thereby serving as a universal transmembrane carrier for intracellular drug delivery and imaging applications. They also have emerged as promising candidates for both passive and active targeted delivery systems and can accumulate in tumor tissues via the EPR effect. Furthermore, specific drug delivery can be achieved via active targeting by the functionalizing of MSNs with targeting ligands, such as folate (FA) or EGF [276]. Antibodies, peptides, and magnetic NPs can also be decorated onto MSNs, thereby acting as a homing device. In the targeting process, particle size and surface modification of MSNs critically influence the particle's cellular uptake, pharmacokinetics, and biodistribution profiles.

Calcium phosphate nanoparticles (CPN): Calcium phosphate nanoparticles (CPN) have long been regarded as potential drug and gene delivery vehicles due to their excellent biocompatibility, biodegradability, and colloidal stability, and they can encapsulate negatively charged therapeutic agents by chelating calcium ions while forming calcium phosphate nanocrystals [277,278]. CPN are the major component of bone and tooth enamel, and both Ca^{2+} and PO_4^{3-} are found in the bloodstream at a relatively high concentration (1–5 mM) [279,280]. Lipid calcium phosphate (LCP) NPs have been found to achieve both systemic delivery of drugs/genes to the lymphatic system and imaging of lymph node metastasis [281]. PEGylated calcium phosphate hybrid micelles enhance the *in vivo* accumulation of siRNA in tumor tissues and promote their gene-silencing activity [282]. Calcium phosphate-based organic–inorganic nanocarriers are known for switching on photodynamic therapy (PDT) in response to acidic environments [283]. Mn^{2+} within CPN of PEG shells has been found to act as an efficient MRI contrast agent that rapidly amplifies magnetic resonance signals in response to pH [284].

Superparamagnetic iron oxide nanoparticles (SPIONs): Superparamagnetic iron oxide nanoparticles (SPIONs) are receiving increased attention for chemotherapy, hypothermia, MRI, tissue engineering, and cell and tissue targeting and transfection due to their intrinsic properties, such as inherent magnetism, visualization by MRI, biocompatibility, guidance to target sites by means of an external magnetic field, heating to provide hyperthermia for cancer therapy, and degradation into nontoxic iron ions *in vivo*. SPIONs are composed of an inner magnetic particle core (usually magnetite, Fe_3O_4, or maghemite, γ-Fe_2O_3) and a hydrophilic coating of polymers, such as polysaccharide, PEG, and poly(vinyl alcohol). Direct use of SPIONs without any polymer coating as an *in vivo* MRI contrast agent results in biofouling of the particles in blood plasma and particle agglomerations that are quickly sequestered by cells of the RES, such as macrophages [285,286]. The coating helps to shield the magnetic particle from the surrounding environment and can also be functionalized by targeting ligands. These magnetic drug-bearing nanocarriers rely on external magnetic field guidance to reach their target tissue. Magnetic albumin microspheres (MM-ADR) in animal tumor models exhibit better responses than adriamycin alone in terms of both tumor size reduction and animal survival [287]. The enhanced efficacy of magnetic albumin microspheres in the targeted delivery of an anticancer agent compared to the pure drug in a rat model is predominantly due to magnetic effects

and is not due to the particle's size or nonmagnetic holding [288]. SPION-based MRI is a very powerful noninvasive tool in biomedical imaging, clinical diagnosis, and therapy. SPIONs potentially provide higher contrast enhancement in MRI and are much more bio-friendly than conventional paramagnetic Gd-based contrast agents [289,290]. Various methods of SPION preparation along with functionalization for targeted therapy and applications in cancer treatment have been reported [291]. Monocrystalline iron oxide nanoparticles (MION) and crosslinked iron oxide nanoparticles (CLIO) are two typical examples of dextran (DEX)-coated SPIONs and have been widely used *in vivo* and *in vitro* MRI [292,293]. Anti-biofouling polymer-coated thermally crosslinked superparamagnetic iron oxide nanoparticles (TCL-SPIONs) act as a novel MR contrast agent for *in vivo* cancer imaging [294], and Cy5.5-conjugated TCL-SPIONs act as a dual (MR/optical) cancer-imaging probe [295]. SPIONs have the potential to cure cancer by generating local heat when exposed to an alternating magnetic field (AMF). Cancer cells are susceptible to hyperthermia when the temperature increases to ~43°C for 30–60 min, which triggers apoptosis [296,297]. Porphyrin-tethered, dopamine (PDA)–oligoethylene glycol ligand-coated bimagnetic Fe/Fe_3O_4 NPs act as a significant antitumor agent on murine B16-F10 mice with three short 10-min AMF exposures (Figure 1.15) [298].

However, hyperthermia alone has not been found to be sufficient for cancer treatment, and it is often used as an adjuvant to other forms of therapy, such as surgery, radiotherapy, and chemotherapy [299]. Thus, recent research in the future has focused on combining chemotherapy and hyperthermia using multifunctional SPIONs. Phospholipid–PEG-coated SPIONs have the potential to concurrently deliver DOX and generate heat for enhanced multimodal cancer treatment [300].

1.11.2 ORGANIC NANOCARRIERS

Polymeric nanoparticles (PNPs) are solid, biocompatible, colloidal, and often biodegradable systems with nanoscale dimensions. PNPs are one of the simplest forms of soft materials for nanomedicine applications due to their facile synthesis and easy structural modification to allow desired properties to be built into the NP, such as surface modifications to improve drug loading efficacy, biodistribution, pharmacokinetic control, and therapeutic efficacy [300,301]. PNPs can be made from synthetic polymers, e.g., poly(lactic acid) (PLA), PCL, poly(lactic-co-glycolic acid), N-(2-hydroxypropyl)methacrylamide copolymer (HPMA), and poly(styrene-maleic anhydride) copolymer, or from natural polymers, such as gelatin, DEX, guar gum, CS, and collagen. Drugs can easily be encapsulated either through dispersion in the polymer matrix or conjugation/attachment to polymer molecules for their controlled delivery through surface or bulk erosion, diffusion through the polymer matrix, swelling followed by diffusion, or as a response to local stimuli. Synthetic polymers have the

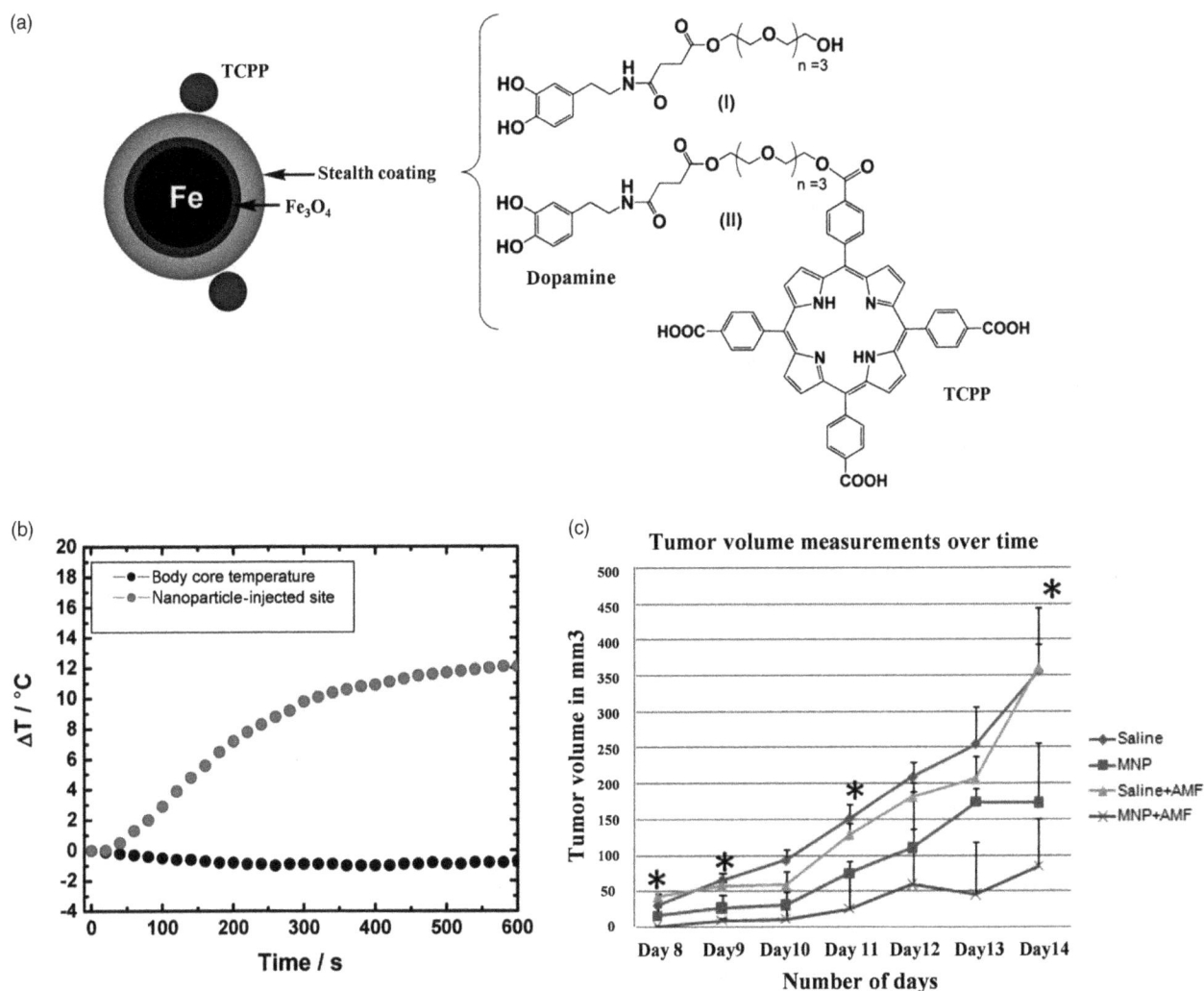

FIGURE 1.15 Effect of surface modification on magnetic nanoparticle on hypothermia to reduce tumor size. (a) Schematic presentation showing the composition of the 4-tetracarboxyphenyl porphyrin (TCPP)-labeled, dopamine-anchored tetraethylene glycol ligand-coated bimagnetic Fe/Fe_3O_4 nanoparticles. (b) Graph illustrating the temperature profiles at the MNP injection site in the body core during alternating magnetic field (AMF) exposure, which is measured with a fiber-optic temperature probe. (c) *In vivo* antitumor response after intratumoral injection of MNPs followed by AMF treatments. The graph demonstrates the relative changes in average tumor volumes over time of B16-F10 tumor-bearing mice that were later injected with either saline or MNPs intratumorally with or without AMF treatments [298].

advantage of sustained release over a period of days to several weeks compared to the relatively shorter duration of drug release of natural polymers; their other benefits include the use of organic solvents and the requirement of typical conditions during encapsulation. PNPs have therefore been widely investigated as drug delivery systems over the last few decades, including the clinical study of Food and Drug Administration (FDA)-approved biodegradable PNPs, such as PLA and PLGA. A drug (DOX) has been conjugated with DEX and subsequently encapsulated in a hydrogel using a reverse microemulsion technique to reduce its cytotoxic effects and improve its therapeutic efficacy in the treatment of solid tumors [302]. Tamoxifen-embedded PLGA NPs, which were prepared using an emulsified nanoprecipitation technique, exhibit DNA cleavage potential and greater *in vitro* anticancer activity than the pure drug [303].

Multifunctional Taxol-loaded PLGA NPs show chemotherapeutic and NIR photothermal destruction of cancer cells *in vitro* and *in vivo* [304]. However, by carefully manipulating the drug-to-polymer ratio, molecular weight, and nature of polymer, the extent and level of drug release from NPs can be fine-tuned for effective cancer treatment.

PNPs are the inventions that relate to a solid micelle with a particle size range of 10–1000 nm [305]. PNPs are collectively known as polymer NPs, nanospheres, nanocapsules, or polymer micelles, and they were the first polymers reported for drug delivery systems. PNPs serve as drug carriers for hydrophobic drugs and are widely used for drug discovery [306–308]. The PNPs constructed from amphiphilic polymers with a hydrophilic and hydrophobic block can perform rapid self-assembly because of the hydrophobic interactions in an aqueous solution [309]. The PNPs can capture the hydrophobic drugs because of a covalent bond or the interaction via a hydrophobic core. Thus, to carry the hydrophilic charged molecules, such as proteins, peptides, and nucleic acids, these blocks are switched to allow interactions in the core and neutralize the charge [307].

The advantages of the higher thermodynamic stability and the smaller volume make the PNPs a suitable drug carrier with good endothelial cell permeability while avoiding kidney rejection [310–313]. The hydrophobic macromolecules and drugs can be transferred to the center of the PNPs; hence, the injection of PNP suspension after being separated in an aqueous solution could achieve a therapeutic effect [313]. Importantly, by oral or parenteral administration, drugs can reach the target cells in different ways, potentially providing alternative ways to lower cytotoxicity in healthy tissues compared to the cancer cells. However, the major challenges in the use of PNPs for cancer nanomedicine still exist in how to effectively deliver the drugs to the target site with limited side effects or drug resistance. Recently, the PNPs have been used widely in the nanotechnology-based cancer drug design due to their excellent potential benefits for patient care. For example, adriamycin-conjugated nanomaterial was used to treat several types of cancers where it achieved therapeutic effects to a decent degree. However, it also presented with many side effects, such as toxicity and heart problems, thereby limiting its use. Such problems are overcome by Doxil (a liposomal form of DOX), which is less associated with cardiotoxicity in patients, and hence may provide a safer nanomaterial synthetic approach for researchers in the future [314–317].

PNPs may represent the most effective nanocarriers for cancer chemotherapy [318,319]. These NPs can be surface-functionalized to target cancer cells specifically and have a prolonged systemic circulating half-life to enhance their therapeutic efficiency. The NP surface is usually sterically stabilized by grafting, conjugating, or adsorbing hydrophilic polymers such as PEG to its surface [320,321]. PNPs can be readily formulated to deliver hydrophilic or hydrophobic small drug molecules, and polymer systems have been developed and used to deliver macromolecules such as proteins [322] and nucleic acids [323]. Biodegradable polymers are typically broken down into individual monomers, which are metabolized and removed from the body via normal metabolic pathways. The rate of polymer degradation and subsequent drug release can be controlled by modification of the polymer side chain, development of novel polymers, or synthesis of copolymers. This subject has been an active area of investigation by our group and other investigators in academic and industry laboratories for several decades [324–327]. The result has been an increasing arsenal of polymers with distinct encapsulation and release characteristics for a myriad of research, industrial, and clinical applications [328,329]. PGA and PLA are common biocompatible polymers that are used for many biomedical applications. PGA is more hydrophilic since it lacks a methyl group and is more susceptible to hydrolysis, making this polymer easily degradable. Alternatively, PLA is relatively more stable

in the body [330]. Through these unique properties, polymers such as PLGA have been derived that are made from both glycolic acid and lactic acid components. The ability to change the ratio of these two components of the polymer can then be used to alter the rate of degradation. Using the PLA and PLGA polymer systems, we have developed proof-of-concept docetaxel-encapsulated targeted NPs, which target the prostate-specific membrane antigen (PSMA) on the surface of prostate cancer cells and are engulfed by cells that express the PSMA protein specifically and efficiently, *in vitro* and *in vivo* [331–333]. We have shown that a single intratumoral injection of these particles results in tumor eradication in five out of seven mice, with the remaining two mice having considerably smaller tumor volumes as compared to controls [333]. These targeted NPs release their payload directly inside the cancer cells, resulting in enhanced efficacy and decreased systemic toxicity [333]. More recently, using the J591 antibody that recognizes the PSMA protein, J591-targeted controlled-release NPs have been developed for effective gene delivery to prostate cancer cells [334,335]. Our group has also developed HER2-targeted NPs that may have utility in the systemic therapy of breast, pancreatic, and ovarian cancers (Figure 1.16). More recently, our group and other investigators have begun to explore computational modeling and screening strategies to identify optimized physicochemical properties of NPs (i.e., size, charge, hydrophilicity, stability, drug release kinetics, and the density of targeting molecules on NP surface) for cancer therapeutic applications [336,337].

Liposomes: Liposomes are small, spherical, self-closed structures with at least one concentric lipid bilayer and an encapsulated aqueous phase in the center. They have been widely used as drug delivery vehicles since their discovery in 1965 due to their biocompatible and biodegradable nature and their unique ability to encapsulate hydrophilic agents (hydrophilic drugs, DNA, RNA, etc.) in their inner aqueous core and hydrophobic drugs within the lamellae, which makes them versatile therapeutic carriers. Furthermore, amphiphilic drugs can also be loaded into the liposome inner aqueous core using remote loading methods, such as the ammonium sulfate method for DOX [338] or the pH gradient method for vincristine [339]. However, one of the major drawbacks of these conventional liposomes was their rapid clearance from the bloodstream. The development of stealth liposomes is underway by utilizing the surface coating of a hydrophilic polymer, usually a lipid derivative of PEG, to extend the circulation half-life of liposomes from less than a few minutes (conventional liposomes) to several hours (stealth liposomes) [340]. Liposomes have the potential to target specific cells through both active and passive targeting strategies. PEGylated liposomes have been found to be more effective at passively targeting cancer cells both *in vitro* and *in vivo* than conventional liposomes, and moreover, PEGylated liposomes exhibit a high degree of nuclear transfection. Liposomal antisense oligonucleotides (ASO) have been found to be effective for the inhibition of pump and nonpump resistance of multidrug-resistant tumors [341]. Ligand-targeted liposomes have been found to

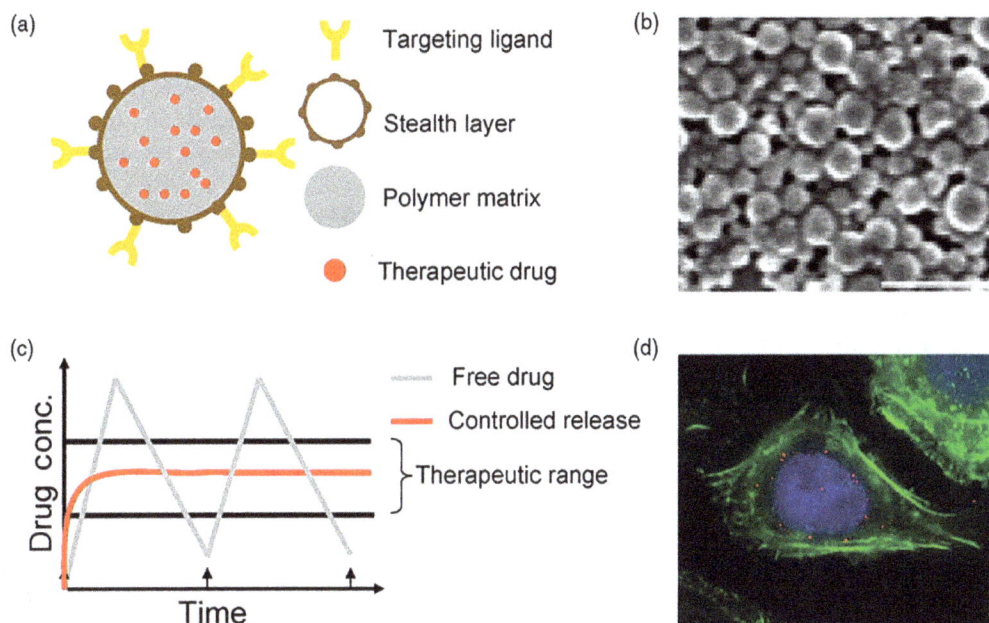

FIGURE 1.16 (a) Schematic representation of a stealth targeted PNP. (b) Scanning electron microscope (SEM) micrograph of PLGA nanoparticles. The white represents 1 μm. (c) Comparative plasma drug concentration of polymeric controlled-release drug delivery system vs. systemic delivery of free drug. (d) Fluorescent micrograph of breast cancer cells treated with HER2-targeted nanoparticles loaded with rhodamine. The cell nuclei and the actin cytoskeleton are stained with blue (DAPI) and green (Alexa Fluor phalloidin), respectively. The intracellular rhodamine-encapsulated HER2-targeted nanoparticle bioconjugates are shown in red.

promote the internalization of liposome–drug conjugates into specific target cells both *in vitro* and *in vivo*, and the vectors can be designed to release their contents in the enzyme-rich, low-pH environment of endosomes and lysosomes using pH-triggered approaches [342,343]. Targeted zwitterionic oligopeptide liposomes exhibit enhanced tumor cell uptake, improved cytoplasmic distribution, and enhanced mitochondrial targeting [344]. A couple of clinically approved liposomal products are on the market, and more are under clinical development. Interestingly, all of these approved liposomal nanocarriers act through passive targeting strategies, whereas few targeted formulations have progressed into the clinic. Ceramide liposomes show an inhibitory effect on peritoneal metastasis in a murine xenograft model of human ovarian cancer and suppress the cell mortality of prometastatic factor, which is promoted by epithelial growth factor [345]. Vascular endothelial growth factors (VEGF), which are often overexpressed in many cancers associated with angiogenesis, are induced at a transcriptional level and suppress VEGF and other genes using RNA interference (RNAi), which is considered to be a novel therapeutic strategy in the silencing of disease-causing genes. CS-coated liposomal formulations, such as the siRNA delivery system, are effective at achieving gene-silencing efficiency [346]. PTX containing A7RC peptide-modified liposomes acts as an antimitotic chemotherapeutic drug, which can be a promising strategy for promoting antitumor and antiangiogenic therapies [347].

Dendrimers: The dendrimers are nanocarriers that have a spherical polymer core with regularly spaced branches [348]. As the dendritic macromolecule diameter increases, the tendency to tilt toward a spherical structure increases

[349]. There are usually two ways to synthesize dendrimers: a divergent method in which the dendrimers can grow outward from the central nucleus, and a convergence method where the dendrimers grow inward from the edges and end up in the central nucleus [350,351]. Various molecules including polyacrylamide, poly(glycerol-succinic acid), polylysine, polyglycerin, poly(2,2-bis(hydroxymethyl)propionic acid), and melamine are commonly used to form dendrimers [352]. These dendritic macromolecules exhibit different chemical structures and properties, such as alkalinity, hydrogen bond capacity, and charge, which can be regulated by growing dendritic macromolecules or changing the groups on the surface of dendritic macromolecules. In general, the dendritic drug conjugates are formed by the covalent binding of antitumor drugs to dendritic peripheral groups [353]. Thus, several drug molecules can attach to each dendritic molecule and the release of these therapeutic molecules is controlled in part by the nature of the attachment. The physicochemical and biological properties of the polymer, including the size, charge, multi-ligand groups, lipid bilayer interactions, cytotoxicity, internalization, plasma retention time, biological distribution, and filtration of dendritic macromolecules, have made dendrimers potential nanoscale carriers [351]. Several studies have further shown that cancer cells with a high expression of folate receptors could form foils from dendritic molecules bound to folate [354–356]. An added advantage of dendrimers is their ability to bind to DNA as seen with the DNA-polyamides clustering DNA–polyamidoamine (DNA-PAMAM), making them highly effective at killing cancer cells that express the folate receptor [357].

Protein-based nanocarriers: Albumin is a protein that can be obtained from a variety of sources, including egg white (ovalbumin), bovine serum (bovine serum albumin, BSA), and human serum (human serum albumin, HSA), and is available in soybeans, milk, and grains. Albumin-based nanocarriers have several advantages, such as easy preparation; a high binding capacity for various drugs; nontoxic, non-immunogenic, biocompatible, and biodegradable properties; and a long half-life in circulating plasma. The presence of functional groups (amino and carboxylic groups) on albumin NP surfaces makes it easy to bind targeting ligands and other surface modifications [358]. DOX-loaded HSA NPs have been found to have better *in vitro* antitumor efficacy than the pure drug against neuroblastoma cell lines (UKF-NB-3 and IMR-32) [359]. PTX-loaded BSA NPs, which are prepared using a desolvation technique, followed by FA decoration, have been found to target human prostate cancer cell line (PC3) effectively [360]. Albumin is a natural carrier of hydrophobic molecules (hormones, vitamins, and other plasma constituents) through favorable, non-covalent reversible binding and helps with their transportation in body fluids and release at the cell surface. Moreover, albumin can bind to the glycoprotein (gp60) receptor and mediate the transcytosis of albumin-bound molecules [361,362]. Abraxane (nab-paclitaxel; PTX–albumin NP), which has an approximate diameter of 130 nm, is the first FDA-approved commercial product based on the nab platform that has shown significant benefits in the treatment of metastatic breast cancer. Several other nab-technology-based chemotherapeutics, such as nab-docetaxel, have already entered into clinical trials.

Micelles as a drug carrier: Micelles are spherical or globular colloidal nanoscale systems formed by self-assembly of amphiphilic block copolymers in an aqueous solution, resulting in a hydrophobic core and a hydrophilic shell. They belong to a group of amphiphilic colloids that can be formed spontaneously under certain concentrations (critical micelle concentration, CMC) and temperatures. The hydrophobic core serves as a reservoir for hydrophobic drugs, whereas the hydrophilic shell stabilizes the hydrophobic core and renders both polymer and hydrophobic drugs water-soluble, making the particle an appropriate candidate for i.v. administration. The drugs are incorporated into a polymeric micelle through physical, chemical, or electrostatic interactions [300]. The first polymeric micelle formulation of PTX, Genexol-PM (PEG-poly(D,L-lactide)-PTX), is Cremophor-free polymeric micelle-formulated PTX, which can be administered without reactions and shows a favorable toxicity profile with advanced refractory malignancies [363]. Multifunctional star-shaped polymeric micelles, based on four-arm disulfide-linked PCL–PEG amphiphilic copolymers coupled with folate ligands, exhibit high stability and sustained release, whereas prompt release can occur in an acidic environment [364]. DOX is encapsulated into cationic 1,2-dioleoyl-3-trimethylammonium propane/methoxy poly(ethylene glycol) (DPP) NPs to form micelles for intravesical drug delivery and has shown an anticancer effect against bladder cancer [365]. Cholesterol-modified mPEG–PLA micelles (mPEG–PLA-Ch) exhibit high encapsulation efficiency and reduce tumor size considerably compared to the pure drug (curcumin, CUR) [366]. Phenylboronic acid (PBA) can selectively recognize sialic acid (SA), showing a high affinity for targeting sialylated epitopes that are overexpressed on cancer cells, and oxaliplatin-incorporated micelles exhibit enhanced tumor-targeting ability through specific interactions with SA (as confirmed using fluorescence spectroscopy), leading to an attractive strategy for increasing the efficiency of chemotherapies [367]. Gilbreth et al. [368] explored the use of lipid- and polyion complex-based micelles for the rapid generation of multivalent agonists targeting tumor necrosis factor (TNF) receptors, and the micelles showed promising therapeutic efficacy.

Self-assembly as a drug carrier: Molecular self-assembly is a free energy-driven process that spontaneously organizes molecules into ordered structures in multiple geometries. Therefore, self-assembly is a very attractive approach to constructing nanoscale-based bioactive materials due to its straightforward use in biomedical applications, including tissue engineering, regenerative medicine, and drug delivery. The great advantage of self-assemblies is their structural features, which can be tuned through molecular chemistry and environmental conditions (pH, ionic strength, solvents, and temperature) [369]. Self-assembly of the photosensitizer (chlorin e6, Ce6) and a chemotherapeutic agent (DOX) linked with electrostatic, π–π stacking, and hydrophobic interactions is designed to inhibit tumor recurrence (Figure 1.17a). Intravenously administered free Ce6 and NPs were distributed throughout the body, whereas the administered self-assembly drugs accumulated in the tumor site exclusively (Figure 1.17b). *Ex vivo* imaging of excised tumors further confirmed higher drug accumulation in tumors with NPs than with free Ce6 solution (Figure 1.17c) [370].

The switchable aptamer–diacyllipid conjugates, formed by the self-assembly of an aptamer switch probe–diacyllipid chimera, showed good results in molecular imaging for bioanalysis, disease diagnosis, and drug delivery [371]. Upon target binding, the conformation of switchable aptamer was altered, resulting in the restoration of a fluorescence signal. The cellular transport of functional D-peptide derivatives relies on the use of taurine-triggered intracellular self-assembly of the D-peptide derivative. Intracellular nanofibers formed by enzyme-instructed self-assembly can disrupt actin filaments and enhance the activity of cisplatin (CP) against drug-resistant ovarian cancer cells by controlling the fate of live cells [372]. Tumor-targeted delivery of siRNA by self-assembled NPs is obtained by mixing carrier DNA, siRNA, protamine, and lipids, followed by post-modification with PEG and a ligand, anisamide. Forty percent of tumor growth inhibition was achieved by treatment with targeted NPs, and complete inhibition lasted for 1 week when combined with CP [373].

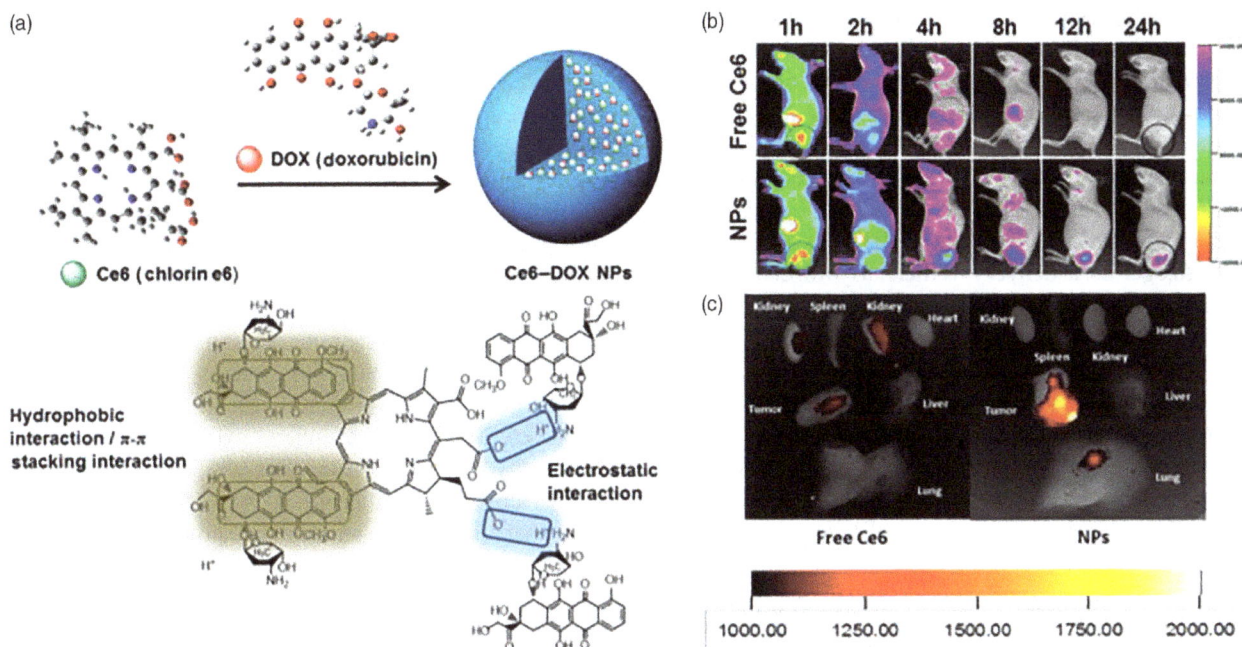

FIGURE 1.17 Co-assembly of drug and photosensitizer for better imaging of tumor size during treatment. (a) Schematic representation of carrier-free nanoparticles (NPs) via co-assembly between DOX and Ce6. (b) *In vivo* fluorescence images of free Ce6 solution and DOX/Ce6 NPs. The areas in the black circles represent tumor tissue. (c) Representative *ex vivo* fluorescence imaging of tumor and organs excised from BALB/c nude mouse xenografted MCF-7 tumor at 24 h post-injection [370].

Supramolecules as a delivery vehicle: Supramolecules are an assembly of two or more molecular entities stabilized by weak and reversible non-covalent interactions, such as hydrogen bonding, metal coordination, hydrophobic attractions, van der Waals forces, and π–π and electrostatic interactions. Therefore, they are expected to function as a carrier in drug delivery designs. Supramolecular systems can provide vehicles for the encapsulation and targeted delivery of therapeutic agents or bioactive materials [374]. The toxicity of traditional anticancer drugs, such as DOX, can be repressed using amphiphilic dendrimers that generate supramolecular micelles for cancer therapy [375]. DOX-loaded supramolecular polymersomes exhibit prolonged circulation in the bloodstream, and *in vivo* studies show that they have better antitumor efficacy toward cancerous HeLa cells with relatively lower cytotoxicity [376]. CD-containing cationic polymer-based supramolecular hydrogels show reduced cytotoxicity compared to their non-CD-containing polymer counterparts [377]. The temperature-responsive behavior of poly(N-isopropylacrylamide) supramolecular micelles and rapid drug release rate are due to induced physical crosslinking; however, these supramolecular micelles demonstrate excellent biocompatibility against most cell lines [378]. Dankers et al. [379] introduced a new concept of transient supramolecular networks in which macroscopic rheological and material properties are tuned by controlled microscopic supramolecular interactions; these interactions are responsible for network formation and lead to promising protein delivery carriers in regenerative medical applications, such as the proof of concept shown in kidney regeneration. Real-time observation of drug distributions

by supramolecular nanocarriers for the treatment of pancreatic tumors has been investigated to obtain feedback on therapeutic efficacy at an early stage. There is no drug accumulation in healthy pancreas, which is supported by the strong diagnostic and anticancer effect of supramolecular micelles [380]. Tumor-targeted drug delivery systems based on supramolecular interactions between iron oxide–carbon nanotubes and polyamidoamine–polyethylene glycol–polyamidoamine (PAMAM–PEG–PAMAM) linear–dendritic copolymers are used as promising systems for future cancer therapy with low drug doses [381]. Porphysome nanovesicles are formed through the self-assembly of porphyrin–lipid bilayers that generate unique fluorescence, photothermal, and photoacoustic properties. The drug loading capacities of porphysomes to destroy tumors by releasing heat are due to their ability to absorb light in the NIR region, which generates a photoacoustic signal that can then be converted into an image. Porphysomes are stable for months when stored in aqueous solutions, but they are prone to enzymatic degradation when incubated with detergent and lipase. The mice in the porphysome- and laser-treated group developed eschars on the tumors (which healed), and their tumors were destroyed [382]. Muhanna et al. [383] demonstrated the effectiveness of porphysome NPs to enhance fluorescence and photoacoustic imaging of oral cavity carcinomas in rabbit and hamster models along with tumor-localized PTT. PTT can be precisely guided by both fluorescence imaging (control of laser placement and tumor delineation) and photoacoustic imaging (tumor margin delineation and assessment of effective PTT doses) for effective therapeutic efficacy. A tailor-made porphyrin-based micelle, self-assembled from a hybrid amphiphilic polymer comprising PEG, poly(D,L-lactide-co-glycolide), and porphyrin, loaded with two chemotherapeutic drugs with synergistic cytotoxicity showed a tendency to accumulate in tumor cells. Drug-loaded micelles improved therapeutic efficacy against triple-negative breast cancer through the synergistic effects of PTT, DOX, and TAX with biocompatible polymers and porphyrin [384].

Hydrogel as a delivery vehicle: Hydrogels are three-dimensional (3D) polymeric and hydrophilic networks that can absorb large amounts of water or biological fluids. Hydrogels are thermodynamically compatible with water, which allows them to swell in aqueous media [385]. Hydrogels are widely used for numerous applications in the pharmaceutical and medical fields, e.g., as biosensors, materials for contact lenses, artificial skin, and lining for artificial hearts. Moreover, they can also be used for 3D cell culture and as drug delivery vehicles [386,387]. Hydrogels are efficient candidates for controlled-release, bioadhesive, and/or targeted drug delivery as they can encapsulate biomacromolecules, including proteins and DNA, and hydrophilic or hydrophobic drugs [388]. Hydrogel-based drug delivery systems can be used in different ways for oral, rectal, ocular, epidermal, and subcutaneous applications [385]. The key success of hydrogel development is *in situ* gelation. Hydrogels can be prepared by introducing non-reversible covalent bonds via self-assembly either through reversible interactions or non-reversible chemical reactions or by UV/photo-polymerization. The gelation process is time- and concentration-dependent and can be triggered by an external stimulus, such as pH, temperature, or light [389]. Hydrogels have been found to be biocompatible with negligible cytotoxicity and can be utilized as a delivery platform when accessed with the normal cell line COS7 and cancer cell lines HepG2 and A549. A variety of innovative semi-interpenetrating polymer network (semi-IPN) hydrogels consisting of Salecan and poly(methacrylic acid) (PMAA) are formed via free-radical polymerization for controlled drug delivery (Figure 1.18a) [390]. Drug release is facilitated under acidic conditions as protonated PMAA disrupts the electrostatic interaction between DOX and the hydrogel (pH < 5.5), favoring drug release compared to the conditions at pH ~ 7.0 (Figure 1.18b). Due to this factor, pH ~ 5 is considered representative of simulated cancer environments. Successive exposure to a different release medium at pH 7.4 and 5.0 causes pH-dependent "off–on" switching of drug release. Cellular uptake of DOX released from drug-loaded hydrogels has effectively been shown in A549 and HepG2 cells, showing great promise for hydrogels to be utilized as a vehicle for anticancer drug delivery (Figure 1.18c).

Polyvinylpyrrolidone-stabilized fluorescent red copper nanoclusters can be converted into hydrogel nanocarriers through crosslinking with poly(vinyl alcohol) to deliver the anticancer drug CP to cervical cancer cells (HeLa), thereby inducing apoptotic cell death [392]. The high encapsulating efficiency is attributed to molecule loading on the surface and inside the hydrogel particle, followed by strong interactions using various functionalities, such as –COOH. The slow release of CP at physiological pH is due to stronger bonding between the drug molecule and the hydrogel, which can be disrupted at acidic pH, favoring fast release. The significant decrease in cell viability in the presence of drug-loaded carriers as opposed to free drug molecules reveals the combination of Cu NC–hydrogel composites and CP as a potential material for the design of new chemotherapeutic agents. DOX-loaded PMAA hydrogel cubes and spheres are capable of both intracellular degradation and pH responsiveness by introducing cystamine crosslinks within networks [393]. The membrane adhesion process in the initial step of cell internalization is greatly affected by the shape of the particles, and hydrogel spheres exhibit 12% higher cell cytotoxicity than cubes using HeLa cells for 10 h. Shape- and pH-sensitive "intelligent" 3D networks with programmable shape-regulating behaviors are promising candidates for the controlled delivery of chemotherapeutics. DOX-encapsulated poly(vinylcaprolactam) (PVCL)-based biodegradable microgels have been designed for stimuli-triggered drug release in acidic or reducing environments [394]. DOX-loaded microgels exhibit efficient antitumor activity to HeLa cells against nontoxic blank microgels. Supramolecular hybrid hydrogels of α-CD and polyethylene-modified gold nanocrystals exhibit pH-dependent sustained release of DOX through host–guest interaction [395]. Tetrapeptide-based thermoreversible, pH-sensitive hydrogels have been prepared for the slow release of anticancer drugs at physiological pH [396]. Hexamethylene diisocyanate (HDI) reacts with Pluronic F127 as a chain extender to form a copolymer, and subsequent incorporation of hyaluronic acid (HA) has been used to develop a composite hydrogel system with a sol–gel transition at 37°C, leading to the formation of a nanocomposite injectable hydrogel for drug delivery with controlled release [397].

Hybrid materials for controlled drug delivery: Nanoscale-dimension hydrogel particles are often called "nanogels" and are formulated by either physically or chemically crosslinked hydrophilic polymers [398,399]. Nanogels have been recently exploited in various fields, including diagnostics, chemical and biochemical sensing, tissue engineering, and cancer imaging, especially as drug delivery vehicle [400–403]. Nanogels offer several advantages in therapeutic delivery in comparison with existing nanocarriers: (i) high drug loading capacity; (ii) higher storage stability than liposomes and micelles; (iii) controlled and sustained drug release; (iv) ease of synthesis; (v) response to external stimuli; and (vi) low inherent toxicity [404,405]. Nanogels act like a soft material when exposed to aqueous media with high water content. Protease/redox/pH stimuli-responsive PEGylated PMAA nanohydrogels have been synthesized using cystamine as crosslinker for targeted anticancer drug delivery [391]. The cumulative release profile indicates greater release in acidic media (pH ~ 5.0) and reducing environments (GSH). Intravital real-time fluorescence image analysis indicates the quick accumulation and maintenance of

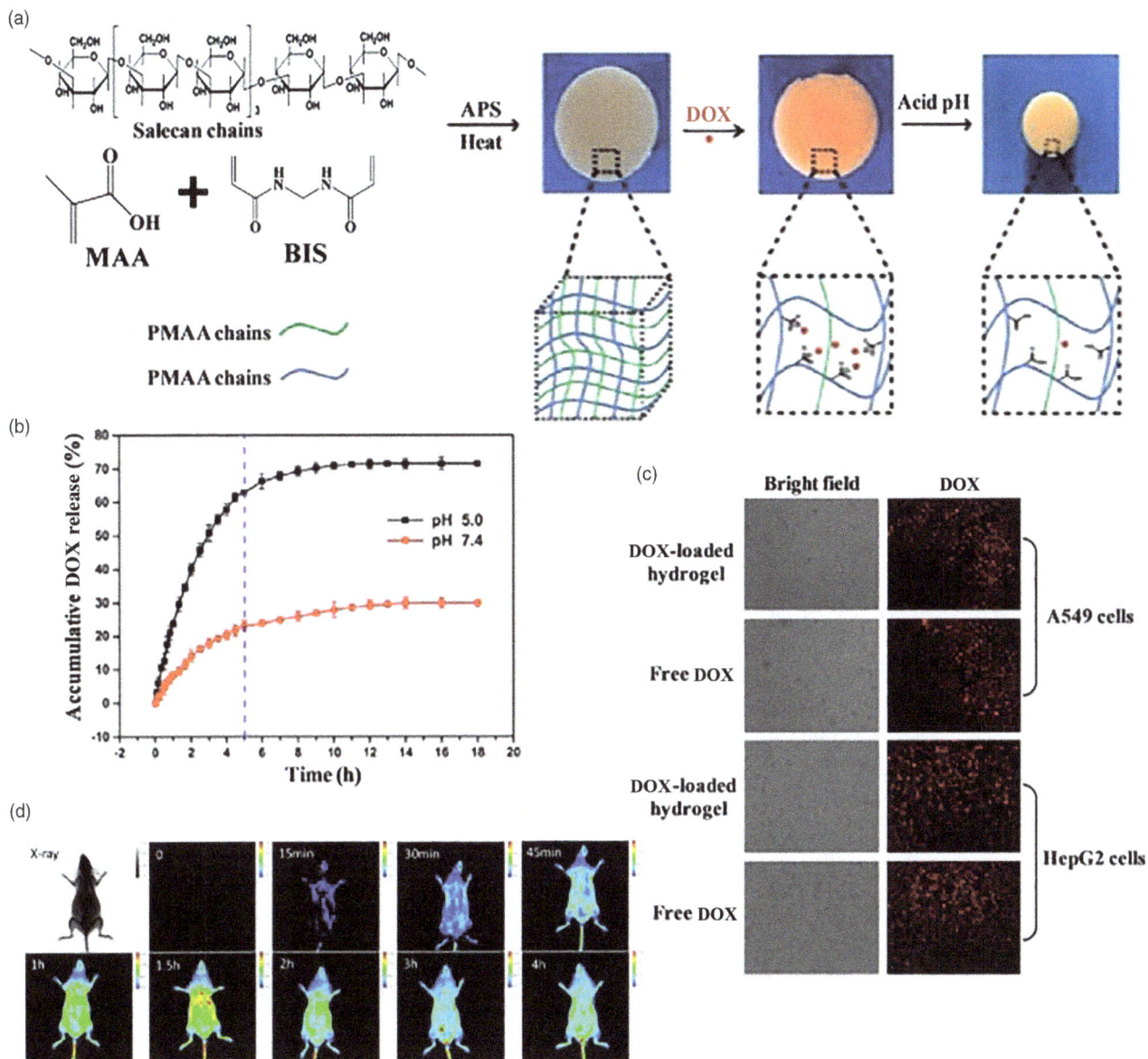

FIGURE 1.18 Controlled delivery of drug using hydrogel as vehicle. (a) Illustration of the preparation and drug release of Salecan/ PMAA semi-IPN hydrogels. (b) *In vitro* DOX release behaviors from the semi-IPN sample at two different pH values of 5.0 and 7.4. (c) Fluorescent microscopy images of A549 and HepG2 cells after 4 h of incubation with 6 μg/mL free DOX solution and the extract liquid of DOX-loaded hydrogel [390]. (d) Intravital real-time fluorescence images of ICR mice injected with FITC-labeled PMAA nanohydrogels [391].

fluorescein isothiocyanate (FITC)-labeled PMAA nano-hydrogels in the kidney, liver, and other organs, such as the heart, lung, and spleen; after 30 min of administration, extended *in vivo* blood circulation lifetimes have been shown using PEGylated FITC-labeled PMAA nanohydrogels (Figure 1.18d). Yang et al. [406] prepared poly(N-isopropylacrylamide)-ss-acrylic acid (P(NIPAM-ss-AA)) nanogels based on NIPAM and AA crosslinked by N,N′-bis(acryloyl)cystamine (BAC) through precipitation polymerization, which exhibited pH/redox dual-responsive DOX release *in vitro* and in tumor cells. Animal studies have demonstrated the efficient penetration of DOX-loaded nanogels with fewer side effects, indicating a prospective platform for intracellular controlled drug release in cancer therapy. BSA and CS nanogels prepared via a green self-assembly technique exhibit slow release with lower cytotoxicity [407,408]. Biocompatible and pH-responsive self-assembled nanogels of CS–graft-poly(N-isopropylacrylamide) have been used as a model tumor-targeting delivery system and had greater activity in acidic media [409]. Alginate–PAMAM dendrimer-based hybrid nanogels have been developed for drug delivery to cancer cells, and they showed pH-dependent release behavior in a sustained way [410]. Nanocarriers have been found to release more drug in acidic environments (mimicking tumor microenvironments) than in physiological conditions.

1.11.3 Quantum Dots

QDs are small particles or nanocrystals of semiconductor materials between 2 and 10 nm in size [411]. The ratio of the height of the surface to the volume of these particles gives the QDs the intermediate electron property which is between a mass semiconductor and a discrete atom [412]. Over the years, various QD-based techniques such as modification of QD conjugates and QD immunostaining have been developed. With the improvement of multiplexing capability, QD conjugation greatly exceeds the monochromatic experiment in both time and cost-effectiveness [413]. Moreover, at low protein expression levels and in a low context, QD immunostaining is more accurate than traditional immunochemical methods. In cancer diagnosis, QD immunostaining is a potential tool for the detection of various tumor biomarkers, such as a cell protein or other components of a heterogeneous tumor sample [414]. QDs can gather in specific parts of the body and transfer the drugs to those parts. The ability of the QDs to concentrate in a single internal organ makes them a potential solution against untargeted drug delivery, and possibly avoid the side effects of chemotherapy. The latest advancement in surface modification of QDs, which combine with biomolecules, including peptides and antibodies, *in vivo*, can be used to target tumors and make possible their potential applications in cancer imaging and treatment. Some studies combine QDs with prostate-specific antigen to label cancer, while others use QDs to make biomarkers that speed up the process with such immune markers having a more stable light intensity than traditional fluorescent immunomarkers [415]. High-sensitivity probes based on QDs have been reported for multicolor fluorescence imaging of cancer cells *in vivo* and can also be used to detect ovarian cancer marker cancer antigen 125 (CA125) in different types of specimens (such as fixed cells, tissue sections, and xenograft) [416]. Besides, the light stability of QD signals is more concrete and brighter than that of traditional organic dyes [417]. Chen et al. successfully detected BC using QD-based probes, confirming that unlike traditional immunohistochemistry (IHC), QD IHC can detect the very low expressions of human epidermal growth factor receptor 2 (HER2) as well as multichannel detection [418, 419].

1.12 CARRIER-FREE NANODRUGS AS ANTICANCER DRUGS

Administration of anticancer drugs, i.e., chemotherapy, remains the most common strategy [420]. Figure 1.19 shows the chemical structures of some example drugs for anticancer therapy. These drugs are used as intravenous therapies for various forms of cancers, requiring them to be ideally dissolvable in water for administration. In general, water

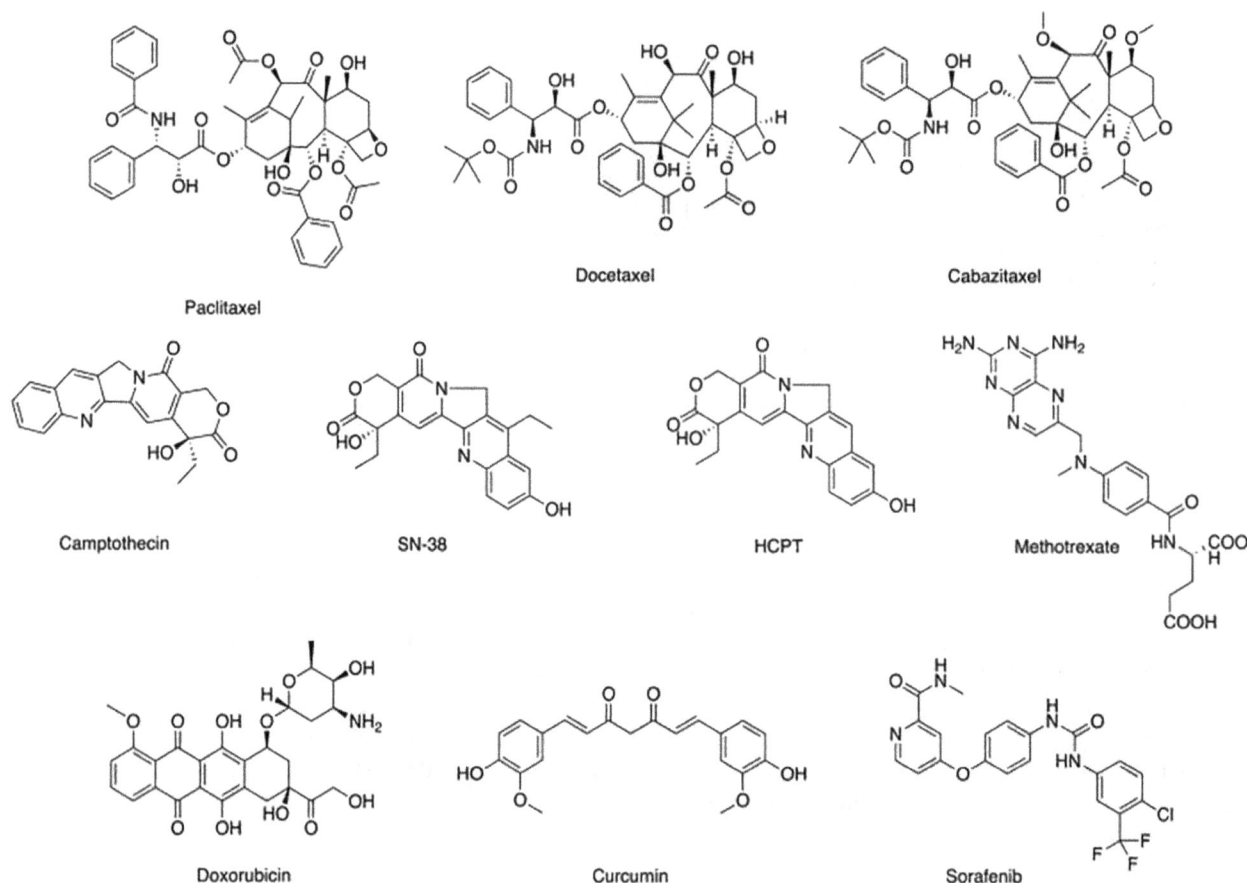

FIGURE 1.19 Chemical structures of example hydrophobic anticancer drugs.

solubility of an organic molecule depends on the balance between its polar (hydrophilic) and nonpolar (hydrophobic) functional groups. In all of the cases in Figure 1.19, this balance tilts toward nonpolar groups due to the molecules' hydrocarbon heavy nature, which is essential to exert their mechanism of anticancer action but makes them poorly soluble in water [421].

Taxanes are among the most promising hydrophobic anticancer drugs. They are anti-microtubule drugs that interfere with cellular mitosis through microtubule stabilization, resulting in apoptosis [422]. Among taxanes, PTX was first isolated from the bark of a Pacific yew tree, Taxus brevifolia, which contains endophytic fungi known to produce PTX [423]. It was approved by the FDA in 1994 and is now widely used to treat breast, prostate, lung, and head and neck carcinomas, malignant melanoma, and Kaposi's sarcoma [423,424]. PTX is a hydrophobic molecule and precipitates into needle-shaped crystals in water due to its low water solubility (0.3 µg/mL). This poses a challenge for its clinical application and necessitates the use of organic solvents such as ethanol, methanol, and dimethylsulfoxide (DMSO) [425]. Taxol, the first commercial formulation of PTX, contains 50% anhydrous ethanol and 50% Cremophor EL®. The latter was shown to cause side effects in the clinic including hypersensitivity, nephrotoxicity, and neurotoxicity, and it was recently reported that Cremophor EL® can even reduce the anticancer efficiency of PTX [426]. Docetaxel (DTX), isolated from Taxus baccata, has twofold greater antimitotic efficacy than PTX and is used for the treatment of lung, breast, and ovarian cancers. The water solubility of DTX is slightly higher compared to PTX (6–7 µg/mL) [427]. Clinical use of PTX and DTX, however, is hindered due to their affinity toward P-glycoprotein (P-gp), a MDR protein [428]. Cabazitaxel (CTX), a semi-synthetic derivative, is another member of this family, approved by the FDA in 2010. CTX poorly binds to P-gp, preventing drug resistance, and demonstrated superior efficacy compared to PTX and DTX [429], but still suffers from the common hydrophobicity of taxanes (8 µg/mL) [430].

Camptothecin (CPT), extracted from Chinese ornamental tree, works by inhibiting the topoisomerase-1 pathway that then prevents DNA re-ligation, resulting in cell death [431]. CPT is mainly used for the treatments of lung, breast, and brain cancers and has a planar pentacyclic ring structure that causes cylindrical-shaped aggregations in water. Biological environment causes the degradation of CPT in only 30 min by hydrolysis of its lactone rings, and CPT has very poor water solubility (2–3 µg/mL) [432,433]. Therefore, derivatives of CPT have been developed in order to increase its solubility and stability in physiological conditions. 7-Ethyl-10-hydroxy-camptothecin (SN-38), a semisynthetic derivative of CPT, is effective on a wide range of solid tumors by inhibiting topoisomerase-1 [434]. SN-38 has two hydroxyl groups that can bond with different molecules and produce more efficient formulations. 10-Hydroxycamptothecin (HCPT), another analogue of CPT, is known to have an antitumor effect against gastric

carcinoma, hepatoma, leukemia, and head and neck tumors [435]. It is demonstrated that compared to CPT, HCPT is more potent and less toxic in animal studies and in human clinical evaluation. However, the clinical applications of both SN-38 and HCPT are limited, again, due to their low water solubility, 11–38 and 7.2 µg/mL, respectively [436–438]. DOX, also a topoisomerase inhibitor which exerts its activity on topoisomerase II, causes DNA damage and prevents mitosis in tumor cells [439,440]. It is widely used to treat breast cancer, urothelial cancer, hematopoietic malignancies, and solid tumors.

Among other anticancer agents suffering from poor water solubility, pemetrexed (PEM) is an antimetabolite agent exhibiting anticancer activity by inhibiting multiple folate-related enzymes, such as thymidylate synthase and dihydrofolate reductase. It was approved by the FDA in 2004 for the treatment of malignant pleural mesothelioma and in 2008 for non-small-cell lung cancer [441]. Bortezomib (BTZ) contains a boronic acid moiety and is approved by the FDA to treat multiple myeloma by targeting proteasomes [442]. Sorafenib (SRF) is a novel small-molecule multi-kinase inhibitor and is used in the treatment of renal cell, liver, and thyroid cancers. SRF has a water-repelling heavy ring structure [443]. Another chemotherapeutic drug, methotrexate (MTX), is a FA antagonist and exerts its effect by interfering with DNA, RNA, and protein formation [444]. MTX is used in cervical, colorectal, lung, and breast cancers as well as leukemia and osteosarcoma [445,446]. BTZ, SRF, and MTX are similarly having low water solubility with 53.2 µg/mL, 1.7 µg/mL, and 0.1 mg/mL, respectively [447–449].

Alongside these FDA-approved anticancer agents, the naturally occurring compound CUR is not clinically approved, but is nevertheless widely investigated in cancer treatment due to its antioxidant properties. CUR, extracted from Curcuma longa, is an antioxidant, anti-inflammatory agent. It has been demonstrated that CUR can exert an anticancer effect by inhibiting transcriptional factor nuclear factor kappa B, which has a key role in inflammation [450]. In particular cases, it was found that CUR has synergistic effects when applied in combination therapy with other anticancer agents overcoming MDR and inhibiting inflammation [451,452]. However, it is extremely hydrophobic with 0.6 µg/mL water solubility and unstable, resulting in inadequate efficiency [453].

As seen from the above examples, poor water solubility is one of the main challenges for clinical applications of many anticancer agents. Beyond this, most anticancer drugs act as antiproliferative agents and have poor selectivity resulting in severe side effects [454]. These anticancer drugs can be taken up by frequently replicating cells, regardless of the cell type, which require high nutrient supply. Therefore, anticancer agents cause serious side effects on healthy tissues dividing rapidly such as mucous membranes of mouth, throat, stomach, and intestines, resulting in gastrointestinal side effects. Hair follicles are also fast-dividing cells, and correspondingly, patients suffer from hair loss including facial and body hair [455]. They also harm bone marrow cells, which are responsible for the production of white and red blood cells. This further reduces the ability of body to fight infections [456]. It is also demonstrated that exhibiting frequently proliferating cell profile in tumor masses can be misleading as this is due to the high number of cells in dividing state. In fact, many of the tumor cells, particularly solid tumor cells, multiply rather slowly [457,458].

Anticancer drugs also often suffer from poor pharmacokinetic properties. First, anticancer agents face rapid blood clearance by the RES which removes foreign substances from the bloodstream. Once anticancer drugs are administered to the body, they exhibit extremely rapid renal clearance and therefore can barely reach cancer cells and have a rather short half-life [458,459]. For example, the half-life of 5-FU and PTX is only 16 min and 5.8 h, respectively [422,460,461]. In addition to these, anticancer drugs are known to create kidney and liver damage. The former arises from excretion of drugs from the body, and the latter results from the detoxification mechanism of liver [462]. All of these side effects limit the maximum tolerated dose and potentially result in early termination of treatment due to their life-threatening toxicities [462,463]. Some of these side effects can cause long-term damage, such as neutropenia, known to remain for years or even permanent in many cases [457]. Anticancer drugs also encounter the issue of MDR being developed by cancer cells, usually after an initial therapy via genetic or non-genetic mechanisms. Second treatment may still have some effect on a minority of patients, but there are few cases who respond to a third administration [457].

To solve these serious problems, nanotechnology has been extensively studied for delivery of anticancer drugs in order to maximize their therapeutic effects and minimize the toxicity and side effects of cancer treatments [464,465]. Many novel nanotechnology-based approaches have been studied for biomedical applications such as liposomes, inorganic NPs, or polymeric micelles [466]. These carrier-based methods bring systematic advantages [467,468]. Firstly, the water solubility is significantly increased. Hydrophobic drugs loaded in amorphous nanocarriers demonstrated higher solubility due to the lack of a lattice energy barrier to dissolution. In addition to that, the surface area of these anticancer drugs is increased by the use of nanoscale formulations [469]. In this way, the characteristics hindering the application of hydrophobic drugs are altered by encapsulating them into nanocarriers [470]. Secondly, the systemic circulation of anticancer drugs can be enhanced. Doxil® (DOX-loaded PEG-surface-modified, PEGylated, liposomes) was one of the first nanomedicines approved by FDA, and it significantly increased the elimination phase of DOX (45.9 h with Doxil®) in the bloodstream compared to free DOX (10.4 h) [471]. Thirdly, these carrier-based drug delivery systems demonstrated an increase in tumor accumulation of NPs. An example of this, Abraxane®, first nanoformulated PTX, bonded with albumin (130 nm), was approved by FDA in 2005, demonstrated fivefold increased transport into cancer via endothelial cells resulting in

higher tumor accumulation [470]. It was demonstrated that NPs between 10 and 200 nm are the most suitable candidates for accumulation at tumor sites [472].

Despite significant progress, carrier-based nanotechnology for anticancer drug delivery still often lacks the required efficiency in terms of pharmacokinetics and biodistribution [473], and the carrier component often comprises the bulk of the mass of these nanosystems. The loading efficiency of anticancer drugs remains low, and their long-term toxicities remain largely unknown [474]. A high amount of carriers is used to reach a required drug doses, resulting in low drug loading (usually ~10% or lower) and high carrier uptake [475–478]. For example, liposomes are cleared from the bloodstream in a relatively short time and accumulate in the liver [479]. On the other hand, some inorganic NPs have an inner core composed of heavy metals which limits clinical application due to their toxicity [470]. In a 2019 study, it was demonstrated that CNTs, an inorganic carrier, can promote metastasis in breast cancer [480].

To combat these new problems, one promising solution is to develop carrier-free nanodrugs. These nanodrugs are made from pure drug molecules without involving any organic or inorganic carriers. It is worth noting that organic molecules may still be used to work as surfactants to stabilize nanodrugs or to tune the physical/chemical properties of drug molecules so they can be self-assembled to nanodrugs, but the amount is generally much smaller in comparison with the cases of using them as carriers. To synthesize carrier-free nanodrugs, coupling two drug molecules (either the same or different anticancer molecules) together or conjugating functional organic molecules, such as vitamins, fatty acids, photosensitizers, and proteins, with drug molecules using covalent bonds and/or physical interactions can be employed to enhance the biostability, targeting ability, and therapeutic efficacy of anticancer drugs. All of the components in this design play active roles, and importantly, the therapeutic drug loading is often over 80% [481]. Such strategies can be further improved by employing tumor microenvironment-responsive linkages. This review highlights the recent progress in the vast and ever-growing area of carrier-free anticancer nanodrugs. We will highlight the various approaches to synthesize NPs directly from pure drug molecules, discuss their advantages over conventional nanomedicines with nanocarriers, and compare the effectiveness and limitations of different approaches. After the comprehensive review, we will provide our insights into the future development of carrier-free nanodrugs for potential clinical applications.

1.13 SYNTHETIC METHODS OF CARRIER-FREE NANODRUGS

1.13.1 Direct Self-Assembly of Drug Molecules

Preparation of nanodrugs via molecular self-assembly without any processing is one of the most convenient strategies for delivery of hydrophobic therapeutics [482–485]. Self-assembly occurs at molecular level with non-covalent interactions, such as hydrophobic interactions, π–π stackings, and CH–π interactions, playing essential roles. In this section, we will review the work of directly self-assembling chemotherapy drug molecules with different molecules to make nanodrugs to solve the problems such as drugs' low solubility in aqueous solution, low anticancer efficiency, and serious side effects.

1.13.1.1 Self-Assembly of Pure Chemotherapy Drug Molecules

As shown in Figure 1.20a, generally, one or multiple types of clinical drug molecules are dissolved in a small amount of organic solvent and then added dropwise into an aqueous solution under vigorous stirring [486]. Due to the interactions between the hydrophobic small molecules, uniform NPs are rapidly obtained [487]. Minimal amounts of surfactants can then be added to stabilize the obtained NPs. The self-assembled nanodrugs tend to exhibit high drug loading capacities, improved water solubility, prolonged blood circulation half-lives, higher drug delivery efficiencies, and reduced side effects [488]. For example, we reported the synthesis of pure DOX NPs solely from DOX-free drug molecules via the self-assembly method. PLGA–PEG was

then added to functionalize the surface of the NPs as a surfactant as shown in Figure 1.20b [489]. After PEGylation of NPs, DOX loading was determined to be 90.47%. DOX has similar chemical properties to surfactants as it has abundant hydroxyl groups and hydrophobic anthracycline rings. Therefore, pure drug NPs can be obtained from DOX which can serve as both the pharmaceutically active ingredient and a surfactant [490]. The prepared NPs resulted in good biocompatibility and stability, and long blood circulation times (Figure 1.20c). Compared to free DOX, the DOX NPs possess fast release in an acidic environment and high accumulation in tumors. Our results showed that the tumor growth in the mice treated with free DOX and DOX NPs was 5.40 ± 0.30-fold and 2.09 ± 0.25-fold, respectively. It was also explored that addition of HCPT (DOX-HCPT NPs) circumvented the MDR in DOX-resistant breast cancer cell lines and showed higher cytotoxicity and tumor inhibition *in vivo* than DOX NPs only.

In a similar manner, we reported carrier-free multidrug nanocrystals (MDNCs) for combination chemotherapy [491]. Three widely used hydrophobic drugs, MTX, HCPT, and PTX, were assembled into nanorods and then conjugated with PEG to improve their bio-environmental

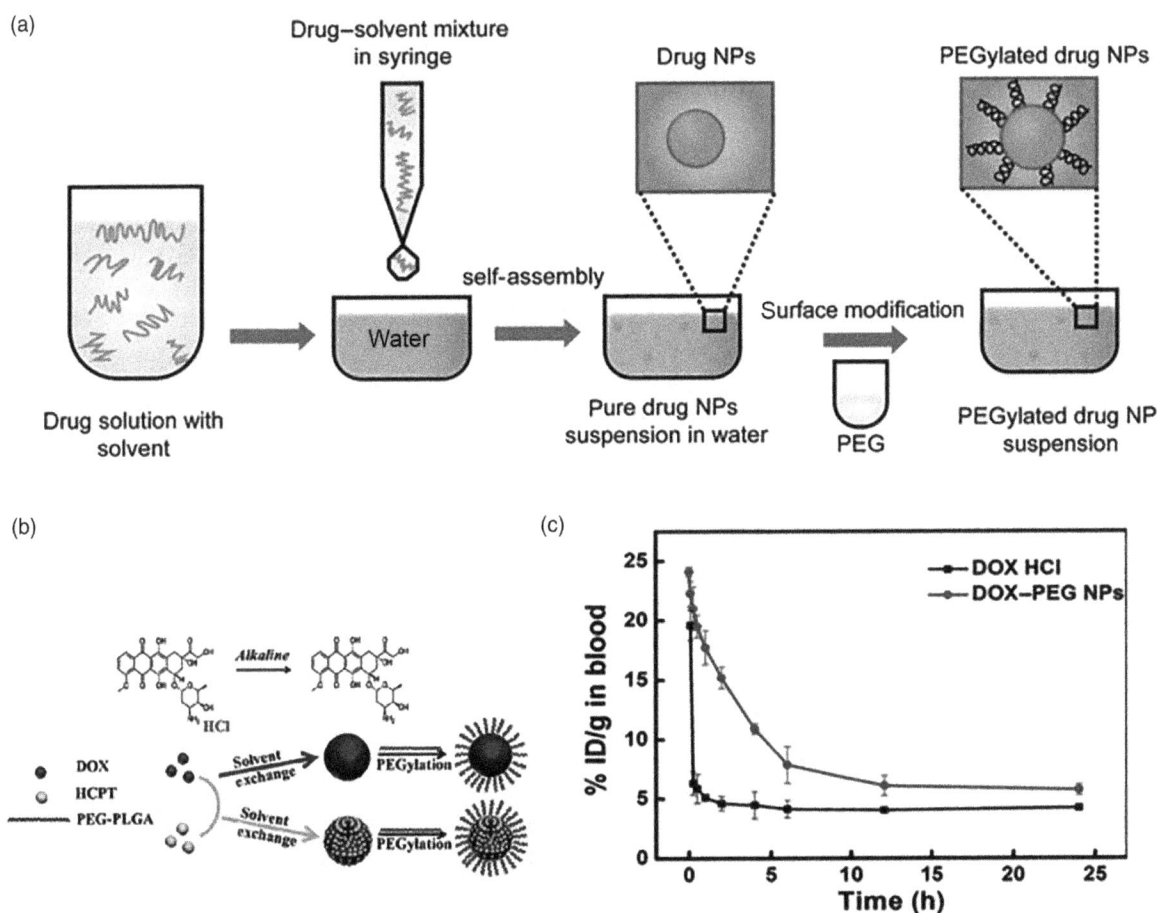

FIGURE 1.20 (a) Schematic illustration of self-assembly of drug molecules and surface modification. (b) Schematic illustration of the preparation and functionalization of DOX and DOX–HCPT NPs. (c) The blood circulation curve of DOX–PEG NPs and DOX·HCl determined by measuring the fluorescence of DOX in the blood at different time points post-injection. (Copyright 2015. Reproduced from Ref. [489] with permission from The Royal Society of Chemistry.)

stability. Our *in vitro* and *in vivo* studies showed that the MDNCs revealed almost threefold higher therapeutic efficacy than free drugs at the same dose and also efficiently suppressed MDR. Some other pure nanodrug formulations have also been achieved with CUR and HCPT by using different solvents and anti-solvents [492]. This technique can also be improved with different therapeutic agents. We have also reported NP synthesis from DOX, triphenylphosphine, and lonidamine which can inhibit energy metabolism by targeting the mitochondria [493]. The prepared NPs increased the half-life of DOX in the bloodstream to 3 h.

1.13.1.2 Self-Assembly of Chemotherapy with PDT or PTT Drug Molecules

Combination of PDT and PTT with chemotherapy is an attractive area of research due to the advantage of increased therapeutic efficacy and alleviated drug resistance. PDT is a light-excited treatment method and shows promising results particularly with anticancer agents [494]. In PDT, a photosensitizer (PS), such as Ce6, di-iodinated borondipyrromethene (BDP-I2), pyropheophorbide-a (PPa), and zinc phthalocyanine (ZnPc), is intravenously administered into the body. These molecules have a tendency to stay longer in tumor cells than healthy cells. After a certain time to ensure minimal damage to the healthy cells, a specific radiation is introduced to the body to activate PS molecules that can convert dissolved oxygen into ROS, resulting in cancer cell apoptosis and tumor eradication [495]. This method can improve the therapy by localizing the treatment to tumor sites and reducing the side effects to normal cells [496]. PTT is another light-excited treatment method, which converts the light energy into heat under specific NIR laser leading to tumor ablation [497]. In spite of these advantages, phototherapeutic agents have some drawbacks such as instability stemming from their insolubility and poor selectivity that weakens the therapeutic effect [495]. To overcome the mentioned disadvantages of both anticancer chemotherapy drugs and phototherapeutic agents, a wide range of PDT and PTT agents were employed to form nanodrugs with anticancer agents via the self-assembly method [498].

Yan et al. reported carrier-free chemo-PDT nanodrugs by using DOX and Ce6 [499]. The molecules self-assembled into NPs via electrostatic, π–π stacking, and hydrophobic interactions. The size of Ce6-DOX NPs was determined as 70 nm with -20 mV zeta potential ensuring stability for 8 days. The encapsulation efficiencies of Ce6 and DOX were more than 95% and 99%, respectively. DOX–Ce6 nanodrugs with high drug loadings demonstrated good cellular uptake and tumor depletion under laser irradiation due to the synergistic chemo-PDT. In a 2020 study, a similar method was also applied with SN-38 and Ce6 which formed carrier-free NPs (154.87±1.82 nm) due to π–π stackings and subordinate hydrogen bonds. SN-38–Ce6 NPs demonstrated enhanced cellular uptake and antitumor efficacy with an 85% inhibition rate with laser irradiation, whereas this ratio was around 65% and <20% for the non-laser-treated and

only drug-injected groups, respectively [500]. The study indicated the importance of combined PDT and chemotherapy. Yan et al. reported a chemo-PDT with HCPT and Ce6, which were mixed to self-assemble into nanorods in water [501]. The prepared nanorods increased both HCPT and Ce6 cell uptake, resulting in enhanced tumor depletion via synergistic action.

In a 2018 study, another PS, BDP-I2, was employed with PTX to self-assemble into nanorods with a size of nearly 200 nm. The NPs were stable for 2 weeks at room temperature [502]. The obtained nanorods exhibited higher cytotoxicity *in vitro* compared to Taxol when irradiated with laser. The authors [420] have reported a carrier-free nanodrug via a simple solvent exchange method by using CUR with a donor–acceptor pair composed of 5,10,15,20-tetra(4-pyridyl)porphyrin (H2TPyP) and perylene, as photosensitizers, allowing PDT [503]. In our nanoplatform, CUR enabled the inhibition of cancer cell growth and the fluorescence state of CUR only became active after its release from the nanoplatform, enabling to self-monitor the drug release. The drug loading of CUR was high at 77.6%. NIR fluorescence emitted from the donor–acceptor pair also achieved real-time tumor imaging via Förster resonance energy transfer.

Anticancer nanodrugs with combinational PTT are also explored due to the aforementioned benefits. Indocyanine green (ICG) is the only FDA-approved PTT agent and is a promising candidate in self-assembly with anticancer drugs, due to its hydrophilic sulfate and hydrophobic indole skeletons [504]. For these reasons, a variety of anticancer nanodrugs conjugated with ICG and its derivatives (IR820, IR780 iodide) were reported. Shao et al. reported the self-assembly of PTX with ICG into uniform NPs, with 53.80±3.79% drug loading content of PTX [505]. The PTX–ICG nanodrug increased the solubility of PTX and tumor accumulation.

1.13.1.3 Self-Assembly of Chemotherapy with Immunotherapy Drugs

Immunotherapy aims to stimulate immune cells to browse and eradicate malignant cells. It has revolutionized cancer treatment [506]. The first example of immunotherapy was reported more than a century ago by William B. Coley who administered streptococcal organisms into a cancer patient to stimulate immune systems and shrink the tumor [507]. This discovery led to bigger developments, and the 2018 Nobel Prize in Physiology or Medicine was awarded for the discovery of cancer therapy by the inhibition of negative immune regulation, i.e., cytotoxic T lymphocyte-associated antigen 4 (CAR T) and programmed death/ligand 1 (PD-1/L1) to enable T cells. Tumor environment is usually immune-suppressed, and crucial responses such as T-cell activation and antigen presentation are inhibited [504]. For these reasons, eight new immunomodulatory drugs based on the blockage of PD-1/L1 and CAR T-cell therapy were approved by the FDA from 2014 to 2018. However, their applications still suffer from low patient response, dose limits, and low stability [508]. NPs can be used to increase the efficacy of immunotherapeutic drugs enabling targeted delivery by releasing their cargo at required sites such as tumor tissues and lymph nodes. With nanodrug formulations, pathophysiological barriers including compact extracellular matrix, renal clearance, and endonuclease degradation can be tackled [509]. For these reasons, numerous immuno-nanodrug delivery systems have been developed, and they showed promising results [510].

Indomethacin (IDM) is a drug that has immunomodulatory effects. IDM is a cyclooxygenase (COX-2) inhibitor and nonsteroidal anti-inflammatory drug that decreases M2 polarization of macrophages by inhibiting the production of prostaglandin E2 (PGE2) which supports immunesuppressant environment in tumor cells. Therefore, the use of IDM alongside chemotherapy may be beneficial. As shown in Figure 1.21, a carrier-free PTX–IDM nanodrug was synthesized via one-pot assembly due to the known strong intermolecular interactions between two drugs including π–π stackings and hydrogen bonds [511]. Diverse morphologies including wirelike, netlike, honeycomb-like, sphere-like, and capsule-like were prepared by changing the weight ratio and initial PTX concentration. The mean size of IDM/PTX nanodrugs was determined as 461.6 ± 57.72 nm, and the zeta potential was -25.5 ± 0.702 mV. IDM/PTX nano-assemblies showed immunoregulatory ability in vivo by having the lowest expression of CD206, an anti-inflammatory macrophage biomarker, and interleukin 10 (IL-10), which has a proliferating effect on cancer cells, and the highest expression of CD86, an inflammatory macrophage biomarker.

Apart from this immunomodulatory agent, it is known that some anticancer drugs such as DOX and PTX can stimulate immune response by inducing immunogenic cell death [512]. To explore the immunotherapeutic effects of

the combinational use of PTX and ICG, Li et al. demonstrated the self-assembly ability of ICG templating strategy by synthesizing stable NPs from a variety of molecules, including PTX, DTX, SRF, and celecoxib, with ICG [513]. Drug solution was added to aqueous solution of ICG, and this mixture self-assembled into NPs with a mean diameter of 112 ± 1.06 nm and a drug loading rate of 90.7%. Using low doses of PTX suppressed the immunosuppressive tumor microenvironment via downregulating T-regulatory (Treg) cells, whereas ICG increased immunogenic cell death under laser irradiation. In vitro and in vivo studies with triple-negative breast cancer cells showed that synergistic therapy elongated the half-life by threefold and increased the intratumoral drug accumulation by 11.2-fold compared to free PTX. The therapy with laser irradiation also showed enhanced antitumor immunity by exhibiting 3.1-fold higher dendritic cell maturation and significantly decreased Treg infiltration due to the killing effect of PTX.

1.13.1.4 Self-Assembly of Chemotherapy Drugs with Other Organic Molecules

DOX and gossypol have been self-assembled with a very small amount of PDA with a weight ratio of 5:5:1 via π–π stacking and hydrogen bonding [514]. Gossypol is an anticancer drug exerting its effect by inducing tumor cell apoptosis. The prepared DOX–PDA–gossypol NPs exhibited the size of 59.6 ± 9.6 nm with a very high drug loading (91%). As shown in Figure 1.22a, in vivo studies demonstrated that free DOX and free DOX–gossypol were quickly cleared from blood, whereas DOX–PDA–gossypol NPs showed 458-fold and 228-fold higher elimination half-lives than free DOX and free gossypol, respectively, due to the strong NP structure. Furthermore, these NPs demonstrated >192 h of blood circulation (Figure 1.22b) and enhanced

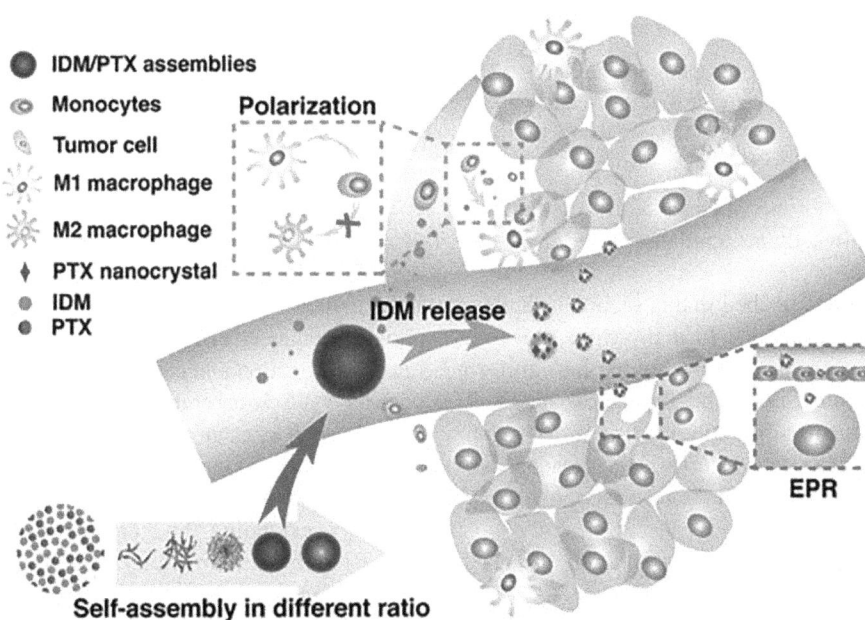

FIGURE 1.21 Schematic illustration of fabrication of IDM/PTX nano-assemblies at different ratios and its mechanism of action. (Copyright 2019. Reproduced from Ref. [511] with permission from the American Chemical Society.)

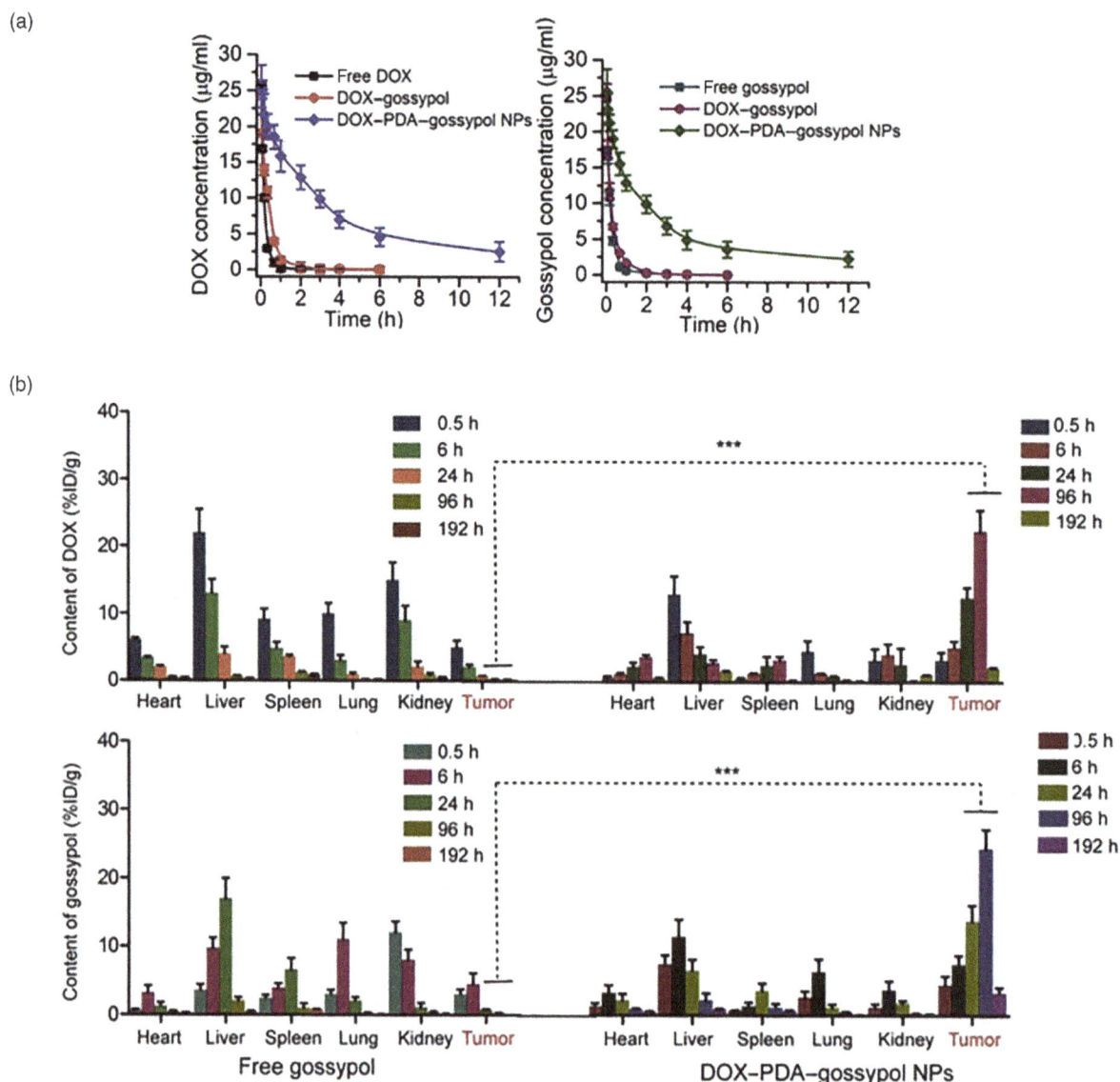

FIGURE 1.22 (a) The pharmacokinetic properties of free DOX, free gossypol, free DOX and gossypol, and DOX–PDA–gossypol NPs in mice after the injection at a drug dose of 2.5 mg/kg over 12 h. (b) Quantitative analysis of drug distribution (DOX—up; gossypol—bottom) over 192 h in major organs and tumors after intravenous injection. (Copyright 2018. Reproduced from Ref. [98] with permission from John Wiley & Sons Inc.)

accumulation at the tumor site when compared to free DOX and gossypol, which mostly accumulated in the liver, kidney, lung, and spleen.

Overall, the method described in this section is facile to use in making carrier-free NPs. In many cases, however, drug molecules cannot simply self-assemble into uniform and stable nanostructures using the above-described self-assembly method due to limitations arising from their structures [511,515]. Therefore, alternative approaches will be required, which are detailed in the next sections.

1.13.2 SELF-ASSEMBLY OF CLINICAL DRUG MOLECULES WITH DIFFERENT CONJUGATION

To solve the problems of many drug molecules not being able to self-assemble to uniform nanodrugs, covalent conjugation of multiple molecules of single anticancer drug or between different drugs or between drug and other organic molecules via different linkages has been widely investigated. These dimeric conjugations can convert hydrophobic anticancer drugs into less rigid molecules, disrupting crystallization and consequently enabling the formation of NPs via self-assembly. By regulating the connecting bridges, such as ester bonds, disulfide bonds, and thioketal bonds, dimeric prodrugs can form stable nanostructures in biological environments, thereby improving drugs' water solubility, extending their blood circulation half-life, and increasing the bioavailability [516,517]. In this section, different conjugations with drug molecules will be reviewed to facilitate their self-assembly to high-quality nanodrugs.

In a 2020 study, Li et al. reported a novel SRF conjugate, employed with hemoglobin (Hb) in combination with

PDT [518]. In addition to be an anticancer agent, SRF can promote ferroptosis, a cell death mechanism dependent on the reaction of iron with excess ROS in tumor. Hb can bind to oxygen due to its iron content, and therefore serve as an oxygen supplement for ferroptosis and PDT. Ce6 was bridged with Hb via an amido bond and mixed with SRF and tumor-sensitive matrix metalloproteinase 2 (MMP2) peptide to self-assemble into SRF@Hb-Ce6 NPs (175 nm) via intermolecular forces. *In vivo* experiments demonstrated that SRF@Hb-Ce6 NPs exhibited tumor-responsive release via MMP2 and high tumor inhibition with synergistic therapy. More examples of tumor-sensitive/targeting peptides will be discussed in detail in later sections.

1.13.2.1 Conjugation of Homodimeric Drug Molecules with Various Linkers

PTX is known to aggregate in aqueous conditions due to the π–π stackings of aromatic rings. This results in the formation of needlelike crystals, instead of self-assembling into uniform NPs [519]. To solve this issue, two PTX molecules were covalently coupled to form a dimer. As shown in Figure 1.23, two PTX molecules were covalently bonded via dicarboxylic acid linkers that contained either an aliphatic carbon chain or a disulfide bond (R: C4, C6, C8, C9, S-S) [520]. The synthesized dimers (PTX2) were then used to form PTX2 NPs in aqueous solution without using any carriers. PTX2 NP formation increased the water solubility of PTX to a maximum of 1000 μg/mL. The NPs containing a disulfide bond were stable in physiological environment, whereas they exhibited a rapid stimuli-responsive release in the tumor tissue due to the cleavage of glutathione (GSH)-sensitive bond. This resulted in enhanced antitumor effects and lowered systemic toxicity [521]. Another connecting bridge with a thioether moiety was also reported for the preparation of PTX2 NPs [522]. PTX loading in

PTX-S-PTX NPs was as high as 94%, and this nanodrug increased the solubility of PTX by 2000-fold. In 2018, Xie and co-workers reported thioketal-linked dimeric PTX NPs [523]. The prepared NPs were coated with red blood cell (RBC) membranes for enhanced circulation, and the mean diameter of NPs was determined to be 168 nm. *In vitro* and *in vivo* experiments showed that the prepared NPs displayed prolonged blood circulation, improved tumor accumulation, and enhanced therapeutic efficacy in cervical cancer cells. The RBC membrane coating also enabled to achieve a 4.6-fold higher concentration of thioketal-linked PTX dimer in tumor compared to the NPs without the coating at 23 h post-treatment.

To further demonstrate the effect of self-assembly of dimeric drugs, Hou et al. reported the synthesis of a CUR dimer via a thioether bond [524]. This CUR-S-CUR prodrug was self-assembled into spherical NPs with 78% drug loading and PEGylated for prolonged circulation. The NP formation increased the water solubility of CUR, thereby enhancing cellular uptake. *In vitro* studies showed that CUR-S-CUR NPs demonstrated comparable cytotoxicity to free CUR, with sustained release arising from thioether bond. Dimer preparation has also been extended to other anticancer drugs such as DOX. In a 2020 study, the synthesis of a DOX dimer was reported via an acid-triggered hydrolyzable carbamate linker with 86% drug loading [525]. DOX dimer was self-assembled into NPs, which exhibited pH-responsive drug release and enhanced antitumor efficacy in liver cancer cells. Kasai et al. reported pure drug NPs below 100 nm by the preparation of SN-38 dimeric nanodrugs [526]. Two SN-38 molecules were coupled together via dicarbamate, diester, and diether linkages. The SN-38 dimers transformed SN-38 molecule into a less planar structure that reduced the risk of crystallization and therefore successfully formed NPs via the nanoprecipitation method.

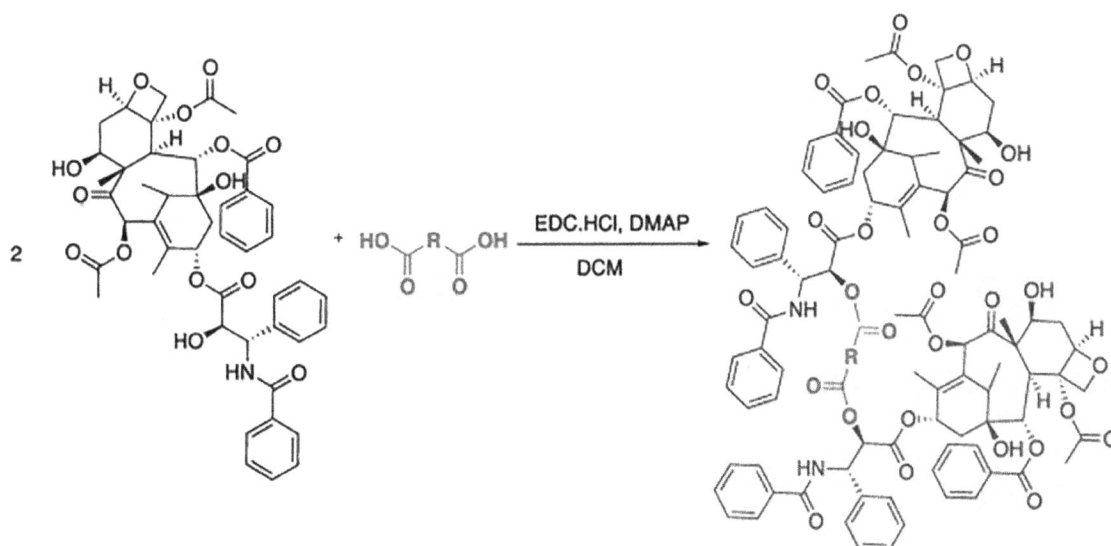

FIGURE 1.23 Schematic illustration of PTX-R-PTX conjugates (R: C4, C6, C8, C9, S-S). (Copyright 2017. Adapted from Ref. [520] with permission from Elsevier Science Ltd.)

1.13.2.2 Conjugation of Heterodimeric Drug Molecules with Various Linkers

1.13.2.2.1 Conjugation of Chemotherapy Drugs

The above approach provides a way to make nanodrugs via preparing homodimeric drug molecules first, followed by self-assembly. However, monotherapies with one type of drug molecule limit their application range due to the drug resistance of tumors [527]. To optimize the efficacy and safety of cancer treatment, a series of nanodrugs based on heterodimeric drug–drug conjugates have been developed [528]. Heterodimeric drugs can be amphiphilic with both hydrophilic and hydrophobic parts and formed by both hydrophobic drugs [529]. In addition to self-assembly into uniform nanostructures, the optimally designed heterodimeric drugs can affect the interaction with cancer cells and release drug molecules in controlled ways at the tumor site, enabling efficient drug delivery to targeted tissues and cells without any external delivery vehicles [530]. Compared to single or sequential administration of anticancer drugs, different drugs in heterodimer drugs result in differences in pharmacokinetics and mechanisms of actions. This can then produce synergistic therapeutic effects and overcome MDR [490,531].

Ni et al. reported the syntheses of alkyne-terminated disulfide (-S-S-) and introduced hydrophobic CPT and azide-modified hydrophilic gemcitabine (GEM). GEM is an FDA-approved chemotherapy drug that works as a pyrimidine nucleoside antimetabolite and is used for the treatment of breast cancer, bladder cancer, pancreatic cancer, and non-small-cell lung cancer [532]. These two molecules were then reacted together in a Cu-catalyzed click reaction to form CPT-S-S-triazole-GEM for combination chemotherapy (Figure 1.24a) [533]. This amphiphilic drug conjugate exhibited a high drug loading content (36.0% CPT, 27.2% GEM) and formed spherical NPs (180 nm) in aqueous solution. In vitro studies showed that CPT-S-S-triazole-GEM NPs released two drugs simultaneously in liver cancer cells due to the cleavage of disulfide bond and exhibited higher toxicity compared to free CPT and free GEM within the 72-h test period. The prodrug NPs demonstrated moderate half-life, high accumulation in tumor tissues, and synergistic therapeutic efficacy in vivo. Condensation reactions can also be used to form amphiphilic drug conjugates. Zhu et al. reported the preparation of MTX–GEM conjugate (MTX–GEM) via an amide bond as shown in Figure 1.24b [534]. MTX–GEM self-assembled into NPs in aqueous solution via the solvent exchange method with 100% drug loading. In vitro studies demonstrated that MTX–GEM NPs achieved an enhanced anticancer effect and inhibited MDR in breast cancer cells compared to free drugs. In another study, MTX and CPT were conjugated via ester linkage for pH-/esterase-responsive cleavage [535]. The MTX–CPT conjugate with amphiphilic and ionic properties self-assembled into MTX–CPT NPs in aqueous solution via hydrogen bonding and hydrophobic interactions.

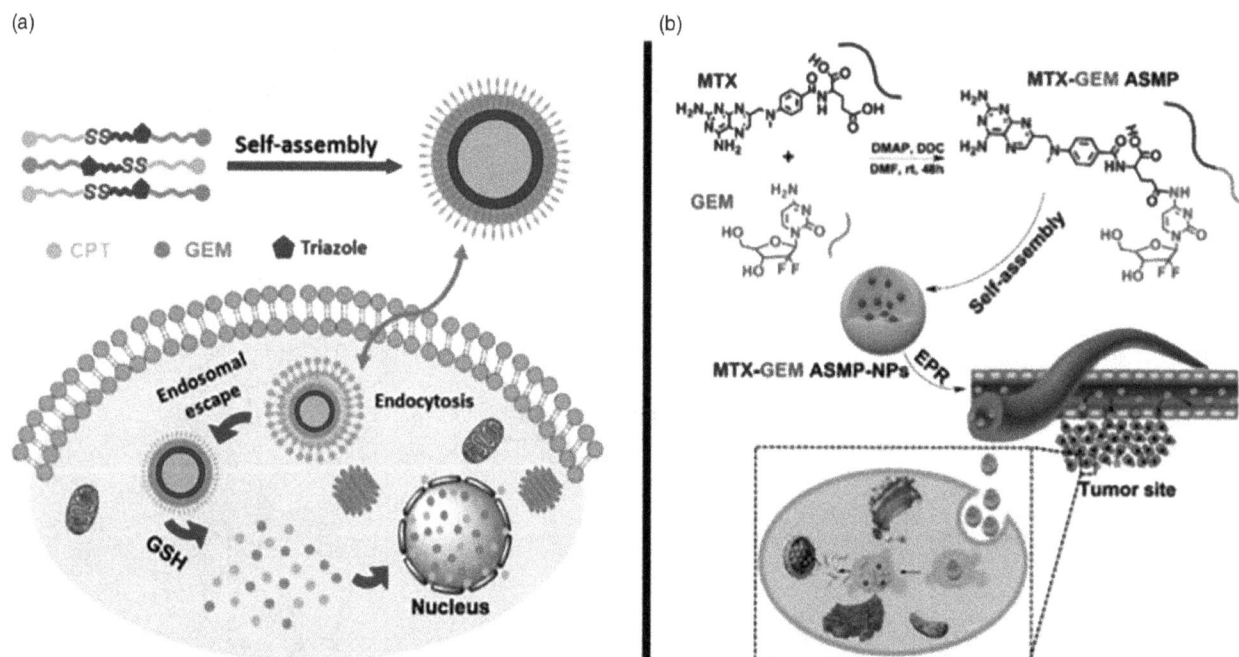

FIGURE 1.24 (a) Illustration of NP formation to form CPT-S-S-triazole-GEM conjugate and its therapeutic mechanism in cells. (Copyright 2019. Reproduced from Ref. [533] with permission from the American Chemical Society.) (b) Schematic of MTX–GEM synthesis and construction of self-assembled MTX–GEM NPs for cancer combination chemotherapy. (Copyright 2016. Reproduced from Ref. [534] with permission from the American Chemical Society.)

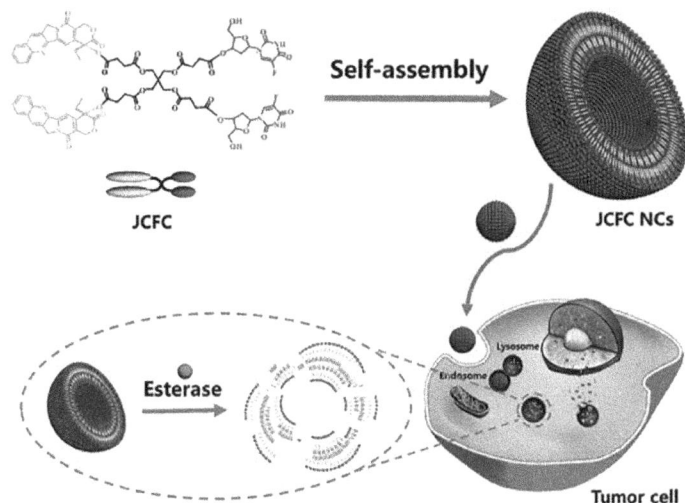

FIGURE 1.25 Schematic illustrations of the preparation of Janus camptothecin–floxuridine conjugate (JCFC) NPs. (Copyright 2017. Reproduced from Ref. [536] with permission from John Wiley & Sons Inc.)

In addition, Dai et al. developed liposome-like nanocapsules based on amphiphilic camptothecin–fluorouridine (CPT–FUDR) molecules as shown in Figure 1.25 [536]. The heterodimeric drug molecules were synthesized by two hydrophilic FUDR molecules and two hydrophobic CPT molecules via hydrolyzable ester linkages. They self-assembled into uniform and stable prodrug NPs in aqueous solution.

In addition to hydrophobic–hydrophilic dimeric drug conjugates, heterodimeric nanodrugs from two poorly water-soluble anticancer drugs have been explored. In a 2019 study, Wang et al. developed PTX–DOX heterodimeric nanodrugs [537]. PTX was conjugated with DOX by using a linking thioether bridge. The resulting conjugates formed uniform NPs via self-assembly. These NPs were further PEGylated for prolonged blood circulation time. The drug loading ratios of PTX and DOX were 46.5% and 30.0%, respectively. The tumor microenvironment triggered the cleavage of thioether bonds in the presence of breast cancer cells, resulting in rapid release of PTX and DOX, thereby synergistic tumor inhibition. We have also reported the conjugation of PTX with pH-responsive cis-aconitic anhydride (CA)-modified DOX [538]. CA modification enabled GSH-responsive DOX release, and the conjugate was modified with a layer of crosslinked surfactant based on HA which can bind to CD44 receptors that are highly expressed in certain tumor cells. Since DOX and PTX have different inhibition mechanisms and antitumor targets, the combination therapy enhanced therapeutic efficacy and inhibited MDR. *In vitro* and *in vivo* studies demonstrated that these CAD–PTX–HA NPs exhibited high stability with a half-life of 4 h, excellent active targeting effect, and controllable intracellular drug release. These NPs achieved significantly enhanced anticancer efficiency when compared with the individual administrations of DOX and PTX.

1.13.2.2.2 Conjugation of Chemotherapy with PDT or PTT Drugs

Sun et al. reported a non-carrier prodrug synthesized by bridging PTX with PPa via a thioether bond [539]. Tumor-responsive nanodrug PPa-S-PTX was prepared by the one-step nanoprecipitation method and PEGylated. The size of these chemo-PDT nanodrugs was around 90 nm with a zeta potential of about −30 mV. In the presence of laser irradiation, these NPs released more than 40% of PTX within 12 h and demonstrated effectiveness in generating ROS. To further increase the sensitivity of PTX, DOX was conjugated with the PS pheophorbide a (Pa), via pH-sensitive hydrazone bond to form Pa-h-DOX (PhD) conjugates [540]. As shown in Figure 1.26, the surface of PhD NPs was further modified with PEG via pH-sensitive Schiff base formation, resulting in NPs with an average size of 79 nm. After the pH-sensitive cleavage of the PEG surface, these NPs transformed into ultra-small strongly positively charged NPs (4 nm) that could achieve deep tumor penetration. PhD NPs remained stable in physiological conditions. Pa exerted both a PDT and PTT effect, and this combinational therapy demonstrated a 100% cure rate as a result of its synergistic effect.

In a 2019 study, a thioether-linked PTX dimer (PTX-S-PTX) was mixed with the photothermal agent IR780 iodide and HSA to form uniform NPs via the self-assembly method [541]. The resulting NPs were stable at 4°C for almost 6 weeks with a size of 129 nm. This approach enhanced the drug loading content of PTX from 6.6 to 48.7 wt% compared to commercially available Abraxane®.

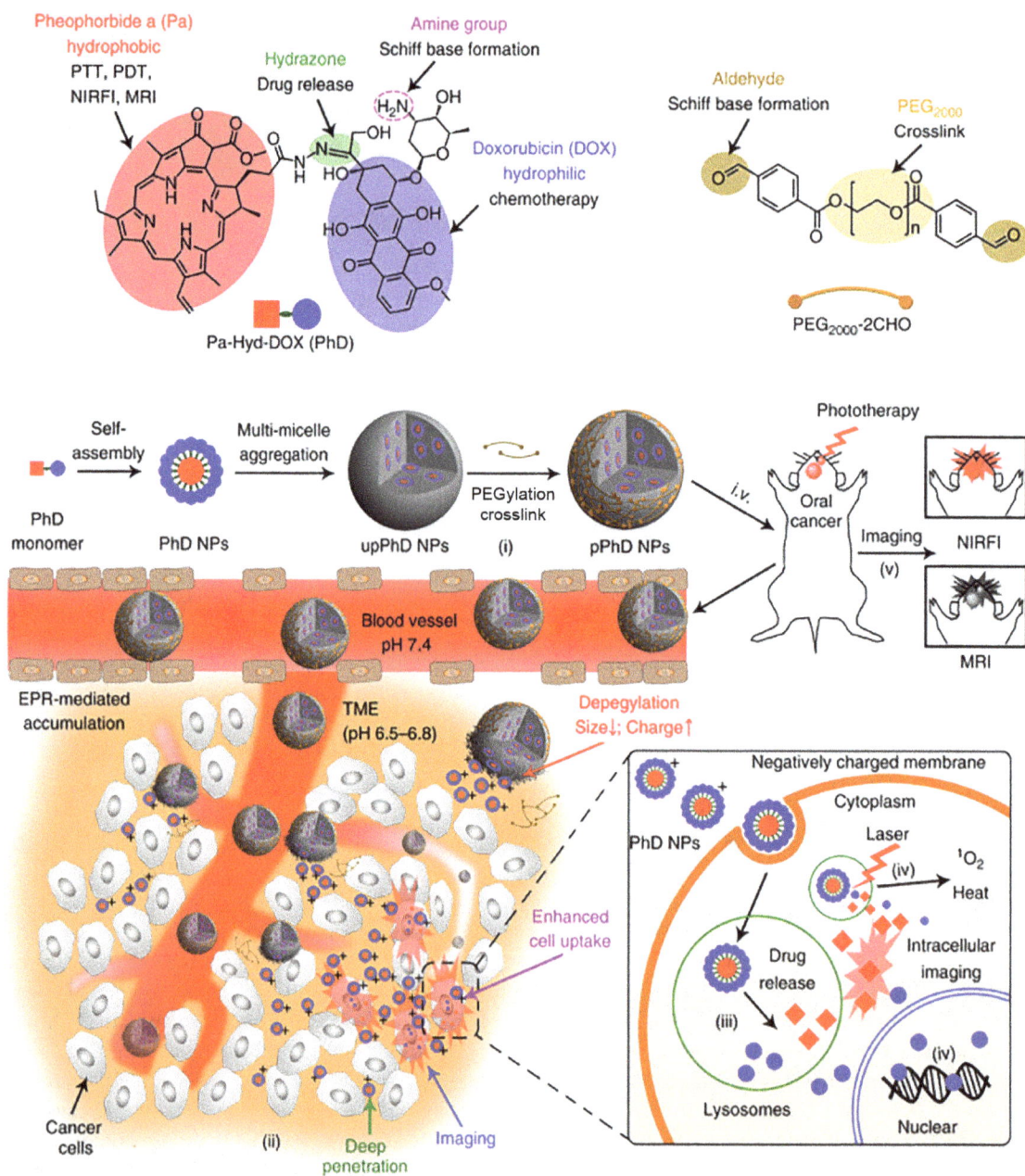

FIGURE 1.26 Schematic illustration of properties of DOX–Pa conjugate nanoparticles. (Copyright 2018. Reproduced from Ref. [540] with permission from Springer Nature.)

1.13.2.2.3 Conjugation of Chemotherapy with Immunotherapy Drugs

A number of recent studies have focused on the synergistic use of immunotherapeutic agents with chemotherapeutics without any carriers via the self-assembly strategy [420,542].

1.13.2.3 Conjugation of Drug Molecules with Various Functional Organic Molecules

1.13.2.3.1 Conjugation with Lipids

In recent years, anticancer drugs have been successfully translated into lipid-based formulations, such as liposomes for the encapsulation of drug molecules. Carrier strategies

based on liposomes have been discussed in detail in the literature and are the subject of the previous review [543]. However, carrier-based liposomal formulations still suffer from problems such as low drug loading and premature drug release. Efficient combination therapy by using two or more different drugs with liposomes as carriers remains challenging due to inefficient co-loading [544].

To explore the rationale behind the self-assembly of anticancer drugs with fatty acids, Zhang et al. studied the effect of lipophilicity and solubility of anticancer agents during self-assembly [545]. First, four different PTX conjugates were reported with different types of fatty acids, each having different extents of saturation. All these

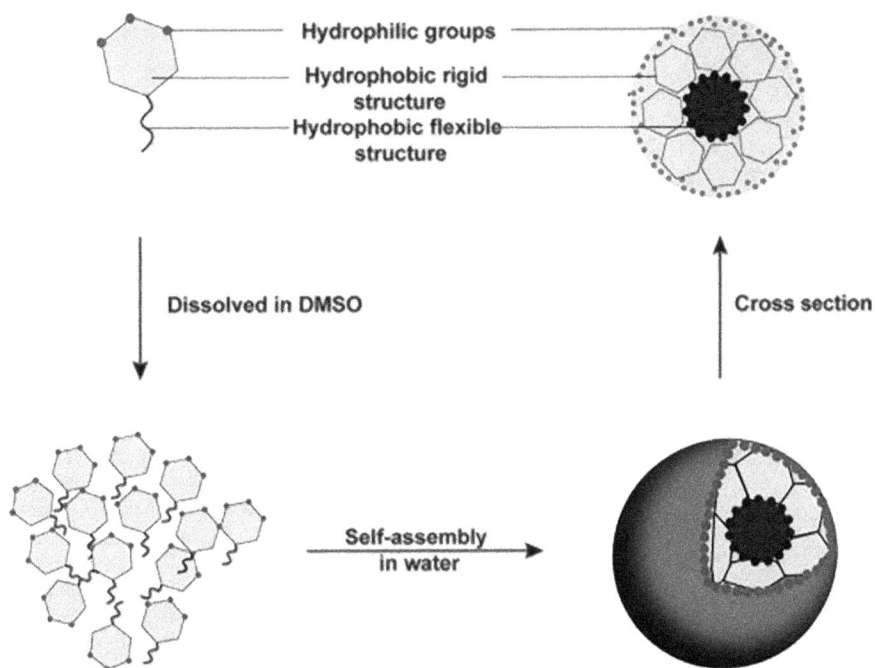

FIGURE 1.27 Self-assembly mechanism of PTX–lipid conjugates. (Copyright 2018. Adapted from Ref. [545] with permission from the American Chemical Society.)

conjugates managed to self-assemble into NPs. Second, the hydrophobicity of the conjugates was determined, and it was revealed that all prepared conjugates had higher hydrophobicity compared to PTX alone. Third, they have calculated the hydrophilicity and lipophilicity values in a variety of PTX conjugates in their study and literature [424,519,546–549] which can self-assemble but were connected with different accessories and linkage. They suggested that when a hydrophobic molecule conjugates with PTX, hydrophobic interactions occur between hydrophobic parts of molecules creating the inner core, whereas the hydroxyl group of PTX places on the outer region of self-assembled NPs (Figure 1.27), which leads to a negative zeta potential.

In a similar study, the same researchers compared the redox-responsive characteristics of thioether (-S-)- and dithioether (-2S-)-bonded PTX–OA conjugates (Figure 1.28), capable of self-assembling into NPs. When PEGylated, they remained stable for 3 months [547]. PTX-S-OA NPs demonstrated increased redox responsiveness *in vitro* and antitumor efficacy *in vivo* when compared to PTX-2S-OA. They have proposed that the single thioether bond near PTX is the key in hydrolysis and the -2S- bond consumes twofold more GSH/ROS compared to -S- and water molecules are unlikely to attack to -2S- due to the longer hydrophobic chain arising from ethylidene between two thioether bonds.

Nanoprecipitation of the PTX-S-S-VE conjugate resulted in the formation of stable NPs with −29.2 mV zeta potential. Molecular simulation studies revealed that the oxygen atom close to the -S-S- linkage has an impact on this negative

charge density and the -S-S- linker acted as a stabilizer (Figure 1.29), enabling the folding of the molecule for self-assembly. NP formation increased the drug loading rate of PTX to 60 wt%, whereas Taxol and Abraxane® have 1% and 10% drug loadings, respectively.

1.13.2.3.2 Conjugation with Carbohydrates

Carbohydrates, such as mannose (MAN), HA, and DEX, are very appealing molecules in nanodrug delivery platforms due to their biodegradable, biocompatible, and low immunogenic properties [550]. Different strategies have been reported to prepare conjugates of hydrophobic anticancer agents and hydrophilic saccharides to form stable nano-assemblies, resulting in enhanced efficiency [551]. In a 2018 study, another HA-based nanodrug was reported. As shown in Figure 1.30, PTX was covalently conjugated to HA and also to ICG-COOH, a derivative of ICG [552].

In a 2019 study, DOX was self-assembled with natural HA–FA conjugates into HA/FA–DOX NPs (labeled as HA/FA-NP-DOX in Figure 1.31) [553]. HA/FA-NP-DOX demonstrated 5.6 h of elimination half-life, whereas it was 0.4 h for free DOX (Figure 1.31a). Furthermore, biodistribution studies revealed that the drug accumulation into the liver, lung, and kidney was lower compared to free DOX (Figure 1.31b) and the DOX uptake with NPs into tumor was fourfold higher (Figure 1.31c) than in the free drug group.

DEX is a carbohydrate known to be useful for drug delivery systems due to its high water solubility and long circulation properties similar to PEG. In a 2020

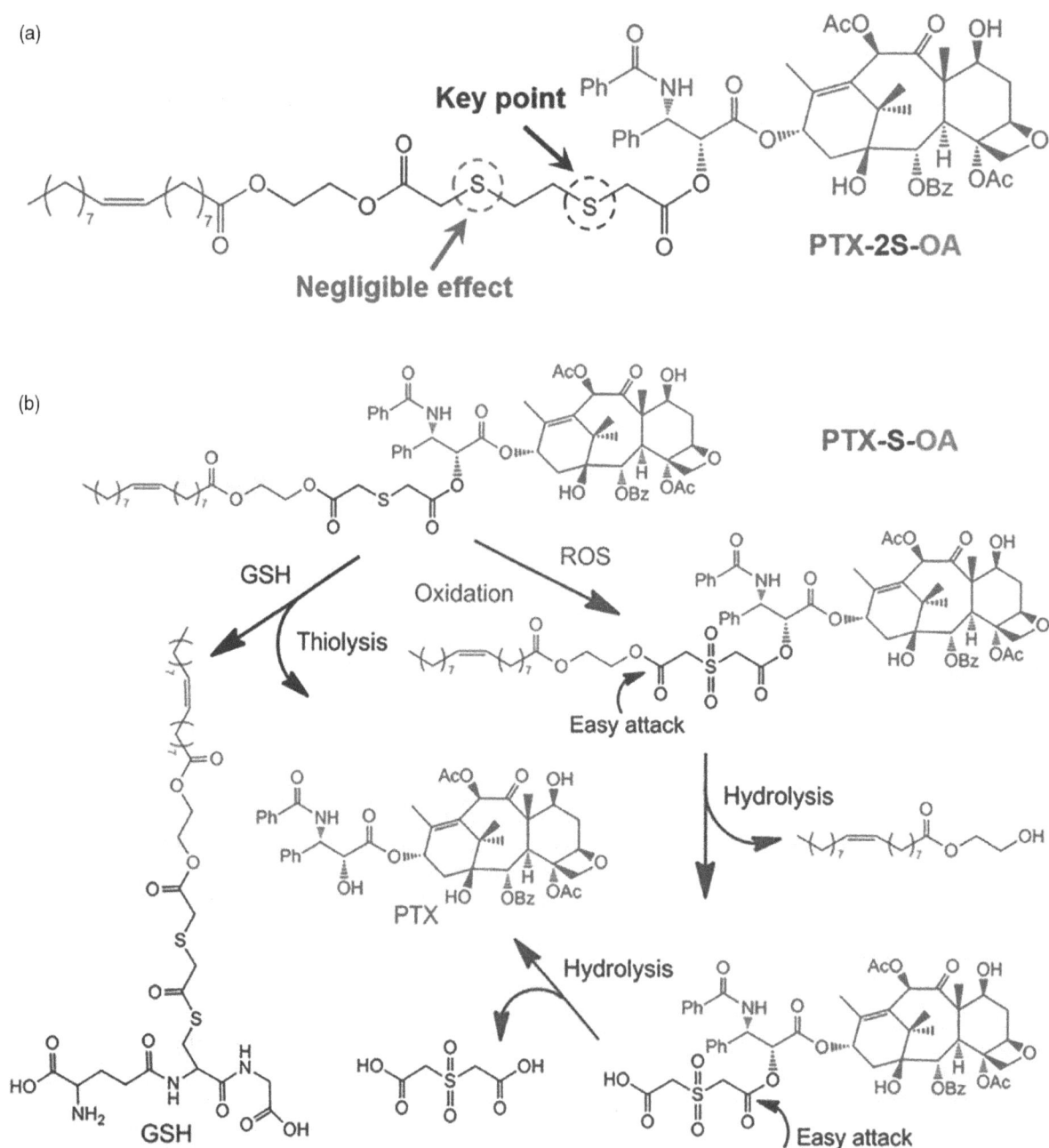

FIGURE 1.28   Redox-responsive release mechanism of PTX-2S-OA (a) and PTX-S-OA (b) conjugates. (Copyright 2016. Reproduced from Ref. [547] with permission from the American Chemical Society.)

study, Yin et al. reported DEX-based self-assembled drug NPs. Amphiphilic DEX–deoxycholic acid (DEX-DOCA) conjugates self-assembled with PTX and silybin (SB), which can enhance the chemosensitivity for synergistic therapy, into NPs [554]. These NPs increased the circulation time from 1.04 h (free PTX) to 5 h. *In vitro* and *in vivo* studies revealed that the NPs enhanced tumor penetration by inducing tumor vascular normalization in a lung cancer model. Li et al. reported the self-assembly of DOX with FA–DEX conjugate, which formed tumor-targeting NPs [555]. DOX@DEX-FA NPs

reduced the side effects arising from DOX and enhanced cellular uptake.

1.13.2.3.3   Conjugation with Peptides

In recent years, peptide-conjugated drug delivery systems have attracted significant research interest due to their biocompatibility, biodegradability, producibility at large scales, and specificity as they can be employed as tumor-targeting moieties by using particular sequences [556]. These sequences can target tumor-specific receptors that play important roles in tumor angiogenesis. Tumor-homing

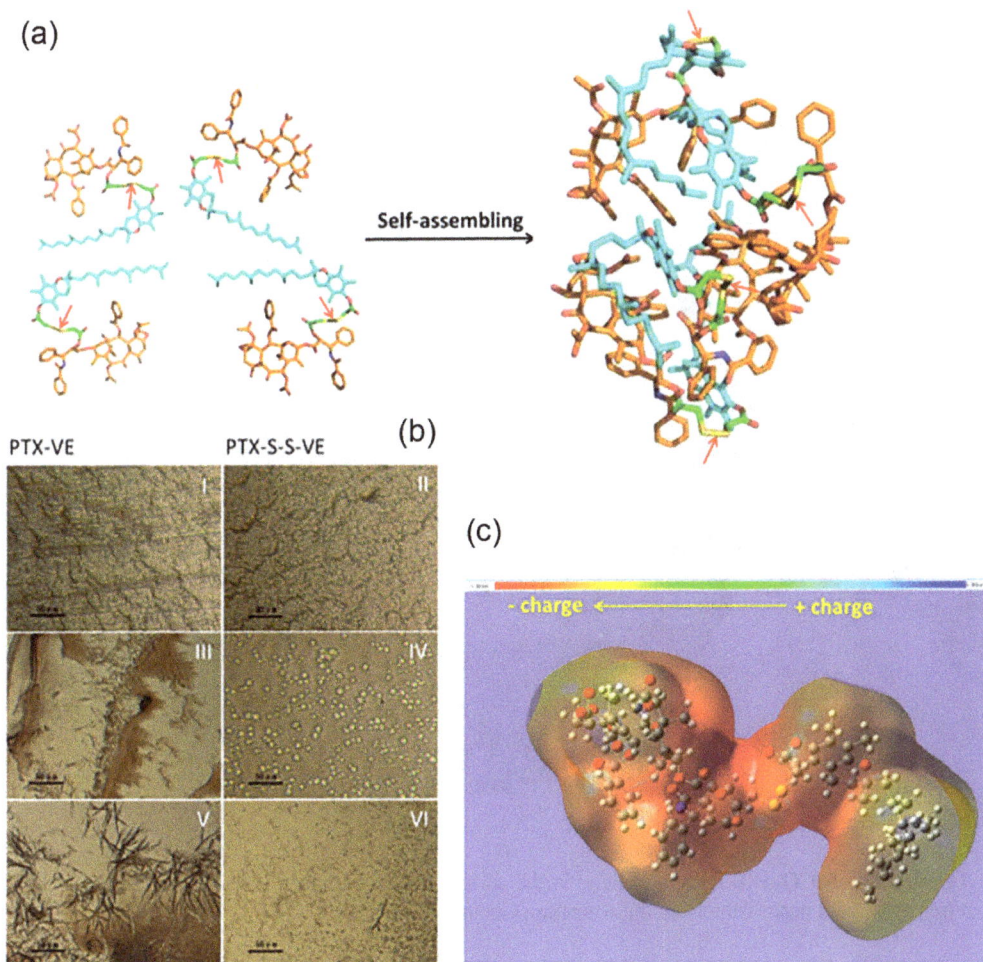

FIGURE 1.29 (a) MD simulation of self-assembled PTX-S-S-VE conjugates. Blue, orange, and yellow represent VE, PTX, and S-S, respectively. (b) Crystallization of PTX–VE and PTX-S-S-VE NPs. (c) Distribution of charges of self-assembled PTX-S-S-VE. (Copyright 2014. Reproduced from Ref. [519] with permission from the American Chemical Society.)

sequences were the subject of a review in 2010 [557]. So far, a variety of tumor-targeting peptide ligands have been discovered, specific to particular cells and receptors such as integrin receptors [558].

Arginine–glycine–aspartic acid (RGD) is a tumor-homing tripeptide that can bind to integrin receptors, expressed in high quantities in tumor cells [559]. There have been many studies focusing on the incorporation of this targeting moiety into anticancer drugs. Zhang et al. prepared tumor-targeting CPT nanodrugs conjugated to the peptide Arg-Gly-Asp-Ser (RGDS) via ester linkage. This cancer biomarker binds to $\alpha v \beta 3$ integrin in cancer cells. Myristic acid was then coupled to the N-terminus of the tumor-targeting moiety, as a hydrophobic group to facilitate prodrug self-assembly. The conjugate was precipitated in cold ether, forming nanofibers that exhibited selective tumor inhibition due to the presence of RGDS tetrapeptide targeting sequence. This study demonstrated that nanofibers are promising therapeutic agents as an alternative to the traditional spherical NP approach.

Different RGD peptides were also used in the literature. Xu et al. reported the conjugation of PTX with iRGD peptide (CRGDKGPDC), forming NPs by dialysis [560]. In another study, Liu et al. reported a simple PTX conjugate by using a tumor-targeting peptide, cyclic Arg-Gly-Asp (cRGDyK), and Ce6, each bonded with HSA separately via amide bonds [561]. The conjugate generated NPs by adding equal amounts of HSA–RGD and HSA–Ce6 in phosphate-buffered saline (PBS) into PTX solution in methanol. This co-assembly mechanism occurred via the hydrophobic interactions between drug molecules and HSA. *In vitro* studies with human glioblastoma cells revealed that the prepared NPs provided superior cytotoxicity under 660 nm light irradiation at 2 mW/cm² for 30 min compared to PDT or chemotherapy alone.

To further increase the targeting ability of RGD, Pan and co-workers reported the preparation of pH-sensitive BTZ nanodrugs with a modified mussel-derived tetrapeptide (DOPA)₄ as shown in Figure 1.32 [562]. Boronic acid and ester groups can degrade in the presence of H_2O_2 [563], and

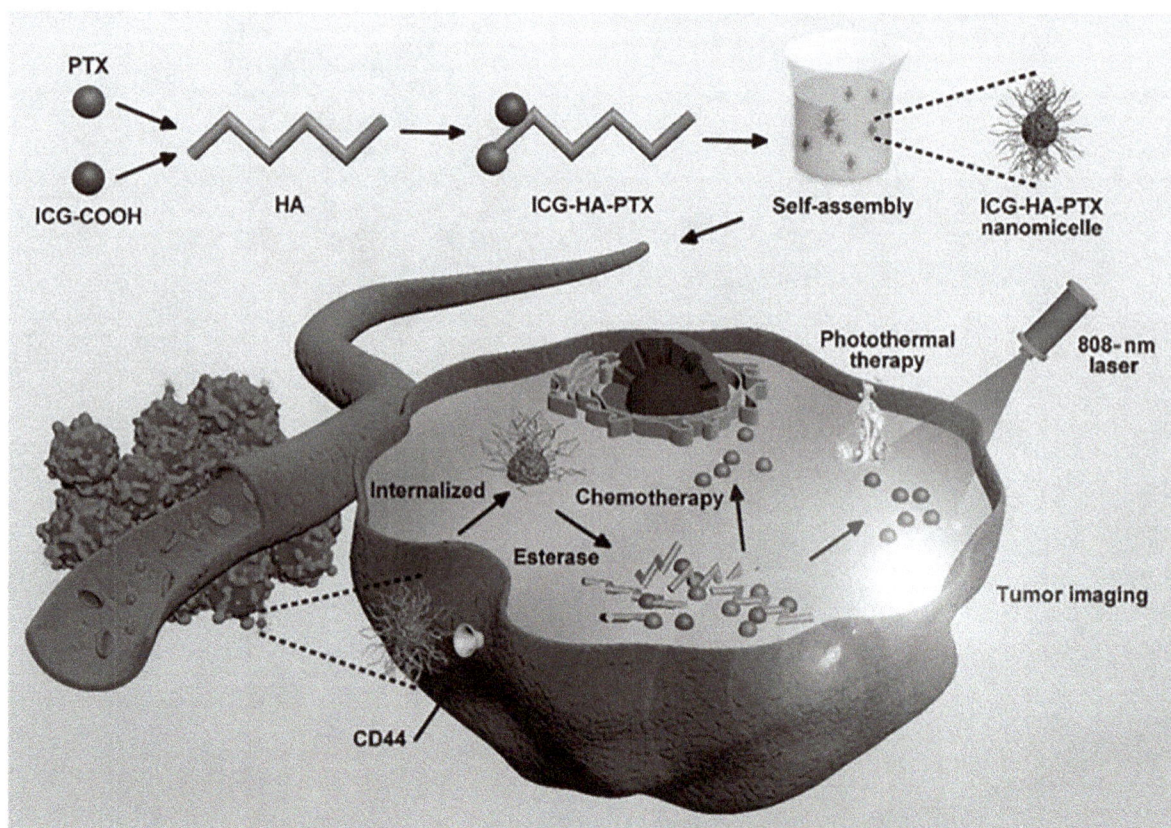

FIGURE 1.30 Preparation of ICG–HA–PTX micelles via the self-assembly method and its therapeutic effect. (Copyright 2018. Reproduced from Ref. [552] with permission from the American Chemical Society.)

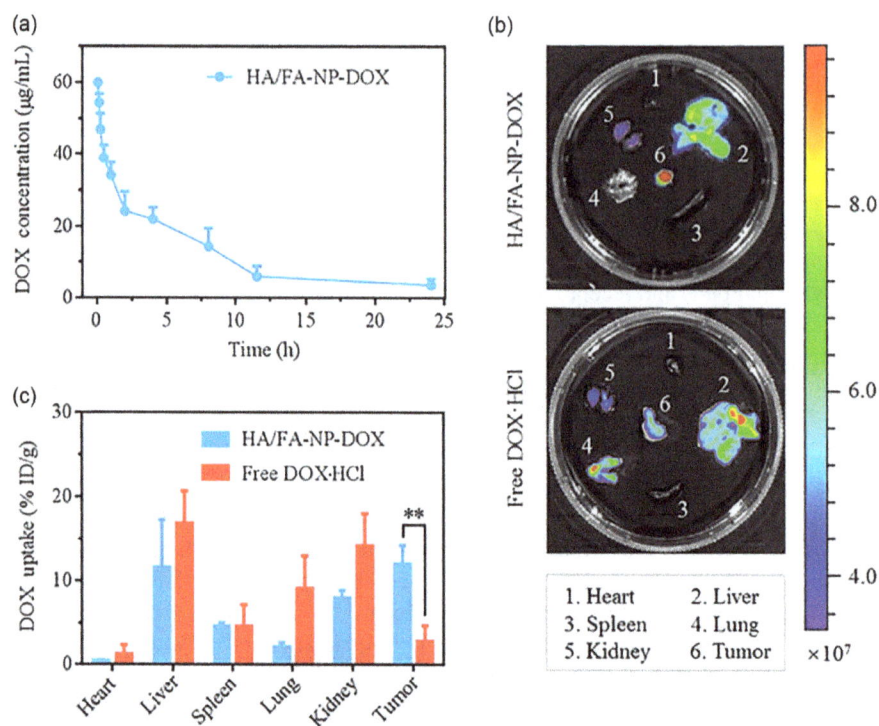

FIGURE 1.31 *In vivo* pharmacokinetics and biodistribution of HA/FA-NP-DOX ($n=3$). (a) Pharmacokinetics in BALB/c mice. (b) Fluorescence images and (c) quantification of DOX in major organs and tumors isolated from SKOV-3 tumor-bearing mice at 8 h after HA/FA-NP-DOX or free DOX·HCl injection. (Copyright 2019. Reproduced from Ref. [553] with permission from the American Chemical Society.)

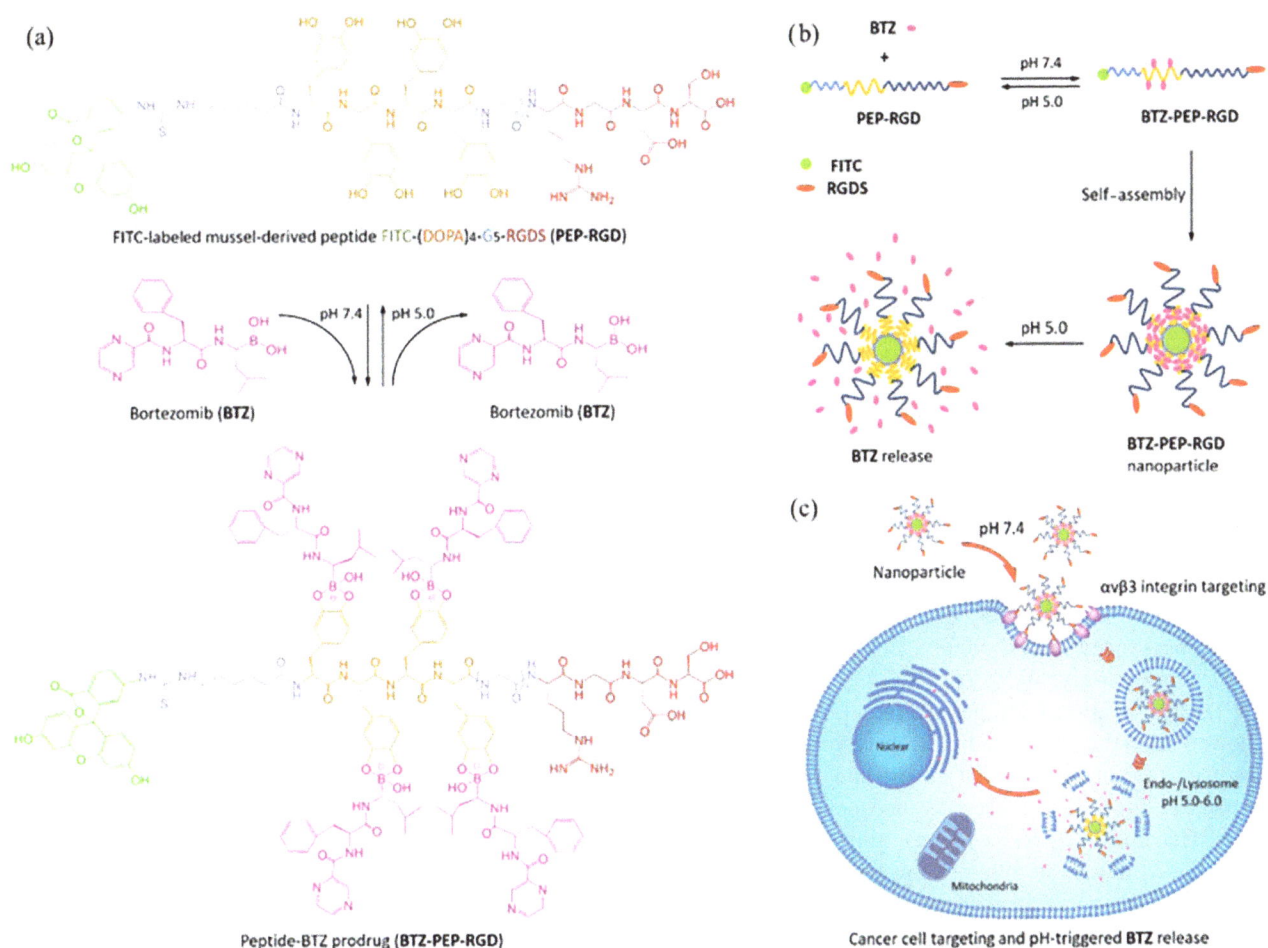

(a)

FITC-labeled mussel-derived peptide FITC-(DOPA)4-G5-RGDS (PEP-RGD)

Bortezomib (BTZ)   Bortezomib (BTZ)

Peptide-BTZ prodrug (BTZ-PEP-RGD)

(b)

BTZ

PEP-RGD   BTZ-PEP-RGD

FITC
RGDS

Self-assembly

BTZ release   BTZ-PEP-RGD nanoparticle

(c)

Nanoparticle   αvβ3 integrin targeting

Nuclear

Mitochondria   Endo-/Lysosome pH 5.0-6.0

Cancer cell targeting and pH-triggered BTZ release

FIGURE 1.32 (a) Conjugation of the mussel-derived cancer-cell-targeting peptide with the antitumor drug BTZ via pH-cleavable linkages. (b and c) Schematic illustration of the peptide-prodrug-based nanoparticle with cancer-cell-targeting and pH-sensitive drug release property. (Copyright 2019. Produced from Ref. [562] with permission from the American Chemical Society.)

BTZ with the boronic acid group (on the drug molecule) was employed for pH-sensitive drug delivery. The tetrapeptide was modified to have the cancer-targeting sequence RGDS; a FITC group, enabling the observation of cellular uptake; and a non-bioactive quintuple glycine G5 spacer. BTZ was conjugated via its boronic acid group to the catechol functionalities on $(DOPA)_4$. The conjugate was able to form NPs with a drug loading capacity of 37.4%. These characteristics enabled an enhanced cellular uptake and specific drug release in endo-/lysosome. The blood circulation time of the NPs was around 24h, whereas free BTZ molecule was cleared from blood almost immediately after administration.

In a 2020 study, CUR was co-assembled with tumor-sensitive Ala-Thr-Lys-Thr-Ala (ATKTA) pentapeptides connected by cysteine [564]. The synthesis of nanodrug was simply achieved by dissolving CUR and the cysteine bridge peptide (CBP) in DMSO, injecting into phosphate buffer at pH 5.5, and removing the sediment. The prepared nanodrug (220 nm) had spherical morphology. *In vitro* and *in vivo* studies on cervical cancer cells demonstrated that CUR–CBP nanodrug has almost twofold higher tumor inhibition rate and showed reduced side effects on healthy cells compared to free CUR.

The effect of various linkers on tumor-homing peptide nanodrugs has also been investigated. In a 2018 study, different DOX conjugates with cRGDfC tumor-targeting peptide were reported by using different linkages, including -S-S-, -S-, and cathepsin B-cleavable valine–citrulline dipeptide (VC). These conjugates were self-assembled into NPs by using the facile nanoprecipitation method [565]. The *in vivo* studies revealed that thioether-linked NPs and VC-linked NPs exhibited superior anticancer activity around 1.5-fold and 2-fold compared to free DOX and disulfide-linked NPs, respectively. It was hypothesized that the reduced activity of disulfide-linked NPs was due to the generation DOX–SH but not DOX, as the prodrug degrades.

Recently, peptide nanodrugs have also been explored to increase the thermodynamic stability of drug NPs [566]. A conjugate of hexadecapeptide modified with a derivative of ICG, three cholic acids, and a pH-sensitive boronate ester moiety was mixed with SN-38. The hexadecapeptide KEKEKEKE, where K and E represent lysine and glutamic acid, respectively, was employed as a shell and formed the hydrophilic segment. This particular peptide has negligible interactions with other proteins and a stronger ability of entangling with water molecules when compared to PEG.

1.14 ADVANTAGES AND CHALLENGES OF CARRIER-FREE NANODRUGS

1.14.1 Drug Loading Capacity

High drug loadings can be achieved in carrier-free nanodrugs. These carrier-free nanodrugs provide remarkably high drug loadings, usually between 50% and 90% [519,567], and even up to 100% in particular studies [513,568]. Dimeric and heterodimeric nanodrugs have demonstrated enhanced drug loading rates, such as 100% for MTX–GEM nanodrugs, 78% with CUR-S-CUR NPs, and 86% with DOX dimer NPs. We have also reported 77.6% drug loading (CUR) with CUR–photosensitizer carrier-free nanodrug. Beyond this high CUR loading percentage, the nanodrug also contained a photosensitizer as a PDT drug. All these values are significantly higher when compared to carrier-based nanoplatforms that usually have ~10% drug loading capacity or lower [490]. In an example study of carrier-based nanodrugs, researchers used block copolymers of either PLA or poly(lactide-co-glycolide) and PEG to encapsulate DTX for the preparation of targeted PNPs [569]. The results showed that the drug loading capacity did not exceed 1% when the nanoprecipitation method was used. This is usually due to the differences between the solubilities of carrier and drug molecule resulting in different precipitation times. In addition to this, the simplicity of the nanoprecipitation method makes large-scale production feasible. Preparation of high-drug-loading carrier-based methodologies requires extensive synthetic work, often hindering their applications. In a rare high drug loading example, Zhao et al. reported a controlled nanoprecipitation method to form drug–core polymer–shell NPs by using multiple solvents together to increase the drug loadings of PNPs [570]. It was shown that this method can reach up to 58.5% drug loading by using a different range of drugs and polymers; however, it requires extensive experimentation and analysis of polymer and drug solubility data to find the "perfect" solvent mixture and drug concentration.

1.14.2 Improved Pharmacokinetic Profile and Stability

Carrier-free nanodrugs increase the half-life of anticancer drugs, remaining stable in systemic circulation and overcoming rapid clearance [504]. Representative examples on how long anticancer drugs remain in circulation are shown in Table 1.2. A dramatic increase in half-life values is clearly observed with nanodrug formulations when compared to free drug solutions. Prolonged systemic circulation time can promote drug accumulation in tumors, which in turn improves the efficacy of chemotherapy. This is in addition to a reduction in side effects on healthy tissues and organs. Addition of covalent linkages between drug molecules and/or functional molecules also enhances their antitumor efficacy by on-target release of the active drug molecules.

Carrier-free nanodrugs also exhibit excellent stability at 2°C–8°C, whereas some carrier-based drug NPs can cause drug leakage in long-term storage due to being physically loaded and the presence of carriers [572,573]. It was also pointed out in a number of *in vivo* studies that premature drug release from carrier-based NPs is a problem of concern [574].

1.14.3 Enhanced Safety Profile

Carrier-free nanodrugs minimize the use of carriers and excipients and therefore overcome the carrier-induced toxicity that is a burden to our body. For instance, although PLA is approved by FDA as a biomaterial, it can produce a local inflammatory response when administered as a NP carrier *in vivo* [575]. Another example, polyethyleneimine, often used in PNPs displayed damage to mitochondrial membrane which further suppresses the electron transportation [576]. There is also a reported case where carrier-based liposomal DOX NPs resulted in unexpected additional side effects, such as hand-foot syndrome [577]. The release of these NPs into tumor sites was unsatisfactory, mainly due to the DOX crystallization in the core of liposomes. Considering long-term clinical applications,

TABLE 1.2

Representative Examples of Half-Life Comparisons between Carrier-Free Nanodrugs and Free Anticancer Drugs

Carrier-Free Nanodrug	Nanodrug $t_{1/2}$	Free Drug $t_{1/2}$	References
PTX-S-S-VE NPs	25.74±7.66 h	1.47±0.16 h (Taxol)	[519]
UA–PTX NPs	6-fold longer	No specific value (PTX)	[571]
hICP NPs	7.97 h	1.44 h (SN-38)	[566]
PTX–ICG NPs	3-fold longer	No specific value (PTX)	[513]
DOX NPs	3 h	<10 min (DOX)	[489]
PhD NPs	31.8 min	4.4 min (DOX)	[540]
DOX–PDA–gossypol NPs	50.381 h	0.110 h (DOX)	[514]

the use of organic nanocarriers will increase the concern of the toxicity of accumulations of nanocarriers in patients. The interaction between unwanted accumulation of carriers and the biomolecules can form aggregation forming a protein corona, disturbing the mechanism of action of nanodrug formulations [578].

When inorganic materials are used as carriers, the side effects may be even more significant. Au-NPs [579], Ag-NPs [580], and iron oxide NPs [580] are found to have toxicities *in vitro* and *in vivo*. The slow degradation of these inorganic nanocarriers also contributes to long-term cytotoxicity [581,582]. In a 2019 study, CNTs were found to induce metastasis in breast cancer by mimicking the toxicity of asbestos, which is a carcinogenic nanofiber [480]. As shown in Figure 1.33, the exposure to CNTs caused strong metastasis signals in three out of five mice, while no signal was detected in the control group at day 4. This number increased to all five mice in the CNT-treated group at days 8 and 12, whereas there was a slightly detectable signal in two of five mice in the control group. It is also important to consider that the drug loadings are generally very low with carrier-based systems, which means a large amount of nanocarriers with no therapeutic role would need to be administered into the body to achieve effective chemotherapy doses. A detailed analysis of the toxicity profiles

of drug delivery nanocarriers was provided in a previous review [471]. On the other hand, carrier-free nanodrugs provide a relatively safe method to avoid carrier-induced toxicity while only requiring simple synthetic procedures, such as the preparation of dimeric and heterodimeric drug conjugates. This increases the safety of nanodrugs and limits the use of non-FDA-approved products [490].

1.14.4 HIGH FLEXIBILITY FOR RESPONSIVE DRUG RELEASE AND SYNERGISTIC COMBINATORIAL THERAPY

The recent studies discussed in this chapter reveal that carrier-free nanodrugs have unique advantages due to their unprecedented synthetic versatility. Anticancer drug molecules containing hydroxyl, carboxyl, amine, or halogen groups can be elegantly conjugated with different drugs or functional molecules including fatty acids, vitamins, photosensitizers, and immunotherapeutic agents. Tumor-responsive carrier-free prodrug NPs can be constructed via using ROS- and GSH-responsive linkages, pH-sensitive bonds, and coupling drug molecules with tumor-targeting peptides. These carrier-free NPs would remain stable until reaching the tumor sites. Upon exposure to tumor microenvironment, tumor-cleavable chemical bonds would break to release their drug loadings.

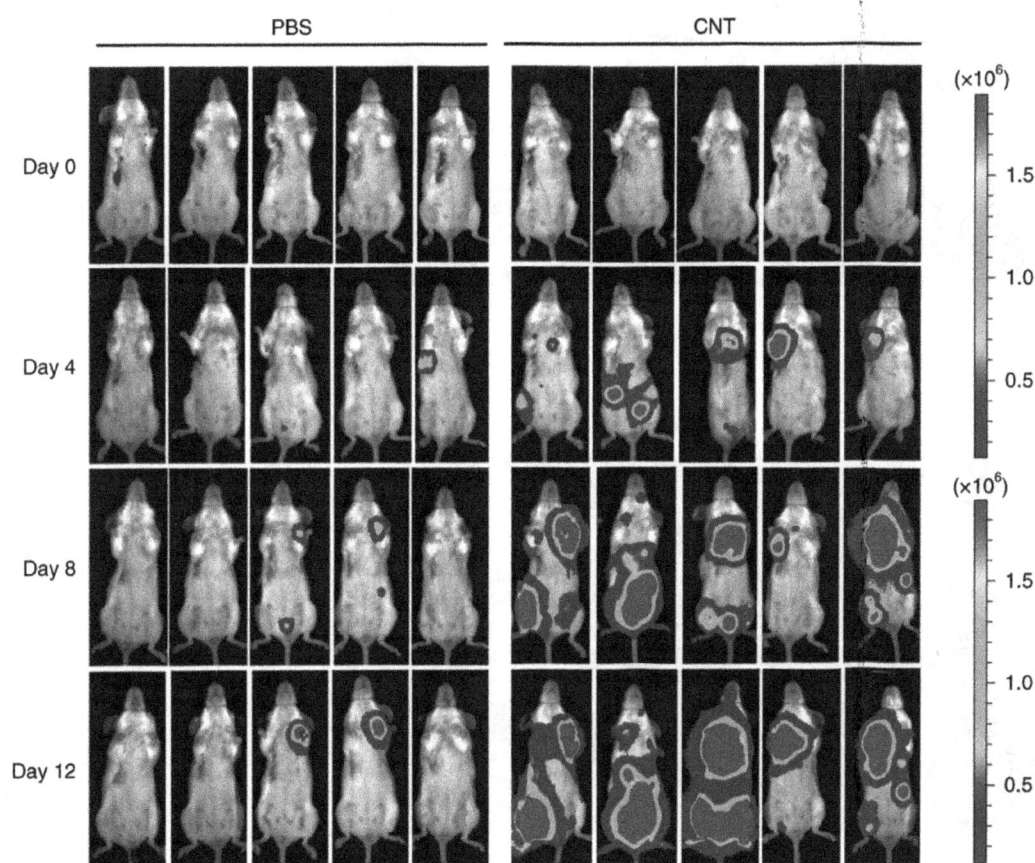

FIGURE 1.33 Metastatic lung lesion formation by bioluminescence imaging at days 0, 4, 8, and 12 after 4T1-Luc cell tumor removal ($n=5$ biologically independent mice for the PBS and CNT groups, respectively.) (Copyright 2019. Adapted from Ref. [480] with permission from Springer Nature.)

In addition, these NPs can be employed as carriers but with a therapeutic role for different drug molecules, paving the way for combinational therapies, such as PDT and PTT, and further enhancing their antitumor efficacy with laser and/or NIR irradiation. Furthermore, carrier-free

nanodrugs can be constructed with immunotherapeutic agents that inhibit the tumor recurrence and strengthen chemotherapy. For instance, as shown in Figure 1.34, the aforementioned PTX–IDM nano-assemblies [511] showed almost twofold higher tumor inhibition compared to the

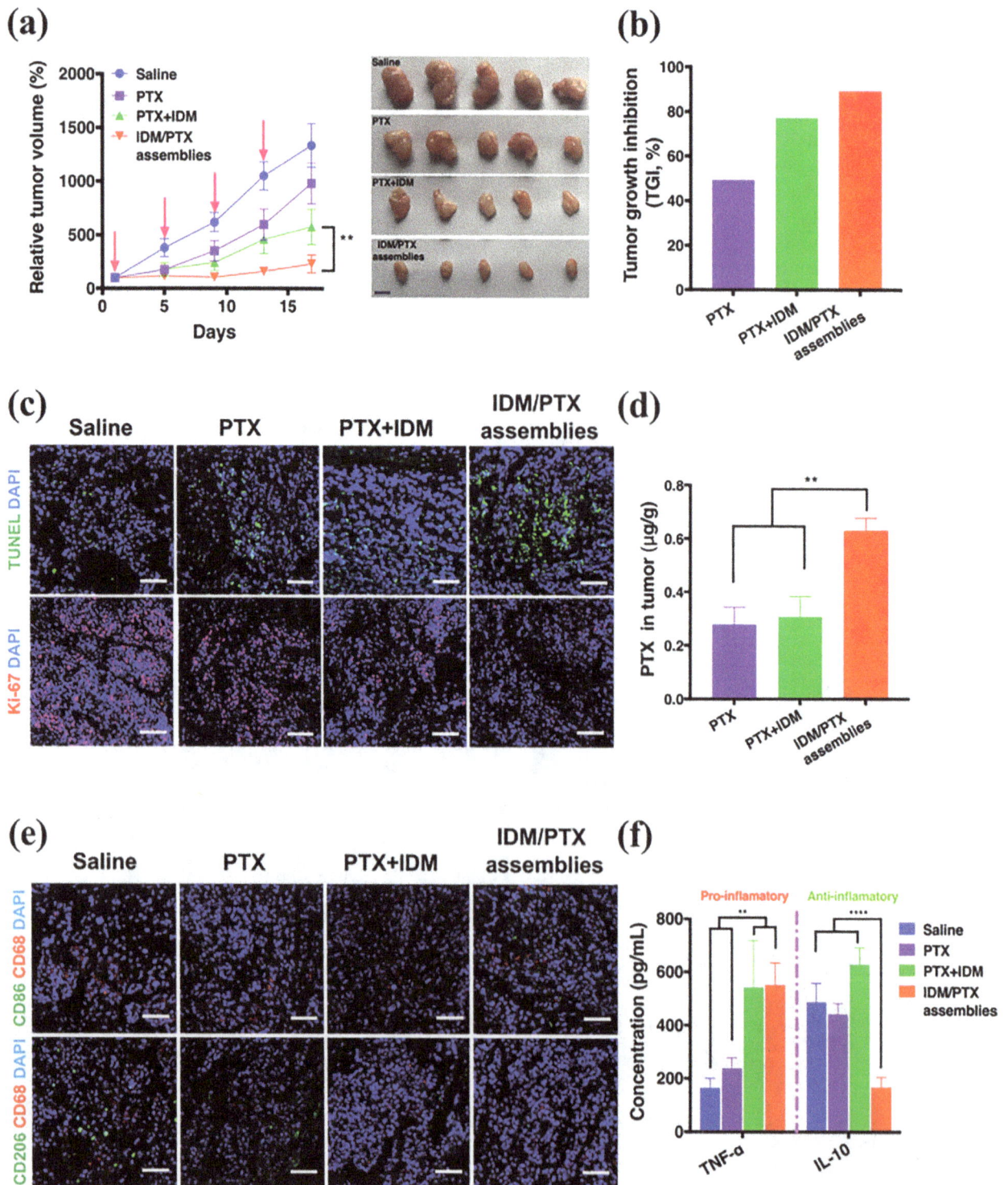

FIGURE 1.34 Antitumor effect of PTX–IDM nano-assemblies. (a) Tumor volumes. (b) Tumor growth inhibition. (c) Representative immunofluorescence images of Ki-67-positive cells (red) and cells undergoing apoptosis (TUNEL stain; green); scale bars represent 50 μm. (d) The amount of PTX in tumor. (e) Macrophage staining results. (f) Concentrations of pro- and anti-inflammatory cytokines. (Copyright 2019. Reproduced from Ref. [511] with permission from the American Chemical Society.)

free PTX- and the IDM–PTX mixture-treated group (a, b). The treatment with PTX–IDM nano-assemblies increased the apoptosis of the tumor cell (TUNEL) resulting in effective inhibition on proliferation (c). It is also demonstrated that the amount of PTX in the tumor site was much higher (d). This efficacy was then demonstrated with analysis of macrophage phenotype in tumor microenvironment (e) by analyzing CD68, CD206 (a biomarker of anti-inflammatory macrophage), and CD86 (a biomarker of pro-inflammatory macrophage). It was shown that the concentration of TNF-α, which has a cytotoxic effect on cancer cells, was higher in the groups treated with PTX–IDM mixture and PTX–IDM nano-assemblies. Attractively, the concentration of IL-10, which can promote angiogenesis and proliferation of cancer cells, was dramatically decreased only in the PTX–IDM nano-assembly-treated group, whereas all the control groups represent high concentrations (f).

1.14.5 Challenges

Despite all these advantages, there are four key points that should be considered for the design of nanodrug platforms. One of the major challenges in these nanoplatforms is long-term nanotoxicity. At present, carrier-free nanodrug research is at its initial stages and we have not witnessed any clinical translation of these nanodrugs due to the lack of safety and toxicity studies [583]. Second, the properties of carrier-free nanodrugs should be consistent every time they are prepared, i.e., the same or similar sizes and shapes, to eliminate batch-to-batch variations [572]. Recently, microfluidic studies were employed to increase the reproducibility of these NPs by precisely controlling the particle size and composition [584]. These microfluidic devices are also advantageous as some of them can mimic physiological conditions. Traditional preclinical studies heavily rely on a high number of animal models due to the lack of poor recapitulation in cell culture dishes [585]. Third, the EPR effect requires a better understanding since tumors grow quickly and blood vessels are leaky in mouse models, resulting in an efficient EPR effect. In reality, tumors in human body are different, usually biologically heterogeneous consisting of a variety of biological barriers such as irregular vascular networks in the same tumor which we have evaluated in another review, causing inefficient therapies [586]. There are only a few clinically approved carrier-based NP formulations, such as Abraxane® and Doxil®.

Finally, most carrier-free nanodrugs reported in the literature were focused on therapeutic outcomes rather than the self-assembly mechanism of hydrophobic anticancer drugs. A variety of small molecules have been extensively studied as a platform to self-assemble numerous anticancer agents. Although there are many successful attempts, the principle for selection of small molecular agents and drugs seems serendipitous [587]. It is important to rationally design nanoplatforms to achieve

efficient cancer therapy, as it becomes clear that all these engineered approaches work in a small percentage of patients. We would like to highlight the importance of the following: (i) π–π stacking interactions, which could occur with the use of anticancer drugs containing heavy aromatic structures; (ii) ionic interactions by using molecules with ionic groups; and (iii) hydrogen bonding between molecules that have oxygen and nitrogen atoms. These interactions should be considered to achieve stable nanoplatforms and also were a subject of another review [588]. Tumor-responsive linkers are dominated by ester; disulfide, and thioether bonds, but selenium and diselenide bonds have been recently emerging.

1.15 THE INVOLVEMENT OF DRUG CHEMICAL STRUCTURE IN NANOCARRIER DESIGN DEVELOPMENT

Although special attention has been paid to the lipid composition (variation in the lipid headgroup and acyl chain), surface charge, particle size of the nanocarrier systems in relation to their serum clearance kinetic, serum protein interaction, and cell interaction [589,590], little is known about the relationship between the structurally relevant physicochemical properties of the drug and the mentioned features of a lipid-based nanocarrier as the data of the control drug-free liposome could not be found in many experiments. For instance, it has that large unilamellar vesicles of about 100 nm in size have the lowest liposomal clearance within a set of liposomes with similar lipid composition than small unilamellar vesicles and larger multilamellar vesicles [591]. Cationic liposomes have the highest serum protein binding affinity (KB). LUVs containing phosphatidylserine (PS), phosphatidic acid (PA), and cardiolipin (CL) exhibited very fast clearance in circulation, while liposomes containing phosphatidylglycerol (PG) and phosphatidylinositol (PI) circulate for longer periods. Liposomes containing bovine PI with the major acyl-chain species being 18:0 have been demonstrated to rapidly remove from the circulation in minutes with KB of 158 g protein/mol lipid, whereas the ones with plant PI with unsaturated acyl chains (18:2) display a half-life of 90 min in the circulation with KB of 27 g protein/mol lipid. Surface coating of liposomes through PEGylation is the most well-known approach to achieve NPs capable of evading RES [591].

All of these findings have been achieved on the presumption that the nanocarrier membrane would be the limiting barrier in restricting the drug transition to serum proteins and cells [592]. However, how a drug molecule structure would influence nanocarrier–cell interaction is far less studied in the drug delivery field using lipid-based nanocarriers.

1.16 CONCLUSIONS AND FUTURE OUTLOOK

Nanotechnology has shown a lot of promise in cancer therapy over the years. Preparing stable nanodrugs at high drug concentrations is among the most important necessities for clinical applications alongside the need for them to be relatively easy to prepare and cost-effective. With the mentioned foundations in this chapter, this field is only expected to grow even more rapidly with exciting novel nanodrugs emerging with an overarching goal of developing a cancer therapy capable of overcoming MDR; achieving prolonged circulation times, enhanced antitumor efficacy, and deep tumor penetration; and possessing safe profiles to facilitate their clinical applications.

Nanotechnology allows targeted drug delivery in affected organs with minimal systemic toxicities due to their specificities. However, as with other therapeutic options, nanotechnology is not completely devoid of toxicities and comes with few challenges with its use including systemic and certain organ toxicities, hence causing setbacks with their clinical applications. Given the limitations with nanotechnology, more advancement must be done to improve drug delivery and maximize their efficacy while keeping the disadvantages to the minimum. By improving the interactions between the physicochemical properties of the nanomaterials employed, safer and more efficacious derivatives for diagnosis and treatment can be made available for cancer management. In sum, we sought to highlight the key advantages of nanotechnology and the shortfalls in their use to meet clinical needs for cancer. Adding to that, the therapeutic benefits of nanotechnology and future advancements could make them a therapeutic potential to be applied in other disease conditions. These may include ischemic stroke and rheumatoid arthritis, which would require targeted delivery of a suitable pharmacologic agent at the affected site. Incorporation of linkers into the anticancer agents enables the preparation of stimuli-responsive nanomedicines with applications in on-target drug release. Tumor-responsive linkers are dominated by ester, disulfide, and thioether bonds, but selenium and diselenide bonds have been recently emerging.

Studies to understand the precise mechanism behind the self-assembly of hydrophobic drugs will help to achieve more rational carrier-free nanodrug designs. It is predicted that a majority of these new formulations will target the tumor microenvironment using various linkers, peptide sequences, and/or other targeting molecules. Such systems have the potential of overcoming side effects on healthy cells and tissues and achieving deep tumor penetration, thereby increasing survival rates.

This chapter has summarized a variety of materials that either are being used or have the potential to be used as drug delivery vehicles for the treatment of cancer (Figure 1.35). Their unique attributes have allowed clinicians to offer them as new treatments (monotherapy) or as adjuncts to existing treatments (combined therapy) to improve therapeutic effectiveness. By their improved pharmacokinetic and pharmacodynamic properties, nanomaterials have contributed to improved cancer diagnosis and treatment.

Although some of the nanomaterials have not been successful upon their clinical translation, several new and

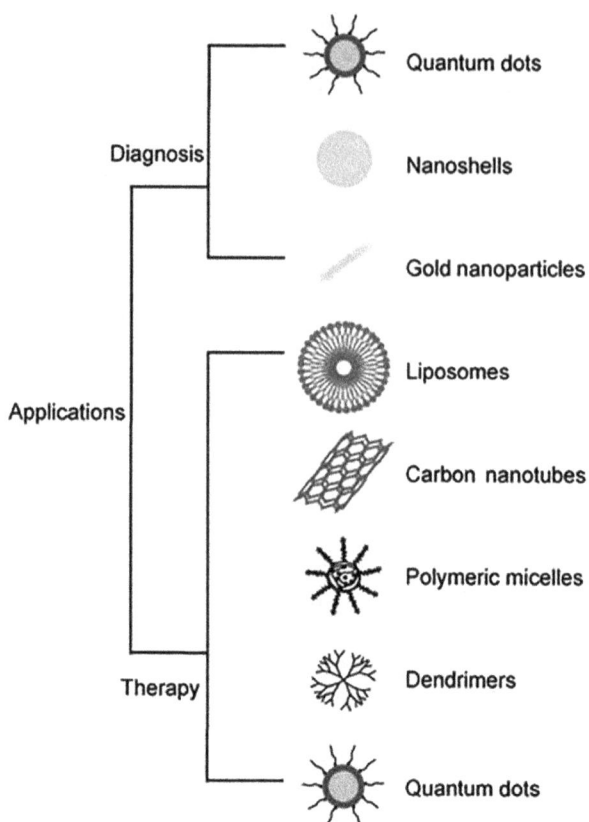

FIGURE 1.35 Application of nanomaterials in cancer diagnosis and therapy.

promising NPs that are currently under development show great promise, thereby providing hope for new treatment options in the near future. Further studies should focus on the clinical safety of both pharmaceutically active ingredients and materials used for surface modifications, enabling their clinical practice in a timely manner.

REFERENCES

1. R.S. Hamida, M.A. Ali, A. Redhwan, M.M. Bin-Meferij, Cyanobacteria: a promising platform in green nanotechnology: a review on nanoparticles fabrication and their prospective applications, *Int. J. Nanomed.* 15 (2020) 6033–6066.
2. S. Dubchak, A. Ogar, J. Mietelski, K. Turnau, Influence of silver and titanium nanoparticles on arbuscular mycorrhiza colonization and accumulation of radiocaesium in Helianthus annuus, *Spanish J. Agri. Res.* 8(1) (2010) 103–108. doi:10.5424/sjar/2010081-1228.
3. D. Mubarak Ali, J. Arunkumar, K.H. Nag, et al. Gold nanoparticles from Pro and eukaryotic photosynthetic microorganisms: comparative studies on synthesis and its application on biolabelling, *Colloids Surf. B Biointerfaces* 103 (2013) 166–173. doi: 10.1016/j.colsurfb.2012. 10.014.
4. X. He, H. Deng, H.-M. Hwang, The current application of nanotechnology in food and agriculture, *J. Food Drug Anal.* 27(1) (2018) 1–21. doi: 10.1016/j.jfda.2018.12.002.
5. Nanotechnology AOo. National Nanotechnology Strategy Annual Report 2008: 2007–2008.

6. M.C. Roco *The Long View of Nanotechnology Development: The National Nanotechnology Initiative at 10 Years*. Springer: Berlin, Germany (2011).

7. K.N. Thakkar, S.S. Mhatre, R.Y. Parikh, Biological synthesis of metallic nanoparticles, *Nanomedicine* 6(2) (2010) 257–262. doi: 10.1016/j.nano.2009.07.002.

8. G. Schmid, *Nanoparticles: From Theory to Application*. John Wiley & Sons: Hoboken, NJ (2011).

9. K. Govindaraju, S.K. Basha, V.G. Kumar, G. Singaravelu, Silver, gold and bimetallic nanoparticles production using single-cell protein (Spirulina platensis) Geitler, *J. Mater. Sci.* 43(15) (2008) 5115–5122. doi: 10.1007/s10853-008-2745-4.

10. N. Durán, M. Durán, M.B. De Jesus, A.B. Seabra, W.J. Fávaro, G. Nakazato, Silver nanoparticles: a new view on mechanistic aspects on antimicrobial activity, *Nanomedicine* 12(3) (2016) 789–799. doi: 10.1016/j.nano.2015.11.016.

11. A. Mohamed, A. Fouda, M. Elgamal, et al. Enhancing of cotton fabric antibacterial properties by silver nanoparticles synthesized by new Egyptian strain Fusarium keratoplasticum A1–3, *Egypt J. Chem.* 60 (2017) 63–71. doi: 10.21608/ejchem.2017.1626.1137.

12. A. Bianco, K. Kostarelos, M. Prato, Applications of carbon nanotubes in drug delivery, *Curr. Opin. Chem. Biol.* 9(6) (2005) 674–679. doi: 10.1016/j.cbpa.2005.10.005.

13. J. Pathak, H. Ahmed, D.K. Singh, A. Pandey, S.P. Singh, R.P. Sinha, Recent developments in green synthesis of metal nanoparticles utilizing cyanobacterial cell factories. In: Durgesh KT, editor. *Nanomaterials in Plants, Algae and Microorganisms*. Elsevier: Amsterdam (2019), 237–265.

14. J.H. Park, G. von Maltzahn, L. Zhang, et al. Magnetic iron oxide nanoworms for tumor targeting and imaging, *Adv. Mater.* 20(9) (2008) 1630–1635. doi: 10.1002/adma.200800004.

15. D. Parial, H.K. Patra, A.K. Dasgupta, R. Pal, Screening of different algae for green synthesis of gold nanoparticles, *Eur. J. Phycol.* 47(1) (2012) 22–29. doi: 10.1080/09670262.2011.653406.

16. S.E.-D. Hassan, A. Fouda, A.A. Radwan, et al. Endophytic actinomycetes Streptomyces spp mediated biosynthesis of copper oxide nanoparticles as a promising tool for biotechnological applications, *JBIC J. Biol. Inorg. Chem.* 24(3) (2019) 377–393. doi:10.1007/s00775-019-01654-5.

17. A. Fouda, E. Saad, S.S. Salem, T.I. Shaheen, *In-vitro* cytotoxicity, antibacterial, and UV protection properties of the biosynthesized Zinc oxide nanoparticles for medical textile applications, *Microb. Pathog.* 125 (2018) 252–261. doi: 10.1016/j.micpath.2018.09.030.

18. S.S. Salem, M.M. Fouda, A. Fouda, et al. Antibacterial, cytotoxicity and larvicidal activity of green synthesized selenium nanoparticles using Penicillium corylophilum, *J. Cluster Sci.* 32 (2021) 351–361. doi.org/10.1007/s10876-020-01794-8

19. A. Gour, N.K. Jain, Advances in green synthesis of nanoparticles, *Artif. Cells Nanomed. Biotechnol.* 47(1) (2019) 844–851. doi:10.1080/21691401.2019.1577878.

20. P. Khanna, A. Kaur, D. Goyal, Algae-based metallic nanoparticles: synthesis, characterization and applications, *J. Microbiol. Methods* 163 (2019) 105656. doi: 10.1016/j.mimet.2019.105656.

21. A. Sharma, S. Sharma, K. Sharma, et al. Algae as crucial organisms in advancing nanotechnology: a systematic review, *J. Appl. Phycol.* 28(3) (2016) 1759–1774. doi: 10.1007/s10811-015-0715-1.

22. N. Asmathunisha, K. Kathiresan, A review on biosynthesis of nanoparticles by marine organisms, *Colloids Surf. B Biointerfaces* 103 (2013) 283–287. doi: 10.1016/j.colsurfb.2012.10.030.

23. S.A. Dahoumane, C. Djediat, C. Yéprémian, et al. Species selection for the design of gold nanobioreactor by photosynthetic organisms, *J. Nanopart. Res.* 14(6) (2012) 883. doi:10.1007/ s11051-012-0883-8.

24. S.A. Dahoumane, E.K. Wujcik, C. Jeffryes, Noble metal, oxide and chalcogenide-based nanomaterials from scalable phototrophic culture systems, *Enzyme Microb. Technol.* 95 (2016) 13–27. doi:10.1016/j.enzmictec.2016.06.008.

25. M.F. Lengke, M.E. Fleet, G. Southam, Biosynthesis of silver nanoparticles by filamentous cyanobacteria from a silver (I) nitrate complex, *Langmuir* 23(5) (2007) 2694–2699.

26. M.F. Lengke, M.E. Fleet, G. Southam, Morphology of gold nanoparticles synthesized by filamentous cyanobacteria from Gold(I)–Thiosulfate and Gold(III)–Chloride complexes, *Langmuir* 22(6) (2006) 2780–2787. doi: 10.1021/la052652c.

27. R.A. Hamouda, M.H. Hussein, R.A. Abo-Elmagd, S.S. Bawazir, Synthesis and biological characterization of silver nanoparticles derived from the cyanobacterium Oscillatoria limnetica, *Sci. Rep.* 9(1) (2019) 13071. doi: 10.1038/s41598-019-49444-y.

28. D. Mubarak Al, V. Gopinath, N. Rameshbabu, N. Thajuddin, Synthesis and characterization of CdS nanoparticles using C-phycoerythrin from the marine cyanobacteria, *Mater. Lett.* 74 (2012) 8–11. doi: 10.1016/j.matlet.2012.01.026.

29. R. Rippka, J. Deruelles, J.B. Waterbury, M. Herdman, R.Y. Stanier, Generic assignments, strain histories and properties of pure cultures of cyanobacteria, *Microbiology* 111(1) (1979) 1–61. doi:10.1099/00221287-111-1-1.

30. R. Tyagi, B. Kaushik, J. Kumar, Antimicrobial activity of some cyanobacteria. In: R.N. Kharwar (ed.) *Microbial Diversity and Biotechnology in Food Security*. Springer: Berlin, Germany (2014), 463–470.

31. S. Mukund, V. Sivasubramanian, Anticancer activity of oscillatoria terebrieormis cyanobacteria in human lung cancer cell line a549, *Int. J. Appl. Biol. Pharm. Technol.* 5(2) (2014) 34–45.

32. R.S. Hamida, N.E. Abdelmeguid, M.A. Ali, M.M. Bin-Meferij, M.I. Khalil, Synthesis of silver nanoparticles using a novel cyanobacteria desertifilum sp. extract: their antibacterial and cytotoxicity effects, *Int. J. Nanomed.* 15 (2020) 49–63. doi: 10.2147/IJN.S238575.

33. M.M. Bin-Meferij, R.S. Hamida, Biofabrication and antitumor activity of silver nanoparticles utilizing novel nostoc sp. Bahar M, *Int. J. Nanomed.* 14 (2019) 9019–9029. doi: 10.2147/IJN.S230457.

34. S. Ahmad, S. Munir, N. Zeb, et al. Green nanotechnology: a review on green synthesis of silver nanoparticles—an ecofriendly approach, *Int. J. Nanomed.* 14 (2019) 5087. doi:10.2147/IJN.S200254.

35. S. Baker, D. Rakshith, K.S. Kavitha, et al. Marine microbes: invisible nanofactories, *Bioimpacts* 3(3) (2013) 111–117. doi: 10.5681/ bi.2013.012.

36. V. Smuleac, R. Varma, B. Baruwati, S. Sikdar, D. Bhattacharyya, Nanostructured membranes for enzyme catalysis and green synthesis of nanoparticles, *ChemSusChem* 4(12) (2011) 1773–1777. doi: 10.1002/cssc.201100211.

37. M.N. Nadagouda, R.S. Varma, Green and controlled synthesis of gold and platinum nanomaterials using vitamin B2: density-assisted self-assembly of nanospheres, wires and rods, *Green Chem.* 8(6) (2006) 516–518. doi: 10.1039/b601271j.

38. S.S. Salem, A. Fouda, Green synthesis of metallic nanoparticles and their prospective biotechnological applications: an overview, *Biol. Trace Elem. Res.* 199 (2020) 344–370. PMID: 32377944. doi: 10.1007/s12011-020-02138-3.

39. X.F. Zhang, Z.G. Liu, W. Shen, S. Gurunathan, Silver nanoparticles: synthesis, characterization, properties, applications, and therapeutic approaches, *Int. J. Mol. Sci.* 17(9) (2016) 1534.

40. K. Patel, B. Bharatiya, T. Mukherjee, T. Soni, A. Shukla, B. Suhagia, Role of stabilizing agents in the formation of stable silver nanoparticles in aqueous solution: characterization and stability study, *J. Dispers Sci. Technol.* 38(5) (2017) 626–631. doi: 10.1080/ 01932691.2016.1185374.

41. V. Amendola, M. Meneghetti, Laser ablation synthesis in solution and size manipulation of noble metal nanoparticles, *Phys. Chem. Chem. Phys.* 11(20) (2009) 3805–3821. doi: 10.1039/b900654k.

42. R. Arbain, M. Othman, S. Palaniandy, Preparation of iron oxide nanoparticles by mechanical milling, *Minerals Eng.* 24(1) (2011) 1–9. doi: 10.1016/j.mineng.2010.08.025.

43. H. Hatakeyama, H. Akita, H. Harashima, A multifunctional envelope type nano device (MEND) for gene delivery to tumours based on the EPR effect: a strategy for overcoming the PEG dilemma, *Adv. Drug Delivery Rev.* 63(3) (2011) 152–160. doi: 10.1016/j. addr.2010.09.001.

44. K. Quester, M. Avalos-Borja, E. Castro-Longoria, Biosynthesis and microscopic study of metallic nanoparticles, *Micron* 54 (2013) 1–27. doi: 10.1016/j.micron.2013.07.003.

45. C. Saravanan, R. Rajesh, T. Kaviarasan, K. Muthukumar, D. Kavitake, P.H. Shetty, Synthesis of silver nanoparticles using bacterial exopolysaccharide and its application for degradation of azo-dyes, *Biotechnol. Rep.* 15 (2017) 33–40. doi: 10.1016/j. btre.2017.02.006.

46. L. Chetia, D. Kalita, G.A. Ahmed, Synthesis of Ag nanoparticles using diatom cells for ammonia sensing, *Sens. Bio-Sens Res.* 16 (2017) 55–61. doi: 10.1016/j.sbsr.2017.11.004.

47. S. Rajeshkumar, C. Malarkodi, K. Paulkumar, M. Vanaja, G. Gnanajobitha, G. Annadurai, Algae mediated green fabrication of silver nanoparticles and examination of its antifungal activity against clinical pathogens, *Int. J. Metals* 2014 (2014) 8 pages. Article ID 692643. doi: 10.1155/2014/692643.

48. H.F. Aritonang, H. Koleangan, A.D. Wuntu, Synthesis of silver nanoparticles using aqueous extract of medicinal plants' (Impatiens balsamina and Lantana camara) fresh leaves and analysis of antimicrobial activity, *Int. J. Microbiol.* 2019 (2019) 8642303. doi: 10.1155/2019/8642303.

49. S. Menon, S. Rajeshkumar, V. Kumar, A review on biogenic synthesis of gold nanoparticles, characterization, and its applications, *Resour. Eff. Technol.* 3(4) (2017) 516–527. doi: 10.1016/j.reffit.2017.08.002.

50. M. Shah, D. Fawcett, S. Sharma, S.K. Tripathy, G.E.J. Poinern, Green synthesis of metallic nanoparticles via biological entities, *Materials (Basel)* 8(11) (2015) 7278–7308. doi: 10.3390/ ma8115377.

51. I. Khan, K. Saeed, K.I. Nanoparticles, Properties, applications and toxicities, *Arab. J. Chem.* 12(7) (2019) 908–931. doi: 10.1016/j. arabjc.2017.05.011.

52. S. Upadhyay, K. Parekh, B. Pandey, Influence of crystallite size on the magnetic properties of Fe_3O_4 nanoparticles, *J. Alloys Compd.* 678 (2016) 478–485. doi: 10.1016/j. jallcom.2016.03.279.

53. T.S. El-Din, A.A. Elzatahry, D.M. Aldhayan, A.M. Al-Enizi, S.S. Al- Deyab, Synthesis and characterization of magnetite zeolite nano composite, *Int. J. Electrochem. Sci.* 6 (2011) 6177–6183.

54. GE.J. Poinern, *A Laboratory Course in Nanoscience and Nanotechnology.* CRC Press: Boca Raton, FL (2014).

55. V. Nikolić, S. Ilić-Stojanović, S. Petrović, A. Tačić A, L. Nikolić, Administration routes for nano drugs and characterization of nano drug loading. In: S.M. Shyam (ed.) *Characterization and Biology of Nanomaterials for Drug Delivery.* Elsevier: Amsterdam (2019), 587–625.

56. C. Dejous, H. Hallil, V. Raimbault, R. Rukkumani, J.V. Yakhmi, Using microsensors to promote the development of innovative therapeutic nanostructures. In: *Nanostructures for Novel Therapy.* Elsevier: Amsterdam (2017), 539–566.

57. R. Russo, E. Esposito, C. Granata, et al. Magnetic nanoparticle characterization using nano-SQUID based on niobium Dayem bridges, *Phys. Procedia* 36 (2012) 293–299. doi: 10.1016/j. phpro.2012.06.162.

58. Y. Yin, X. Yang, L. Hu, et al. Superoxide-mediated extracellular biosynthesis of silver nanoparticles by the fungus Fusarium oxysporum, *Environ. Sci. Technol. Lett.* 3(4) (2016) 160–165. doi: 10.1021/acs.estlett.6b00066.

59. V. Patel, D. Berthold, P. Puranik, M. Gantar, Screening of cyanobacteria and microalgae for their ability to synthesize silver nanoparticles with antibacterial activity, *Biotechnol. Rep. (Amst)* 5 (2015) 112–119. doi: 10.1016/j. btre.2014.12.001.

60. S. Husain, M. Sardar, T. Fatma, Screening of cyanobacterial extracts for synthesis of silver nanoparticles. *World J. Microbiol. Biotechnol.* 31(8) (2015) 1279–1283. doi:10.1007/ s11274-015-1869-3.

61. P. Mukherjee, S. Senapati, D. Mandal, et al. Extracellular synthesis of gold nanoparticles by the fungus Fusarium oxysporum, *Chembiochem* 3(5) (2002) 461–463. doi: 10.1002/1439-7633(20020503)3:5<461::AID-CBIC461>3.0.CO;2-X.

62. T. Kalabegishvili, E. Kirkesali, A. Rcheulishvili, Synthesis of gold nanoparticles by blue-green algae spirulina platensis, *J. Appl. Microbiol. Biotechnol.* (2012). E 14-2012-31. https://inis.iaea.org/collection/ NCLCollectionStore/_Public/43/108/43108872.pdf?r=1

63. J. Jena, N. Pradhan, B.P. Dash, L.B. Sukla, P.K. Panda, Biosynthesis and characterization of silver nanoparticles using microalga Chlorococcum humicola and its antibacterial activity, *Int. J. Nanomater. Biostruct.* 3(1) (2013) 1–8.

64. D.D. Merin, S. Prakash, B.V. Bhimba, Antibacterial screening of silver nanoparticles synthesized by marine micro algae, *Asian Pac. J. Trop. Med.* 3(10) (2010) 797–799. doi:10.1016/S1995-7645(10)60191-5.

65. M. Focsan, I.I. Ardelean, C. Craciun, S. Astilean, Interplay between gold nanoparticle biosynthesis and metabolic activity of cyanobacterium Synechocystis sp. PCC 6803, *Nanotechnology* 22(48) (2011) 485101. doi:10.1088/0957-4484/22/48/485101.

66. C. Jeffryes, S.N. Agathos, G. Rorrer, Biogenic nanomaterials from photosynthetic microorganisms, *Curr. Opin. Biotechnol.* 33 (2015) 23–31. doi: 10.1016/j. copbio.2014.10.005.

67. M.F. Lengke, B. Ravel, M.E. Fleet, G. Wanger, R.A. Gordon, G. Southam, Mechanisms of gold bioaccumulation by filamentous cyanobacteria from gold(III)-chloride complex, *Environ. Sci. Technol.* 40(20) (2006) 6304–6309. doi: 10.1021/es061040r.

68. K. Kalishwaralal, V. Deepak, S. Ram Kumar Pandian, et al. Biosynthesis of silver and gold nanoparticles using Brevibacterium casei, *Colloids Surf. B Biointerfaces* 77(2) (2010) 257–262. doi: 10.1016/j. colsurfb.2010.02.007.

69. G. Oza, S. Pandey, A. Mewada, et al. Facile biosynthesis of gold nanoparticles exploiting optimum pH and temperature of fresh water algae Chlorella pyrenoidusa, *Adv. Appl. Sci. Res.* 3(3) (2012) 1405–1412.

70. N. Shabnam, P. Pardha-Saradhi, Photosynthetic electron transport system promotes synthesis of Au-nanoparticles, *PLoS One* 8(8) (2013) e71123. doi: 10.1371/journal.pone.0071123.

71. S.A. Dahoumane, C. Yéprémian, C. Djédiat, et al. A global approach of the mechanism involved in the biosynthesis of gold colloids using micro-algae, *J. Nanopart. Res.* 16(10) (2014) 2607. doi:10.1007/s11051-014-2607-8.

72. S.S. Sudha, K. Rajamanickam, J. Rengaramanujam, Microalgae mediated synthesis of silver nanoparticles and their antibacterial activity against pathogenic bacteria, *Indian J. Exp. Biol.* 51(5) (2013) 393–399.

73. N.E. El-Naggar, M.H. Hussein, A.A. El-Sawah, Biofabrication of silver nanoparticles by phycocyanin, characterization, in vitro anticancer activity against breast cancer cell line and in vivo cytotoxicity, *Sci. Rep.* 7(1) (2017) 10844. doi:10.1038/s41598-017-11121-3.

74. Y.N. Mata, E. Torres, M.L. Blazquez, A. Ballester, F. Gonzalez, J.A. Munoz, Gold(III) biosorption and bioreduction with the brown alga Fucus vesiculosus, *J. Hazard. Mater.* 166(2–3), 612–618 (2009). doi: 10.1016/j.jhazmat.2008.11.064.

75. S.R. Vijayan, P. Santhiyagu, M. Singamuthu, N. Kumari Ahila, R. Jayaraman, K. Ethiraj, Synthesis and characterization of silver and gold nanoparticles using aqueous extract of seaweed, Turbinaria conoides, and their antimicrofouling activity, *Sci. World J.* 2014 (2014) 938272. doi: 10.1155/2014/938272.

76. S. Keskin, N. Oya, N. Koçberber Kılıç, G. Dönmez, T. Tekinay, Green synthesis of silver nanoparticles using cyanobacteria and evaluation of their photocatalytic and antimicrobial activity, *J. Nano Res.* 40 (2016) 120–127. doi: 10.4028/www.scientific.net/JNanoR.40.120.

77. H. Singh, J. Du, P. Singh, T.H. Yi, Extracellular synthesis of silver nanoparticles by Pseudomonas sp. THG-LS1.4 and their antimicrobial application, *J. Pharm. Anal.* 8(4) (2018) 258–264. doi: 10.1016/j.jpha.2018.04.004.

78. S. Shivaji, S. Madhu, Shashi Singh, Extracellular synthesis of antibacterial silver nanoparticles using psychrophilic bacteria. *Process Biochem.* 46(9) (2011) 1800–1807. doi: 10.1016/j.procbio.2011.06.008.

79. S. Al Rashed, S. Al Shehri, N.M. Moubayed, Extracellular biosynthesis of silver nanoparticles from cyanobacteria, *Biomed. Res.* 29(13) (2018) 2859–2862. ISSN 0970-938X www.biomedres.info. doi: 10.4066/biomedicalresearch.29-17-3209.

80. H. Sowani, P. Mohite, S. Damale, M. Kulkarni, S. Zinjarde, Carotenoid stabilized gold and silver nanoparticles derived from the Actinomycete Gordonia amicalis HS-11 as effective free radical scavengers, *Enzyme Microb. Technol.* 95 (2016) 164–173. doi:10.1016/j.enzmictec.2016.09.016.

81. O. Bekasova, A. Brekhovskikh, A. Revina, V. Dubinchuk, Preparation and optical properties of silver nanoparticles in R-phycoerythrin, a protein matrix, *Inorg. Mater.* 44(8) (2008) 835. doi:10.1134/S0020168508080098.

82. A.N. Glazer, Phycobiliproteins: a family of valuable, widely used fluorophores, *J. Appl. Phycol.* 6(2) (1994) 105–112. doi: 10.1007/ BF02186064.

83. R. MacColl, Cyanobacterial phycobilisomes, *J. Struct. Biol.* 124(2–3) (1998) 311–334. doi:10.1006/jsbi.1998.4062.

84. E. Gelagutashvili, Binding of heavy metals with C-phycocyanin: a comparison between equilibrium dialysis, fluorescence and absorption titration, *Am. J. Biomed. Life Sci.* 1 (2013) 12–16. doi: 10.11648/j.ajbls.20130101.13.

85. S.S. Chen, D.S. Berns, Effect of plastocyanin and phycocyanin on the photosensitivity of chlorophyll-containing bilayer membranes, *J. Membr. Biol.* 47(2) (1979) 113–127. doi:10.1007/BF01876112.

86. N. Wei, Y. Hou, Z. Lu, H. Yu, Wang Q Synthesis of silver nanoparticles stabilized with C-phycocyanin and for fluorimetric detection of copper ions. *Paper Presented at: IOP Conference Series: Earth and Environmental Science*, Banda Aceh, Indonesia (2018).

87. N.E. El-Naggar, M.H. Hussein, A.A. El-Sawah, Phycobiliprotein- mediated synthesis of biogenic silver nanoparticles, characterization, in vitro and in vivo assessment of anticancer activities, *Sci. Rep.* 8(1) (2018) 8925. doi: 10.1038/s41598-018-27276-6.

88. A. Bharde, D. Rautaray, V. Bansal, et al. Extracellular biosynthesis of magnetite using fungi, *Small* 2(1) (2006) 135–141. doi: 10.1002/ smll.200500180.

89. A.S. Reddy, C.Y. Chen, C.C Chen, et al. Biological synthesis of gold and silver nanoparticles mediated by the bacteria Bacillus subtilis, *J. Nanosci. Nanotechnol.* 10(10) (2010) 6567–6574. doi: 10.1166/ jnn.2010.2519.

90. K. Khalifa, R. Hamouda, D. Hanafy, A. Hamza, In vitro antitumor activity of silver nanoparticles biosynthesized by marine algae, *Digest. J. Nanomater. Biostruct.* 11(1) (2016) 213–221.

91. D.M. Ali, M. Sasikala, M. Gunasekaran, N. Thajuddin, Biosynthesis and characterization of silver nanoparticles using marine cyanobacterium, Oscillatoria willei NTDM01, *Digest. J. Nanomater. Biostruct.* 6(2) (2011) 385–390.

92. A. Rahman, A. Ismail, D. Jumbianti, S. Magdalena, H. Sudrajat, Synthesis of copper oxide nano particles by using Phormidium cyanobacterium, *Indonesian J. Chem.* 9(3) (2009) 355–360. doi: 10.22146/ijc.21498.

93. L.M. Rosken, F. Cappel, S. Korsten, et al. Time-dependent growth of crystalline Au(0)-nanoparticles in cyanobacteria as self-reproducing bioreactors: 2. Anabaena cylindrica, *Beilstein J. Nanotechnol.* 7 (2016) 312–327. doi: 10.3762/bjnano.7.30.

94. J. Ali, N. Ali, L. Wang, H. Waseem, G. Pan. Revisiting the mechanistic pathways for bacterial mediated synthesis of noble metal nanoparticles, *J. Microbiol. Methods* 159 (2019) 18–25. doi: 10.1016/j.mimet.2019.02.010.

95. R. Brayner, H. Barberousse, M. Hemadi, et al. Cyanobacteria as bioreactors for the synthesis of Au, Ag, Pd, and Pt nanoparticles via an enzyme-mediated route, *J. Nanosci. Nanotechnol.* 7(8) (2007) 2696–2708. doi: 10.1166/jnn.2007.600.

96. F.M. Morsy, N.A. Nafady, M.H. Abd-Alla, D.A. Elhady, Green synthesis of silver nanoparticles by water soluble fraction of the extracellular polysaccharides/matrix of the cyanobacterium Nostoc commune and its application as a potent fungal surface sterilizing agent of seed crops, *Univ. J. Microbiol. Res.* 2(2) (2014) 36–43.

97. M. Mankad, G. Patil, D. Patel, P. Patel, A. Patel, Comparative studies of sunlight mediated green synthesis of silver nanoparaticles from Azadirachta indica leaf extract and its antibacterial effect on Xanthomonas oryzae pv. Oryzae, *Arab. J. Chem.* 13(1) (2018). 2865–2872, doi:10.1016/j.arabjc.2018.07.016.

98. M.F. Lengke, M.E. Fleet, G. Southam, Synthesis of platinum nanoparticles by reaction of filamentous cyanobacteria with platinum(IV)-chloride complex, *Langmuir* 22(17) (2006) 7318–7323. doi: 10.1021/la060873s.

99. S. Zada, A. Ahmad, S. Khan, et al. Biogenic synthesis of silver nanoparticles using extracts of Leptolyngbya JSC-1 that induce apoptosis in HeLa cell line and exterminate pathogenic bacteria, *Artif. Cells Nanomed. Biotechnol.* 46(sup3) (2018) S471–S480. doi: 10.1080/21691401.2018.1499663.

100. G. Singh, P.K. Babele, A. Kumar, A. Srivastava, R.P. Sinha, M.B. Tyagi, Synthesis of ZnO nanoparticles using the cell extract of the cyanobacterium, Anabaena strain L31 and its conjugation with UV-B absorbing compound shinorine, *J. Photochem. Photobiol. B.* 138 (2014) 55–62. doi: 10.1016/j.jphotobiol.2014.04.030.

101. A.S. Sonker, J. Pathak, V.K. Kannaujiya, R.P. Sinha, Characterization and in vitro antitumor, antibacterial and antifungal activities of green synthesized silver nanoparticles using cell extract of Nostoc sp. strain HKAR-2, *Can. J. Biotechnol.* 1(1) (2017) 26. doi:10.24870/cjb.2017-000103.

102. B. Vashishta, *Botany for Degree Student.* S. Chand: New Delhi (1978).

103. M. Ebadi, M.R. Zolfaghari, S.S. Aghaei, et al. A bio-inspired strategy for the synthesis of zinc oxide nanoparticles (ZnO NPs) using the cell extract of cyanobacterium Nostoc sp. EA03: from biological function to toxicity evaluation, *RSC Adv.* 9(41) (2019) 23508–23525. doi: 10.1039/C9RA03962G.

104. T. Saran, G. Sharma, M. Kumar, M. Ali, Biosynthesis of copper oxide nanoparticles using cyanobacteria spirulina platensis and its antibacterial activity, *Int. J. Pharm. Sci. Res.* 8 (2017) 3887.

105. K. Vijayaraghavan, S.K. Nalini, Biotemplates in the green synthesis of silver nanoparticles, *Biotechnol J.* 5(10) (2010) 1098–1110. doi:10.1002/biot.201000167.

106. P. Manivasagan, S.Y. Nam, J. Oh, Marine microorganisms as potential biofactories for synthesis of metallic nanoparticles, *Crit. Rev. Microbiol.* 42(6) (2016) 1007–1019. doi: 10.3109/1040841X.2015.1137860.

107. D. Kim, S. Jeong, J. Moon, Synthesis of silver nanoparticles using the polyol process and the influence of precursor injection, *Nanotechnology* 17(16) (2006) 4019. doi: 10.1088/0957-4484/17/16/004.

108. G. Kratošová, Z. Konvičková, I. Vávra, E. Zapomělová, A. Schröfel, Noble metal nanoparticles synthesis mediated by the genus Dolichospermum: perspective of green approach in the nanoparticles preparation, *Adv. Sci. Lett.* 22(3) (2016) 637–641. doi: 10.1166/ asl.2016.6993.

109. R. Jin, Y.C. Cao, E. Hao, G.S. Métraux, G.C. Schatz, C.A. Mirkin, Controlling anisotropic nanoparticle growth through plasmon excitation, *Nature* 425(6957) (2003) 487–490. doi: 10.1038/ nature02020.

110. M.F. Lengke, M.E. Fleet, G. Southam, Biosynthesis of silver nanoparticles by filamentous cyanobacteria from a silver(I) nitrate complex, *Langmuir* 23(5) (2007) 2694–2699.

111. J.B Vines, J.H. Yoon, N.E. Ryu, D.J. Lim, H. Park, Gold nanoparticles for photothermal cancer therapy, *Front Chem.* 7 (2019) 167. doi: 10.3389/fchem.2019.00167.

112. M. Lenartowicz, P.H. Marek, I.D. Madura, J. Lipok, Formation of variously shaped gold nanoparticles by Anabaena laxa, *J. Cluster. Sci.* 28(5) (2017) 3035–3055. doi: 10.1007/s10876-017-1275-0.

113. L.M. Rösken, S. Körsten, C.B. Fischer, et al. Time-dependent growth of crystalline Au 0-nanoparticles in cyanobacteria as self-reproducing bioreactors: 1. Anabaena sp, *J. Nanopart. Res.* 16(4) (2014) 2370. doi:10.1007/s11051-014-2370-x.

114. S. Geetha, Z. Sathakkathul, R. Aarthi, B. Heizline, Green synthesis of gold nanoparticle using marine cyanobacteria Gloeocapsa sp and the antitumor potential, *J. Chem. Pharm. Sci.* 4 (2014) 172–174.

115. N. Fu, Y. Hu, S. Shi, S. Ren, W. Liu, S. Su, et al. Au nanoparticles on two-dimensional MoS(2) nanosheets as a photoanode for efficient photoelectrochemical miRNA detection, *Analyst* 143 (2018) 1705–1712.

116. C. Jin, K. Wang, A. Oppong-Gyebi, J. Hu, Application of nanotechnology in cancer diagnosis and therapy: a mini-review, *Int. J. Med. Sci.* 17(18) (2020) 2964–2973. doi: 10.7150/ijms.49801.

117. F. Fu, L. Li, Q. Luo, Q. Li, T. Guo, M. Yu, et al. Selective and sensitive detection of lysozyme based on plasmon resonance light-scattering of hydrolyzed peptidoglycan stabilized-gold nanoparticles, *Analyst* 143 (2018) 1133–1140.

118. K. Shrivas, N. Nirmalkar, S.S. Thakur, M.K. Deb, S.S. Shinde, R. Shankar, Sucrose capped gold nanoparticles as a plasmonic chemical sensor based on non-covalent interactions: application for selective detection of vitamins B(1) and B(6) in brown and white rice food samples, *Food Chem.* 250 (2018) 14–21.

119. M.F. Lengke, M.E. Fleet, G. Southam, Synthesis of palladium nanoparticles by reaction of filamentous cyanobacterial biomass with a palladium(II) chloride complex, *Langmuir* 23(17) (2007) 8982–8987. doi: 10.1021/la7012446.

120. A. Ahmad, P. Mukherjee, D. Mandal, et al. Enzyme mediated extracellular synthesis of CdS nanoparticles by the fungus, Fusarium oxysporum, *J. Am. Chem. Soc.* 124(41) (2002) 12108–12109. doi: 10.1021/ja027296o.

121. C. Dameron, R. Reese, R. Mehra, et al. Biosynthesis of cadmium sulphide quantum semiconductor crystallites, *Nature* 338(6216) (1989) 596–597. doi: 10.1038/338596a0.

122. K. Prasad, A.K. Jha. Biosynthesis of CdS nanoparticles: an improved green and rapid procedure, *J. Colloid Interface Sci.* 342(1) (2010) 68–72. doi: 10.1016/j.jcis.2009.10.003.

123. R. Brayner, C. Yéprémian, C. Djediat, et al. Photosynthetic microorganism-mediated synthesis of akaganeite (β-FeOOH) nanorods, *Langmuir* 25(17) (2009) 10062–10067. doi: 10.1021/la9010345.

124. S.A. Dahoumane, C. Djediat, C. Yéprémian, A. Couté, F. Fiévet, R. Brayner, Design of magnetic akaganeite-cyanobacteria hybrid biofilms, *Thin Solid Films* 518(19) (2010) 5432–5436. doi: 10.1016/j.tsf.2010.04.001.

125. P. Roychoudhury, S. Ghosh, R. Pal, Cyanobacteria mediated green synthesis of gold-silver nanoalloy, *J. Plant Biochem. Biotechnol.* 25(1) (2016) 73–78. doi:10.1007/s13562-015-0311-0.

126. S.R. Grobmyer, B.M. Moudgil, *Book Cancer Nanotechnology Methods and Protocols.* Springer: New York, Dordrecht Heidelberg, London (2010) (www.springer.com).

127. F. Alexis, J.W. Rhee, J.P. Richie, A.F. Radovic-Moreno, R. Langer, O.C Farokhzad, New frontiers in nanotechnology for cancer treatment, *Urol. Oncol.* 26(1) (2008) 74–85.

128. K. Cho, X. Wang, S. Nie, Z.G. Chen, D.M. Shin, Therapeutic nanoparticles for drug delivery in cancer, *Clin. Cancer Res.* 14(5) (2008) 1310–1316.

129. J.R. Heath, M.E. Davis, Nanotechnology and cancer, *Annu. Rev. Med.* 59 (2008) 251–265.

130. D. Peer, J.M. Karp, S. Hong, O.C. Farokhzad, R. Margalit, R. Langer, Nanocarriers as an emerging platform for cancer therapy, *Nat. Nanotechnol.* 2(12) (2007) 751–760.

131. M.A. Maurer-Jones, K.C. Bantz, S.A. Love, B.J. Marquis, C.L. Haynes, Toxicity of therapeutic nanoparticles, *Nanomediciean* 4(2) (2009) 219–241.

132. K.W. Powers, S.C. Brown, V.B. Krishna, S.C. Wasdo, B.M. Moudgil, S.M. Roberts, Research strategies for safety evaluation of nanomaterials. Part VI. Characterization of nanoscale particles for toxicological evaluation, *Toxicol. Sci.* 90(2) (2006) 296–303.

133. M.A. Dobrovolskaia, S.E. McNeil, Immunological properties of engineered nanomaterials, *Nat. Nanotechnol.* 2(8) (2007) 469–478.

134. B.J. Marquis, S.A. Love, K.L. Braun, C.L. Haynes, Analytical methods to assess nanoparticle toxicity, *Analyst* 134(3) (2009) 425–439.

135. T. Lammers, W.E Hennink, G. Storm, Tumour-targeted nanomedicines: principles and practice, *Br. J. Cancer* 99(3) (2008) 392–397.

136. H. Maeda, Y. Matsumura, Tumoritropic and lymphotropic principles of macromolecular drugs, *Crit. Rev. Ther. Drug Carr. Syst.* 6(3) (1989) 193–210.

137. F. Yuan, M. Dellian, D. Fukumura, M. Leunig, D.A. Berk, V.P. Torchilin, R.K. Jain, Vascular permeability in a human tumor xenograft: molecular size dependence and cutoff size, *Cancer Res.* 55(17) (1995) 3752–3756.

138. G. Kong, R.D. Braun, M.W. Dewhirst, Hyperthermia enables tumor-specific nanoparticle delivery: effect of particle size, *Cancer Res.* 60(16) (2000) 4440–4445.

139. W.H. De Jong, P.J. Borm, Drug delivery and nanoparticles: applications and hazards, *Int. J. Nanomed.* 3(2) (2008) 133–149.

140. T.M. Allen, Ligand-targeted therapeutics in anticancer therapy, *Nat. Rev. Cancer* 2(10) (2002) 750–763.

141. K.C. Black, N.D. Kirkpatrick, T.S. Troutman, L. Xu, J. Vagner, R.J. Gillies, J.K. Barton, U. Utzinger, M. Romanowski, Gold nanorods targeted to delta opioid receptor: plasmon-resonant contrast and photothermal agents, *Mol. Imaging* 7(1) (2008) 50–57.

142. K. Cho, X. Wang, S. Nie, Z. Chen, D.M. Shin, Therapeutic nanoparticles for drug delivery in cancer, *Clin. Cancer Res.* 14(5) (2008) 1310–1315.

143. S. Santra, B. Liesenfeld, D. Dutta, D. Chatel, C.D. Batich, W. Tan, B.M. Moudgil, R.A. Mericle, Folate conjugated fluorescent silica nanoparticles for labeling neoplastic cells, *J. Nanosci. Nanotechnol.* 5(6) (2005) 899–904.

144. S.K. Sahoo, W. Ma, V. Labhasetwar, Efficacy of transferrin-conjugated paclitaxel-loaded nanoparticles in a murine model of prostate cancer, *Int. J. Cancer* 112(2) (2004) 335–340.

145. B.R. Smith, Z. Cheng, A. De, A.L. Koh, R. Sinclair, S.S. Gambhir, Real-time intravital imaging of RGD-quantum dot binding to luminal endothelium in mouse tumor neovasculature, *Nano Lett.* 8(9) (2008) 2599–2606.

146. D.B. Kirpotin, D.C. Drummond, Y. Shao, M.R. Shalaby, K. Hong, U.B. Nielsen, J.D. Marks, C.C. Benz, J.W. Park, Antibody targeting of longcirculating lipidic nanoparticles does not increase tumor localization but does increase internalization in animal models, *Cancer Res.* 66(13) (2006) 6732–6740.

147. J.W. Park, C.C. Benz, F.J. Martin, Future directions of liposome- and immunoliposome-based cancer therapeutics, *Semin. Oncol.* 31(6 Suppl 13) (2004) 196–205.

148. F. Alexis, J.W. Rhee, J.P. Richie, A.F. Radovic-Moreno, R. Langer, O.C. Farokhzad. New frontiers in nanotechnology for cancer treatment, *Urol. Oncol. Semin. Original Invest.* 26 (2008) 74–85.

149. J. Kost, R. Langer, Responsive polymeric delivery systems, *Adv. Drug Delivery Rev.* 46 (2001) 125–148.

150. D.B. Shenoy, M.M. Amiji, Poly(ethylene oxide)-modified poly(ε-caprolactone) nanoparticles for targeted delivery of tamoxifen in breast cancer, *Int. J. Pharmacol.* 293 (2005) 261–270.

151. H. Shmeeda, L. Mak, D. Tzemach, et al. Intracellular uptake and intracavitary targeting of folate-conjugated liposomes in a mouse lymphoma model with up-regulated folate receptors, *Mol. Cancer Ther.* 5 (2006) 818–824.

152. X. Yin, A.S. Hoffman, P.S. Stayton, Poly(N-isopropylacrylamide-copropylacrylic acid) copolymers that respond sharply to temperature and pH, *Biomacromolecules* 7 (2006) 1381–1385.

153. D.Y. Furgeson, M.R. Dreher, A. Chilkoti, Structural optimization of a "smart" doxorubicin polypeptide conjugate for thermally targeted delivery to solid tumors, *J. Controlled Release* 110 (2006) 362–369.

154. L.R. Brown, E.R. Edelman, F. Fischel-Ghodsian, et al. Characterization of glucose-mediated insulin release from implantable polymers. *J. Pharmacol. Sci.* 85 (1996) 1341–1345.

155. J.S. Ross, D.P. Schenkein, R. Pietrusko, et al. Targeted therapies for cancer 2004, *Am. J. Clin. Pathol.* 122 (2004) 598–609.

156. K. Cho, X. Wang, S. Nie, et al. Therapeutic nanoparticles for drug delivery in cancer, *Clin. Cancer Res.* 14 (2008) 1310–1316.

157. H. Maeda, The enhanced permeability and retention (EPR) effect in tumor vasculature: the key role of tumor-selective macromolecular drug targeting, *Adv. Enzyme Regul.* 41 (2001) 189–207.

158. T.M. Allen, Ligand-targeted therapeutics in anticancer therapy, *Nat. Rev. Cancer* 2 (2002) 750–763.

159. A. Dadwal, A. Baldi, R.K. Narang, Nanoparticles as carriers for drug delivery in cancer, *Artif. Cells Nanomed. Biotechnol.* 46(S2) (2018) S295–S305. doi: 10.1080/21691401.2018.1457039.

160. A.C. Society, *Breast Cancer Facts & Figures.* American Cancer Society: Atlanta, GA (2007).

161. R. Duncan, Polymer conjugates as anticancer nanomedicines, *Nat. Rev. Cancer* 6 (2006) 688–701.

162. M. Ferrari, Cancer nanotechnology: opportunities and challenges, *Nat. Rev. Cancer* 5 (2005) 161–171.

163. E. Hood, Nanotechnology: looking as we leap, *Environ. Health Perspect.* 112(13) (2004) A740–A749.

164. L.S. Jabr-Milane, L.E. van Vlerken, S. Yadav, M.M. Amiji, Multifunctional nanocarriers to overcome tumor drug resistance, *Cancer Treat. Rev.* 34(7) (2008) 592–602.

165. P. Sharma, S. Brown, G. Walter, S. Santra, B. Moudgil, Nanoparticles for bioimaging, *Adv. Colloid Interface Sci.* 123–126 (2006) 471–485.

166. Y.W. Jun, J.T. Jang, J. Cheon, Magnetic nanoparticle assisted molecular MR imaging, *Adv. Exp. Med. Biol.* 620 (2007) 85–106.

167. O. Will, S. Purkayastha, C. Chan, T. Athanasiou, A.W. Darzi, W. Gedroyc, P.P. Tekkis, Diagnostic precision of nanoparticle-enhanced MRI for lymph-node metastases: a meta-analysis, *Lancet Oncol.* 7(1) (2006) 52–60.

168. A. Pope-Harman, M.M. Cheng, F. Robertson, J. Sakamoto, M. Ferrari, Biomedical nanotechnology for cancer, *Med. Clin. North Am.* 91(5) (2007) 899–927.

169. C. Sun, J.S. Lee, M. Zhang, Magnetic nanoparticles in MR imaging and drug delivery, *Adv. Drug Delivery Rev.* 60(11) (2008) 1252–1265.

170. A. Jurj, C. Braicu, L.A. Pop, C. Tomuleasa, C.D. Gherman, I. Berindan-Neagoe, The new era of nanotechnology, an alternative to change cancer treatment, *Drug Design Dev. Ther.* 11 (2017) 2871–2890.

171. Rosenzweig SA. Acquired resistance to drugs targeting receptor tyrosine kinases, *Biochem. Pharmacol.* 83(8) (2012) 1041–1048.

172. M. Gultekin, P. Dursun, B. Vranes, et al. Gynecologic oncology training systems in Europe: a report from the European network of young gynaecological oncologists, *Int. J. Gynecol. Cancer.* 21(8) (2011) 1500–1506.

173. C. Braicu, R. Chiorean, A. Irimie, et al. Novel insight into triple-negative breast cancers, the emerging role of angiogenesis, and antiangiogenic therapy, *Expert. Rev. Mol. Med.* 18 (2016) e18.

174. C. Vlad, P. Kubelac, D. Vlad, A. Irimie, P. Achimas Cadariu, Evaluation of clinical, morphopathological and therapeutic prognostic factors in rectal cancer: experience of a tertiary oncology center, *J. BUON* 20(1) (2015) 92–99.

175. M. Herbrink, B. Nuijen, J.H. Schellens, J.H. Beijnen, Variability in bioavailability of small molecular tyrosine kinase inhibitors, *Cancer Treat Rev.* 41(5) (2015) 412–422.

176. H. Banu, D.K. Sethi, A. Edgar, et al. Doxorubicin loaded polymeric gold nanoparticles targeted to human folate receptor upon laser photo thermal therapy potentiates chemotherapy in breast cancer cell lines, *J. Photochem. Photobiol. B* 149 (2015) 116–128.

177. Y. Fujita, K. Kuwano, T. Ochiya, Development of small RNA delivery systems for lung cancer therapy, *Int. J. Mol. Sci.* 16(3) (2015) 5254–5270.

178. C. Kleinstreuer, E. Childress, A. Kennedy, Chapter 10 – Targeted drug delivery: Multifunctional nanoparticles and direct micro-drug delivery to tumors. In: S.M. Becker, A.V. Kuznetsov (eds.) *Transport in Biological Media*. Elsevier: Boston, MA (2013), 391–416.

179. A.Z. Wilczewska, K. Niemirowicz, K.H. Markiewicz, H. Car, Nanoparticles as drug delivery systems, *Pharmacol. Rep.* 64(5) (2012) 1020–1037.

180. M. Shahin, R. Soudy, H. El-Sikhry, J.M. Seubert, K. Kaur, A. Lavasanifar, Engineered peptides for the development of actively tumor targeted liposomal carriers of doxorubicin, *Cancer Lett.* 334(2) (2013) 284–292.

181. B.S. Lee, A.T. Yip, A.V. Thach, A.R. Rodriguez, T.J. Deming, D.T. Kamei, The targeted delivery of doxorubicin with transferrin-conjugated block copolypeptide vesicles, *Int. J. Pharm.* 496(2) (2015) 903–911.

182. S. Senapati, A.K. Mahanta, S. Kumar, P. Maiti, Controlled drug delivery vehicles for cancer treatment and their performance, *Signal Transduction Targeted Ther.* 3(7) (2018) 1–19. doi: 10.1038/s41392-017-0004-3.

183. S. Lokina, A. Stephen, V. Kaviyarasan, C. Arulvasu, V. Narayanan, Cytotoxicity and antimicrobial activities of green synthesized silver nanoparticles, *Eur. J. Med. Chem.* 76 (2014) 256–263.

184. O.S. Wolfbeis, An overview of nanoparticles commonly used in fluorescent bioimaging, *Chem. Soc. Rev.* 44 (2015) 4743–4768.

185. S. Rajendran, et al. Ce^{3+}-ion-induced visible-light photocatalytic degradation and electrochemical activity of ZnO/CeO$_2$ nanocomposite, *Sci. Rep.* 6 (2016) 31641.

186. R. Singh, J.W. Lillard, Nanoparticle-based targeted drug delivery, *Exp. Mol. Pathol.* 86 (2009) 215–223.

187. M. Rasoulzadeh, H. Namazi, Carboxymethyl cellulose/graphene oxide bionanocomposite hydrogel beads as anticancer drug carrier agent, *Carbohydr. Polym.* 168 (2017) 320–326.

188. K.M. Rao, S. Nagappan, D.J. Seo, C.S. Ha, pH sensitive halloysite-sodium hyaluronate/poly(hydroxyethyl methacrylate) nanocomposites for colon cancer drug delivery, *Appl. Clay Sci.* 97–98 (2014) 33–42.

189. F.F. Azhar, A. Olad, A study on sustained release formulations for oral delivery of 5-fluorouracil based on alginate–chitosan/montmorillonite nanocomposite systems, *Appl. Clay Sci.* 101 (2014) 288–296.

190. R. Nanda, A. Sasmal, P.L. Nayak, Preparation and characterization of chitosan polylactide composites blended with cloisite 30B for control release of the anticancer drug paclitaxel, *Carbohydr. Polym.* 83 (2011) 988–994.

191. N.K. Singh, et al. Nanostructure controlled anti-cancer drug delivery using poly (ε-caprolactone) based nanohybrids, *J. Mater. Chem.* 22 (2012) 17853–17863.

192. A. Mishra, et al. Self-assembled aliphatic chain extended polyurethane nanobiohybrids: emerging hemocompatible biomaterials for sustained drug delivery, *Acta Biomater.* 10 (2014) 2133–2146.

193. D.K. Patel, et al. Superior biomaterials using diamine modified graphene grafted polyurethane, *Polym. (Guildf)* 106 (2016) 109–119.

194. D.K. Patel, et al. Graphene as a chain extender of polyurethanes for biomedical applications, *RSC Adv.* 6 (2016) 58628–58640.

195. D.K. Patel, et al. Functionalized graphene tagged polyurethanes for corrosion inhibitor and sustained drug delivery, *ACS Biomater. Sci. Eng.* 3 (2017) 3351–3363.

196. S. Dhanavel, E.A.K. Nivethaa, V. Narayanan, A. Stephen, In vitro cytotoxicity study of dual drug loaded chitosan/palladium nanocomposite towards HT-29 cancer cells, *Mater Sci. Eng. C.* 75 (2017) 1399–1410.

197. H. Lei, et al. Chitosan/sodium alginate modified graphene oxide-based nanocomposite as a carrier for drug delivery, *Ceram Int.* 42 (2016) 17798–17805.

198. D.M. Seema, M. Datta, MMT-PLGA nanocomposites as an oral and controlled release carrier for 5-fluorouracil: a novel approach, *Int. J. Pharm. Pharm. Sci.* 5 (2013) 332–341.

199. S. Rasouli, S. Davaran, F. Rasouli, M. Mahkam, R. Salehi, Synthesis, characterization and pH-controllable methotrexate release from biocompatible polymer/silica nanocomposite for anticancer drug delivery, *Drug Deliv.* 21 (2014) 155–163.

200. F.B. Zeynabad, et al. pH-controlled multiple-drug delivery by a novel antibacterial nanocomposite for combination therapy, *RSC Adv.* 5 (2015) 105678–105691.

201. S.M. Moghimi, A.C. Hunter, J.C. Murray, Long-circulating and targetspecific nanoparticles: theory to practice, *Pharmacol. Rev.* 53 (2001) 283–318.

202. S.M. Moghimi, J. Szebeni, Stealth liposomes and long circulating nanoparticles: critical issues in pharmacokinetics, opsonization and protein-binding properties, *Prog. Lipid. Res.* 42 (2003) 463–478.

203. J.M. Harris, N.E. Martin, M. Modi, Pegylation: a novel process for modifying pharmacokinetics, *Clin. Pharmacokinet* 40 (2001) 539–551.

204. E. Wisse, F. Braet, D. Luo, et al. Structure and function of sinusoidal lining cells in the liver, *Toxicol. Pathol.* 24 (1996) 100–111.

205. F. Yuan, M. Dellian, D. Fukumura, et al. Vascular permeability in a human tumor xenograft: molecular size dependence and cutoff size, *Cancer Res.* 55 (1995) 3752–3756.

206. K. Jain, N.K. Mehra, N.K. Jain, Potentials and emerging trends in nano pharmacology, *Curr. Opin. Pharmacol.* 15 (2014) 97–106.

207. C. Tomuleasa, C. Braicu, A. Irimie, L. Craciun, I. Berindan-Neagoe, Nanopharmacology in translational hematology and oncology, *Int. J. Nanomed.* 9 (2014) 3465–3479.

208. P.S. Kim, S. Djazayeri, R. Zeineldin, Novel nanotechnology approaches to diagnosis and therapy of ovarian cancer, *Gynecol. Oncol.* 120(3) (2011) 393–403.

209. G. Ajnai, A. Chiu, T. Kan, C.C. Cheng, T.H. Tsai, J. Chang, Trends of gold nanoparticle-based drug delivery system in cancer therapy, *J. Exp. Clin. Med.* 6(6) (2014) 172–178.

210. Y. Gao, J. Xie, H. Chen, et al. Nanotechnology-based intelligent drug design for cancer metastasis treatment, *Biotechnol. Adv.* 32(4) (2014) 761–777.

211. G. Song, T.K. Tarrant, T.F. White, et al. Roles of chemokines CCL2 and CCL5 in the pharmacokinetics of PEGylated liposomal doxorubicin in vivo and in patients with recurrent epithelial ovarian cancer, *Nanomedicine* 11(7) (2015) 1797–1807.

212. Y. Wang, L. Chen, Quantum dots, lighting up the research and development of nanomedicine, *Nanomedicine* 7(4) (2011) 385–402.

213. S.C. Baetke, T. Lammers, F. Kiessling, Applications of nanoparticles for diagnosis and therapy of cancer, *Br. J. Radiol.* 88(1054) (2015) 20150207.

214. A.I. Irimie, C. Braicu, R. Cojocneanu-Petric, I. Berindan-Neagoe, R.S. Campian, Novel technologies for oral squamous carcinoma biomarkers in diagnostics and prognostics, *Acta Odontol. Scand.* 73(3) (2015) 161–168.

215. N.T.K. Thanh, L.A.W. Green, Functionalisation of nanoparticles for biomedical applications, *Nano Today* 5 (2010) 213–230.

216. B. Petrushev, S. Boca, T. Simon, et al. Gold nanoparticles enhance the effect of tyrosine kinase inhibitors in acute myeloid leukemia therapy, *Int. J. Nanomed.* 11 (2016) 641–660.

217. T. Nagy-Simon, A.S. Tatar, A.M. Craciun, et al. Antibody conjugated, Raman tagged hollow gold-silver nanospheres for specific targeting and multimodal darkfield/SERS/two photon-FLIM imaging of CD19(+) B lymphoblasts, *ACS Appl. Mater. Interfaces* 9(25) (2017) 21155–21168.

218. A.S. Tatar, T. Nagy-Simon, C. Tomuleasa, S. Boca, S. Astilean, Nanomedicine approaches in acute lymphoblastic leukemia, *J. Controlled Release* 238 (2016) 123–138.

219. S. Suarasan, T. Simon, S. Boca, C. Tomuleasa, S. Astilean, Gelatin-coated gold nanoparticles as carriers of FLT3 inhibitors for acute myeloid leukemia treatment, *Chem. Biol. Drug Des.* 87(6) (2016) 927–935.

220. T. Simon, C. Tomuleasa, A. Bojan, I. Berindan-Neagoe, S. Boca, S. Astilean, Design of FLT3 inhibitor – gold nanoparticle conjugates as potential therapeutic agents for the treatment of acute myeloid leukemia, *Nanoscale Res. Lett.* 10(1) (2015) 466.

221. Y. Schilt, T. Berman, X. Wei, Y. Barenholz, U. Raviv, Using solution X-ray scattering to determine the high-resolution structure and morphology of PEGylated liposomal doxorubicin nanodrugs, *Biochim. Biophys. Acta* 1860(1 Pt A) (2016) 108–119.

222. H. Shibata, H. Yoshida, K. Izutsu, et al. Interaction kinetics of serum proteins with liposomes and their effect on phospholipase-induced liposomal drug release, *Int. J. Pharm.* 495(2) (2015) 827–839.

223. A.K. Varkouhi, M. Scholte, G. Storm, H.J. Haisma, Endosomal escape pathways for delivery of biological, *J. Controlled Release* 151(3) (2011) 220–228.

224. L. Kou, J. Sun, Y. Zhai, Z. He, The endocytosis and intracellular fate of nanomedicines: implication for rational design, *Asian J. Pharm. Sci.* 8(1) (2013) 1–10.

225. E. Rascol, M. Daurat, A. Da Silva, et al. Biological fate of Fe(3)O(4) core-shell mesoporous silica nanoparticles depending on particle surface chemistry, *Nanomaterials* 7(7) (2017) 162.

226. J.P. Peñaloza, V. Márquez-Miranda, M. Cabana-Brunod, et al. Intracellular trafficking and cellular uptake mechanism of PHBV nanoparticles for targeted delivery in epithelial cell lines, *J. Nanobiotechnol.* 15(1) (2017) 1.

227. P. Couvreur, C. Vauthier, Nanotechnology: intelligent design to treat complex disease, *Pharm. Res.* 23 (2006) 1417–1450.

228. M.J. Alonso, Nanomedicines for overcoming biological barriers, *Biomed. Pharmacother* 58 (2004) 168–172.

229. Y. Matsumura, H. Maeda, A new concept for macromolecular therapeutics in cancer chemotherapy: mechanism of tumoritropic accumulation of proteins and the antitumor agent smancs, *Cancer Res.* 46 (1986) 6387–6392.

230. V.P. Torchilin, Recent advances with liposomes as pharmaceutical carriers, *Nat. Rev. Drug Discov.* 4 (2005) 145–160.

231. S.K. Hobbs, W.L. Monsky, F. Yuan, et al. Regulation of transport pathways in tumor vessels: role of tumor type and microenvironment, *Proc. Natl. Acad Sci U S A.* 95 (1998) 4607–4612.

232. M.M. Gottesman, T. Fojo, S.E. Bates, Multidrug resistance in cancer: role of ATP-dependent transporters, *Nat. Rev. Cancer* 2 (2002) 48–58.

233. D. Peer, R. Margalit, Fluoxetine and reversal of multidrug resistance, *Cancer Lett*, 237 (2006) 180–187.

234. R.K. Jain, Barriers to drug delivery in solid tumors, *Sci. Am.* 271 (1994) 58–65.

235. D.E.L. de Menezes, L.M. Pilarski, T.M. Allen, In vitro and in vivo targeting of immunoliposomal doxorubicin to human B-cell lymphoma, *Cancer Res.* 58 (1998) 3320–3330.

236. J.W. Park, K. Hong, D.B. Kirpotin, et al. Anti-HER2 immunoliposomes, *Clin. Cancer Res.* 8 (2002) 1172–1181.

237. I. Pastan, R. Hassan, D.J. Fitzgerald, et al. Immunotoxin therapy of cancer, *Nat. Rev Cancer* 6 (2006) 559–565.

238. D. Peer, P. Zhu, C.V. Carman, et al. Selective gene silencing in activated leukocytes by targeting siRNAs to the integrin lymphocyte function-associated antigen-1, *Proc. Natl. Acad Sci U. S. A.* 104 (2007) 4095–4100.

239. P. Sapra, T.M. Allen, Internalizing antibodies are necessary for improved therapeutic efficacy of antibody-targeted liposomal drugs, *Cancer Res.* 62 (2002) 7190–7194.

240. T.M. Allen, Long-circulating (sterically stabilized) liposomes for targeted drug delivery, *Trends Pharmacol. Sci.* 15 (1994) 215–220.

241. S. Hong, P.R. Leroueil, I.J. Majoros, et al. The binding avidity of a nanoparticle-based multivalent targeted drug delivery platform, *Chem. Biol.* 14 (2007) 107–115.

242. D.J. Bharali, D.W. Lucey, H. Jayakumar, H.E. Pudavar, P.N. Prasad, Folatereceptor-mediated delivery of InP quantum dots for bioimaging using confocal and two-photon microscopy, *J. Am. Chem. Soc.* 127 (2005) 11364–11371.

243. P. Zrazhevskiy, M. Sena, X. Gao, Designing multifunctional quantum dots for bioimaging, detection, and drug delivery, *Chem. Soc. Rev.* 39 (2010) 4326–4354.

244. B.A. Kairdolf, et al. Semiconductor quantum dots for bioimaging and biodiagnostic applications, *Annu. Rev. Anal. Chem.* 6 (2013) 143–162.

245. A. Bianco, K. Kostarelos, M. Prato, Opportunities and challenges of carbonbased nanomaterials for cancer therapy, *Expert Opin. Drug Delivery* 5 (2008) 331–342.

246. C.B. Murray, D.J. Norris, M.G. Bawendi, Synthesis and characterization of nearly monodisperse CdE (E=sulfur, selenium, tellurium) semiconductor nanocrystallites, *J. Am. Chem. Soc.* 115 (1993) 8706–8715.

247. R. Bilan, I. Nabiev, A. Sukhanova, Quantum dot-based nanotools for bioimaging, diagnostics, and drug delivery, *Chembiochem* 17 (2016) 2103–2114.

248. B. Dubertret, et al. In vivo imaging of quantum dots encapsulated in phospholipid micelles, *Science* 298 (2002) 1759–1762.

249. G.J. Halder, C.J. Kepert, B. Moubaraki, K.S. Murray, J.D. Cashion, Guestdependent spin crossover in a nanoporous molecular framework material, *Science* 298 (2002) 1762–1765.

250. X. Zhao, H. Li, R.J. Lee, Targeted drug delivery via folate receptors, *Expert Opin. Drug Delivery* 5 (2008) 309–319.

251. X. Gao, Y. Cui, R.M. Levenson, L.W.K. Chung, S. Nie, In vivo cancer targeting and imaging with semiconductor quantum dots, *Nat. Biotechnol.* 22 (2004) 969–976.

252. M.S. Muthu, S.A. Kulkarni, A. Raju, S.S. Feng, Theranostic liposomes of TPGS coating for targeted co-delivery of docetaxel and quantum dots, *Biomaterials* 33 (2012) 3494–3501.

253. C.L. Huang, et al. Application of paramagnetic graphene quantum dots as a platform for simultaneous dual-modality bioimaging and tumor-targeted drug delivery, *J. Mater. Chem. B* 3 (2012) 651–664.

254. Z. Li, et al. Quantum dots loaded nanogels for low cytotoxicity, pH-sensitive fluorescence, cell imaging and drug delivery. *Carbohydr. Polym.* 121 (2015) 477–485.

255. N. Huang, et al. Single-wall carbon nanotubes assisted photothermal cancer therapy: animal study with a murine model of squamous cell carcinoma, *Lasers Surg. Med.* 42 (2010) 798–808.

256. N. Ahmed, H. Fessi, A. Elaissari, Theranostic applications of nanoparticles in cancer, *Drug Discov. Today* 17 (2012) 928–934.

257. Y. Lin, et al. Advances toward bioapplications of carbon nanotubes, *J. Mater. Chem.* 14 (2004) 527–541.

258. A. Bianco, K. Kostarelos, M. Prato, Applications of carbon nanotubes in drug delivery, *Curr. Opin. Chem. Biol.* 9 (2005) 674–679.

259. T.R. Fadel, T.M. Fahmy, Immunotherapy applications of carbon nanotubes: from design to safe applications, *Trends Biotechnol.* 32 (2014) 198–209.

260. C.H. Villa, et al. Single-walled carbon nanotubes deliver peptide antigen into dendritic cells and enhance IgG responses to tumor-associated antigens, *ACS Nano* 5 (2011) 5300–5311.

261. S. Senapati, et al. Layered double hydroxides as effective carrier for anticancer drugs and tailoring of release rate through interlayer anions, *J Control Release* 224 (2016) 186–198.

262. N.T. Whilton, P.J. Vickers, S. Mann, Bioinorganic clays: synthesis and characterization of amino- and polyamino acid intercalated layered double hydroxides, *J. Mater. Chem.* 7 (1997) 1623–1629.

263. M. Del Arco, S. Gutiérrez, C. Martín, V. Rives, J. Rocha, Synthesis and characterization of layered double hydroxides (LDH) intercalated with non-steroidal anti-inflammatory drugs (NSAID). *J. Solid State Chem.* 177 (2004) 3954–3962.

264. V. Rives, M. del Arco, C. Martín. Intercalation of drugs in layered double hydroxides and their controlled release: a review, *Appl. Clay Sci.* 88–89 (2014) 239–269.

265. K.M. Tyner, S.R. Schiffman, E.R. Giannelis, Nanobiohybrids as delivery vehicles for camptothecin, *J. Controlled Release* 95 (2004) 501–514.

266. L. Li, W. Gu, J. Chen, W. Chen, Z.P. Xu, Co-delivery of siRNAs and anti-cancer drugs using layered double hydroxide nanoparticles, *Biomaterials* 35 (2014) 3331–3339.

267. P. Kesharwani, A.K. Iyer, Recent advances in dendrimer-based nanovectors for tumor-targeted drug and gene delivery, *Drug Discovery Today* 20 (2015) 536–547.

268. A. Bianco, K. Kostarelos, M. Prato, Applications of carbon nanotubes in drug delivery, *Curr Opin. Chem. Biol.* 9 (2005) 674–679.

269. M.E. Brennan, J.N. Coleman, A. Drury, B. Lahr, T. Kobayashi, W.J. Blau, Nonlinear photoluminescence from van Hove singularities in multiwalled carbon nanotubes, *Optics Lett.* 28 (2003) 266–268.

270. N.W. Kam, M. O'Connell, J.A. Wisdom, H. Dai, Carbon nanotubes as multifunctional biological transporters and near-infrared agents for selective cancer cell destruction, *Proc. Nat. Acad. Sci. U. S. A.* 102 (2005) 11600–11605.

271. A. Burlaka, S. Lukin, S. Prylutska, O. Remeniak, Y. Prylutskyy, M. Shuba, et al. Hyperthermic effect of multiwalled carbon nanotubes stimulated with near infrared irradiation for anticancer therapy: in vitro studies, *Exp. Oncol.* 32 (2010) 48–50.

272. X. Yu, D. Gao, L. Gao, J. Lai, C. Zhang, Y. Zhao, et al. Inhibiting metastasis and preventing tumor relapse by triggering host immunity with tumor-targeted photodynamic therapy using photosensitizer-loaded functional nanographenes, *ACS Nano* 11 (2017) 10147–10158.

273. K.R. Karnati, Y. Wang, Understanding the co-loading and releasing of doxorubicin and paclitaxel using chitosan functionalized single-walled carbon nanotubes by molecular dynamics simulations, *Phys. Chem. Chem. Phys. PCCP* 20 (2018) 9389–9400.

274. B.C. Yadav, R. Kumar, Structure, properties and applications of fullerenes, *Int. J. Nanotechnol. Appl.* 2 (2008) 15–24.

275. C.-Y. Lai, et al. A mesoporous silica nanosphere-based carrier system with chemically removable CdS nanoparticle caps for stimuli-responsive controlled release of neurotransmitters and drug molecules, *J. Am. Chem. Soc.* 125 (2003) 4451–4459.

276. V. Mamaeva, et al. Mesoporous silica nanoparticles as drug delivery systems for targeted inhibition of Notch signaling in cancer, *Mol. The.r* 19 (2011) 1538–1546.

277. M. Okazaki, Y. Yoshida, S. Yamaguchi, M. Kaneno, J.C. Elliott, Affinity binding phenomena of DNA onto apatite crystals, *Biomaterials* 22 (2001) 2459–2464.

278. M.S. Lee, et al. Target-specific delivery of siRNA by stabilized calcium phosphate nanoparticles using dopa–hyaluronic acid conjugate, *J. Controlled Release* 192 (2014) 122–130.

279. S. Wang, E.H. McDonnell, F.A. Sedor, J.G. Toffaletti, pH effects on measurements of ionized calcium and ionized magnesium in blood, *Arch Pathol. Lab. Med.* 126 (2002) 947–950.

280. T.T. Morgan, et al. Encapsulation of organic molecules in calcium phosphate nanocomposite particles for intracellular imaging and drug delivery, *Nano Lett.* 8 (2008) 4108–4115.

281. Y.C. Tseng, Z. Xu, K. Guley, H. Yuan, L. Huang, Lipid–calcium phosphate nanoparticles for delivery to the lymphatic system and SPECT/CT imaging of lymph node metastases, *Biomaterials* 35 (2014) 4688–4698.

282. F. Pittella, et al. Systemic siRNA delivery to a spontaneous pancreatic tumor model in transgenic mice by PEGylated calcium phosphate hybrid micelles, *J. Controlled Release* 178 (2014) 18–24.

283. T. Nomoto, et al. Calcium phosphate-based organic–inorganic hybrid nanocarriers with pH-responsive on/off switch for photodynamic therapy, *Biomater. Sci.* 4 (2016) 826–838.

284. P. Mi, et al. A pH-activatable nanoparticle with signal-amplification capabilities for non-invasive imaging of tumour malignancy, *Nat. Nanotechnol.* 11 (2016) 724–730.

285. I. Raynal, et al. Macrophage endocytosis of superparamagnetic iron oxide nanoparticles: mechanisms and comparison of ferumoxides and ferumoxtran-10, *Invest. Radiol.* 39 (2004) 56–63.

286. W.J. Rogers, P. Basu, Factors regulating macrophage endocytosis of nanoparticles: implications for targeted magnetic resonance plaque imaging, *Atherosclerosis* 178 (2005) 67–73.

287. K.J. Widder, A.E. Senyei, D.F. Ranney, In vitro release of biologically active adriamycin by magnetically responsive albumin microspheres, *Cancer Res.* 40 (1980) 3512–3517.

288. P.K. Gupta, C.T. Hung, Targeted delivery of low dose doxorubicin hydrochloride administered via magnetic albumin microspheres in rats, *J. Microencapsul.* 7 (1990) 85–94.

289. S. Aime, et al. Insights into the use of paramagnetic Gd(III) complexes in MRmolecular imaging investigations. *J. Magn. Reson. Imaging* 16 (2002) 394–406.

290. A.S. Arbab, et al. Characterization of biophysical and metabolic properties of cells labeled with superparamagnetic iron oxide nanoparticles and transfection agent for cellular MR imaging, *Radiology* 229 (2003) 838–846.

291. S. Laurent, A.A. Saei, S. Behzadi, A. Panahifar, M. Mahmoudi, Superparamagnetic iron oxide nanoparticles for delivery of therapeutic agents: opportunities and challenges, *Expert Opin. Drug Delivery* 11 (2014) 1449–1470.

292. H. Choi, S.R. Choi, R. Zhou, H.F. Kung, I.W. Chen, Iron oxide nanoparticles as magnetic resonance contrast agent for tumor imaging via folate receptortargeted delivery, *Acad Radiol.* 11 (2004) 996–1004.

293. L. Josephson, C.H. Tung, A. Moore, R. Weissleder, High-efficiency intracellular magnetic labeling with novel superparamagnetic-Tat peptide conjugates, *Bioconjug. Chem.* 10 (1999) 186–191.

294. H. Lee, et al. Antibiofouling polymer-coated superparamagnetic iron oxide nanoparticles as potential magnetic resonance contrast agents for in vivo cancer imaging, *J. Am. Chem. Soc.* 128 (2006) 7383–7389.

295. H. Lee, et al. Thermally cross-linked superparamagnetic iron oxide nanoparticles: synthesis and application as a dual imaging probe for cancer in vivo, *J. Am. Chem. Soc.* 129 (2007) 12739–12745.

296. C.A. Quinto, P. Mohindra, S. Tong, G. Bao, Multifunctional superparamagnetic iron oxide nanoparticles for combined chemotherapy and hyperthermia cancer treatment, *Nanoscale* 7 (2015) 12728–12736.

297. J.P. Fortin, et al. Size-sorted anionic iron oxide nanomagnets as colloidal mediators for magnetic hyperthermia, *J. Am. Chem. Soc.* 129 (2007) 2628–2635.

298. S. Balivada, et al. A/C magnetic hyperthermia of melanoma mediated by iron(0)/iron oxide core/shell magnetic nanoparticles: a mouse study, *Bmc Cancer* 10 (2010) 119.

299. B. Hildebrandt, et al. The cellular and molecular basis of hyperthermia, *Crit. Rev. Oncol. Hematol.* 43 (2002) 33–56.

300. J.H. Park, et al. Polymeric nanomedicine for cancer therapy, *Prog. Polym. Sci.* 33 (2008) 113–137.

301. S. Parveen, S.K. Sahoo, Polymeric nanoparticles for cancer therapy, *J. Drug Target* 16 (2008) 108–123.

302. S. Mitra, U. Gaur, P.C. Ghosh, A.N. Maitra, Tumour targeted delivery of encapsulated dextran–doxorubicin conjugate using chitosan nanoparticles as carrier, *J Control Release* 74 (2001) 317–323.

303. S.K. Pandey, et al. Controlled release of drug and better bioavailability using poly(lactic acid-co-glycolic acid) nanoparticles, *Int. J. Biol. Macromol.* 89 (2016) 99–110.

304. F.Y. Cheng, C.H. Su, P.C. Wu, C.S. Yeh, Multifunctional polymeric nanoparticles for combined chemotherapeutic and near-infrared photothermal cancer therapy in vitro and in vivo, *Chem. Commun.* 46 (2010) 3167–3169.

305. P. Couvreur, Polyalkylcyanoacrylates as colloidal drug carriers, *Crit. Rev. Ther. Drug Carrier Syst.* 5 (1988) 1–20.

306. R. Duncan, The dawning era of polymer therapeutics, *Nat. Rev. Drug Discov.* 2 (2003) 347–360.

307. K. Miyata, R.J. Christie, K.J.R. Kataoka, F. Polymers, Polymeric micelles for nano-scale drug delivery, *React Funct. Polym.* 71 (2011) 227–234.

308. E. Blanco, E.A. Bey, C. Khemtong, S.G. Yang, J. Setti-Guthi, H. Chen, et al. Beta-lapachone micellar nanotherapeutics for non-small cell lung cancer therapy, *Cancer Res.* 70 (2010) 3896–3904.

309. C. Tian, J. Feng, H.J. Cho, S.S. Datta, Prud'homme RK. Adsorption and denaturation of structured polymeric nanoparticles at an interface, *Nano Lett.* 18 (2018) 4854–4860.

310. T. Nakanishi, S. Fukushima, K. Okamoto, M. Suzuki, Y. Matsumura, M. Yokoyama, et al. Development of the polymer micelle carrier system for doxorubicin, *J. Controlled Release Off J. Controlled Release Soc.* 74 (2001) 295–302.

311. R. Savic, L. Luo, A. Eisenberg, D. Maysinger, Micellar nanocontainers distribute to defined cytoplasmic organelles, *Science (New York, NY)* 300 (2003) 615–618.

312. M. Jones, J. Leroux, Polymeric micelles: a new generation of colloidal drug carriers, *Eur. J. Pharm. Biopharm. Off J. Arbeitsgemeinschaft fur Pharmazeutische Verfahrenstechnik eV* 48 (1999) 101–111.

313. J.C. Sung, B.L. Pulliam, D.A. Edwards, Nanoparticles for drug delivery to the lungs, *Trends Biotechnol.* 25 (2007) 563–570.

314. M.E Davis, Z.G. Chen, D.M. Shin, Nanoparticle therapeutics: an emerging treatment modality for cancer, *Nat. Rev. Drug Discov.* 7 (2008) 771–782.

315. G. Berry, M. Billingham, E. Alderman, P. Richardson, F. Torti, B. Lum, et al. The use of cardiac biopsy to demonstrate reduced cardiotoxicity in AIDS Kaposi's sarcoma patients treated with pegylated liposomal doxorubicin, *Ann. Oncol. Off. J. Eur. Soc. Med. Oncol.* 9 (1998) 711–716.

316. M.S. Ewer, F.J. Martin, C. Henderson, C.L. Shapiro, R.S. Benjamin, A.A. Gabizon, Cardiac safety of liposomal anthracyclines, *Semin. Oncol.* 31 (2004) 161–181.

317. G. Sharma, S. Anabousi, C. Ehrhardt, M.N. Ravi Kumar, Liposomes as targeted drug delivery systems in the treatment of breast cancer, *J. Drug Targeting* 14 (2006) 301–310.

318. R. Gref, Y. Minamitake, M.T. Peracchia, et al. Biodegradable longcirculating polymeric nanospheres, *Science* 263 (1994) 1600–1603.

319. Moghimi SM, Hunter AC, Murray JC. Long-circulating and targetspecific nanoparticles: theory to practice, *Pharmacol. Rev.* 53 (2001) 283–318.

320. R. Gref, M. Luck, P. Quellec, et al. "Stealth" corona-core nanoparticles surface modified by polyethylene glycol (PEG): influences of the corona (PEG chain length and surface density) and of the core composition on phagocytic uptake and plasma protein adsorption, *Colloids Surf. B Biointerfaces* 18 (2000) 301–313.

321. D.E. Owens DE III, Peppas NA. Opsonization, biodistribution, and pharmacokinetics of polymeric nanoparticles, *Int. J. Pharmacol.* 307 (2006) 93–102.

322. M. Tobio, R. Gref, A. Sanchez, et al. Stealth PLA-PEG nanoparticles as protein carriers for nasal administration, *Pharmacol. Res.* 15 (1998) 270–275.

323. C. Perez, A. Sanchez, D. Putnam, et al. Poly(lactic acid)-poly(ethylene glycol) nanoparticles as new carriers for the delivery of plasmid DNA, *J. Controlled Release* 75 (2001) 211–224.

324. R. Langer, D.A. Tirrell, Designing materials for biology and medicine, *Nature* 428 (2004) 487–492.

325. R. Langer, J. Folkman, Polymers for the sustained release of proteins and other macromolecules, *Nature* 263 (1976) 797–800.

326. R. Langer, Drug delivery and targeting, *Nature* 392 (1998) 5–10.

327. R. Langer, New methods of drug delivery, *Science* 249 (1990) 1527–1533.

328. R. Langer, Drug delivery: drugs on target, *Science* 293 (2001) 58–59.

329. R. Langer, N.A. Peppas, Advances in biomaterials, drug delivery, and bionanotechnology, *AICHE J.* 49 (2003) 2990–3006.

330. Y. Matsusue, S. Hanafusa, T. Yamamuro, et al. Tissue reaction of bioabsorbable ultra high strength poly (L-lactide) rod. A long-term study in rabbits, *Clin. Orthop. Relat. Res.* (1995) 246–253.

331. O.C. Farokhzad, J.M. Karp, R. Langer, Nanoparticle-aptamer bioconjugates for cancer targeting, *Expert Opin. Drug Delivery* 3 (2006) 311–324.

332. O.C. Farokhzad, S. Jon, A. Khademhosseini, et al. Nanoparticleaptamer bioconjugates: a new approach for targeting prostate cancer cells, *Cancer Res.* 64 (2004) 7668–7672.

333. O.C. Farokhzad, J. Cheng, B.A. Teply, et al. Targeted nanoparticleaptamer bioconjugates for cancer chemotherapy in vivo, *Proc. Natl. Acad. Sci. U. S. A.* 103 (2006) 6315–6320.

334. S. Moffatt, C. Papasakelariou, S. Wiehle, et al. Successful in vivo tumor targeting of prostate-specific membrane antigen with a highly efficient J591/PEI/DNA molecular conjugate, *Gene Ther.* 13 (2006) 761–772.

335. S. Moffatt, R.J. Cristiano, Pegylated J591 mAb loaded in PLGA-PEGPLGA tri-block copolymer for targeted delivery: in vitro evaluation in human prostate cancer cells, *Int. J. Pharmacol.* 317 (2006) 10–13.

336. R. Weissleder, K. Kelly, K.Y. Sun, et al. Cell-specific targeting of nanoparticles by multivalent attachment of small molecules, *Nat. Biotechnol.* 23 (2005) 1418–1423.

337. P. Decuzzi, S. Lee, B. Bhushan, et al. A theoretical model for the margination of particles within blood vessels, *Ann. Biomed. Eng.* 33 (2005) 179–190.

338. K.M. Bolotin, et al. Ammonium sulfate gradients for efficient and stable remote loading of amphipathic weak bases into liposomes and ligandoliposomes, *J. Liposome Res.* 4 (1994) 455–479.

339. N.L. Boman, D. Masin, L.D. Mayer, P.R. Cullis, M.B. Bally, Liposomal vincristine which exhibits increased drug retention and increased circulation longevity cures mice bearing P388 tumors, *Cancer Res.* 54 (1994) 2830–2833.

340. P. Sapra, T.M. Allen, Ligand-targeted liposomal anticancer drugs, *Prog. Lipid Res.* 42 (2003) 439–462.

341. R.I. Pakunlu, et al. In vitro and in vivo intracellular liposomal delivery of antisense oligonucleotides and anticancer drug, *J. Controlled Release* 114 (2006) 153–162.

342. T. Jiang, et al. Dual-functional liposomes based on pH-responsive cell-penetrating peptide and hyaluronic acid for tumor-targeted anticancer drug delivery, *Biomaterials* 33 (2012) 9246–9258.

343. X. Guo, F.C. Szoka, Steric stabilization of fusogenic liposomes by a low-pH sensitive PEG–diortho ester–lipid conjugate, *Bioconjug. Chem.* 12 (2001) 291–300.

344. R. Mo, et al. Multistage pH-responsive liposomes for mitochondrial-targeted anticancer drug delivery, *Adv. Mater.* 24 (2012) 3659–3665.

345. K. Kitatani, et al. Ceramide limits phosphatidylinositol-3-kinase C2β-controlled cell motility in ovarian cancer: potential of ceramide as a metastasis-suppressor lipid, *Oncogene* 35 (2016) 2801–2812.

346. Şalva E, S.O. Turan, F. Eren, J. Akbuğa, The enhancement of gene silencing efficiency with chitosan-coated liposome formulations of siRNAs targeting HIF-1α and VEGF, *Int. J. Pharm.* 478 (2015) 147–154.

347. J. Cao, et al. A7RC peptide modified paclitaxel liposomes dually target breast cancer, *Biomater. Sci.* 3 (2015) 1545–1554.

348. S. Svenson, D.A. Tomalia, Dendrimers in biomedical applications--reflections on the field, *Adv. Drug Delivery Rev.* 57 (2005) 2106–2129.

349. S.N. Svenson, D.A.J.A.D.D.R. Tomalia, Dendrimers in biomedical applications: reflections on the field, *Adv. Drug Delivery Rev.* 57 (2005) 2106–2129.

350. D.A. Tomalia, H. Baker, J. Dewald, M. Hall, G. Kallos, S. Martin, et al. Dendritic macromolecules: synthesis of starburst dendrimers. *Macromolecules* 19 (1986) 2466–2468.

351. D.A.H. Tomalia, H. Baker, J.R. Dewald, M.J. Hall, P.B.J.P.J. Smith, A new class of polymers: starburst-dendritic macromolecules, *Polymer J.* 17 (1985) 117–132.

352. L. Palmerston Mendes, J. Pan, V.P. Torchilin, Dendrimers as nanocarriers for nucleic acid and drug delivery in cancer therapy, *Molecules (Basel, Switzerland)* 22 (2017) 1401–1421. doi: 10.3390/molecules22091401.

353. A.P. Sherje, M. Jadhav, B.R. Dravyakar, D. Kadam, Dendrimers: a versatile nanocarrier for drug delivery and targeting, *Int. J. Pharm.* 548 (2018) 707–720.

354. E.C. Wiener, S. Konda, A. Shadron, M. Brechbiel, O. Gansow, Targeting dendrimer-chelates to tumors and tumor cells expressing the high-affinity folate receptor, *Invest. Radiol.* 32 (1997) 748–754.

355. A. Quintana, E. Raczka, L. Piehler, I. Lee, A. Myc, I. Majoros, et al. Design and function of a dendrimer-based therapeutic nanodevice targeted to tumor cells through the folate receptor, *Pharm. Res.* 19 (2002) 1310–1316.

356. K. Kono, M. Liu, J.M. Fréchet, Design of dendritic macromolecules containing folate or methotrexate residues, *Bioconjugate Chem.* 10 (1999) 1115–1121.

357. R. Roy, M.G. Baek, Glycodendrimers: novel glycotope isosteres unmasking sugar coding. case study with T-antigen markers from breast cancer MUC1 glycoprotein, *J. Biotechnol.* 90 (2002) 291–309.

358. A.O. Elzoghby, W.M. Samy, N.A. Elgindy, Albumin-based nanoparticles as potential controlled release drug delivery systems, *J. Controlled Release* 157 (2012) 168–182.

359. S. Dreis, et al. Preparation, characterisation and maintenance of drug efficacy of doxorubicin-loaded human serum albumin (HSA) nanoparticles, *Int. J. Pharm.* 341 (2007) 207–214.

360. D. Zhao, et al. Preparation, characterization, and in vitro targeted delivery of folate-decorated paclitaxel-loaded bovine serum albumin nanoparticles, *Int. J. Nanomed.* 5 (2010) 669–677.

361. M.J. Hawkins, P. Soon-Shiong, N. Desai, Protein nanoparticles as drug carriers in clinical medicine, *Adv. Drug Delivery Rev.* 60 (2008) 876–885.

362. D.A. Yardley, nab-Paclitaxel mechanisms of action and delivery, *J. Controlled Release* 170 (2013) 365–372.

363. T.Y. Kim, et al. Phase I and pharmacokinetic study of Genexol-PM, a cremophor-free, polymeric micelle-formulated paclitaxel, in patients with advanced malignancies, *Clin. Cancer Res.* 10 (2004) 3708–3716.

364. C. Shi, et al. Actively targeted delivery of anticancer drug to tumor cells by redox-responsive star-shaped micelles, *Biomaterials* 35 (2014) 8711–8722.

365. X. Jin, et al. Efficient intravesical therapy of bladder cancer with cationic doxorubicin nanoassemblies, *Int. J. Nanomed.* 11 (2016) 4535–4544.

366. P. Kumari, et al. Cholesterol-conjugated poly(D, L-lactide)-based micelles as a nanocarrier system for effective delivery of curcumin in cancer therapy, *Drug Delivery* 24 (2017) 209–223.

367. S. Deshayes, et al. Phenylboronic acid-installed polymeric micelles for targeting sialylated epitopes in solid tumors, *J. Am. Chem. Soc.* 135 (2013) 15501–15507.

368. R.N. Gilbreth, et al. Lipid- and polyion complex-based micelles as agonist platforms for TNFR superfamily receptors, *J. Controlled Release* 234 (2016) 104–114.

369. H. Cui, M.J. Webber, S.I. Stupp, Self-assembly of peptide amphiphiles: from molecules to nanostructures to biomaterials, *Biopolymers* 94 (2010) 1–18.

370. R. Zhang, et al. Carrier-free, chemophotodynamic dual nanodrugs via self-assembly for synergistic antitumor therapy, *ACS Appl. Mater. Interfaces* 8 (2016) 13262–13269.

371. C. Wu, et al. Engineering of switchable aptamer micelle flares for molecular imaging in living cells, *ACS Nano* 7 (2013) 5724–5731.

372. J. Zhou, X. Du, J. Li, N. Yamagata, B. Xu, Taurine boosts cellular uptake of small D-peptides for enzyme-instructed intracellular molecular self-assembly, *J. Am. Chem. Soc.* 137 (2015) 10040–10043.

373. S.D. Li, Y.C. Chen, M.J. Hackett, L. Huang, Tumor-targeted delivery of siRNA by self-assembled nanoparticles, *Mol. Ther.* 16 (2008) 163–169.

374. H.J. Yoon, W.D. Jang, Polymeric supramolecular systems for drug delivery, *J. Mater. Chem.* 20 (2010) 211–222.

375. T. Wei, et al. Anticancer drug nanomicelles formed by self-assembling amphiphilic dendrimer to combat cancer drug resistance, *Proc. Natl. Acad. Sci. U. S. A.* 112 (2015) 2978–2983.

376. G. Yu, et al. Fabrication of a targeted drug delivery system from a Pillar5.arenebased supramolecular diblock copolymeric amphiphile for effective cancer therapy, *Adv. Funct. Mater.* 26 (2016) 8999–9008.

377. J. Li, X. Loh, Cyclodextrin-based supramolecular architectures: syntheses, structures, and applications for drug and gene delivery. *Adv. Drug Delivery Rev.* 60 (2008) 1000–1017.

378. C.C. Cheng, et al. Highly efficient drug delivery systems based on functional supramolecular polymers: in vitro evaluation, *Acta Biomater.* 33 (2016) 194–202.

379. P.Y.W. Dankers, et al. Hierarchical formation of supramolecular transient networks in water: a modular injectable delivery system, *Adv. Mater.* 24 (2012) 2703–2709.

380. S. Kaida, et al. Visible drug delivery by supramolecular nanocarriers directing to single-platformed diagnosis and therapy of pancreatic tumor model, *Cancer Res.* 70 (2010) 7031–7041.

381. M. Adeli, M. Ashiri, B.K. Chegeni, P. Sasanpour, Tumor-targeted drug delivery systems based on supramolecular interactions between iron oxide–carbon nanotubes PAMAM–PEG–PAMAM linear-dendritic copolymers, *J. Iran Chem. Soc.* 10 (2013) 701–708.

382. J.F. Lovell, et al. Porphysome nanovesicles generated by porphyrin bilayers for use as multimodal biophotonic contrast agents, *Nat. Mater.* 10 (2011) 324–332.

383. N. Muhanna, et al. Phototheranostic porphyrin nanoparticles enable visualization and targeted treatment of head and neck cancer in clinically relevant models, *Theranostics* 5 (2015) 1428–1443.

384. S. Su, Y. Ding, Y. Li, Y. Wu, G. Nie, Integration of photothermal therapy and synergistic chemotherapy by a porphyrin self-assembled micelle confers chemosensitivity in triple-negative breast cancer, *Biomaterials* 80 (2016) 169–178.

385. N. Peppas, P. Bures, W. Leobandung, H. Ichikawa, Hydrogels in pharmaceutical formulations, *Eur. J. Pharm. Biopharm.* 50 (2000) 27–46.

386. N. Peppas, R. Langer, New challenges in biomaterials, *Science* 263 (1994) 1715–1720.

387. A.S. Hoffman, B.D Ratner, Synthetic hydrogels for biomedical applications. In: J.D. Andrade (ed) *Hydrogels for Medical and Related Applications*, ACS Symposium Series. American Chemical Society: Washington, DC (1976), 1–36. doi: 10.1021/bk-1976-0031.

388. C.C. Lin, A.T. Metters, Hydrogels in controlled release formulations: network design and mathematical modeling, *Adv. Drug Delivery Rev.* 58 (2006) 1379–1408.

389. S.R.V. Tomme, G. Storm, W.E. Hennink, In situ gelling hydrogels for pharmaceutical and biomedical applications. *Int. J. Pharm.* 355 (2008) 1–18.

390. X. Qi, et al. Fabrication and characterization of a novel anticancer drug delivery system: salecan/poly(methacrylic acid) semi-interpenetrating polymer network hydrogel, *ACS Biomater. Sci. Eng.* 1 (2015) 1287–1299.

391. S. Jin, et al. Biodegradation and toxicity of protease/redox/pH stimuli-responsive PEGlated PMAA nanohydrogels for targeting drug delivery, *ACS Appl. MaterInterfaces* 7 (2015) 19843–19852.

392. R. Ghosh, U. Goswami, S.S. Ghosh, A. Paul, A. Chattopadhyay, Synergistic anticancer activity of fluorescent copper nanoclusters and cisplatin delivered through a hydrogel nanocarrier, *ACS Appl. Mater. Interfaces* 7 (2015) 209–222.

393. B. Xue, et al. Intracellular degradable hydrogel cubes and spheres for anti-cancer drug delivery, *ACS Appl. Mater. Interfaces* 7 (2015) 13633–13644.

394. Y. Wang, J. Nie, B. Chang, Y. Sun, W. Yang, Poly(vinylcaprolactam)-based biodegradable multiresponsive microgels for drug delivery, *Biomacromolecules* 14 (2013) 3034–3046.

395. J. Yu, W. Ha, J.N. Sun, Y.P. Shi, Supramolecular hybrid hydrogel based on host–guest interaction and its application in drug delivery, *ACS Appl. Mater. Interfaces* 6 (2014) 19544–19551.

396. J. Naskar, G. Palui, A. Banerjee, Tetrapeptide-based hydrogels: for encapsulation and slow release of an anticancer drug at physiological pH, *J. Phys. Chem. B* 113 (2009) 11787–11792.

397. Y.Y. Chen, H.C. Wu, J.S. Sun, G.C. Dong, T.W. Wang, Injectable and thermoresponsive self-assembled nanocomposite hydrogel for long-term anticancer drug delivery, *Langmuir* 29 (2013) 3721–3729.

398. Y. Li, D. Maciel, J. Rodrigues, X. Shi, H. Tomás, Biodegradable polymer nanogels for drug/nucleic acid delivery, *Chem. Rev.* 115 (2015) 8564–8608.

399. A.V. Kabanov, S.V. Vinogradov, Nanogels as pharmaceutical carriers: finite networks of infinite capabilities, *Angew Chem. Int. Ed. Engl.* 48 (2009) 5418–5429.

400. M. Oishi, S. Sumitani, Y. Nagasaki, On–off regulation of 19F magnetic resonance signals based on pH-sensitive PEGylated nanogels for potential tumor-specific smart 19F MRI probes, *Bioconjug. Chem.* 18 (2007) 1379–1382.

401. H.-S. Peng, J.A. Stolwijk, L.-N. Sun, J. Wegener, O.S. Wolfbeis, A nanogel for ratiometric fluorescent sensing of intracellular pH values, *Angew Chem.* 122 (2010) 4342–4345.

402. T. Miyahara, et al. Exploitation of a novel polysaccharide nanogel cross-linking membrane for guided bone regeneration (GBR), *J. Tissue Eng. Regen Med.* 6 (2012) 666–672.

403. W. Wu, et al. *In-situ* immobilization of quantum dots in polysaccharide-based nanogels for integration of optical pH-sensing, tumor cell imaging, and drug delivery, *Biomaterials* 31 (2010) 3023–3031.

404. D.M. Eckmann, R.J. Composto, A. Tsourkas, V.R. Muzykantov, Nanogel carrier design for targeted drug delivery, *J. Mater. Chem. B* 2 (2014) 8085–8097.

405. W.H. Chiang, et al. Dual stimuli-responsive polymeric hollow nanogels designed as carriers for intracellular triggered drug release, *Langmuir* 28 (2012) 15056–15064.

406. H. Yang, et al. Smart pH/Redox dual-responsive nanogels for on-demand intracellular anticancer drug release, *ACS Appl. Mater. Interfaces* 8 (2016) 7729–7738.

407. Y. Wang, et al. Nanogels fabricated from bovine serum albumin and chitosan via self assembly for delivery of anticancer drug. *Colloids Surf. B Biointerfaces* 146 (2016) 107–113.

408. A.K. Mahanta, S. Senapati, P. Maiti, A polyurethane–chitosan brush as an injectable hydrogel for controlled drug delivery and tissue engineering. *Polym. Chem.* 8 (2017) 6233–6249.

409. C. Duan, et al. Chitosan-g-poly(N-isopropylacrylamide) based nanogels for tumor extracellular targeting, *Int. J. Pharm.* 409 (2011) 252–259.

410. I. Matai, P. Gopinath, Chemically cross-linked hybrid nanogels of alginate and PAMAM dendrimers as efficient anticancer drug delivery vehicles, *ACS Biomater. Sci. Eng.* 2 (2016) 213–223.

411. A.I. Ekimov, A.A.J.J.L. Onushchenko, Quantum size effect in three-dimensional microscopic semiconductor crystals, *J. Exp. Theor Phys. Lett.* 34 (1981) 363.

412. M.A.J.P.T. Kastner, Artificial atoms, *Phys. Today* 46 (1993) 24.

413. A. Shiohara, A. Hoshino, K. Hanaki, K. Suzuki, K. Yamamoto, On the cyto-toxicity caused by quantum dots, *Microbiol. Immunol.* 48 (2004) 669–675.

414. Q.M. Xiang, L.M. Wang, J.P. Yuan, J.M. Chen, F. Yang, Y. Li, Quantum dot-based multispectral fluorescent imaging to quantitatively study co-expressions of Ki67 and HER2 in breast cancer, *Exp. Mol. Pathol.* 99 (2015) 133–138.

415. Y. Ruan, W. Yu, F. Cheng, X. Zhang, T. Rao, Y. Xia, et al. Comparison of quantum-dots- and fluorescein-isothiocyanate-based technology for detecting prostate-specific antigen expression in human prostate cancer, *IET Nanobiotechnol.* 5 (2011) 47.

416. I.L. Medintz, H.T. Uyeda, E.R. Goldman, H. Mattoussi, Quantum dot bioconjugates for imaging, labelling and sensing, *Nat. Mater.* 4 (2005) 435–446.

417. H.Z. Wang, H.Y. Wang, R.Q. Liang, K.C. Ruan, Detection of tumor marker CA125 in ovarian carcinoma using quantum dots, *Acta Biochimica et Biophysica Sinica* 36 (2004) 681–686.

418. S.Y. Sung, Y.L. Su, W. Cheng, P.F. Hu, C.S. Chiang, W.T. Chen, et al. Graphene quantum dots-mediated theranostic penetrative delivery of drug and photolytics in deep tumors by targeted biomimetic nanosponges, *Nano Lett* 19 (2019) 69–81.

419. C. Chen, J. Peng, H.S. Xia, G.F. Yang, Q.S. Wu, L.D. Chen, et al. Quantum dots-based immunofluorescence technology for the quantitative determination of HER2 expression in breast cancer, *Biomaterials* 30 (2009) 2912–2918.

420. S. Karaosmanoglu, M. Zhou, B. Shi, X. Zhang, G.R. Williams, X. Chen, Carrier-free nanodrugs for safe and effective cancer treatment, *J. Controlled Release* 329 (2021) 805–832. doi: 10.1016/j.jconrel.2020.10.014.

421. H. Wang, K. Wang, B. Tian, R. Revia, Q.X. Mu, M. Jeon, F.C. Chang, M.Q. Zhang, Preloading of hydrophobic anticancer drug into multifunctional nanocarrier for multimodal imaging, NIR-responsive drug release, and synergistic therapy, *Small* 12 (2016) 6388–6397. doi: 10.1002/smll.201602263.

422. N.I. Marupudi, J.E. Han, K.W. Li, V.M. Renard, B.M. Tyler, H. Brem, Paclitaxel: a review of adverse toxicities and novel delivery strategies, *Expert Opin. Drug Saf.* 6 (2007) 609–621. doi: 10.1517/14740338.6.5.609.

423. S.B. Horwitz, Reflections on my life with taxol, *Cell* 177 (2019) 502–505. doi: 10.1016/j.cell.2019.03.031.

424. C. Luo, J. Sun, B.J. Sun, D. Liu, L. Miao, T.J. Goodwin, L. Huang, Z.G. He, Facile fabrication of tumor redox-sensitive nanoassemblies of small-molecule oleate prodrug as potent chemotherapeutic nanomedicine, *Small* 12 (2016) 6353–6362. doi: 10.1002/smll.201601597.

425. S.C. Lee, K.M. Huh, J. Lee, Y.W. Cho, R.E. Galinsky, K. Park, Hydrotropic polymeric micelles for enhanced paclitaxel solubility: in vitro and in vivo characterization, *Biomacromolecules* 8 (2007) 202–208. doi: 10.1021/bm060307b.

426. M. Skwarczynski, Y. Hayashi, Y. Kiso, Paclitaxel prodrugs: toward smarter delivery of anticancer agents, *J. Med. Chem.* 49 (2006) 7253–7269. doi: 10.1021/jm0602155.

427. J.S. Choi, J.S. Park, Development of docetaxel nanocrystals surface modified with transferrin for tumor targeting, *Drug Des. Dev. Ther.* 11 (2017) 17–26. doi: 10.2147/dddt.s122984.

428. U. Baisch, L. Vella-Zarb, Towards understanding P-gp resistance: a case study of the antitumour drug cabazitaxel. *Crystengcomm* 16 (2014) 10161–10164. doi: 10.1039/c4ce01279h.

429. P. Xue, D. Liu, J. Wang, N. Zhang, J.H. Zhou, L. Li, W.L. Guo, M.C. Sun, X.F. Han, Y.J. Wang, Redox-sensitive citronellol-cabazitaxel conjugate: maintained in vitro cytotoxicity and self-assembled as multifunctional nanomedicine, *Bioconjug. Chem.* 27 (2016) 1360–1372. doi: 10.1021/acs. bioconjchem.6b00155.

430. X.X. Han, F.R. Gong, J. Sun, Y.Q. Li, X.F. Liu, D. Chen, J.W. Liu, Y.L. Shen, Glutathione-responsive core cross-linked micelles for controlled cabazitaxel delivery, *J. Nanopart. Res.* 20 (2018). doi: 10.1007/s11051-018-4128-3.

431. Y. Li, T.Y. Kang, Y.J. Wu, Y.W. Chen, J. Zhu, M.L. Gou, Carbonate esters turn camptothecin-unsaturated fatty acid prodrugs into nanomedicines for cancer therapy, *Chem. Commun.* 54 (2018) 1996–1999. doi: 10.1039/ c8cc00639c.

432. Z.P. Guo, L. Lin, K. Hao, D.W. Wang, F. Liu, P.J. Sun, H.Y. Yu, Z.H. Tang, M. W. Chen, H.Y. Tian, X.S. Chen, Helix self-assembly behavior of amino acid-modified camptothecin prodrugs and its antitumor effect, *ACS Appl. Mater. Interfaces* 12 (2020) 7466–7476. doi: 10.1021/acsami.9b21311.

433. H. Su, P.C. Zhang, A.G. Cheetham, J.M. Koo, R. Lin, A. Masood, P. Schiapparelli, A. Quinones-Hinojosa, H.G. Cui, Supramolecular crafting of self-assembling camptothecin prodrugs with enhanced efficacy against primary cancer cells, *Theranostics* 6 (2016) 1065–1074. doi: 10.7150/thno.15420.

434. Y.X. Zheng, X.L. Yan, Y.L. Wang, X. Duan, X.M. Wang, C.R. Chen, D.M. Tian, Z. H. Luo, Z.L. Zhang, Y.C. Zeng, Hydrophobized SN38 to redox-hypersensitive nanorods for cancer therapy, *J. Mater. Chem. B* 7 (2019) 265–276. doi: 10.1039/c8tb02319k.

435. B.L. Lian, Y. Li, X.H. Zhao, Y.G. Zu, Y. Wang, Y. Zhang, Y.Y. Li, Preparation and optimization of 10-hydroxycamptothecin nanocolloidal particles using antisolvent method combined with high pressure homogenization, *J. Chem.* (2017). doi: 10.1155/2017/5752090.

436. H.D. Wang, J.L. Feng, G.J. Liu, B.Q. Chen, Y.B. Jiang, Q.L. Xie, In vitro and in vivo anti-tumor efficacy of 10-hydroxycamptothecin polymorphic nanoparticle dispersions: shape-and polymorph-dependent cytotoxicity and delivery of 10- hydroxycamptothecin to cancer cells, *Nanomed. Nanotechnol. Biol. Med.* 12 (2016) 881–891. doi: 10.1016/j.nano.2015.12.373.

437. G.F. Li, C.F. Cai, Y.J. Qi, X. Tang, Hydroxyethyl starch-10-hydroxy camptothecin conjugate: synthesis, pharmacokinetics, cytotoxicity and pharmacodynamics research, *Drug Delivery* 23 (2016) 277–284. doi: 10.3109/10717544.2014.911394.

438. Y.P. Fang, C.H. Chuang, Y.J. Wu, H.C. Lin, Y.C. Lu, SN38-loaded < 100 nm targeted liposomes for improving poor solubility and minimizing burst release and toxicity: in vitro and in vivo study, *Int. J. Nanomed.* 13 (2018) 2789–2802. doi: 10.2147/ijn.s158426.

439. N. Duhem, F. Danhier, V. Pourcelle, J.M. Schumers, O. Bertrand, C.S. LeDuff, S. Hoeppener, U.S. Schubert, J.F. Gohy, J. Marchand-Brynaert, V. Preat, Self-assembling doxorubicin-tocopherol succinate prodrug as a new drug delivery system: synthesis, characterization, and in vitro and in vivo anticancer activity, *Bioconjug. Chem.* 25 (2014) 72–81. doi: 10.1021/bc400326y.

440. M. Li, L.W. Zhao, T. Zhang, Y. Shu, Z.G. He, Y. Ma, D. Liu, Y.J. Wan, Redox-sensitive prodrug nanoassemblies based on linoleic acid-modified docetaxel to resist breast cancers, *Acta Pharm. Sin. B* 9 (2019) 421–432. doi: 10.1016/j. apsb.2018.08.008.

441. T. Min, H. Ye, P. Zhang, J. Liu, C. Zhang, W.B. Shen, W. Wang, L.S. Shen, Water-soluble Poly(ethylene glycol) prodrug of pemetrexed: synthesis, characterization, and preliminary cytotoxicity, *J. Appl. Polym. Sci.* 111 (2009) 444–451. doi: 10.1002/app.29047.

442. F. Accardi, D. Toscani, M. Bolzoni, B.D. Palma, F. Aversa, N. Giuliani, Mechanism of action of bortezomib and the new proteasome inhibitors on myeloma cells and the bone microenvironment: impact on myeloma-induced alterations of bone remodeling, *Biomed. Res. Int.* (2015). doi: 10.1155/2015/172458.

443. A. Clavreul, E. Roger, M. Pourbaghi-Masouleh, L. Lemaire, C. Tetaud, P. Menei, Development and characterization of sorafenib-loaded lipid nanocapsules for the treatment of glioblastoma, *Drug Delivery* 25 (2018) 1756–1765. doi: 10.1080/10717544.2018.1507061.

444. A.M. dos Santos, F.C. Carvalho, D.A. Teixeira, D.L. Azevedo, W.M. de Barros, M.P.D. Gremiao, Computational and experimental approaches for development of methotrexate nanosuspensions by bottom-up nanoprecipitation, *Int. J. Pharm.* 524 (2017) 330–338. doi: 10.1016/j. ijpharm.2017.03.068.

445. E. Attari, H. Nosrati, H. Danafar, H.K. Manjili, Methotrexate anticancer drug delivery to breast cancer cell lines by iron oxide magnetic based nanocarrier, *J. Biomed. Mater. Res. A* 107 (2019) 2492–2500. doi: 10.1002/jbm. a.36755.

446. X. Duan, X. Yang, C.F. Li, L.H. Song, Highly water-soluble methotrexate-polyethyleneglycol-rhodamine prodrug micelle for high tumor inhibition activity, *AAPS Pharm. Sci. Technol.* 20 (2019). doi: 10.1208/s12249-019-1462-4.

447. R.M. Moshikur, M.R. Chowdhury, R. Wakabayashi, Y. Tahara, M. Moniruzzaman, M. Goto, Ionic liquids with methotrexate moieties as a potential anticancer prodrug: synthesis, characterization and solubility evaluation, *J. Mol. Liq.* 278 (2019) 226–233. doi: 10.1016/j.molliq.2019.01.063.

448. C.Y. Liu, Z. Chen, Y.J. Chen, J. Lu, Y. Li, S.J. Wang, G.L. Wu, F. Qian, Improving oral bioavailability of sorafenib by optimizing the "Spring" and "Parachute" based on molecular interaction mechanisms, *Mol. Pharm.* 13 (2016) 599–608. doi: 10.1021/acs.molpharmaceut.5b00837.

449. A.K. Deshantri, J.M. Metselaar, S. Zagkou, G. Storm, S.N. Mandhane, M.H.A. M. Fens, R.M. Schiffelers, Development and characterization of liposomal formulation of bortezomib, *Int. J. Pharm. X* 1 (2019) 100011. doi: 10.1016/j.ijpx.2019.100011.

450. C. Buhrmann, A. Mobasheri, F. Busch, C. Aldinger, R. Stahlmann, A. Montaseri, M. Shakibaei, Curcumin modulates nuclear factor kappa B (NF-kappa B)- mediated inflammation in human tenocytes in vitro role of the phosphatidylinositol 3-kinase/Akt pathway, *J. Biol. Chem.* 286 (2011) 28556–28566. doi: 10.1074/jbc.M111.256180.

451. S. Ganta, M. Amiji, Coadministration of paclitaxel and curcumin in nanoemulsion formulations to overcome multidrug resistance in tumor cells, *Mol. Pharm.* 6 (2009) 928–939. doi: 10.1021/mp800240j.

452. Y.L. Lu, S.M. Wu, B.D. Xiang, L.Q. Li, Y.Z. Lin, Curcumin attenuates oxaliplatin-induced liver injury and oxidative stress by activating the Nrf2 pathway, *Drug Des. Dev. Ther.* 14 (2020) 73–85. doi: 10.2147/dddt.s224318.

453. G.H. Shin, J. Li, J.H. Cho, J.T. Kim, H.J. Park, Enhancement of curcumin solubility by phase change from crystalline to amorphous in Cur-TPGS nanosuspension. *J. Food Sci.* 81 (2016) N494–N501. doi: 10.1111/ 1750-3841.13208.

454. C. Souza, D.S. Pellosi, A.C. Tedesco, Prodrugs for targeted cancer therapy, *Expert Rev. Anticancer Ther.* 19 (2019) 483–502. doi: 10.1080/ 14737140.2019.1615890.

455. Z.G. Wang, Z.Q. Deng, G.Y. Zhu, Emerging platinum(IV) prodrugs to combat cisplatin resistance: from isolated cancer cells to tumor microenvironment, *Dalton Trans.* 48 (2019) 2536–2544. doi: 10.1039/c8dt03923b.

456. L. Zitvogel, L. Apetoh, F. Ghiringhelli, G. Kroemer, Immunological aspects of cancer chemotherapy, *Nat. Rev. Immunol.* 8 (2008) 59–73. doi: 10.1038/nri2216.

457. B.Y. Liu, L. Ezeogu, L. Zellmer, B.F. Yu, N.Z. Xu, D.J. Liao, Protecting the normal in order to better kill the cancer, *Cancer Med.* 4 (2015) 1394–1403. doi: 10.1002/cam4.488.

458. K.B. Sutradhar, M.L. Amin, Nanotechnology in cancer drug delivery and selective targeting. *ISRN Nanotechnol.* 2014 (2014) 939378. doi: 10.1155/ 2014/939378.

459. S. Dragojevic, J.S. Ryu, D. Raucher, Polymer-based prodrugs: improving tumor targeting and the solubility of small molecule drugs in cancer therapy, *Molecules* 20 (2015) 21750–21769. doi: 10.3390/molecules201219804.

460. F. Di Costanzo, S. Gasperoni, V. Rotella, Targeted delivery of albumin bound paclitaxel in the treatment of advanced breast cancer, *Oncotargets Ther.* 2 (2009) 179–188. doi: 10.2147/OTT.S3863.

461. M.W. Saif, L.S. Rosen, K. Saito, C. Zergebel, L. Ravage-Mass, D.S. Mendelson, A phase I study evaluating the effect of CDHP as a component of S-1 on the pharmacokinetics of 5-fluorouracil, *Anticancer Res.* 31 (2011) 625–632.

462. R. Oun, Y.E. Moussa, N.J. Wheate, The side effects of platinum-based chemotherapy drugs: a review for chemists, *Dalton Trans.* 47 (2018) 6645–6653. doi: 10.1039/ c8dt00838h.

463. J. Delahousse, C. Skarbek, A. Paci, Prodrugs as drug delivery system in oncology, *Cancer Chemother Pharmacol.* 84 (2019) 937–958. doi: 10.1007/ s00280-019-03906-2.

464. Q. Zhou, C. Dong, W. Fan, H. Jiang, J. Xiang, N. Qiu, Y. Piao, T. Xie, Y. Luo, Z. Li, F. Liu, Y. Shen, Tumor extravasation and infiltration as barriers of nanomedicine for high efficacy: the current status and transcytosis strategy, *Biomaterials* 240 (2020). doi: 10.1016/j.biomaterials.2020.119902.

465. J. Zhou, A.V. Kroll, M. Holay, R.H. Fang, L. Zhang, Biomimetic nanotechnology toward personalized vaccines, *Adv. Mater* 32 (2020). doi: 10.1002/ adma.201901255.

466. X. Qi, X. Liu, L. Matiski, R.R. Del Villar, T. Yip, F. Zhang, S. Sokalingam, S. Jiang, L. Liu, H. Yan, Y. Chang, RNA origami nanostructures for potent and safe anticancer immunotherapy, *ACS Nano* 14 (2020) 4727–4740. doi: 10.1021/acsnano.0c00602.

467. S.G. Carvalho, V.H. Sousa Araujo, A.M. dos Santos, J.L. Duarte, A.L. Polli Silvestre, B. Fonseca-Santos, J.C. Oliveira Villanova, M.P. Daflon Gremiao, M. Chorilli, Advances and challenges in nanocarriers and nanomedicines for veterinary application, *Int. J. Pharm.* 580 (2020). doi: 10.1016/j. ijpharm.2020.119214.

468. M.C. Scicluna, L. Vella-Zarb, Evolution of nanocarrier drug-delivery systems and recent advancements in covalent organic framework-drug systems, *ACS Appl. Nano Mater.* 3 (2020) 3097–3115. doi: 10.1021/acsanm.9b02603.

469. F.L.O. Da Silva, M.B.D. Marques, K.C. Kato, G. Carneiro, Nanonization techniques to overcome poor water-solubility with drugs, *Expert Opin. Drug Discovery* (2020). doi: 10.1080/17460441.2020.1750591.

470. Y. Saadeh, T. Leung, A. Vyas, L.S. Chaturvedi, O. Perumal, D. Vyas, Applications of nanomedicine in breast cancer detection, imaging, and therapy, *J. Nanosci. Nanotechnol.* 14 (2014) 913–923. doi: 10.1166/jnn.2014.8755.

471. X.S. Liu, I.V. Tang, Z.A. Wainberg, H. Meng, Safety considerations of cancer nanomedicine-a key step toward translation, *Small* (2020). doi: 10.1002/smll.202000673.

472. N. Hoshyar, S. Gray, H.B. Han, G. Bao, The effect of nanoparticle size on in vivo pharmacokinetics and cellular interaction, *Nanomedicine* 11 (2016) 673–692. doi: 10.2217/ nnm.16.5.

473. P. Ma, R.J. Mumper, Paclitaxel nano-delivery systems: a comprehensive review, *J. Nanomed. Nanotechnol.* 4 (2013) 1000164. doi: 10.4172/2157-7439.1000164.

474. A. Zugic, V. Tadic, S. Savic, Nano- and microcarriers as drug delivery systems for usnic acid: review of literature, *Pharmaceutics* 12 (2020). doi: 10.3390/ pharmaceutics12020156.

475. S.H. Shen, Y.S. Wu, Y.C. Liu, D.C. Wu, High drug-loading nanomedicines: progress, current status, and prospects, *Int. J. Nanomed.* 12 (2017) 4085–4109. doi: 10.2147/ijn. s132780.

476. L. Yan, M. Zhou, X. Zhang, L. Huang, W. Chen, V.A.L. Roy, W. Zhang, X. Chen, A novel type of aqueous dispersible ultrathin-layered double hydroxide nanosheets for in vivo bioimaging and drug delivery, *ACS Appl. Mater. Interfaces* 9 (2017) 34185–34193. doi: 10.1021/acsami.7b05294.

477. L. Yan, S. Gonca, G. Zhu, W. Zhang, X. Chen, Layered double hydroxide nanostructures and nanocomposites for biomedical applications. *J. Mater Chem. B* 7 (2019) 5583–5601. doi: 10.1039/c9tb01312a.

478. R. Ma, Z. Wang, L. Yan, X. Chen, G. Zhu, Novel Pt-loaded layered double hydroxide nanoparticles for efficient and cancer-cell specific delivery of a cisplatin prodrug. *J. Mater Chem. B* 2 (2014) 4868–4875. doi: 10.1039/c4tb00645c.

479. U. Wais, A.W. Jackson, T. He, H.F. Zhang, Nanoformulation and encapsulation approaches for poorly water-soluble drug nanoparticles, *Nanoscale* 8 (2016) 1746–1769. doi: 10.1039/ c5nr07161e.

480. X.F. Lu, Y. Zhu, R. Bai, Z.S. Wu, W.C. Qian, L.Y. Yang, R. Cai, H. Yan, T. Li, V. Pandey, Y. Liu, P.E. Lobie, C.Y. Chen, T. Zhu, Long-term pulmonary exposure to multi-walled carbon nanotubes promotes breast cancer metastatic cascades, *Nat. Nanotechnol.* 14 (2019) 719. doi: 10.1038/ s41565-019-0472-4.

481. M.J. Ramalho, S. Andrade, J.A. Loureiro, M.D.C. Pereira, Nanotechnology to improve the Alzheimer's disease therapy with natural compounds, *Drug Del. Transl. Res.* 10 (2020) 380–402. doi: 10.1007/s13346-019-00694-3.

482. Y. Zheng, X. You, S. Guan, J. Huang, L. Wang, J. Zhang, J. Wu, Poly(ferulic acid) with an anticancer effect as a drug nanocarrier for enhanced colon cancer therapy, *Adv. Funct. Mater.* 29 (2019). doi: 10.1002/ adfm.201808646.

483. X. Nan, X. Zhang, Y. Liu, M. Zhou, X. Chen, X. Zhang, Dual-targeted multifunctional nanoparticles for magnetic resonance imaging guided cancer diagnosis and therapy, *ACS Appl. Mater. Interfaces* 9 (2017) 9986–9995. doi: 10.1021/acsami.6b16486.

484. M. Zhou, X. Zhang, C. Yu, X. Nan, X. Chen, X. Zhang, Shape regulated anticancer activities and systematic toxicities of drug nanocrystals in vivo, *Nanomedicine* 12 (2016) 181–189. doi: 10.1016/j.nano.2015.09.006.

485. W. Wei, X. Zhang, X. Chen, M. Zhou, R. Xu, X. Zhang, Smart surface coating of drug nanoparticles with cross-linkable polyethylene glycol for bio-responsive and highly efficient drug delivery, *Nanoscale* 8 (2016) 8118–8125. doi: 10.1039/c5nr09167e.

486. Z. Gao, T. He, P. Zhang, X. Li, Y. Zhang, J. Lin, J. Hao, P. Huang, J. Cui, Polypeptide-based theranostics with tumor-microenvironment-activatable cascade reaction for chemo-ferroptosis combination therapy, *ACS Appl. Mater. Interfaces* 12 (2020) 20271–20280. doi: 10.1021/acsami.0c03748.

487. R. Zhu, L. Su, J. Dai, Z.-W. Li, S. Bai, Q. Li, X. Chen, J. Song, H. Yang, Biologically responsive plasmonic assemblies for second near-infrared window photoacoustic imaging-guided concurrent chemo-immunotherapy, *ACS Nano* 14 (2020) 3991–4006. doi: 10.1021/acsnano.9b07984.

488. S.Y. Qin, A.Q. Zhang, S.X. Cheng, L. Rong, X.Z. Zhang, Drug self-delivery systems for cancer therapy, *Biomaterials* 112 (2017) 234–247. doi: 10.1016/j.biomaterials.2016.10.016.

489. C. Yu, M. Zhou, X. Zhang, W. Wei, X. Chen, X. Zhang, Smart doxorubicin nanoparticles with high drug payload for enhanced chemotherapy against drug resistance and cancer diagnosis, *Nanoscale* 7 (2015) 5683–5690. doi: 10.1039/c5nr00290g.

490. C. Gao, P. Bhattarai, M. Chen, N.S. Zhang, S. Hameed, X.L. Yue, Z.F. Dai, Amphiphilic drug conjugates as nanomedicines for combined cancer therapy, *Bioconjug. Chem.* 29 (2018) 3967–3981. doi: 10.1021/acs.bioconjchem.8b00692.

491. M. Zhou, X. Zhang, Y. Yang, Z. Liu, B. Tian, J. Jie, X. Zhang, Carrier-free functionalized multidrug nanorods for synergistic cancer therapy, *Biomaterials* 34 (2013) 8960–8967. doi: 10.1016/j.biomaterials.2013.07.080.

492. J.F. Zhang, S.L. Li, F.F. An, J. Liu, S.B. Jin, J.C. Zhang, P.C. Wang, X.H. Zhang, C. S. Lee, X.J. Liang, Self-carried curcumin nanoparticles for in vitro and in vivo cancer therapy with real-time monitoring of drug release, *Nanoscale* 7 (2015) 13503–13510. doi: 10.1039/c5nr03259h.

493. Y.Q. Liu, X.J. Zhang, M.J. Zhou, X.Y. Nan, X.F. Chen, X.H. Zhang, Mitochondrial-targeting lonidamine-doxorubicin nanoparticles for synergistic chemotherapy to conquer drug resistance, *ACS Appl. Mater. Interfaces* 9 (2017) 43498–43507. doi: 10.1021/acsami.7b14577.

494. I.M. Tynga, H. Abrahamse, Nano-mediated photodynamic therapy for cancer: enhancement of cancer specificity and therapeutic effects, *Nanomaterials* 8 (2018). doi: 10.3390/nano8110923.

495. Z.T. Zhang, R.Y. Wang, X.X. Huang, R.J. Luo, J.W. Xue, J. Gao, W.Y. Liu, F.L. Liu, F. Feng, W. Qu, Self-delivered and self-monitored chemo-photodynamic nanoparticles with light-triggered synergistic antitumor therapies by downregulation of HIF-1 alpha and depletion of GSH, *ACS Appl. Mater. Interfaces* 12 (2020) 5680–5694. doi: 10.1021/acsami.9b23325.

496. D. Dolmans, D. Fukumura, R.K. Jain, Photodynamic therapy for cancer, *Nat. Rev. Cancer* 3 (2003) 380–387. doi: 10.1038/nrc1071.

497. Y. Wang, P.F. Yang, X.R. Zhao, D. Gao, N. Sun, Z.M. Tian, T.Y. Ma, Z. Yang, Multifunctional cargo-free nanomedicine for cancer therapy, *Int. J. Mol. Sci.* 19 (2018). doi: 10.3390/ijms19102963.

498. M. Sivasubramanian, Y.C. Chuang, L.W. Lo, Evolution of nanoparticle-mediated photodynamic therapy: from superficial to deep-seated cancers, *Molecules* 24 (2019). doi: 10.3390/molecules24030520.

499. R.Y. Zhang, R.R. Xing, T.F. Jiao, K. Ma, C.J. Chen, G.H. Ma, X.H. Yan, Carrier-free, chemophotodynamic dual nanodrugs via self-assembly for synergistic antitumor therapy, *ACS Appl. Mater. Interfaces* 8 (2016) 13262–13269. doi: 10.1021/acsami.6b02416.

500. Y. Zhao, Y. Zhao, Q. Ma, H. Zhang, Y. Liu, J. Hong, Z. Ding, M. Liu, J. Han, Novel carrier-free nanoparticles composed of 7-ethyl-10-hydroxycamptothecin and chlorin e6: self-assembly mechanism investigation and in vitro/in vivo evaluation, *Colloids Surf. B Biointerfaces* 188 (2020) 110722. doi: 10.1016/j.colsurfb.2019.110722.

501. Y. Wen, W. Zhang, N.Q. Gong, Y.F. Wang, H.B. Guo, W.S. Guo, P.C. Wang, X. J. Liang, Carrier-free, self-assembled pure drug nanorods composed of 10- hydroxycamptothecin and chlorin e6 for combinatorial chemo-photodynamic antitumor therapy in vivo, *Nanoscale* 9 (2017) 14347–14356. doi: 10.1039/c7nr03129g.

502. Y.Y. Li, X.L. Hu, X.H. Zheng, Y. Liu, S. Liu, Y. Yue, Z.G. Xie, Self-assembled organic nanorods for dual chemo-photodynamic therapies, *RSC Adv.* 8 (2018) 5493–5499. doi: 10.1039/c8ra00067k.

503. J.F. Zhang, Y.C. Liang, X.D. Lin, X.Y. Zhu, L. Yan, S.L. Li, X. Yang, G.Y. Zhu, A. L. Rogach, P.K.N. Yu, P. Shi, L.C. Tu, C.C. Chang, X.H. Zhang, X.F. Chen, W. J. Zhang, C.S. Lee, Self-monitoring and self-delivery of photosensitizer-doped nanoparticles for highly effective combination cancer therapy in vitro and in vivo, *ACS Nano* 9 (2015) 9741–9756. doi: 10.1021/acsnano.5b02513.

504. X.B. Zhang, N. Li, S.W. Zhang, B.J. Sun, Q. Chen, Z.G. He, C. Luo, J. Sun, Emerging carrier-free nanosystems based on molecular self-assembly of pure drugs for cancer therapy, *Med. Res. Rev.* (2020). doi: 10.1002/med.21669.

505. J.F. Lin, C. Li, Y. Guo, J.J. Zou, P.Y. Wu, Y.Q. Liao, B.C. Zhang, J.Q. Le, R.R. Zhao, J.W. Shao, Carrier-free nanodrugs for in vivo NIR bioimaging and chemo-photothermal synergistic therapy, *J. Mater. Chem. B.* 7 (2019) 6914–6923. doi: 10.1039/c9tb00687g.

506. Y.J. Li, C. Ayala-Orozco, P.R. Rauta, S. Krishnan, The application of nanotechnology in enhancing immunotherapy for cancer treatment: current effects and perspective, *Nanoscale* 11 (2019) 17157–17178. doi: 10.1039/c9nr05371a.

507. B. Wiemann, C.O. Starnes, Coleys toxins, tumor-necrosis-factor and cancer-research: a historical-perspective, *Pharmacol. Ther.* 64 (1994) 529–564. doi: 10.1016/0163-7258(94)90023-x.

508. Y. Zhu, L. Xing, X. Zheng, C.X. Yang, Y.J. He, T.J. Zhou, Q.R. Jin, H.L. Jiang, Amplification of tumor antigen presentation by NLGplatin to improve chemoimmunotherapy, *Int. J. Pharm.* 573 (2020). doi: 10.1016/j.ijpharm.2019.118736.

509. M. Saeed, J. Gao, Y. Shi, T. Lammers, H.J. Yu, Engineering nanoparticles to reprogram the tumor immune microenvironment for improved cancer immunotherapy, *Theranostics* 9 (2019) 7981–8000. doi: 10.7150/thno.37568.

510. J. Gao, W.Q. Wang, Q. Pei, M.S. Lord, H.J. Yu, Engineering nanomedicines through boosting immunogenic cell death for improved cancer immunotherapy, *Acta Pharmacol. Sin.* (2020). doi: 10.1038/s41401-020-0400-z.

511. C. Zhang, L. Long, Y. Xiong, C. Wang, C. Peng, Y. Yuan, Z. Liu, Y. Lin, Y. Jia, X. Zhou, X. Li, Facile engineering of indomethacin-induced paclitaxel nanocrystal aggregates as carrier-free nanomedicine with improved synergetic antitumor activity, *ACS Appl. Mater. Interfaces* 11 (2019) 9872–9883. doi: 10.1021/acsami.8b22336.

512. F.Y. Huang, J. Lei, Y. Sun, F. Yan, B. Chen, L.M. Zhang, Z.X. Lu, R. Cao, Y.Y. Lin, C.C. Wang, G.H. Tan, Induction of enhanced immunogenic cell death through ultrasound-controlled release of doxorubicin by liposome-microbubble complexes, *Oncoimmunology* 7 (2018). doi: 10.1080/2162402x.2018.1446720.

513. B. Feng, Z.F. Niu, B. Hou, L. Zhou, Y.P. Li, H.J. Yu, Enhancing triple negative breast cancer immunotherapy by ICG-templated self-assembly of paclitaxel nanoparticles, *Adv. Funct. Mater.* 30 (2020). doi: 10.1002/adfm.201906605.

514. Y. Wang, Y. Wu, K. Li, S. Shen, Z. Liu, D. Wu, Ultralong circulating lollipop-like nanoparticles assembled with gossypol, doxorubicin, and polydopamine via π-π stacking for synergistic tumor therapy, *Adv. Funct. Mater.* 29 (2019). doi: 10.1002/adfm.201805582.

515. Y. He, M. Wang, X. Li, T. Yu, X. Gao, Targeted MIP-3beta plasmid nanoparticles induce dendritic cell maturation and inhibit M2 macrophage polarisation to suppress cancer growth, *Biomaterials* 249 (2020). doi: 10.1016/j.biomaterials.2020.120046, 120046.

516. S. Fang, Y. Hou, L. Ling, D. Wang, M. Ismail, Y. Du, Y. Zhang, C. Yao, X. Li, Dimeric camptothecin derived phospholipid assembled liposomes with high drug loading for cancer therapy, *Colloids Surf B: Biointerfaces* 166 (2018) 235–244. doi: 10.1016/j.colsurfb.2018.02.046.

517. X. He, J. Zhang, C. Li, Y. Zhang, Y. Lu, Y. Zhang, L. Liu, C. Ruan, Q. Chen, X. Chen, Q. Guo, T. Sun, J. Cheng, C. Jiang, Enhanced bioreduction-responsive diselenide-based dimeric prodrug nanoparticles for triple negative breast cancer therapy, *Theranostics* 8 (2018) 4884–4897. doi: 10.7150/thno.27581.

518. T. Xu, Y.Y. Ma, Q.L. Yuan, H.X. Hu, X.K. Hu, Z.Y. Qian, J.K. Rolle, Y.Q. Gu, S. W. Li, Enhanced ferroptosis by oxygen-boosted phototherapy based on a 2-in-1 nanoplatform of ferrous hemoglobin for tumor synergistic therapy, *ACS Nano* 14 (2020) 3414–3425. doi: 10.1021/acsnano.9b09426.

519. Y.J. Wang, D. Liu, Q.C. Zheng, Q. Zhao, H.J. Zhang, Y. Ma, J.K. Fallon, Q. Fu, M. T. Haynes, G.M. Lin, R. Zhang, D. Wang, X.G. Yang, L.X. Zhao, Z.G. He, F. Liu, Disulfide bond bridge insertion turns hydrophobic anticancer prodrugs into self-assembled nanomedicines, *Nano Lett.* 14 (2014) 5577–5583. doi: 10.1021/nl502044x.

520. Q. Pei, X. Hu, S. Liu, Y. Li, Z. Xie, X. Jing, Paclitaxel dimers assembling nanomedicines for treatment of cervix carcinoma, *J. Controlled Release* 254 (2017) 23–33. doi: 10.1016/j.jconrel.2017.03.391.

521. F. Seidi, R. Jenjob, D. Crespy, Designing smart polymer conjugates for controlled release of payloads, *Chem. Rev.* 118 (2018) 3965–4036. doi: 10.1021/acs.chemrev.8b00006.

522. Q. Pei, X.L. Hu, J.L. Zhou, S. Liu, Z.G. Xie, Glutathione-responsive paclitaxel dimer nanovesicles with high drug content, *Biomater. Sci.* 5 (2017) 1517–1521. doi: 10.1039/c7bm00052a.

523. Q. Pei, X. Hu, X. Zheng, S. Liu, Y. Li, X. Jing, Z. Xie, Light-activatable red blood cell membrane-camouflaged dimeric prodrug nanoparticles for synergistic photodynamic/chemotherapy, *ACS Nano* 12 (2018) 1630–1641. doi: 10.1021/acsnano.7b08219.

524. H.B. Zhang, Y.B. Zhang, Y.L. Chen, Y. Zhang, Y.G. Wang, Y.Y. Zhang, L. Song, B. L. Jiang, G.H. Su, Y. Li, Z.Q. Hou, Glutathione-responsive self-delivery nanoparticles assembled by curcumin dimer for enhanced intracellular drug delivery, *Int. J. Pharm.* 549 (2018) 230–238. doi: 10.1016/j.ijpharm.2018.07.061.

525. J.G. Li, X.M. Li, P. Liu, Doxorubicin-doxorubicin conjugate prodrug as drug self-delivery system for intracellular pH-triggered slow release, *Colloids Surf B: Biointerfaces* 185 (2020). doi: 10.1016/j.colsurfb.2019.110608.

526. H. Kasai, T. Murakami, Y. Ikuta, Y. Koseki, K. Baba, H. Oikawa, H. Nakanishi, M. Okada, M. Shoji, M. Ueda, H. Imahori, M. Hashida, Creation of pure nanodrugs and their anticancer properties, *Angew Chem. Int. Ed.* 51 (2012) 10315–10318. doi: 10.1002/anie.201204596.

527. Y. Li, J. Lin, Z. Fan, Y. Li, L. Song, Z. Hou, A small molecule nanodrug consisting of amphiphilic drug-drug conjugate for self-targeted multi-drug delivery and synergistic anticancer effect, *J. Controlled Release* 259 (2017). doi: 10.1016/j.jconrel.2017.03.375. E191.

528. W. Qu, Q. Yang, G. Wang, Z. Wang, P. Huang, W. Huang, R. Zhang, D. Yan, Amphiphilic irinotecan-melampomagnolide B conjugate nanoparticles for cancer chemotherapy, *RSC Adv.* 10 (2020) 8958–8966. doi: 10.1039/ d0ra00912a.

529. T. Idowu, G. Arthur, G.G. Zhanel, F. Schweizer, Heterodimeric Rifampicin- Tobramycin conjugates break intrinsic resistance of Pseudomonas aeruginosa to doxycycline and chloramphenicol in vitro and in a Galleria mellonella in vivo model, *Eur. J. Med. Chem.* 174 (2019) 16–32. doi: 10.1016/j. ejmech.2019.04.034.

530. J. Xi, H. Liu, Recent advances in the design of self-delivery amphiphilic drugs and vaccines, *Adv. Ther.* 3 (2019). doi: 10.1002/adtp.201900107.

531. H. Mao, Y. Xie, H. Ju, H. Mao, L. Zhao, Z. Wang, L. Hua, C. Zhao, Y. Li, R. Yu, H. Liu, Design of tumor microenvironment-responsive drug-drug micelle for cancer radiochemotherapy, *ACS Appl. Mater. Interfaces* 10 (2018) 33923–33935. doi: 10.1021/acsami.8b11159.

532. J. Zhang, P. Zhang, Q. Zou, X. Li, J.J. Fu, Y. Luo, X.L. Liang, Y. Jin, Co-delivery of gemcitabine and paclitaxel in cRGD-modified long circulating nanoparticles with asymmetric lipid layers for breast cancer treatment, *Molecules* 23 (2018). doi: 10.3390/molecules23112906.

533. S. Dong, J. He, Y. Sun, D. Li, L. Li, M. Zhang, P. Ni, Efficient click synthesis of a protonized and reduction-sensitive amphiphilic small-molecule prodrug containing camptothecin and gemcitabine for a drug self-delivery system, *Mol. Pharm.* 16 (2019) 3770–3779. doi: 10.1021/acs.molpharmaceut.9b00349.

534. Y. Wang, P. Huang, M.X. Hu, W. Huang, X.Y. Zhu, D.Y. Yan, Self-delivery nanoparticles of amphiphilic methotrexate-gemcitabine prodrug for synergistic combination chemotherapy via effect of deoxyribonucleotide pools, *Bioconjug. Chem.* 27 (2016) 2722–2733. doi: 10.1021/acs.bioconjchem.6b00503.

535. Y. Li, J. Lin, J. Ma, L. Song, H. Lin, B. Tang, D. Chen, G. Su, S. Ye, X. Zhu, F. Luo, Z. Hou, Methotrexate-camptothecin prodrug nanoassemblies as a versatile nanoplatform for

biomodal imaging-guided self-active targeted and synergistic chemotherapy, *ACS Appl. Mater. Interfaces* 9 (2017) 34650–34665. doi: 10.1021/acsami.7b10027.

536. X. Liang, C. Gao, L. Cui, S. Wang, J. Wang, Z. Dai, Self-assembly of an amphiphilic janus camptothecin-floxuridine conjugate into liposome-like nanocapsules for more efficacious combination chemotherapy in cancer, *Adv. Mater.* 29 (2017). doi: 10.1002/adma.201703135.

537. Y. Wang, J. Wang, L. Yang, W. Wei, B. Sun, K. Na, Y. Song, H. Zhang, Z. He, J. Sun, Y. Wang, Redox dual-responsive paclitaxel-doxorubicin heterodimeric prodrug self-delivery nanoaggregates for more effective breast cancer synergistic combination chemotherapy, *Nanomedicine* 21 (2019) 102066. doi: 10.1016/j.nano.2019.102066.

538. M. Zhou, W. Wei, X. Chen, X. Xu, X. Zhang, X. Zhang, pH and redox dual responsive carrier-free anticancer drug nanoparticles for targeted delivery and synergistic therapy, *Nanomedicine* 20 (2019) 102008. doi: 10.1016/j. nano.2019.04.011.

539. C. Luo, B.J. Sun, C. Wang, X.B. Zhang, Y. Chen, Q. Chen, H. Yu, H.Q. Zhao, M. C. Sun, Z.B. Li, H.T. Zhang, Q.M. Kan, Y.J. Wang, Z.G. He, J. Sun, Self-facilitated ROS-responsive nanoassembly of heterotypic dimer for synergistic chemo-photodynamic therapy, *J. Controlled Release* 302 (2019) 79–89. doi: 10.1016/j.jconrel.2019.04.001.

540. X.D. Xue, Y. Huang, R.N. Bo, B. Jia, H. Wu, Y. Yuan, Z.L. Wang, Z. Ma, D. Jing, X. B. Xu, W.M. Yu, T.Y. Lin, Y.P. Li, Trojan Horse nanotheranostics with dual transformability and multifunctionality for highly effective cancer treatment, *Nat. Commun.* 9 (2018). doi: 10.1038/s41467-018-06093-5.

541. Q. Pei, X.L. Hu, X.H. Zheng, R. Xia, S. Liu, Z.G. Xie, X.B. Jing, Albumin-bound paclitaxel dimeric prodrug nanoparticles with tumor redox heterogeneity-triggered drug release for synergistic photothermal/chemotherapy, *Nano Res.* 12 (2019) 877–887. doi: 10.1007/s12274-019-2318-7.

542. S.Y. Han, K.Q. Huang, Z.P. Gu, J. Wu, Tumor immune microenvironment modulation-based drug delivery strategies for cancer immunotherapy, *Nanoscale* 12 (2020) 413–436. doi: 10.1039/c9nr08086d.

543. T.O.B. Olusanya, R.R.H. Ahmad, D.M. Ibegbu, J.R. Smith, A.A. Elkordy, Liposomal drug delivery systems and anticancer drugs, *Molecules* 23 (2018). doi: 10.3390/molecules23040907.

544. S. Li, X. Shan, Y. Wang, Q. Chen, J. Sun, Z. He, B. Sun, C. Luo, Dimeric prodrug-based nanomedicines for cancer therapy, *J. Controlled Release* 326 (2020) 510–522. doi: 10.1016/j.jconrel.2020.07.036.

545. T. Zhong, Y.L. Hao, X. Yao, S. Zhang, X.C. Duan, Y.F. Yin, M.Q. Xu, Y. Guo, Z.T. Li, X.C. Zheng, H. Li, X. Zhang, Effect of XlogP and hansen solubility parameters on small molecule modified paclitaxel anticancer drug conjugates self-assembled into nanoparticles, *Bioconjug. Chem.* 29 (2018) 437–444. doi: 10.1021/acs.bioconjchem.7b00767.

546. F. Dosio, L.H. Reddy, A. Ferrero, B. Stella, L. Cattel, P. Couvreur, Novel nanoassemblies composed of squalenoyl-paclitaxel derivatives: synthesis, characterization, and biological evaluation, *Bioconjug. Chem.* 21 (2010)1349–1361. doi: 10.1021/bc100154g.

547. C. Luo, J. Sun, D. Liu, B.J. Sun, L. Miao, S. Musetti, J. Li, X.P. Han, Y.Q. Du, L. Li, L. Huang, Z.G. He, Self-assembled redox dual-responsive prodrug-nanosystem formed by single thioether-bridged paclitaxel-fatty acid conjugate for cancer chemotherapy, *Nano Lett.* 16 (2016) 5401–5408. doi: 10.1021/acs. nanolett.6b01632.

548. Y. Jiang, X.Z. Wang, X. Liu, W. Lv, H.J. Zhang, M.W. Zhang, X.R. Li, H.L. Xin, Q.W. Xu, Enhanced antiglioma efficacy of ultrahigh loading capacity paclitaxel prodrug conjugate self-assembled targeted nanoparticles, *ACS Appl. Mater. Interfaces* 9 (2017) 211–217. doi: 10.1021/acsami.6b13805.

549. X.F. Han, J.L. Chen, M.J. Jiang, N. Zhang, K.X. Na, C. Luo, R.S. Zhang, M.C. Sun, G.M. Lin, R. Zhang, Y. Ma, D. Liu, Y.J. Wang, Paclitaxel-paclitaxel prodrug nanoassembly as a versatile nanoplatform for combinational cancer therapy, *ACS Appl. Mater Interfaces* 8 (2016) 33506–33513. doi: 10.1021/ acsami.6b13057.

550. D. Dheer, D. Arora, S. Jaglan, R.K. Rawal, R. Shankar, Polysaccharides based nanomaterials for targeted anticancer drug delivery. *J. Drug Target* 25 (2017) 1–16. doi: 10.3109/1061186x.2016.1172589.

551. B. Posocco, E. Dreussi, J. de Santa, G. Toffoli, M. Abrami, F. Musiani, M. Grassi, R. Farra, F. Tonon, G. Grassi, B. Dapas, Polysaccharides for the delivery of antitumor drugs, *Materials* 8 (2015) 2569–2615. doi: 10.3390/ma8052569.

552. Y.J. Su, Y. Liu, X.T. Xu, J.P. Zhou, L. Xu, X.L. Xu, D. Wang, M. Li, K.R. Chen, W. Wang, On-demand versatile prodrug nanomicelle for tumor-specific bioimaging and photothermal-chemo synergistic cancer therapy, *ACS Appl. Mater. Interfaces* 10 (2018) 38700–38714. doi: 10.1021/ acsami.8b11349.

553. Y. Yan, Y.Y. Dong, S.J. Yue, X.Y. Qiu, H.L. Sun, Z.Y. Zhong, Dually active targeting nanomedicines based on a direct conjugate of two purely natural ligands for potent chemotherapy of ovarian tumors, *ACS Appl. Mater. Interfaces* 11 (2019) 46548–46557. doi: 10.1021/acsami.9b17223.

554. M.R. Huo, H.L. Wang, Y. Zhang, H. Cai, P. Zhang, L.C. Li, J.P. Zhou, T.J. Yin, Co-delivery of silybin and paclitaxel by dextran-based nanoparticles for effective anti-tumor treatment through chemotherapy sensitization and microenvironment modulation, *J. Controlled Release* 321 (2020) 198–210. doi: 10.1016/j. jconrel.2020.02.017.

555. Y.X. Tang, Y.H. Li, R. Xu, S. Li, H. Hu, C. Xiao, H.L. Wu, L. Zhu, J.X. Ming, Z. Chu, H.Q. Xu, X.L. Yang, Z.F. Li, Self-assembly of folic acid dextran conjugates for cancer chemotherapy, *Nanoscale* 10 (2018) 17265–17274. doi: 10.1039/c8nr04657c.

556. L. Rong, S.Y. Qin, C. Zhang, Y.J. Cheng, J. Feng, S.B. Wang, X.Z. Zhang, Biomedical applications of functional peptides in nano-systems, *Mater Today Chem.* 9 (2018) 91–102. doi: 10.1016/j.mtchem.2018.06.001.

557. P. Laakkonen, K. Vuorinen, Homing peptides as targeted delivery vehicles, *Integr. Biol.* 2 (2010) 326–337. doi: 10.1039/c0ib00013b.

558. X.X. Zhang, H.S. Eden, X.Y. Chen, Peptides in cancer nanomedicine: drug carriers, targeting ligands and protease substrates, *J. Controlled Release* 159 (2012) 2–13. doi: 10.1016/j.jconrel.2011.10.023.

559. S.Y. Qin, A.Q. Zhang, X.Z. Zhang, Recent advances in targeted tumor chemotherapy based on smart nanomedicines, *Small* 14 (2018). doi: 10.1002/smll.201802417.

560. H. Hu, B. Wang, C. Lai, X.J. Xu, Z.H. Zhen, H. Zhou, D.F. Xu, iRGD-paclitaxel conjugate nanoparticles for targeted paclitaxel delivery, *Drug Dev. Res.* (2019). doi: 10.1002/ ddr.21589.

561. Q. Chen, X. Wang, C. Wang, L.Z. Feng, Y.G. Li, Z. Liu, Drug-induced self-assembly of modified albumins as nanotheranostics for tumor-targeted combination therapy, *ACS Nano.* 9 (2015) 5223–5233. doi: 10.1021/acsnano.5b00640.

562. Y. Ma, P.Y. He, X.H. Tian, G.L. Liu, X.W. Zeng, G.Q. Pan, Mussel-derived, cancer-targeting peptide as ph-sensitive prodrug nanocarrier, *ACS Appl. Mater. Interfaces* 11 (2019) 23948–23956. doi: 10.1021/acsami.9b09031.

563. X. Peng, V. Gandhi, ROS-activated anticancer prodrugs: a new strategy for tumor-specific damage, *Ther. Deliv.* 3 (2012) 823–833. doi: 10.4155/tde.12.61.

564. Y.M. Dai, Z.L. Jiang, J.Y. Li, M.F. Wang, C. Liu, W. Qi, R.X. Su, Z.M. He, Co-assembly of curcumin and a cystine bridged peptide to construct tumor-responsive nanomicelles for efficient chemotherapy, *J. Mater. Chem. B* 8 (2020) 1944–1951. doi: 10.1039/c9tb02625h.

565. Y.Q. Liang, S.X. Li, X.L. Wang, Y. Zhang, Y.N. Sun, Y.Q. Wang, X.Y. Wang, B. He, W.B. Dai, H. Zhang, X.Q. Wang, Q. Zhang, A comparative study of the antitumor efficacy of peptide-doxorubicin conjugates with different linkers, *J. Controlled Release* 275 (2018) 129–141. doi: 10.1016/j.jconrel.2018.01.033.

566. Z.Q. Cong, L. Zhang, S.Q. Ma, K.S. Lam, F.F. Yang, Y.H. Liao, Size-transformable hyaluronan stacked self-assembling peptide nanoparticles for improved transcellular tumor penetration and photo-chemo combination therapy, *ACS Nano* 14 (2020) 1958–1970. doi: 10.1021/acsnano.9b08434.

567. B.J. Sun, C. Luo, H. Yu, X.B. Zhang, Q. Chen, W.Q. Yang, M.L. Wang, Q.M. Kan, H. T. Zhang, Y.J. Wang, Z.G. He, J. Sun, Disulfide bond-driven oxidation- and reduction-responsive prodrug nanoassemblies for cancer therapy, *Nano Lett.* 18 (2018) 3643–3650. doi: 10.1021/acs.nanolett.8b00737.

568. T. Zhong, X. Yao, S. Zhang, Y. Guo, X.C. Duan, W. Ren, D. Huang, Y.F. Yin, X. Zhang, A self-assembling nanomedicine of conjugated linoleic acid-paclitaxel conjugate (CLA-PTX) with higher drug loading and carrier-free characteristic, *Sci. Rep.* 6 (2016). doi: 10.1038/srep36614.

569. J. Hrkach, D. Von Hoff, M.M. Ali, E. Andrianova, J. Auer, T. Campbell, D. De Witt, M. Figa, M. Figueiredo, A. Horhota, S. Low, K. McDonnell, E. Peeke, B. Retnarajan, A. Sabnis, E. Schnipper, J.J. Song, Y.H. Song, J. Summa, D. Tompsett, G. Troiano, T.V. Hoven, J. Wright, P. LoRusso, P.W. Kantoff, N. H. Bander, C. Sweeney, O.C. Farokhzad, R. Langer, S. Zale, Preclinical development and clinical translation of a PSMA-targeted docetaxel nanoparticle with a differentiated pharmacological profile, *Sci. Transl. Med.* 4 (2012). doi: 10.1126/scitranslmed.3003651.

570. Y. Liu, G.Z. Yang, T. Baby, Tengjisi, D. Chen, D.A. Weitz, C.X. Zhao, Stable polymer nanoparticles with exceptionally high drug loading by sequential nanoprecipitation, *Angew Chem. Int. Ed.* (2020). doi: 10.1002/anie.201913539.

571. J.C. Wang, H.T. Zhao, K.K. Zhi, X. Yang, Exploration of the natural active small-molecule drug-loading process and highly efficient synergistic antitumor efficacy, *ACS Appl. Mater. Interfaces* 12 (2020) 6827–6839. doi: 10.1021/acsami.9b18443.

572. P. Xue, J. Wang, X.F. Han, Y.J. Wang, Hydrophobic drug self-delivery systems as a versatile nanoplatform for cancer therapy: a review, *Colloids Surf B: Biointerfaces* 180 (2019) 202–211. doi: 10.1016/j.colsurfb.2019.04.050.

573. S.Y. Qin, Y.J. Cheng, Q. Lei, A.Q. Zhang, X.Z. Zhang, Combinational strategy for high-performance cancer chemotherapy, *Biomaterials* 171 (2018) 178–197. doi: 10.1016/j.biomaterials.2018.04.027.

574. S. Taurin, H. Nehoff, K. Greish, Anticancer nanomedicine and tumor vascular permeability; where is the missing link? *J. Controlled Release* 164 (2012) 265–275. doi: 10.1016/j.jconrel.2012.07.013.

575. K.A. Athanasiou, G.G. Niederauer, C.M. Agrawal, Sterilization, toxicity, biocompatibility and clinical applications of polylactic acid polyglycolic acid copolymers, *Biomaterials* 17 (1996) 93–102. doi: 10.1016/0142-9612(96)85754-1.

576. J. Wolfram, M.T. Zhu, Y. Yang, J.L. Shen, E. Gentile, D. Paolino, M. Fresta, G. J. Nie, C.Y. Chen, H.F. Shen, M. Ferrari, Y.L. Zhao, Safety of nanoparticles in medicine, *Curr. Drug Targets* 16 (2015) 1671–1681. doi: 10.2174/1389 450115666140804124808.

577. S. Bun, M. Yunokawa, Y. Tamaki, A. Shimomura, T. Shimoi, M. Kodaira, C. Shimizu, K. Yonemori, Y. Fujiwara, Y. Makino, H. Terakado, K. Tamura, Symptom management: the utility of regional cooling for hand-foot syndrome induced by pegylated liposomal doxorubicin in ovarian cancer, *Support Care Cancer* 26 (2018) 2161–2166. doi: 10.1007/s00520-018-4054-z.

578. P.N. Navya, A. Kaphle, S.P. Srinivas, S.K. Bhargava, V.M. Rotello, H.K. Daima, Current trends and challenges in cancer management and therapy using designer nanomaterials, *Nano Converg.* 6 (2019). doi: 10.1186/s40580-019-0193-2.

579. Y. Pan, S. Neuss, A. Leifert, M. Fischler, F. Wen, U. Simon, G. Schmid, W. Brandau, W. Jahnen-Dechent, Size-dependent cytotoxicity of gold nanoparticles, *Small* 3 (2007) 1941–1949. doi: 10.1002/smll.200700378.

580. A. Pratsinis, P. Hervella, J.C. Leroux, S.E. Pratsinis, G.A. Sotiriou, Toxicity of silver nanoparticles in macrophages, *Small* 9 (2013) 2576–2584. doi: 10.1002/smll.201202120.

581. N. Feliu, D. Docter, M. Heine, P. del Pino, S. Ashraf, J. Kolosnjaj-Tabi, P. Macchiarini, P. Nielsen, D. Alloyeau, F. Gazeau, R.H. Stauber, W.J. Parak, In vivo degeneration and the fate of inorganic nanoparticles, *Chem. Soc. Rev.* 45 (2016) 2440–2457. doi: 10.1039/c5cs00699f.

582. S. Roy, Z.Y. Liu, X. Sun, M. Gharib, H.J. Yan, Y.L. Huang, S. Megahed, M. Schnabel, D.C. Zhu, N. Feliu, I. Chalcraborty, C. Sanchez-Cano, A.M. Alkilany, W.J. Parak, Assembly and degradation of inorganic nanoparticles in biological environments, *Bioconjug. Chem.* 30 (2019) 2751–2762. doi: 10.1021/acs.bioconjchem.9b00645.

583. Z.P. Zhang, L. Mei, S.S. Feng, Paclitaxel drug delivery systems, *Expert Opin. Drug Delivery* 10 (2013) 325–340. doi: 10.1517/17425247.2013.752354.

584. J. Ahn, J. Ko, S. Lee, J. Yu, Y. Kim, N.L. Jeon, Microfluidics in nanoparticle drug delivery; from synthesis to pre-clinical screening, *Adv Drug Delivery Rev.* 128 (2018) 29–53. doi: 10.1016/j.addr.2018.04.001.

585. J. Wei, L.C. Cheng, J.M. Li, Y.C. Liu, S.Q. Yin, B. Xu, D. Wang, H.Y. Lu, C. Liu, A microfluidic platform culturing two cell lines paralleled under *in-vivo* like fluidic microenvironment for testing the tumor targeting of nanoparticles, *Talanta* 208 (2020). doi: 10.1016/j.talanta.2019.120355.

586. X. Feng, H. Dixon, H. Glen-Ravenhill, S. Karaosmanoglu, Q. Li, L. Yan, X.F. Chen, Smart nanotechnologies to target tumor with deep penetration depth for efficient cancer treatment and imaging, *Adv. Ther.* 2 (2019). doi: 10.1002/adtp.201900093.

587. B. Yang, K.Y. Wang, D. Zhang, B. Ji, D.Y. Zhao, X. Wang, H.T. Zhang, Q.M. Kan, Z. G. He, J. Sun, Polydopamine-modified ROS-responsive prodrug nanoplatform with enhanced stability for precise treatment of breast cancer, *RSC Adv.* 9 (2019) 9260–9269. doi: 10.1039/c9ra01230c.

588. S. Yadav, A.K. Sharma, P. Kumar, Nanoscale self-assembly for therapeutic delivery, *Front Bioeng. Biotechnol.* 8 (2020). doi: 10.3389/fbioe.2020.00127.

589. G. Wang, J. Wang, W. Wu, S.S. Tony To, H. Zhao, J. Wang, Advances in lipid-based drug delivery: enhancing efficiency for hydrophobic drugs, *Expert Opin. Drug Delivery* 12 (2015) 1475–1499.

590. V. Torchilin, Liposomes in drug delivery. In: J. Siepmann, R.A. Siegel, and Rathbone, Michael J. (eds.) *Fundamentals and Applications of Controlled Release Drug Delivery.* Springer: Berlin, Germany (2012), 289–328.

591. S.C. Semple, A. Chonn, P.R. Cullis, Interactions of liposomes and lipid-based carrier systems with blood proteins: relation to clearance behaviour in vivo, *Adv Drug Delivery Rev.* 32 (1998) 3–17.

592. M. Teymouri, M. Mashreghi, E. Saburi, A. Hejazi, A.R. Nikpoor, The trip of a drug inside the body: from a lipid-based nanocarrier to a target cell, *J. Controlled Release* 309 (2019) 59–71.

2 Strategies, Design, and Chemistry in Small Interfering RNA Delivery Vehicle Systems for Cancer Therapy

After validation of the *in vitro* potency and specificity, small interfering RNA (siRNA) strands are further stabilized via optimization of chemically modified nucleotides. Finally, a variety of different delivery formulation strategies can be implemented, as described below. This chapter will discuss the strategies and design of nonviral siRNA therapeutics from a chemical perspective.

2.1 EXTRACELLULAR AND INTRACELLULAR BARRIERS IN SYSTEMIC siRNA DELIVERY TO SOLID TUMORS

Various delivery vehicles have been developed for systemic delivery of therapeutic siRNA into solid tumors [1]. They need to protect vulnerable siRNAs from enzymatic degradation and avoid rapid renal filtration as well as entrapment by phagocytes and further extravasate from the blood to tumor tissues (Figure 2.1a). Once siRNAs reach the tumor tissue, they need to (i) be internalized by cancer cells, (ii) escape from the endosome into the cytoplasm, and (iii) finally release the siRNA payload to form the RNA-induced silencing complex (RISC) (Figure 2.1b).

2.2 DESIGN CRITERIA TO OVERCOME EXTRACELLULAR BARRIERS

Kidney glomeruli work as a physical filtration barrier that allows water and small molecules to pass into urine while larger molecules are retained in the circulation [2]. The pore size of the glomerular basement membrane (GBM) is reported to be approximately 6–10 nm. Thus, naked siRNAs with a size of approximately 7 nm in length and 2 nm in diameter [3], as well as their degraded products, can be readily filtered within 10 min through the GBM and passed into the urine [4,5]. These facts generate the lower size limitation of approximately 10 nm for design of delivery vehicles. Meanwhile, it is believed that various solid tumors have defective "leaky" vascular structures associated with immature lymphatic ducts, compared with healthy organs/tissues, permitting the accumulation of nanoparticles with several tens to hundred nm in tumor tissues. This size-mediated tumor accumulation mechanism of nanoparticles (or macromolecular drugs) was originally observed by Y. Matsumura and H. Maeda in 1986 and was termed the enhanced permeability and retention (EPR) effect [6]. To date, the size-mediated tumor accumulation

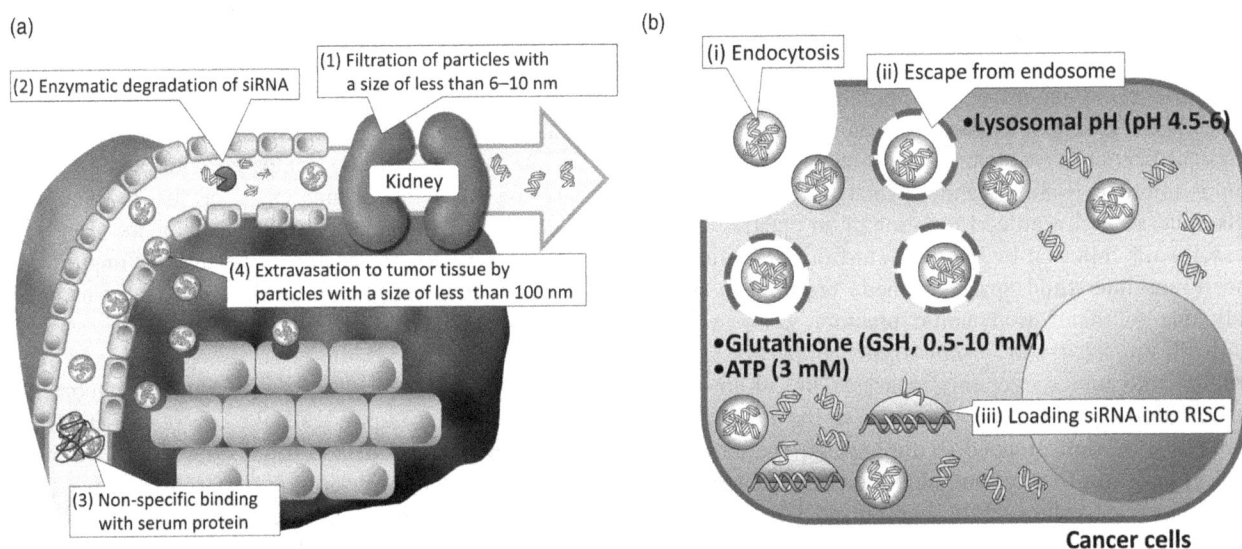

FIGURE 2.1 Schematic illustration of delivery barriers in extracellular (a) and intracellular (b) regions.

DOI: 10.1201/9781003229674-2

of nanoparticles has been widely demonstrated in various tumor-bearing murine models using polymeric micelles, inorganic nanoparticles, and lipid nanoparticles (LNPs) [7–9]. Of importance in this regard is that the tumor accumulation behavior of nanoparticles is significantly affected by the pathophysiology of tumor tissues [10]. In 11 canine cancer patients with spontaneous solid tumors, a 110-nm-sized nanoparticle displayed high uptake levels in six of seven carcinomas, whereas the same nanoparticle accumulated only one of four sarcomas [11]. Highly permeable tumor models, such as the colon adenocarcinoma LS174T model, are reported to allow significant accumulation of nanoparticles that are even 400 nm in diameter [12]. On the other hand, subcutaneous pancreatic BxPC3 tumors are reported to have thick fibrotic stroma and hypovascularity, hampering the tumor accumulation of N50-nm-sized nanoparticles, but not 30-nm-sized ones. Eventually, only 30-nm-sized nanoparticles accomplished significant antitumor activity in the pancreatic tumor model [13]. These facts have encouraged researchers to engineer smaller delivery vehicles with a size of less than 50 nm for enhanced accumulation in heterogeneous tumor tissues. Meanwhile, the EPR effect in human patients has been observed in a handful of examples and is noteworthy [14,15]. A polymer–drug conjugate with a molecular weight of approximately 15 kDa, termed SMANCS, which is able to bind to blood albumin and thereby shows significantly increased blood circulation, was found to accumulate in clinical hepatocellular and renal cell carcinomas with a high vascular density through arterial infusion [16]. With a diameter of approximately 90 nm, PEGylated (poly(ethylene glycol)) liposomal doxorubicin or Doxil® has a circulation half-life of 21–90 h [17–20], exhibiting a 10-fold greater selective accumulation in the metastatic breast carcinoma tissue compared to tumor-free skeletal muscle in two patients [21]. The EPR effect observed in animal models needs to be carefully interpreted for the translation to clinical settings as described in other reviews [22–24].

Transports of nanoparticles from blood vessels to cancer cells are governed by particle dynamics regarding the physical barrier of stroma. The recent observation onto tumor microenvironment showed that tumor blood vessels undergo time-limited formation of an opening in the vessel walls followed by brief outward flow of fluid into the tumor interstitial space (termed "eruptions") probably due to the hydrodynamic pressure gradient [25]. Both 30-nm-sized and 70-nm-sized nanoparticles were erupted into tumor interstitial spaces. The 30-nm-sized nanoparticles quickly diffused away, but the 70-nm-sized nanoparticles were trapped in stroma-rich barriers [25]. Cancer cells mostly surround blood vessels in some clinical tumor (e.g., kidney, brain, liver, thyroid, ovarian, and head and neck cancers), whereas stroma surrounds vessel in other clinical tumor (e.g., breast, pancreatic, colorectal and non–small-cell lung cancers) [26,27]. Thus, in case of stroma-rich tumors, nanoparticles need to penetrate into (or distribute across) the stroma tissue to reach the cancer cells nests. In this regard, the penetrability of nanoparticles is reported to significantly depend on their particle size as follows: 20-nm-sized PEGylated gold nanoparticles (AuNPs) permeated to 40–50 μm depth from vessel centers in a subcutaneous MDA-MB-435 tumor, which was deeper than 60 and 100-nm-sized nanoparticles [28]. Also, 12-nm-sized PEGylated nanoparticles diffused to approximately 80 μm depths from vessel centers in the subcutaneous melanoma tumor [29]. These results indicate that smaller nanoparticles are preferred to diffuse into a stroma-rich extracellular matrix. On the other hand, rapid proliferation of cancer cells and the resulting blood and lymphatic vessel compression can induce higher interstitial fluid pressure in the tumor area, preventing efficient diffusion of nanoparticles from the vessel to cancer cells [30]. Treatment of transforming growth factor-β inhibitor and collagenase can reduce the pericyte coverage of endothelium and fibrosis in the tumor microenvironment, respectively, allowing the enhanced penetration of nanoparticles [31,32]. Of note, the majority of tumor xenograft model in mice relatively lacks of stroma, compared to human patients' tumors. This indicates that the delivery efficacy of a nanoparticle is likely overestimated using inadequate animal tumor models [27].

It is important that the aforementioned size of delivery vehicles must be maintained even in the bloodstream including a huge amount of biomacromolecules and cells. Thus, delivery vehicles should be carefully designed to avoid undesired aggregation and rapid dissociation in the biological milieu until the target tumor region is reached. In particular, positively charged delivery vehicles may electrostatically bind to negatively charged serum proteins and proteoglycans, such as albumin and heparan sulfate, resulting in their aggregation and/or dissociation. Transmission electron microscopy has shown that the intravenously injected CALAA-01 has a zeta-potential of 10–30 mV and was entrapped with GBMs, which have a high density of heparan sulfate [33], resulting in the loss of their structural integrity. In another study, siRNA-loaded cationic polysaccharide nanoparticles were transferred from the kidney to the bladder more slowly compared with naked siRNA. Considering that the original size of the nanoparticles (220–230 nm in diameter) was larger than the pore size of GBMs, the siRNA transfer to the bladder implies that siRNA payloads were gradually released from the nanoparticles and that the GBM partially contributes to disassembly of the intravenously administered nanoparticles. Of note, nanoparticles with a size of several hundred nanometers can be engulfed by Kupffer cells through phagocytosis and entrapped by the reticuloendothelial system in the liver and spleen [34–36]. Thus, absorption of serum proteins on to delivery vehicles likely reduces the blood circulation property of delivery vehicles [37]. An effective approach to limit protein absorption is surface coating with nonionic, hydrophilic, and flexible polymer brushes, e.g., PEG, poly(N-vinyl pyrrolidone) (PVP), poly(N-(2-hydroxypropyl) methacrylamide) (PHPMA), and poly(oxazoline), which all generate steric repulsive forces on the nanoparticle surface [38]. The impact of these polymer brushes on circulation kinetics and biodistribution of delivery vehicles was well explained in other reviews [39–41]. Among these polymer brushes, PEG has been most widely used over many years and approved as an injectable material by the Food and Drug Administration (FDA) in the United States [42,43]. On the other hand, a few reports on the limitations of PEG, e.g., immunogenicity, have been published after two decades of clinical usage [41,44]. Although the immunogenicity of PEG in patients was not reported after treatment with PEGylated liposomes or micelles, PEGylated phenylalanine ammonia lyase tested in Phase I trials induced antibodies against PEG within 6 weeks after single subcutaneous administration [45]. This anti-PEG antibody reduced the efficacy of PEGylated asparaginase because it may eliminate the PEGylated protein from the bloodstream [46,47].

2.3 DESIGN CRITERIA TO OVERCOME INTRACELLULAR BARRIERS

Once target tissues or cancer cells have been reached, delivery vehicles should interact with the cellular surface for internalization into cells. The main parameters that determine endocytosis of delivery vehicles are shape, size, and surface chemistry. These parameters are believed to affect not only the cellular uptake efficiency but also the endocytotic route [48]. The shape effect of delivery vehicles is not described in this review because most delivery vehicles for cancer therapy are constructed to possess a spherical morphology through simple self-assembly procedures or natural growth of seed inorganic particles (see the reference [49,50] on the shape effect). Multimolecular delivery vehicles, e.g., polymeric micelles and LNPs, are generally constructed to be 30–100 nm in size, to promote the EPR effect. Inorganic nanoparticles are also reported to demonstrate a size effect on endocytosis; bare AuNPs with a diameter of 20–50 nm have demonstrated that the most efficient cellular uptake between 10 nm and 100 nm size ranges in cultured cancer cells because AuNPs with these size ranges may balance between the elevated elastic energy associated with increased curvature of the cell membrane and reduced entropy associated with receptor/ligand immobilization [51–53]. Surface chemistries of delivery vehicles are apparently more critical for their endocytosis, compared to the size and shape. Positively charged nanoparticles have a high affinity to negatively charged proteoglycans expressed on the surface of most cells, resulting in more efficient adsorptive endocytosis, compared with neutral and negatively charged nanoparticles. Of note, heparin sulfate proteoglycans, comprising transmembrane proteins termed syndecans, are considered major binding sites for cationic delivery vehicles [54]. However, such cationic nanoparticles are not able to take advantage of systemic administration due to nonspecific interactions with negatively charged blood components before reaching target cells. PEGylation of delivery vehicles is a standard strategy, which suppresses

such aggregate formation [38]. Nevertheless, PEGylation of delivery vehicles concurrently generates disadvantages for cellular entry due to weakened interactions with the surface of target cells (termed PEG dilemma) [55].

To overcome this PEG dilemma, ligand-mediated targeting strategies have been explored for delivery vehicles to selectively bind to receptor molecules that are overexpressed on targeted cancer cells (other reviews summarize promising ligand candidates, including small molecules, peptides, antibody, and aptamers [56,57]). Arginine–glycine–aspartic acid (RGD) peptide and folate are typical ligands used in siRNA delivery for various types of cancers because these ligands are closely related to angiogenesis of tumor development and metabolism of fast-growing cancer cells. The RGD peptide can strongly and specifically bind to $\alpha_v\beta_3$ and $\alpha_v\beta_5$ integrin receptors, which are overexpressed on many cancerous and neovascular endothelial cell surfaces [58,59]. A cyclic form of the RGD peptide (cRGD) provides the rigid structure for enhanced affinity to the target integrins (KD = approximately 40 nM for $\alpha_v\beta_3$ integrin [60]) and prevents degradation of the highly susceptible aspartic acid residue [58]. Folate is a low molecular weight vitamin required by all eukaryotic cells for 1-carbon metabolism and the synthesis of purines and pyrimidines. It has a high affinity (KD = approximately 10 nM) for folate receptor isoform α (FR-α), which is highly overexpressed on the surface of ovarian, uterine, brain, and central nervous system (CNS) cancers, whereas a high to moderate level of the FR-α expression is detected in lung, kidney, and breast cancers [56,61]. Monoclonal antibodies and their fragments are also utilized to recognize specific molecules (i.e., antigens) on the surface of cancer cells. The structure of antibody divides into two different biofunctional subdomains. The antigen-binding fragment (Fab) mediates antigen recognition via complementarity-determining regions, and the crystallizable fragment (Fc) recruits the Fc receptor on the immune cell or the other antibody recognition [62]. Trastuzumab, an antibody for FDA-approved antibody-drug conjugate trastuzumab emtansine, has equilibrium dissociation constant, KD = 1–7 nM for the transmembrane tyrosine kinase receptor (HER2) [63–65]. Fabs can be used to reduce the bulky size of a full antibody (approximately 15 nm), alleviating immunogenicity and improving the pharmacokinetic profile of delivery vehicles [61,66]. Nucleic acid aptamers, which are single-stranded oligonucleotides with a specific 3D structure, also exert high binding specificity to their target molecules [61]. To date, no ligand-installed multimolecular delivery vehicle containing oligonucleotides or small molecular drug goes to markets [67]. On the other hand, two antibody-drug conjugates are approved by the FDA for treatment of lymphoma and HER2-positive breast cancer [63]. In the subcutaneous folate receptor-positive tumor mice model, folate-conjugated Vinca alkaloid, EC145, showed complete cures without a relapse for > 90 days post-tumor implantation in 4/5 mice [68]. However, in Phase II trials combined with PEGylated liposomal doxorubicin (PLD), median progression-free survival (PFS) of EC145 plus PLD marginally increased from 2.7 to 5.0 months compared to PLD-alone control in ovarian cancer [69]. In the recent report, the Phase III study was stopped because EC145 did not demonstrate efficacy regarding PFS in patients. One plausible explanation is that receptor properties in an animal's tumor did not represent properties of the primary cancer cell found in a patient's tumor [23]. Other gaps between the laboratory animal model and human patients in tumor targeting were well explained in interesting perspectives [23,70].

After endocytosis, siRNA-loaded delivery vehicles encounter a sequential pH drop in the early endosome (pH: 6.5), late endosome (pH: 6.0), and lysosome (pH: 4.5–5.0) [71,72]. In this way, the endocytosed delivery vehicles (and siRNA payloads) are subjected to lysosomal hydrolysis and inactivated for RNA interference (RNAi) machinery. Thus, delivery vehicles need to contain a functionality to breach the endosomal membranes for translocation to the cytoplasm. Many previous studies have demonstrated that polycations containing low pKa amines and their poly-ion complexes (PICs) with nucleic acids can induce endosome disruption (or endosomal escape), resulting in high transfection efficiency [73,74]. Endosomal escape induced by low pKa amines has been explained by two possible mechanisms. One is the proton sponge hypothesis based on increased osmotic pressure [75,76]. Low pKa amines can protonate in acidic endosomal compartments and induce proton influx into endo/lysosomal compartments accompanied by counter ions, mainly chloride ions. This ion influx increases the osmotic pressure in endo/lysosomal compartments, possibly eliciting the membrane destabilization. Of note, the endosomal escape of siRNA elicited by a huge excess of cationic polymers in cultured cells does not predict *in vivo* efficacy in animal experiments because unbound cationic polymers may not accumulate in the same cancer cells as delivery vehicles do. In addition, it has gradually been believed that this hypothesis does not work well. Polycations with high pKa still induce comparatively high endosomal escape in cultured cells [74]. The other mechanism is direct membrane destabilization by highly charged polycations [74,77]. As aforementioned, polycations can bind to the oppositely charged cellular membrane and perturb membrane integrity. In particular, polycations bearing low pKa amines can significantly elevate their positive charge density through amine protonation in endo/lysosomal compartments and consequently perturb the endo/lysosomal membrane integrity for membrane destabilization. The design strategies of delivery vehicles, which are capable of endosome disruption, will be described later in this chapter.

2.4 DESIGN OF siRNA DELIVERY VEHICLES

Delivery vehicles have been developed (i) to stabilize their multimolecular structures in the bloodstream; (ii) to selectively release siRNA from the stabilized structures into the cytoplasm; (iii) to specifically recognize the target cellular surface; and (iv) to allow efficient endosomal escape (Table 2.1). Various technologies (or strategies) have been applied to mainly elaborate three compartments of multimolecular structures, which are surface, intermediate layer, and core. In this review, multimolecular structures are defined as polymer- and lipid-based nanoparticles (LPNs). Both nanoparticles comprise cationic monomer components to efficiently encapsulate negatively charged siRNA and increase the siRNA load in nanoparticles. In addition,

TABLE 2.1
Summary of Design Strategies in This Section

Position in Multimolecular Structures	Functionalities	Introduction Methods in Monomer Components
Surface	• Peptide installation for extracellular pH responsiveness.	Ligand and peptide are conjugated into terminal end of monomer.
	• Ligand installation for high cell-specific recognition	
Intermediate	• Hydrophobic layer for high stability	Carbon chain and head group modification in lipid monomers
	• High endosome escapability	
	• GSH response for selective release of siRNA	Thiol group is introduced into triblock copolymer.
	• MMP response for high cell specific recognition	Peptide is introduced between PEG and cationic segments.
Core region	• Hydrophobic interaction for high stability	Individual moiety is introduced into block copolymer or cationic homopolymer.
	• GSH, endosomal acidic pH, ATP response for selective release of siRNA	
	• High cell-specific recognition responsive on extracellular acidic pH	PEI in triblock copolymer
	• High endosome escapability	Cationic moiety in block copolymer or cationic homopolymer has secondary/tertiary amines.

these components drive the electrostatic interaction with siRNA and spontaneously assemble into a multimolecular structure in the aqueous milieu [78,79].

2.5 CARRIER DESIGN FOR STABILITY AND RELEASE

Multimolecular delivery vehicles are stabilized by various driving forces, e.g., electrostatic interaction, hydrophobic interaction, and hydrogen bonding. The design of building components to maintain multimolecular structures is a key point to increase delivery efficacy. Various features in building components, e.g., chemical structures and length of building components (cationic moieties, nonionic/hydrophilic moieties, and hydrocarbon tail of lipid), contribute to vehicle stability [80–82]. These features need to be optimized in the individual delivery vehicles. Among them, pKa of cationic building components is generally well studied in terms of vehicle stability and particle formulation. An ionizable cationic lipid in stabilized nucleic acid lipid particles (SNALP) contains a dimethylamino headgroup (pKa=6.7±0.1), efficiently formulating a multimolecular assembly with siRNA at pH 4. At physiological pH, this vehicle maintains a neutral or low cationic surface charge density to avoid nonspecific disruption of plasma membranes. The polymeric complex delivery vehicle is also significantly influenced by pKa of the functional group in cationic components. The primary amines ($-NH_2$) in polylysine have pKa of 10.5 and are protonated into $-NH_3^+$ at 99% in pH 7.4, whereas the secondary amines in polyethyleneimine (PEI) have pKa of 6.6 and are protonated at approximately 50% in the neutral pH condition [77]. Thus, two-fold quantities of secondary amines in PEI are necessary to neutralize single negatively charged siRNA compared with primary amines in polylysine.

Meanwhile, internalized delivery vehicles need to release siRNA payloads into the cytoplasm for siRNA loading into RISC proteins for RNAi. The target site-selective release of siRNA can be accomplished by designing the vehicles that respond to different gradients of biological signals between intracellular and extracellular regions. As stabilizing/releasing strategies, multimolecular structures can dissociate to release encapsulated siRNAs in response to three representative biological signals: redox potential, pH, and adenosine triphosphate (ATP) concentration. The design strategies of the multimolecular structure for these kinds of biosignals are divided into two categories. The first category is covalent conjugation of siRNA into delivery vehicles through biosignal-responsive crosslinkers. The terminal end of siRNA is readily modified with biosignal-responsive chemical moieties and then associates with the vehicles. These vehicles can release siRNA through cleavage of the crosslinks in the presence of higher amounts of biosignals. The other category is construction of the multimolecular assembly using biosignal responsive components. In this way, the multimolecular structure can dissociate into

building components and simultaneously releases encapsulated siRNAs. This biosignal responsive disassembly of the multimolecular structure elicits the rapid siRNA release in the target site.

2.5.1 HYDROPHOBICITY-STABILIZED DELIVERY VEHICLES

Stabilization of delivery vehicles by hydrophobic interaction in aqueous solutions has been investigated in the early development of vehicles because of simple chemistry for introduction of hydrophobic moieties into component materials [83,84]. Hydrophobic moieties, such as alkyl chains and cholesterol, installed into cationic components can assist the spontaneous assembly of multimolecular structures with siRNA through hydrophobic interactions, rendering delivery vehicles more resistant to dissociation (Figure 2.2a). This increase in the association number (e.g., the number of building components in single delivery vehicle) between hydrophobic cationic components and siRNA results in a higher resistance against serum-containing media compared with unmodified cationic components [85,86]. Consequently, the hydrophobized delivery vehicles permitted a more efficient cellular uptake of siRNA payloads, leading to enhanced endogenous gene silencing in cultured cancer cells. However, the higher stability of delivery vehicles in serum-containing media does not guarantee the stability in the bloodstream. When hydrophobized PEG-polycations formulated with siRNA, blood circulation property increased for only 10 min after tail vein administration [87,88]. The resulting delivery vehicles exerted inefficient tumor growth inhibition in a subcutaneous model of tumor, indicating that simple hydrophobic moiety introduction into cationic components is not enough to generate the stability of vehicles in bloodstream. In this regard, a previous study demonstrated that vehicle stability could be further improved by compartmentalizing the hydrophobic moieties within the multimolecular structure [89] (Figure 2.2b). The exclusion of hydrophilic siRNA payload as well as cationic segments from the hydrophobic core allowed for more stable assembly because the hydrophobic components were more tightly packaged in the core without interferences of hydrophilic siRNAs and polycations. This vehicle had better stability in the bloodstream compared with the control vehicle without the compartmentalization of hydrophobic moieties. The intermediate layer in the multimolecular structure can also be stabilized by hydrophobic moieties (Figure 2.2c). This type of delivery vehicles (e.g., mostly LPNs) contains siRNA in the core and exhibits longer blood circulation properties compared with the core-hydrophobized delivery vehicles [90,91]. The cationic lipid-based core was coated with siRNA and further formulated with anionic PEG-lipid as the outer bilayer, utilizing the alkyl chain-constituted intermediate bilayer, stabilized the delivery vehicle [90]. This delivery vehicle (a particle size of 100 nm) has a plasma half-life of approximately 18 h and tumor accumulation of siRNA peaked at 24 h after systemic administration.

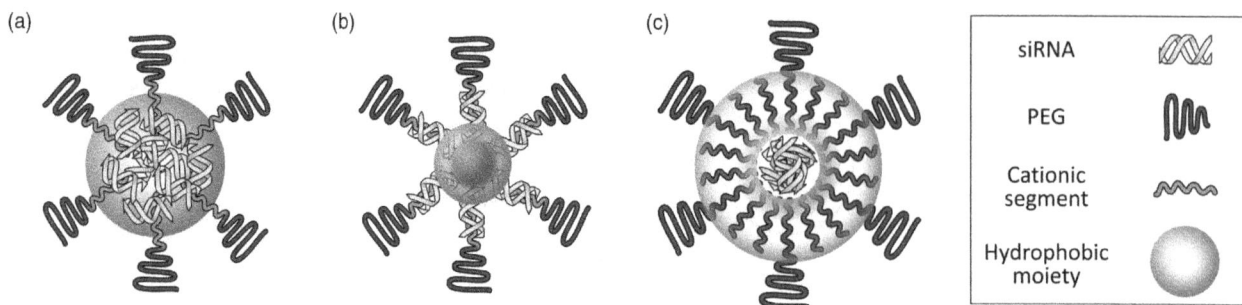

FIGURE 2.2 Platform structures for the design of delivery vehicles with high stabilies. Multimolecular structures have hydrophobized core (a, b) or intermediate layer (c).

Furthermore, significant fluorescence of fluorescent-dye-labeled siRNA could be detected in the tumor tissue until 72 h after administration. Another delivery vehicle is composed of the cationic lipid, azide-modified cholesterol, and anionic alkyne-modified hyaluronic acid (HA) [92]. The cationic LNP contains siRNA and azide-modified cholesterol in the core and intermediate layer, respectively. Interestingly, the anionic alkyne-modified HA was covalently conjugated to the azide-modified cholesterol, reducing interference of integrity of the intermediate bilayer. The delivery vehicle had a particle size of 130 nm and exhibited a plasma half-life of 3–4 h. The vehicle showed better tumor growth inhibition, compared to controls, e.g., LNP electrostatically coated with HA and cationic LNP without HA. This result probably indicates that the integrity of the hydrophobic intermediate layer affects stability of multimolecular structures. However, these delivery vehicles with longer blood circulation properties exhibited dose ranges of siRNA between 1.2 and 7.5 mg/kg for tumor growth inhibition in animal models. These values are similar to those with other vehicles with shorter blood circulation properties, implying that selective release of siRNA and better endosomal escape ability may be further required for reducing the dose amount of siRNA and increasing the gene silencing efficiency.

2.5.2 Delivery Carrier Design for Selective Release of siRNA

2.5.2.1 Redox Potential Responsive Delivery Vehicles

Glutathione is a thiol-containing tripeptide composed of glutamic acid, cysteine, and glycine and works as the main antioxidant in cells. Glutathione is distinguished from other common peptides by the unique structure of γ-glutamate, rendering glutathione inert to normal intracellular peptidase-mediated degradation [93]. The cell maintains reduced glutathione (GSH) by de novo synthesis from the three amino acids and reduction of oxidized glutathione (GSSG) by glutathione reductase, which induces the concentration of GSH to be 50–1000 times higher than that of GSSG in cells [94,95]. In this way, GSH concentrations can be distinguished between the intracellular and extracellular environment. The GSH concentration within cells is 0.5–10 mM but decreases to 10–30 μM in the blood plasma [93–95]. Thus, the disulfide linkage can be preferably cleaved in the cytoplasm or intracellular compartments while it is slowly degraded during blood circulation. The payload drug release from disulfide crosslinked nanoparticles was observed from 2 to 4 h after internalization by the cells in cultured cells [96].

Thiol functionality greatly contributes to reversible stability of delivery vehicles when disulfide bonds are introduced into the intermediate layer or the core. The multimolecular structure maintains (or slowly dissociate) its preformed structure in the bloodstream, facilitates tumor accumulation by EPR effects or ligand-mediated targeting, disassembles in the GSH-rich cell interior, and eventually delivers the amount of siRNA in the RISC to induce desired RNAi. As a representative, the primary amine group in the side chain of PEG-polycations was modified with 2-iminothiolane to introduce a free thiol group as well as an amine group [97]. The resulting disulfide crosslinked delivery vehicle had a thiolate core structure with a 40–50 nm diameter size and neutrally charged with a zeta-potential of 0.1 mV (Figure 2.3a). The vehicle improved blood circulation property of half-life (approximately 10 min) compared to naked siRNA and noncrosslinked vehicle control (both half-lives 3–4 min). The improved blood circulation affected the biodistribution of fluorescent-dye-labeled siRNA in the animal experiment. The similar amount of siRNA was accumulated in the kidney administered by naked siRNA and the noncrosslinked vehicle at 24 h after injection of vehicles, whereas half of the siRNA amount was observed in the kidney administered by the crosslinked vehicle. Moreover, a crosslinked vehicle with ligand installation delivered approximately a two-fold higher amount of siRNA in the tumor compared to the controls (e.g., naked siRNA, a noncrosslinked vehicle, and crosslinked vehicles without ligand installation). Finally, this crosslinked vehicle improved tumor growth inhibition in subcutaneous cervical tumor (25 μg siRNA/mice, 6 injections), demonstrating that the selective release of siRNA in the tumor was successfully accomplished. Stability of disulfide crosslinked delivery vehicles can be further increased when hydrophobic moieties are simultaneously formulated in the core through additional hydrophobic interaction. In this term, ligand-installed and thiolated PEG-polycations

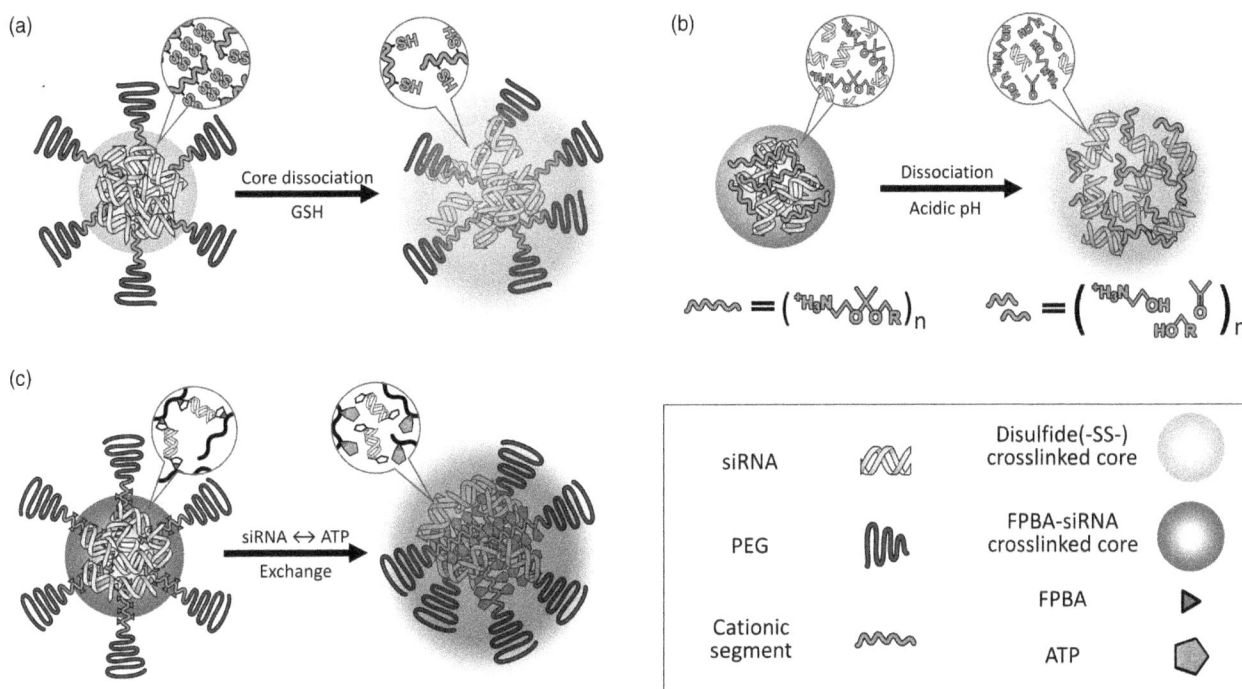

FIGURE 2.3 Illustration of delivery vehicles for selective release of siRNA. Multimolecular structures introduce redox-responsive thiol bonds in the core region (a). The delivery vehicle contains acidic pH responsiveness for faster dissocation (b) and introduce ATP-responsiveness in the core region for selective dissociation (c).

were formulated with cholesterol-modified siRNA [98]. The resulting delivery vehicles were stabilized by additional cholesterol-mediated hydrophobic interactions as well as by thiol crosslinking. The vehicle increased blood circulation properties with a half-life ≤ 20 min compared to naked siRNA/ligand-installed and thiolated PEG-polycations control, leading to higher tumor accumulation of siRNA and enhanced RNAi efficacy in subcutaneous cervical tumor. These researches clearly showed that increased stability/selective release of siRNA can achieve higher RNAi efficacy in an animal tumor model.

The thiol crosslinking strategy in the core of the multimolecular structure needs to consider an innate phenomenon of preferable intermolecular disulfide linkages. When large quantities of the thiol group are introduced into the core region or intermediate layer, the possibility of intramolecular disulfide linkage is higher than that of intermolecular disulfide linkage. Thus, the current disulfide crosslinked nanoparticles showed restricted redox responsive stability, indicating that the increase in intermolecular disulfide crosslinking will be a key factor to improve RNAi efficacy of delivery vehicles in passive or ligand-mediated targeting.

Disulfide linkages are introduced into a clinically ongoing polymer/siRNA conjugate vehicle (named Dynamic PolyConjugate) for systemic delivery of siRNA into viral-infected hepatocytes [99]. This conjugate vehicle consists of an endosomolytic backbone polymer conjugated with thiolated siRNA, N-acetylgalactosamine as a targeting ligand and PEG. In a Phase I clinical trial in healthy volunteers, a single dose of Dynamic PolyConjugates was well tolerated up to 2 mg/kg when administered intravenously [100].

Adverse events were reported to be mild or moderate. The serum hepatitis B surface antigen was reduced by up to 50% after a single dose of 2 mg/kg, and significant reductions were detected between 43 and 57 days in a Phase IIa trial.

2.5.2.2 Acidic pH Responsive Delivery Vehicles

Acidic pH (pH: 4.5–6) in late endosomes has frequently been highlighted as a representative biosignal for triggering the site-specific drug release from delivery vehicles because a large pH change from extracellular neutral pH to endosomal acidic pH allows us to utilize acid-labile chemistry [101]. Various acid-labile bonds, such as acetals [102], hydrazones [103], β-thiopropionate [104], phosphoramidate [105], orthoesters [106], and citraconic amide [107,108], have been applied to construct multimolecular structures that elicit acidic pH-responsive release of drug payloads, including anticancer drugs and biomacromolecules (Figure 2.4). For instance, amino ketal linkages were installed into a polycation backbone and the resulting ketalized polycations formulated siRNA into nanoparticles, which is highly charged with a zeta-potential of 16–22 mV (Figure 2.3b) [109]. The ketalized vehicles efficiently disassembled and released more quantities of siRNA into the cytoplasm whereas unmodified control vehicles exhibited delayed dissociation and captured siRNA at 4 h of incubation in cultured cells. Furthermore, the unmodified control vehicles (and loaded siRNA) were observed both in the cytoplasm and the nucleus because their high surface charge probably induced a nonspecific interaction with the membrane of the nucleus. This ketalized delivery vehicle improved RNAi efficiency in cultured cell condition and clearly showed advantages of

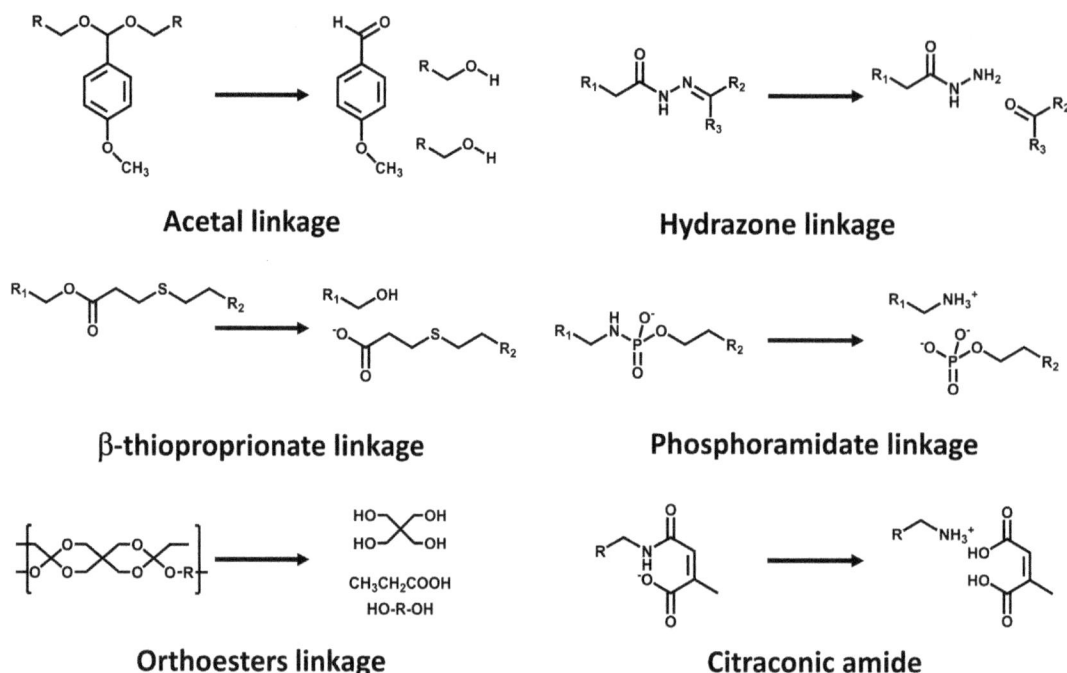

FIGURE 2.4 Cleavage of acidic pH-sensitive linkages.

selective siRNA release. In other example, siRNA is conjugated with a maleic acid derivative amide into anionic polymer, and the resulting anionic polymer/siRNA was further formulated with cationic polymers [110]. Released siRNA from the vehicle was not detected at pH 7.4 in 1 h incubation whereas approximately 30% of released siRNA was observed at pH 5.0. However, RNAi efficiency of the vehicle was moderately improved in cultured cancer cells compared with a pH-unresponsive control. One research reported that cholesterol was conjugated with acetal linkage into PEG-poly(vinyl alcohol) (termed Chol-PVA-PEG) [111]. This Chol-PVA-PEG was further formulated with siRNA and cationic cyclodextrin, rendering a nanoparticle in the size of 120–170 nm. Cholesterol moiety facilitated the compaction of siRNA into the nanoparticle through hydrophobic interaction. The acetal linkage of the cholesterol moiety was degraded in late endosome, promoting decondensation of the nanoparticle and release of siRNA. The size of the nanoparticle was not changed at pH 7.4 for up to 24 h, but the polydispersity of the nanoparticle started to increase after 4 h at pH 5.5. The nanoparticle showed similar RNAi efficiency to PEI and Lipofectamine 2000 in cultured cancer cells. Acid-labile chemistry has also frequently applied to the responses of other components in multimolecular structures for the delivery of biomacromolecules, e.g., detachment of PEG [112], ligand [99], and cationic polymer [113].

2.5.2.3 ATP Concentration-responsive Delivery Vehicles

ATP, the most abundant ribonucleotide, is a responsive signal for cell-specific release of siRNA. Although ATP is present in the extracellular environment at approximately

0.4 mM, its concentration is dramatically higher up to 3 mM within the intracellular matrix [114]. Similar to the aforementioned environment-responsive delivery vehicles, delivery vehicles can be designed to release payload siRNA into the ATP-abundant cytosol by utilizing phenylboronic acid (PBA) chemistry. PBA can form reversible covalent esters with 1,2-cis-diols on a ribose ring, which is present at the 3′ end of siRNA and ATP [115]. As a representative, 3-fluoro-4-carboxyphenylboronic acid (FPBA) was conjugated into primary amino groups in the side chain in PEG-polycations and complexed with the ribose-terminated siRNA as an intermolecular crosslinker (Figure 2.3c). This delivery vehicle was stabilized by the covalent conjugation between siRNA ribose and ionized FPBA moiety, hydrophobic interaction derived from nonionized FPBA moieties, and ion-pair formation between siRNA phosphates and residual amino groups in the polycation. Consequently, the delivery vehicle containing the ribose-terminated siRNA showed better stability against counter polyanion exchange with dextran sulfate, compared to control containing deoxyribose-terminated siRNA at either or both ends. On the other hand, this delivery vehicle dissociated in the ATP concentration range of more than 1 mM. Compared to disulfide crosslinking, this crosslinking further needs to be clarified in terms of (i) difference of on–off responsiveness between ATP concentration and GSH concentration, and (ii) although the thiol group does not affect initial electrostatic association between the polycations and siRNA, the relatively hydrophobic and bulky PBA group may prevent efficient crosslinking between diol and PBA. More precise design of block copolymer can improve delivery vehicle performance. The payload release dependent on the gradient of the ATP concentration was also attained by using an ATP-binding aptamer-incorporated DNA motif for anticancer drug delivery [116,117]. The Gu group (guideline for mouse model experiments) designed a doxorubicin-incorporated aptamer/single stranded DNA duplex, where the aptamer changed its tertiary structure in the presence of ATP and lost binding affinity for doxorubicin. The doxorubicin-incorporated aptamer/DNA duplex forms a nanogel with additions of protamine and HA. Finally, the nanogels successfully obtained moderate ATP-responsive growth inhibition in subcutaneous breast tumors.

2.6 DELIVERY CARRIER DESIGN FOR HIGH CELL SPECIFIC RECOGNITION

Delivery vehicles enter the tumor microenvironment from neighboring blood vessels. Multimolecular structures that are stable enough in the bloodstream can arrive at the tumor tissue from the leaky vessels. As described above, the vehicle can be further elaborated to possess higher selectivity to individual cancer cells or have more efficient uptake into cells. The tumor microenvironment is composed of many types of cells, including malignant cancer cells, fibroblasts, immune cells, and endothelial cells [118]. The delivery vehicle should be designed to recognize its target cells to increase the delivery efficiency. This can be accomplished by the ligand–receptor interaction (or active targeting). For efficient recognition, cell-specific ligands are installed onto the surface of delivery vehicles or the distal ends of neutral and hydrophilic spacers. Alternatively, the delivery vehicle is designed to selectively expose the positive charges near target cells, facilitating the binding to the cellular surface. The vehicle detaches neutral and hydrophilic layers or alters its charge to positive charge in response to tumor-specific biosignals. The tumor environment-specific biosignals include acidic pH and specific enzymes, which trigger the chemical reaction in delivery vehicles to alter their multimolecular structures.

2.6.1 BIOLOGICAL STIMULI-RESPONSIVE DELIVERY VEHICLES

The lowered pH (pH: 6.5–7.0) in the deep tumor tissue has gradually paid attentions as acidic pH signals [119]. This slight pH drop in the tumor extracellular matrix originates from the high metabolic rate of cancer cells in poorly perfused regions. Inadequate oxygen delivery to some regions of tumors generates hypoxic condition, which restricts oxidative phosphorylation of pyruvate in the mitochondria. Hypoxic cancer cells shift their glycolysis metabolism from generation of pyruvate to lactate. The increased oncogenic metabolism also generates an excess of protons and carbon dioxide, which are kept in equilibrium with carbonic acid by the enzyme, carbonic anhydrase. These weak acids and protons are exported out of the cells, inducing enhanced acidification of the extracellular milieu [119]. The protonation degree of amino groups in cationic components of the delivery vehicle is a key for utilization of the lowered

tumoral pH as a biosignal. In this regard, the amine pKa value of cationic components has been highlighted as an indicator for their protonation behavior and regulated to convert the surface charge of multimolecular structures from negative to positive in response to the acidic pH in deep tumor tissues. This strategy expects that a higher cellular uptake of positively charged vehicles occurs in tumors, whereas negatively charged vehicles suppress nonspecific cellular uptake in healthy tissues. For instance, the delivery vehicle was prepared from branched PEI, which increased a protonation degree when the solution pH decreased from 7.4 to 6.8 [120] (Figure 2.5a). The mixing ratios between cationic PEI and anionic siRNA were carefully selected in gel retardation assays to formulate multimolecular vehicles that had negative surface charges at pH 7.4 and positive surface charges at pH 6.8, associated with the facilitated protonation of PEI. The resulting surface charge-reversible vehicles had higher tumor accumulation of fluorescent-dye-labeled siRNA than non–charge-reversible negative and positive control vehicles. A similar surface charge conversional vehicle was also developed using peptides comprising histidine and glutamic acid residues [121] (Figure 2.5b). Considering that the pKa value of histidine is approximately 6.0, glutamic acid residues were utilized as neighbors of histidine in the peptide sequence for increasing the pKa value of the basic amino acid via stabilization of the protonated form. Delivery vehicles integrated with this peptide exhibited an increase in the surface charge at pH 6.5, compared to pH 7.4, and enhanced the cellular uptake in cultured cancer cells. These studies fully utilized an advantage of multimolecular assembly by amplifying a subtle change in the protonation degree of component amino groups for a dramatic change in the surface charge of the assembly.

An alternative strategy for high cellular internalization is that the neutral and hydrophilic shielding layer is torn off in the extracellular matrix near the tumor whereas it protects the delivery vehicle in the bloodstream. Increased surface charges or exposure of a ligand moiety induces higher cellular uptake of delivery vehicles [122]. Acidic pH and specific enzymes in the extracellular matrix can trigger the detachment of the shielding layer. The detachable strategy has widely been used for delivery of biomacromolecules such as plasmid DNA and antisense oligonucleotide, but more researches regarding enzyme response than acidic pH response have been investigated for systemic delivery of siRNA. The vehicle responding to the subtle pH difference between the extracellular matrix and neutral pH may not have significantly increased RNAi efficiency compared with the vehicle responding to the pH difference between late endosome and neutral pH.

The invasive nature of malignant tumors has long been associated with the ability to degrade the collagen in the extracellular matrix, a three-dimensional noncellular structure that is present in all tissues and provides physical support for tissue integrity and elasticity [123]. The matrix metalloproteinase (MMP) family is involved in tissue invasion, angiogenesis, regulation of inflammation,

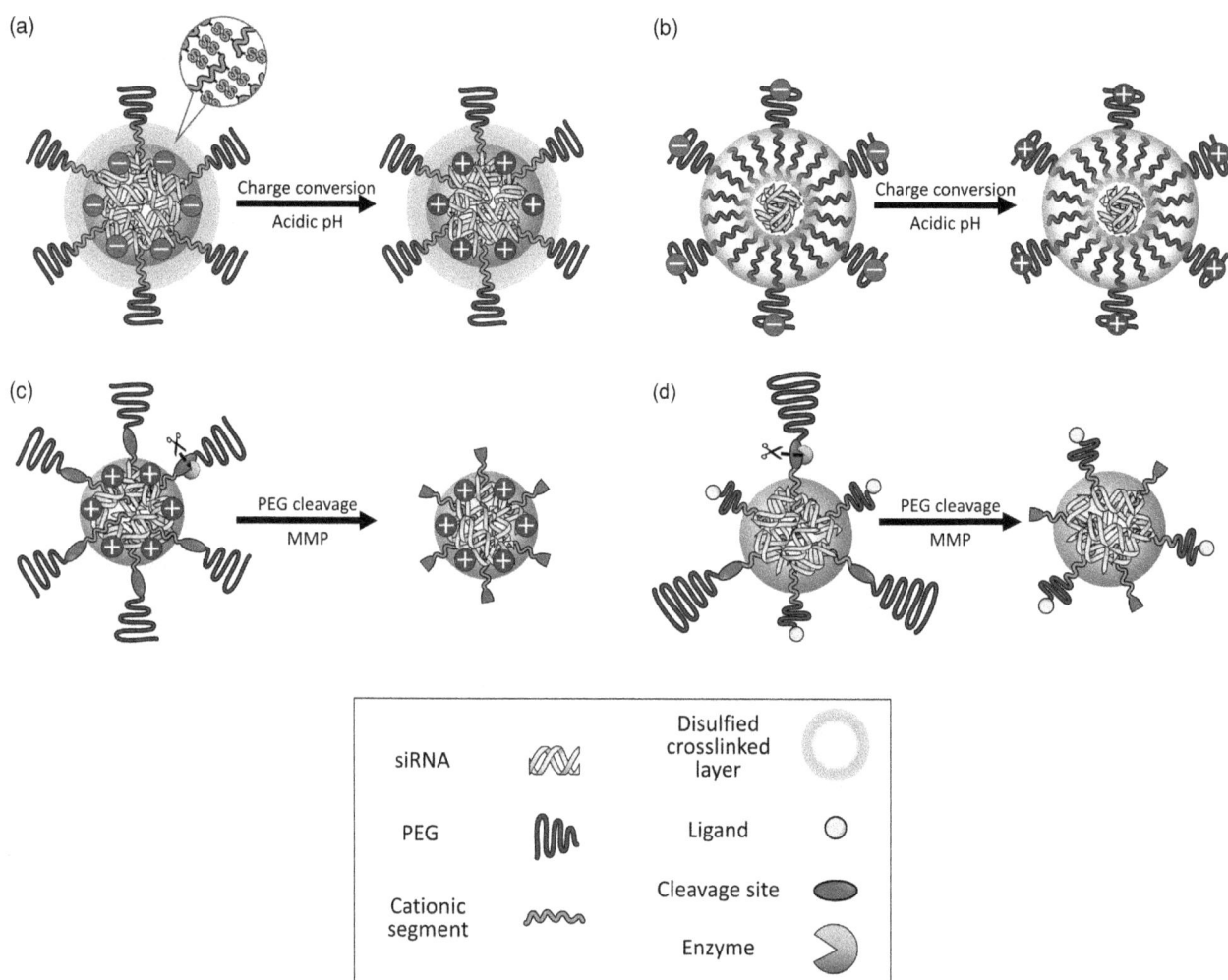

FIGURE 2.5 Illustration of delivery vehicles for cell-specific recognition in tumor microenviroment. Multimolecular structures contain charge-conversion moieties in the core (a) or on to the surface (b). Enzymes (e.g., MMPs) cleave PEG layers, which exposes positive charges in the core (c) or cell-specific ligands (d).

and formation of metastatic niche [124,125]. MMPs include 23 zinc-dependent endopeptidases and have been overexpressed from tumor cells or stromal cells infiltrating the tumor. Therefore, MMPs with a higher concentration in the tumor environment can also represent biosignals, which can be used to design intelligent vehicles. An MMP-cleavable peptide (VPLSLYSGCG) is placed between PEG and the polycations [126] (Figure 2.5c). When the delivery vehicle was treated with 50 nM MMP-7, a similar concentration in the metastatic tumor microenvironment, the zeta-potential of the delivery vehicle gradually increased over 6.5 h and MMP-7 efficiently cleaved PEG layers. Using MMP-7 treatment at 1–5 nM concentrations relevant to normal and healthy tissue, the vehicle showed a slower rate of increase in zeta-potentials, indicating a dose-dependent response to the MMP-7 concentration. The MMP-7-pretreated vehicle was internalized at 2.5-fold higher amounts in cultured cancer cells than nontreated controls due to the increase in its surface charges. In luciferase overexpressing cancer cells, the MMP-7-pretreated vehicle also showed better endogenous luciferase gene silencing than nontreated controls,

implying that PEG-peptide-polycation has the potential to function in an animal tumor model. It is notable that the VPLSLYSGCG peptide can also be efficiently cleaved by other enzymes, MMP-2 and MMP-9. This PEG-peptide-polycation was further improved with a folate-conjugated polymer to increase cellular uptake in the tumor microenvironment [127]. PEG20K-peptide-polycation and folate-PEG2K-polycation were synthesized, and micellar nanoparticles were prepared using a 1:1 mixing ratio of each polymer. When the micellar nanoparticle arrived at the MMP-rich environment, the longer PEG shield was cleaved by MMP-7 and the underlying folate ligand exposed (Figure 2.5d). Thus, the nanoparticles can internalize into target cells by ligand-mediated endocytosis. These nanoparticles achieved greater than 50% protein-level knockdown in cultured folate receptor expressing breast cancer cells. The MMP responsive delivery vehicle was further evaluated in an animal model [122]. A PEG-sheddable delivery vehicle through MMP-2-cleavable peptide (PLGLAGR9) significantly enhanced growth inhibition in the subcutaneous breast tumor (20 μg siRNA/mice, 7–8 injections).

TABLE 2.2
List of MMP Cleavable Peptide Sequences and Delivery Vehicles

Cleavable Peptide Sequences	Enzyme	Delivery Vehicles
GGGV	MMP-2, MMP-9	Lipid-based nanoparticle [128]
PLSLYSGGGG		
GPLGIAGQ	MMP-2	Lipid-based nanoparticle [129]
VPLSLYSGCG	MMP-2, MMP-7, and MMP-9	Polymeric micelles [126,127]
PLGLAGR9	MMP-2	Polymeric micelles [122], Dendrimer [130]
RSWMGLP	MMP-9	Silica particle [131]
GPLGVRG	MMP-2	Polymeric micelles [132]
PVGLIG	MMP-2, MMP-9	Lipid-based nanoparticle [133]

However, moderate inhibition of tumor growth compared with controls indicated that MMP of high molecular weight cannot easily access the target peptide in the intermediate layer of the delivery vehicle, probably inducing a delayed responsiveness in the tumor environment. The high-dense PEG layer in the current delivery vehicles probably guarantees reduction of nonspecific absorption of serum proteins in the bloodstream but simultaneously reduces the MMP approaches. Thus, biosignals of large Molecular weight (Mw) such as MMP may not fully induce desired responses in multimolecular structures. Other MMP-cleavable peptides and their applicable delivery vehicles are summarized in Table 2.2.

2.6.2 Ligand Installed Delivery Vehicles

To optimize the ligand-mediated active targeting functionality, several parameters, including ligand density and length/density of spacer, should be considered for construction of actively targeted multimolecular structures. The underlying mechanism of active targeting is the recognition of the ligand by its target receptors, and thus, a higher density of both ligand and receptor generally guarantees higher opportunities of their binding. For example, conjugates of chemically modified siRNA and tri-N-acetylgalactosamine (GalNAc) resulted in a higher cellular uptake in primary mouse hepatocytes than bi-GalNAc siRNA conjugates [134]. This result demonstrates a multivalent binding effect of ligands for the enhanced cellular uptake efficiency, at least in cultured cells. Similarly, a higher number of ligands on the multimolecular vehicle surface exhibit more efficient internalization in cultured cells. However, such enhanced uptakes through the binding of the multivalent ligands were not always observed for active targeting in systemic administration. The receptors are expressed not only on the target cellular surface but also on nontarget ones at lower levels. Thus, a higher number of ligands can generate the higher affinity (or avidity) to target cellular surface, but concurrently increase the risk for nonspecific binding to such nontargeted cells. Intercellular adhesion molecule-1 (ICAM-1) is constitutively expressed at a basal level on endothelial cells in quiescent vasculature, but its expression is markedly elevated in pathologically activated endothelium.

Introduction of the reduced quantity of the ICAM-1-specific antibody onto a particle surface enhanced the selectivity for binding to inflamed vasculature compared with normal tissues [135]. The length of spacer between the ligand and a nanoparticle surface affects the binding chances due to flexibility of the spacer. Antibody-installed nanoparticles equipped with PEG_{2000} or PEG_{3000} exhibited greater binding to cultured dendritic cells, compared to those with PEG_{6000}, PEG_{10000}, or PEG_{20000} [136]. The optimal PEG length depends on the individual delivery vehicle. A peptide ligand-installed liposome with a PEG_{350} linker dramatically enhanced the cellular uptake in cultured cancer cells with appropriate density of the peptide, whereas control liposome with a PEG_{2000} linker showed the similar level of cellular uptake to nontargeted controls [137]. The density of PEG onto nanoparticles also affects the cellular uptake amount by active targeting. cRGD installed nanoparticle tailored with 5% PEG_{2000} density exhibited the highest relative internalization amounts in cultured cancer cells and animal experiments compared to no ligand-installed control with the same PEG density [138]. Other nanoparticles tailored with 10%–50% PEG_{2000} densities showed less active targeting effects. There are other factors such as charges of the ligand/delivery vehicle and the size of the delivery vehicle to obtain efficient active targeting, and these are precisely described in other researches [8,56].

Interestingly, delivery vehicles can utilize blood components for active targeting. Cholesterol-conjugated siRNA with a partial phosphorothioate backbone and 2′-O-methyl-modified nucleotides binds to low-density lipoprotein (LDL) (KD = 100 μM) and obtained a plasma half-life of approximately 100–120 min (dose amount: 50 mg/kg), accompanied by significant gene silencing in the liver through LDL receptor-mediated endocytosis [139,140]. Some LPNs are also believed to exchange their components with serum and adsorb lipoproteins, leading to enhanced internalization into hepatocytes through lipoprotein receptors [141].

2.7 DELIVERY VEHICLES FOR HIGH ENDOSOMAL ESCAPABILITY

Delivery vehicles potentially contain endosomal escapability and facilitate their escape from endo/lysosomal acidification. In cultured cells, this enhanced endosomal escapability of vehicles greatly increases gene silencing efficiency compared with controls without escapability. In systemic administration, the functional chemical groups of endosomal escapability, e.g., secondary/tertiary amines or histidine should be carefully tailored in multimolecular structures because those possess a low pKa value and unprotonated amino groups do not participate in electrostatic association with siRNA.

PEI is a representative cationic polymer eliciting endosomal escapability through the proton sponge hypothesis [75,76]. PEI shows partial protonation of nitrogens at physiological pH (45% in linear PEIDP520) and augmented protonation at endo/lysosomal acidification (55% in linear PEIDP520) in 150 mM NaCl [77,142]. One notable disadvantage of PEI is cytotoxicity. It is known that the cytotoxicity is substantially elevated with an increase in the molecular weight of PEI. However, low molecular weight PEI cannot maintain a stable multimolecular structure under physiological milieu because of its less ion-pairing sites to nucleic acids, compromising the transfection efficacy. Thus, the low molecular weight PEI (e.g., molecular weight 800 Da) was conjugated with each other to have a higher molecular weight (e.g., average molecular weight: 10–20 kDa) through biodegradable linkages for maintaining higher transfection efficiency associated with lower cytotoxicity [143,144].

A low-toxic and pH-dependent cationic moiety was alternately developed by fine-tuning the number of the repeating aminoethylene unit, $-(CH_2CH_2NH)n-$ in the side chain of polyaspartamide [74]. The polymers were synthesized by direct aminolysis of PEG-b-poly(β-benzyl-L-aspartate) with diethylenetriamine $[-(CH_2CH_2NH)_2-,$ DET] or tetraethylenepentamine $[-(CH_2CH_2NH)_4-,$ TEP] [termed as PEGPAsp(DET) and PEG-PAsp(TEP), respectively] [145]. PAsp(DET) contained 51% and 82% protonated amino groups at pH 7.4 and pH 5.5, respectively, thereby eliciting a large change in the protonation degree ($\Delta\alpha =31\%$) [77]. PAsp(DET) had a monoprotonated structure $(-CH_2CH_2NH-CH_2CH_2NH_3^+)$ to induce a low membrane destabilization effect at pH 7.4, whereas the diprotonated structure of PAsp(DET) $(-CH_2CH_2NH_2^+-CH_2CH_2NH_3^+)$ had a high membrane destabilization effect at pH 5.5. PAsp(TEP) also exhibited acidic pH-selective membrane destabilization ability, which is only possessed by even numbered aminoethylene units: PAsp(DET) and PAsp(TEP) had two and four aminoethylene units, respectively. Further detailed and comprehensive mechanisms regarding the endosomal escape moiety are explained in other review papers [77]. Derivatives of these polymers, PEGPAsp(DET) and PEG-PAsp(TEP), successfully delivered therapeutic siRNA into the subcutaneous and spontaneous model of cancers [87,88,146].

Other chemical structures in the cationic polymer also facilitated pH-mediated membrane disruption. For example, poly(dimethylaminoethyl methacrylate-co-propyl acrylic acid-co-butyl methacrylate) [termed as p(DMAEMA-co-PAA-co-BMA)] was ampholytic under physiological pH in that positive DMAEMA and negative PAA residues masked hydrophobic BMA [147]. At endosomal pH, PAA underwent hydrophilic to hydrophobic transition of carboxylate groups and DMAEMA (pKa=7.4) increased the positive charge in the residues. This changed the polymer from a hydrophilic polyampholyte to hydrophobic polycations that were capable of disrupting the endosomal membrane. In addition, the imidazole ring (pKa=6.0) of histidine induces a proton sponge effect in an acidic condition and poly(histidine) has been utilized as an endosomal escape moiety [148].

Although some cationic lipids were synthesized by linking the alkyl chain or lipid components with PEI to provide a buffering effect [149,150], the LPN had its own endosomal escape mechanism, which was first proposed by the Szoka group [151,152]. Cationic components of LPNs are associated with anionic phospholipid in the endosomal membranes, promoting the formation of the inverted hexagonal (HII) phase. The HII phase involves six cylindrical fused structures of two oppositely charged lipid components, where the head group of the lipid components faces inward and the hydrocarbon tail faces outward. Cationic lipids promoting these nonbilayer structures lead to disruption of the endosomal membrane and release of siRNA from nanoparticles into the cytoplasm [151,153]. Dioleoylphosphatidylethanolamine is known as a "fusogenic" cationic lipid because it can place this nonbilayer structure, whereas dioleylphosphatidylcoline (DOPC) forms a stable lamellar structure that dramatically decreases LPN fusion with the endosomal membrane.

2.8 DELIVERY CARRIER DESIGN IN OTHER CATEGORY

2.8.1 LAYER-BY-LAYER DELIVERY VEHICLE

Delivery vehicles constructed by the layer-by-layer (LbL) technology for high loading of siRNA have been an attractive strategy for local administration because the vehicle has superior gene silencing efficiency even at picomolar siRNA concentrations in cultured cells [154,155]. Nevertheless, its larger particle size (> 100 nm) and wide size distribution have been believed to be drawbacks for passive/active targeting by systemic route. Very recently, a systemically injected LbL particle was developed to exhibit comparative tumor growth inhibition in animal models when the particle was carefully engineered to possess building components for tumor targeting (Figure 2.6a). LbL nanoparticle construction, which alternately deposits siRNA and polycations on to template, has a unique advantage over other multimolecular structures because a single nanoparticle can load much larger amounts of siRNAs (approximately 3500 siRNA molecules) and exhibit a long period of siRNA release time (approximately 3 weeks) in cultured cells [156]. When an LbL nanoparticle codelivered multidrug resistance protein 1 (MRP1) siRNA with doxorubicin

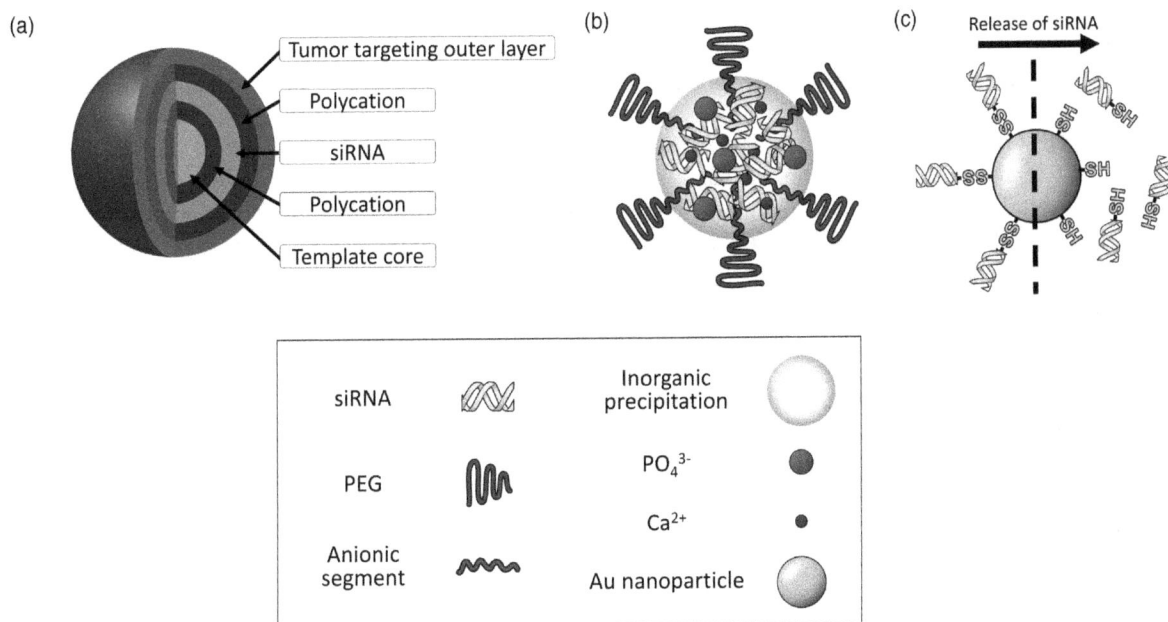

FIGURE 2.6 Illustration of delivery vehicles for other categories. An LbL particle is constructed by alternative deposition of anionic and cationic components (a). A calcium phosphate particle stably formulates siRNA and PEG-polyanions in the core region (b). Thiolated siRNA is attached to Au nanoparticles and released in the response of GSH concentration (c).

into a subcutaneous animal model of triple-negative breast cancer, MDA-MB-468 cancer, it showed the synergistic inhibition of tumor growth (1 mg/kg siRNA and 1 mg/kg doxorubicin) [157]. Of note, MRP1 is a cell-surface efflux pump involved in redox regulation of multidrug resistance by clearing the intracellular concentration of xenobiotics and toxins [158,159]. Because MRP1 siRNA treatment did not show any tumor inhibitory effects, this result demonstrated that siRNA as supplements can be applied for combination therapy with clinically approved anticancer drugs. At present, to reduce cancer drug resistance, two combination therapies regarding ERCC1 siRNA/cisplatin and mutated KRAS siRNA/gemcitabine are being conducted in Phase I and Phase II studies, respectively. Design strategies of delivery vehicles to increase the efficiency of combination therapy and the targeting gene/cancer drug combination are well described in a previous review [160]. The LbL nanoparticle provides clues in the design of delivery vehicles. High loading of siRNA in the single delivery vehicle is also a critical factor for efficient gene silencing. Another point to consider is that altering the size of LbL nanoparticles loaded with a high amount of siRNA will increase the performance of the delivery vehicles.

2.8.2 Calcium Phosphate-formulated Delivery Vehicles

Deposition and coprecipitation of inorganic materials on multimolecular structures can facilitate to formulate siRNA [161]. These inorganic material-stabilized vehicles have been developed for better size control of the particles and higher encapsulation of siRNA. Calcium phosphate (CaP) is one of the most commonly used component materials

because CaP is a mineral of human bone and generally considered to be biocompatible. CaP precipitates were used as transfection reagents of plasmid DNA because they can bind and encapsulate polyanions/ nucleic acids and protect the nucleic acid from enzymatic degradation. The major limitation of CaP precipitates was the uncontrollable and rapid growth of CaP crystals after preparation, resulting in the formation of micrometer-sized agglomerates. Size-controlled nanoparticles with high colloidal stability were obtained when CaP was precipitated with a mixture of PEG-polyanions and siRNA [162]. CaP precipitation simultaneously formulates phosphate of siRNA and the carboxyl group of the PEG-polyanions (Figure 2.6b). Precipitated nanoparticles carefully need to be examined so that single particles encapsulate both building components because there is a possibility that one component is favored in CaP precipitates. The resulting nanoparticle can dissolve under highly dilute conditions for payload release, based on the equilibrium shift toward calcium and phosphate ions. The resulting CaP nanoparticle has approximately 40 nm diameter size and maintained its initial size in the serum containing medium while the nanoparticle rapidly dissociated in the medium mimicking the cytoplasm [146,163]. CaP nanoparticles showed better endogenous vascular endothelial growth factor (VEGF) messenger RNA (mRNA) silencing in cultured pancreatic cancer cells and did not induce significant toxicity at concentrations of up to 25-fold higher concentrations than RNAi-induced concentrations. A high dose of unbound calcium ions can apparently affect the heart because cardiac excitation–contraction is based on regulation of the intracellular calcium ion concentration in heart muscle cells [164]. Thus, for systemic delivery of therapeutic siRNA, the CaP nanoparticle was further purified by an ultrafiltration method, and approximately, 80% of the original calcium contents were removed [146]. VEGF siRNA delivered by the purified CaP nanoparticles (25 μg siRNA/mice, four injections) inhibited subcutaneous tumor growth with negligible acute toxicity, indirectly indicating that CaP nanoparticles are stable enough in the bloodstream to attain gene silencing in remote tumors. While CaP precipitates contribute to increased stability of block copolymer-based nanoparticles, CaP precipitates can enhance endosomal escape ability. Delivery vehicles containing CaP precipitates disassemble at low pH in the endosome, which cause endosome swelling and eruption, releasing the entrapped siRNA due to a high concentration of ions [165]. This nanoparticle has been coformulated with three different siRNAs against MDM2, c-myc, and VEGF at the weight ratio of 1:1:1 and significantly reduced lung metastases of B16F10 at a relatively low dose (0.36 mg/kg siRNA, four injections) [166]. Delivery efficiency of the current delivery vehicles stabilized with inorganic materials may increase with more precise design of vehicle components. When inorganic materials/siRNA are further encapsulated within the hydrophobic intermediate layer in the core, this structure may prevent rapid dissociation in the bloodstream.

2.8.3 Gold Nanoparticle-templated Delivery Vehicles

The AuNP is widely selected for siRNA delivery because the bonding of gold-thiol group exhibits GSH concentration-responsive cleavage. Thus, thiolated building components (e.g., siRNA or polymers)-conjugated AuNP is also relatively stable under the extracellular condition, but these thiolated components can be competed off the AuNP in the cell interior. In this term, siRNA is designed to be released from the delivery vehicle in response to GSH concentration (Figure 2.6c). Thiol-terminated RNA duplexes are loaded into a 13-nm AuNP and further treated with oligoethylene glycol-thiol or PEG-thiol, as an additional surface passivating ligand [167]. The resulting spherical nucleic acid (SNA) nanoparticles contained approximately 90 sense strand and approximately 38 antisense strands per AuNP. Pharmacokinetic analyses using a two-compartment model showed that the blood circulation properties of the SNA nanoparticles had a half-life of approximately 1 min in the first phase and approximately 8.5 h half-life in the second phase. This data suggests that thiol-gold coordination is stable enough to maintain thiol-terminated RNA duplexes in the bloodstream. The SNA nanoparticle successfully penetrates the blood–brain barrier and blood–tumor barrier, and reduced Bcl2L12 expression in intracerebral glioblastoma multiforme. The reduction in Bcl2L12 mRNA and the subsequent protein level compared with controls indicates that the thiol-terminated RNA duplexes can be efficiently released in GSH-rich cytoplasm and exert appropriate gene silencing. Other example is that thiol-terminated PEG-polycations were complexed with siRNA

and then the resulting thiolated complex was conjugated into a 20-nm AuNP [168]. This delivery vehicle had 40 nm diameter size and was loaded with approximately 20 siRNAs per a particle. The blood circulation property of this vehicle showed that 10% amount of the initial dose continued to circulate at 3 h and higher tumor accumulation of siRNA was obtained in subcutaneous cervical tumor compared to controls, e.g., naked siRNA, thiolated complex, and nonthiolated complex-loaded AuNP. Finally, this vehicle obtained luciferase gene silencing in an animal tumor model.

2.9 SYNTHESIS OF siRNA AND CHEMICAL MODIFICATION OF NUCLEOTIDES

The presence of endogenous RNAi pathways in mammalian cells provides a powerful mechanism for the regulation of cellular signaling pathways by enabling precise modulation of the gene expression [169]. As one component of the RNAi complex, siRNAs are able to "silence" expression of specific genes with complementary sequences. In contrast to traditional drugs, the sequence of a siRNA therapeutic can be identified based on the knowledge of the sequence of the mRNA that would encode for the protein target. While siRNA has the potential to target essentially any gene, function requires methods to deliver these molecules inside of target cells safely and effectively. The FDA recently approved the first ever siRNA therapeutic, which is a LNP, called Onpattro™ (Patisiran) that encapsulates and delivers siRNA against mutant and wild-type transthyretin (TTR) to treat TTR-mediated amyloidosis [170]. We believe that Onpattro is the first of many RNAi medicines, but that additional development is required to achieve the broadest clinical application of siRNA. Below, we describe how chemistry has played a critical role in improving the efficacy, specificity, and safety of siRNA therapeutics, since the initial description of RNAi in 1998 [169].

In 2006, the Nobel Prize was awarded for the discovery and characterization of RNAi [169]. RNAi is mediated by small double-stranded RNA molecules, or siRNAs, which associate with the RISC inside of cells. After loading, the strands are separated, leaving the antisense (or guide) strand to bind complementary mRNA (Figure 2.7a) [171–173]. The Argonaute endoribonuclease cleaves the mRNA, which prevents it from being translated to protein [173]. The antisense strand stays bound to the RISC and is able to act catalytically to cleave additional mRNA strands. Although siRNA is generally double-stranded, it can be single-stranded, hairpin, or dumbbell shaped as long as the antisense strand can become loaded into the RNAi machinery [174]. For example, single-stranded siRNA is able to activate RNAi in mice, albeit less efficiently than the canonical double-stranded forms [175,176].

Delivery of siRNA has been the major challenge to application of siRNA therapeutics in humans

[172,177–180]. One key challenge to delivery is the pharmacological properties of siRNA. For example, siRNAs are relatively large (~13 kDa) in molecular weight in comparison to small molecule drugs. They are highly anionic with approximately thirty-eight to fifty phosphate groups, which make them difficult to diffuse across cellular membranes. Furthermore, unmodified siRNAs are unstable in the bloodstream and can induce immune responses through interaction with Toll-like receptors [174]. Intravenously administered siRNA must cross the vascular endothelial barrier and then diffuse through the extracellular matrix to function. They must also avoid filtration by kidneys and uptake by nontargeted cells. After cellular internalization, siRNAs need to be released from endosomal compartments, decomplex, and access the RNAi machinery. Throughout this whole process, siRNAs need to have sufficient resistance to nuclease degradation to enable function [4]. Therefore, siRNAs have significant delivery challenges that do not exist for small molecule drugs [173]. Nevertheless, significant progress has been made, and there are currently >20 ongoing clinical trials with siRNA-based therapeutics [1,181–183].

Figure 2.7b describes a typical process for the development of siRNA therapeutics [182]. First, for a specific biological target, many RNA strands need to be designed and synthesized to identify the most potent sequences along the target mRNA strand. This is generally done both experimentally and computationally [184].

Chemically modified nucleotides can improve chemical stability and efficacy, increase cell specificity, reduce immunological effects, and decrease off-target effects [174]. siRNA conjugation is one important method to achieve efficacious RNAi both *in vitro* and *in vivo*. This section will focus on the chemical modification of nucleotides and synthesis of siRNA.

2.9.1 Nucleotides Modification

Nucleotides are the basic building blocks for both DNA and RNA. In general, natural nucleotides are composed of a ribose or 2′-deoxyribose sugar with 1′-nucleobase and 3′-phosphate groups (Figure 2.8). Chemical modification of nucleotides dates back to the 1960s [185]. In recent years, the effects of modified nucleotides on siRNA activity have been extensively examined [186,187]. As illustrated in Figure 2.8, four major sites have been explored for modification: the 2′-position, phosphate linkage, ribose, and nucleobase [174].

The 2′-position is the most common modification site in nucleotides. In 1959, Smith and Dunn isolated 2′-O-methyladenosine from the wheat germ and rat liver [188]. The selective synthesis of this compound using diazomethane and 1,2-dimethoxyethane was described by Robins and coworkers [189]. Because chemical modification can potentially inhibit activity, Rana and coworkers performed a chemical modification analysis for siRNA function [187].

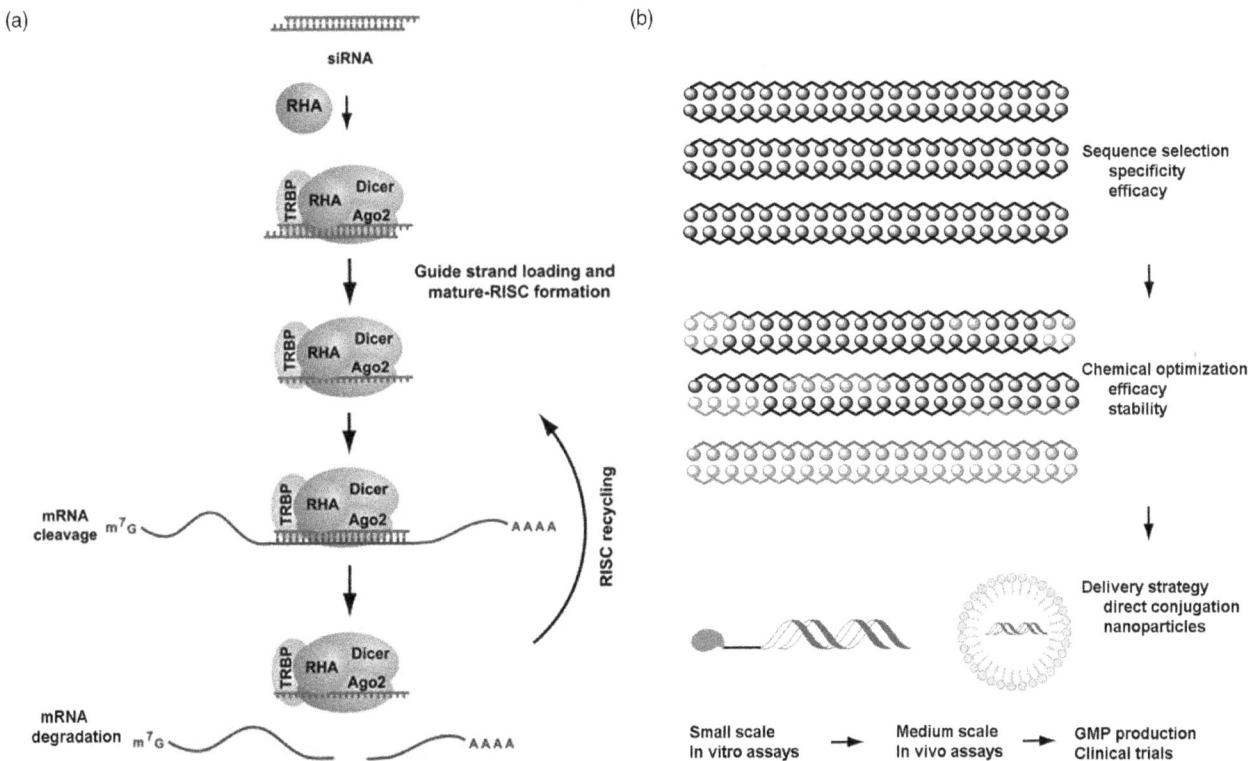

FIGURE 2.7 Mechanism of RNA interference and strategies for siRNA synthesis and delivery. (a). An illustration of RNA interference process [171]. (b). Strategies and procedures for siRNA development and delivery.

Their results indicated that 2'-OHs are not required for the siRNA activity and that 2' modification could significantly improve the stability of siRNA and extend their half-life [187]. The 2'-position has been modified with a number of residues including 2'-Omethyl, 2'-O-methoxyethyl, and fluoro (Figure 2.8). Conformational constrained nucleotides such as locked nucleic acid (LNA) were developed by Imanishi and Wengel independently [190,191]. Introduction of LNA bases not only improves the stability of siRNA but can also increase the binding affinity to RNA [186]. Recently, an α-L-tricyclic nucleic acid was developed, which is also highly constrained (Figure 2.8) [192].

With regard to the phosphate linkage, chemical synthesis using nucleotide phosphorothioate (including the relevant diastereomers) was the earliest exploration of nucleotide modification [185]. These linkages significantly stabilize the RNA to nuclease degradation such as those found in the human serum, but may lead to increased toxicity [186]. Interestingly, DNA phosphorothioation was discovered in 2007 as an endogenous process in bacteria [193]. Recently, Wu and coworkers explored different types of phosphorodithioate on siRNAs and their antitumor activity in mouse models [194]. In addition, a polyamide-based peptide nucleic acid (PNA) was reported by Nielsen and coworkers in 1991 [195]. Later, PNA modification was installed at the end of RNA strands [196]. This PNA-siRNA was reported to inhibit the activity of telomerase and introduce cell death of human tumor cells. Boron-containing nucleotide analogs were reported in the early 1990s [197]. A recent study reports that boranophosphate siRNAs can be more potent than native siRNA and phosphorothioate siRNAs [198]. However, PNA and boranophosphate siRNAs have not been investigated as extensively in animal models as phosphorothioate modified siRNAs, which are in human clinical trials [182].

Modification of the ribose ring has also been investigated (Figure 2.8). A morpholino nucleoside was developed in 1989, which has been examined in a number of antisense applications [199]. Morpholino nucleotide oligomers are being examined clinically as a therapy for Duchenne muscular dystrophy [200]. Also of note, Wengel and coworkers developed unlocked nucleic acid (UNA) in 2009 [201]. These acyclic UNA-based siRNAs were shown to induce silencing *in vitro* and *in vivo* [202]. Moreover, UNA modification was reported to reduce off-target effects and improve biostability in mice. At the same time, hexitol- and anitrol-based nucleotides were reported and show potential for use as siRNA modifications [203]. Bramsen and coworkers performed an analysis of chemically modified siRNA for their silencing activity, stability, and toxicity in human tumor cells [204]. They report that the sense strand can tolerate diverse chemical modifications, while the antisense strand can be moderately modified under certain conditions. siRNA stabilization does not require the modification of the whole siRNA duplex, but only on a few selected positions.

They also reported that UNA modification introduced less toxicity and retained the silencing activity [204]. In 2018, oxabicyclic nucleoside phosphonates were chemically synthesized [205] and might be incorporated into siRNA sequences for gene silencing.

Finally, modification of the nucleobase has been examined to improve the nuclease resistance of siRNA duplexes in serum. For instance, siRNAs containing several 2-thiouracil modified units were thermally stable and showed similar silencing activity compared with the unmodified siRNAs [206]. Other representative examples include 5-bromouracil, 6-diaminopurine, and 2,4-difluorotoluene [187,206–208]. In general, base modifications are not widely applied for siRNA modification, but nevertheless offer an additional opportunity for chemical manipulation.

2.9.2 Synthesis of siRNA

The synthesis of siRNA is based on the research that originated in 1950s [209]. In 1978, Zamecnik and Stephenson reported that a synthetic oligonucleotide complementary to Rous sarcoma virus 35S RNA could inhibit protein expression [210,211]. This work reported that a synthetic antisense oligonucleotide (ASO) could bind to a target mRNA through Watson-Crick base pairing led to substantial research development of ASOs as therapeutics. In 2013, the FDA approved mipomersen, an ASO against apolipoprotein B, for the treatment of homozygous familial hypercholesterolemia [212]. Nusinersen (Spinraza) was later approved by the FDA in 2016 for the indication of spinal muscular atrophy [213]. In general, ASOs do not function *in vivo* through the RNAi pathway and therefore are not considered siRNAs [214]. Nonetheless, research on ASOs provided the basis for much of the chemistry used in siRNA synthesis and chemical modification today.

Solid-phase synthesis is currently the primary approach used to make synthetic RNA [215,216]. As shown in Figure 2.8b, RNA synthesis is a repetitive chemical cycle in which each nucleotide is added on a solid support. This cycle starts with a deprotection step to remove the protective group on 5'-hydroxyl of the solid support bound nucleotide. The resulting 5'-hydroxyl is then coupled with an activated 3'-phosphorous ester, followed by a capping step to remove the unreacted nucleotides from the reaction system. The intermediate undergoes another step to oxidize phosphite to phosphorous ester. After the chain assembly, the oligomer is released from the solid support, deprotected, and purified by Pressure Liquid Chromatography (HPLC). Two types of building blocks were later developed for the efficient synthesis of RNA including 2'-O-TOM and 2'-O-ACE modified nucleotides (Figure 2.7c) [215]. Both methods provide a coupling yield of over 99% [215]. The whole process has been successfully automated by utilizing oligonucleotide synthesizers [215].

(a)

(b)

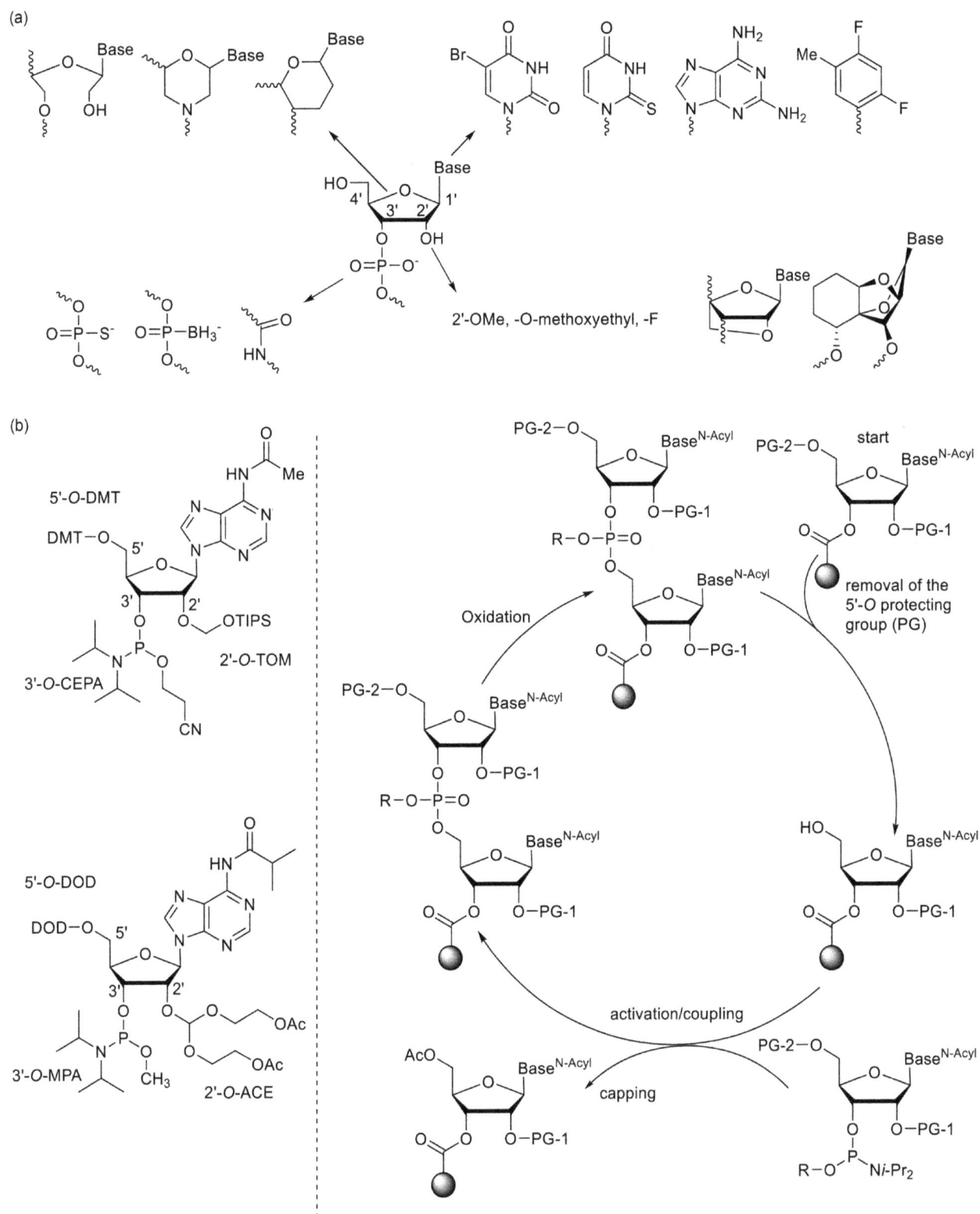

FIGURE 2.8 siRNA synthesis. (a). Chemical modification of nucleic acids including the 2′-position, phosphate linkage, ribose, and nucleobase. (b). Solid-phase synthesis of RNA strands using automated RNA synthesizer [215].

2.10 sIRNA-LIGAND CONJUGATES

Direct ligand conjugation to siRNA is a promising delivery strategy. Diverse ligands including small molecules, carbohydrates, aptamers, peptides, and antibodies have been covalently linked to siRNA in order to improve cellular uptake and target-specific cell types (Figure 2.9a) [217–221]. An advantage of siRNA conjugates is that they reduce the

need for extra delivery materials and may thereby improve the tolerability and safety profile of the delivery formulation [222]. Because the 5′-end of the antisense strand is required for silencing activity, conjugation is typically performed on the sense strand or 3′-end of antisense strand [217]. Two synthetic approaches have been applied: parallel synthesis and linear synthesis.

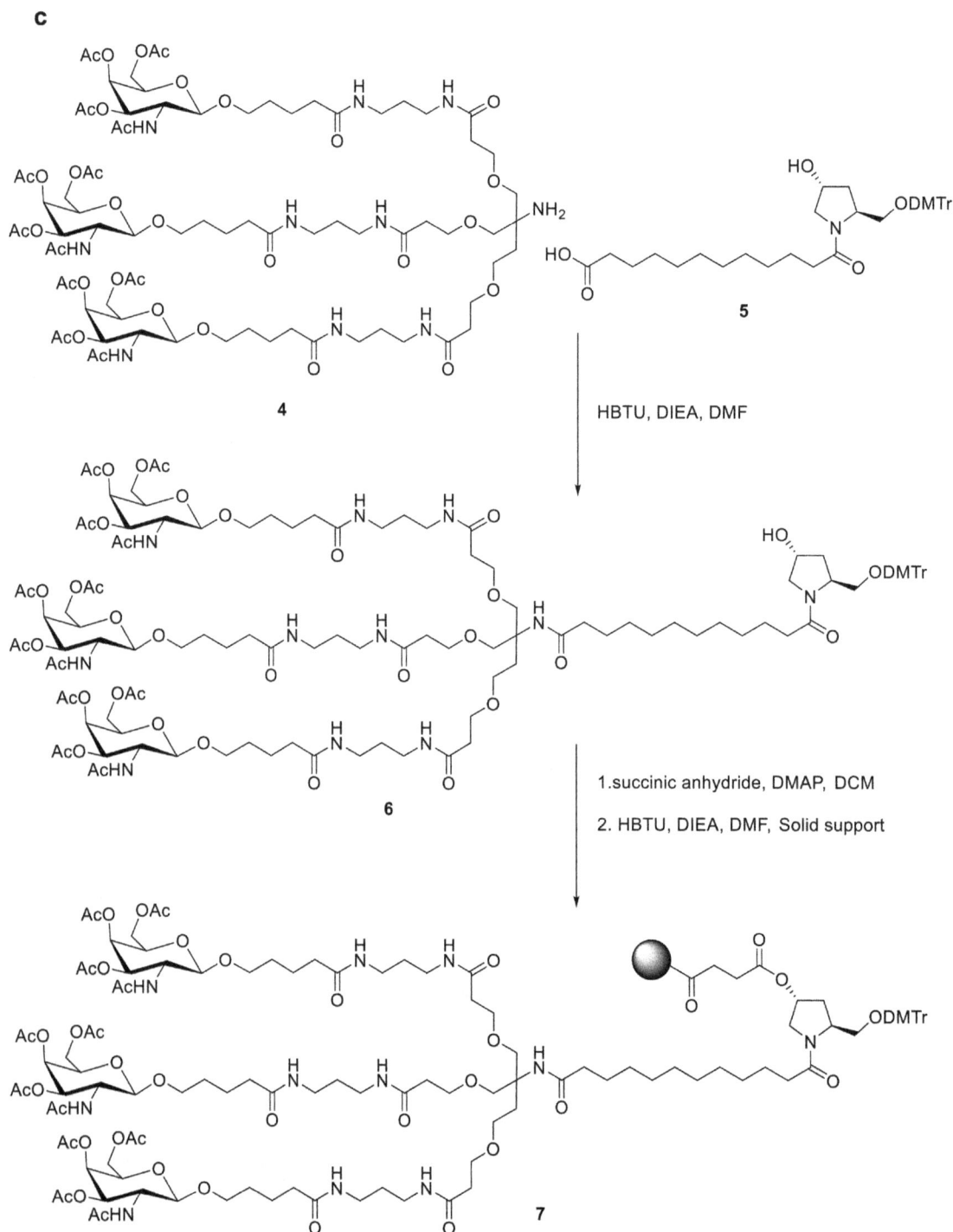

FIGURE 2.9 Chemical strategies for synthesis of siRNA conjugates. (a). siRNA conjugates with ligands including small molecules, carbohydrates peptides, antibodies, and aptamers. (b). Parallel and linear synthesis siRNA-peptide and siRNA-cholesterol conjugates. (c). An example of linear synthesis of GalNAc-siRNA conjugates.

For parallel synthesis (Figure 2.9b), siRNA and its relevant conjugate ligand are synthesized in separate synthetic routes and then are conjugated with each other usually through biodegradable bonds [217]. For example, conjugation of membrane permanent peptides (MPPs, 1) and anti-green fluorescent protein (GFP) siRNA was achieved through a disulfide bond using a diamide oxidizing reagent [223]. Rana and coworkers applied a similar strategy to conjugate trans-activated transcription (TAT) peptide (2), a cell penetrating peptide and siRNA through a succinimidyl 4-[p-maleimidophenyl] butyrate based linker [224]. Condensation of insulin receptor substrate 1 (3) and siRNA was also achieved through an amide linkage [225]. The above siRNA conjugates were reported to show silencing effects in different human cell lines.

Linear synthesis (functional groups are added sequentially) is also widely used for a variety of chemical conjugations to siRNA (Figure 2.9b). In 1989, Letsinger and coworkers reported the synthesis of amide-linked, cholesterol-modified oligonucleotides [226]. In 2004, cholesterol- and lipid-modified siRNAs were created using a pyrrolidine-based linkage [140]. These lipophilic siRNA conjugates were shown to silence apolipoprotein B through intravenous injection in mice [139], via a lipoprotein-dependent mechanism. Both the low-density lipoprotein receptor and scavenger receptor class B Type I are required for the uptake of siRNA conjugates by the liver and other tissues.

A similar conjugation strategy was applied to develop hepatocyte-targeted delivery using the asialoglycoprotein receptor (ASGPR) targeted ligand, N-acetyl-D-galactosamine (GalNAc) [227]. As shown in Figure 2.9c, pyrrolidine derivative 4 and GalNAc derivative 5 were condensed to afford an intermediate 6 [227]. A solid support was installed on the intermediate through a succinic acid linker and gave the substrate 7 that could then be used to generate the siRNA strand (Figure 2.9c). Finally, the GalNAc-siRNA strand was synthesized by adding the nucleotide one by one through the solid phase–based approach as discussed above. This GalNAc-siRNA conjugate is able to significantly silence target gene in hepatocytes via subcutaneous administration at a dose of single digit mg/kg in mice [222]. Results from a clinical trial of this conjugate demonstrate significant reduction of serum TTR protein for treating TTR-mediated amyloidosis [228]. Currently, a series of these GalNAc-siRNA conjugates are in the early or late stage of clinical trials [170,183]. Cemdisiran is in Phase II clinical investigation for patients with complement-mediated diseases [170,183]. In addition, several promising candidates including Vutrisiran (indication: TTR-mediated amyloidosis), Fitusiran (indication: hemophilia and rare bleeding disorders), Inclisiran (indication: hypercholesterolemia), and Lumasiran (indication: primary hyperoxaluria type 1) are in Phase III clinical trials [170,183]. In addition to the clinical advance, a wide variety of new chemical approaches were reported to optimize the GalNAc-siRNA conjugate. For example, GalNAc can be conjugated on the 2′-position of the ribose

[229]. Matsuda et al. systematically explored the effects of GalNAc on different sites of siRNA strands and identified several potent sequences [229]. Most recently, Parmar and coworkers incorporated (E)-vinylphosphonate at the 5′-end of the antisense strand, which stabilized the siRNA and improved its potency [230]. These findings provide new insights into next generation siRNA conjugates.

2.11 NUCLEOTIDES DERIVED NANOPARTICLES

Nucleotides have long been utilized as building blocks to assemble a wide variety of nanoparticles [231]. For example, DNA nanostructures, also called DNA origami, have been explored for over 30 years [231]. A number of two-dimensional and three-dimensional nanostructures have been self-assembled through branched DNA motifs and crystalized for characterization and visualization. In 2012, self-assembled DNA-siRNA tetrahedral nanoparticles were developed for siRNA delivery [232]. The 28.6 nm tetrahedron nanoparticles were composed of 186 Watson-Crick base pairs. Each edge is 30 base pairs long and contains a nick in the middle (Figure 2.10). This nick is complementary to the overhang of siRNA strands to serve as a siRNA carrier, which was also applied for aptamer-based siRNA delivery [221]. In order to differentiate tumor cells from normal cells, a cancer-targeting ligand, folate, was installed on the nanoparticle surface. The targeted siRNA-DNA origami showed significant silencing in tumor cells at a dose of 2.5 mg/kg (antiluciferase siRNA) in a mouse xenograft model. It also displayed a longer blood circulation time ($t_{1/2} \approx 24.2$ min) compared with free siRNA ($t_{1/2} \approx 6$ min). Different from the DNA origami, Mirkin and coworkers first reported SNA conjugates in 1996, which were made with gold cores and DNA shells [233]. SNA nanostructures are determined by the shape of the cores, and the shells can accommodate both single and double-stranded nucleic acids with sequences of interest. To construct functional SNA, three components were necessary: a particle attachment moiety, a spacer region, and a programmable recognition region [233]. In the past decade, a number of inorganic cores and nucleic acids shells have been investigated for diverse applications including diagnosis, small molecular drug delivery, and DNA and siRNA delivery [233]. By conjugating different siRNA sequences, SNA achieved gene silencing of a variety of biological targets including luciferase, epidermal growth factor receptor, and Bcl2Like12 [167]. Currently, this platform is in the clinical trial for treating glioblastoma. In addition, RNA nanostructures were also applied to siRNA delivery [234,235]. For example, Guo and coworkers constructed multifunctional RNA nanoparticles based on RNA three-way junctions, which showed effective delivery of siRNA targeting survivin [236]. Later on, a diverse set of RNA-based nanomaterials were created for gene silencing and other applications [234,237]. In 2012, Hammond and coworkers developed self-assembled RNAi microsponges

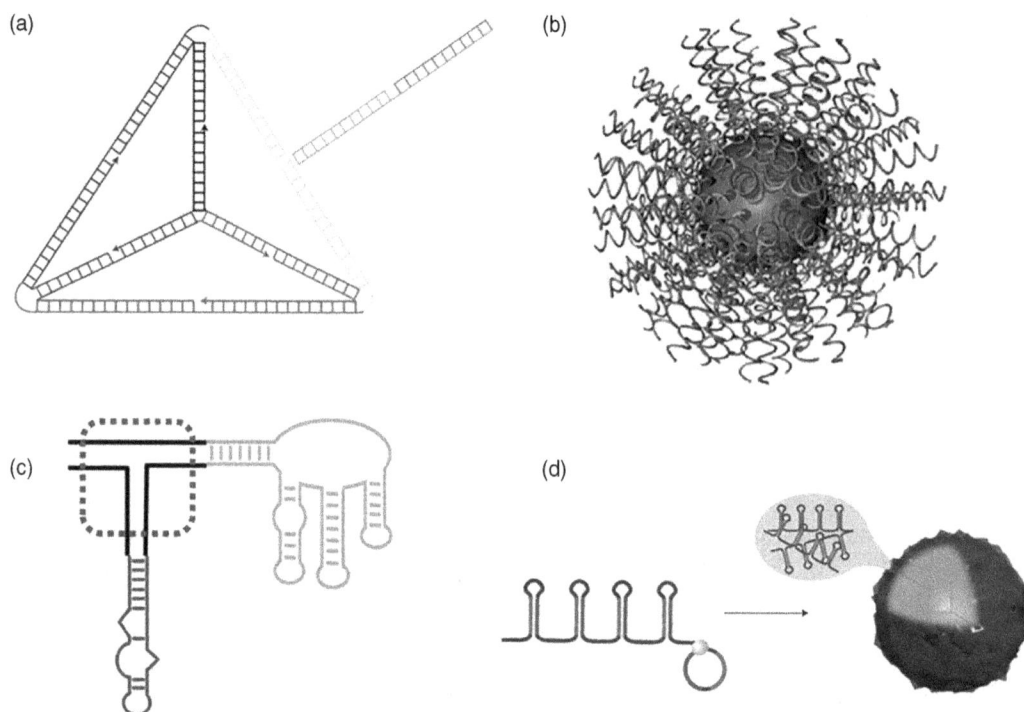

FIGURE 2.10 Nucleotides derived nanoparticles. (a). Tetrahedron DNA origami [232]. (b). Spherical nucleic acid (SNA) conjugates with a gold core and siRNA shell [233]. (c). Three-way junction RNA nanoparticles [237]. (d). RNAi microsponges with multiple copies of shRNA [238].

via rolling circle replication, which was applied by viruses to amplify their genes [238]. To achieve this process, they constructed a linear DNA strand encoding the antisense and sense sequences. Also, their ends were partially complementary to the T7 promoter. After hybridization with a T7 promoter, this linear DNA formed a circular DNA with its nick closed by a T4 DNA ligase. During the RNA transcription, T7 RNA polymerase can produce multiple copies of antisense and sense sequences to form hairpin RNA structures. As the concentration of circular DNA increased from 3 nM to 100 nM, RNA products grow from fiber-like structures to sponge-like structures. A single sponge contains approximately five hundred thousand copies of siRNA. After condensation with PEI, the microsponge size reduced from 2 μm to 200 nm [238].

2.12 LIPID-BASED DELIVERY SYSTEMS

Phospholipids are natural components of cell membranes that form lipid bilayers [239]. Liposomes have been developed as drug delivery carriers using a variety of synthetic lipids [239]. They have been widely used to encapsulate small molecule drugs for treating diseases in humans, most notably Doxil for breast cancer and AmBisome for fungal infection [239]. For example, the formulation of Doxil is composed of doxorubicin, methoxypolyethylene glycol 2000–1,2- distearoyl-sn-glycero-3 phosphoethanolamine (MPEG-DSPE), hydrogenated soy phosphatidylcholine, and cholesterol [239]. These previous studies provide important guidance for the development of lipid-based siRNA delivery systems.

2.12.1 LIPID ANALOGS WITH CATIONIC HEAD GROUPS AND HYDROPHOBIC TAILS

LPNs, particularly lipids with single or multiple cationic centers (Figure 2.11), are highly effective carriers of siRNA [3]. In 2005, SNALPs for intracellular delivery of siRNA were reported [240]. SNALPs are typically composed of a formulation consisting of an amine-based lipid, cholesterol, a PEG-lipid, as well as helper phospholipids [240]. Early SNALPs were formulated from DlinDMA, 1,2-distearoyl-sn-glycero-3-phosphocholine (DSPC) as a helper lipid, mPEG-C-DMA, and cholesterol (DlinDMA:DSPC:Chol:PEG-C-DMA 30:20:48:2 M percent) [240]. DlinDMA is composed of an ionizable amino head group, a glycerol-based ether linker, and two unsaturated carbon tails (Figure 2.11) [240]. Amino lipids are central components of SNALPs as they play a role in the assembly of the nanoparticles, by binding the siRNA through electrostatic interactions [241]. These amino groups also facilitate endosomal escape, through interaction with endosomal components during acidification [242]. The common structure of this type of lipids includes a cationic head group, a linker, and two long hydrophobic domains (Figure 2.11).

In vivo, SNALPs have shown the ability to deliver siRNA to tumor tissues. A Phase I clinical trial using DlinDMA-based ALN-VSP to target VEGF and kinesin family member **11** (KIF11 or KSP) demonstrated antitumor activity in patients with advanced solid tumors (dose > 0.7 mg/kg). To improve the delivery efficiency, the ether linker in DlinDMA was replaced by a ketal linker to afford DLin-KC2-DMA [243]. This chemical alteration reduces the transition temperatures of DLin-KC2-DMA and facilitates its ability to form hexagonal structures when it interacts with naturally occurring anionic phospholipids in the endosomal membrane. This process is believed to promote endosomal release [239]. DLin-KC2-DMA showed improved delivery efficiency with an efficacious dose of 0.01 mg/kg for hepatocyte silencing of Factor VII in mice. Recently, it was reported that DLin-KC2-DMA SNALPs can transfect leukemia cells *in vivo* as well [244].

The structure–activity relationship (SAC) for DLin-KC2-DMA derivatives has been investigated systematically (Figure 2.11) [241]. Head groups were substituted by amino

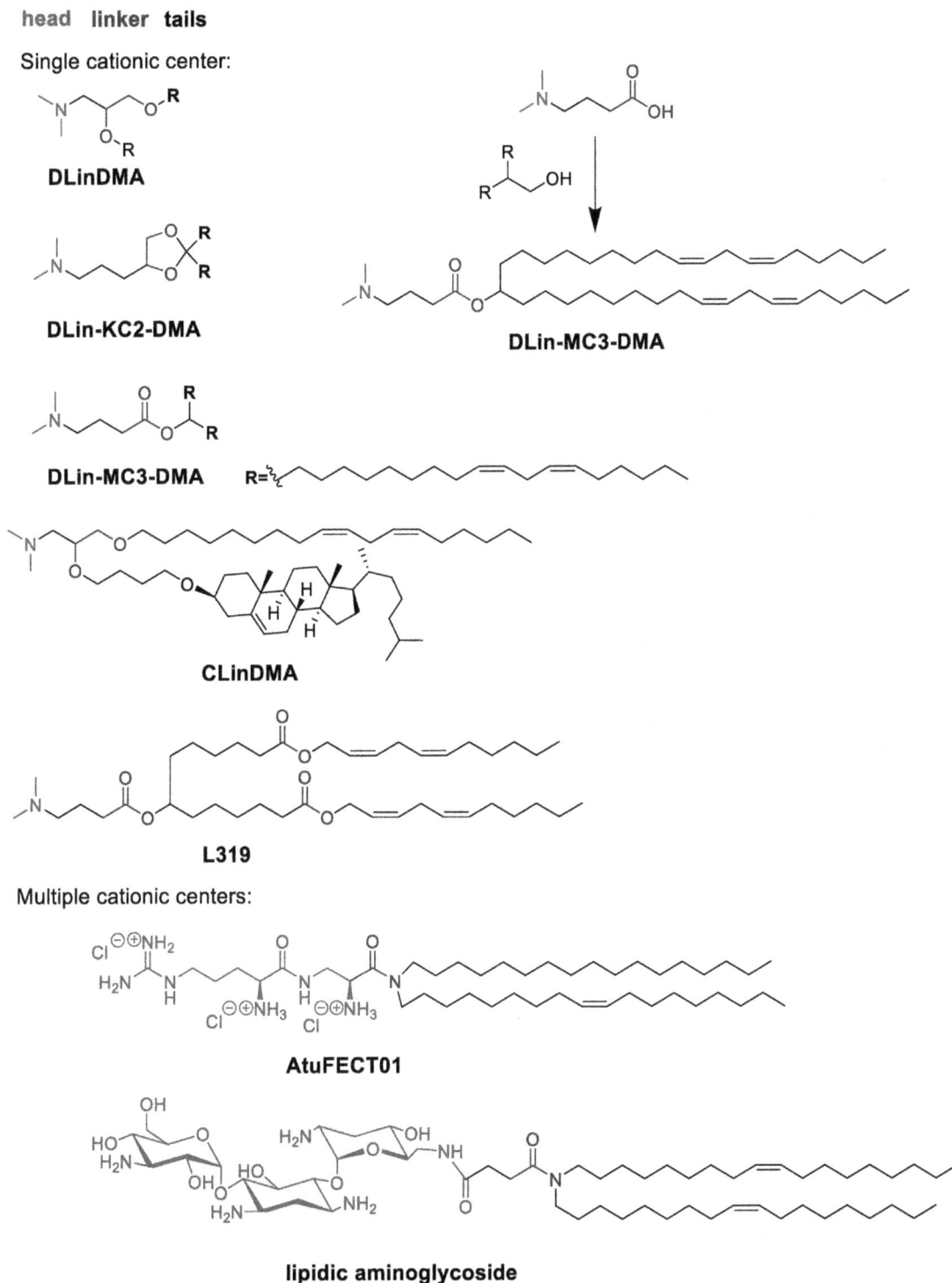

FIGURE 2.11 Lipid analogs with cationic head groups, linker, and hydrophobic tails and a representative synthetic route to DLin-MC3-DMA. Cationic head groups can be single or multiple cationic centers. Linkers span from ester, amide to ketal. Hydrophobic tails can accommodate unsaturated bonds, cholesterol, and ester groups.

groups with different size and ring structures. SAR studies of 56 amino lipids *in vivo* indicate that a dimethyl substitution on the amine head group was preferred to diethyl, diisopropyl, and ringed structures. The linkers ranged from ester, amide, ketal, ether, and carbamate. Efficacy was generally retained for ester, ketal, and carbamate linkers, though the length and functional groups of the linker could significantly affect the activity. For example, both DLin-KC2-DMA and DLin-MC3-DMA displayed significant silencing of FVII in mice [241]. Lipids with amide and ether linkers possessed reduced delivery performance when formulated. The author's show that pKa is an important factor for delivery efficiency and an optimum pKa value of the nanoparticles was between 6.2 and 6.5. Consistent with this report, a recent study investigated the correlation between nanoparticle properties and siRNA delivery efficiency [245]. In this study, pKa was also identified as a key determinant of nanoparticle delivery efficacy [245]. Hydrophobic tails can accommodate diverse functional groups, including unsaturated carbon bonds and small molecules [246]. Maier and coworkers report that an ester bond can be installed in the middle of hydrophobic tails (Figure 2.11, L319), which retain delivery efficiency and improve biodegradability [247]. In this collection, DLin-MC3-DMA was reported to be the most potent lipid with siRNA formulations having an ED50 around 0.005 mg/kg in mice (Figure 2.11) [241]. Onpattro™ (Patisiran) formulated from DLin-MC3-DMA was approved by the FDA for the treatment of TTR-mediated amyloidosis in August 2018 [170,248]. A simple substitution reaction was used to prepare the DLin-MC3-DMA (Figure 2.11) [246].

In addition to lipids with a single cationic center, numerous lipid derivatives and lipid-like materials with multiple cationic centers have been developed [249]. Here, we discuss two representative examples: aminoglycoside and amino acid derivatives. Aminoglycoside-based lipids are composed of an aminoglycosides head, an amide linker, and two unsaturated tails [250] (Figure 2.11). Formulated with

1,2-dioleoyl-snglycero-3-phosphoethanolamine (DOPE), lipidic aminoglycoside derivatives are capable of delivering siRNA in various human tumor cell lines [250]. In 2006, an arginine-based lipid, AtuFECT01, was reported, which consists of arginine-derived head, anamide linker, and two different carbon tails [251]. AtuFECT01 siRNA-lipoplexes were reported to silence in the vasculature of mice via systemic administration. Recently, a similar arginine-based liposomal delivery system was developed for hepatic silencing [252,253]. The lead material was reported to have dose-dependent silencing with an ED50 of 0.1 mg/kg in mice [246]. Both SNALP- and AtuFECT01-based siRNA delivery systems were in clinical trials for treating solid tumors [1].

2.13 CONCLUSIONS

Several multimolecular delivery vehicles are under clinical trial for RNAi-based cancer therapy, but the dose amounts of siRNA (0.1–1.5 mg/kg) are comparatively higher than levels observed in diseases of other organs (e.g., 0.15–0.3 mg/kg in the liver). This may indicate that the highest expected RNAi efficacy in tumor is similar with that in the liver. RNAi efficacy in rapid-growing cancer cells is not comparable to relatively slow-growing hepatocytes because siRNA concentration in the cytoplasm will dilute in divided cells. But more efficient delivery vehicles for tumor may contribute to increase RNAi rather than the present efficacies. Compared to a clinically approved Trastuzumab emtansine (half-life: 1–4 days) and clinically tested anticancer drug-loaded polymeric micelles (half-life: 16–80 h), the current clinically tested vehicles showed shorter circulation properties (half-life < 2 h) (Table 2.3).

This indicated that the current delivery vehicle needs better performance. The clinical trial results and new biological evidences provide the clues for development of the next vehicle design. (i) The vehicle should exhibit long blood circulation properties (half-life ≥2 h). The higher amounts of the circulating delivery vehicle (containing

TABLE 2.3
Summary of Blood Circulation and Size of Delivery Vehicles in This Chapter [254]

Delivery Formulation	Half-Life in Mouse or Patient	Hydrodynamic Diameter (nm)
Naked siRNA [4,5]	3–10 min	7 (length)×2 (diameter)
ALN-VSP02 [255]	≤2 h in patient	80–100
Atu027 [251,256]	≤2 h in patient	120
CALAA-01 [257,258]	≤30 min in patient	60–150
Hydrophobic interaction [87]	10 min	140
Hydrophobic interaction [90]	18 h	100
Hydrophobic interaction [92]	3–4 h	130
Redox potential responsiveness [98]	20 min	40
Extracellular pH responsiveness [120]	5 h	150
MMP responsiveness [122]	≤1 h	80
High quantity of siRNA [157]	4 min in the first phase, 27 h in the second phase	300
Gold nanoparticle [167]	1 min in the first phase, 8.5 h in the second phase	31–34
Gold nanoparticle [168]	30 min	40

siRNA) will increase possibility that the vehicle diffuses/accumulates into tumor microenvironment. Some vehicles introduced in this review showed longer than half-life =2 h, but their doses for tumor growth inhibition in the animal model were not significantly lower than other vehicles. These results indicate that other aspects in vehicle design should be considered. (ii) The vehicle should be smaller than 30 nm diameter size to enhance diffusion/ accumulation in tumor because the nanoparticle with this diameter size penetrated in thick fibrotic stroma and hypovascular tumor in animal models. This research indicates that less number of examples of Doxil (diameter size 90 nm) in clinical tumor accumulation may be hampered by this size limitation. Eventually, the behavior of the delivery vehicle inside the tumor is governed by diffusion, implicating that smaller particles with less than 30 nm size are also preferred to reach cancer cells. Fabrication of these small nanoparticles has gradually been realized by various materials and techniques [259–262], e.g., unimer PIC/AuNPs and polymers [168,263–265]. Repeatedly, we emphasize that size distribution of the vehicle in buffer or fetal bovine serum does not guarantee the same size distribution in bloodstream. (iii) Other functionalities (e.g., selective release of siRNA, high cell-specific recognition, and high endosome escapability) must endow the delivery vehicle which simultaneously satisfied with both (i) and (ii). To date, it is not clear which functionality is the most critical factor to enhance RNAi in patients. Furthermore, the delivery vehicle satisfied with (i) and (ii) but not (iii) does not expect to exhibit superior RNAi than the current vehicles in clinical trials. Ultimately, simpler formulation of delivery vehicles can be more easily translated to their clinical use because of better quality control as well as lower possibility of unexpected adverse effects.

REFERENCES

1. R. Kanasty, J.R. Dorkin, A. Vegas, D. Anderson, Delivery materials for siRNA therapeutics, *Nat. Mater.* 12 (2013) 967–977.
2. H.S. Choi, W. Liu, P. Misra, E. Tanaka, J.P. Zimmer, B. Itty Ipe, M.G. Bawendi, J.V. Frangioni, Renal clearance of quantum dots, *Nat. Biotechnol.* 25 (2007) 1165–1170.
3. A. Schroeder, C.G. Levins, C. Cortez, R. Langer, D.G. Anderson, Lipid-based nanotherapeutics for siRNA delivery, *J. Intern. Med.* 267 (2010) 9–21.
4. S. Gao, F. Dagnaes-Hansen, E.J.B. Nielsen, J. Wengel, F. Besenbacher, K.A. Howard, J. Kjems, The effect of chemical modification and nanoparticle formulation on stability and biodistribution of siRNA in mice, *Mol. Ther.* 17 (2009) 1225–1233.
5. J.J. Turner, S.W. Jones, S.A. Moschos, M.A. Lindsay, M.J. Gait, MALDI-TOF mass spectral analysis of siRNA degradation in serum confirms an RNAse A-like activity, *Mol. BioSyst.* 3 (2007) 43–50.
6. Y. Matsumura, H. Maeda, A new concept for macromolecular therapeutics in cancer chemotherapy: mechanism of tumoritropic accumulation of proteins and the antitumor agent smancs, *Cancer Res.* 46 (1986) 6387–6392.
7. H. Cabral, J. Makino, Y. Matsumoto, P. Mi, H. Wu, T. Nomoto, K. Toh, N. Yamada, Y. Higuchi, S. Konishi, M.R. Kano, H. Nishihara, Y. Miura, N. Nishiyama, K. Kataoka, Systemic targeting of lymph node metastasis through the blood vascular system by using size-controlled nanocarriers, *ACS Nano* 9 (2015) 4957–4967.
8. E.A. Sykes, J. Chen, G. Zheng, W.C.W. Chan, Investigating the impact of nanoparticle size on active and passive tumor targeting efficiency, *ACS Nano* 8 (2014) 5696–5706.
9. X. Zhu, Y. Xu, L.M. Solis, W. Tao, L. Wang, C. Behrens, X. Xu, L. Zhao, D. Liu, J. Wu, N. Zhang, I.I. Wistuba, O.C. Farokhzad, B.R. Zetter, J. Shi, Long-circulating siRNA nanoparticles for validating prohibitin1-targeted non-small cell lung cancer treatment, *Proc. Natl. Acad. Sci. U. S. A.* 112 (2015) 7779–7784.
10. M.R. Kano, Nanotechnology and tumor microcirculation, *Adv. Drug Deliv. Rev.* 74 (2014) 2–11.
11. A.E. Hansen, A.L. Petersen, J.R. Henriksen, B. Berresen, P. Rasmussen, D.R. Elema, P.M. Rosenschöld, A.T. Kristensen, A. Kjær, T.L. Andresen, Positron emission tomography based elucidation of the enhanced permeability and retention effect in dogs with cancer using copper-64 liposomes, *ACS Nano* 9 (2015) 6985–6995.
12. F. Yuan, M. Dellian, D. Fukumura, M. Leunig, D.A. Berk, V.P. Torchilin, R.K. Jain, Vascular permeability in a human tumor xenograft: molecular size dependence and cutoff size, *Cancer Res.* 55 (1995) 3752–3756.
13. H. Cabral, M. Murakami, H. Hojo, Y. Terada, M.R. Kano, U.-.I. Chung, N. Nishiyama, K. Kataoka, Targeted therapy of spontaneous murine pancreatic tumors by polymeric micelles prolongs survival and prevents peritoneal metastasis, *Proc. Natl. Acad. Sci. U. S. A.* 110 (2013) 11397–11402.
14. H. Maeda, Toward a full understanding of the EPR effect in primary and metastatic tumors as well as issues related to its heterogeneity, *Adv. Drug Deliv. Rev.* 91 (2015) 3–6.
15. Ó. Arrieta, L.A. Medina, E. Estrada-Lobato, N. Hernández-Pedro, G. Villanueva-Rodríguez, L. Martínez-Barrera, E.O. Macedo, V. López-Rodríquez, D. Motola-Kuba, J.F. Corona-Cruz, First-line chemotherapy with liposomal doxorubicin plus cisplatin for patients with advanced malignant pleural mesothelioma: phase II trial, *Br. J. Cancer* 106 (2012) 1027–1032.
16. J.W. Nicholas, Y.H. Bae, EPR: evidence and fallacy, *J. Control. Release* 190 (2014) 451–464.
17. N.M. Marina, D. Cochrane, E. Harney, K. Zomorodi, S. Blaney, N. Winick, M. Bernstein, M.P. Link, Dose escalation and pharmacokinetics of pegylated liposomal doxorubicin (doxil) in children with solid tumos: a pediatric oncology group study, *Clin. Cancer Res.* 8 (2002) 413–418.
18. A. Hubert, O. Lyass, D. Pode, A. Gabizon, Doxil (Caelyx): an exploratory study with pharmacokinetics in patients with hormone-refractory prostate cancer, *Anti-Cancer Drugs* 11 (2000) 123–127.
19. O. Lyass, B. Uziely, R. Ben-Yosef, D. Tzemach, N.I. Heshing, M. Lotem, G. Brufman, A. Gabizon, Correlation of toxicity with pharmacokinetics of pegylated liposomal doxorubicin (Doxil) in metastatic breast carcinoma, *Cancer* 89 (2000) 1037–1047.
20. M.J. Boers-Sonderen, C.M. van Herpen, W.T. van der Graaf, I.M. Desar, M.G. van der Logt, Y.M. de Beer, P.B. Ottevanger, N.P. van Erp, Correlation of toxicity and efficacy with pharmacokinetics (PK) of pegylated liposomal doxorubicin (PLD) (Caelyx®), *Cancer Chemother. Pharmacol.* 74 (2014) 457–463.

21. Z. Symon, A. Peyser, D. Tzemach, O. Lyass, E. Sucher, E. Shezen, A.A. Gabizon, Selective delivery of doxorubicin to patients with breast carcinoma metastases by stealth liposomes, *Cancer* 86 (1999) 72–78.

22. T. Lammers, F. Kiessling, W.E. Hennink, G. Storm, Drug targeting to tumors: principles, pitfalls, and (pre-) clinical progress, *J. Control. Release* 161 (2012) 175–187.

23. Y.H. Bae, K. Park, Targeted drug delivery to tumors: myths, reality, and possibility, *J. Control. Release* 153 (2011) 198–205.

24. S. Taurin, H. Nehoff, K. Greish, Anticancer nanomedicine and tumor vascular permeability; where is the missing link? *J. Control. Release* 164 (2012) 265–275.

25. Y. Matsumoto, J.W. Nichols, K. Toh, T. Nomoto, H. Cabral, Y. Miura, R.J. Christie, N. Yamada, T. Ogura, M.R. Kano, Y. Matsumura, N. Nishiyama, T. Yamasoba, Y.H. Bae, K. Kataoka, Vascular bursts enhance permeability of tumour blood vessels and improve nanoparticle delivery, *Nat. Nanotechol.* 11(6) (2016) 533–538. doi: 10.1038/nnano.2015.342. Epub 2016 Feb 15. PMID: 26878143.

26. V.P. Chauhan, R.K. Jain, Strategies for advancing cancer nanomedicine, *Nat. Mater.* 12 (2013) 958–962.

27. N.R. Smith, D. Baker, M. Farren, A. Pommier, R. Swann, X. Wang, S. Mistry, K. McDaid, J. Kendrew, C. Womack, S.R. Wedge, S.T. Barry, Tumor stromal architecture can define the intrinsic tumor response to VEGF-targeted therapy, *Clin. Cancer Res.* 19 (2013) 6943–6956.

28. S.D. Perrault, C. Walkey, T. Jennings, H.C. Fischer, W.C. Chan, Mediating tumor targeting efficiency of nanoparticles through design, *Nano Lett.* 9 (2009) 1909–1915.

29. Z. Popović, W. Liu, V.P. Chauhan, J. Lee, C.Wong, A.B. Greytak, N. Insin, D.G. Nocera, D. Fukumura, R.K. Jain, M.G. Bawendi, A nanoparticle size series for in vivo fluorescence imaging, *Angew. Chem. Int. Ed.* 49 (2010) 8649–8652.

30. R.K. Jain, J.D. Martin, T. Stylianopoulos, The role of mechanical forces in tumor growth and therapy, *Annu. Rev. Biomed. Eng.* 16 (2014) 321–346.

31. M.R. Kano, Y. Bae, C. Iwata, Y. Morishita, M. Yashiro, M. Oka, T. Fujii, A. Komuro, K. Kiyono, M. Kaminishi, K. Hirakawa, Y. Ouchi, N. Nishiyama, K. Kataoka, K. Miyazono, Improvement of cancer-targeting therapy, using nanocarriers for intractable solid tumors by inhibition of TGF-β signaling, *Proc. Natl. Acad. Sci. U. S. A.* 104 (2007) 3460–3465.

32. T.D. Mckee, P. Grandi, W. Mok, G. Alexandrakis, N. Insin, J.P. Zimmer, M.G. Bawendi, Y. Boucher, X.O. Breakefield, R.K. Jain, Degradation of fibrillary collagen in a human melanoma xenograft improves the efficacy of an oncolytic herpes simplex virus vector, *Cancer Res.* 66 (2006) 2509–2513.

33. Y.S. Kanwar, M.G. Farquhar, Presence of heparan sulfate in the glomerular basement membrane, *Proc. Natl. Acad. Sci. U. S. A.* 76 (1979) 1303–1307.

34. T. Soji, Y. Murata, A. Ohira, H. Nishizono, M. Tanaka, D.C. Herbert, Evidence that hepatocytes can phagocytize exogenous substances, *Anat. Rec.* 233 (1992) 543–546.

35. K. Elvevold, B. Smedsrød, I. Martinez, The liver sinusoidal endothelial cell: a cell type of controversial and confusing identity, *Am. J. Physiol. Gastrointest. Liver Physiol.* 294 (2008) G391–G400.

36. H.H. Gustafson, D. Holt-Casper, D.W. Grainger, H. Ghandehari, Nanoparticle uptake: the phagocyte problem, *Nano Today* 10 (2015) 487–510.

37. K. Braeckmans, K. Buyens, W. Bouquet, C. Vervaet, P. Joye, F. De Vos, L. Plawinski, L. Doeuvre, E. Angles-Cano, N.N. Sanders, J. Demeester, S.C. De Smedt, Sizing nanomatter in biological fluids by fluorescence single particle tracking, *Nano Lett.* 10 (2010) 4435–4442.

38. A. Akinc, G. Battaglia, Exploiting endocytosis for nanomedicines, *Cold Spring Harb. Perspect. Biol.* 5 (2013) a016980.

39. E.M. Pelegri-O'Day, E.-W. Lin, H.D. Maynard, Therapeutic protein-polymer conjugates: advancing beyond PEGylation, *J. Am. Chem. Soc.* 136 (2014) 14323–14332.

40. K. Knop, R. Hoogenboom, D. Fischer, U.S. Schubert, Poly(ethylene glycol) in drug delivery:pros and cons as well as potential alternatives, *Angew. Chem. Int. Ed.* 49 (2010) 6288–6308.

41. Y. Qi, A. Chilkoti, Protein-polymer conjugation-moving beyond PEGylation, *Curr. Opin. Chem. Biol.* 28 (2015) 181–193.

42. Y. Barenholz, Doxil®-the first FDA-approved nano-drug: lessons learned, *J. Control. Release* 160 (2012) 117–134.

43. E. Pérez-Herrero, A. Fernández-Medarde, Advanced targeted therapies in cancer: drug nanocarriers, the future of chemotherapy, *Eur. J. Pharm. Biopharm.* 93 (2015) 52–79.

44. H. Schellekens, W.E. Hennink, V. Brinks, The immunogenicity of polyethylene glycol: facts and fiction, *Pharm. Res.* 30 (2013) 1729–1734.

45. N. Longo, C.O. Harding, B.K. Burton, D.K. Grange, J. Vockley, M. Wasserstein, G.M. Rice, A. Dorenbaum, J.K. Neuenburg, D.G.Musson, Z. Gu, S. Sile, Single-dose, subcutaneous recombinant phenylalanine ammonia lyase conjugated with polyethylene glycol in adult patients with phenylketonuria: an open-label, multicenter, phase 1 dose-escalation trial, *Lancet* 384 (2014) 37–44.

46. Q. Yang, S.K. Lai, Anti-PEG immunity: emergence, characteristics, and unaddressed questions, *Wiley Interdiscip. Rev. Nanomed. Nanobiotechnol.* 7 (2015) 655–677.

47. J.K. Armstrong, G. Hempel, S. Koling, L.S. Chan, T. Fisher, H.J. Meiselman, G. Garratty, Antibody against poly(ethylene glycol) adversely affects PEG-asparaginase therapy in acute lymphoblastic leukemia patients, *Cancer* 110 (2007) 103–111.

48. C.M. Beddoes, C.P. Case, W.H. Briscoe, Understanding nanoparticle cellular entry: a physicochemical perspective, *Adv. Colloid Interf. Sci.* 218 (2015) 48–68.

49. I. Canton, G. Battaglia, Endocytosis at the nanoscale, *Chem. Soc. Rev.* 41 (2012) 2718–2739.

50. S. Venkataraman, J.L. Hedrick, Z.Y. Ong, C. Yang, P.L. Ee, P.T. Hammond, Y.Y. Yang, The effects of polymeric nanostructure shape on drug delivery, *Adv. Drug Deliv. Rev.* 63 (2011) 1228–1246.

51. J.D. Trono, K. Mizuno, N. Yusa, T. Matsukawa, K. Yokoyama, M. Uesaka, Size, concentration and incubation time dependence of gold nanoparticle uptake into pancreas cancer cells and its future application to X-ray drug delivery system, *J. Radiat. Res.* 52 (2011) 103–109.

52. D.B. Chithrani, Intracellular uptake, transport, and processing of gold nanostructures, *Mol. Membr. Biol.* 27 (2010) 299–311.

53. H. Gao, W. Shi, L.B. Freund, Mechanics of receptor-mediated endocytosis, *Proc. Natl. Acad. Sci. U. S. A.* 102 (2005) 9469–9474.

54. Z.U. Rehman, I.S. Zuhorn, D. Hoekstra, How cationic lipids transfer nucleic acids into cells and across cellular membranes: recent advances, *J. Control. Release* 166 (2013) 46–56.

55. K. Itaka, K. Kataoka, Recent development of nonviral gene delivery systems with virus-like structures and mechanism, *Eur. J. Pharm. Biopharm.* 71 (2009) 475–483.

56. N. Bertrand, J. Wu, X. Xu, N. Kamaly, O.C. Farokhzad, Cancer nanotechnology: the impact of passive and active targeting in the era of modern cancer biology, *Adv. Drug Deliv. Rev.* 66 (2014) 2–25.

57. Y. Zhong, F. Meng, C. Deng, Z. Zhong, Ligand-directed active tumor-targeting polymeric nanoparticles for cancer chemotherapy, *Biomacromolecules* 15 (2014) 1955–1969.

58. K. Temming, R.M. Schiffelers, G. Molema, R.J. Kok, RGD-based strategies for selective delivery of therapeutics and imaging agents to the tumor vasculature, *Drug Resist. Updat.* 8 (2005) 381–402.

59. M. Sutherland, A. Gordon, S.D. Shnyder, L.H. Patterson, H.M. Sheldrake, RGDbinding integrins in prostate cancer: expression patterns and therapeutic prospects against bone metastasis, *Cancers* 4 (2012) 1106–1145.

60. L. Sancey, E. Garanger, S. Foilard, G. Schoehn, A. Hurbin, C. Albiges-Rizo, D. Boturyn, C. Souchier, A. Grichine, P. Dumy, J.L. Coll, Clustering and internalization of integrin αvβ3 with a tetrameric RGD-synthetic peptide, *Mol. Ther.* 17 (2009) 837–843.

61. G. Trapani, N. Denora, A. Trapani, V. Laquintana, Recent advances in ligand targeted therapy, *J. Drug Target.* 20 (2012) 1–22.

62. K.E. Tiller, P.M. Tessier, Advances in antibody design, *Annu. Rev. Biomed. Eng.* 17 (2015) 191–216.

63. C. Peters, S. Brown, Antibody-drug conjugates as novel anti-cancer chemotherapeutics, *Biosci. Rep.* 35 (2015) e00225.

64. N. Zhang, L. Liu, C.D. Dumitru, N.R. Cummings, M. Cukan, Y. Jiang, Y. Li, F. Li, T. Mitchell, M.R. Mallem, Y. Ou, R.N. Patel, K. Vo, H. Wang, I. Burnina, B.-K. Choi, H. Huber, T.A. Stadheim, D. Zha, Glycoengineered pichia produced anti-HER2 is comparable to trastuzumab in preclinical study, *mAbs* 3 (2011) 289–298.

65. L. Elmlund, C. Käck, T. Aastrup, I.A. Nicholls, Study of the interaction of trastuzumab and SKOV3 epithelial cancer cells using a quartz crystal microbalance sensor, *Sensors* 15 (2015) 5884–5894.

66. H. Tong, L. Zhang, A. Kaspar, M.J. Rames, L. Huang, G. Woodnutt, G. Ren, Peptideconjugation induced conformational changes in human IgG1 observed by optimized negative-staining and individual-particle electron tomography, *Sci. Rep.* 3 (2013) 1089.

67. R. van der Meel, L.J. Vehmeijer, R.J. Kok, G. Storm, E.V. van Gaal, Ligand-targeted particulate nanomedicines undergoing clinical evaluation: current status, *Adv. Drug Deliv. Rev.* 65 (2013) 1284–1298.

68. J.A. Reddy, R. Dorton, E. Westrick, A. Dawson, T. Smith, L.-C. Xu, M. Vetzel, P. Kleindl, I.R. Vlahov, C.P. Leamon, Preclinical evaluation of EC145, a folate-Vinca alkaloid conjugate, *Cancer Res.* 67 (2007) 4434–4442.

69. R.W. Naumann, R.L. Coleman, R.A. Burger, E.A. Sausville, E. Kutarska, S.A. Ghamande, N.Y. Gabrail, S.E. DePasquale, E. Nowara, L. Gilbert, R.H. Gersh, M.G. Teneriello, W.A. Harb, P.A. Konstantinopoulos, R.T. Penson, J.T. Symnowski, C.D. Lovejoy, C.P. Leamon, D.E. Morgenstern, R.A. Messmann, Precedent: a randomized phase II trial comparing vintafolide (EC145) and pegylated liposomal doxorubicin (PLD) in combination versus PLD alone in patient with platinum-resistant ovarian cell, *J. Clin. Oncol.* 31 (2013) 4400–4406.

70. K. Park, Facing the truth about nanotechnology in drug delivery, *ACS Nano* 7 (2013) 7442–7447.

71. J.A. Mindell, Lysosomal acidification mechanisms, *Annu. Rev. Physiol.* 74 (2012) 69–86.

72. H. Appelqvist, P. Wäster, K. Kågedal, K. Öllinger, The lysosome: from waste bag to potential therapeutic target, *J. Mol. Cell Biol.* 5 (2013) 214–226.

73. S. Höbel, A. Aigner, Polyethylenimines for siRNA andmiRNA delivery in vivo, *Wiley Interdiscip. Rev. Nanomed. Nanobiotechnol.* 5 (2013) 484–501.

74. K. Miyata, M. Oba, M. Nakanishi, S. Fukushima, Y. Yamasaki, H. Koyama, N. Nishiyama, K. Kataoka, Polyplexes from poly(aspartamide) bearing 1,2-diaminoethane side chains induce pH-selective endosomalmembrane destabilization with amplified transfection and negligible cytotoxicity, *J. Am. Chem. Soc.* 130 (2008) 16287–16294.

75. J.P. Behr, The proton sponge: a trick to enter cells the viruses did not exploit, *Chimia* 51 (1997) 34–36.

76. N.D. Sonawane, F.C. Szoka, A.S. Verkman, Chloride accumulation and swelling in endosomes enhances DNA transfer by polyamine–DNA polyplexes, *J. Biol. Chem.* 278 (2003) 44826–44831.

77. K. Miyata, N. Nishiyama, K. Kataoka, Rational design of smart supramolecular assemblies for gene delivery: chemical challenges in the creation of artificial viruses, *Chem. Soc. Rev.* 41 (2012) 2562–2574.

78. N.M. Rao, Cationic lipid-mediated nucleic acid delivery: beyond being cationic, *Chem. Phys. Lipids* 163 (2010) 245–252.

79. K. Kataoka, A. Harada, Y. Nagasaki, Block copolymer micelles for drug delivery: design, characterization and biological significance, *Adv. Drug Deliv. Rev.* 47 (2001) 113–131.

80. Y. Dong, K.T. Love, J.R. Dorkin, S. Sirirungruang, Y. Zhang, D. Chen, R.L. Bogorad, H. Yin, Y. Chen, A.J. Vegas, C.A. Alabi, G. Sahay, K.T. Olejnik, W. Wang, A. Schroeder, A.K.R. Lytton-Jean, D.J. Siegwart, A. Akinc, C. Barnes, S.A. Barros, M. Carioto, K. Fitzgerald, J. Hettinger, V. Kumar, T.I. Novobrantseva, J. Qin, W. Querbes, V. Koteliansky, R. Langer, D.G. Anderson, Lipopeptide nanoparticles for potent and selective siRNA delivery in rodents and nonhuman primates, *Proc. Natl. Acad. Sci. U. S. A.* 111 (2014) 3955–3960.

81. D. Schaffert, C. Troiber, E.E. Salcher, T. Fröhlich, I. Martin, N. Badgujar, C. Dohmen, D. Edinger, R. Kläger, G. Maiwald, K. Farkasova, S. Seeber, K. Jahn-Hofmann, P. Hadwiger, E. Wagner, Solid-phase synthesis of sequence-defined T-, i-, and U-shape polymers for pDNA and siRNA delivery, *Angew. Chem. Int. Ed.* 50 (2011) 8986–8989.

82. T.K. Endres, M. Beck-Broichsitter, O. Samsonova, T. Renette, T.H. Kissel, Selfassembled biodegradable amphiphilic PEG-PCL-lPEI triblock copolymers at the borderline between micelles and nanoparticles designed for drug and gene delivery, *Biomaterials* 32 (2011) 7721–7731.

83. T.-M. Sun, J.-Z. Du, Y.-D. Yao, C.-Q. Mao, S. Dou, S.-Y. Huang, P.-Z. Zhang, K.W. Leong, E.-W. Song, J. Wang, Simultaneous delivery of siRNA and paclitaxel via a "two-in-one" micelleplex promotes synergistic tumor suppression, *ACS Nano* 5 (2011) 1483–1494.

84. H. Yu, Y. Zou, Y. Wang, X. Huang, G. Huang, B.D. Sumer, D.A. Boothman, J. Gao, Overcoming endosomal barrier by amphotericin B-loaded dual pH-responsive PDMA-b-PDPA micelleplexes for siRNA delivery, *ACS Nano* 5 (2011) 9246–9255.

85. H.J. Kim, A. Ishii, K. Miyata, Y. Lee, S. Wu, M. Oba, N. Nishiyama, K. Kataoka, Introduction of stearoylmoieties into a biocompatible cationic polyaspartamide derivative, PAsp(DET), with endosomal escaping function for enhanced siRNA-mediated gene knockdown, *J. Control. Release* 145 (2010) 141–148.

86. A. Philipp, X. Zhao, P. Tarcha, E. Wagner, A. Zintchenko, Hydrophobically modified oligoethylenimines as highly efficient transfection agents for siRNA delivery, *Bioconjug. Chem.* 20 (2009) 2055–2061.

87. H.J. Kim, M. Oba, F. Pittella, T. Nomoto, H. Cabral, Y. Matsumoto, K. Miyata, N. Nishiyama, K. Kataoka, PEG-detachable cationic polyaspartamide derivatives bearing stearoyl moieties for systemic siRNA delivery toward subcutaneous BxPC3 pancreatic tumor, *J. Drug Target.* 20 (2012) 33–42.

88. H.J. Kim, T. Ishii, M. Zheng, S.Watanabe, K. Toh, Y. Matsumoto, N. Nishiyama, K. Miyata, K. Kataoka, Multifunctional polyion complex micelle featuring enhanced stability, targetability, and endosome escapability for systemic siRNA delivery to subcutaneous model of lung cancer, *Drug Deliv. Transl. Res.* 4 (2014) 50–60.

89. H.J. Kim, K. Miyata, T. Nomoto, M. Zheng, A. Kim, X. Liu, H. Cabral, R.J. Christie, N. Nishiyama, K. Kataoka, siRNA delivery from triblock copolymer micelles with spatially-ordered compartments of PEG shell, siRNA-loaded intermediate layer, and hydrophobic core, *Biomaterials* 35 (2014) 4548–4556.

90. N. Yagi, I. Manabe, T. Tottori, A. Ishihara, F. Ogata, J.H. Kim, S. Nishimura, K. Fujiu, Y. Oishi, K. Itaka, Y. Kato, M. Yamauchi, R. Nagai, A nanoparticle system specifically designed to deliver short interfering RNA inhibits tumor growth in vivo, *Cancer Res.* 69 (2009) 6531–6538.

91. B.L. Mui, Y.K. Tam, M. Jayaraman, S.M. Ansell, X. Du, Y.Y.C. Tam, P.J.C. Lin, S. Chen, J.K. Narayanannair, K.G. Rajeev, M. Manoharan, A. Akinc, M.A. Maier, P. Cullis, T.D. Madden, M.J. Hope, Influence of polyethylene glycol lipid desorption rates on pharmacokinetics and pharmacodynamics of siRNA lipid nanoparticles, *Mol. Ther. Nucleic Acids* 2 (2013), e139.

92. Q. Sun, Z. Kang, L. Xue, Y. Shang, Z. Su, H. Sun, Q. Ping, R. Mo, C. Zhang, A collaborative assembly strategy for tumor-targeted siRNA delivery, *J. Am. Chem. Soc.* 137 (2015) 6000–6010.

93. J.M. Hansen, C. Harris, Glutathione during embryonic development, *Biochim. Biophys. Acta* (2014) (Epub ahead of print).

94. M.L. Circu, T.Y. Aw, Glutathione andmodulation of cell apoptosis, *Biochim. Biophys. Acta* 1823 (2012) 1767–1777.

95. M. Smeyne, R.J. Smeyne, Glutathione metabolism and Parkinson's disease, *Free Radic. Biol. Med.* 62 (2013) 13–25.

96. J.H. Ryu, R.T. Chacko, S. Jiwpanich, S. Bickerton, R.P. Babu, S. Thayumanavan, Self-cross-linked polymer nanogels: a versatile nanoscopic drug delivery platform, *J. Am. Chem. Soc.* 132 (2010) 17227–17235.

97. S. Matsumoto, R.J. Christie, N. Nishiyama, K. Miyata, A. Ishii, M. Oba, H. Koyama, Y. Yamasaki, K. Kataoka, Environment-responsive block copolymer micelles with a disulfide cross-linked core for enhanced siRNA delivery, *Biomacromolecules* 10 (2009) 119–127.

98. Y. Oe, R.J. Christie, M. Naito, S.A. Low, S. Fukushima, K. Toh, Y. Miura, Y. Matsumoto, N. Nishiyama, K. Miyata, K. Kataoka, Actively-targeted polyion complex micelles stabilized by cholesterol and disulfide cross-linking for systemic delivery of siRNA to solid tumors, *Biomaterials* 35 (2014) 7887–7895.

99. D.B. Rozema, D.L. Lewis, D.H. Wakefield, S.C. Wong, J.J. Klein, P.L. Roesch, S.L. Bertin, T.W. Reppen, Q. Chu, A.V. Blokhin, J.E. Hagstrom, J.A. Wolff, Dynamic polyconjugates for targeted in vivo delivery of siRNA to hepatocytes, *Proc. Natl. Acad. Sci. U. S. A.* 104 (2007) 12982–12987.

100. R.G. Gish, M.-F. Yuen, H.L.Y. Chan, B.D. Given, C.-L. Lai, S.A. Locarnini, J.Y.N. Lau, C.I. Wooddell, T. Schluep, D.L. Lewis, Synthetic RNAi triggers and their use in chronic hepatitis B therapies with curative intent, *Antivir. Res.* 121 (2015) 97–108.

101. T. Stauber, T.J. Jentsch, Chloride in vesicular trafficking and function, *Annu. Rev. Physiol.* 75 (2013) 453–477.

102. N. Murthy, Y.X. Thng, S. Schuck, M.C. Xu, J.M.J. Fréchet, A novel strategy for encapsulation and release of proteins: hydrogels and microgels with acid-labile acetal cross-linkers, *J. Am. Chem. Soc.* 124 (2002) 12398–12399.

103. Y. Bae, S. Fukushima, A. Harada, K. Kataoka, Design of environment-sensitive supramolecular assemblies for intracellular drug delivery: polymeric micelles that are responsive to intracellular pH change, *Angew. Chem. Int. Ed.* 42 (2003) 4640–4643.

104. M. Oishi, Y. Nagasaki, K. Itaka, N. Nishiyama, K. Kataoka, Lactosylated poly(ethylene glycol)-siRNA conjugate through acid-labile β-thiopropionate linkage to construct pH-sensitive polyion complex micelles achieving enhanced gene silencing in hepatoma cells, *J. Am. Chem. Soc.* 127 (2005) 1624–1625.

105. J.H. Jeong, S.W. Kim, T.G. Park, Novel intracellular delivery system of antisense oligonucleotide by self-assembled hybrid micelles composed of DNA/PEG conjugate and cationic fusogenic peptide, *Bioconjug. Chem.* 14 (2003) 473–479.

106. J. Heller, J. Barr, S.Y. Ng, K.S. Abdellauoi, R. Gurny, Poly(ortho esters): synthesis, characterization, properties and uses, *Adv. Drug Deliv. Rev.* 54 (2002) 1015–1039.

107. Y. Lee, S. Fukushima, Y. Bae, S. Hiki, T. Ishii, K. Kataoka, A protein nanocarrier from charge-conversion polymer in response to endosomal pH, *J. Am. Chem. Soc.* 129 (2007) 5362–5363.

108. Y. Lee, T. Ishii, H. Cabral, H.J. Kim, J.H. Seo, N. Nishiyama, H. Oshima, K. Osada, K. Kataoka, Charge-conversional polyionic complex micelles—efficient nanocarriers for protein delivery into cytoplasm, *Angew. Chem. Int. Ed.* 48 (2009) 5309–5312.

109. M.S. Shim, Y.J. Kwon, Acid-responsive linear polyethyleneimine for efficient, specific, and biocompatible siRNA delivery, *Bioconjug. Chem.* 20 (2009) 488–499.

110. H. Takemoto, K. Miyata, S. Hattori, T. Ishii, T. Suma, S. Uchida, N. Nishiyama, K. Kataoka, Acidic pH-responsive siRNA conjugate for reversible carrier stability and accelerated endosomal escape with reduced IFNα-associated immune response, *Angew. Chem. Int. Ed.* 52 (2013) 6218–6221.

111. A. Kulkarni, K. DeFrees, S.-H. Hyun, D.H. Tompson, Pendant polyer:amino-β-cyclodextrin: siRNA guest:host nanoparticles as efficient vectors for gene silencing, *J. Am. Chem. Soc.* 134 (2012) 7596–7599.

112. Y. Nie, M. Günther, Z. Gu, E. Wagner, Pyridylhydrazone-based PEGylation for pH-reversible lipopolyplex shielding, *Biomaterials* 32 (2011) 858–869.

113. X.Z. Yang, J.Z. Du, S. Dou, C.Q. Mao, H.Y. Long, J. Wang, Sheddable ternary nanoparticles for tumor acidity-targeted siRNA delivery, *ACS Nano* 6 (2012) 771–781.

114. M.W. Gorman, E.O. Feigl, C.W. Buffington, Human plasma ATP concentration, *Clin. Chem.* 53 (2007) 318–325.

115. M. Naito, T. Ishii, A. Matsumoto, K. Miyata, Y. Miyahara, K. Kataoka, A phenylboronate-functionalized polyion complex micelle for ATP-triggered release of siRNA, *Angew. Chem. Int. Ed.* 51 (2012) 1–6.

116. R. Mo, T. Jiang, R. DiSanto, W. Tai, Z. Gu, ATP-triggered anticancer drug delivery, *Nat. Commun.* 5 (2014) 3364.

117. R. Mo, T. Jiang, Z. Gu, Enhanced anticancer efficacy by ATP-mediated liposomal drug delivery, *Angew. Chem.* 126 (2014) 5925–5930.

118. D.F. Quail, J.A. Joyce, Microenvironmental regulation of tumor progression andmetastasis, *Nat. Med.* 19 (2013) 1423–1437.

119. D. Neri, C.T. Supuran, Interfering with pH regulation in tumours as a therapeutic strategy, *Nat. Rev. Drug Discov.* 10 (2011) 767–777.

120. J. Li, X. Yu, Y. Wang, Y. Yuan, H. Xiao, D. Cheng, X. Shuai, A reduction and pH dualsensitive polymeric vector for long-circulating and tumor-targeted siRNA delivery, *Adv. Mater.* 26 (2014) 8217–8224.

121. S. Hama, S. Itakura, M. Nakai, K. Nakayama, S. Morimoto, S. Suzuki, K. Kogure, Overcoming the polyethylene glycol dilemma via pathological environment-sensitive change of the surface property of nanoparticles for cellular entry, *J. Control. Release* 206 (2015) 67–74.

122. H.-X. Wang, X.-Z. Yang, C.-Y. Sun, C.-Q. Mao, Y.-H. Zhu, J. Wang, Matrixmetalloproteinase 2-responsive micelle for siRNA delivery, *Biomaterials* 35 (2014) 7622–7634.

123. L.A. Shuman Moss, S. Jensen-Taubman, W.G. Stetler-Stevenson, Matrix metalloproteinases: changing roles in tumor progression and metastasis, *Am. J. Pathol.* 181 (2012) 1895–1899.

124. J. Decock, S. Thirkettle, L. Wagstaff, D.R. Edwards, Matrix metalloproteinases: protective roles in cancer, *J. Cell. Mol. Med.* 6 (2011) 1254–1265.

125. K. Kessenbrock, V. Plaks, Z. Werb, Matrix metalloproteinases: regulators of the tumor microenvironment, *Cell* 141 (2010) 52–67.

126. H. Li, S.S. Yu, M. Miteva, C.E. Nelson, T. Werfel, T.D. Giorgio, C.L. Duvall, Matrix metalloproteinase responsive, proximity-activated polymeric nanoparticles for siRNA delivery, *Adv. Funct. Mater.* 23 (2013) 3040–3052.

127. H. Li, M. Miteva, K.C. Kirkbride, M.J. Cheng, C.E. Nelson, E.M. Simpson, M.K. Gupta, C.L. Duvall, T.D. Giorgio, Dual MMP7-proximity-activated and folate receptor-targeted nanoparticles for siRNA delivery, *Biomacromolecules* 16 (2015) 192–201.

128. H. Hatakeyama, H. Akita, E. Ito, Y. Hayashi, M. Oishi, Y. Nagasaki, R. Danev, K. Nagayama, N. Kaji, H. Kukuchi, Y. Baba, H. Harashima, Systemic delivery of siRNA to tumors using a lipid nanoparticle containing a tumor-specific cleavable PEG-lipid, *Biomaterials* 32 (2011) 4306–4316.

129. L. Zhu, T. Wang, F. Perche, A. Taigind, V.P. Torchilin, Enhanced anticancer acitivty of nanopreparation containing an MMP2-sensitive PEG-drug conjugate and cellpenetrating moiety, *Proc. Natl. Acad. Sci. U. S. A.* 110 (2013) 17047–17052.

130. S. Huang, K. Shao, Y. Kuang, Y. Liu, J. Li, S. An, Y. Guo, H. Ma, X. He, C. Jiang, Tumor targeting and microenvironment-responsive nanoparticles for gene delivery, *Biomaterials* 34 (2013) 5294–5302.

131. S.H. van Rijt, D.A. Bölükbas, C. Argyo, S. Datz, M. Lindner, O. Eickelberg, M. Königshoff, T. Bein, S. Meiners, Protease-mediated release of chemotherapeutics from mesoporous silica nanoparticles to ex vivo human and mouse lung tumors, *ACS Nano* 9 (2015) 2377–2389.

132. J. Le, Z. Ge, S. Liu, PEG-sheddable polyplexmicelles as smart gene carriers based on MMP-cleavable peptide-linked block copolymers, *Chem. Commun.* 49 (2013) 6974–6976.

133. W. Gao, B. Xiang, T.-T. Meng, F. Liu, X.-R. Qi, Chemotherapeutic drug delivery to cancer cells using a combination of folate targeting and tumor microenvironment-sensitive polypeptides, *Biomaterials* 34 (2013) 4137–4149.

134. J.K. Nair, J.L.S. Willoughby, A. Chan, K. Charisse, M.R. Alam, Q. Wang, M. Hoekstra, P. Kandasamy, A.V. Kel'in, S. Milstein, N. Taneja, J. O'Shea, S. Shaikh, L. Zhang, R.J. van der Sluis, M.E. Jung, A. Akinc, R. Hutabarat, S. Kuchimanchi, K. Fitzgerald, T. Zimmermann, T.J.C. van Berkel, M.A. Maier, K.G. Rajeev, M. Manoharan, Multivalent N-acetylgalactosamine-conjugated siRNA localizes in hepatocytes and elicits robust RNAi-mediated gene silencing, *J. Am. Chem. Soc.* 136 (2014) 16958–16961.

135. B.J. Zern, A.-M. Chacko, J. Liu, C.F. Greineder, E.R. Blankemeyer, R. Radhakrishnan, V. Muzykantov, Reduction of nanoparticle avidity enhances the selectivity of vascular targeting and PEG detection of pulmonary inflammation, *ACS Nano* 7 (2013) 2461–2469.

136. L.J. Cruz, P.J. Tacken, R. Fokkink, C.G. Figdor, The influence of PEG chain length and targeting moiety on antibody-mediated delivery of nanoparticle vaccines to human dendritic cells, *Biomaterials* 32 (2011) 6791–6803.

137. J.F. Stefanick, J.D. Ashley, T. Kiziltepe, B. Bilgicer, A systemic analysis of peptide linker length and liposomal polyethylene glycol coating on cellular uptake of peptide-targeted liposomes, *ACS Nano* 7 (2013) 2935–2947.

138. S. Hak, E. Helgesen, H.H. Hektoen, E.M. Huuse, P.A. Jarzyna, W.J. Mulder, O. Haraldseth, C. de L. Davies, The effect of nanoparticle polyethylene glycol surface density on ligand-directed tumor targeting studied in vivo by dual-modality imaging, *ACS Nano* 6 (2012) 5648–5658.

139. C. Wolfrum, S. Shi, K.N. Jayaprakash, M. Jayaraman, G. Wang, F.K. Pandey, K.G. Rajeev, T. Nakayama, K. Charrise, E.M. Ndungo, T. Zimmermann, V. Koteliansky, M. Manoharan, M. Stoffel, Mechanisms and optimization of in vivo delivery of lipophilic siRNAs, *Nat. Biotechnol.* 25 (2007) 1149–1157.

140. J. Soutschek, A. Akinc, B. Bramlage, K. Charisse, R. Constien, M. Donoghue, S. Elbashir, A. Geick, P. Hadwiger, J. Harborth, M. John, V. Kesavan, G. Lavine, R.K. Pandey, T. Racie, K.G. Rajeev, I. Röhl, I. Toudjarska, G. Wang, S. Wuschko, D. Bumcrot, V. Koteliansky, S. Limmer, M. Manoharan, H.-P. Vornlocher, Therapeutic silencing of an endogenous gene by systemic administration of modified siRNAs, *Nature* 432 (2004) 173–178.

141. O.F. Khan, E.W. Zaia, H. Yin, R.L. Bogorad, J.M. Pelet, M.J. Webber, I. Zhuang, J.E. Dahlman, R. Langer, D.G. Anderson, Ionizable amphiphilic dendrimer-based nanomaterials with alkyl-chain-substitutcd amines for tunable siRNA delivery to the liver endothelium in vivo, *Angew. Chem. Int. Ed.* 53 (2014) 1–6.

142. R.G. Smits, G.J.M. Koper, M. Mandel, The influence of nearest- and next-neearestneighbor interactions on the potentiometric titration of linear poly(ethylenimine), *J. Phys. Chem.* 97 (1993) 5745–5751.

143. Y. Lee, H. Mo, H. Koo, J.Y. Park, M.Y. Cho, G.W. Jin, J.S. Park, Visualization of the degradation of a disulfide polymer, linear poly(ethylenimine sulfide), for gene delivery, *Bioconjug. Chem.* 18 (2007) 13–18.

144. M.A. Gosselin, W. Guo, R.J. Lee, Efficient gene transfer using reversible cross-linked low molecular weight polyethylenimine, *Bioconjug. Chem.* 12 (2001) 989–994.

145. H. Uchida, K. Miyata, M. Oba, T. Ishii, T. Suma, K. Itaka, N. Nishiyama, K. Kataoka, Odd-even effect of repeating aminoethylene units in the side chain of N-substituted polyaspartamides on gene transfection profiles, *J. Am. Chem. Soc.* 133 (2011) 15524–15532.

146. F. Pittella, K. Miyata, Y. Maeda, T. Suma, S. Watanabe, Q. Chen, R.J. Christie, K. Osada, N. Nishiyama, K. Kataoka, Pancreatic cancer therapy by systemic administration of VEGF siRNA contained in calcium phosphate/charge-conversional polymer hybrid nanoparticles, *J. Control. Release* 161 (2012) 868–874.

147. A.J. Convertine, D.S.W. Benoit, C.L. Duvall, A.S. Hoffman, P.S. Stayton, Development of a novel endosomolytic diblock copolymer for siRNA delivery, *J. Control. Release* 133 (2009) 221–229.

148. P. Midoux, C. Pichon, J.J. Yaouanc, P.A. Jaffrés, Chemical vectors for gene delivery: a current review on polymers, peptides and lipids containing histidine or imidazole as nucleic acids carriers, *Br. J. Pharmacol.* 157 (2009) 166–178.

149. J.E. Dahlman, C. Barnes, O.F. Khan, A. Thiriot, S. Jhunjunwala, T.E. Shaw, Y. Xing, H.B. Sager, G. Sahay, L. Speciner, A. Bader, R.L. Bogorad, H. Yin, T. Racie, Y. Dong, S. Jiang, D. Seedorf, A. Dave, K.S. Sandhu, M.J. Webber, T. Novobrantseva, V.M. Ruda, A.K.R. Lytton-Jean, C.G. Levins, B. Kalish, D.K. Mudge, M. Perez, L. Abezgauz, P. Dutta, L. Smith, K. Charisse, M.W. Kieran, K. Fitzgerald, M. Nahrendorf, D. Danino, R.M. Tuder, U.H. von Andrian, A. Akinc, D. Panigrahy, A. Schroeder, V. Koteliansky, R. Langer, D.G. Anderson, In vivo endothelial siRNA delivery using polymeric nanoparticles with low molecular weight, *Nat. Biotechnol.* 9 (2014) 648–655.

150. F. Perche, S. Biswas, T. Wang, L. Zhu, V.P. Torchilin, Hypoxia-targeted siRNA delivery, *Angew. Chem. Int. Ed.* 53 (2014) 3362–3366.

151. Y. Xu, F.C. Szoka Jr., Mechanism of DNA release from cationic liposome/DNA complexes used in cell transfection, *Biochemistry* 35 (1996) 5616–5623.

152. H. Hatakeyama, H. Akita, H. Harashima, A multifunctional envelope type nano device (MEND) for gene delivery to tumours based on the EPR effect: a strategy for overcoming the PEG dilemma, *Adv. Drug Deliv. Rev.* 63 (2011) 152–160.

153. I.M. Hafez, N. Maurer, P.R. Cullis, On the mechanism whereby cationic lipids promote intracellular delivery of polynucleic acids, *Gene Ther.* 8 (2001) 1188–1196.

154. C.E. Ashley, E.C. Carnes, K.E. Epler, D.P. Padilla, G.K. Phillips, R.E. Castillo, D.C. Wilkinson, B.S. Wilkinson, C.A. Burgard, R.M. Kalinich, J.L. Townson, B. Chackerian, C.L. Willman, D.S. Peabody, W. Wharton, C.J. Brinker, Delivery of small interfering RNA by peptide-targeted mesoporous silica nanoparticlesupported lipid bilayers, *ACS Nano* 6 (2012) 2174–2188.

155. A. Elbakry, A. Zaky, R. Liebl, R. Rachel, A. Geopferich, M. Breunig, Layer-by-layer assembled gold nanoparticles for siRNA delivery, *Nano Lett.* 9 (2009) 2059–2064.

156. S.K. Lee, C.-H. Tung, A Fabricated siRNA nanoparticle for ultralong gene silencing in vivo, *Adv. Funct. Mater.* 23 (2013) 3488–3493.

157. Z.J. Deng, S.W. Morton, E. Ben-Akiva, E.C. Dreaden, K.E. Shopsowitz, P.T. Hammond, Layer-by-layer nanoparticles for systemic codelivery of an anticancer drug and siRNA for potential triple-negative breast cancer treatment, *ACS Nano* 7 (2013) 9571–9584.

158. H.M. Coley, Mechanisms and strategies to overcome chemotherapy resistance in metastatic breast cancer, *Cancer Treat. Rev.* 34 (2008) 378–390.

159. M. Taheri, F. Mahjoubi, MRP1 but not MDR1 is associated with response to neoadjuvant chemotherapy in breast cancer patients, *Dis. Markers* 34 (2013) 387–393.

160. N.S. Gandhi, R.K. Tekade, M.B. Chougule, Nanocarrier mediated delivery of siRNA/miRNA in combination with chemotherapeutic agents for cancer therapy: current progress and advances, *J. Control. Release* 194 (2014) 238–256.

161. T. Suma, K. Miyata, Y. Anraku, S. Watanabe, R.J. Christie, H. Takemoto, M. Shioyama, N. Gouda, T. Ishii, N. Nishiyama, K. Kataoka, Smart multilayered assembly for biocompatible siRNA delivery featuring dissolvable silica, endosome-disrupting polycations, and detachable PEG, *ACS Nano* 6 (2012) 6693–6705.

162. Y. Kakizawa, S. Furukawa, A. Ishii, K. Kataoka, Organic–inorganic hybridnanocarrier of siRNA constructing through the self-assembly of calciumphosphate and PEG-based block aniomer, *J. Control. Release* 111 (2006) 368–370.

163. F. Pittella, M. Zhang, Y. Lee, H.J. Kim, T. Tockary, K. Osada, T. Ishii, K. Miyata, N. Nishiyama, K. Kataoka, Enhanced endosomal escape of siRNA-incorporating hybrid nanoparticles from calcium phosphate and PEG-block charge-conversional polymer for efficient gene knockdown with negligible cytotoxicity, *Biomaterials* 32 (2011) 3106–3114.

164. M. Yamaguchi, Regulatory role of regucalcin in heart calciumsignaling: insight into cardiac failure (Review), *Biomed. Rep.* 2 (2014) 303–308.

165. J. Li, Y.-C. Chen, Y.-C. Tseng, S. Mozumdar, L. Huang, Biodegradable calcium phosphate nanoparticle with lipid coating for systemic siRNA delivery, *J. Control. Release* 142 (2010) 416–421.

166. Y. Yang, J. Li, F. Liu, L. Huang, Systemic delivery of siRNA via LCP nanoparticle efficiently inhibits lung metastasis, *Mol. Ther.* 20 (2012) 609–615.

167. S.A. Jensen, E.S. Day, C.H. Ko, L.A. Hurley, J.P. Luciano, F.M. Kouri, T.J. Merkel, A.J. Luthi, P.C. Patel, J.I. Cutler, W.L. Daniel, A.W. Scott, M.W. Rotz, T.J. Meade, D.A. Giljohann, C.A. Mirkin, A.H. Stegh, Spherical nucleic acid nanoparticle conjugates as an RNAi-based therapy for glioblastoma, *Sci. Transl. Med.* 5 (2013), 209ra152.

168. H.J. Kim, H. Takemoto, Y. Yi, M. Zheng, Y. Maeda, H. Chaya, K. Hayashi, P. Mi, F. Pittella, R.J. Christie, K. Toh, Y. Matsumoto, N. Nishiyama, K. Miyata, K. Kataoka, Precise engineering of siRNA delivery vehicles to tumors using polyion complexes and gold nanoparticles, *ACS Nano* 8 (2014) 8979–8991.

169. A. Fire, et al., Potent and specific genetic interference by double-stranded RNA in Caenorhabditis elegans, *Nature* 391 (1998) 806–811.

170. K. Garber, Alnylam launches era of RNAi drugs, *Nat. Biotechnol.* 36 (2018) 777–778.

171. G.B. Robb, T.M. Rana, RNA helicase a interacts with RISC in human cells and functions in RISC loading, *Mol. Cell* 26 (2007) 523–537.

172. K.A. Whitehead, R. Langer, D.G. Anderson, Knocking down barriers: advances in siRNA delivery, *Nat. Rev. Drug Discov.* 8 (2009) 129–138.

173. J.W. Gaynor, B.J. Campbell, R. Cosstick, RNA interference: a chemist's perspective, *Chem. Soc. Rev.* 39 (2010) 4169–4184.

174. J.K. Watts, G.F. Deleavey, M.J. Damha, Chemically modified siRNA: tools and applications, *Drug Discov. Today* 13 (2008) 842–855.

175. W.F. Lima, et al., Single-stranded siRNAs activate RNAi in animals, *Cell* 150 (2012) 883–894.

176. T.P. Prakash, et al., Identification of metabolically stable 5′-phosphate analogs that support single-stranded siRNA activity, *Nucleic Acids Res.* 43 (2015) 2993–3011.

177. R. Juliano, J. Bauman, H. Kang, X. Ming, Biological barriers to therapy with antisense and siRNA oligonucleotides, *Mol. Pharm.* 6 (2009) 686–695.

178. D. Castanotto, J.J. Rossi, The promises and pitfalls of RNA-interference-based therapeutics, *Nature* 457 (2009) 426–433.

179. J.B. Miller, D.J. Siegwart, Design of synthetic materials for intracellular delivery of RNAs: from siRNA-mediated gene silencing to CRISPR/Cas gene editing, *Nano Res.* 11 (2018) 5310–5337.

180. Y. Lu, A.A. Aimetti, R. Langer, Z. Gu, Bioresponsive materials, *Nat. Rev. Mater.* 2 (2017) 16075. doi: 10.1038/natrevmats.2016.75.

181. J.C. Burnett, J.J. Rossi, K. Tiemann, Current progress of siRNA/shRNA therapeutics in clinical trials, *Biotechnol. J.* 6(9) (2011) 1130–1146. doi: 10.1002/biot.201100054.

182. A. de Fougerolles, H.P. Vornlocher, J.Maraganore, J. Lieberman, Interfering with disease: a progress report on siRNA-based therapeutics, *Nat. Rev. Drug Discov.* 6 (2007) 443–453.

183. J.C. Kaczmarek, P.S. Kowalski, D.G. Anderson, Advances in the delivery of RNA therapeutics: from concept to clinical reality, *Genome Med.* 9 (2017) 1–6.

184. J.E. Zuckerman, M.E. Davis, Clinical experiences with systemically administered siRNA-based therapeutics in cancer, *Nat. Rev. Drug Discov.* 14 (2015) 843–856.

185. F. Eckstein, Nucleoside phosphorothioates, *Annu. Rev. Biochem.* 54 (1985) 367–402.

186. D.A. Braasch, et al., RNA interference in mammalian cells by chemically-modified RNA, *Biochemistry* 42 (2003) 7967–7975.

187. Y.L. Chiu, T.M. Rana, siRNA function in RNAi: a chemical modification analysis, *RNA* 9 (2003) 1034–1048.

188. J.D. Smith, D.B. Dunn, An additional sugar component of ribonucleic acids, *Biochim. Biophys. Acta* 31 (1959) 573–575.

189. A.D. Broom, R.K. Robins, The direct preparation of 2′-O-Methyladenosine from adenosine, *J. Am. Chem. Soc.* 87 (1965) 1145–1146.

190. S. Obika, et al., Synthesis of 2′-O, 4′-C-methyleneuridine and -cytidine. Novel bicyclic nucleosides having a fixed C3′-endo sugar puckering, *Tetrahedron Lett.* 38 (1997) 8735–8738.

191. A.A. Koshkin, et al., LNA (locked nucleic acids): synthesis of the adenine, cytosine, guanine, 5-methylcytosine, thymine and uracil bicyclonucleoside monomers, oligomerization, and unprecedented nucleic acid recognition, *Tetrahedron* 54 (1998) 3607–3630.

192. S. Hanessian, et al., Structure-based design of a highly constrained nucleic acid analogue: improved duplex stabilization by restricting sugar pucker and torsion angle gamma, *Angew. Chem. Int. Ed.* 51 (2012) 11242–11245.

193. L. Wang, et al., Phosphorothioation of DNA in bacteria by dnd genes, *Nat. Chem. Biol.* 3 (2007) 709–710.

194. S.Y. Wu, et al., 2′-OMe-phosphorodithioate-modified siRNAs show increased loading into the RISC complex and enhanced anti-tumour activity, *Nat. Commun.* 5 (2014) 1–2.

195. P.E. Nielsen, M. Egholm, R.H. Berg, O. Buchardt, Sequence-selective recognition of DNA by strand displacement with a thymine-substituted polyamide, *Science* 254 (1991) 1497–1500.

196. B. Herbert, et al., Inhibition of human telomerase in immortal human cells leads to progressive telomere shortening and cell death, *Proc. Natl. Acad. Sci. U. S. A.* 96 (1999) 14276–14281.

197. P. Li, Z.A. Sergueeva, M. Dobrikov, B.R. Shaw, Nucleoside and oligonucleoside boranophosphates: chemistry and properties, *Chem. Rev.* 107 (2007) 4746–4796.

198. A.H. Hall, J. Wan, E.E. Shaughnessy, B. Ramsay Shaw, K.A. Alexander, RNA interference using boranophosphate siRNAs: structure-activity relationships, *Nucleic Acids Res.* 32 (2004) 5991–6000.

199. E.P. Stirchak, J.E. Summerton, D.D. Weller, Uncharged stereoregular nucleic acid analogs: 2. Morpholino nucleoside oligomers with carbamate internucleoside linkages, *Nucleic Acids Res.* 17 (1989) 6129–6141.

200. J. Alter, et al., Systemic delivery of morpholino oligonucleotide restores dystrophin expression bodywide and improves dystrophic pathology, *Nat. Med.* 12 (2006) 175–177.

201. N. Langkjaer, A. Pasternak, J. Wengel, UNA (unlocked nucleic acid): a flexible RNA mimic that allows engineering of nucleic acid duplex stability, *Bioorg. Med. Chem.* 17 (2009) 5420–5425.

202. M.B. Laursen, et al., Utilization of unlocked nucleic acid (UNA) to enhance siRNA performance in vitro and in vivo, *Mol. BioSyst.* 6 (2010) 862–870.

203. M. Fisher, et al., Biological effects of hexitol and altritol-modified siRNAs targeting B-Raf, *Eur. J. Pharmacol.* 606 (2009) 38–44.

204. J.B. Bramsen, et al., A large-scale chemical modification screen identifies design rules to generate siRNAs with high activity, high stability and low toxicity, *Nucleic Acids Res.* 37 (2009) 2867–2881.

205. J.C. Salinas, J. Yu, M. Ostergaard, P.P. Seth, S. Hanessian, Conception and synthesis of Oxabicyclic nucleoside Phosphonates as Internucleotidic phosphate surrogates in antisense oligonucleotide constructs, *Org. Lett.* 20 (2018) 5296–5299.

206. K. Sipa, et al., Effect of base modifications on structure, thermodynamic stability, and gene silencing activity of short interfering RNA, *RNA* 13 (2007) 1301–1316.

207. J. Xia, et al., Gene silencing activity of siRNAs with a ribo-difluorotoluyl nucleotide, *ACS Chem. Biol.* 1 (2006) 176–183.

208. S.R. Suter, et al., Controlling miRNA-like off-target effects of an siRNA with nucleobase modifications, *Org. Biomol. Chem.* 15 (2017) 10029–10036.

209. A.F. Turner, H.G. Khorana, Studies on polynucleotides. VI. Experiments on the chemical polymerization of mononucleotides. Oligonucleotides derived from thymidine-3′-phosphate, *J. Am. Chem. Soc.* 81 (1959) 4651–4656.

210. P.C. Zamecnik, M.L. Stephenson, Inhibition of Rous-sarcoma virus-replication and cell transformation by a specific Oligodeoxynucleotide, *Proc. Natl. Acad. Sci. U. S. A.* 75 (1978) 280–284.

211. M.L. Stephenson, P.C. Zamecnik, Inhibition of Rous-sarcoma viral-Rna translation by a specific Oligodeoxyribonucleotide, *Proc. Natl. Acad. Sci. U. S. A.* 75 (1978) 285–288.

212. F.J. Raal, et al., Mipomersen, an apolipoprotein B synthesis inhibitor, for lowering of LDL cholesterol concentrations in patients with homozygous familial hypercholesterolaemia: a randomised, double-blind, placebo-controlled trial, *Lancet* 375 (2010) 998–1006.

213. C.F. Bennett, Therapeutic antisense oligonucleotides are coming of age, *Annu. Rev. Med.* 70 (2019) 307–321.

214. J.K. Watts, D.R. Corey, Silencing disease genes in the laboratory and the clinic, *J. Pathol.* 226 (2012) 365–379.

215. R. Micura, Small interfering RNAs and their chemical synthesis, *Angew. Chem. Int. Ed.* 41 (2002) 2265–2269.

216. W.S. Marshall, R.J. Kaiser, Recent advances in the high-speed solid phase synthesis of RNA, *Curr. Opin. Chem. Biol.* 8 (2004) 222–229.

217. J.H. Jeong, H. Mok, Y.K. Oh, T.G. Park, siRNA conjugate delivery systems, *Bioconjug. Chem.* 20 (2009) 5–14.

218. A.A. Turanov, et al., RNAi modulation of placental sFLT1 for the treatment of preeclampsia, *Nat. Biotechnol.* 36 (2018) 1164–+.

219. J. Zhou, et al., Receptor-targeted aptamer-siRNA conjugate-directed transcriptional regulation of HIV-1, *Theranostics* 8 (2018) 1575–1590.

220. S. Kruspe, P.H. Giangrande, Aptamer-siRNA chimeras: discovery, Progress, and future prospects, *Biomedicines* 5 (2017).

221. J.P. Dassie, et al., Systemic administration of optimized aptamer-siRNA chimeras promotes regression of PSMA-expressing tumors, *Nat. Biotechnol.* 27 (2009) 839–849.

222. A. Sehgal, et al., An RNAi therapeutic targeting antithrombin to rebalance the coagulation system and promote hemostasis in hemophilia, *Nat. Med.* 21 (2015)492–497.

223. A. Muratovska, M.R. Eccles, Conjugate for efficient delivery of short interfering RNA (siRNA) into mammalian cells, *FEBS Lett.* 558 (2004) 63–68.

224. Y.L. Chiu, A. Ali, C.Y. Chu, H. Cao, T.M. Rana, Visualizing a correlation between siRNA localization, cellular uptake, and RNAi in living cells, *Chem. Biol.* 11 (2004) 1165–1175.

225. G. Cesarone, O.P. Edupuganti, C.P. Chen, E.Wickstrom, Insulin receptor substrate 1 knockdown in human MCF7 ER+ breast cancer cells by nuclease-resistant IRS1 siRNA conjugated to a disulfide-bridged D-peptide analogue of insulin-like growth factor 1, *Bioconjug. Chem.* 18 (2007) 1831–1840.

226. R.L. Letsinger, G.R. Zhang, D.K. Sun, T. Ikeuchi, P.S. Sarin, Cholesteryl-conjugated oligonucleotides: synthesis, properties, and activity as inhibitors of replication of human immunodeficiency virus in cell culture, *Proc. Natl. Acad. Sci. U. S. A.* 86 (1989) 6553–6556.

227. K.G. Rajeev, T. Zimmermann, M. Manoharan, M. Maier, K. Fitzgerald, Inhibitory RNA Interference AgentsModified with Saccharide Ligands, Alnylam Pharmaceuticals, Inc, USA, 2018 (WO 2012/037254, 2012).

228. http://investors.alnylam.com/news-releases/news-release-details/alnylam-provides-rd-updates-and-announces-2019-product-and-2018.

229. S. Matsuda, et al., siRNA conjugates carrying sequentially assembled trivalent Nacetylgalactosamine linked through nucleosides elicit robust gene silencing in vivo in hepatocytes, *ACS Chem. Biol.* 10 (2015) 1181–1187.

230. R.G. Parmar, et al., Facile synthesis, geometry, and 2'-substituent-dependent in vivo activity of 5'-(E)- and 5'-(Z)-Vinylphosphonate-modified siRNA conjugates, *J. Med. Chem.* 61 (2018) 734–744.

231. N.C. Seeman, Nanomaterials based on DNA, *Annu. Rev. Biochem.* 79 (2010) 65–87.

232. H. Lee, et al., Molecularly self-assembled nucleic acid nanoparticles for targeted in vivo siRNA delivery, *Nat. Nanotechnol.* 7 (2012) 389–393.

233. J.I. Cutler, E. Auyeung, C.A. Mirkin, Spherical nucleic acids, *J. Am. Chem. Soc.* 134 (2012) 1376–1391.

234. D. Jasinski, F. Haque, D.W. Binzel, P. Guo, Advancement of the emerging field of RNA nanotechnology, *ACS Nano* 11 (2017) 1142–1164.

235. P. Guo, The emerging field of RNA nanotechnology, *Nat. Nanotechnol.* 5 (2010) 833–842.

236. D. Shu, Y. Shu, F. Haque, S. Abdelmawla, P. Guo, Thermodynamically stable RNA three-way junction for constructing multifunctional nanoparticles for delivery of therapeutics, *Nat. Nanotechnol.* 6 (2011) 658–667.

237. Y. Shu, et al., Stable RNA nanoparticles as potential new generation drugs for cancer therapy, *Adv. Drug Deliv. Rev.* 66 (2014) 74–89.

238. J.B. Lee, J. Hong, D.K. Bonner, Z. Poon, P.T. Hammond, Self-assembled RNA interference microsponges for efficient siRNA delivery, *Nat. Mater.* 11 (2012) 316–322.

239. T.M. Allen, P.R. Cullis, Liposomal drug delivery systems: from concept to clinical applications, *Adv. Drug Deliv. Rev.* 65 (2013) 36–48.

240. J. Heyes, L. Palmer, K. Bremner, I. MacLachlan, Cationic lipid saturation influences intracellular delivery of encapsulated nucleic acids, *J. Control. Release* 107 (2005) 276–287.

241. M. Jayaraman, et al., Maximizing the potency of siRNA lipid nanoparticles for hepatic gene silencing in vivo, *Angew. Chem. Int. Ed.* 51 (2012) 8529–8533.

242. T.M. Allen, P.R. Cullis, Drug delivery systems: entering themainstream, *Science* 303 (2004) 1818–1822.

243. S.C. Semple, et al., Rational design of cationic lipids for siRNA delivery, *Nat. Biotechnol.* 28 (2010) 172–176.

244. W. He, et al., Discovery of siRNA lipid nanoparticles to transfect suspension Leukemia cells and provide in vivo delivery capability, *Mol. Ther.* 22 (2014) 359–370.

245. C.A. Alabi, et al., Multiparametric approach for the evaluation of lipid nanoparticles for siRNA delivery, *Proc. Natl. Acad. Sci. U. S. A.* 110 (2013) 12881–12886.

246. M.T. Abrams, et al., Evaluation of efficacy, biodistribution, and inflammation for a potent siRNA nanoparticle: effect of dexamethasone co-treatment, *Mol. Ther.* 18 (2010) 171–180.

247. M.A. Maier, et al., Biodegradable lipids enabling rapidly eliminated lipid nanoparticles for systemic delivery of RNAi therapeutics, *Mol. Ther.* 21 (2013) 1570–1578.

248. T. Coelho, et al., Safety and efficacy of RNAi therapy for transthyretin amyloidosis, *N. Engl. J. Med.* 369 (2013) 819–829.

249. D. Zhi, et al., The headgroup evolution of cationic lipids for gene delivery, *Bioconjug. Chem.* 24 (2013) 487–519.

250. L. Desigaux, et al., Self-assembled lamellar complexes of siRNA with lipidic aminoglycoside derivatives promote efficient siRNA delivery and interference, *Proc. Natl. Acad. Sci. U. S. A.* 104 (2007) 16534–16539.

251. A. Santel, et al., A novel siRNA-lipoplex technology for RNA interference in the mouse vascular endothelium, *Gene Ther.* 13 (2006) 1222–1234.

252. R.C. Adami, et al., An amino acid-based amphoteric liposomal delivery system for systemic administration of siRNA, *Mol. Ther.* 19 (2011) 1141–1151.

253. Y. Dong, D.J. Siegwart, D.G. Anderson. Strategies, design, and chemistry in siRNA delivery systems, *Adv. Drug Deliv. Rev.* 144 (2019) 133–147.

254. H. Jin Kim, A. Kim, K. Miyata, K. Kataoka, Recent progress in development of siRNA delivery vehicles for cancer therapy, *Adv. Drug Deliv. Rev.* 104 (2016) 61–77.

255. J. Tabernero, G.I. Shapiro, P.M. LoRusso, A. Cervantes, G.K. Schwartz, G.J. Weiss, L. Paz-Ares, D.C. Cho, J.R. Infante, M. Alsina, M.M. Gounder, R. Falzone, J. Harrop, A.C.S. White, I. Toudjarska, D. Bumcrot, R.E. Meyers, G. Hinkle, N. Svrzikapa, R.M. Hutabarat, V.A. Clausen, J. Cehelsky, S.V. Nochur, C. Gamba-Vitalo, A.K. Vaishnaw, D.W.Y. Sah, J.A. Gollob, H.A. Burris III, First-in-humans trial of an RNA interference therapeutic targeting VEGF and KSP in cancer patients with liver involvement, *Cancer Discov.* 3 (2013) 406–417.

256. B. Schultheis, D. Strumberg, A.C. Vank, F. Gebhardt, O. Keil, C. Lange, K. Giese, J. Kaufmann, M. Khan, J. Drevs, First-in-human phase I study of the liposomal RNA interference therapeutic Atu027 in patients with advanced solid tumors, *J. Clin. Oncol.* 32 (2014) 4141–4148.

257. D.W. Bartlett, M.E. Davis, Physiochemical and biological characterization of targeted, nucleic acid-containing nanoparticles, *Bioconjug. Chem.* 18 (2007) 456–468.

258. J.E. Zuckerman, I. Gritli, A. Tolcher, J.D. Heidel, D. Lim, R.Morgan, B. Chmielowski, A. Ribas, M.E. Davis, Y. Yen, Correlating animal and human phase Ia/Ib clinical data with CALAA-01, a targeted, polymer-based nanoparticle containing siRNA, *Proc. Natl. Acad. Sci. U. S. A.* 111 (2014) 11449–11454.

259. Loutfy H. Madkour, *Reactive Oxygen Species (ROS), Nanoparticles, and Endoplasmic Reticulum (ER) Stress-Induced Cell Death Mechanisms.* Paperback ISBN: 9780128224816. Imprint: Academic Press Published Date: 1st August 2020. https://www.elsevier.com/books/reactive-oxygen-species-ros-nanoparticles-and-endoplasmic-reticulum-er-stress-induced-cell-death-mechanisms/madkour/978-0-12-822481-6.

260. Loutfy H. Madkour, *Nanoparticles Induce Oxidative and Endoplasmic Reticulum Antioxidant Therapeutic Defenses.* Copyright 2020 Publisher Springer International Publishing. Copyright Holder Springer Nature Switzerland AG eBook ISBN 978-3-030-37297-2 DOI 10.1007/978-3-030-37297-2 Hardcover ISBN 978-3-030-37296-5 Series ISSN 2194-0452 Edition Number 1. https://www.springer.com/gp/book/9783030372965?utm_campaign=3_pier05_buy_print&utm_content=en_08082017&utm_medium=referral&utm_source=google_books#otherversion=9783030372972.

261. Loutfy H. Madkour, *Nucleic Acids as Gene Anticancer Drug Delivery Therapy.* 1st Edition. Publishing house: Elsevier, (2020). Paperback ISBN: 9780128197776 Imprint: Academic Press Published Date: 2nd January 2020 Imprint: Academic Press Copyright: Paperback ISBN: 9780128197776 © Academic Press 2020 Published: 2nd January 2020 Imprint: Academic Press Paperback ISBN: 9780128197776. https://www.elsevier.com/books/nucleic-acids-as-gene-anticancer-drug-deliverytherapy/madkour/978-0-12-819777-6.

262. Loutfy H. Madkour, *Nanoelectronic Materials: Fundamentals and Applications (Advanced Structured Materials)* 1st ed. 2019 Edition: https://link.springer.com/book/10.1007%2F978-3-030-21621-4 Series Title Advanced Structured Materials Series Volume 116 Copyright 2019 Publisher Springer International Publishing Copyright Holder Springer Nature Switzerland AG. eBook ISBN 978-3-030-21621-4 DOI 10.1007/978-3-030-21621-4 Hardcover ISBN 978-3-030-21620-7 Series ISSN 1869-8433 Edition Number 1 Number of Pages XLIII, 783 Number of Illustrations 122 b/w illustrations, 494 illustrations in colour Topics. ISBN-10: 3030216209 ISBN-13: 978-3030216207 #117 in Nanotechnology (Books) #725 in Materials Science (Books) #187336 in Textbooks. https://books.google.com.eg/books/about/Nanoelectronic_Materials.html?id=YQXCxAEACAAJ&source=kp_book_description&redir_esc=y; https://www.springer.com/gp/book/9783030216207.

263. H. Shimizu, Y. Hori, S. Kaname, K. Yamada, N. Nishiyama, S. Matsumoto, K. Miyata, M. Oba, A. Yadama, K. Kataoka, T. Fujita, siRNA-based therapy ameliorates glomerulonephritis, *J. Am. Soc. Nephrol.* 21 (2010) 622–633.

264. A. Sizovs, X. Song, M.N. Waxham, Y. Jia, F. Feng, J. Chen, A.C. Wicker, J. Xu, Y. Yu, J. Wang, Precisely tunable engineering of sub-30 nm monodisperse oligonucleotide nanoparticles, *J. Am. Chem. Soc.* 136 (2014) 234–240.

265. C. Dohmen, D. Edinger, T. Fröhlich, L. Schreiner, U. Lächelt, C. Troiber, J. Rädler, P. Hadwiger, H. Vornlocher, E. Wagner, Nanosized multifunctional polyplexes for receptor-mediated siRNA delivery, *ACS Nano* 6 (2012) 5198–5208.

3 DNA/RNA Nanoparticles Structures for siRNA Delivery Applications

In order to activate the RNA interference (RNAi) pathway, double-stranded small interfering RNA (siRNA) must travel through the bloodstream and gain access to the cytosol of target cells. The hydrophilic nature and large molecular weight of siRNAs prevent the molecules from diffusing across the cellular membrane into the cell; therefore, modifications to the nucleic acid and generation of clever delivery strategies are necessary for the creation of siRNA therapeutics.

3.1 STRUCTURAL DNA-/RNA-BASED RNAi SYSTEMS

RNAi has been recognized as the sequence-specific silencing of target messenger RNA (mRNA) by a long double-stranded RNA (dsRNA), enabling efficient suppression of gene and protein expression [1]. After the first report on *Caenorhabditis elegans* in 1998, this phenomenon has been verified in plant, insect, fungi, and mammalian cells [2]. RNAi is now considered to be a highly preserved natural mechanism for the regulation of the gene expression in many organisms. Once a long dsRNA is introduced into the cytoplasm, it is processed by an RNase type-III enzyme (dicer) to generate a short dsRNA fragment of 21–25 base pairs [3]. The processed dsRNA fragment can be loaded onto the RNA-induced silencing complex (RISC), and an antisense RNA strand serves as a sequence-specific guide for targeted mRNA cleavage [4,5]. After the dicer process, a short, double-stranded, small interfering RNA (ds-siRNA) shows more specific cleavage of target mRNA with improved off-targeting effects.

In 2001, synthetic siRNAs drew much attention as novel therapeutic drugs to treat various genetic diseases as well as cancer [6,7]. Synthetic dsRNAs can be easily designed and customized for any gene silencing applications. A synthetic siRNA is composed of 21–23 bp dsRNA with a 2-nucleotide overhang at the 3′-end of both strands, and there have been numerous studies to prepare more stable siRNAs with modified bases [8]. It is considered that the presence of a 5′-monophosphate is required to induce proper RNAi, while the phosphodiester backbone, internal, or 3′-ends of the 2′-OH in sugar residues can be modified to improve the chemical stability and reduce the immunostimulation. However, siRNAs still show poor pharmacological properties due to their physical characteristics including low molecular weight (LMW), high anionic charge, and a relatively rigid rod-like helical structure.

To overcome the critical hurdles of siRNA delivery, various delivery systems have been proposed, such as viral and synthetic cationic carrier systems. To date, various viral systems have been developed to endogenously express short hairpin RNAs (shRNAs) for gene silencing, and these systems include retrovirus, adenovirus, adeno-associated virus (AAV), and lentivirus [9]. The viral systems have the clear advantage of a high transduction efficiency and stable expression of shRNAs for a prolonged period. However, many studies have shown the potential drawbacks of viral systems such as risk of mutation, high initial immune response, nonspecific tissue distribution, and undesirable inflammation. Nonviral and synthetic cationic carriers are another class of the siRNA delivery system.

Positively charged polymers, peptides, and lipids have been widely utilized to formulate siRNAs into a compact nanoparticle (NP), facilitating the intracellular uptake of siRNAs [10]. The main mechanism of preparation of NP complexes is an electrostatic charge interaction between anionic nucleic acids and cationic carriers in aqueous solution. It is similar to that of cationic delivery systems for plasmid DNA (pDNA); however, there is a huge difference in the physical behavior of siRNA compared with long pDNA. siRNA is known to be more rigid due to its rod-like helical structure, having a relatively low charge density, and it remains difficult to formulate compact and stable siRNA complexes with conventional cationic carriers [11,12]. To simply achieve enhanced particle stability, the addition of an excess amount of cationic condensing agent is often carried out to formulate uncompromising siRNAs. However, this nonspecific and excessive positive charge on nanocomplexes can cause severe cytotoxicity and immune responses.

Recently, a variety of structural DNA-/RNA-based RNAi systems (structural RNAi systems) have been suggested to resolve the aforementioned problems of siRNA delivery. Structural RNAi systems mimic endogenous long dsRNA but are prepared by synthetic or equivalent methods to resemble the therapeutic efficacy of siRNAs. The preparation of structural RNAi systems can be as simple as base-pair hybridization and bioconjugation, or as complicated as 3D nucleic acid nanotechnology (Table 3.1). The concept of structural RNAi systems is to overcome the physical drawbacks of siRNAs, while providing structural flexibility to generate more condensed and stable polyelectrolyte complexes. In addition, some of the suggested structural RNAi systems aim to act as carrier-free delivery systems for siRNAs. This approach is particularly unique due to the fact

TABLE 3.1

Pros and Cons of Structural DNA/RNA-based RNAi Systems

Types of siRNA Structure		Pros/Cons
Long linear siRNA and branched siRNA delivery	Linear siRNAs [13]	High charge density for polyplex formation, enhanced serum stability, and cellular uptake.
		Only one gene target and relatively fast degradation of long siRNAs.
	Linear siRNAs having two different RNA sequences [14,15]	Effective dual-target gene knockdown.
		Multigene targeting at the same time and the synergistic effect of codelivery.
		Gene silencing of different target genes at the same time.
	Branched siRNAs [16]	Higher charge density than long linear siRNAs.
		Sustanance of RNAi effects *in vivo*.
	siRNA microhydrogels [17]	Enhanced cellular uptake compared with multi-siRNA *in vitro*.
		Higher binding capacity with low molecular weight (LMW) cationic carriers compared with linear siRNAs.
	Linear siRNAs with aptamers [18,19]	Active targeting effect and minimization of immune response problem.
		Endolytic activity of aptamers is not clear.
Three-dimensional oligonucleotide structures for siRNA delivery	RNA nanoparticles [20–22]	Thermodynamically stable and good resistance to serum ribonuclease *in vivo*.
		High cost and size limit of RNA synthesis.
		Difficulty in RNA NP synthesis and low retention time in serum of patients.
	pRNA structures [23–26]	Generally stable to changes in temperature, salt, and pH.
		Can deliver various molecules to cell-surface receptors.
		Higher gene silencing effect than the naked siRNAs.
		Degradation by RNase *in vivo*.
	DNA nanostructures [27]	Chemically modified oligonucleotides are used to increase the plasma stability, as well as to reduce the immune stimulation.
		Defined three-dimensional structure can govern the density and spatial orientation of the ligands.
		Good for delivery of siRNA-ligand conjugates.
DNA/RNA ball technology	RNA microsponge/ball [28,29]	Enhanced cellular uptake of siRNA with a high cargo capacity.
		Good silencing effects *in vitro* and *in vivo*.
		RNA structures with various shapes can be prepared.
	DNA scaffolds [30,31]	Enhanced stability for microscopic DNA structures.
		Shape of DNA structures can facilitate the endosomal release of siRNAs.

that the structural DNA or RNA itself can serve as a delivery carrier in addition to functioning as a therapeutic drug. In this chapter, we have focused and emphasized the current advances and technological developments in structural RNAi systems. The structural RNAi systems are beginning to show promise; however, the impact on the RNAi field and gene therapy will be realized shortly through the persistent interdisciplinary research in diverse fields.

RNAi is a process by which RNA molecules, with sequences complementary to a gene's coding sequence, induce degradation of corresponding mRNAs, thus blocking the translation of the mRNA into protein [32,33]. RNAi is initiated by exposing cells to long dsRNA via transfection or endogenous expression. dsRNAs are processed into smaller fragments (usually 21–23 nucleotides) of siRNAs [34], which form a complex with the RISCs [35]. Introduction of siRNA into mammalian cells leads to downregulation of target genes without triggering interferon responses [34]. Molecular therapy using siRNA has shown great potential for diseases caused by abnormal gene overexpression or mutation, such as various cancers, viral

infections, and genetic disorders, as well as for pain management. In the last 10 years, a tremendous effort has been made in biomedical therapeutic application of gene silencing in humans. Phase I studies of siRNA for the treatment of age-related macular degeneration and respiratory syncytial virus provided promising data with no sign of nonspecific toxicity [36,37]. However, there are many challenges to be overcome for siRNA cancer therapeutics, including safety, stability, and effective siRNA delivery.

The major barrier facing siRNA therapeutics is the efficiency of delivery to the desired cell type, tissue, or organ. siRNAs do not readily pass through the cell membrane due to their size and negative charge. Cationic liposome-based strategies are usually used for the cellular delivery of chemically synthesized or *in vitro* transcribed siRNA [38]. However, there are many problems with lipid-based delivery systems *in vivo*, such as rapid clearance by the liver and lack of target tissue specificity. Delivery systems can be categorized into physical methods, conjugation methods, and natural carrier (viruses and bacteria) and nonviral carrier methods [39]. DNA-based expression cassettes that express shRNA are usually delivered to target cells *ex vivo* by viruses and bacteria, and these modified cells are then reinfused back into the patient [40]. The popular adenovirus-derived vectors and AAV-derived vectors provide efficient delivery for the shRNA expression [9]. However, there are problems with delivery using viral vectors, such as insertional mutagenesis and immunogenicity [41]. Nonviral gene delivery systems are highly attractive for gene therapy because they are safer and easier to produce than viral vectors.

Nanotechnology has made significant advances in the development of efficient siRNA delivery systems. Current nonviral delivery systems can be categorized as organic and inorganic [42]. Organic complexes include lipid complexes, conjugated polymers, and cationic polymers, whereas inorganic NPs include magnetic NPs, quantum dots, carbon nanotubes, and gold NPs (AuNPs).

3.2 POLY/MULTIMERIC siRNA DELIVERY APPLICATIONS

In order to properly induce systemic *in vivo* gene silencing, a large amount of siRNA (3–9 mg/kg) has often been required [43]. However, due to the immune response triggered by excessive RNA materials and cationic carriers, practical applications of RNAi gene therapy have been hampered [44–46]. High molecular weight siRNAs were first proposed in 2007 to improve the physical drawbacks of short rigid dsRNA [47]. For polyelectrolyte complexation, a more flexible chain of dsRNA is favorable to form condensed and compact NPs with cationic carriers. However, as compared with pDNA that shows a very flexible nature, siRNA has a rigid rod-like structure with an estimated length of 7 nm. Since the persistent length of dsRNA is over 260 bp [48–50], siRNA cannot be easily formulated using conventional cationic carriers that are designed for the delivery of pDNA. The physical problems of short dsRNA have been well-documented in various studies, and the advantages of high molecular weight siRNAs have been highlighted [47,51].

3.2.1 Long Linear siRNA

Previously, various methods for preparing long linear siRNA have been investigated. Simple sticky overhang hybridization and bioconjugation of each sense and antisense strand of siRNA has mainly been proposed to generate multimeric blocks of siRNA. Among these, a cleavable disulfide linkage between siRNA strands has been popularly utilized [52–54]. The 5′-ends of the sense and antisense siRNA strand were functionalized with free thiol groups, and these thiol-modified RNA strands were utilized to form a disulfide-polymerized poly-siRNA. The polymerized siRNA had a broad range of bp length in the order of 50–1000 bp [13]. In the complexation experiment with an LMW polyethylenimine (MW: 1800), poly-siRNA formed

condensed and compact nanocomplexes at a weight ratio of 1.25 and a size of 235 nm, while mono-siRNA or naked siRNA generated large and loose particles with a size over 1000 nm. The stability of poly-siRNA was also confirmed by a heparin competition assay and serum stability assay. The results revealed that poly-siRNA was far more condensed, overcoming the serum degradation and being more ionically stable than mono-siRNA. In addition, *in vitro* cellular uptake and gene silencing experiments verified that poly-siRNA has a greater efficiency over mono-siRNA due to its high charge density and stability under formulated conditions.

Mok *et al.* highlighted the *in vivo* efficacy of long linear siRNA (Figure 3.1). Multimerized siRNA (multi-siRNA) was prepared by utilizing a cleavable and noncleavable crosslinker [14]. The 3′-end of each RNA strand had a thiol functional group, which later reacted with a short crosslinker to produce a multi-siRNA. Since this study utilized both cleavable and noncleavable linkers, a detailed study of the gene silencing mechanism of multi-siRNA was accomplished. For multi-siRNA with a cleavable linker, once it is internalized, it can dissociate to mono-siRNA due to the reducing conditions in the cytoplasm as a result of glutathione. However, in the case of multi-siRNA with a noncleavable linker, dicer is needed to process the multi-siRNA to generate short dsRNAs by random cleavage. Therefore, the cleavable linker provided a more sequence-specific degradation of mRNA. *In vivo* experiments have revealed that multi-siRNA show far enhanced gene silencing efficacy as compared with naked siRNA. Immunostimulation upon the injection of multi-siRNA has also been investigated, and both cleavable and noncleavable multi-siRNA showed a relatively low level of interferon alpha (IFN-α) when formulated with linear PEI (LPEI). It is important to note that when noncleavable multi-siRNA was formulated with N-[1-(2,3-dioleoyloxy)propyl]-N, N, N-trimethylammonium methylsulfate, a massive increase in IFN-α was observed. This suggests that immunostimulation is highly affected not only by the genetic material itself but also by the delivery carriers.

Dual gene targeted multimeric siRNA conjugates (DGT multi-siRNA) were developed to induce simultaneous gene knockdown of two selective proteins (green fluorescent protein (GFP) and vascular endothelial growth factor [VEGF]). Using either cleavable or noncleavable crosslinkers, an anti-GFP and anti-VEGF sequence containing multimeric siRNA was prepared by the thiol-maleimide reaction of the 3′-end of the thiol functional group of the RNA and crosslinker [15]. It is interesting to note that, at the same concentration, the DGT multi-siRNA induced enhanced gene silencing of target proteins as compared with the mixture of single gene–targeted multimeric siRNA. Since simultaneous silencing of multiple upregulated genes is highly attractive for anticancer treatment, the survivin and Bcl-2 genes have been dual-targeted, and a synergistic apoptotic effect on cancer cells was achieved. To further evaluate the

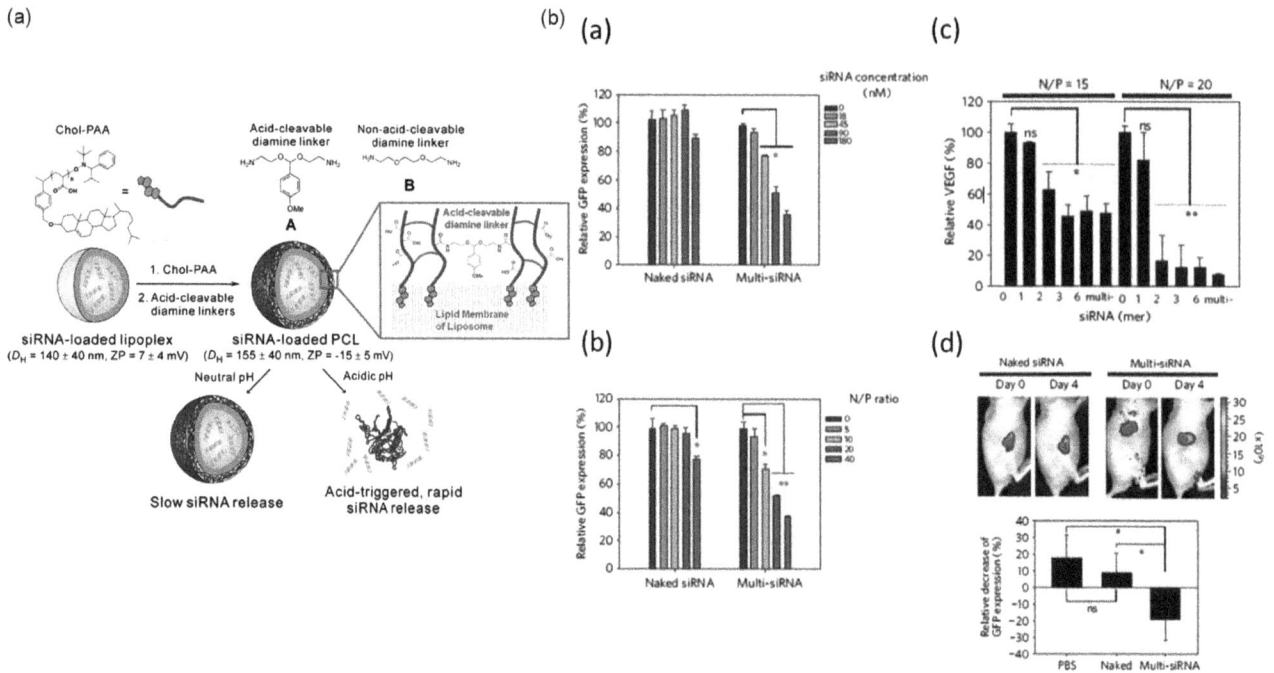

FIGURE 3.1 Preparation of an acid-degradable siRNA-loaded polymer-caged lipoplex (PCL) nanocarrier and its acid-triggered release of siRNA.

enhanced gene silencing on dual-targeted siRNA delivery, dimerized siRNA was synthesized with a cleavable disulfide bond [55]. Unlike multi-siRNA, that is the mixture of various long dsRNAs, such as a mixed population of multimers, the dimerized siRNA can offer better quality control for synthesis. As compared with monomer siRNA, dimerized siRNA showed far enhanced complexation behaviors with cationic polymers. In addition, enhanced intracellular delivery and gene silencing could be achieved with the dimerized siRNA with a polyethylene glycol (PEG) modification to improve the serum stability of nanocomplexes.

Multi-siRNA systems have been utilized as a scaffold carrier for the delivery of aptamer–siRNA conjugates (Figure 3.2). An aptamer is a short oligonucleotide with a high binding affinity for various target molecules, including small molecules, peptides, and oligonucleotides. Aptamers have been widely used as novel ligands for targeted gene delivery due to their various advantages such as high specificity and binding affinity, low immunostimulation, and the ease of preparation [18]. A mucin 1 (MUC1) DNA aptamer was used as a targeting ligand for cancer cells because MUC1 is highly overexpressed in malignant adenocarcinoma [10,18]. To prepare the comb-type aptamer–siRNA (Comb-Apt–siR) conjugates, antisense strands of siRNA were first multimerized with a cleavable disulfide linkage and later, MUC1 aptamer sense strands were hybridized to form a linear multimerized dsRNA structure with repeated introduction of MUC1 aptamers. As compared with the direct one-to-one conjugate of MUC1 aptamer and

siRNA, the enhanced uptake of the Comb-Apt–siR conjugates was achieved in MCF-7 cells. It is likely that this enhanced intracellular uptake of multivalent Comb-Apt–siR conjugates is attributed to a more favorable chance of contact with MUC1 and/or the synergistic effects of multivalent aptamers for endocytosis. However, gene silencing of Comb-Apt–siR without an additional cationic carrier was not achieved due to the lack of endosomal escaping properties. This study highlighted that the multivalent ligands can greatly enhance the intracellular delivery efficiency of Comb-Apt–siR [19].

3.2.2 Branched siRNA

As an alternative to long linear siRNA, branched and dendrimer-like siRNA structures have been developed. Unlike the natural RNA strands that are quickly degraded in the biological fluid, functional RNA structures may provide a prolonged RNAi effect due to their increased serum stability and charge density [56]. Nakashima et al. reported the synthesis of a branched siRNA structure with three- or four-way junctions [16]. By simple base-pair hybridization, trimer and tetramer RNA were efficiently self-assembled (Figure 3.3). To evaluate their prolonged RNAi effects, these branched RNA structures were incubated with the dicer, and their stability against nuclease was investigated. Compared with the linear RNA substrate, the branched RNA structures produced active 21 bp siRNAs at a much slower rate. The prolonged generation of siRNAs under

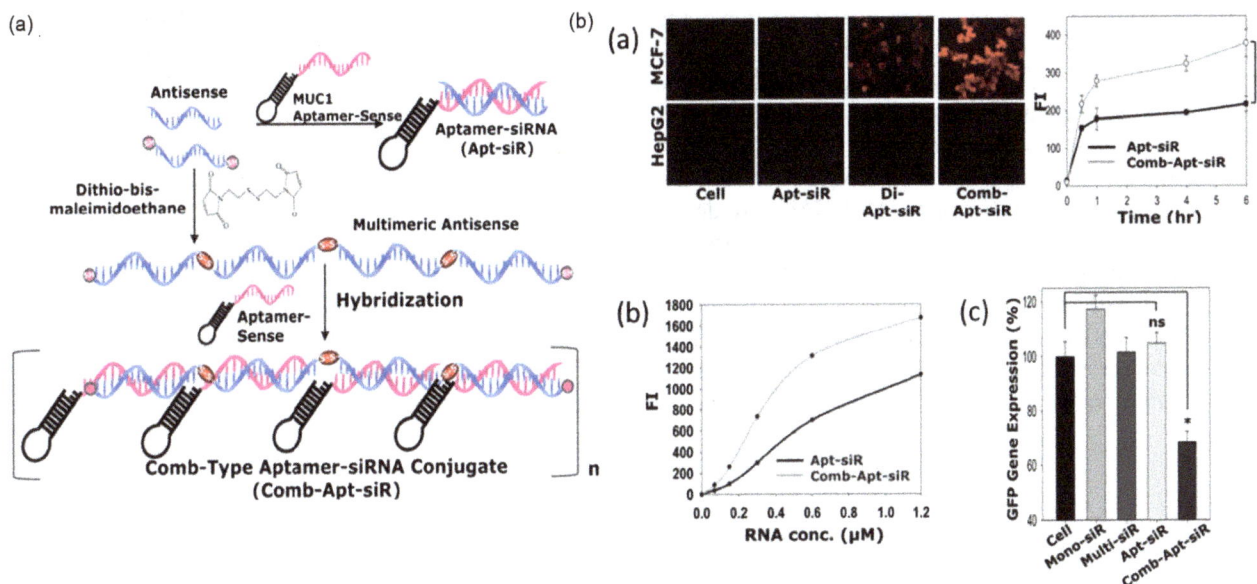

FIGURE 3.2 A. Schematic illustration of the synthesis process of multivalent comb-type aptamer–siRNA conjugates (Comb-Apt-siR). B. Gene expression effects of Comb-Apt-siRs. (a) Gene expression effect analysis of Comb-Apt-siRs using confocal microscopy. (b) Fluorescence intensity of Comb-Apt-siRs in MCF-7 cells. (c) Relative GFP expression of Comb-Apt-siRs in A549 cells (*p<0.01; ns=not significant). (Reprinted with permission from Ref. [19]. Copyright 2014, Royal Society of Chemistry.) - Multivalent comb-type aptamer–siRNA conjugates for efficient and selective intracellular delivery.

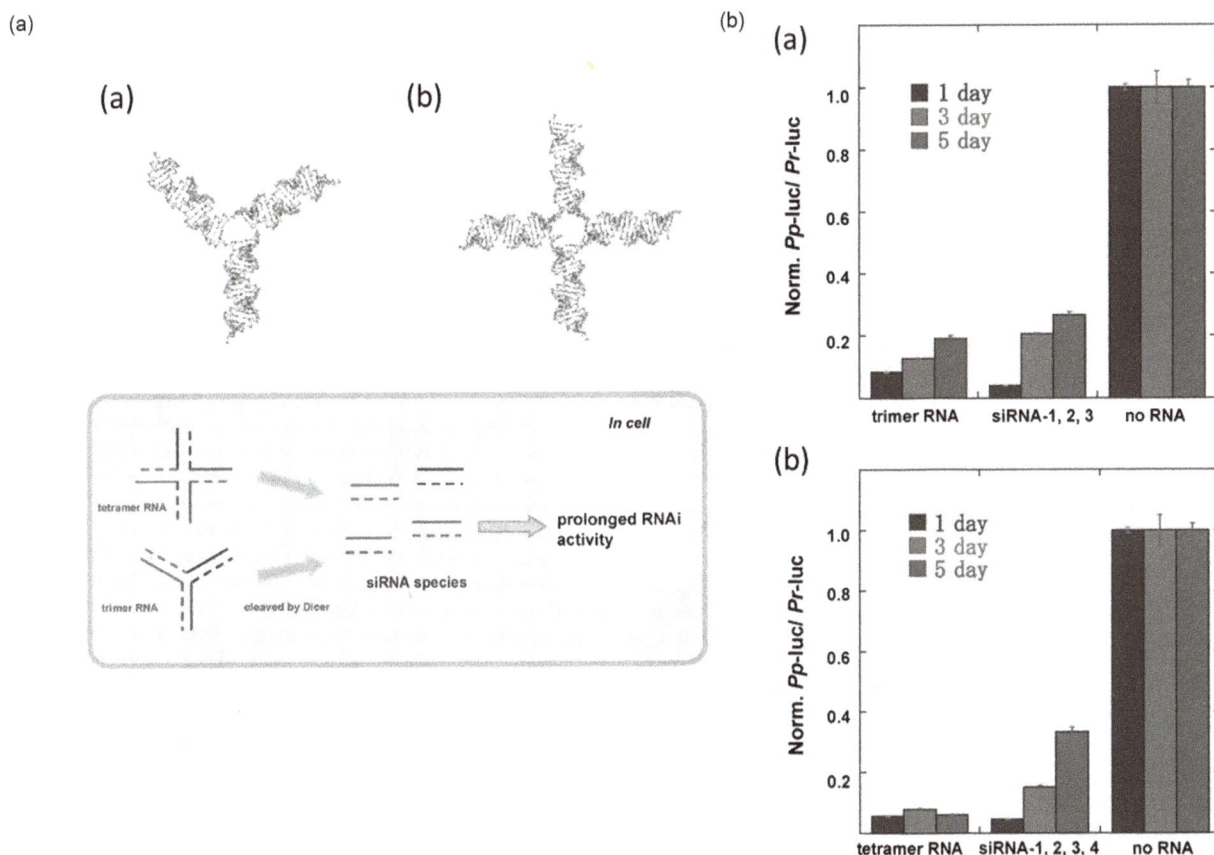

FIGURE 3.3 A. Schematic illustration of the branched RNA structure with siRNA and RNAi process of structures. (a) Trimer RNA. (b) Tetramer RNA. B. Gene silencing effects of branched RNA structures. (a) Trimer RNA. (b) Tetramer RNA. Effects of branched RNA analysis after 1, 3, and 5 days in HeLa cells (RNA concentraion=25 nM). (Reprinted with permission from Ref. [16]. Copyright 2011, Royal Society of Chemistry.) - Branched RNA nanostructures for RNA interference.

cytosolic conditions can enhance the overall duration of the RNAi effect, thereby maximizing gene regulation under various applications. The tetramer RNA resulted in stable luciferase gene silencing over a period of 5 days without chemical modification of RNA bases.

In addition to the simple branched RNA structure, more complex dendrimer-like structures of siRNAs were developed by Hong et al. [17]. Two types of RNA dendrimers were prepared by the simple hybridization of dimeric siRNA and Y-shaped siRNA (Figure 3.4). The dimeric and Y-shaped siRNAs were synthesized by the use of a noncleavable crosslinker of 1,8-bis(maleimidodiethylene) glycol and tri-[2-maleimidoethyl]-amine. Depending on the mixture of dimeric and Y-shaped siRNA, highly branched and dendrimer-like structures were generated, and this networked structure could form RNA microhydrogel. The porosity and networked structure of RNA microhydrogel could be controlled by simply increasing the ratio of Y shaped siRNA over dimeric RNA. The size of RNA microhydrogel is roughly 2 μm in the dried state and 8 μm in the well-swollen state in aqueous solution. The highly networked structure of siRNA microhydrogel offers a greater charge density that facilitates the complexation with a weakly charged cationic carrier such as LPEI (MW: 2500). At a nitrogen/phosphate (N/P) ratio of 60, highly condensed nanocomplexes could be prepared with a size

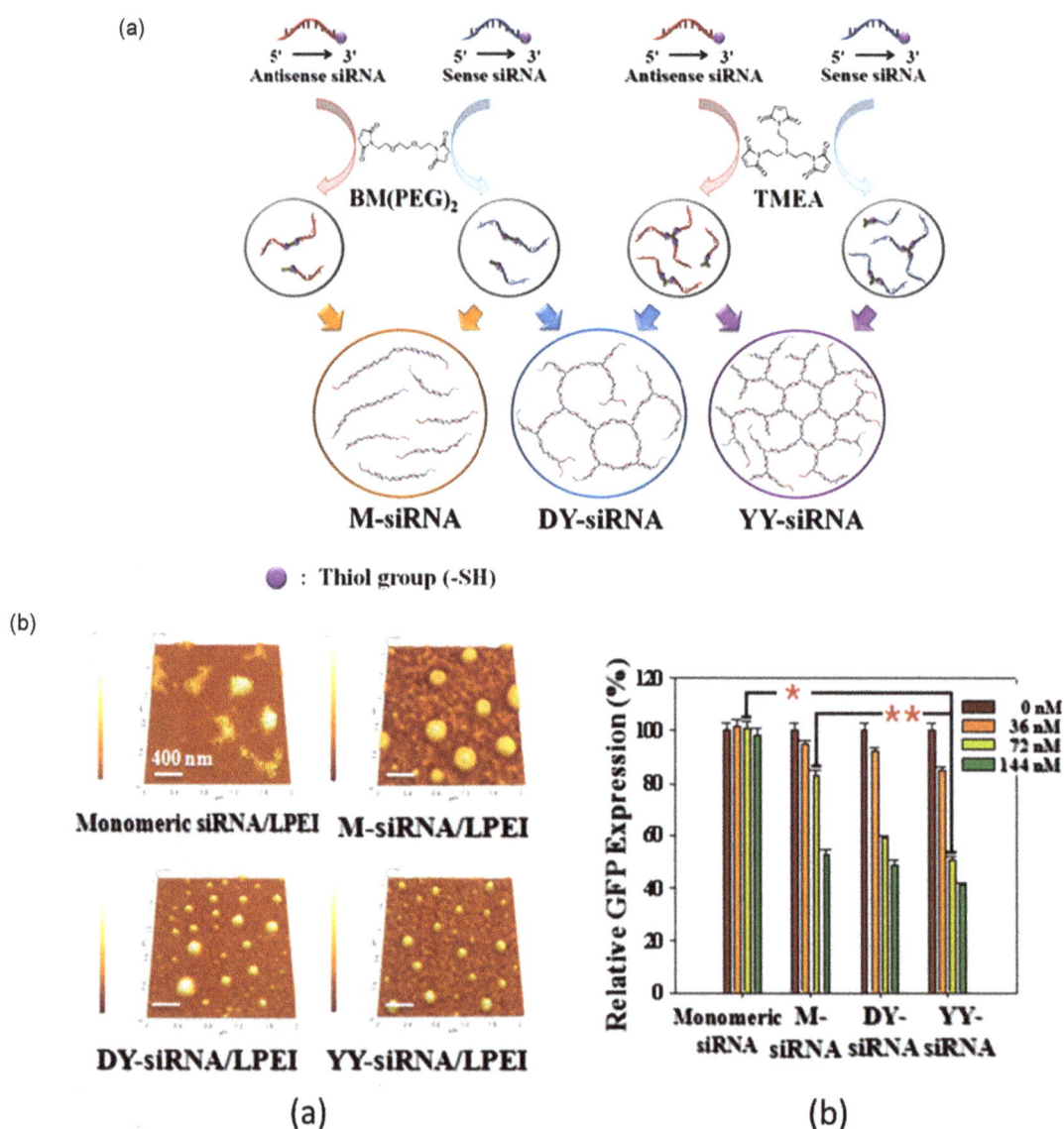

FIGURE 3.4 A. Scheme of the synthesis of multimeric siRNA (multi-siRNA), dimeric by Y-shaped siRNAs (DY-siRNA), and branched by Y-shaped siRNAs (YYsiRNA). B. AFM images of siRNA/LPEI complexes and gene silencing effects. (a) Monomeric siRNA/LPEI, M-siRNA/LPEI, DY-siRNA/LPEI, and YY-siRNA/LPEI (scale bar = 400 nm). (b) GFP gene silencing effects of siRNAs/LPEI complexes. (Reprinted with permission from Ref. [17]. Copyright 2011, American Chemical Society.) - Gene silencing by siRNA microhydrogels via polymeric nanoscale condensation.

of 120 nm. The compact nanocomplexes of RNA hydrogel and LPEI under 150 nm in size were highly efficient for inducing the internalization of these particles into cells via an endocytic pathway. In addition, due to more favorable condensation with mild cationic polymers, the siRNA microhydrogel exhibited far enhanced gene silencing compared with the monomeric and multi-siRNA, with negligible cytotoxicity. At a siRNA concentration of 72 nM, the siRNA microhydrogel/LPEI complexes showed significant gene silencing effects (52.8% reduction in GFP expression) over the monomeric siRNA/LPEI (37.7% reduction in GFP expression). Dicer processing of a highly networked structure of RNA has been verified. Random ds-siRNA fragments could be generated from siRNA hydrogel, and the processed short ds-siRNA participated in the RNAi mechanism.

AuNPs can also be used to prepare multimerized and highly branched RNA structures [57]. AuNPs have received much attention as an excellent nanoplatform for biomolecule conjugation due to their excellent biocompatibility, controllable morphology, and ease of surface functionalization [1–4,58]. Since AuNPs can readily react with thiol-containing RNA molecules, siRNA-immobilized AuNPs have been investigated for efficient cellular uptake and gene inhibition [58–61]. Kong and coworkers utilized 5 nm AuNPs as a platform to build multimeric/branched RNA structures. The 3′-ends of thiolfunctionalized RNA strands were immobilized to prepare the sense- and antisense-AuNPs. Once the two different AuNPs were mixed together, they formed multi-siRNA crosslinked by AuNPs. Due to the distinct optical properties of AuNPs, formation of multi-siRNA can be verified by Ultra Violet–Visible (UV–VIS) measurement, exhibiting a blue shift in the absorbance spectrum. Under reducing conditions, thiolmodified siRNAs were released from the surface of AuNPs ready for the formation of the RISC without dicer processing in the cytoplasm. The prepared multi-siRNA by AuNPs with LPEI (25 kDa) showed enhanced intracellular uptake of nanocomplexes as measured by computed tomography imaging, and efficient targeted GFP and VEGF gene silencing were achieved in MDA-MB-435 cells.

3.2.3 Novel Carriers for Poly/Multimeric siRNA Delivery

Various cationic carriers for poly/multimeric siRNA have been developed. Unlike monomeric siRNA that requires a high cationic charge density for stable polyelectrolyte complexation, lower cationically charged and relatively small molecular weight carriers have been utilized for the delivery of poly/multimeric siRNA [14]. Due to reduced cationic charges on carriers, the serum stability and cytotoxicity of siRNA/carrier complexes have been resolved with more potent gene silencing as compared with that of monomeric siRNA delivery [62,63]. For instance, the thiolated glycol chitosan (TGC) polymer has been developed to formulate a stable NP structure with poly-siRNA through the charge–charge interaction and chemical crosslinking [64]. Upon weak-charge interaction with poly-siRNA, the TGC first formed loosely bound structures, enabling the tight crosslinking of glycol chitosan (GC) polymers for the generation of more condensed nanostructures (size: ~300 nm). The condensed nanocomplexes were sensitive to reducing conditions, and 10 mM dithiothreitol (DTT) treatment allowed the total dissociation of monomeric siRNA from the complexes. There were several advantages of TGC polymers as compared with strong cationic polymers such as PEI. When TGC polymers formed nanocomplexes with poly-siRNA, their surface was slightly positive (zeta-potential of 3.55 mV) and showed enhanced stability against physiological anionic proteins or carbohydrates. This allowed the effective passive targeting of tumors by systemic injection of poly-siRNA/TGC complexes. Unlike the strong cationic PEI carriers that tend to accumulate in the liver, the TGC carriers exhibited reduced nonspecific accumulation in the liver and other organs and extremely high accumulation in the tumor tissue. The therapeutic efficacy of poly-siRNA/TGC has been tested in tumor-bearing mice, and effective tumor suppression has been achieved upon systemic injection of anti-VEGF poly-siRNA.

Transferrin (TF), a serum protein, is considered to be a good candidate for an efficient siRNA carrier due to its biocompatibility and tumor targeting ability. Since TF receptors (TFRs) are highly overexpressed in many types of cancer cells, the active targeting of TFR and the intracellular delivery of therapeutics to tumor tissue have been attempted [65]. However, natural TF does not have sufficient binding affinity for the short nucleic acid drugs such as siRNA, thus is unable to serve as a carrier for genetic drugs. To improve the molecular interaction between RNA drugs and TF, poly-siRNA has been utilized along with thiolated TF (tTF). Due to the increase in charge interaction of poly-siRNA and tTF, poly-siRNA/tTF could generate a loosely conjugated state followed by a tight condensation process to form NPs through the disulfide crosslinking of tTF. To prepare tTF, TF was functionalized with 2-iminothiolanes under oxygen-limiting conditions, and approximately 8.7 free thiol groups were introduced on TF. Poly-siRNA and tTF formed stable complexes with a mixing ratio of 1:10 (w/w). The particle size before and after the crosslinking process was measured by dynamic light scattering (DLS), and the size of complexes was decreased to 343 nm. The formulated poly-siRNA/tTF complexes were systemically introduced to tumor bearing mice, and their biodistribution was obtained by real-time in vivo near-infrared fluorescence imaging. The results confirmed that siRNA/tTF complexes showed tumor-specific active targeting as well as moderate accumulation of these particles in the liver, spleen, and kidney. Since TF served as both an active targeting ligand and a carrier, there was no use of additional cationic materials in this study of this chapter, and effective target-gene silencing in vitro and in vivo was achieved without cytotoxicity.

Similar to TF, human serum albumin (HSA) has been widely utilized as a drug carrier, owing to its excellent physical and biological properties such as water solubility, plasma stability, low toxicity, and reduced immunogenicity [66,67]. It is also known that HSA shows a relatively high uptake in tumor and inflamed tissue. Abraxane is the best example of a commercialized albumin-based formulation for anticancer drug delivery, and under cellular stress-inducing conditions, HAS been preferentially taken up by fast-growing tumors as the main energy source for growth and maintenance. For successful encapsulation of poly-siRNA within HSA, the thiolated HSA (tHSA) was synthesized by reacting the amine groups of albumin with Traut's reagent [68]. tHSA was utilized to encapsulate the poly-siRNA by self-crosslinking via disulfide bond formation, generating stable poly-siRNA/HSA NPs. The optimized formulation resulted with NPs under a size of 200 nm, which showed an enhanced cellular uptake by albumin transcytosis, and effective *in vitro* gene silencing was achieved at a siRNA concentration as low as 50 nM. *In vivo* systemic gene silencing testing has revealed tumor-specific accumulation of poly-siRNA/tHSA complexes and the induction of effective tumor suppression over a period of 30 days. Therefore, along with poly-siRNA, the self-crosslinked HSA nanocarrier system could be a potential candidate for the systemic delivery of siRNA therapeutics for safe and effective anticancer gene therapy.

3.3 THREE-DIMENSIONAL RNA/DNA STRUCTURES FOR siRNA DELIVERY APPLICATIONS

Although the conventional formulation of siRNA delivery using cationic materials has shown some promise in *in vivo* animal studies, nonspecific charge interaction–driven complexation of cationic carriers and anionic siRNAs have shown multiple drawbacks. These include the heterogeneous size, composition, and surface chemistry of the formulation. Due to the lack of precise control of such properties, varied *in vivo* biodistribution and pharmacokinetics have been observed, as well as a lack of correlation between *in vitro* and *in vivo* studies. Consequently, undesirable and unpredictable *in vivo* performance of cationic carriers has been reported elsewhere [2,63,69]. To overcome the current problems of cationic delivery carriers, various self-assembled structures of short oligonucleotides have been explored. DNA and RNA molecules are genetic and informative materials; however, they can also serve as an excellent genuine material to prepare more complex and higher ordered structures for various applications [70]. As a result of the good biocompatibility and biodegradability of DNA and RNA molecules, multifunctional self-assembled NPs were prepared for drug delivery by a simple programmable hybridization of complementary strands. These nucleic acid NPs clearly show structural and compositional advantages over the conventional carriers, and various siRNA delivery applications are highlighted in this chapter.

3.3.1 RNA-BASED NANOPARTICLES FOR siRNA DELIVERY

Various naturally occurring RNA structures have been utilized in living cells as gene regulatory materials for mRNA transcription, maturation, translation, degradation, and the catalytic activity of ribozymes [71,72]. For synthetic RNA-based NPs, multiple advantages can be attained as a nanocarrier such as a compact and defined size for tumor targeting, multivalent characteristics for various conjugation, and ease of chemical modification. Naturally or synthetically generated RNA motifs and modulus can be utilized for assembling NPs with various structural diversities [73–77]. This is particularly attractive to biomedical and clinical applications, since the *in vivo* fate of NPs is governed by their size, structure, and composition [21,23,24,78–86]. The self-assembled nucleic acid NPs can offer modulation of the therapeutic half-life, biodistribution, cell-specific internalization, and excretion [87]. Moreover, high affinity aptamers can be incorporated into the nucleic acid structures for targeted delivery, and the intracellular uptake process can be more precisely controlled [88].

Among various RNA NPs, self-assembling RNA nanorings, by inverse kissing loop complexation, have been reported for the delivery of siRNA (Figure 3.5) [20]. Among the polygons, a hexamer nanoring structure was selected to provide a thermodynamically stable structure at a relatively low RNA concentration. Assembled nanorings have a distinct size and shape that can be later loaded with six siRNAs by simple hybridization on helical stems. Interestingly, the assembled nanoring structures show improved serum stability, but are also processed by the dicer to release the loaded siRNAs. When RNA kissing loop complexes with siRNAs were delivered to MDA-MB-231 cells, efficient GFP gene silencing was achieved [22]. Although there exist various advantages of functional RNA NPs, there remain three major drawbacks for siRNA delivery: 1) cost of long synthetic RNA, 2) complexity and difficulty in generating 3D RNA NPs, and 3) short blood half-life due to serum nuclease and renal filtration. To resolve the aforementioned matter, RNA NPs are enzymatically prepared by an *in vitro* transcription process using T7 RNA polymerase. To optimize the self-assembly conditions, Mn^{2+} was additionally applied to the incubation solution to result in a high yield preparation of RNA NPs. Lastly, 2′-F-dUMPs can be utilized to generate a 2′-F modification on RNA strands in order to highly improve the serum stability against nucleases [22].

To further apply RNA nanorings, multifunctional RNA NPs have been developed for broad applications in nanomedicine. dsRNAs are utilized to generate a nanoring scaffold by the toehold interaction. The nanoring scaffold can be further functionalized with various molecules such as siRNAs, aptamers, fluorescence dyes, and proteins. The multifunctional RNA NPs show an enhanced uptake and gene silencing as compared with an equal concentration of duplex RNA molecules. These results are similar to the report of multi-siRNA delivery, and prolonged gene

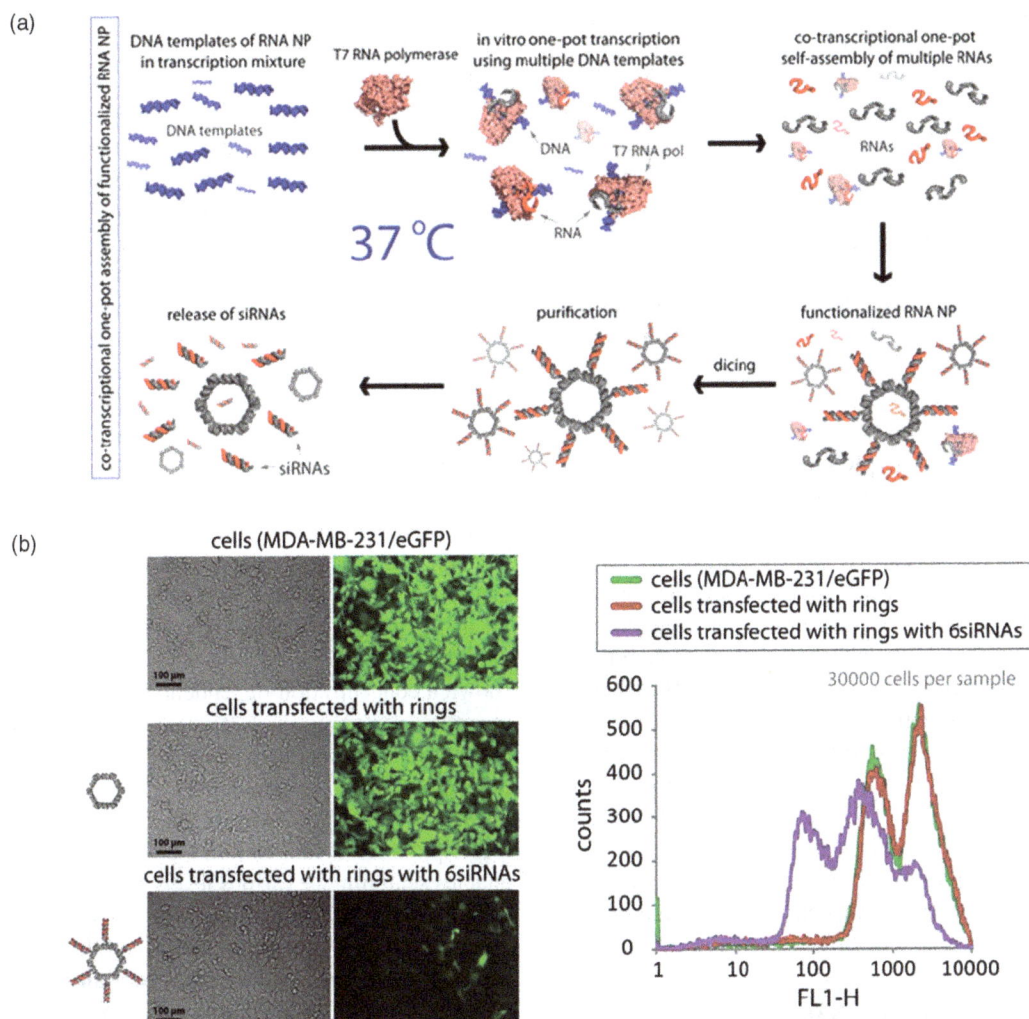

FIGURE 3.5 A. Synthesis process of functionalized RNA NP (nanoring) and release of siRNAs. B. Analysis of gene expression effects using fluorescence microscopy and flow cytometry inMDAMB-231/GFP cells. (Reprinted with permission from Ref. [22]. Copyright 2012, American Chemical Society.) - Cotranscriptional assembly of chemically modified RNA nanoparticles functionalized with siRNAs.

silencing was also achieved using the multifunctional RNA NPs. It is likely that the multivalency of RNA nanorings can be attributed to the enhanced and prolonged effect of RNAi *in vitro*. Similarly, for *in vivo* tumor suppression experiments, the intratumoral injection of multifunctional RNA NPs was conducted, achieving up to a sixfold enhanced GFP gene silencing as compared with ds-siRNA. Finally, functional nanorings have been prepared against HIV-1, and their site-specific cleavage against six different regions of HIV-1 has been verified. Complete viral inhibition was obtained at 1 nM concentrations of nanorings. Another bottom-up approach of RNA nanotechnology, to generate functional NPs for siRNA delivery, is the use of the DNA-packaging motor of the bacterial virus, phi29 [25]. Six copies of packaging RNA (pRNA) molecules can form a hexameric ring as a critical part of the motor. These molecules can be utilized as a building block to form supramolecular structures such as RNA twins, tetramers, and arrays by the intermolecular self-assembly of palindromic

sequences at the 3'-ends of the left and right loop [89–91]. It is known that these self-assembled RNA nanostructures show good stability against changes in temperature, salt, and pH [25]. Due to the small size of these pRNA nanostructures, they have advantages in the cell surface interaction as well as internalization. This physical property is particularly pertinent to the delivery of therapeutics and molecular imaging agents, and the bottom-up assembly of pRNA has been applied to the preparation of appropriate delivery scaffolds for such applications.

The trimer pRNA structure, harboring siRNA or other therapeutic molecules, has been fabricated through the interaction of engineered right and left interlocking RNA loops [26]. pRNA with a single-strand stem loop does not require additional linkers to incorporate cargo materials within the structure [92]. In fact, the trimer pRNA is multifunctionalized by incorporating aptamers for cell surface targeting, heavy metals, fluorescence dyes, and radioisotopes for molecular imaging and diagnostics [26].

The pRNA/aptamer (CD4) has shown enhanced binding and accumulation of these chimeras on a CD4-overexpressing thymic T cell line. The intracellular entry of the pRNA/aptamer has been confirmed as endocytosis of membrane-bound molecules. Effective *in vitro* gene regulation by anti-CD4 siRNA has also been achieved in a targeted manner.

Although 117 nt long pRNA has shown effective intracellular delivery of various therapeutics into specific cancer or viral-infected cells, the chemical synthesis of such long RNA is not commercially feasible. To overcome the synthetic drawback, Yi Shu et al. developed a bipartite approach to prepare a pRNA structure from two synthetic RNA fragments with variable modification [93]. The two individual synthetic RNA strands are self-assembled and readily formed a dimeric pRNA structure similar to that of wild-type pRNA. The viral assembly and DNA packaging activity of bipartite pRNA were compared with wild-type pRNA, and their ability was similar. In addition, an *in vitro* gene silencing test confirmed that the bipartite pRNA/siRNA could induce effective gene silencing in a targeted manner, with the incorporation of a folate ligand. To improve the multivalency of pRNA, a pRNA-X motif was developed by opening the right-hand loop and introducing further nine nucleotides within the system [24]. An X motif provides functional arms for four guest molecules and is prepared by assembling four different RNA oligonucleotide strands. The pRNA-X motif is thermodynamically stable at ambient temperature and can provide multimodule functionalities to carry four different cargo materials such as aptamers, targeting ligands, and siRNA.

3.3.2 DNA Polyhedron Nanoparticles for siRNA Delivery

Various polyhedron DNA nanostructures have been developed by A. J. Turberfield and C. Mao. These include tetrahedron, cube, dodecahedron, and buckyball structures [94,95]. Similar to that of RNA nanostructures, 3D DNA nanostructures have been explored for imaging and delivery applications [96–98]. Due to the programmable assembly of DNA strands, the size and shape of NPs can be easily controlled. In addition, various polyhedron particles allow precise control of spatial orientation and density of targeting ligands, which cannot be controlled by any other synthetic NP system.

Lee et al. have reported the use of tetrahedron DNA NPs for the targeted *in vivo* delivery of folic acid (FA)–conjugated siRNA (Figure 3.6). The DNA tetrahedron, consisting of 186 bp, self-assembled from six DNA strands to prepare molecularly identical oligonucleotide NPs (ONPs). The six edges of the tetrahedron are 30 bp long, with an estimated size of 10 nm. Each edge contains a nick in the middle, where each end of the 5′- and 3′- oligonucleotides meets. To properly incorporate siRNAs into this system, 21-bp overhangs are added to the 3′-end of each DNA strand. As a result, six siRNA strands can be applied to each tetrahedron DNA NP (one per edge). In addition, for

in vivo applications, RNA strands are chemically modified with 2′-OMe to reduce the potential immune response as well as to improve the serum stability [99].

The resultant ONPs have a hydrodynamic diameter of ~28.6 nm, which is suitable for the avoidance of renal filtration, while passively being delivered to tumors via the enhanced permeability and retention (EPR) effect. Since the hybrid DNA/RNA NPs show strong negative surface charges, the intracellular uptake of these particles is not favorable by charge-repulsion between the particles and cell membrane. To enhance the interfacial interaction, various targeting and cell-penetrating ligands have been introduced to the ONP system to facilitate the intracellular uptake of the particles. Targeting ligands are selected from broad materials such as peptides, small molecules, and sugars. Many cationic peptides show false positive enhanced uptake data due to their nonspecific interaction with ONPs through electrostatic interactions, forming larger aggregates. Very few cationic peptides allowed particle stability at neutral pH; however, these did not show enhanced uptake of the ONPs. Among the screened ligands, FA has shown a concentration-dependent gene silencing effect. FA receptor-overexpressing KB cells were utilized to verify the receptor-mediated uptake of these particles. "KB cells" is a descriptor in the National Library of Medicine's controlled vocabulary thesaurus, MeSH (Medical Subject Headings). Descriptors are arranged in a hierarchical structure, which enables searching at various levels of specificity.

This line KB is now known to be a subline of the ubiquitous KERATIN-forming tumor cell line HeLa. It was originally thought to be derived from an epidermal carcinoma of the mouth, but was subsequently found, based on isoenzyme analysis, HeLa marker chromosomes, and DNA fingerprinting, to have been established via contamination by HeLa cells. The cells are positive for keratin by immunoperoxidase staining. KB cells have been reported to contain human papillomavirus 18 (HPV-18) sequences.

Since polyhedron ONPs can precisely control the ligand density and location, structure function studies of various ligand densities and orientations on ONPs have been conducted. It has been shown that at least three FA ligands are required to induce appropriate GFP gene silencing and that their ligand orientation also affects the gene silencing efficiency. It is likely that a higher local FA ligand density may influence the intracellular trafficking pathway of ONPs and the corresponding gene silencing [27].

3.3.3 Large-scale Preparation of DNA Nanostructures for Translational Study

There has been much interest in utilizing oligonucleotide-based drug carriers for gene delivery. Despite the advantages of precise size control, superior intracellular delivery efficiency, and good biocompatibility and biodegradability, many oligonucleotide nanostructures require multiple long nucleotide strands for self-assembly [17]. The cost and synthetic problems in preparing long nucleotides clearly hamper

(a)

Single-strand oligonucleotides

siRNA with 3' overhang

One-step self-assembly

Molecularly identical oligonucleotide nanoparticle

(b)

siRNA alone (5 mg kg⁻¹)

ONPs (2.5 mg kg⁻¹)

ONPs (5 mg kg⁻¹)

(a)   (b)

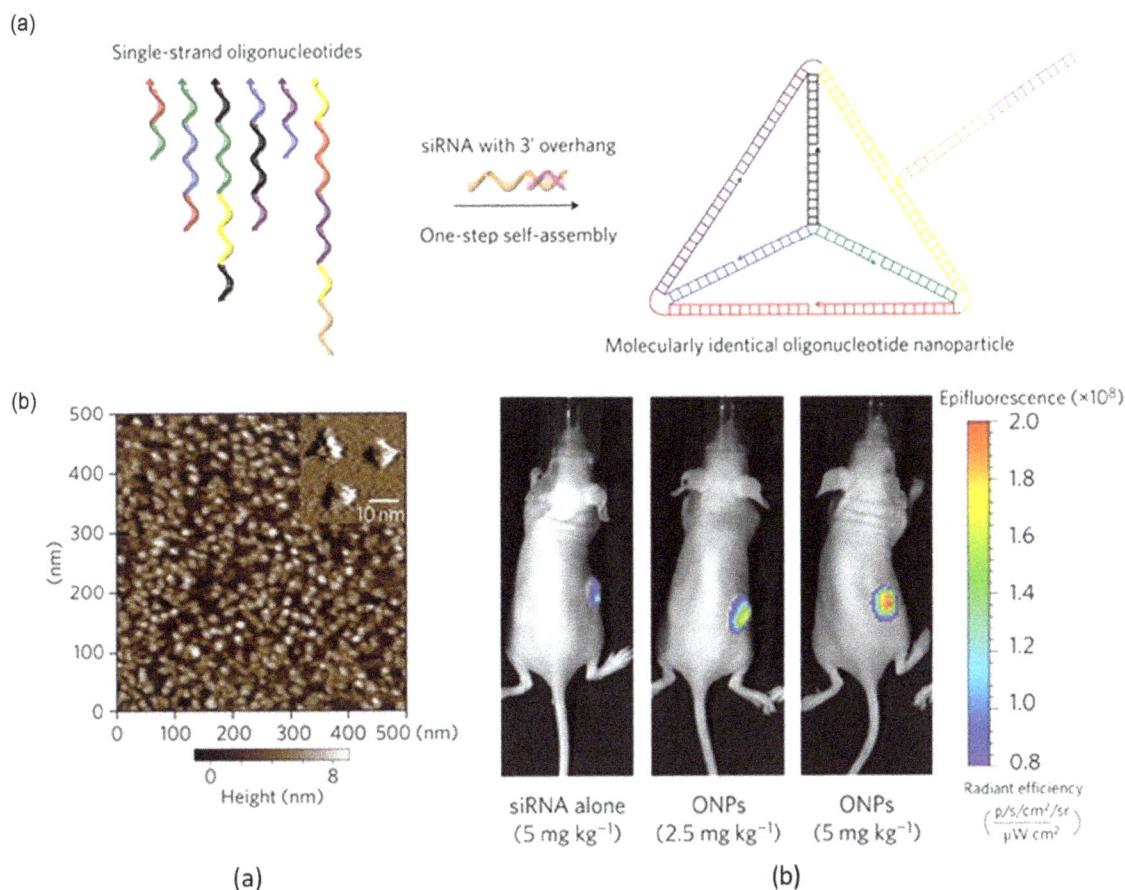

FIGURE 3.6 A. Preparation of tetrahedron DNA nanostructure. B. (a) AFM image of tetrahedron nanostructure. (b) Analysis of gene silencing effects after intravenous injection of ONPs in a tumor mouse model (n=3). (Reprinted with permission from Ref. [27]. Copyright 2012, rights managed by Nature Publishing Group.) -Molecularly self-assembled nucleic acid nanoparticles for targeted *in vivo* siRNA delivery, Nature Nanotechnology.

the practical use of DNA- or RNA-based NPs. In addition to the synthetic method of preparing long oligonucleotides, there is an enzymatic approach to prepare theses strands that self-assemble to generate DNA nanostructures [100]. Rolling circle amplification (RCA) is one of the examples of enzymatic preparation of DNA nanostructures. This method is a robust technique to generate elongated single-stranded (ss) DNA around a circular ss DNA template under isothermal conditions [101–103].

Hong et al. demonstrated RCA-based enzymatic amplification of DNA nanostructures for the delivery of siRNAs (Figure 3.7). A self-assembled Y shaped DNA structure (159 nt) was used as the closed circular template for RCA to generate long amplified DNA products. Site-specific cleavage can be achieved by containing PstI endonuclease-specific sequences in the open loop of the Y-DNA junction. Intermolecular and intramolecular self-assembly of an elongated ss DNA product can form hybridization of palindromic PstI sites without the addition of helper DNA strands. The occurrence of the PstI palindromes in two otherwise unrelated DNA species is consistent with the hypothesis that they are related to mobile DNA sequences

that either propagate or were once capable of propagating within mitochondria. The Neurospora PstI palindromes are found flanking genetic elements (e.g. the small and large rRNA genes, protein genes, and tRNA genes) as well as within the large rRNA gene new opposite end of the 2.3-kilobase intervening sequence. The presence of PstI palindromic sequences in two otherwise unrelated DNA species, Neurospora mtDNA and the Mauriceville plasmid, could be accounted for by common ancestry, by a common mechanism for intramolecular repetition of DNA sequences, or by some type of recombination event (e.g. transposition). Further insight into the function of the PstI elements may come when the Mauriceville plasmid has been more fully characterized with respect to genetic function and location of genetic elements such as the DNA replication origin and promoters. After treatment with PstI enzymes, the long ss DNA product is site-specifically cleaved to generate individual DNA fragments, which can later self-assemble to form Y-DNA nanostructures. The overhang sequences on each arm have been designed to form stable hybridization with FA-conjugated siRNAs. In this study, 1 pmol DNA template was amplified to approximately 1068 pmol

(a)

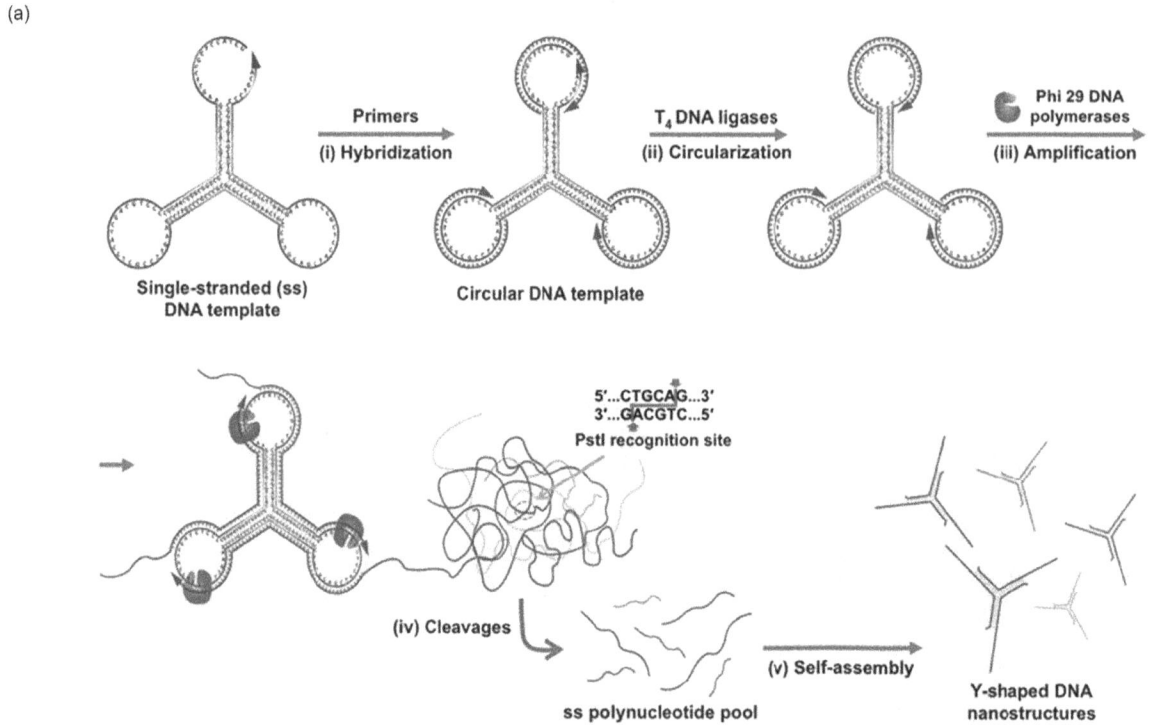

(b)

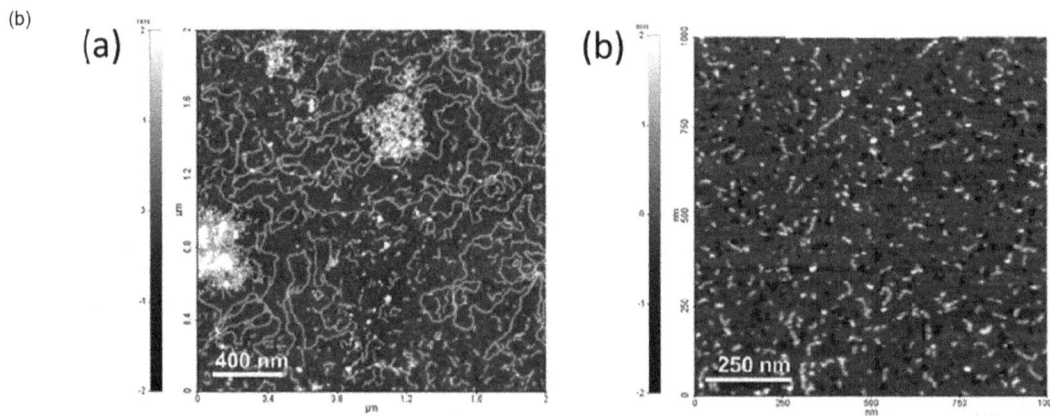

(c)

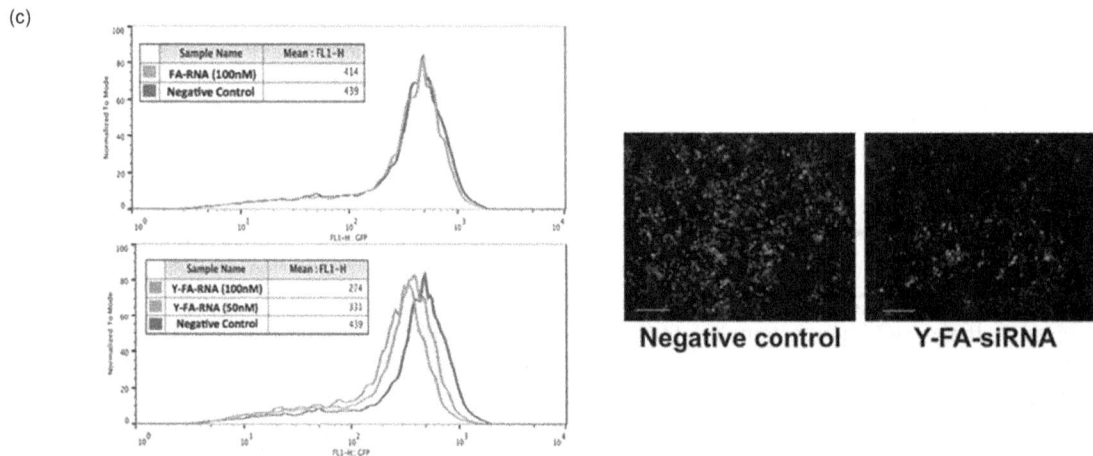

FIGURE 3.7   A. Synthesis of Y-shaped DNA (Y-DNA) nanostructure via rolling circle amplification (RCA). B. AFM images. (a) Elongated RCA products. (b) Cleaved RCA products C. Gene silencing effects of FA-siRNA and Y-FA-siRNA conjugates using flow cytometry and fluorescence microscopy in GFP-KB cells (siRNA concentration = 100 nM). (Reprinted with permission from Ref. [104]. Copyright 2014, Royal Society of Chemistry.) - Self-assembled DNA nanostructures prepared by rolling circle amplification for the delivery of siRNA conjugates.

elongated ss DNA, and 213 pmol of Y-DNA structure was produced. This approach is widely useful as a simple platform for the large-scale synthesis of various DNA nanostructures for therapeutic applications [104].

3.4 DNA/RNA BALL TECHNOLOGY FOR siRNA DELIVERY APPLICATIONS

Rolling circle replication (RCR) has been extensively explored to overcome the instability of RNA and the low packing efficiency of the carriers. While a conventional polymerase chain reaction requires a thermal cycling process and is limited to amplification of short DNA segments, RCR is an isothermal process and is used for the exponential synthesis of long concatameric DNA/RNA strands by a processive rolling mechanism [105,106]. Rolling circle mechanisms have been widely adapted to different areas including genomics [107], proteomics [108], biosensing [109,110], drug delivery [111,112], and structure building [113,114]. The RCR technique used for gene delivery applications is of special interest. Specifically, rolling circle transcription (RCT) involves T7 RNA polymerase that can continuously generate multiple ss RNA copies from the template circular DNA. A number of studies have shown that RCT can be used for continued RNA synthesis with high efficiency [106,115,116].

3.4.1 RNA MICROSPONGE/BALL TECHNOLOGY FOR siRNA DELIVERY

By taking advantage of enzymatic RNA polymerization, condensed RNA structures with predetermined sequences for RNAi were synthesized [112]. According to the formation process of RNA structures, long replicated RNA strands show similar behavior to traditional synthetic polymers, which is a key factor for efficient siRNA delivery and high cargo capacity. In the early stage of polymerization, a fiber-like structure is gradually entangled and forms a sheet-like structure. As these structures grow larger, RNA strands eventually self-assemble into sponge-like spherical structures called RNAi-microsponges (Figure 3. 8). Due to the fact that RNAi-microsponges consist of multiple copies of tandem RNA units, a large amount of siRNA can be loaded onto a single microsponge. Moreover, it is possible that PEI, as a polymeric transfection agent, can be used to condense the microsponge for enhancement of the cellular uptake of the particle. Indeed, the RNAi-microsponge/PEI complex showed reasonable silencing efficiency under *in vitro* and *in vivo* conditions.

This study demonstrated a new platform for the synthesis of self-assembled RNA structures. By using polymeric RNA strands, sponge-like spherical RNA structures can be synthesized, which can achieve a high loading efficiency. Furthermore, RNAi-microsponges which consist entirely of RNA strands are able to rapidly deliver a large amount

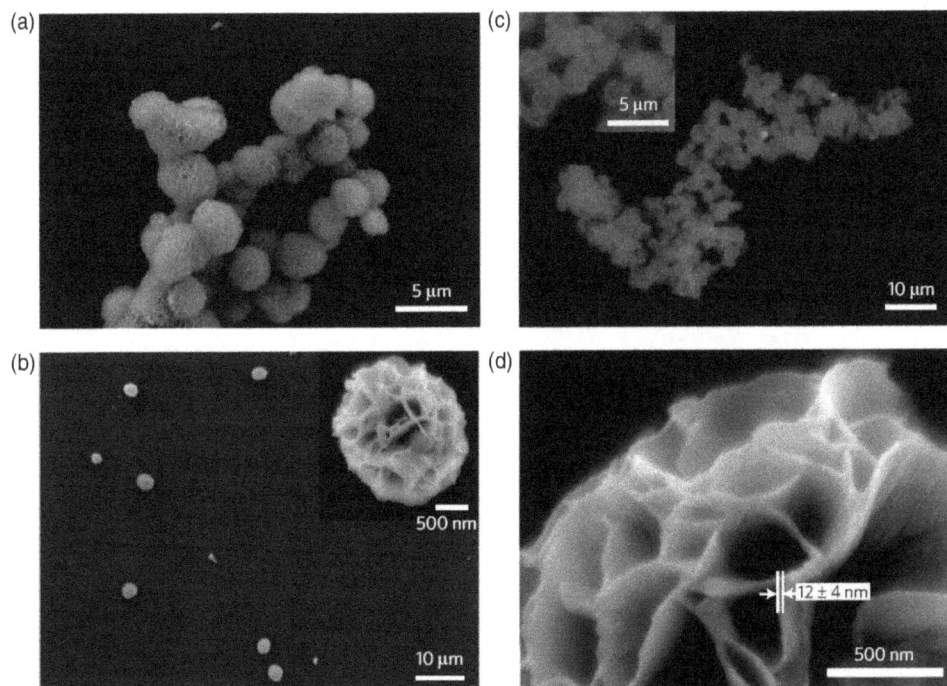

FIGURE 3.8   A. SEM image of RNAi-microsponges, having a porous nanoscopic structure. B. Fluorescence microscopy image of SYBR II (RNA-specific dye)-stained RNAi-microsponges, showing bright green fluorescence, which confirms that RNAi-microsponges are composed of RNA. C. Low magnification and high magnification SEM image (inset) of the monodispersed RNAi-microsponges with a uniform size of 2 μm after brief sonication. D. Higher magnification SEM image reveals that RNAi-microsponges are composed of a sheet-like structure, having a thickness of 12±4 nm. (Reprinted with permission from Ref. [112]. Copyright 2012, rights managed by Nature Publishing Group.) - Self-assembled RNA interference microsponges for efficient siRNA delivery.

of siRNA to target cells by simply coating with positively charged polyions. This novel approach can reduce the limitations of siRNA therapeutics and also be applied to the synthesis of various RNA structures.

Since RCT has drawn a great deal of attention, the complementary rolling circle transcription (cRCT) method also emerged. Without any assistance from a synthetic polycation for condensing, enzymatic size control was feasible with a recently introduced cRCT method [28]. Extension of RNA strands from two complementary circular DNAs results in two strands that hybridize with each other, leading to the formation of RNA particles (Figure 3.9). Resulting dsRNA is rationally designed to function as a substrate for the dicer enzyme to induce RNAi. In the synthesis of RNA particles, the T7 RNA polymerase is used to generate RNA strands, and the concentration of the enzyme was found to be critical to the size of the resulting RNA particles. By controlling the concentration of the enzyme in the cRCT reaction, the size of RNA NPs was shrunk from 5 μm to 600 nm in diameter.

By taking advantage of cRCT, RNA membranes were also developed by J. B. Lee's group in 2014 [29]. RNA membranes are designed to contain siRNA sequences to be cleaved by the dicer enzyme for siRNA release and are the first example of a macroscopic RNA membrane composed solely of RNA strands. Furthermore, its structural and functional properties can be rationally controlled by adjusting the RNA base-pairing, thus controlled release of chemical molecules and sequence-specific drug release are feasible.

3.4.2 MICROSCOPIC DNA SCAFFOLDS FOR GENE DELIVERY

By utilizing RCR, DNA structures for gene delivery applications have also been introduced. For instance, self-assembled hierarchical DNA nanoflowers (NFs) with densely packed DNA and built-in multifunctional moieties for versatile biomedical applications were developed by W. Tan's research group (Figure 3.10) [30]. The assembly of DNA NFs is independent of the traditional Watson-Crick base-pairing between DNA strands. Instead, it is driven by dense packaging of the resulting long building blocks generated via RCA and liquid crystallization, an anisotropic process for orderly alignment of highly concentrated polymers. In virtue of this distinctive characteristic, templates for RCA can be flexibly designed to include aptamers, antisense nucleotides, and drug loading sequences. Furthermore, the NFs were featured by size tunability and stability toward nuclease treatment, dilution to low concentration, or denaturation by heating or urea treatment.

In addition, a layer-by-layer (LbL) assembly strategy offering a potent delivery method for nucleic acid therapeutics for cancer treatment was introduced by P. Hammond's group in 2014 [31]. Oligonucleotide antisense microsponge particles (ODN-MSs) were generated by RCA, then cationic polymers (poly-L-lysine [PLL]) were added for condensing (Figure 3.11). By electrostatic interaction and

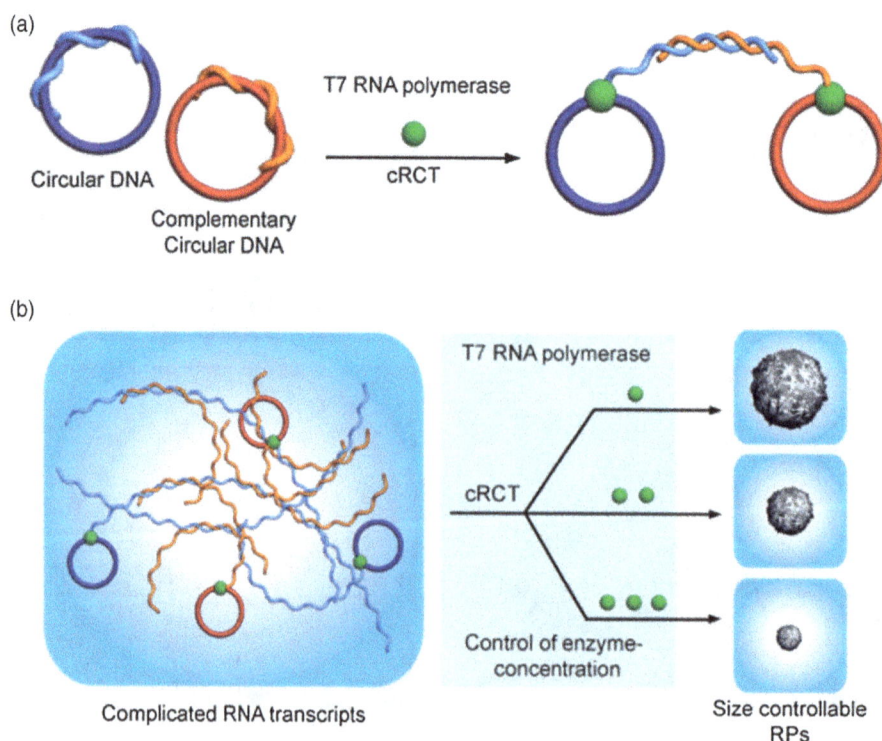

FIGURE 3.9 A. Schematic illustration showing two predesigned complementary circular DNA templates for the complementary rolling circle transcription (cRCT) process by T7 RNA polymerase, and the hybridization process of the resulting RNA strands. B. By adjusting the concentration of enzyme, the size of the resulting RNA particles from cRCT is controllable. (Reprinted with permission from Ref. [28]. Copyright 2014, Royal Society of Chemistry.) - Enzymatic size control of RNA particles using complementary rolling circle transcription (cRCT) method for efficient siRNA production.

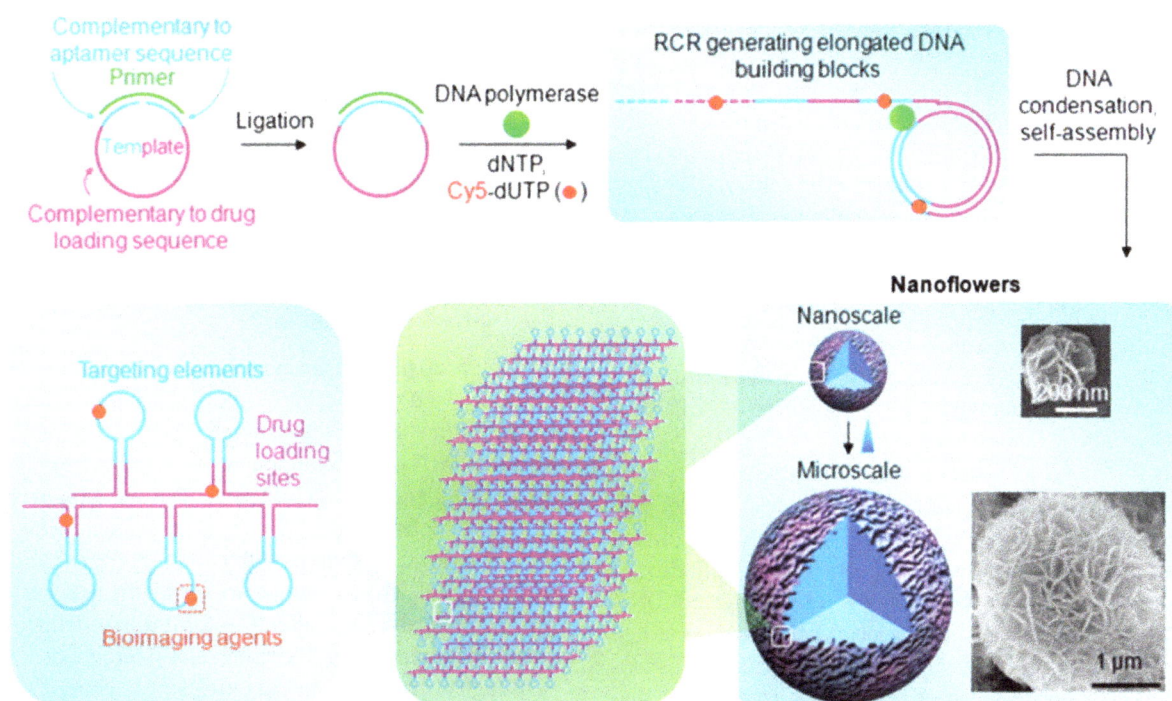

FIGURE 3.10 Schematic illustration of the synthesis of multifunctional DNA nanoflowers (DNA NFs) by noncanonical self-assembly. Circularized DNA template is first ligated, then DNA building blocks are elongated via the RCR process by Φ29 DNA polymerase. The resulting DNA NFs have adjustable sizes from several hundred nanometers to several micrometers and can serve as targeting, bioimaging, and drug delivery agents with a predesigned DNA sequence. (Reprinted with permission from Ref. [30]. Copyright 2013, American Chemical Society.) – Noncanonical self-assembly of multifunctional DNA NFs for biomedical applications.

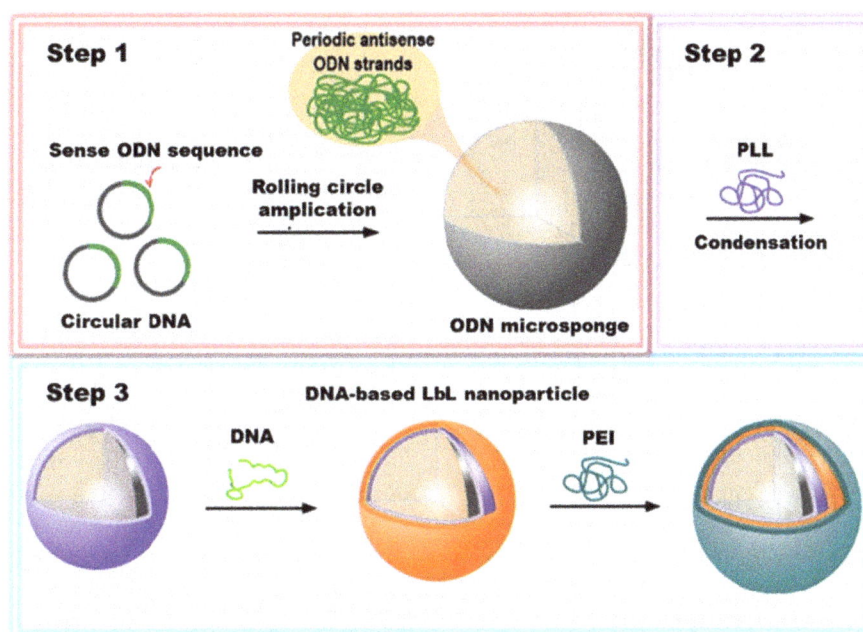

FIGURE 3.11 Stepwise assembly of multifunctional antisense oligonucleotide microsponge particles (ODN-MS). First, periodic antisense ODN strands are generated from the circular DNA template having sense ODN sequence by the rolling circle amplification process (Step 1). By adding poly-L-lysine (PLL) for condensation, ODN-MS is reconstructed into nanoscopic particles covered with PLL (Step 2). Through the layer-by-layer (LbL) technique, DNA-based LbL nanoparticles (LbL-ODN-NPs) are generated with given multifunctionality. (Reprinted with permission from Ref. [31]. Copyright 2014, American Chemical Society.) - LbL assembled antisense DNA microsponge particles for efficient delivery of cancer therapeutics.

physical agitation, the average size of ODN-MS decreased from 2 μm to 200 nm, which is a desirable size for efficient cellular uptake. Condensing with PLL also increased the stability of the ODN particles and changed the surface charge from negative to positive. Similarly, additional layers such as ssDNA and PEI could also be achieved by electrostatic interaction. The LbL assembly has advantages for controlling surface charge and fine-tuning of their multifunctional properties. This study implies that the spherical ODN NPs could be nucleic acid carriers for gene delivery applications with negligible cytotoxicity. Moreover, this approach can achieve multifunctionality by adding layers of different functional DNAs and selecting different biomaterials.

Another novel approach to synthesize DNA structures is a cocoon-like self-degradable anticancer drug system that fully utilizes the RCA mechanism [117]. RCA was carried out with the template DNA that incorporates a palindromic sequence to facilitate self-assembly. The elongated DNA strands have multiple GC-pair sequences, achieving a high doxorubicin (DOX) loading capacity. Furthermore, this bioinspired drug delivery carrier is functionalized by FA, and pH-responsive polymeric nanocapsules encapsulate DNase I. FA conjugated to the surface of the carrier promotes internalization of nanoclew into target cells and enters the acidic endolysosome. Subsequently, the acidic cellular environment activates the degradation of nanocapsules embedded into the nanoclew, thus triggering escape of DNase I from the nanocage. As a result, the DNA-based delivery vehicle can release intercalated DOX in target cells due to degradation of DNA by DNase I. This study demonstrated that RCA could be applied to long DNA synthesis, facilitating self-assembly of DNA-based structures. As a further step, the DNA structure was improved by adopting simple methods such as controlling DNA sequences and combining DNA with targetable or stimuli-responsive materials.

DNA nanoribbon (DNR), having a periodically repeating sequence, was also synthesized via RCA by the Y. Weizmann's group [118]. While the conventional DNA origami strategy involves hundreds of staple strands, only three short staple strands are required in RCA-based DNR with three staple stands (DNR-T) production. Furthermore, because staple strands and scaffold strands are sequentially assembled by incorporating nicking processes into RCA, it is possible to generate DNR in a one-pot process. Despite the negative electric charge of DNR, its unique rigidity and ribbon-like structure enable DNR to easily pass through the cell membrane. Moreover, the rigidity of DNR is maintained after penetration, and the high aspect ratio allows DNR to easily escape from endosomal entrapment. In virtue of these characteristics, DNR can be used for effective siRNA delivery. siRNA-DNR-T, which has a high loading capacity, can deliver siRNA into the cytoplasm without requiring the proton sponge mechanism and effectively mediates gene silencing in human cancer cells.

3.5 DNA/RNA NANOPARTICLES

DNA or RNA nanotechnology is the design, construction, and application of nucleic acid nanostructures using specific base paring and programmability of nucleic acids [78,119]. The bottom-up self-assembly based on DNA/RNA nanotechnology has been used for various therapeutic applications [81].

3.5.1 pRNA NANOPARTICLES

The Guo group has constructed RNA NPs based on pRNA engineering and tried to apply the RNA NPs to biomedical applications through functionalization with therapeutic molecules. pRNA is a component of bacteriophage phi29 DNA packing motor possessing two distinct domains. One is a dsRNA helical domain with 3'- and 5'-ends, and the other is interlocking domain with two loops (right hand and left hand) [120]. The two loops are complementary to each other, which enables the pRNA to form dimer, trimer, and oligomeric structures by intermolecular interactions.

Through utilization of interlocking loops, trimeric pRNA NPs were prepared (Figure 3.12A) [26]. Chimeric pRNAs were produced by replacing the helical domain with siRNA, aptamer, or folate. The reengineering of the helical domain did not hinder formation of trimeric pRNA NPs. Trimeric pRNA NPs harboring pRNAsiRNA, pRNA-CD4 aptamer, and pRNA-fluorescent molecules were treated to CD4 overexpressing cells to examine target-specific codelivery of all the components at the same time. All the three functional molecules were target-specifically delivered at one time and showed gene silencing activities. Dicer treatment of chimeric pRNA-siRNA also resulted in ~21 nt siRNA, which suggested that gene silencing was achieved through intracellular dicer processed siRNAs. The advantage of the trimeric pRNA NP is the ability to carry multiple siRNAs or other functional moieties at the same time.

3.5.2 RNA NANORING

RNA nanorings functionalized with siRNAs were constructed with high yield using RNAI and RNAII modules [22,121]. RNAI and RNAII are transcripts of plasmid that control the replication of ColE1 plasmid of Escherichia coli [122]. The RNAI/II can form so called an inverse kissing-loop complex, mediated by specific loop–loop interaction. The Shapiro group carefully designed 6 loop sequence-modified RNA modules that were able to self-assemble into ~15 nm hexameric nanoring (Figure 3.12B). The RNA nanoring further functionalized with 6 siRNAs to use as a siRNA delivery system. Dicer treatment of the nanoring harboring siRNA produced siRNA of ~21 nt in length which could enter the RNAi pathway. When the RNA nanoring with siRNAs was transfected into cells, efficient target gene inhibition was achieved. Because 6 siRNAs could be incorporated into a single RNA nanoring, multiple genes could be targeted at

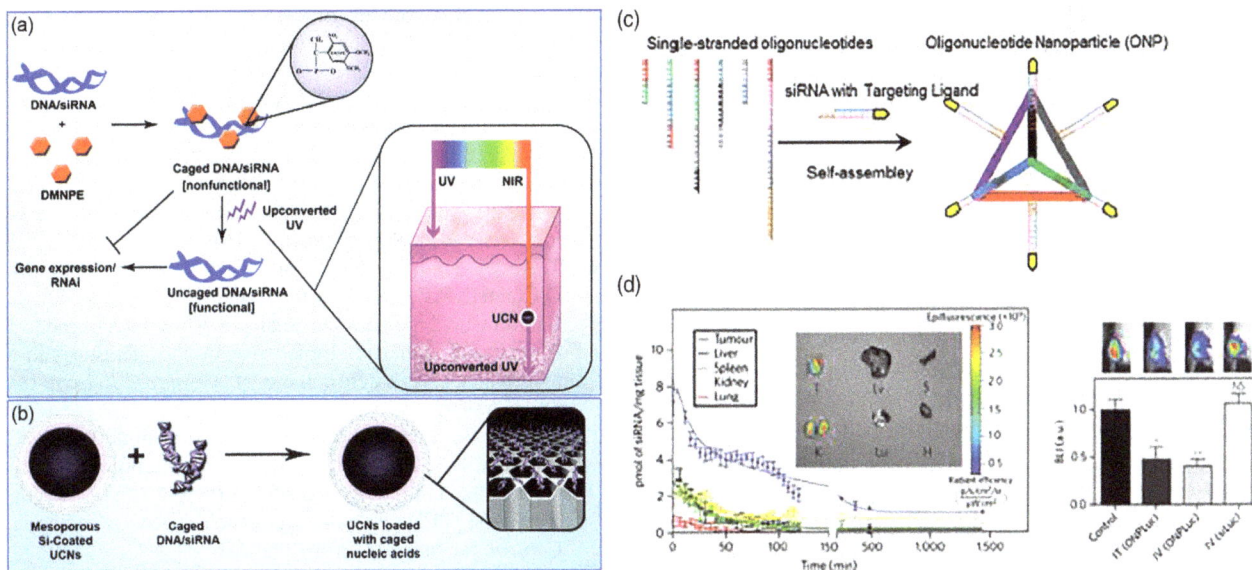

FIGURE 3.12 siRNAs are caged with DMNPE and uncaged by upconverted UV light from NIR-to-UV UCNPs.

the same time for synergistic effects or 6 different regions of one gene could be targeted for more efficient gene silencing. Precise stoichiometric control of siRNA is another attractive quality of RNA nanotechnology-based delivery systems.

3.5.3 Tetrahedron Oligonucleotide Nanoparticles

Conventional drug delivery systems based on polymers or lipids have a heterogeneous size, shape, and composition which make it difficult to predict *in vivo* pharmacokinetics and pharmacodynamics of drugs [87]. To overcome these limitations, Lee et al. proposed siRNA delivery NPs which are molecularly identical in size and shape by utilizing DNA nanotechnology [27]. Carefully designed 6 DNA strands were self-assembled into homogeneous tetrahedron ONP using sequence-specific complementary base paring. Each edge of the ONP had a ss overhang which was complementary to overhang sequence of siRNA; thereby, 6 siRNAs can be accommodated in a single ONP (Figure 3.12C). The ONP showed a homogeneous structure of ~26.8 nm in size when measured using DLS. This size of the ONP was expected not only to be accumulated near tumor tissues by taking advantage of EPR effects but also to avoid renal clearance. ONPs harboring 6 siRNAs which were functionalized with folate at the end were treated into folate overexpressing KB cells *in vitro* without any cationic carriers. They exhibited efficient gene silencing in spite of the absence of cationic carriers. ONPs were intravenously injected into KB xenograft mouse to examine *in vivo* behavior of the particles. ONPs showed ~4 times longer blood circulation time than parental siRNA and mainly accumulated in the tumor site (Figure 3.12D). Furthermore, effective target gene silencing in the tumor was achieved without cationic carriers, and no significant increased production of INF-α was observed. The influence of targeting

ligand spatial orientation and density on cellular uptake and gene silencing was also investigated by taking advantage of precise structural control of ONPs. Although it is important to understand the relationship between cellular uptake and ligand density and orientation, it was difficult to figure out experimentally with conventional NPs.

The DNA/RNA nanotechnology-based siRNA delivery particles have several outstanding features than conventional polymeric or liposomal delivery systems. First, the uniform size and shape of nanostructures could be constructed on demand. Second, stoichiometry and geometry of ligands or therapeutic molecules can be precisely controlled. Third, multiple siRNAs could be incorporated in one NP for targeting multiple genes or several regions of one gene, which will improve therapeutic efficacy. Lastly, DNA and RNA are biomaterials and considered less toxic and immunogenic. Although there are some challenges, such as endosomal escape, production cost, stability, and more precise understanding of DNA/RNA folding, the DNA/RNA nanostructure-based particles are a promising new type of delivery systems.

3.6 CONCLUSIONS

RNAi therapeutics has unique advantages over conventional pharmaceutical drugs. RNAi is an endogenous gene regulation process; thus, almost all genes can be modulated by siRNAs. The identification and selection of highly potent siRNA sequences has already been accomplished for many gene targets, and the synthesis of siRNAs on a large scale has been achieved. In addition, RNAi therapeutics has demonstrated promise in the treatment of cancers, viral diseases, and genetic disorders. Although significant progress has been made in the field of siRNA delivery, there remain challenges to be overcome. These challenges include (i) the minimization of off-target effects and immune stimulation, (ii) target-specific accumulation of RNAi therapeutics after systemic administration, and (iii) the induction of a potent RNAi effect at an acceptable dose level. The key to therapeutic achievement using an RNAi approach depends on delivery issues; thus, advanced delivery strategies are critical to fully optimize the power of siRNAs.

Engineered design of synthetic DNA/RNA molecules [123–126] can generate predefined structures that can easily self-assemble to form NPs with multiple functionalities. The field of oligonucleotide-based nanotechnology for biomedical applications is just emerging, but will play an important role in the delivery of siRNA. In particular, oligonucleotide-based structural RNAi systems described in this chapter are promising as a new generation of gene delivery carriers for cancer therapy. To realize clinical application of structural RNAi systems, the potency of the delivery systems needs to be optimized. One of the solutions may be the incorporation of highly specific ligands within the system. Preclinical data from various biopharmaceutical companies have suggested that the delivery of ligand-conjugated siRNA can be highly improved by the utilization of the engineered design of structural RNAi systems [127]. Another considerable issue in the delivery of structural RNAi systems is the facilitated endosomal release of these materials. It is important to understand the endosomal escape mechanism of structural RNAi systems and endeavor to use the endolytic properties to accelerate the transfer of active siRNAs into the cytoplasm. Future prospects of multi-siRNA/branched siRNA structures and oligonucleotide-based structural RNAi systems with defined size and functionality will continue to improve the precision and efficacy of siRNA delivery.

REFERENCES

1. S.M. Hammond, E. Bernstein, D. Beach, G.J. Hannon, An RNA-directed nuclease mediates post-transcriptional gene silencing in Drosophila cells, *Nature* 404 (2000) 293–296.
2. Y.K. Oh, T.G. Park, siRNA delivery systems for cancer treatment, *Adv. Drug Deliv. Rev.* 61 (2009) 850–862.
3. T. Holen, Mechanisms of RNAi: mRNA cleavage fragments may indicate stalled RISC, *J. RNAi Gene Silenc.* 1 (2005) 21–25.
4. G.B. Robb, T.M. Rana, RNA helicase A interacts with RISC in human cells and functions in RISC loading, *Mol. Cell* 26 (2007) 523–537.
5. J. Wang, Z. Lu, M.G. Wientjes, J.L. Au, Delivery of siRNA therapeutics: barriers and carriers, *AAPS J.* 12 (2010) 492–503.
6. R.J. Lee, P.S. Low, Delivery of liposomes into cultured KB cells via folate receptor mediated endocytosis, *J. Biol. Chem.* 269 (1994) 3198–3204.
7. J. Yang, H. Chen, I.R. Vlahov, J.X. Cheng, P.S. Low, Characterization of the pH of folate receptor-containing endosomes and the rate of hydrolysis of internalized acid-labile folate-drug conjugates, *J. Pharmacol. Exp. Ther.* 321 (2007) 462–468.
8. S.D. Patil, D.G. Rhodes, D.J. Burgess, DNA-based therapeutics and DNA delivery systems: a comprehensive review, *AAPS J.* 7 (2005) E61–E77.
9. Y.P. Liu, B. Berkhout, miRNA cassettes in viral vectors: problems and solutions, *Biochim. Biophys. Acta* 1809 (2011) 732–745.
10. J.C. Burnett, J.J. Rossi, RNA-based therapeutics: current progress and future prospects, *Chem. Biol.* 19 (2012) 60–71.
11. S.H. Lee, B.H. Chung, T.G. Park, Y.S. Nam, H. Mok, Small-interfering RNA (siRNA)-based functional micro- and nanostructures for efficient and selective gene silencing, *Acc. Chem. Res.* 45 (2012) 1014–1025.
12. T. Andey, S. Marepally, A. Patel, T. Jackson, S. Sarkar, M. O'Connell, R.C. Reddy, S. Chellappan, P. Singh, M. Singh, Cationic lipid guided short-hairpin RNA interference of annexin A2 attenuates tumor growth and metastasis in a mouse lung cancer stem cell model, *J. Control. Release* 184 (2014) 67–78.
13. S.Y. Lee, M.S. Huh, S. Lee, S.J. Lee, H. Chung, J.H. Park, Y.K. Oh, K. Choi, K. Kim, I.C. Kwon, Stability and cellular uptake of polymerized siRNA (poly-siRNA)/ polyethylenimine (PEI) complexes for efficient gene silencing, *J. Control. Release* 141 (2010) 339–346.
14. H. Mok, S.H. Lee, J.W. Park, T.G. Park, Multimeric small interfering ribonucleic acid for highly efficient sequence-specific gene silencing, *Nat. Mater.* 9 (2010) 272–278.
15. S.H. Lee, H. Mok, S. Jo, C.A. Hong, T.G. Park, Dual gene targeted multimeric siRNA for combinatorial gene silencing, *Biomaterials* 32 (2011) 2359–2368.
16. Y. Nakashima, H. Abe, N. Abe, K. Aikawa, Y. Ito, Branched RNA nanostructures for RNA interference, *Chem. Commun.* 47 (2011) 8367–8369.
17. C.A. Hong, S.H. Lee, J.S. Kim, J.W. Park, K.H. Bae, H. Mok, T.G. Park, H. Lee, Gene silencing by siRNA microhydrogels via polymeric nanoscale condensation, *J. Am. Chem. Soc.* 133 (2011) 13914–13917.
18. J. Zhou, Y. Shu, P. Guo, D.D. Smith, J.J. Rossi, Dual functional RNA nanoparticles containing phi29 motor pRNA and anti-gp120 aptamer for cell-type specific delivery and HIV-1 inhibition, *Methods* 54 (2011) 284–294.
19. H. Yoo, H. Jung, S.A. Kim, H. Mok, Multivalent comb-type aptamer–siRNA conjugates for efficient and selective intracellular delivery, *Chem. Commun.* 50 (2014) 6765–6767.
20. W.W. Grabow, P. Zakrevsky, K.A. Afonin, A. Chworos, B.A. Shapiro, L. Jaeger, Selfassembling RNA nanorings based on RNAI/II inverse kissing complexes, *Nano Lett.* 11 (2011) 878–887.
21. K.A. Afonin, W.W. Grabow, F.M. Walker, E. Bindewald, M.A. Dobrovolskaia, B.A. Shapiro, L. Jaeger, Design and self-assembly of siRNA-functionalized RNA nanoparticles for use in automated nanomedicine, *Nat. Protoc.* 6 (2011) 2022–2034.
22. K.A. Afonin, M. Kireeva, W.W. Grabow, M. Kashlev, L. Jaeger, B.A. Shapiro, Cotranscriptional assembly of chemically modified RNA nanoparticles functionalized with siRNAs, *Nano Lett.* 12 (2012) 5192–5195.
23. Y. Shu, F. Haque, D. Shu, W. Li, Z. Zhu, M. Kotb, Y. Lyubchenko, P. Guo, Fabrication of 14 different RNA nanoparticles for specific tumor targeting without accumulation in normal organs, *RNA* 19 (2013) 767–777.
24. F. Haque, D. Shu, Y. Shu, L.S. Shlyakhtenko, P.G. Rychahou, B.M. Evers, P. Guo, Ultrastable synergistic tetravalent RNA nanoparticles for targeting to cancers, *Nano Today* 7 (2012) 245–257.
25. D. Shu, W.D. Moll, Z. Deng, C. Mao, P. Guo, Bottom-up assembly of RNA arrays and superstructures as potential parts in nanotechnology, *Nano Lett.* 4 (2004) 1717–1723.

26. A. Khaled, S. Guo, F. Li, P. Guo, Controllable self-assembly of nanoparticles for specific delivery of multiple therapeutic molecules to cancer cells using RNA nanotechnology, *Nano Lett.* 5 (2005) 1797–1808.

27. H. Lee, A.K. Lytton-Jean, Y. Chen, K.T. Love, A.I. Park, E.D. Karagiannis, A. Sehgal, W. Querbes, C.S. Zurenko, M. Jayaraman, C.G. Peng, K. Charisse, A. Borodovsky, M. Manoharan, J.S. Donahoe, J. Truelove, M. Nahrendorf, R. Langer, D.G. Anderson, Molecularly self-assembled nucleic acid nanoparticles for targeted in vivo siRNA delivery, *Nat. Nanotechnol.* 7 (2012) 389–393.

28. J. BumáLee, Enzymatic size control of RNA particles using complementary rolling circle transcription (cRCT) method for efficient siRNA production, *Chem. Commun.* 50 (2014) 11665–11667.

29. D. Han, Y. Park, H. Kim, J.B. Lee, Self-assembly of free-standing RNA membranes, *Nat. Commun.* 5 (2014) 4367.

30. G. Zhu, R. Hu, Z. Zhao, Z. Chen, X. Zhang, W. Tan, Noncanonical self-assembly of multifunctional DNA nanoflowers for biomedical applications, *J. Am. Chem. Soc.* 135 (2013) 16438–16445.

31. Y.H. Roh, J.B. Lee, K.E. Shopsowitz, E.C. Dreaden, S.W. Morton, Z. Poon, J. Hong, I. Yamin, D.K. Bonner, P.T. Hammond, Layer-by-layer assembled antisense DNA microsponge particles for efficient delivery of cancer therapeutics, *ACS Nano* 8 (2014) 9767–9780.

32. G.J. Hannon, RNA interference, *Nature* 418(6894) (2002) 244–251.

33. P.A. Sharp, RNAi and double-strand RNA, *Genes Dev.* 13(2) (1999) 139–141.

34. S.M. Elbashir, J. Harborth, W. Lendeckel, A. Yalcin, K. Weber, T. Tuschl, Duplexes of 21-nucleotide RNAs mediate RNA interference in cultured mammalian cells, *Nature* 411(6836) (2001) 494–498.

35. E. Bernstein, A.A. Caudy, S.M. Hammond, G.J. Hannon, Role for a bidentate ribonuclease in the initiation step of RNA interference, *Nature* 409(6818) (2001) 363–366.

36. E. Check, Acrucial test, *Nat. Med.* 11(3) (2005) 243–244.

37. J. DeVincenzo, J.E. Cehelsky, R. Alvarez et al., Evaluation of the safety, tolerability and pharmacokinetics of ALN-RSV01, a novel RNAi antiviral therapeutic directed against respiratory syncytial virus (RSV), *Antivir. Res.* 77(3) (2008) 225–231.

38. L. Aagaard, J.J. Rossi, RNAi therapeutics: principles, prospects and challenges, *Adv. Drug Deliv. Rev.* 59(2–3) (2007) 75–86.

39. X. Yuan, S. Naguib, Z. Wu, Recent advances of siRNA delivery by nanoparticles, *Expert Opin. Drug Deliv.* 8(4) (2011) 521–536.

40. J.C. Burnett, J.J. Rossi, K. Tiemann, Current progress of siRNA/shRNA therapeutics in clinical trials, *Biotechnol. J.* 6(9) (2011) 1130–1146.

41. P.L. Sinn, S.L. Sauter, P.B. McCray Jr., Gene therapy progress and prospects: development of improved lentiviral and retroviral vectors-design, biosafety, and production, *Gene Ther.* 12(14) (2005) 1089–1098.

42. Y. Wang, Z. Li, Y. Han, L.H. Liang, A. Ji, Nanoparticle based delivery system for application of siRNA in vivo, *Curr Drug Metab.* 11(2) (2010) 182–196.

43. J.D. Heidel, Z. Yu, J.Y. Liu, S.M. Rele, Y. Liang, R.K. Zeidan, D.J. Kornbrust, M.E. Davis, Administration in non-human primates of escalating intravenous doses of targeted nanoparticles containing ribonucleotide reductase subunit M2 siRNA, *Proc. Natl. Acad. Sci. U. S. A.* 104 (2007) 5715–5721.

44. D. Castanotto, J.J. Rossi, The promises and pitfalls of RNA-interference-based therapeutics, *Nature* 457 (2009) 426–433.

45. A.D. Judge, V. Sood, J.R. Shaw, D. Fang, K. McClintock, I. MacLachlan, Sequence dependent stimulation of the mammalian innate immune response by synthetic siRNA, *Nat. Biotechnol.* 23 (2005) 457–462.

46. S.H. Kim, J.H. Jeong, S.H. Lee, S.W. Kim, T.G. Park, Local and systemic delivery of VEGF siRNA using polyelectrolyte complex micelles for effective treatment of cancer, *J. Control. Release* 129 (2008) 107–116.

47. A.L. Bolcato-Bellemin, M.E. Bonnet, G. Creusat, P. Erbacher, J.P. Behr, Sticky overhangs enhance siRNA-mediated gene silencing, *Proc. Natl. Acad. Sci. U. S. A.* 104 (2007) 16050–16055.

48. D.J. Gary, N. Puri, Y.Y. Won, Polymer-based siRNA delivery: perspectives on the fundamental and phenomenological distinctions from polymer-based DNA delivery, *J. Control. Release* 121 (2007) 64–73.

49. S.A. Shah, A.T. Brunger, The 1.8 A crystal structure of a statically disordered 17 base-pair RNA duplex: principles of RNA crystal packing and its effect on nucleic acid structure, *J. Mol. Biol.* 285 (1999) 1577–1588.

50. P. Kebbekus, D.E. Draper, P. Hagerman, Persistence length of RNA, *Biochemistry* 34 (1995) 4354–4357.

51. S. Tumova, A. Woods, J.R. Couchman, Heparan sulfate proteoglycans on the cell surface: versatile coordinators of cellular functions, *Int. J. Biochem. Cell Biol.* 32 (2000) 269–288.

52. A.M. Derfus, A.A. Chen, D.H. Min, E. Ruoslahti, S.N. Bhatia, Targeted quantum dot conjugates for siRNA delivery, *Bioconjug. Chem.* 18 (2007) 1391–1396.

53. S.H. Kim, J.H. Jeong, S.H. Lee, S.W. Kim, T.G. Park, PEG conjugated VEGF siRNA for anti-angiogenic gene therapy, *J. Control. Release* 116 (2006) 123–129.

54. J.H. Jeong, H. Mok, Y.K. Oh, T.G. Park, siRNA conjugate delivery systems, *Bioconjug. Chem.* 20 (2009) 5–14.

55. H.J. Chung, C.A. Hong, S.H. Lee, S.D. Jo, T.G. Park, Reducible siRNA dimeric conjugates for efficient cellular uptake and gene silencing, *Bioconjug. Chem.* 22 (2011) 299–306.

56. S.J. Lee, S. Son, J.Y. Yhee, K. Choi, I.C. Kwon, S.H. Kim, K. Kim, Structural modification of siRNA for efficient gene silencing, *Biotechnol. Adv.* 31 (2013) 491–503.

57. W.H. Kong, K.H. Bae, C.A. Hong, Y. Lee, S.K. Hahn, T.G. Park, Multimerized siRNA cross-linked by gold nanoparticles, *Bioconjug. Chem.* 22 (2011) 1962–1969.

58. A.P. Alivisatos, K.P. Johnsson, X. Peng, T.E. Wilson, C.J. Loweth, M.P. Bruchez Jr., P.G. Schultz, Organization of 'nanocrystal molecules' using DNA, *Nature* 382 (1996) 609–611.

59. C.A. Mirkin, R.L. Letsinger, R.C. Mucic, J.J. Storhoff, A DNA-based method for rationally assembling nanoparticles into macroscopic materials, *Nature* 382 (1996) 607–609.

60. F.A. Aldaye, H.F. Sleiman, Dynamic DNA templates for discrete gold nanoparticle assemblies: control of geometry, modularity, write/erase and structural switching, *J. Am. Chem. Soc.* 129 (2007) 4130–4131.

61. P. Ghosh, G. Han, M. De, C.K. Kim, V.M. Rotello, Gold nanoparticles in delivery applications, *Adv. Drug Deliv. Rev.* 60 (2008) 1307–1315.

62. K. Gao, L. Huang, Nonviral methods for siRNA delivery, *Mol. Pharm.* 6 (2009) 651–658.

63. H. Lv, S. Zhang, B. Wang, S. Cui, J. Yan, Toxicity of cationic lipids and cationic polymers in gene delivery, *J. Control. Release* 114 (2006) 100–109.

64. S.J. Lee, M.S. Huh, S.Y. Lee, S.Min, S. Lee, H. Koo, J.U. Chu, K.E. Lee, H. Jeon, Y. Choi, K. Choi, Y. Byun, S.Y. Jeong, K. Park, K. Kim, I.C. Kwon, Tumor-homing poly-siRNA/glycol chitosan self-cross-linked nanoparticles for systemic siRNA delivery in cancer treatment, *Angew. Chem.* 51 (2012) 7203–7207.

65. J.Y. Yhee, S.J. Lee, S. Lee, S. Song, H.S. Min, S.W. Kang, S. Son, S.Y. Jeong, I.C. Kwon, S.H. Kim, K. Kim, Tumor-targeting transferrin nanoparticles for systemic polymerized siRNA delivery in tumor-bearing mice, *Bioconjug. Chem.* 24 (2013) 1850–1860.

66. A.J. Kuijpers, P.B. van Wachem, M.J. van Luyn, L.A. Brouwer, G.H. Engbers, J. Krijgsveld, S.A. Zaat, J. Dankert, J. Feijen, In vitro and in vivo evaluation of gelatinchondroitin sulphate hydrogels for controlled release of antibacterial proteins, *Biomaterials* 21 (2000) 1763–1772.

67. H. Ishikawa, Y. Nakamura, J. Jo, Y. Tabata, Gelatin nanospheres incorporating siRNA for controlled intracellular release, *Biomaterials* 33 (2012) 9097–9104.

68. S. Son, S. Song, S.J. Lee, S.Min, S.A. Kim, J.Y. Yhee, M.S. Huh, I. Chan Kwon, S.Y. Jeong, Y. Byun, S.H. Kim, K. Kim, Self-crosslinked human serum albumin nanocarriers for systemic delivery of polymerized siRNA to tumors, *Biomaterials* 34 (2013) 9475–9485.

69. K.A. Whitehead, R. Langer, D.G. Anderson, Knocking down barriers: advances in siRNA delivery, *Nat. Rev. Drug Discov.* 8 (2009) 129–138.

70. R.J. Boado, Blood-brain barrier transport of non-viral gene and RNAi therapeutics, *Pharm. Res.* 24 (2007) 1772–1787.

71. T.E. LaGrandeur, A. Huttenhofer, H.F. Noller, N.R. Pace, Phylogenetic comparative chemical footprint analysis of the interaction between ribonuclease P RNA and tRNA, *EMBO J.* 13 (1994) 3945–3952.

72. C. Chen, C. Zhang, P. Guo, Sequence requirement for hand-in-hand interaction in formation of RNA dimers and hexamers to gear phi29 DNA translocation motor, *RNA* 5 (1999) 805–818.

73. K.A. Afonin, W.K. Kasprzak, E. Bindewald, M. Kireeva, M. Viard, M. Kashlev, B.A. Shapiro, In silico design and enzymatic synthesis of functional RNA nanoparticles, *Acc. Chem. Res.* 47 (2014) 1731–1741.

74. K.A. Afonin, E. Bindewald, A.J. Yaghoubian, N. Voss, E. Jacovetty, B.A. Shapiro, L. Jaeger, In vitro assembly of cubic RNA-based scaffolds designed in silico, *Nat. Nanotechnol.* 5 (2010) 676–682.

75. I. Severcan, C. Geary, A. Chworos, N. Voss, E. Jacovetty, L. Jaeger, A polyhedron made of tRNAs, *Nat. Chem.* 2 (2010) 772–779.

76. W.W. Grabow, L. Jaeger, RNA self-assembly and RNA nanotechnology, *Acc. Chem. Res.* 47 (2014) 1871–1880.

77. A. Chworos, I. Severcan, A.Y. Koyfman, P. Weinkam, E. Oroudjev, H.G. Hansma, L. Jaeger, Building programmable jigsaw puzzles with RNA, *Science* 306 (2004) 2068–2072.

78. P. Guo, The emerging field of RNA nanotechnology, *Nat. Nanotechnol.* 5 (2010) 833–842.

79. G.C. Shukla, F. Haque, Y. Tor, L.M. Wilhelmsson, J.J. Toulme, H. Isambert, P. Guo, J.J. Rossi, S.A. Tenenbaum, B.A. Shapiro, A boost for the emerging field of RNA nanotechnology, *ACS Nano* 5 (2011) 3405–3418.

80. A.Y. Koyfman, G. Braun, S. Magonov, A. Chworos, N.O. Reich, L. Jaeger, Controlled spacing of cationic gold nanoparticles by nanocrown RNA, *J. Am. Chem. Soc.* 127 (2005) 11886–11887.

81. Y. Shu, F. Pi, A. Sharma, M. Rajabi, F. Haque, D. Shu, M. Leggas, B.M. Evers, P. Guo, Stable RNA nanoparticles as potential new generation drugs for cancer therapy, *Adv. Drug Deliv. Rev.* 66 (2014) 74–89.

82. E.F. Khisamutdinov, D.L. Jasinski, P. Guo, RNA as a boiling-resistant anionic polymer material to build robust structures with defined shape and stoichiometry, *ACS Nano* 8 (2014) 4771–4781.

83. C. Hao, X. Li, C. Tian, W. Jiang, G. Wang, C. Mao, Construction of RNA nanocages by re-engineering the packaging RNA of Phi29 bacteriophage, *Nat. Commun.* 5 (2014) 3890.

84. H. Ohno, T. Kobayashi, R. Kabata, K. Endo, T. Iwasa, S.H. Yoshimura, K. Takeyasu, T. Inoue, H. Saito, Synthetic RNA-protein complex shaped like an equilateral triangle, *Nat. Nanotechnol.* 6 (2011) 116–120.

85. E. Osada, Y. Suzuki, K. Hidaka, H. Ohno, H. Sugiyama, M. Endo, H. Saito, Engineering RNA-protein complexes with different shapes for imaging and therapeutic applications, *ACS Nano* 8 (2014) 8130–8140.

86. P. Tarapore, Y. Shu, P. Guo, S.M. Ho, Application of phi29 motor pRNA for targeted therapeutic delivery of siRNA silencing metallothionein-IIA and survivin in ovarian cancers, *Mol. Ther.* 19 (2011) 386–394.

87. R.A. Petros, J.M. DeSimone, Strategies in the design of nanoparticles for therapeutic applications, *Nat. Rev. Drug Discov.* 9 (2010) 615–627.

88. J. Kaur, K. Tikoo, Ets1 identified as a novel molecular target of RNA aptamer selected against metastatic cells for targeted delivery of nano-formulation, *Oncogene* 34 (2015) 5216–5228.

89. G. Baneyx, L. Baugh, V. Vogel, Fibronectin extension and unfolding within cell matrix fibrils controlled by cytoskeletal tension, *Proc. Natl. Acad. Sci. U. S. A.* 99 (2002) 5139–5143.

90. P. Hyman, R. Valluzzi, E. Goldberg, Design of protein struts for self-assembling nanoconstructs, *Proc. Natl. Acad. Sci. U. S. A.* 99 (2002) 8488–8493.

91. J. Goldberger, R. He, Y. Zhang, S. Lee, H. Yan, H.J. Choi, P. Yang, Single-crystal gallium nitride nanotubes, *Nature* 422 (2003) 599–602.

92. D. Shu, Y. Shu, F. Haque, S. Abdelmawla, P. Guo, Thermodynamically stable RNA three-way junction for constructing multifunctional nanoparticles for delivery of therapeutics, *Nat. Nanotechnol.* 6 (2011) 658–667.

93. Y. Shu, M. Cinier, S.R. Fox, N. Ben-Johnathan, P. Guo, Assembly of therapeutic pRNA-siRNA nanoparticles using bipartite approach, *Mol. Ther.* 19 (2011) 1304–1311.

94. R.P. Goodman, I.A. Schaap, C.F. Tardin, C.M. Erben, R.M. Berry, C.F. Schmidt, A.J. Turberfield, Rapid chiral assembly of rigid DNA building blocks for molecular nanofabrication, *Science* 310 (2005) 1661–1665.

95. Y. He, T. Ye, M. Su, C. Zhang, A.E. Ribbe, W. Jiang, C. Mao, Hierarchical self-assembly of DNA into symmetric supramolecular polyhedra, *Nature* 452 (2008) 198–201.

96. D. Bhatia, S. Surana, S. Chakraborty, S.P. Koushika, Y. Krishnan, A synthetic icosahedral DNA-based host-cargo complex for functional in vivo imaging, *Nat. Commun.* 2 (2011) 339.

97. A.S. Walsh, H. Yin, C.M. Erben, M.J. Wood, A.J. Turberfield, DNA cage delivery to mammalian cells, *ACS Nano* 5 (2011) 5427–5432.

98. J.W. Keum, J.H. Ahn, H. Bermudez, Design, assembly, and activity of antisense DNA nanostructures, *Small* 7 (2011) 3529–3535.

99. M. Gaglione, A. Messere, Recent progress in chemically modified siRNAs, *Mini Rev. Med. Chem.* 10 (2010) 578–595.

100. Z. Li, B. Wei, J. Nangreave, C. Lin, Y. Liu, Y. Mi, H. Yan, A replicable tetrahedral nanostructure self-assembled from a single DNA strand, *J. Am. Chem. Soc.* 131 (2009) 13093–13098.

101. A. Fire, S.Q. Xu, Rolling replication of short DNA circles, *Proc. Natl. Acad. Sci. U. S. A.* 92 (1995) 4641–4645.

102. D. Liu, S.L. Daubendiek, M.A. Zillman, K. Ryan, E.T. Kool, Rolling circle DNA synthesis: small circular oligonucleotides as efficient templates for DNA polymerases, *J. Am. Chem. Soc.* 118 (1996) 1587–1594.

103. C. Lin, M. Xie, J.J. Chen, Y. Liu, H. Yan, Rolling-circle amplification of a DNA nanojunction, *Angew. Chem.* 45 (2006) 7537–7539.

104. C.A. Hong, B. Jang, E.H. Jeong, H. Jeong, H. Lee, Self-assembled DNA nanostructures prepared by rolling circle amplification for the delivery of siRNA conjugates, *Chem. Commun.* 50 (2014) 13049–13051.

105. M.M. Ali, F. Li, Z. Zhang, K. Zhang, D.K. Kang, J.A. Ankrum, X.C. Le, W. Zhao, Rolling circle amplification: a versatile tool for chemical biology, materials science and medicine, *Chem. Soc. Rev.* 43 (2014) 3324–3341.

106. S.L. Daubendiek, K. Ryan, E.T. Kool, Rolling-circle RNA synthesis: circular oligonucleotides as efficient substrates for T7 RNA polymerase, *J. Am. Chem. Soc.* 117 (1995) 7818–7819.

107. D. Zhang, J. Wu, F. Ye, T. Feng, I. Lee, B. Yin, Amplification of circularizable probes for the detection of target nucleic acids and proteins, *Clinica chimica acta, Int. J. Clin. Chem.* 363 (2006) 61–70.

108. N.O. Fischer, T.M. Tarasow, J.B. Tok, Protein detection via direct enzymatic amplification of short DNA aptamers, *Anal. Biochem.* 373 (2008) 121–128.

109. J. Jarvius, J. Melin, J. Göransson, J. Stenberg, S. Fredriksson, C. Gonzalez-Rey, S. Bertilsson, M. Nilsson, Digital quantification using amplified single-molecule detection, *Nat. Methods* 3 (2006) 725–727.

110. C. Larsson, I. Grundberg, O. Soderberg, M. Nilsson, In situ detection and genotyping of individual mRNA molecules, *Nat. Methods* 7 (2010) 395–397.

111. Z. Zhang, M.M. Ali, M.A. Eckert, D.K. Kang, Y.Y. Chen, L.S. Sender, D.A. Fruman, W. Zhao, A polyvalent aptamer system for targeted drug delivery, *Biomaterials* 34 (2013) 9728–9735.

112. J.B. Lee, J. Hong, D.K. Bonner, Z. Poon, P.T. Hammond, Self-assembled RNA interference microsponges for efficient siRNA delivery, *Nat. Mater.* 11 (2012) 316–322.

113. H. Qi, M. Ghodousi, Y. Du, C. Grun, H. Bae, P. Yin, A. Khademhosseini, DNA-directed self-assembly of shape-controlled hydrogels, *Nat. Commun.* 4 (2013) 2275.

114. J.B. Lee, S. Peng, D. Yang, Y.H. Roh, H. Funabashi, N. Park, E.J. Rice, L. Chen, R. Long, M. Wu, A mechanical meta-material made from a DNA hydrogel, *Nat. Nanotechnol.* 7 (2012) 816–820.

115. S.L. Daubendiek, E.T. Kool, Generation of catalytic RNAs by rolling transcription of synthetic DNA nanocircles, *Nat. Biotechnol.* 15 (1997) 273–277.

116. A.A. Seyhan, A.V. Vlassov, B.H. Johnston, RNA interference from multimeric shRNAs generated by rolling circle transcription, *Oligonucleotides* 16 (2006) 353–363.

117. W. Sun, T. Jiang, Y. Lu, M. Reiff, R. Mo, Z. Gu, Cocoon-like self-degradable DNA nanoclew for anticancer drug delivery, *J. Am. Chem. Soc.* 136 (2014) 14722–14725.

118. G. Chen, D. Liu, C. He, T.R. Gannett, W. Lin, Y. Weizmann, Enzymatic synthesis of periodic DNA nanoribbons for intracellular pH sensing and gene silencing, *J. Am. Chem. Soc.* 137 (2015) 3844–3851.

119. A.V. Pinheiro, D.R. Han, W.M. Shih, H. Yan, Challenges and opportunities for structural DNA nanotechnology, *Nat. Nanotechnol.* 6 (2011) 763–772.

120. P.X. Guo, S. Erickson, D. Anderson, A small viral-RNA is required for in vitro packaging of bacteriophage-Phi-29 DNA, *Science* 236 (1987) 690–694.

121. W.W. Grabow, P. Zakrevsky, K.A. Afonin, A. Chworos, B.A. Shapiro, L. Jaeger, Selfassembling RNA nanorings based on RNAI/II inverse kissing complexes, *Nano Lett.* 11 (2011) 878–887.

122. Y. Eguchi, J. Tomizawa, Complex formed by complementary RNA stem-loops and its stabilization by a protein - function of Cole1 rom protein, *Cell* 60 (1990) 199–209.

123. Loutfy H. Madkour. *Reactive Oxygen Species (ROS), Nanoparticles, and Endoplasmic Reticulum (ER) Stress-Induced Cell Death Mechanisms.* Paperback ISBN: 9780128224816. Imprint: Academic Press Published Date: 1st August 2020. https://www.elsevier.com/books/reactive-oxygen-species-ros-nanoparticles-and-endoplasmic-reticulum-er-stress-induced-cell-death-mechanisms/madkour/978-0-12-822481-6.

124. Loutfy H. Madkour, *Nanoparticles Induce Oxidative and Endoplasmic Reticulum Antioxidant Therapeutic Defenses.* Copyright 2020 Publisher Springer International Publishing. Copyright Holder Springer Nature Switzerland AG eBook ISBN 978-3-030-37297-2 DOI 10.1007/978-3-030-37297-2 Hardcover ISBN 978-3-030-37296-5 Series ISSN 2194–0452 Edition Number 1. https://www.springer.com/gp/book/9783030372965?utm_campaign=3_pier05_buy_print&utm_content=en_08082017&utm_medium=referral&utm_source=google_books#otherversion=9783030372972.

125. Loutfy H. Madkour, *Nucleic Acids as Gene Anticancer Drug Delivery Therapy.* 1st Edition. Publishing house: Elsevier, (2020). Paperback ISBN: 9780128197776 Imprint: Academic Press Published Date: 2nd January 2020 Imprint: Academic Press Copyright: Paperback ISBN: 9780128197776 © Academic Press 2020 Published: 2nd January 2020 Imprint: Academic Press Paperback ISBN: 9780128197776. https://www.elsevier.com/books/nucleic-acids-as-gene-anticancer-drug-deliverytherapy/madkour/978-0-12-819777-6.

126. Loutfy H. Madkour, *Nanoelectronic Materials: Fundamentals and Applications (Advanced Structured Materials)* 1st ed. 2019 Edition: https://link.springer.com/book/10.1007%2F978-3-030-21621-4 Series Title Advanced Structured Materials Series Volume 116 Copyright 2019 Publisher Springer International Publishing Copyright Holder Springer Nature Switzerland AG. eBook ISBN 978-3-030-21621-4 DOI 10.1007/978-3-030-21621-4 Hardcover ISBN 978-3-030-21620-7 Series ISSN 1869-8433 Edition Number 1 Number of Pages XLIII, 783

Number of Illustrations 122 b/w illustrations, 494 illustrations in colour Topics. ISBN-10: 3030216209 ISBN-13: 978-3030216207 #117 in Nanotechnology (Books) #725 in Materials Science (Books) #187336 in Textbooks. https://books.google.com.eg/books/about/Nanoelectronic_Materials.html?id=YQXCxAEACAAJ&source=kp_book_description&redir_esc=y; https://www.springer.com/gp/book/9783030216207.

127. J.K. Nair, J.L. Willoughby, A. Chan, K. Charisse, M.R. Alam, Q. Wang, M. Hoekstra, P. Kandasamy, A.V. Kel'in, S. Milstein, N. Taneja, J. O'Shea, S. Shaikh, L. Zhang, R.J. van der Sluis, M.E. Jung, A. Akinc, R. Hutabarat, S. Kuchimanchi, K. Fitzgerald, T. Zimmermann, T.J. van Berkel, M.A. Maier, K.G. Rajeev, M. Manoharan, Multivalent N-acetylgalactosamine-conjugated siRNA localizes in hepatocytes and elicits robust RNAi-mediated gene silencing, *J. Am. Chem. Soc.* 136 (2014) 16958–16961.

4 Codelivery in Nanoparticle-based siRNA for Cancer Therapy

Important progress in nanotechnology has led to the development of efficient short interfering RNA (siRNA) delivery systems. In this chapter, we discuss recent advances in nanoparticle-mediated siRNA delivery and the application of siRNA in clinical trials for cancer therapy. Furthermore, we offer perspectives on future applications of siRNA therapeutics.

4.1 NANOCARRIERS TO DELIVER RNA (siRNA) CHAINS

Chemotherapeutical agents present many limitations that hinder the effectiveness of chemotherapy: poor solubility in aqueous solutions (making them difficult to administer) [1], nonspecific distribution throughout the body (which causes insufficient penetration to tumors) [2], toxicity to healthy tissues [3] (which limits the dose and frequency of the treatment), and cancer cell resistance [4].

There are two main mechanisms by which cells become multidrug resistant (MDR): by increasing drug efflux pumps on the cell membrane and by increasing antiapoptotic pathways [5]. An increase in efflux pumps causes a decrease in the intracellular concentration of the drug, compromising the efficiency of the treatment [6]. The onset of nanotechnology has fostered the ability to provide solutions to these limitations, by encapsulating drugs in hydrophilic nanocarriers, which increases the solubility of the drug, decreases the toxicity to healthy tissues, and bypasses the effect of the efflux pumps [7,8].

Although the initial limitations of antineoplastic drugs have been mitigated through the use of nanocarriers [9,10], new limitations have arisen. Cells have developed strategies to avoid death, increasing their resistance to chemotherapy, by the activation of antiapoptotic pathways [11]. siRNA has the ability to disrupt cellular pathways by knocking down genes, opening the door for new treatments of diseases caused by aberrant gene expression [12,13]. However, siRNA chains exhibit a short half-life in blood if injected intravenously due to intravascular degradation by the catalytic activity of ribonuclease (RNase) enzymes present in the bloodstream [13]. Rapid systemic clearance of siRNA through the renal system, low selectivity for the desired tissue, and poor cellular uptake have been reported for intravenous injection of siRNA in chemotherapeutic studies, decreasing the effectiveness of the therapy.

The use of nanocarriers for siRNA encapsulation can prevent both renal clearance and RNase degradation, effectively increasing its half-life in blood [14,15]. Promising results have been shown in which resistant cancer cells were sensitized to chemotherapy by knocking down one of the multidrug resistance mechanisms [16]. While some types of cancer cells were completely sensitized to antineoplastic drugs by siRNA therapy, others maintained their resistance to the treatment, compensating the loss of one type of resistance mechanism by increasing other multidrug resistance mechanisms.

Even though cotreatment of cancer cells with nano delivery systems carrying either siRNA or drugs proved to be important in decreasing resistance of cancer cells [17–20], it has been proposed that codelivering drugs and siRNA together in the same delivery system would be more effective in overcoming resistance of cancer cells [21]. In this chapter, we discuss the progress of nanoscale codelivery systems in overcoming multidrug cancer resistance.

4.2 MECHANISMS OF CANCER DRUG RESISTANCE

The treatment of cancer cells has evolved from general drugs targeting DNA, such as doxorubicin (DOX) or cisplatin, to more specific molecules that target overexpressed proteins or upregulated pathways present in cancer cells [22]. The specificity of DNA binding chemotherapy slightly directed toward cancer cells rather than healthy cells has improved cancer treatment. However, due to the high toxicity of most chemotherapeutical agents and the severity of the secondary effects, cancer treatment with chemotherapy requires convalescence time to allow patients to recover from treatment to treatment [23]. Since tumors have heterogeneous populations of cancer cells [24], only sensitive cancer cells within the tumor will die due to chemotherapy, and those that are drug resistant remain intact. This allows for a population of almost exclusively nonresistant cancer cells to become a resistant population, making each chemotherapy session less effective (Figure 4.1). The lack of effectiveness of chemotherapy to treat cancer is due to several factors, but mostly due to the low concentration of drug reaching its target and/or poor effectiveness in killing cancer cells, even when the target its reached [25].

The vast majority of tumors (85%) in cancer patients are solid tumors [26]. The first line of treatment for solid tumors is surgery, when possible, followed by radiation and chemotherapy. Drugs that are injected systemically need to reach the cells within the tumor. Because tumors are highly irrigated with abnormal vasculature that leave gaps between the endothelial cells, but poorly irrigated with

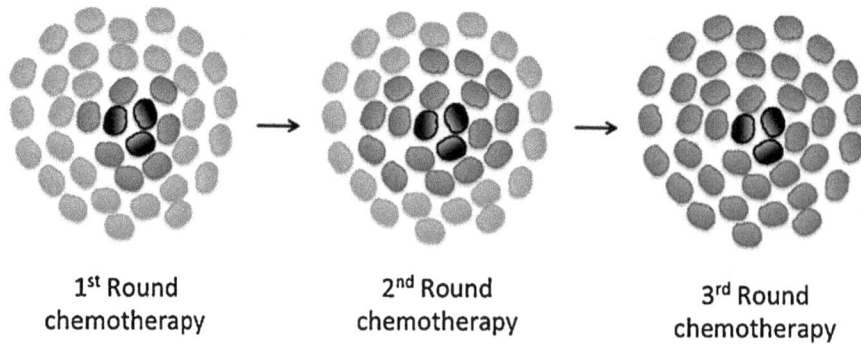

FIGURE 4.1 Acquired resistance of a cancer cell population after intervals of chemotherapy. After the first round of chemotherapy, cell population decreases significantly due to the death of sensitive cancer cells. Recovery time between chemotherapy sessions allows for resistant cells to grow and take over the entire population.

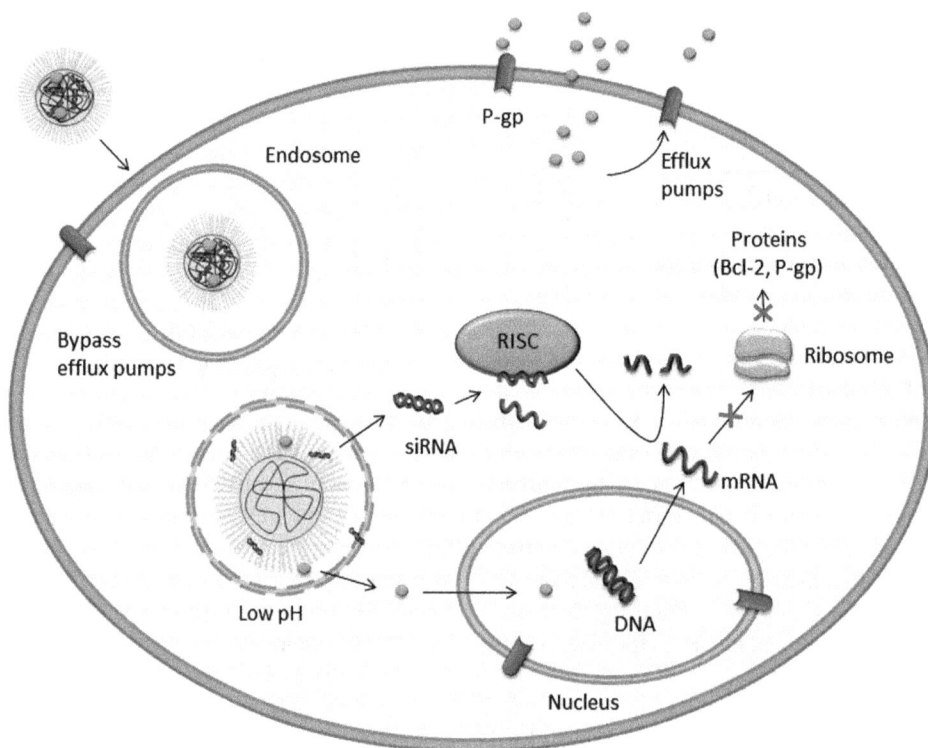

FIGURE 4.2 Mechanism of drug resistance and sensitization of cancer cells by co-delivering siRNA and an antineoplastic agent. Drugs encapsulated in nanoparticles evade the efflux pump, by endosomal internalization. Once in the endosome, specifically designed nanoparticles, release siRNA and drug to the cytosol.

lymphatic vessels, drugs can easily leak from the blood vessels to the interstitial space within the tumor minimizing clearance through the lymphatic system. This is known as the enhanced permeability and retention (EPR) effect [27]. Drugs that reach the tumor must be taken up by cancer cells [28].

Transport across the cell membrane depends on the type of molecule. Alterations in the transport of drugs across the membrane and/or efflux of internalized drugs from the intracellular compartment to the extracellular matrix are one of the major causes of cancer resistance [29]. Drugs that reach their target within the cell start a cascade of reactions that lead cells to enter programmed cell death, known

as apoptosis [30]. A wide variety of cells, from many types of cancers, present different strategies to prevent apoptosis induced by chemotherapy, *i.e.*, by upregulating antiapoptosis pathways, altering cell cycle checkpoints, increasing repair mechanism, *etc.* [5]. Here, we describe the two major mechanism of cancer resistance (Figure 4.2).

4.3 ALTERATIONS IN THE MEMBRANE TRANSPORTERS OR EFFLUX PUMPS

Cancer cells can develop resistance to specific drugs or type of drugs. For example, several types of cancer cells present resistance to folate, such as methotrexate [31]. Loss of cell surface receptors or transporters for the drug, increased metabolism of the drug, or alteration of the drug's target are some of the strategies that cells use to avoid cell death [32–34]. By combining several different types of chemotherapy agents, treatments can overcome this type of resistance. However, a wide variety of cancer cells are resistant to a multiple of drugs. This phenomenon is known as multidrug resistance [33].

The primary protein known to be involved in MDR is P-gp, an ATP-dependent transporter of the ATP-binding cassette family (ABC), and encoded by the gene MDR1 in humans [6]. P-gp can be present in the cell membrane as well as in the nuclear membrane. P-gp binds to neutral and positively charged molecules. A great number of antineoplastic drugs are either neutral or positive at physiological pH, and hence act as a substrate for P-gp, which pumps the drug across the membrane. This decreases the concentration of the drug inside the cell and the nucleus by removing the drug to the extracellular matrix or the cytoplasm, respectively. This mechanism of self-defense is widely known as efflux pump–related cell resistance. In healthy cells, P-gp is involved not only in the efflux of undesirable molecules but also in the transport of beneficial molecules and nutrients across the cell membrane and intracellular membranes in the cell [35]. P-gp is expressed in many cancers including, but not limited to, small and large intestine, liver, pancreas, kidney, ovary, and testicle. Other important ABC is the MDR protein 1 (MRP1) and 2 (MRP2) [36]. MRP1 has been found to be expressed in a great variety of cancers. MRP1 binds to negatively charged molecules or molecules that have been modified by the cell through glycosylation, sulfonation, or other post-translational modifications. Other ABC transporters with implications in cancer resistance have been reported [37].

4.4 ACTIVATION OF ANTIAPOPTOTIC PATHWAYS

Among nondrug pump–related mechanisms, the most important is the activation of antiapoptotic pathways; a defense mechanism that rescues cells from cell death [38]. Apoptosis is the most common type of programmed cell death and is an essential part of the cell cycle. Apoptosis is activated by a series of cascade signals in which many proteins are involved. Bcl-2 is a protein of the Bcl-2 family, encoded by the gene BCL-2, which has a major role in preventing apoptosis in healthy cells [11]. Bcl-2 overexpression prevents cells from entering apoptosis. It is correlated with cancer cell survival and cancer cell resistance. Other members of the Bcl-2 family, such as Mcl-1, a protein encoded by the gene MCL-1, have been identified as inhibitors of apoptosis [39].

Another protein involved in cancer resistance is the protein Plk-1, encoded by the Plk-1 gene. Plk-1 is a protooncogene overexpressed in some types of cancer cells, such as breast and colon [40,41]. The loss of Plk-1 has been associated with activation of apoptosis [42]. c-Myc is a gene encoding for a transcription factor that is constitutively expressed in cancer cells. c-Myc overexpression has been linked to breast [38], ovarian [43], and lung [44] cancer resistance.

4.5 SENSITIZATION STRATEGIES FOR siRNA-BASED THERAPEUTICS

In order to activate the RNAi pathway, double-stranded siRNA must travel through the bloodstream and gain access to the cytosol of target cells. The hydrophilic nature and large molecular weight of siRNAs prevent the molecules from diffusing across the cellular membrane into the cell; therefore, modifications to the nucleic acid and generation of clever delivery strategies are necessary for the creation of siRNA therapeutics.

Considerable efforts have been made recently to suppress multidrug resistance; both in efflux pump– and nonefflux pump–related multidrug resistance. Sensitization strategies include targeting membrane transporters [45–47], inhibition of cell survival pathways [48,49], altering transcription factors [19], and silencing antiapoptotic pathways [17,50].

4.6 EFFLUX PUMP–RELATED SENSITIZATION STRATEGIES

Several sensitization strategies have been tested by using selective inhibitors of the ABC transporters, such as verapamil [46]. Poly(D, L-lactide-coglycolide) (PLGA) nanoparticles were synthesized to simultaneously deliver verapamil and vincristine, a potent chemotherapeutical agent, to cancer cells to reverse the cell's resistance to the latter [47]. Results have shown the resistance to certain chemotherapy agents by inhibition of efflux transporters can only be achieved for certain cancer cell types. A strategy to increase the success of sensitization is by using a broader inhibitor of the transporter, such as depharantine [51]. This, however, resulted in an increase in toxicity in vivo [5]. These results seem to indicate that sensitization of cancer cells by inhibitors of ABC transporters is not only cell specific but also drug specific.

Nanoparticles are not affected by efflux pumps, and they can be used as carriers for drugs that are affected by efflux [52]. Encapsulation of drugs in nanoparticles that are specifically designed to release their cargo in the cytoplasm has been proved to increase drug concentration inside cells [52].

Classic chemotherapeutical drugs such as DOX, cisplatin, and paclitaxel (PAC) must reach DNA preserved within the nucleus to decrease cell viability. The use of nanoparticles to bypass transporters present in the surface of cell membranes has increased the drug concentration in the cytoplasm, but drugs also must cross the nuclear membrane. The presence of efflux pumps in the nuclear membrane decreases the intranuclear concentration of the drug, compromising the efficacy of the treatment. The use of siRNA against genes encoding for efflux pump proteins has been employed as a promising strategy to sensitize cells to cancer drugs. For example, Yadav et al. [20] synthesized poly(ethylene oxide)-modified poly(beta aminoester) (PEO-PbAE) to deliver siRNA against P-gp in PAC-resistant SKOV3 human ovarian adenocarcinoma cells. The cell membrane P-gp protein was targeted by using monoclonal antibodies to increase sensitization of human ovarian carcinoma cells A2780/AD to DOX [53].

4.7 NONEFFLUX PUMP–RELATED SENSITIZATION STRATEGIES

A wide variety of sensitization strategies have been used by inhibition of cell survival pathways, altering transcription factors and silencing antiapoptotic pathways. Among these strategies, some involved the use of nanocarriers to deliver cargo to either block or inhibit pathways or silence genes. For example, poly(ethylene glycol) lipoplexes were used to deliver siRNA to silence Bcl-2 genes (siBcl-2), which sensitized cancer cells to 5-fluoracil [18]. Nanogels were used to deliver siRNA against the gene encoding for epidermal growth factor receptor (EGFR) to sensitize SKOV3 human ovarian adenocarcinoma cells to docetaxel [54]. Liposomes were used to sensitize temozolomide resistant glioblastoma mutiforme (GM) cancer cells by delivering siRNA against the gene encoding for Methyl Guanine Methyl Transferase (MGMT), a DNA repair protein that is overexpressed in GM cancer cells [17]. An inhibitor of the nuclear factor kappa B and downregulator of ABC transporters, curcumin, was delivered with PAC using nanoemulsions to sensitize PAC resistant SKOV3 human ovarian adenocarcinoma cells [48].

4.8 NANOCARRIERS TO CODELIVER siRNA AND SMALL DRUGS

Nanocarriers have been successfully used as platforms for delivery of the cargo to sensitize cells to chemotherapy. A promising sensitization strategy is using siRNA to silence genes encoding for proteins involved in cancer resistance. Cotreatment of resistant cancer cells by using siRNA and drugs, administered separately, has been shown to increase efficacy of cancer treatment. However, codelivery of siRNA and drugs would be more efficient in overcoming cancer resistance to chemotherapy [21]. Several different codelivery systems have been synthesized, but all can be grouped into three categories: polymer based, lipid based, and inorganic based.

4.9 POLYMERIC NANOPARTICLES

Incorporation of siRNAs into nanoparticles is widely used to overcome limitations of nucleic acid formulations. Biodegradable polymeric nanoparticles synthesized via a variety of methods have shown significant therapeutic

potential allowing improved stability in serum, better delivery, and controlled release. Nanoparticles used in siRNA delivery studies are divided into two categories—natural polymers and synthetic polymers. Cyclodextrin, chitosan, atelocollagen, albumin, gelatin and others are promising natural polymer candidates for siRNA delivery in cancer and other diseases [55–57]. Synthetic polymers such as polyethylene glycol (PEG), polyethyleneimine (PEI), PLGA, and others have also been extensively investigated as siRNA delivery agents.

The cyclodextrin polymer (CDP) was used as a raw material for first nanoparticles delivery system for siRNA used in clinical trials [58]. The CDP is a polycationic oligosaccharide produced during bacterial digestion of cellulose and used by the pharmaceutical industry to deliver small molecules [59]. As a siRNA delivery formulation, self-assembled CDP with PEG and human transferrin (Tf), denoted as CALAA-01, has demonstrated improved targeting ability for cancer cells in preclinical tests. Subsequently, this system was tested in a clinical phase trial 1. Another polymeric nanoparticle class frequently used in nanomedicine is chitosan-based systems. Chitosan, a polysaccharide originally derived from chitin, comprises β-(1-4)-linked D-glucosamine (deacetylated unit) and N-acetyl-D-glucosamine (acetylated unit). The cationic nature of the resulting nanoparticle allows electrostatic interactions with negatively charged siRNAs facilitating formulation into the delivery system. Various modifications of chitosan, such as PEGylation and thiolation, have also shown potential in cancer models via a variety of routes of administration [60–63]. Atelocollagen/siRNA complexes have also exhibited anticancer effects in several xenograft cancer models. Collagen is a fibrous structural protein in the connective tissue. By pepsin treatment, the telopeptide of collagen is removed to reduce immunogenicity generating highly purified type I collagen, also known as atelocollagen. Atelocollagen particles have shown improved cellular uptake, nuclease resistance, and controlled release of nucleic acids [64]. Inhibition in tumor growth of an orthotopic xenograft cancer model has been seen when atelocollagen/siRNA complexes were intratumorally administered [65]. Several factors, such as low toxicity, biodegradability, reduction in immunostimulation, and facile condensation with nucleic acids, contribute to advantages of using natural polymers as delivery agents for siRNA.

Synthetic polymers have been extensively investigated in the drug delivery field because of their well-defined chemistries and the high degree of molecular diversity obtainable via chemical modifications [66]. PEI is considered the most potent in its ability to form stable complexes with nucleic acids due to its highly positive charged nature. Branched PEI (bPEI), which has been found to have lower toxicity than linear PEI, and its derivatives have demonstrated successful siRNA delivery to the tumor sites with resultant anticancer effects in preclinical studies. In addition to PEI/siRNA complexes, PEGylation is often incorporated into nanoparticles to increase stability in biological fluids and lend protection against nucleases. Several groups have demonstrated a PEI-PEG platform for effective siRNA delivery in various cancer models [67–69]. Another widely studied synthetic polymer is PLGA. PLGA is a copolymer made from lactic acid and glycolic acid that is approved in therapeutic applications due to its high biodegradability and biocompatibility. With a sustained drug release profile due to slow hydrolytic degradation, PLGA was linked with siRNA through disulfide linkage to form spherical micelles which showed gene silencing effects in breast cancer cells [70].

Though other delivery strategies are gaining attention, particularly including lipid-based siRNA delivery, many investigators continue to use and seek to improve polymeric nanoparticles, based on their stability, flexibility of modification, and high targetability. Nevertheless, deeper understanding into the toxicity and immunogenicity of these delivery methods is necessary to develop polymers as a siRNA delivery strategy for clinical use.

Polymeric nanoparticles are solid, biodegradable, colloidal systems that have been widely investigated as drug or gene carriers [71]. Polymeric nanoparticles are classified into two major categories, natural polymers and synthetic polymers. Natural polymers for siRNA delivery include cyclodextrin, chitosan, and atelocollagen [57]. Of the synthetic polymers, PEI, PLGA, and dendrimers have been intensively investigated [72].

4.9.1 Cyclodextrin Nanoparticle

Cyclodextrins are natural polymers generated during the bacterial digestion of cellulose and can form water-soluble inclusion complexes with small molecules and portions of large compounds [59]. Hu-Lieskoven et al. developed the cyclodextrin-containing polycation system for the targeted delivery of siRNA [73]. This system consists of a cyclodextrin-containing polymer, PEG for stability, and Tf as the targeting ligand for binding to transferrin receptors, which are often overexpressed on cancer cells. This targeted nanoparticle system, called CALLA-01, was developed for the first siRNA phase I trial by Calando Pharmaceuticals (Pasadena, CA, USA) [74]. The siRNA in CALLA-01 is designed to inhibit tumor growth via a mechanism to reduce expression of the M2 subunit of RNase reductase (R2). Patients with solid cancers refractory to standard-of-care therapies were administered targeted nanoparticles via IV infusion on days 1, 3, 8, and 10 of a 21-day cycle [74]. Successful delivery of targeted nanoparticles was confirmed by the presence of intracellular nanoparticles in tumor biopsies from melanoma patients after treatment. Furthermore, knockdown of the M2 subunit of R2 was confirmed in tumor biopsies from these patients by quantitative reverse transcription-polymerase chain reaction (qRT-PCR) and by immunohistochemical staining in the patients treated with the highest dosage. This study demonstrated that siRNA administered systemically to humans may result in specific gene inhibition by an RNAi-mediated mechanism of action.

4.9.2 Chitosan Nanoparticles

Chitosan, a type of naturally occurring polysaccharide, has been extensively studied for the delivery of plasmid DNA and siRNA in vitro and in vivo [75–77]. The advantages of chitosan include mucoadhesivity, biocompatibility, biodegradability, and low cost of production. However, results of studies of siRNA delivery have been inconsistent due to discrepancies between experiments [75,78]. In addition, high molecular weight chitosans are cytotoxic, thus limiting their use in clinical trials [79]. They still also lack the buffering capacity needed for endosomolysis, which is essential to siRNA release from the endosome [66].

4.9.3 Polyethyleneimine

PEI, a commonly used cationic polymeric drug carrier with high transfection efficiency, has been widely investigated for siRNA delivery [57,66,72,]. PEI forms small and compact structures, spontaneously forming polyplexes, with negatively charged siRNA through a simple and short polycation process [57]. The PEI-siRNA complexes protect siRNA from nuclease degradation, resulting in prolonged half-life. In addition, complete encapsulation of siRNA prevents avoid off-target effects such as immune activation by a toll-like receptor–dependent mechanism [80]. However, PEI complexes have been associated with significant toxicity issues limiting their broad use in clinical trials [79]. Molecular mechanisms of PEI cytotoxicity include membrane damage and activation of a mitochondria-mediated apoptotic program due to PEI-induced channel formation in the outer mitochondrial membrane [81,82].

4.9.4 PLGA

PLGA is a copolymer of glycolic acid and lactic acid and a US Food and Drug Administration (FDA)–approved biodegradable polymer [83]. PLGA has been used as a nanocarrier for plasmid DNA and siRNA delivery in recent years. The advantages of PLGA-based siRNA delivery include high stability, facile cellular uptake by endocytosis, ability to target specific tissues or organs by adsorption or ligand binding, biodegradability, low toxicity, and sustained release characteristics [15]. However, PLGA could not be applied efficiently in siRNA delivery due to the lower electrostatic interaction between PLGA and siRNA and less efficient endosomal escape and release of siRNA [15,72]. To overcome these problems, the surface of PLGA can be decorated with various cationic nanoparticles such as 1,2-dioleoyl-3-trimethylammonium-propane (DOTAP), PEI, or polyamine [66].

4.9.5 Dendrimers

Dendrimers are synthetic, highly branched monodisperse and usually highly symmetric, spherical macromolecules with a three-dimensional nanometric structure. The unique structural features such as the tunable structure and molecular size, large number of accessible terminal functional groups, and ability to encapsulate cargos add to their potential as drug carriers [84]. Polycationic dendrimers such as poly(amidoamine) (PAMAM) and poly(propylenimine) (PPI) dendrimers have been studied for siRNA delivery in recent years. PAMAM dendrimers have become the most used dendrimer-based carriers for gene delivery because of the ease of synthesis and commercial availability. However, PAMAMs were demonstrated to be cytotoxic, predominately related to apoptosis mediated by mitochondrial dysfunction [85]. Cytotoxicity can be reduced by various modifications without compromising gene silencing. Surface-modified and cationic PAMAM dendrimers show very low cytotoxicity, even at high concentrations and efficiently penetrated cancer cells *in vitro* [86]. PPI dendrimers were also used to formulate siRNA nanoparticles, and these nanoparticles showed efficient gene silencing [87]. Dendrimer-conjugated magnetofluorescent nanoworms (dendriworms) were developed to achieve siRNA delivery in a transgenic murine model of glioblastoma [88]. These siRNA-carrying dendriworms maximized endosomal escape to robustly produce protein target knockdown and were tolerated well in the mouse brain.

4.10 INORGANIC NANOPARTICLES

A number of inorganic nanoparticles have been emerging as potential siRNA delivery systems devised for simultaneous imaging and therapeutic purposes. They include carbon nanotubes (CNTs) and metals such as iron oxide, quantum dots (QDs), and gold. CNTs are nanomaterials, with interesting physical and chemical properties, and have recently emerged as a new option for cancer treatment, bioengineering, and gene therapy. It has been proposed that CNTs easily cross the plasma membrane and translocate directly into the cytoplasm of target cells due to their nanoneedle structure, using an endocytosis-independent mechanism without inducing cell death [89,90]. CNTs are classified as single-walled CNTs and multiwalled CNTs [91]. Several functionalized CNTs have been designed and tested for the purpose of siRNA delivery. Zhang et al. used single-walled CNTs functionalized with $-CONH-(CH_2)_6-NH_3^+Cl-$ as siRNA carriers [92]. They released the siRNA from the nanotube sidewall to silence telomerase reverse transcriptase expression, which considerably suppressed tumor growth. CNTs functionalized with amine-terminated PEG (phospholipid (PL)-PEG2000-NH_2) were shown to be efficient in siRNA delivery into human T cells [93]. Ammonium-functionalized CNTs and dendron-CNTs have also been reported to be efficient in siRNA delivery with low cytotoxicity [94,95]. A comparative study of antitumor activity of the proprietary cytotoxic siRNA sequence delivered either by cationic liposomes (DOTAP: cholesterol) or amino-functionalized MWNT-NH^{+3} in a human lung xenograft model demonstrated that only MWNT-NH^{+3}: siRNA complexes administered intratumorally could elicit delayed

tumor growth and increased survival of xenograft-bearing animals [96]. However, several studies have discussed the potential toxicity of CNTs although the underlying mechanisms are uncertain [97,98].

Magnetic nanoparticles, including superparamagnetic iron oxide nanoparticles (SPIOs) and magnetic iron tetroxide particles, emerged as feasible nanotheranostics for tumor imaging and drug delivery due to their distinct characteristics [99]. The large surface area of SPIOs makes their functional modification feasible, enabling the conjugation of targeting molecules, drugs, and imaging agents [100]. Moore et al. reported the synthesis and characterization of a new dual-purpose probe for the simultaneous noninvasive imaging and delivery of siRNAs to tumors [101]. This probe consists of magnetic nanoparticles (SPIOs for magnetic resonance imaging) conjugated with Cy5.5 dye (for near-infrared fluorescence imaging (NIRF)) and myristoylated polyarginine peptide for membrane translocation. A nanoparticle probe (MN-NIRF-siSurvivin) targeting the antiapoptotic gene Birc5, which encodes survivin, significantly increased cancer cell apoptosis and necrosis *in vitro* and in xenograft mouse models. Therefore, use of MN-NIRF-siSurvivin conjugates combining siRNA delivery with a dual imaging modality (magnetic resonance imaging and NIRF) was feasible for multimodality imaging and targeted gene delivery. Lee et al. developed manganese-doped magnetism engineered iron oxide (MnMEIO) nanoparticles conjugated to a cancer-specific targeting moiety the Arg-Gly-Asp (RGD) peptide, which specifically binds to tumors expressing $\alpha v\beta3$ integrin, and Cy5-dye-labeled siGFP, which inhibits the expression of green fluorescent protein (GFP) [102]. The constructed nanoparticle (MnMEIO-siGFP-Cy5/PEG-RGD) showed specific internalization and target gene silencing in $\alpha v\beta3$ integrin-expressing breast cancer MDA-MB-435 cells. An additional advantage of iron oxide nanoparticle delivery systems is that they can be delivered in a targeted manner to a desired region by applying an external magnetic field [103].

Semiconductor QDs, which are light-emitting nanoparticles, have been increasingly used as biological imaging and labeling probes [104]. QDs also have the potential of serving as photostable beacons for siRNA delivery and imaging [105–107]. However, the major problem in using QDs as multifunctional imaging probes and delivery systems is their toxicity because most well-established QDs are composed of highly toxic elements, such as cadmium, selenium, or tellurium [108]. Recently, nontoxic QDs, which were developed by a novel sonochemical approach for the high-throughput synthesis of a library of biocompatible ZnS-AgInS2 QDs, showed great potential for imaging and siRNA delivery *in vitro* with negligible cytotoxicity [109]. However, a more thorough investigation of their long-term cytotoxicity is necessary before they can be used *in vivo*.

Gold nanoparticles (AuNPs) have emerged as a promising siRNA delivery carrier due to their excellent biocompatibility, ease of synthesis, high surface-to-volume ratio, and facile surface functionalization [110]. Recently, various types of AuNPs have been widely investigated for siRNA delivery. These include AuNPs functionalized with cationic quaternary ammonium or bPEI, cationic lipid bilayer coated AuNPs, and oligonucleotide-modified AuNPs [110–112]. Gold nanorods also have the potential to deliver siRNA to target cells or tissues. The Prasad group developed gold nanorod-DARPP-32 siRNA complexes to target and reduce expression of the key proteins (DARPP-32, extracellular signal-regulated kinase [ERK], and protein phosphatase 1 [PP-1]) in the dopaminergic signaling pathway in the brain for therapy of drug addiction [113]. Using dark-field imaging and confocal microscopy, they demonstrated that the siRNA was efficiently delivered into dopaminergic neuronal (DAN) cells after treatment with the gold nanorod-siRNA conjugates. Moreover, the delivery of nanoplexes containing siRNA targeted to the DARPP-32 gene in DAN cells resulted in the silencing not only of DARPP-32 but also of other key downstream effector molecules in this pathway, such as ERK and PP-1, with greater efficiency than commercial transfection agents. Recently, Kim et al. reported that AuNPs stably functionalized with covalently attached oligonucleotides activate immune-related genes and pathways in human peripheral blood mononuclear cells, but not an immortalized, lineage-restricted cell line [114]. These later findings suggest that assessment of the toxic potential of engineered nanoparticles in immortalized, lineage-restricted cell lines may not predict their phenotypic effects in relevant biological systems.

4.11 INORGANIC-BASED NANOPARTICLES

Increasing use of inorganic-based nanoparticles in biological applications has been observed due to their tunable specific properties [115–117]. Silica-based nanoparticles have been used for several applications, such as delivery systems to deliver either drugs or siRNA [118,119]. Its high surface area to volume ratio and large pore volume make them ideal for loading large amounts of drugs and conjugation/complexation of other components on the surface [119,120].

The use of silica nanoparticles for simultaneous codelivery of a hydrophobic drug (DOX) and siRNA (siBcl-2) was explored by Chen et al. [121]. Silica macroporous nanoparticles were conjugated with 3-isocyanatopropyltriethoxysilane to obtain an isocyanatopropyl-modified surface that could be further functionalized with a polyamidoamine dendrimer (PAMA) to confer nanoparticles with positive surface charge. DOX was encapsulated within the silica pores and siRNA was complexed to PAMA. They successfully delivered DOX and siRNA into A2780/AD ovarian cancer cells. Cell viability of cells treated with a low concentration of DOX (0.01 μM) encapsulated within silica particles complexed to siBcl-2 decreased down to 50% compared to cells treated with the same concentration of free DOX. These encouraging results showed that at a nontoxic concentration of DOX, cell viability can be reduced

down to 50% when DOX is encapsulated and codelivered with siBcl-2.

To confer good particle dispersion and biocompatibility to mesoporous silica nanoparticles, Meng et al. [122] coated them with phosphonate groups. This also allowed for adsorption of molecules such as PEI for complexing siRNA. To improve hydrophilicity of PEI-coated nanoparticles, they were treated with a solution of bovine serum albumin before being transferred to the culture media. Silica particles were coated with various molecular weights PEI, and toxicity, cell uptake, and siRNA complexation were studied. Particles coated with high molecular weight PEI (25 kD) presented greater cell uptake and better knock down efficiency (90%) but also greater toxicity, compared with lower molecular weight PEI (1.8 and 10 kD). PEI 10 kD nanoparticles were nontoxic when the concentration was kept below 100 μg/mL and presented the same cellular uptake as PEI 25 kD nanoparticles when cultured with KB-V1 resistant cancer cells at various concentrations for 24 h. DOX was encapsulated in the mesoporous silica pores through electrostatic complexation to negatively charged silica. DOX was released intracellularly due to the lysosomal low pH due to the sponge proton effect of PEI that disrupts the lysosome, compared to the physiological 7.4 pH.

When using PEI 10 kD coated nanoparticles loaded with DOX (PEI-DOX), more DOX was found inside cells compared to cells cultured with free DOX. However, no presence of DOX was found in the nucleus, suggesting a need to suppress P-gp protein to avoid rapid extrusion of DOX from the cell before the drug can penetrate the nucleus. When PEI-coated silica particles loaded with DOX and complexed to siP-gp (PEI-DOX-siPgp) were cultured with KB-V1 cells, a significant increase of DOX in the nucleus was observed. The IC_{50} of KB-V1 cells was 2.5 times lower when treated with PEI-DOX-siPgp compared to cells treated with free DOX, even though it was not as low as the IC_{50} of nonresistant cells. Experiments targeting simultaneously Bcl-2 and P-gp while administering DOX on KB-V1 cells did not seem to improve cytotoxicity of DOX and failed in restoring sensitivity of resistant cancer cells to normal levels. This indicates that the dual targeting (Bcl-2 and P-gp) strategy to overcome cancer resistance is cell type specific. Mesoporous silica nanoparticles for the inhalatory administration route to treat lung cancer cells were synthesized. This route is favored because it avoids systemic toxicity and first-pass metabolic degradation [21]. DOX and cisplatin were loaded into the nanoparticle pores. Two different reduced siRNAs were conjugated to pyridylthiolsilica nanoparticles via disulfide bonds. Nanoparticles were decorated with LHRH peptide to target A549 human adenocarcinoma cells. LHRH was conjugated to HS-PEG-COOH to obtain LHRH-PEG-SH, which was then covalently linked to silica nanoparticles. The hydrodynamic diameter of the fully functionalized nanoparticle measured by dynamic light scattering was ≈200 nm. Cell viability of cells cultured with silica nanoparticles for 24 h decreased down to 95%

at a concentration of 1 mg/mL. This low cytotoxicity, compared with other formulations used for delivery of siRNA, is probably due to the lack of positively charged polymer on the surface. Confocal experiments showed release of DOX in the perinuclear region. According to RT-PCR results, the effectiveness of siBcl-2-silica and siMRP1-silica nanoparticles in silencing genes in the condition mentioned above was of 56% for Bcl-2 and 58% for MRP1. Cell viability of cells treated with a mixture of targeted nanoparticles carrying siBcl-2, siMRP1, DOX, and cisplatin for 24 h at a drug concentration of 1 µg/mL decreased down to 25% compared to a decrease down to 85% when treated with a mixture of free cisplatin and DOX. The IC_{50} dose of a mixture of free drugs was 30 times greater when compared to cells treated with the aforementioned mixture.

To be able to track the fate of the codelivery system once in contact with cells, Li et al. [123] opted to use QDs. QDs have been widely used in biomedicine as imaging and delivery systems [32,124–126]. CdSe/ZnSe QDs were coated with β-cyclodextrin, which was previously functionalized with L-arginine or L-histidine to confer positive charge and biocompatibility. DOX was encapsulated within the β-cyclodextrin rings. siRNA against MRP1 was complexed onto the nanoparticle surface. A release study of DOX from the QD-DOX showed that more DOX was released at endosomal pH (5.0) compared to physiological pH (7.4). The authors attributed this to the fact that DOX is protonated at low pH, leading to increased solubility. siRNA-DOX-QD were internalized by DOX resistant HeLa cells (HeLa/Dox) within 1 h of incubation. The nanoparticles were confined to vesicles and attached to the membrane, probably due to its positive charge. Within 3 h, nanoparticles were released to the cytosol after rupture of the vesicles and rapidly dispersed throughout the cytoplasm. By using confocal, they observed that DOX was able to reach the nucleus when cells were incubated with siMRP1-DOX-QD, indicating that these particles were also able to silence the gene encoding for the P-gp protein. Cell viability of DOX-resistant HeLa cells was assessed by treatment with various formulations maintaining the concentration of DOX fixed at 1 µg/mL during 72 h. Cytotoxicity of siMDR1-DOX-QD presented a 3-fold increase compared to DOX-QD and a 5-fold increase when compared to free DOX.

4.12 POLYMER-BASED NANOPARTICLES

Polymer-based nanoparticles have been used as delivery systems for a variety of drugs, proteins, and nucleotides [9,10,127,128]. Due to the tunability, biocompatibility, and high transfection rate of DNA and siRNA, polymeric nanoparticles are the preferred nanosystem to codeliver a drug and siRNA (Table 4.1). PEI is a cationic polymer, and it has been widely used as a major component for nonviric delivery carriers of siRNA due to its high siRNA complexation and its proton sponge effect for endosomal escape of the cargo to the cytosol [129]. Since high molecular weight PEI nanocarriers are toxic, Cao et al. [130] incorporated

polycaprolactone (PCL) biodegradable structures containing disulfide or ester covalent linkages between low molecular weight PEI chains. Phosphate species negatively charged in the siRNA were complexed onto the positively charged nitrogen species of the nanoparticles by electrostatic interactions. They studied cytotoxicity of siRNA conjugated PEI-PCL polyplexes at different nitrogen (N)/phosphate (P) ratios and found an optimum N/P ratio of 30, which decreased viability down to 65%. To improve cytotoxicity, the carrier surface was modified with PEG chains, which has been proved to provide stability and reduce toxicity of nanoparticles.

It has also been reported that PEG can hinder the complexation of siRNA; hence, Cao et al. [130] proposed a hierarchical assembly strategy, in which PEGylation is performed after complexation of siRNA to the nanocarrier. DOX was loaded to PEI-PCL micelles using a chloroform/water mixture under sonication. The treatment of hepatic cancer cells with DOX causes an increase in the production of BCl-2 protein as a defense mechanism that leads to resistance of cancer cells to the drug. They studied the ability of the nanocarriers to diminish the upregulation of BCl-2 protein caused by the administration of DOX. Bcl-2 siRNA—DOX loaded nanocarriers were capable of decreasing the overexpression of Bcl-2 protein induced by DOX. The 3-[4,5-dimethylthiazole-2-yl]-2,5-diphenyltetrazolium bromide (MTT) assay is a colorimetric assay for assessing cell metabolic activity. NAD(P)H-dependent cellular oxidoreductase enzymes may, under defined conditions, reflect the number of viable cells present. These enzymes are capable of reducing the tetrazolium dye MTT to its insoluble formazan, which has a purple color. The MTT assay (succinate dehydrogenase activity) has been widely used to assess cell viability. However, one must consider that the enzymatic reduction of MTT to MTT formazan is catalyzed by mitochondrial succinate dehydrogenase. Hence, the MTT assay is dependent on mitochondrial respiration and indirectly serves to assess the cellular energy capacity of a cell. The MTT assay is a colorimetric reaction that can easily be measured from cell monolayers that have been plated in 35 mm dishes or multiwell plates. The MTT assay is a sensitive and reliable indicator of the cellular metabolic activity and is preferred over the other methods measuring this endpoint like the ATP and ^{3}H-thymidine incorporation assay. The MTT assay is done to evaluate the cell viability of all cells in culture, namely, the peripheral blood mononuclear cells (PBMCs)-derived monocytes, brain microvascular endothelial cells, and national homelessness advice service. Cell viability is also tested in the monocytes prior to being infected by HIV-1 as well as at 7 days postinfection. The ability of the codelivery system in reducing cell viability was measured using MTT assay. Nanocarriers loaded with BCl-2 siRNA and DOX were incubated for 96 h with hepatic cancer cells. Cell viability was reduced down to 40% at the highest concentration of DOX (1 µM) when using Bcl-2 siRNA; however, for scrambled siRNA, cell viability was reduced down to 60%. When using folate receptor–targeted

TABLE 4.1
Nanosystems to Codeliver siRNA and Drugs to Overcome Multidrug Resistance in Cancer Therapy

System	Type of Nanoparticle	SiRNA	Drug	Size and Zeta Potential	Cell Line	Targeting	Reference
FA-PEG-PGA coated onto PEI-PCL	Cationic biodegradable polymeric	Bcl-2 electrostatic complexed	DOX encapsulated	150 nm, −5 mV	Bcl-7402 hepatoma	FA	[130]
FA-PEG-PGA coated onto PEI-PCL	Cationic biodegradable polymeric	Bcl-2 electrostatic complexed	DOX encapsulated	150 nm, −5 mV	C6 glioma	FA	[131]
PEI-SA	Cationic polymeric	VEGF complexed	DOX encapsulated	303 nm, 64 mV	HUH-7		[132]
Octasilsesquioxanep(L-Lys)	Cationic biodegradable polymeric	Cye3 complexed	DOX conjugate biodegradable disulfide spacer.		Hepatocarcinoma U87 Glioblastoma	RGD	[133]
Dendritic polyamine-β-CD	Cationic biodegradable polymeric	EGFR complexed	Erlotinib or SAHA encapsulated	200–400 nm	U78 glioblastoma	mAb-EGFR	[49]
PLGA-PEI-Biotin	Cationic biodegradable polymeric	P-gp complexed	PAC encapsulated	237 nm, −12.2 mV	JC breast adenocarcinoma	Biotin	[134]
mPEG-PCL-PPEEA	Cationic biodegradable polymeric	Plk1 complexed	PAC encapsulated	50 nm	MDA-MB-435 breast carcinoma		[40]
P(MDS-co-CES)	Cationic biodegradable polymeric	Bcl-2 complexed	PAC encapsulated	160 nm, 44 mV	MDA-MB-231 breast carcinoma		[135]
PEO-b-PCL	Biodegradable polymeric	MDR-1 complexed	DOX conjugate pH-sensitive hydrazone linkage	103 nm, 4 mV	MDA-MB-435 breast carcinoma	RGD TAT	[136]
PDMAEMA—PCL—PDMAEMA	Cationic biodegradable polymeric	VEGF GFP	PAC encapsulated	95 nm, 35 mV	PC3 prostate adenocarcinoma		[137]
mono-Pal-MTO di-Pal-MTO	Cationic mono-di lipidic	Mcl-1 complexed	MTO conjugated	210 nm	KB nasopharynx carcinoma		[138]
LPD LPD-II	Cationic liposome Anionic liposome	VEGF c-Myc complexed	Dox Dox complexed	Cationic liposome 135 nm, 35 mV Anionic liposome 62 nm, −19 mV.	HT-1080 fibrosarcoma	AA	[139]

nanocarriers loaded with Bcl-2 siRNA, cell viability was reduced down to 5% at the same DOX concentration. This indicates the synergistic effect a codelivery system has on cell metabolism and the importance of developing targeted codelivery systems. Further investigations *in vivo* using the same system were carried out [131]. By using Western blot and Tunel assay, they studied the effect of different treatments on apoptotic response of C6 glioma cells. They concluded that the synthesis of Bcl-2 protein is DOX dose dependent. They also noticed that at high DOX concentration (15 µg/mL), the protein Bax is inhibited and there is a higher presence of cleaved caspase 3.

Another strategy to reduce cytotoxicity of high molecular weight PEI is by grafting stearic acid (SA) to PEI through carbodiimide conjugation using 1-ethyl-3-(3-dimethylamino-propyl) carbodiimide (EDC) reaction [132]. PEI-SA micelles were formed using the oil in water (o/w) solvent evaporation method, obtaining small ($\approx$51 nm) and cationic ($\approx$64 mV) micelles. These micelles contain both a hydrophobic core that can encapsulate a hydrophobic drug and a hydrophilic cationic shell capable of complexing siRNA. DOX was encapsulated into the micelles by mild agitation. siRNA against the vascular endothelial growth factor (VEGF) was complexed onto the nanoparticle surface. VEGF is a growth factor over secreted by tumors to force the formation of new blood vessels by stimulating the growth and division of endothelial cells to provide oxygen-rich blood to tumor cells. This process is known as angiogenesis, and it has been proven to be necessary for the tumor to survive. By blocking the formation of new blood vessels irrigating the tumor with oxygen, tumor growth can be stopped. PEI-SA/DOX reduced the volume of the tumor down to 13% relative to the control. When using PEI-SA/DOX/viVEGF, the tumor was reduced down to 56.7%.

Another strategy to obtain biodegradable nanoparticles is by introducing the biodegradable polymer poly(ε-caprolactone) into the formulation [40]. Micelleplexes were synthesized using tri-block copolymers of poly(ethylene glycol)-b-poly(ε-caprolactone)-b-poly(2-aminoethylethylene phosphate) (mPEG-b-PCL-b-PPEE). PAC was encapsulated through hydrophobic–hydrophobic interactions. siRNA to silence Plk-1, a serine/threonine protein kinase overexpressed in some tumors, was complexed on the positive surface of the micelle. They studied MDA-MB-435 cell viability *in vitro* and *in vivo* when codelivering PAC and siPlk-1. They concluded that the use of a codelivery system requires one thousand-fold less PAC required for monotherapy. Micelleplexes carrying PAC were administered along with micelleplexes complexed to siPlk-1 to mice bearing an MDA-MB-435 tumor. Micelleplexes carrying PAC and complexed to siPlk-1 showed a great decrease in tumor volume when compared to the control. These results clearly indicate that it is necessary to codeliver both the drug and the siRNA in the same system.

A different strategy to achieve biodegradability is by incorporating hydrophilic cholesterol into a hydrophobic cationic polymer [135]. Poly[(N-methyldietheneamine

sebacate)-co-[(cholesteryl oxocarbonylamido ethyl) methyl bis(ethylene) ammonium bromide] sebacate] (P(MDS-co-CES)) was self-assembled into a cationic biodegradable nanoparticle. The hydrophobic drug PAC was added into the solution at the moment of self-assembly in order to be encapsulated in the nanoparticle through hydrophobic–hydrophobic interactions. siBcl-2 was complexed onto the nanoparticle surface *via* electrostatic interaction. Synergistic effects between siBcl-2 and the encapsulated drug were studied in breast adenocarcinoma MDA-MB-231 cells. Cell viability decreased from 78% to 59% and from 58% to 39% in the presence of siRNA at PAC concentrations of 100 and 400 nM, respectively. As the cytotoxicity of the siRNA was only 8%, there was indeed a synergistic effect associated with the codelivery of PAC and siRNA, possibly because the suppression of the antiapoptotic activity of Bcl-2 by the siRNA made cells more sensitive to PAC.

The biodegradable polymer PLGA was mixed with PEI to form micelles using a water-in-oil (W/O) emulsion [134]. PAC was encapsulated during the emulsion. SiPgp was complexed through electrostatic interactions to the nanoparticle and increased PAC uptake by resistant breast cancer cells. P-gp silencing increased intracellular PAC accumulation *in vitro*, and it enhanced *in vivo* activity of PAC, which translated in a reduction of tumor growth.

Another strategy to complex negative siRNA onto a nanoparticle is by grafting a positive polymer chain onto a biodegradable neutral nanoparticle after it is formed [136]. The poly(ethylene oxide)-block-poly(ε-caprolactone) (PEOb-PCL) polymer was used as a backbone to ensemble a biodegradable polymer that could further be functionalized with different moieties. Polyamine was attached to the PCL block to allow complexation of the siRNA through electrostatic interactions. A pH-sensitive hydrazone link was conjugated to other PCL blocks to covalently conjugate DOX. The cell penetrating peptide TAT and the integrin $R_v\beta_3$-specific ligand (RGD4C) were attached to the PEO block to facilitate cell internalization and uptake. The functionalized polymers self-assembled into micelles of $\approx$103 nm and $\approx$4.23 mV.

Previous studies from the same group [136], in which they delivered DOX using nanoparticles, showed that DOX released in the cytoplasm was pumped out of the cells and failed to accumulate in the nucleus of P-gp-overexpressing DOX-resistant cells. It has been demonstrated that nanocarriers bypass the P-gp pump efflux system expressed on the surface of the cell membrane [8], increasing the concentration of the drug in the cytoplasm. However, once the drug is released inside the cytoplasm, it still has to reach its site of action, the nucleus. By developing nanoparticles that release the drug in the cytoplasm and block the efflux pump present in the nuclear membrane, Xiong and Lavasanifar [136] increased the drug concentration in the nucleus of MDA-MB-435/LCC6MDR1-resistant cells. This increase translated in a greater decrease in cell viability.

A promising polymer used to deliver siRNA is the poly(2-(N, N-dimethyl aminoethyl) methacrylate), designated as

P(DMAEMA), due to its high efficiency in complexing and transfecting siRNA. However, P(DMEAMEA) is highly toxic to cells, limiting its use for biological applications. One strategy to decrease its toxicity is by adding a biodegradable polymer in the backbone. To do so, Zhu et al. [137] synthesized the block copolymer 2-(N, N-dimethyl aminoethyl) methacrylate-b-poly(ε-caprolactone)-b-2-(N, N-dimethyl aminoethyl) methacrylate (PDMAEMA-PCL-PDMAEMA) by free radical reversible addition-fragmentation chain transfer polymerization and assembled it into biodegradable cationic micelles. Nile red, a hydrophobic molecule used as a drug model, was encapsulated using hydrophobic–hydrophobic interactions after the micelle was formed. siRNA to silence GFP was complexed onto the nanoparticle surface. Codelivery of siGFP and Nile red into PC3 human prostate cancer cells was successfully achieved *in vitro*, according to confocal microscopy studies. PAC and siVEGF were both successfully incorporated into the micelle, which opens the possibility to use a biodegradable PDMAEMA carrier to codeliver siRNA and hydrophobic drugs.

A different approach to codeliver siRNA and a drug is by using a three-dimensional octasilsesquioxane cage as a backbone to grow poly(L-lysine) chains to create a nanoglobular system [133]. Two different moieties were conjugated to the p(L-Lys) chains to confer polyfunctionality to the nanoparticle. A biodegradable disulfide spacer was used to conjugate DOX. A PEG chain was used as a linker to attach RGD, a cyclic peptide that binds specifically to $\alpha_v\beta_3$ integrin, conferring the nanoparticle with specificity toward cancer cells that overexpress $\alpha_v\beta_3$ integrin. U78 glioblastoma cancer cells treated with free DOX reduced cell viability down to 50% at 6.50 µg/mL of DOX. Cells treated with conjugated DOX, reduced viability down to 50% at 0.7µg/mL of DOX, probably due to the ability of these nanoparticles to bypass the efflux effect. Colocalization studies showed that the siRNA was found mostly in the cytoplasm and not in endosomes and/or lysosomes.

Due to the heterogeneity of cells in tumors, a promising strategy to overcome cancer resistance of a heterogeneous population of cells is to target multiple signaling elements. The synthesis of a carrier capable of codelivering multiple therapeutic agents is required to achieve a cooperative effect. Kim et al. [49] developed a low toxicity, high transfection efficiency, and high solubility system capable of encapsulating hydrophobic drugs, complexing with siRNA and attaching to proteins. To do so, they synthesized a dendritic polyamine, which was further conjugated to a β-cyclodextrin to confer solubility to hydrophobic drugs [140]. In this case, erlotinib and suberoylanilide hydroxamic acid (SAHA) were encapsulated *via* hydrophobic–hydrophobic interactions with β-cyclodextrin. Furthermore, the presence of β-cyclodextrin decreased the cytotoxicity of the dendritic polyamines. The free amines in the dendritic polyamine served to complex siRNA and to conjugate an antibody to target EGFR. The final DexAM nanoparticle had significantly less amines available on its surface compared to commercially available transfection systems such as PEI,

lipofectamine 2000 (LF), and X-treme GENE (Xgene). Cytotoxicity of these compounds has been attributed to the presence of positive charge due to the amine groups, which are necessary for siRNA complexation and for endosomal escape once the nanoparticle is internalized in the cell. Cell viability of U87 glioblastoma cells was determined after incubation with DexMA, PEI, LF, and Xgene. Cell viability was decreased down to 90% for DexMA, 60% for PEI, and 25% for LF and Xgene, showing that DexMA is a highly biocompatible system compared to other commonly used transfection systems.

U78 glioblastoma cells were treated with EGFR targeted DexMA-siEGFR conjugated with and without erlotinib and SAHA. Targeting EGFR with nanoparticles has proven to be effective in increasing internalization of nanoparticles and in improving treatment of EGFR overexpressing cancer cells [141]. EGFR overexpression is correlated with cell survival and response to therapy. Erlotinib and SAHA have been shown to enhance the efficacy of other EGFR antagonists [142]. EGFR targeted DexMA-siEGFR without erlotinib reduced cell viability down to 50%; when using erlotinib conjugated nanoparticles, cell viability was reduced down to 30%. A similar trend was observed when comparing nanoparticles with and without SAHA.

4.13 LIPID-BASED NANOPARTICLES

Lipidic nanoparticles have been widely used for different biomedical and pharmaceutical applications [143–146]. Liposomes as drug delivery systems gain a lot of attention after DoxilR, a PEGylated liposome, was FDA approved to deliver DOX [147].

An interesting approach to incorporate an antineoplastic drug within a lipidic nanoparticle is by covalently attaching a positively charged drug to a lipidic chain to create an amphiphilic molecule that can be further used to self-assemble into a multilayer cationic nanoparticle. To do so, Chang et al. [138] covalently conjugated mitoxantrone (MTO) to either one or two chains of palmitoleyl to create monopalmitoleys-MTO (mono-Pal-MTO) and dipalmitoleys-MTO (di-Pal-MTO), respectively. The positive charge of the MTO confers cationic properties to the nanoparticle and allows complexation of siRNA by the electrostatic interaction within the layers of the nanoparticle (Figure 4.2). They studied the ability of this multilayer system to codeliver MTO and siRNA against Mcl-1, a Bcl-2-related gene, into human epithelial carcinoma KB cells. After 24 h of incubation, they observed a 68% reduction when using pal-MTO and 81% when using siRNA-pal-MTO compared to controls. Efficacy of the codelivery treatment in reducing tumor growth *in vivo* in mice bearing KB cell tumors was studied. A reduction in tumor volume after 20 days of starting the treatment down to 53.9% when using pal-MTO and 83.4% when using siRNApal-MTO compared to controls was observed (Figure 4.3).

The possibility of functionalizing lipids with molecules leads to a great variety of applications. For example,

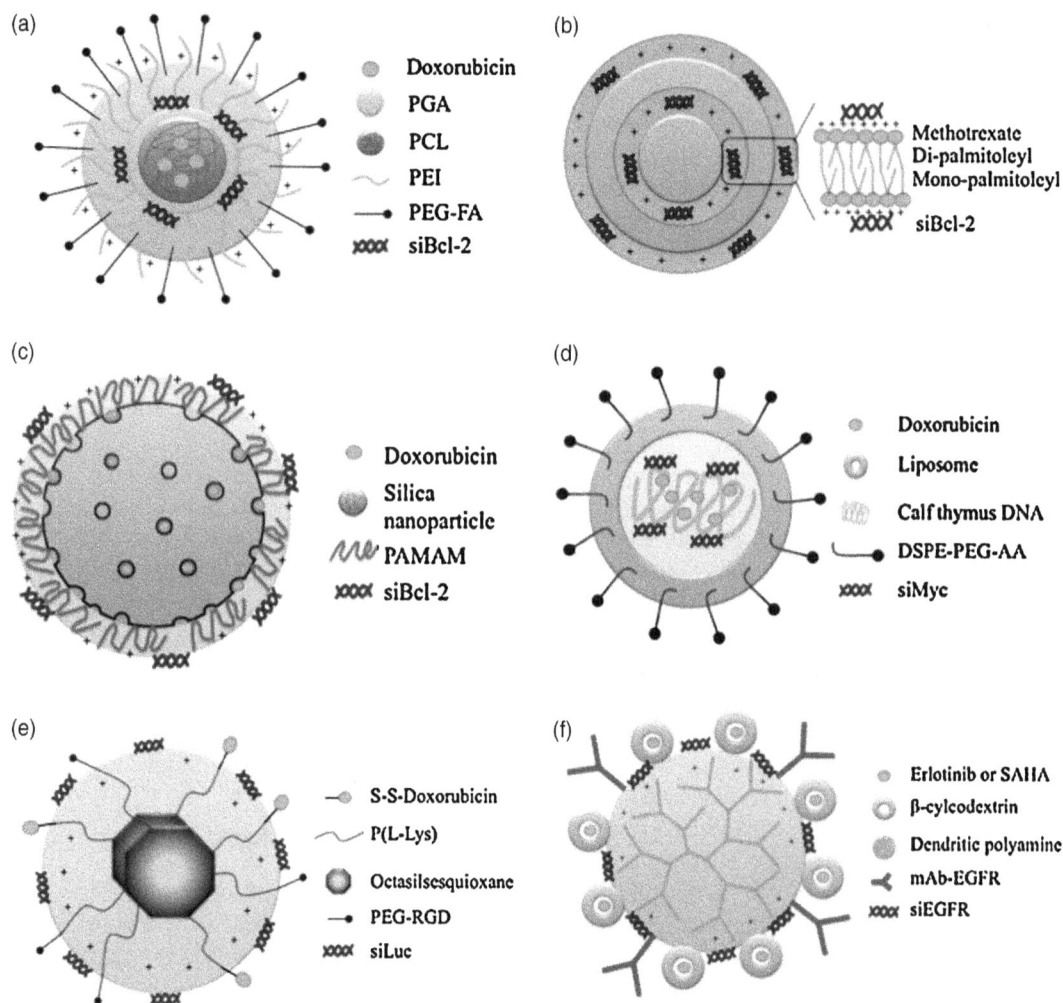

FIGURE 4.3 schematic representations of various types of nanoparticles to co-deliver siRNA and a chemotherapeutical agent. (a) Biodegradable nanoparticle [131], (b) cationic mono-, di-lipidic nanoparticle [138], (c) mesoporous silica nanoparticle [121], (d) liposome [139], (e) octasilesquioxane nanoparticle [133], (f) dendritic nanoparticle [49].

cationic liposome-DNA (LPD) was synthesized using the guanidine containing cationic lipid N, N-distearyl-N-methyl-N-2-(N-arginyl) aminoethyl ammonium chloride (DSAA) [139]. DOX was complexed to the negatively charged DNA and encapsulated within the liposome as cargo. siVEGF was complexed onto the liposome surface. Anionic liposome-DNA (LPD-II) was synthesized using the anionic lipid 2-di-(9Z-octadecenoyl)-sn-glycero-3-phosphate (DOPA) and cholesterol. DOX was complexed to the DNA and encapsulated within the liposome as cargo. The entrapment efficiency of DOX was low (10%) for LPD nanoparticles compared with LPD-II nanoparticles (90%). Leakage of DOX from LPD nanoparticles was reported, most likely due to the competition of cationic lipids for the negatively charged DNA, displacing the positively charged DOX. Small interference molecules siVEGF and siMyc, respectively, were complexed onto the liposome surface. Transfection efficiency of siRNA *in vitro* was high for LPD and low for LPD-II. Cytotoxicity studies showed that anionic liposomes, LPD-II, were nontoxic at every

concentration studied. However, cationic liposomes, LPD, were cytotoxic by increasing interleucine-2 (IL-12) and decreasing white blood cells and platelets. Both systems were capable of inhibiting tumor growth significantly when compared to the untreated group after systemic intravenous injection in mice.

PEGylated LPD [148] were decorated with NGR (aspargine-glycine-arginine) moiety to target amino peptidase N (CD13) expressed in tumor cells and tumor vascular endothelium. Delivery and efficiency of siMyc in mice by LPD-PEG-NGR was studied in CD13 expressing cells HT-1080 and CD13 nonexpressing HT-29 cells. siRNA was efficiently delivered to the cytoplasm and c-Myc was downregulated in HT-1080 cells but not in HT-29 cells. When codelivering siMyc and DOX using LPD-PEG-NGR, an accumulation of siRNA and DOX in the tumor tissue was observed which translated in an enhanced therapeutic effect.

As new lipids are synthesized, new liposomic formulations become available. In this case, cationic liposomes (DGL) were synthesized using a new N′,N″-dioleylglutamide

(DG) cationic lipid [40], 1,2-dioleoyl-sn-glycero-3- phosphoethanolamine (DOPE), and cholesterol [149]. The mitogen-activated protein kinase (MEK) inhibitor PD0325901 was encapsulated through hydrophobic–hydrophobic interactions in the liposome. The inhibition of MEK results in inhibition of phosphorylation and inactivation of the MAPK/ERK signaling pathway that in cancer is known to be involved in proliferation and resistance to apoptosis. The myeloid cell leukemia sequence 1 (Mcl-1) gene has been reported to be overexpressed in tumor cells that presented resistance to chemotherapeutical agents. siRNA against Mcl-1, was complexed to the cationic liposomes. PD0325901 containing liposomes (PDGL) and siMcdl-1 were incubated with KB tumor cells to study the ability of this carrier to codeliver both cargos. PDGL liposomes were capable of codelivering ERK inhibitor and siMcl-1 in KB tumor cells. Western blot shows inhibition of both phosphorylated ERK1/2 protein and MCl-1 protein when treated with PDGL-siMcl-1, indicating not only the feasibility of codelivery but also the therapeutic effect of downregulating both proteins. Cytotoxicity of KB tumor cells was studied when treated with free PD0325901. At a low concentration (0.72 µg/mL) of PD0325901, cell viability was not affected by the MEK inhibitor. However, when the same concentration was delivered using the cationic liposome with siMcl-1, cell viability was reduced down to 10%. Codelivery of siMcl-1and the drug using cationic liposomes (PDGL-siMcl-1) in BALB/c mice injected with KB cells resulted in suppression of the tumor size by 79% when compared to the control. Suppression of the tumor growth was greater when using PDGL-siMcl-1 compared to any other cotreatment studied.

The results of tumor growth suppression using liposomes as a codelivery system are promising and encouraging. However, due to the lack of systemic delivery systems currently available, Shim et al. [150] developed new cationic liposomes using oligolysine-based lipids and studied their suitability as systemic codelivery systems. Different formulations using varying amounts of lysine, DOPE, cholesterol, and PEG were synthesized. The final multilayer cationic liposomes were systematically studied to determine their ability to complex siRNA and their cytotoxicity when cultured with cancer cells.

In order to increase the transfection efficiency of liposomes, Yu et al. [151] synthesized 1,2-dioleoyl-snglycero-3-ethylphosphocholine (EDOPC)-based cationic lipid nanoparticles (cSLN), which have been shown to have higher transfection efficiency than formulations using other lipids [152]. The structure of liposomes allows the encapsulation of poorly soluble drugs, such as PAC, in the core of the cSLN matrix without altering the chemical structure of the drug. This type of encapsulation allows a gradual release of the drug, instead of a burst release. The cationic nature of the lipids that form the liposome allow for negative moieties, such as siMcl-1, to complex onto the liposome surface through electrostatic interactions. KB cancer cells treated with free PAC and free siMcl-1 show a small decrease in cell viability down to approximately 90%. Cells treated with cSLN liposomes carrying siMcl-1 decreased viability down to 58%. When cells were treated with cSLN liposomes carrying both siMCl-1 and PAC, viability was decreased down to 38%. Mice bearing a KB tumor were treated with free PAC and cSLN liposomes carrying siMcl-1. Tumor volume was reduced 48% compared to the control. When mice were treated with cSLN liposomes carrying both PAC and siMcl-1, the volume was reduced 88% compared to the control.

Saad et al. [153] studied the possibility of codelivering DOX and two different siRNA: siBcl-2 and siMRP1. They synthesized a liposome using DOTAP, encapsulated DOX *via* hydrophobic–hydrophobic interactions, and complexed siRNA through electrostatic interactions. They observed that the mere use of liposome-siMRP1 caused a decrease in small cell lung carcinoma cancer cells. A decrease in an effective efflux mechanism caused cell death, probably due to the fact that MRP1 proteins are involved not only in the efflux of drugs from the cell but also in detoxifying cells of their own metabolic products. An accumulation of undesired products could cause cells to enter apoptosis. When DOX was added to the liposome-siMRP1, cell viability was significantly decreased. As reported before, liposomes-siBcl-2 reduce cell viability to a certain extent by promoting cells to enter apoptosis. However, liposomes-siBcl-2 carrying DOX decreased cell viability to a greater extent. Liposomes-siBcl-2-siMRP1 carrying DOX decreased cell viability down to 5%, the most effective treatment. By blocking two resistance mechanisms at the same time while administering DOX, in a single carrier, higher levels of effectiveness can be achieved. However, due to the nonspecificity of this system to target cancer cells, adverse effects of DOX toward healthy cells when used *in vivo* may be significant.

4.14 LIPID-BASED DELIVERY

Among various strategies to overcome challenges of siRNA therapeutics, lipid-based nanoparticles have great potential due to their biocompatibility and low toxicity in comparison to inorganic, viral, and synthetic polymers. In particular, cationic lipids have emerged as attractive siRNA delivery vehicles owing to their electrostatic interaction with nucleic acids, high transfection efficiency into mammalian cells, and improved pharmacokinetic profiles. DOTAP is a type of cationic lipid that is commonly used in laboratories and is also commercially available. Kim et al. demonstrated a liposomal siRNA/DOTAP/Cholesterol platform for liver-targeting delivery of siRNAs against HBV [154]. Yagi et al. demonstrated a siRNA delivery complex utilizing cationic DOTAP attached to egg phosphatidylcholine and PEG lipid in a weight ratio of 24:14.8. This complex has been shown to inhibit tumor growth in a xenograft cancer model via systemic injection [155].

For *in vivo* delivery studies, stable nucleic acid-lipid particles (SNALPs) have been formulated and tested in multiple disease models. SNALPs consist of a lipid bilayer of fusogenic and cationic lipids entrapping nucleic acids in the core. The surface of the SNALP is coated with PEG to provide enhanced hydrophilicity for improved stability in the serum. The half-life of a siRNA-SNALP complex is much longer compared to unformulated siRNA. An HBV targeted siRNA-SNALP has shown specific reduction in HBV mRNA when intravenously administered in a mouse model of HBV replication at a dosage of 3 mg/kg/day [156]. A siRNA-SNALP delivery complex was also tested against Ebola virus–related genes in a guinea pig model [157]. Furthermore, an ApoB-specific siRNA encapsulated in a SNALP has shown to have N90% maximal silencing effect of ApoB mRNA in the liver upon a single systemic dosage of 2.5 mg/kg in cynomolgus monkeys [158]. Thus, RNAi-mediated gene silencing in nonhuman primates has clearly demonstrated the therapeutic potential of this new class of drug using SNALP technology.

Although cationic lipid-based siRNA delivery has demonstrated potential in therapy in various disease models, several hurdles remain to enter commercialization of this class of drugs. Toxicity and immediate immune responses elicited by lipid-based delivery designs must be further investigated, and it is likely that further thoughtful modifications will need to be devised.

4.15 BIOCONJUGATED siRNAs

In addition to chemically modifying siRNA or incorporating it into nanoparticles, covalently conjugating biological agents to siRNA cargo is an alternative method to overcome barriers to siRNA efficacy *in vivo*. Such conjugated delivery systems currently include cholesterol, various peptides, antibodies, aptamers, and biopolymers with various physicochemical profiles, as summarized in Table 4.2.

Cholesterol conjugation of siRNA facilitates cellular import and improves intracellular activity of siRNA when injected systemically. Cholesterol in circulation is transported by lipoproteins in serum and taken up by hepatocytes through low density lipoprotein receptor-mediated endocytosis. Apolipoprotein B (apoB) targeted siRNA conjugated with cholesterol showed enhanced stability in serum and greater suppression in apoB mRNA levels in the liver [159].

Biofunctional or cell-penetrating peptides can be covalently conjugated to siRNA for improved targeting of cancer cells. In a study by Choi et al., siRNA conjugated with branched PEG was functionalized with a cell penetrating peptide, Hph1, as well as a cationic self-crosslinked fusogenic KALA peptide to form a polyelectrolyte complex micelle for gene silencing in MDA-MB-435 breast cancer cells [180]. In an attempt to reduce innate immune responses, siRNAs directed against the p38MAP kinase conjugated to the HIV TAT cell penetrating peptide were intratracheally administered into the lung [160].

For targeted delivery of siRNA to specific tissues or cell types, antibodies or aptamers are being conjugated directly to siRNAs. A considerable number of antibody-based drugs including trastuzumab, pertuzumab, and cetuximab are currently given to cancer patients with great success. Antibodies conjugated to chemotherapeutic small molecules have also shown successful therapeutic results, with TDM-1 serving as a prominent example of this class of antibody conjugate [181]. Recently, an anti-EGFR antibody conjugated to a siRNA targeted to KRAS has shown activity *in vitro* and *in vivo* in colon cancer resistant to EGFR inhibitors [173].

An alternative target agent that can be conjugated to siRNA is the nucleic acid–based aptamer. These aptamers consist of synthetic short single-stranded RNA or DNA ligands that have been selected for target binding with high affinity and specificity. Ever since the generation of aptamers that target the extracellular domains of transmembrane receptors overexpressed in cancer cells, aptamers have gained extensive attention as active targeting moieties for cancer therapeutic agents including siRNA [182]. Meyerholz et al. developed an aptamer conjugated RNA-only approach for prostate cancer therapy. When siRNAs targeting the prosurvival genes, Plk1 and Bcl2, were conjugated with aptamers that specifically binds to prostate-specific membrane antigen (PSMA) and injected intratumorally in a xenograft cancer model, inhibition in tumor growth was observed [174]. Despite the high specificity and binding affinity of aptamers, aptamer-siRNA conjugation faces barriers arising from, among other causes, stability issues due to unprotected negative charge.

In addition to being used as for direct coupling to siRNAs both antibodies and aptamers can be used to target nanoparticles containing siRNAs. As a surface targeting moiety, different types of aptamer facilitate nanoparticle delivery to the specific tumor sites.

4.16 TARGETED DELIVERY

Significant advances have been made in the development of efficient siRNA delivery in nonviral vector systems, such as cationic lipids and polymers. However, a major problem with these approaches is that a large amount of siRNA has to be administered for efficient gene silencing. Moreover, cell type-specific targeting can prevent off-target effects, thus reducing the side effects of the therapeutics. A common approach for targeted delivery of siRNA to specific cells or tissues is conjugation to ligands such as antibodies, aptamers, and peptides which specifically bind to the corresponding moieties on target cells. Song and colleagues developed a protamine-antibody fusion protein for systemic and targeted siRNA delivery [170]. They fused protamine, a protein that binds nucleic acids, to a Fab directed against the human immunodeficiency virus type 1 (HIV-1) envelope protein and mixed the siRNA with the fusion protein. Treatment with the fusion protein mixed with siRNA targeted to the HIV-1 gag protein suppressed viral replication in infected primary T cells. Kumar et al. demonstrated T cell-specific siRNA delivery in a preclinical animal model

TABLE 4.2
Types of Conjugated siRNA

Conjugation	Structure	Function	Example
Cholesterol		Increases hydrophobicity for stability, free nucleases resistance of siRNA in serum, and mRNA suppression by polyplexes	Cholesterol (C27) [159–162] Cholesteryloxypropan-1-amine (COPA) and cholesteryl-2 aminoethylcarbamate (CAEC) [163]
Peptide		Cell-penetration peptides (CPP) is able to cross the biological membrane for intracellular delivery	TAT [164,165] MPG8 [166] Pep-3 [167] Penetratin [160] Transportan [168]
Antibody		Antibody increases the target ability by ligand binding to specific receptors of cancer	Trastuzumab anti-TENB2, anti-NaPi2b [169] F105-P [170] F5-P [171] HIRMAb, TfRMAb [172] Anti-EGFR [173]
Aptamer		Aptamer selectively deliver siRNA to affected tissue via specific binding with reduced side effects	PSMA aptamer [174–177] BAFF-R aptamer [178] HER2 aptamer [179]

[183]. In this chapter, a CD7-specific single-chain antibody was conjugated to oligo-9-arginine peptide (scFvCD7-9R) for T cell-specific siRNA delivery in humanized mice. Antiviral siRNAs complexed to scFvCD7-9R were shown to be delivered to naïve T cells and suppressed HIV replication in HIV-infected mice.

Nucleic-acid aptamers, which are normally selected from a large random-sequence pool to bind to a specific target molecule, have been explored for targeted siRNA delivery as an alternative to antibodies. Aptamers have advantages, such as high selective binding to proteins and receptors, ready-to-use chemical synthesis, process-compatible storability, and low immunogenicity [57]. McNamara II et al. have developed aptamer-siRNA chimeric RNAs for targeted delivery of siRNA [175]. The aptamer portions of the chimeras were introduced for specific binding to PSMA, a cell-surface receptor overexpressed in prostate cancer cells and tumor endothelium, whereas the siRNA portion targeted the expression of survival genes. The chimeric RNA was demonstrated to bind only PSMA-expressing cells, resulting in depletion of siRNA target proteins and cell death. In addition, treatment with the chimeric RNA specifically inhibited tumor growth and mediated tumor regression in a xenograft model of prostate cancer. The aptamer-siRNA chimera is a promising targeted approach for siRNA delivery because RNA is not recognized by antibodies. However, more RNA and DNA aptamers must be developed for specific cancer or disease markers to expand the use of aptamer delivery approach. Recently, extensive studies have been performed to develop an RNA nanoparticle-based siRNA vector [184]. Packaging RNA is a 117-nt RNA molecule that constitutes one of the six packaging RNA subunits of the phi29 bacteriophage DNA packaging motor [185]. Chemically modified and folate receptor-targeted packaging RNA nanoparticles for siRNA delivery showed high *in vivo* stability with a blood half-life of 5 to 10h and were retained in cancer tissue for more than 8h. Tumor targeted delivery and efficacy of gene silencing have also been in xenograft tumor models [185–187].

Another strategy for enhanced delivery of siRNA involves covalent conjugates to cell penetrating peptides (CPPs) or protein transduction domains [188]. The cationic nature of CPPs is crucial for their ability to bind and pass through the anionic cellular membrane. CPP conjugates of siRNA exhibited gene-silencing effects on target receptor proteins in various mammalian cell lines. However, conjugations of cationic peptides to anionic siRNA may neutralize and reduce the penetrating efficacy of these peptides [188]. In addition, CPP-siRNA conjugates may exhibit cytotoxicity caused by cell membrane perturbation or immunogenicity [160].

Recently, we have developed a new approach for targeted delivery and expression of siRNAs *in vivo* using DNA based siRNA expression nanocassettes and receptor-targeted nanoparticles [189]. This new nanoparticle consists of an amphiphilic polymer-coated QD conjugated to 10 to 20 DNA nanocassettes that contain a U6 promoter and shRNA gene for *in vivo* siRNA gene expression following delivery to target cells. The nanoparticle was conjugated to the amino terminal fragment of urokinase plasminogen activator (uPA), which targets its cellular receptor, uPAR. This receptor is highly expressed in tumor, angiogenic endothelial and stromal cells in many types of human cancers [190,191]. Targeted delivery and gene-silencing efficiency of firefly luciferase siRNA nanogenerators were demonstrated in tumor cells and in animal tumor models. Moreover, delivery of survivin siRNA expressing nanocassettes into tumor cells induced apoptotic cell death and sensitized cells to chemotherapeutic drugs. In cultured cells, the extent of targeted gene knockdown by survivin siRNA-expressing DNA nanocassettes using the uPAR-targeted nanoparticle delivery system was similar to that achieved with SV40-nuclear localization signal- (NLS-) mediated internalization of the QD-survivin siRNA nanocassettes. However, SV40-NLS-QD-siRNA nanocassettes could not be used for *in vivo* delivery due to their lack of specificity. These findings suggest that a receptor-targeted nanoparticle carrier allows efficient delivery into target tissues as well as intracellular delivery.

4.17 CLINICAL TRIALS

Currently, there are six cancer clinical trials underway using nanoparticle-based siRNA delivery, all in Phase I, evaluating the initial safety and utility of these treatments. All the nanoparticle-formulated siRNA delivery systems for cancer therapy that are currently in clinical trials are based on polymers or liposomes. Since CALLA-01 was developed for the first siRNA phase I trial by Calando Pharmaceuticals, several other companies, including Tekmira, Alnylam, Silence Therapeutics, Marina, and others, have introduced siRNA nanoparticle products in either the preclinical or clinical phases. Silenseed Ltd (Jerusalem, Israel) initiated a phase I dose-escalation trial for siG12D LODER local drug eluter (LODER) (http://www.clinicaltrials.gov/ct2/show/NCT01188785).

The siG12D LODER is a miniature biodegradable polymeric matrix that encompasses siRNA target to KRASG12D mRNA (siG12D) drug, designed to release the drug locally within a pancreatic tumor, for a prolonged period of 8 weeks. The siG12D LODER is injected into the patient's tumor with needle during an endoscopic ultrasound biopsy procedure. The majority of pancreatic ductal adenocarcinomas involves mutations in the KRAS oncogene with the most common being G12D; therefore, administration of KRASG12D siRNA has the potential to silence KRAS, leading to apoptosis of the cancer cells and, thereby, slowing and halting tumor growth. In an upcoming Phase II study, a single dose of 3,000 μg (eight 375-μg siG12D LODERs) will be administered to patients with unresectable, locally advanced pancreatic cancer, in combination with chemotherapy treatment (http://www.clinicaltrials.gov/ct2/show/NCT01676259).

4.18 CONCLUSIONS

Due to the tunable size of the nanocarriers, they can be formulated to penetrate tumors from the blood stream by the EPR effect while evading renal clearance from the body. This decreases the nonspecific distribution by increasing penetration to the tumor, increasing efficiency of the treatment. Even though the initial limitations of antineoplastic drugs were improved by the use of nanocarriers, new limitations have arisen. Cells have developed strategies to avoid cell death [192–195] by increasing their resistance to chemotherapy through the activation of efflux pumps to clear drugs from inside the cell and by increasing antiapoptotic pathways. By encapsulating drugs into nanoparticles that bypass the efflux pumps [8], drug efflux is reduced, hence increasing the intracellular concentration of the drug. The activation of antiapoptotic pathways is a defense mechanism that rescues cells from cell death. siRNA has the ability to disrupt cellular pathways by knocking down genes, opening the door to new treatments of diseases caused by aberrant gene expression. Rapid systemic clearances of siRNA by the renal system, lack of selectivity toward the desired tissue, and poor cell uptake have been reported, decreasing the effectiveness of gene therapy. The use of nanocarriers prevents both renal clearance and RNase degradation by protecting siRNA chains, increasing their half-life in blood. However, to be able to sensitize cancer cells, while retaining all the aforementioned advantages of using nanocarriers, both the siRNA and drug must be delivered in the same device. While some types of cancer cells were completely sensitized to antineoplastic drugs by siRNA therapy, others maintained their resistance to the treatment by compensating for the loss of one type of resistance mechanism by increasing other multidrug resistance mechanisms. Double sensitization, targeting two multidrug resistance mechanisms simultaneously while administering the drug, is a promising strategy to overcome multidrug resistance, but also prevents healthy cells from protecting themselves from antineoplastic agents, increasing the toxicity of the drug. Moreover, it appears that the effectiveness of decreasing cell viability by double sensitization is cell specific. Even though these strategies have been effective for sensitizing cancer cells, they target machinery that is common to both cancer and healthy cells. Specific targeting strategies to treat only cancer cells would be needed in order to reduce side effects of drugs *in vivo* when double-sensitizing cells. By functionalizing nanocarriers with different types of polymers, antibodies, ligands or small molecules, selectivity and cellular uptake can be significantly increased. It has been well established that cancer cells have the ability to avoid cell death by activating different antiapoptotic pathways. These pathways seem to be cell type specific and assault type specific. Due to the heterogeneity of tumors and the diversity of cancer cells, a "one type fits all" method of treatment seems unlikely to eradicate prove viable. However, a multi-sensitization individualized therapy designed specifically for each type of cancer cell may be more likely to prove viable to overcome cancer cell resistance.

REFERENCES

1. L. Mu, S.S. Feng, A novel controlled release formulation for the anticancer drug paclitaxel (Taxol®): PLGA nanoparticles containing vitamin E TPGS, *J. Control. Release* 86 (2003) 33–48. doi:10.1016/S0168-3659(02)00320-6.
2. A.J. Primeau, A. Rendon, D. Hedley, L. Lilge, I.F. Tannock, The distribution of the anticancer drug doxorubicin in relation to blood vessels in solid tumors, *Clin. Cancer Res.* 11 (2005) 8782–8788. doi:10.1158/1078-0432.CCR-05-1664.
3. T.W. Hambley, The influence of structure on the activity and toxicity of Pt anti-cancer drugs, *Coord. Chem. Rev.* 166 (1997) 181–223. doi:10.1016/S0010-8545(97)00023-4.
4. M.A. Izquierdo, R.H. Shoemaker, M.J. Flens, G.L. Scheffer, L. Wu, T.R. Prather, R.J. Scheper, Overlapping phenotypes of multidrug resistance among panels of human cancer-cell lines, *Int. J. Cancer* 65 (1996) 230–237. doi: 10.1002/(SICI)1097-0215(19960117)65:2<230::AID-IJC17>3.0.CO;2-H.
5. M.M. Gottesman, Mechanisms of cancer drug resistance, *Annu. Rev. Med.* 53 (2002) 615–627. doi:10.1146/annurev.med.53.082901.103929.
6. E.M. Leslie, R.G. Deeley, S.P.C. Cole, Multidrug resistance proteins: role of P-glycoprotein, MRP1, MRP2, and BCRP (ABCG2) in tissue defense, *Toxicol. Appl. Pharmacol.* 204 (2005) 216–237. doi:10.1016/j.taap.2004.10.012.
7. A. Shapira, Y.D. Livney, H.J. Broxterman, Y.G. Assaraf, Nanomedicine for targeted cancer therapy: towards the overcoming of drug resistance, *Drug Resist. Updat.* 14 (2011) 150–163. doi:10.1016/j.drup.2011.01.003.
8. T.-G. Iversen, T. Skotland, K. Sandvig, Endocytosis and intracellular transport of nanoparticles: Present knowledge and need for future studies, *Nano Today* 6 (2011) 176–185.
9. M.A. Phillips, M.L. Gran, N.A. Peppas, Targeted nanodelivery of drugs and diagnostics, *Nano Today* 5 (2010) 143–159. doi:10.1016/j.nantod.2010.03.003.
10. W.B. Liechty, N.A. Peppas, Expert opinion: responsive polymer nanoparticles in cancer therapy, *Eur. J. Pharm. Biopharm.* 80 (2012) 241–246. doi:10.1016/j.ejpb.2011.08.004.
11. J.M. Adams, S. Cory, Bcl-2-regulated apoptosis: mechanism and therapeutic potential, *Curr. Opin. Immunol.* 19 (2007) 488–496. doi:10.1016/j.coi.2007.05.004.
12. J.C. Burnett, J.J. Rossi, RNA-Based Therapeutics: Current Progress and Future Prospects, *Chem. Biol.* 19(1) (2012) 60–71. doi:10.1016/j.chembiol.2011.12.008.
13. S.-H. Chen, G. Zhaori, Potential clinical applications of siRNA technique: benefits and limitations, *Eur. J. Clin. Invest.* 41 (2011) 221–232. doi:10.1111/j.1365-2362.2010.02400.x.
14. H.M. Aliabadi, B. Landry, C. Sun, T. Tang, H. Uluda, Supramolecular assemblies in functional siRNA delivery: where do we stand?, *Biomaterials* 33(8) (2011) 2546–2569. doi:10.1016/j.biomaterials.2011.11.079.
15. K. Singha, R. Namgung, W.J. Kim, Polymers in small-interfering RNA delivery, Polymers in small interfering RNA delivery, *Nucleic Acid Ther.* 21(3) (2011) 133–147. doi:10.1089/nat.2011.0293.
16. G.R. Devi, siRNA-based approaches in cancer therapy, *Cancer Gene Ther.* 13 (2006) 819–829.

17. T. Kato, A. Natsume, H. Toda, H. Iwamizu, T. Sugita, R. Hachisu, R. Watanabe, K. Yuki, K. Motomura, K. Bankiewicz, T. Wakabayashi, Efficient delivery of liposome-mediated MGMT-siRNA reinforces the cytotoxity of temozolomide in GBM-initiating cells, *Gene Ther.* 17 (2010) 1363–1371. doi: 10.1038/gt.2010.88.

18. K. Nakamura, A.S. Abu Lila, M. Matsunaga, Y. Doi, T. Ishida, H. Kiwada, Functional lipid nanosystems in cancer, *Mol. Ther.* 19 (2011) 2040–2047, CRC Press, ISBN: 1000093166, 9781000093162.

19. A. Singh, S. Boldin-Adamsky, R.K. Thimmulappa, S.K. Rath, H. Ashush, J. Coulter, A. Blackford, S.N. Goodman, F. Bunz, W.H. Watson, E. Gabrielson, E. Feinstein, S. Biswal, RNAi-mediated silencing of nuclear factor erythroid-2-related factor 2 gene expression in non-small cell lung cancer inhibits tumor growth and increases efficacy of chemotherapy, *Cancer Res.* 68 (2008) 7975–7984. doi:10.1158/0008-5472.CAN-08-1401.

20. S. Yadav, L.E. van Vlerken, S.R. Little, M.M. Amiji, Evaluations of combination MDR-1 gene silencing and paclitaxel administration in biodegradable polymeric nanoparticle formulations to overcome multidrug resistance in cancer cells, *Cancer Chemother. Pharmacol.* 63(4) (2009) 711–722. doi: 10.1007/s00280-008-0790-y.

21. O. Taratula, O.B. Garbuzenko, A.M. Chen, T. Minko, Innovative strategy for treatment of lung cancer: targeted nanotechnology-based inhalation co-delivery of anticancer drugs and siRNA, *J. Drug Target.* 19 (2011) 900–914. doi:10.3109/1061186X.2011.622404.

22. D. Galmarini, C.M. Galmarini, F.C. Galmarini, Cancer chemotherapy: A critical analysis of its 60 years of history, *Crit. Rev. Oncol. Hematol.* 84(2) (2012) 181–199. doi:10.1016/j.critrevonc.2012.03.002.

23. R.S. Kerbel, G. Klement, K.I. Pritchard, B. Kamen, Continuous low-dose anti-angiogenic/ metronomic chemotherapy: from the research laboratory into the oncology clinic, *Ann. Oncol.* 13(1) (2002) 12–15. doi:10.1093/annonc/mdf093.

24. M. Shipitsin, L.L. Campbell, P. Argani, S. Weremowicz, N. Bloushtain-Qimron, J. Yao, T. Nikolskaya, T. Serebryiskaya, R. Beroukhim, M. Hu, M.K. Halushka, S. Sukumar, L.M. Parker, K.S. Anderson, L.N. Harris, J.E. Garber, A.L. Richardson, S.J. Schnitt, Y. Nikolsky, R.S. Gelman, K. Polyak, Molecular definition of breast tumor heterogeneity, *Cancer Cell* 11(3) (2007) 259–273. doi:10.1016/j.ccr.2007.01.013.

25. J.-P. Gillet, M.M. Gottesman, Mechanisms of multidrug resistance in cancer, *Methods Mol. Biol.* 596 (2010) 47–76. doi:10.1007/978-1-60761-416-6_4.

26. S.H. Jang, M.G. Wientjes, D. Lu, J.L.-S. Au, Drug delivery and transport to solid tumors *Pharm. Res.* 20(9) (2003) 1337–1350. doi:10.1023/a:1025785505977.

27. H. Maeda, J. Wu, T. Sawa, Y. Matsumura, K. Hori, Tumor vascular permeability and the EPR effect in macromolecular therapeutics: a review, *J. Control. Release* 65(1–2) (2000) 271–284. doi:10.1016/S0168-3659(99)00248-5.

28. T.M. Allen, P.R. Cullis, Drug delivery systems: entering the mainstream, *Science* 303(5665) (2004) 1818–1822. doi:10.1126/science.1095833.

29. A. Persidis, Cancer multidrug resistance. Progress in understanding the molecular basis of drug resistance in cancer promises more effective treatments, *Nat. Biotechnol.* 18 (2000) IT18–IT20, Springer Nature. doi:10.1038/80051, https://www.nature.com/articles/nbt0199_94.

30. S.W. Lowe, H.E. Ruley, T. Jacks, D.E. Housman, p53-dependent apoptosis modulates the cytotoxicity of anticancer agents, *Cell* 74(6) (1993) 957–967. doi:10.1016/0092-8674(93)90719-7.

31. G. Longo-Sorbello, Bertino, Current understanding of methotrexate pharmacology and efficacy in acute leukemias. Use of newer antifolates in clinical trials, *Haematologica* 86(2) (2001) 121–127. doi:10.3324/%25x.

32. J.G. Huang, T. Leshuk, F.X. Gu, Emerging nanomaterials for targeting subcellular organelles, *Nano Today* 6(5) (2011) 478–492. doi:10.1016/j.nantod.2011.08.002.

33. P. Borst, R. Evers, M. Kool, J. Wijnholds, A family of drug transporters: the multidrug resistance-associated proteins, *J. Natl. Cancer Inst.* 92(16) (2000) 1295–1302. doi:10.1093/jnci/92.16.1295.

34. X.-Q. Zhao, J.-D. Xie, X.-G. Chen, H.M. Sim, X. Zhang, Y.-J. Liang, S. Singh, T.T. Talele, Y. Sun, S.V. Ambudkar, Z.-S. Chen, L.-W. Fu, Neratinib reverses ATP-binding cassette B1-mediated chemotherapeutic drug resistance in vitro, in vivo, and ex vivo, *Mol. Pharmacol.* 82(1) (2012) 47–58. doi:10.1124/mol.111.076299.

35. Y. Wang, Q. Chen, S. Jin, W. Deng, S. Li, Q. Tong, Y. Chen, Up-regulation of P-glycoprotein is involved in the increased paclitaxel resistance in human esophageal cancer radioresistant cells, *Scand. J. Gastroenterol.* 47(7) (2012) 802–808. doi:10.3109/00365521.2012.683042.

36. S.P. Ebert, R.L. Myette, B.G. Wetzel, G. Conseil, S.P.C. Cole, G.A. Sawada, T.W. Loo, M.C. Bartlett, D.M. Clarke, M.R. Detty, Chalcogenopyrylium compounds as modulators of the ATP-binding cassette transporters P-glycoprotein (P-gp/ABCB1) and multidrug resistance protein 1 (MRP1/ABCC1), *J. Med. Chem.* 55 (2012) 4683–4699. doi:10.1021/jm3004398.

37. N. Setia, O. Abbas, Y. Sousa, J.L. Garb, M. Mahalingam, *Mod. Pathol.* (2012), ISSN: 1530-0285.

38. C.M. McNeil, C.M. Sergio, L.R. Anderson, C.K. Inman, S.A. Eggleton, N.C. Murphy, E.K.A. Millar, P. Crea, J.G. Kench, M.C. Alles, M. Gardiner-Garden, C.J. Ormandy, A.J. Butt, S.M. Henshall, E.A. Musgrove, R.L. Sutherland, c-Myc overexpression and endocrine resistance in breast cancer, *J. Steroid Biochem. Mol. Biol.* 102(1–5) (2006) 147–155. doi:10.1016/j.jsbmb.2006.09.028.

39. D. Nijhawan, M. Fang, E. Traer, Q. Zhong, W. Gao, F. Du, X. Wang, Elimination of Mcl-1 is required for the initiation of apoptosis following ultraviolet irradiation, *Genes Dev.* 17 (2003) 1475–1486. doi:10.1101/gad.1093903.

40. T.-M. Sun, J.-Z. Du, Y.-D. Yao, C.-Q. Mao, S. Dou, S.-Y. Huang, P.-Z. Zhang, K.W. Leong, E.-W. Song, J. Wang, Simultaneous delivery of siRNA and paclitaxel via a "two-in-one" micelleplex promotes synergistic tumor suppression, *ACS Nano* 5(2) (2011) 1483–1494. doi:10.1021/nn103349h.

41. J. Luo, M.J. Emanuele, D. Li, C.J. Creighton, M.R. Schlabach, T.F. Westbrook, K.-K. Wong, S.J. Elledge, A genome-wide RNAi screen identifies multiple synthetic lethal interactions with the Ras oncogene, *Cell* 137(5) (2009) 835–848. doi:10.1016/j.cell.2009.05.006.

42. K. Strebhardt, A. Ullrich, Targeting polo-like kinase 1 for cancer therapy, *Nat. Rev. Cancer* 6 (2006) 321–330. https://www.nature.com/articles/nrc1841.

43. R.L. Baldwin, H. Tran, B.Y. Karlan, Loss of c-myc repression coincides with ovarian cancer resistance to transforming growth factor β growth arrest independent of transforming growth factor β/Smad signaling, *Cancer Res.* 63 (2003) 1413–1419. https://cancerres.aacrjournals.org/content/63/6/1413.short.

44. D.C. Knapp, J.E. Mata, M.T. Reddy, G.R. Devi, P.L. Iversen, Resistance to chemotherapeutic drugs overcome by c-Myc inhibition in a Lewis lung carcinoma murine model, *Anticancer Drugs* 14(1) (2003) 39–47. https://journals.lww.com/anti-cancerdrugs/Abstract/2003/01000/Resistance_to_chemotherapeutic_drugs_overcome_by.6.aspx.

45. Y. Huang, P. Anderle, K.J. Bussey, C. Barbacioru, U. Shankavaram, Z. Dai, W.C. Reinhold, A. Papp, J.N. Weinstein, J.N. Weinstein, W. Sadee, Membrane transporters and channels, *Cancer Res.* 64 (2004) 4294–4301. doi:10.1158/0008-5472.CAN-03-3884.

46. J. Wu, Y. Lu, A. Lee, X. Pan, X. Yang, X. Zhao, R.J. Lee, Reversal of multidrug resistance by transferrin-conjugated liposomes co-encapsulating doxorubicin and verapamil, *J. Pharm. Pharm. Sci.* 10(3) (2007) 350–357.

47. X.R. Song, Z. Cai, Y. Zheng, G. He, F.Y. Cui, D.Q. Gong, S.X. Hou, S.J. Xiong, X.J. Lei, Y.Q. Wei, Reversion of multidrug resistance by co-encapsulation of vincristine and verapamil in PLGA nanoparticles, *Eur. J. Pharm. Sci.* 37(3–4) (2009) 300–305. doi:10.1016/j.ejps.2009.02.018.

48. S. Ganta, M. Amiji, Coadministration of paclitaxel and curcumin in nanoemulsion formulations to overcome multidrug resistance in tumor cells, *Mol. Pharm.* 6(3) (2009) 928–939. doi:10.1021/mp800240j.

49. C. Kim, B.P. Shah, P. Subramaniam, K.-B. Lee, Synergistic induction of apoptosis in brain cancer cells by targeted codelivery of siRNA and anticancer drugs, *Mol. Pharm.* 8(5) (2011) 1955–1961. doi:10.1021/mp100460h.

50. C.W. Beh, W.Y. Seow, Y. Wang, Y. Zhang, Z.Y. Ong, P.L.R. Ee, Y.-Y. Yang, Efficient delivery of Bcl-2-targeted siRNA using cationic polymer nanoparticles: downregulating mRNA expression level and sensitizing cancer cells to anticancer drug, *Biomacromolecules* 10(1) (2009) 41–48. doi:10.1021/bm801109g.

51. P. Zahedi, R. De Souza, L. Huynh, M. Piquette-Miller, C. Allen, Combination drug delivery strategy for the treatment of multidrug resistant ovarian cancer, *Mol. Pharm.* 8(1) (2011) 260–269.

52. M.E. Davis, Z. Chen, D.M. Shin, Nanoparticle therapeutics: an emerging treatment modality for cancer, *Nat. Rev. Drug Discov.* 7 (2008) 771–782. doi:10.1142/9789814287005_0025.

53. K.D. Fowers, J. Kopeček, Targeting of multidrug-resistant human ovarian carcinoma cells with anti-P-glycoprotein antibody conjugates, *Macromol. Biosci.* 12(4) (2012) 502–514. doi:10.1002/mabi.201100350.

54. E. Dickerson, W. Blackburn, M. Smith, L. Kapa, L.A. Lyon, J. McDonald, Chemosensitization of cancer cells by siRNA using targeted nanogel delivery, *BMC Cancer* 10 (2010) 10. doi:10.1186/1471-2407-10-10.

55. S.J. Lee, J.Y. Yhee, S.H. Kim, I.C. Kwon, K. Kim, Biocompatible gelatin nanoparticles for tumor-targeted delivery of polymerized siRNA in tumor-bearing mice, *J. Control. Release* 172 (2013) 358–366.

56. S. Son, S. Song, S.J. Lee, S. Min, S.A. Kim, J.Y. Yhee, M.S. Huh, I. Chan Kwon, S.Y. Jeong, Y. Byun, S.H. Kim, K. Kim, Self-crosslinked human serum albumin nanocarriers for systemic delivery of polymerized siRNA to tumors, *Biomaterials* 34 (2013) 9475–9485.

57. Y. Wang, Z. Li, Y. Han, L.H. Liang, A. Ji, Nanoparticle-based delivery system for application of siRNA in vivo, *Curr. Drug Metab.* 11 (2010) 182–196.

58. M.E. Davis, The first targeted delivery of siRNA in humans via a self-assembling, cyclodextrin polymer-based nanoparticle: from concept to clinic, *Mol. Pharm.* 6 (2009) 659–668.

59. M.E. Davis, M.E. Brewster, Cyclodextrin-based pharmaceutics: past, present and future, *Nat. Rev. Drug Discov.* 3 (2004) 1023–1035.

60. H.D. Han, E.M. Mora, J.W. Roh, M. Nishimura, S.J. Lee, R.L. Stone, M. Bar-Eli, G. Lopez-Berestein, A.K. Sood, Chitosan hydrogel for localized gene silencing, *Cancer Biol. Ther.* 11 (2011) 839–845.

61. Z. Ma, C. Yang, W. Song, Q. Wang, J. Kjems, S. Gao, Chitosan hydrogel as siRNA vector for prolonged gene silencing, *J. Nanobiotechnol.* 12 (2014) 23.

62. E. Salva, L. Kabasakal, F. Eren, N. Ozkan, F. Cakalagaoglu, J. Akbuga, Local delivery of chitosan/VEGF siRNA nanoplexes reduces angiogenesis and growth of breast cancer in vivo, *Nucleic Acid Ther.* 22 (2012) 40–48.

63. H. de Martimprey, J.R. Bertrand, A. Fusco, M. Santoro, P. Couvreur, C. Vauthier, C. Malvy, siRNA nanoformulation against the ret./PTC1 junction oncogene is efficient in an in vivo model of papillary thyroid carcinoma, *Nucleic Acids Res.* 36 (2008) e2.

64. T. Ochiya, S. Nagahara, A. Sano, H. Itoh, M. Terada, Biomaterials for gene delivery: atelocollagen-mediated controlled release of molecular medicines, *Curr. Gene Ther.* 1 (2001) 31–52.

65. S. Inaba, S. Nagahara, N. Makita, Y. Tarumi, T. Ishimoto, S. Matsuo, K. Kadomatsu, Y. Takei, Atelocollagen-mediated systemic delivery prevents immunostimulatory adverse effects of siRNA in mammals, *Mol. Ther.* 20 (2012) 356–366.

66. Z.W. Wu, C.T. Chien, C.Y. Liu, J.Y. Yan, S.Y. Lin, Recent progress in copolymermediated siRNA delivery, *J. Drug Target.* 20 (2012) 551–560.

67. J. DeRouchey, C. Schmidt, G.F. Walker, C. Koch, C. Plank, E. Wagner, J.O. Radler, Monomolecular assembly of siRNA and poly(ethylene glycol)-peptide copolymers, *Biomacromolecules* 9 (2008) 724–732.

68. A. Malek, F. Czubayko, A. Aigner, PEG grafting of polyethylenimine (PEI) exerts different effects on DNA transfection and siRNA-induced gene targeting efficacy, *J. Drug Target.* 16 (2008) 124–139.

69. S. Mao, M. Neu, O. Germershaus, O. Merkel, J. Sitterberg, U. Bakowsky, T. Kissel, Influence of polyethylene glycol chain length on the physicochemical and biological properties of poly(ethylene imine)-graft-poly(ethylene glycol) block copolymer/SiRNA polyplexes, *Bioconjug. Chem.* 17 (2006) 1209–1218.

70. S.H. Lee, H. Mok, Y. Lee, T.G. Park, Self-assembled siRNA-PLGA conjugate micelles for gene silencing, *J. Control. Release* 152 (2011) 152–158.

71. S.P. Egusquiaguirre, M. Igartua, R.M. Hernandez, J.L. Pedraz, Nanoparticle delivery systems for cancer therapy: advances in clinical and preclinical research, *Clin. Transl. Oncol.* 14(2) (2012) 83–93.

72. X. Yuan, S. Naguib, Z. Wu, Recent advances of siRNA delivery by nanoparticles, *Expert Opin. Drug Deliv.* 8(4) (2011) 521–536.

73. S. Hu-Lieskovan, J.D. Heidel, D.W. Bartlett, M.E. Davis, T.J. Triche, Sequence-specific knockdown of EWS-FLI1 by targeted, nonviral delivery of small interfering RNA inhibits tumor growth in a murine model of metastatic Ewing's sarcoma, *Cancer Res.* 65(19) (2005) 8984–8992.

74. M.E. Davis, J.E. Zuckerman, C.H.J. Choi et al., Evidence of RNAi in humans from systemically administered siRNA via targeted nanoparticles, *Nature* 464(7291) (2010) 1067–1070.

75. K.A. Howard, U.L. Rahbek, X. Liu et al., RNA interference in vitro and in vivo using a novel chitosan/siRNA nanoparticle system, *Mol. Ther.* 14(4) (2006) 476–484.
76. X. Liu, K.A. Howard, M. Dong et al., The influence of polymeric properties on chitosan/siRNA nanoparticle formulation and gene silencing, *Biomaterials* 28(6) (2007) 1280–1288.
77. M. Jean, F. Smaoui, M. Lavertu et al., Chitosan-plasmid nanoparticle formulations for IM and SC delivery of recombinant FGF-2 and PDGF-BB or generation of antibodies, *Gene Ther.* 16(9) (2009) 1097–1110.
78. H. Katas, H.O. Alpar, Development and characterisation of chitosan nanoparticles for siRNA delivery, *J. Control. Release* 115(2) (2006) 216–225.
79. M. Alameh, D. Dejesus, M. Jean et al., Low molecular weight chitosan nanoparticulate system at low N:P ratio for nontoxic polynucleotide delivery, *Int. J. Nanomed.* 7 (2012) 1399–1414.
80. O.M. Merkel, A. Beyerle, B.M. Beckmann et al., Polymerrelated off-target effects in non-viral siRNA delivery, *Biomaterials* 32(9) (2011) 2388–2398.
81. S.M. Moghimi, P. Symonds, J.C. Murray, A.C. Hunter, G. Debska, A. Szewczyk, A two-stage poly(ethylenimine)-mediated cytotoxicity: implications for gene transfer/therapy, *Mol. Ther.* 11(6) (2005) 990–995.
82. A.C. Hunter, S.M. Moghimi, Cationic carriers of genetic material and cell death: a mitochondrial tale, *Biochimica et Biophysica Acta* 1797(6–7) (2010) 1203–1209.
83. K.A. Woodrow, Y. Cu, C.J. Booth, J.K. Saucier-Sawyer, M.J. Wood, W.M. Saltzman, Intravaginal gene silencing using biodegradable polymer nanoparticles densely loaded with small-interfering RNA, *Nat. Mater.* 8(6) (2009) 526–533.
84. P. Kesharwani, R.K. Tekade, V. Gajbhiye, K. Jain, N.K. Jain, Cancer targeting potential of some ligand-anchored poly(propylene imine) dendrimers: a comparison, *Nanomedicine* 7(3) (2011) 295–304.
85. J.-H. Lee, K.E. Cha, M.S. Kim et al., Nanosized polyamidoamine (PAMAM)dendrimer-induced apoptosis mediated by mitochondrial dysfunction, *Toxicol. Lett.* 190(2) (2009) 202–207.
86. M.L. Patil, M. Zhang, O. Taratula, O.B. Garbuzenko, H. He, T. Minko, "Internally cationic polyamidoamine PAMAMOH dendrimers for siRNA delivery: effect of the degree of Quaternization and cancer targeting, *Biomacromolecules* 10(2) (2009) 258–266.
87. O. Taratula, O.B. Garbuzenko, P. Kirkpatrick et al., Surface engineered targeted PPI dendrimer for efficient intracellular and intratumoral siRNA delivery, *J. Control. Release* 140(3) (2009) 284–293.
88. A. Agrawal, D.-H. Min, N. Singh et al., Functional delivery of siRNA in mice using dendriworms, *ACS Nano* 3(9) (2009) 2495–2504.
89. D. Pantarotto, R. Singh, D. McCarthy et al., Functionalized carbon nanotubes for plasmid DNA gene delivery, *Angewandte Chemie* 43(39) (2004) 5242–5246.
90. D. Cai, J.M. Mataraza, Z.-H. Qin et al., Highly efficient molecular delivery into mammalian cells using carbon nanotube spearing, *Nat. Methods* 2(6) (2005) 449–454.
91. P. Kesharwani, V. Gajbhiye, N.K. Jain, A review of nanocarriers for the delivery of small interfering RNA, *Biomaterials* 33(29) (2012) 7138–7150.
92. Z. Zhang, X. Yang, Y. Zhang et al., Delivery of telomerase reverse transcriptase small interfering RNA in complex with positively charged single-walled carbon nanotubes suppresses tumor growth, *Clin. Cancer Res.* 12(16) (2006) 4933–4939.
93. Z. Liu, M. Winters, M. Holodniy, H. Dai, siRNA delivery into human T cells and primary cells with carbon-nanotube transporters, *Angewandte Chemie* 46(12) (2007) 2023–2027.
94. H. Wang, J. Wang, X. Deng et al., Biodistribution of carbon single-wall carbon nanotubes in mice, *J. Nanosci. Nanotechnol.* 4(8) (2004) 1019–1024.
95. K.T. Al-Jamal, F.M. Toma, A. Yilmazer et al., Enhanced cellular internalization and gene silencing with a series of cationic dendron-multiwalled carbon nanotube:siRNA complexes, *FASEB J.* 24(11) (2010) 4354–4365.
96. J.E. Podesta, K.T. Al-Jamal, M.A. Herrero et al., Antitumor activity and prolonged survival by carbon-nanotube-mediated therapeutic sirna silencing in a human lung xenograft model, *Small* 5(10) (2009) 1176–1185.
97. A.A. Shvedova, E.R. Kisin, D. Porter et al., Mechanisms of pulmonary toxicity and medical applications of carbon nanotubes: two faces of Janus? *Pharmacol. Ther.* 121(2) (2009) 192–204.
98. C.P. Firme III, P.R. Bandaru, Toxicity issues in the application of carbon nanotubes to biological systems, *Nanomedicine* 6(2) (2010) 245–256.
99. Y. Yu, D. Sun, Superparamagnetic iron oxide nanoparticle 'theranostics' for multimodality tumor imaging, gene delivery, targeted drug and prodrug delivery, *Expert Rev. Clin. Pharmacol.* 3(1) (2010) 117–130.
100. X.-H. Peng, X. Qian, H. Mao et al., "Targeted magnetic iron oxide nanoparticles for tumor imaging and therapy, *Int. J. Nanomed.* 3(3) (2008) 311–321.
101. Z. Medarova, W. Pham, C. Farrar, V. Petkova, A. Moore, In vivo imaging of siRNA delivery and silencing in tumors, *Nat. Med.* 13(3) (2007) 372–377.
102. J.-H. Lee, K. Lee, S.H. Moon, Y. Lee, T.G. Park, J. Cheon, All-in-one target-cell-specific magnetic nanoparticles for simultaneous molecular imaging and siRNA delivery, *Angewandte Chemie.* 48(23) (2009) 4174–4179.
103. Y.-S. Cho, T.-J. Yoon, E.-S. Jang et al., Cetuximab-conjugated magneto-fluorescent silica nanoparticles for in vivo colon cancer targeting and imaging, *Cancer Lett.* 299(1) (2010) 63–71.
104. A.M. Smith, H. Duan, A.M. Mohs, S. Nie, Bioconjugated quantum dots for in vivo molecular and cellular imaging, *Adv. Drug. Deliv. Rev.* 60(11) (2008) 1226–1240.
105. A.M. Derfus, A.A. Chen, D.-H. Min, E. Ruoslahti, S.N. Bhatia, Targeted quantum dot conjugates for siRNA delivery, *Bioconjug. Chem.* 18(5) (2007) 1391–1396.
106. W.B. Tan, S. Jiang, Y. Zhang, Quantum-dot based nanoparticles for targeted silencing of HER2/neu gene via RNA interference, *Biomaterials* 28(8) (2007) 1565–1571.
107. M.V. Yezhelyev, L. Qi, R.M. O'Regan, S. Nie, X. Gao, Proton-sponge coated quantum dots for siRNA delivery and intracellular imaging, *J. Am. Chem. Soc.* 130(28) (2008) 9006–9012.
108. Y. Su, Y. He, H. Lu et al., The cytotoxicity of cadmium based, aqueous phase—synthesized, quantumdots and its-modulation by surface coating, *Biomaterials* 30(1) (2009) 19–25.

109. P. Subramaniam, S.J. Lee, S. Shah, S. Patel, V. Starovoytov, K.B. Lee, Generation of a library of non-toxic quantum dots for cellular imaging and siRNA delivery, *Adv. Mater.* 24(29) (2012) 4014–4019.

110. P. Ghosh, G. Han, M. De, C.K. Kim, V.M. Rotello, Gold nanoparticles in delivery applications, *Adv. Drug Deliv. Rev.* 60(11) (2008) 1307–1315.

111. N.L. Rosi, D.A. Giljohann, C.S. Thaxton, A.K.R. Lytton-Jean, M.S. Han, C.A. Mirkin, Oligonucleotide-modified gold nanoparticles for infracellular gene regulation, *Science* 312(5776) (2006) 1027–1030.

112. W.H. Kong, K.H. Bae, S.D. Jo, J.S. Kim, T.G. Park, Cationic lipid-coated gold nanoparticles as efficient and noncytotoxic intracellular siRNA delivery vehicles, *Pharm. Res.* 29(2) (2012) 362–374.

113. A.C. Bonoiu, S.D. Mahajan, H. Ding et al., Nanotechnology approach for drug addiction therapy: gene silencing using delivery of gold nanorod-siRNA nanoplex in dopaminergic neurons, *Proc. Natl. Acad. Sci. U. S. A.* 106(14) (2009) 5546–5550. doi:10.1073/pnas.0901715106.

114. E.-Y. Kim, R. Schulz, P. Swantek, K. Kunstman, M.H. Malim, S.M. Wolinsky, Gold nanoparticle-mediated gene delivery induces widespread changes in the expression of innate immunity genes, *Gene Ther.* 19(3) (2012) 347–353. doi:10.1038/gt.2011.95.

115. G. Liu, M. Swierczewska, S. Lee, X. Chen, Functional nanoparticles for molecular imaging guided gene delivery, *Nano Today* 5(6) (2010) 524–539. doi:10.1016/j.nantod.2010.10.00.

116. N.T.K. Thanh, L.A.W. Green, Functionalisation of nanoparticles for biomedical applications, *Nano Today* 5(3) (2010) 213–230. doi:10.1016/j.nantod.2010.05.003.

117. L. Yildirimer, N.T.K. Thanh, M. Loizidou, A.M. Seifalian, Toxicology and clinical potential of nanoparticles, *Nano Today* 6(6) (2011) 585–607. doi:10.1016/j.nantod.2011.10.001

118. P. Rigby, Silica nanoparticles target cancer cells, *Nano Today* 2(4) (2007) 12. doi:10.1016/S1748-0132(07)70110-X.

119. C. Sealy, Shocking prediction for light source: optical materials, *Nano Today* 9(3) (2006) 19. doi:10.1016/S1369-7021(06)71383-9.

120. S.J. Soenen, P. Rivera-Gil, J.-M. Montenegro, W.J. Parak, S.C. De Smedt, K. Braeckmans, Cellular toxicity of inorganic nanoparticles: Common aspects and guidelines for improved nanotoxicity evaluation, *Nano Today* 6(5) (2011) 446–465. doi:10.1016/j.nantod.2011.08.001.

121. A.M. Chen, M. Zhang, D. Wei, D. Stueber, O. Taratula, T. Minko, H. He, Co-delivery of doxorubicin and Bcl-2 siRNA by mesoporous silica nanoparticles enhances the efficacy of chemotherapy in multidrug-resistant cancer cells, *Small* 5(23) (2009) 2673–2677. doi:10.1002/smll.200900621.

122. H. Meng, M. Liong, T. Xia, Z. Li, Z. Ji, J.I. Zink, A.E. Nel, Engineered design of mesoporous silica nanoparticles to deliver doxorubicin and P-glycoprotein siRNA to overcome drug resistance in a cancer cell line, *ACS Nano* 4(8) (2010) 4539–4550. doi:10.1021/nn100690m.

123. J.-M. Li, Y.-Y. Wang, M.-X. Zhao, C.-P. Tan, Y.-Q. Li, X.-Y. Le, L.-N. Ji, Z.-W. Mao, Multifunctional QD-based co-delivery of siRNA and doxorubicin to HeLa cells for reversal of multidrug resistance and real-time tracking, *Biomaterials* 33(9) (2012) 2780–2790. doi:10.1016/j.biomaterials.2011.12.035.

124. P. Zrazhevskiy, X. Gao, Multifunctional quantum dots for personalized medicine, *Nano Today* 4 (2009) 414–428. doi:10.1016/j.nantod.2009.07.004.

125. H. Hong, Y. Zhang, J. Sun, W. Cai, Molecular imaging and therapy of cancer with radiolabeled nanoparticles, *Nano Today* 4(5) (2009) 399–413. doi:10.1016/j.nantod.2009.07.001.

126. H. Koo, M.S. Huh, J.H. Ryu, D.-E. Lee, I.-C. Sun, K. Choi, K. Kim, I.C. Kwon, Nanoprobes for biomedical imaging in living systems, *Nano Today* 6(2) (2011) 204–220. doi:10.1016/j.nantod.2011.02.007.

127. M. Caldorera-Moore, N.A. Peppas, Micro- and nanotechnologies for intelligent and responsive biomaterial-based medical systems, *Adv. Drug Deliv. Rev.* 61(15) (2009) 1391–1401. doi:10.1016/j.addr.2009.09.002.

128. M.E. Caldorera-Moore, W.B. Liechty, N.A. Peppas, Responsive theranostic systems: integration of diagnostic imaging agents and responsive controlled release drug delivery carrier, *Acc. Chem. Res.* 44(10) (2011) 1061–1070. doi:10.1021/ar2001777.

129. W.B. Liechty, D.R. Kryscio, B.V. Slaughter, N.A. Peppas, Polymers for drug delivery systems, *Annu. Rev. Chem. Biomol. Eng.* 1 (2010) 149–173. doi:10.1146/annurev-chembioeng-073009-100847.

130. N. Cao, D. Cheng, S. Zou, H. Ai, J. Gao, X. Shuai, The synergistic effect of hierarchical assemblies of siRNA and chemotherapeutic drugs co-delivered into hepatic cancer cells, *Biomaterials* 32(8) (2011) 2222–2232. doi:10.1016/j.biomaterials.2010.11.061.

131. D. Cheng, N. Cao, J. Chen, X. Yu, X. Shuai, Multifunctional nanocarrier mediated co-delivery of doxorubicin and siRNA for synergistic enhancement of glioma apoptosis in rat, *Biomaterials* 33(4) (2012) 1170–1179. doi:10.1016/j.biomaterials.2011.10.057.

132. H.-Y. Huang, W.-T. Kuo, M.-J. Chou, Y.-Y. Huang, Co-delivery of anti-vascular endothelial growth factor siRNA and *doxorubicin* by multifunctional polymeric micelle for tumor growth suppression, *J. Biomed. Mater. Res. Part A* 97A(3) (2011) 330–338. doi:10.1002/jbm.a.33055.

133. T.L. Kaneshiro, Z.-R. Lu, Targeted intracellular codelivery of chemotherapeutics and nucleic acid with a well-defined dendrimer-based nanoglobular carrier, *Biomaterials* 30(29) (2009) 5660–5666. doi:10.1016/j.biomaterials.2009.06.026.

134. Y.B. Patil, S.K. Swaminathan, T. Sadhukha, L. Ma, J. Panyam, The use of nanoparticle-mediated targeted gene silencing and drug delivery to overcome tumor drug resistance *Biomaterials* 31(2) (2010) 358–365. doi:10.1016/j.biomaterials.2009.09.048.

135. Y. Wang, S. Gao, W.-H. Ye, H.S. Yoon, Y.-Y. Yang, Co-delivery of drugs and DNA from cationic core–shell nanoparticles self-assembled from a biodegradable copolymer, *Nat. Mater.* 5 (2006) 791–796. https://www.nature.com/articles/nmat1737.

136. X.-B. Xiong, A. Lavasanifar, Traceable multifunctional micellar nanocarriers for cancer-targeted co-delivery of MDR-1 siRNA and doxorubicin, *ACS Nano* 5(6) (2011) 5202–5213. doi:10.1021/nn2013707.

137. C. Zhu, S. Jung, S. Luo, F. Meng, X. Zhu, T.G. Park, Z. Zhong, Co-delivery of siRNA and paclitaxel into cancer cells by biodegradable cationic micelles based on PDMAEMA–PCL–PDMAEMA triblock copolymers, *Biomaterials* 31(8) (2010) 2408–2416. doi:10.1016/j.biomaterials.2009.11.077.

138. R.S. Chang, M.S. Suh, S. Kim, G. Shim, S. Lee, S.S. Han, K.E. Lee, H. Jeon, H.-G. Choi, Y. Choi, C.-W. Kim, Y.-K. Oh, Cationic drug-derived nanoparticles for multifunctional delivery of anticancer siRNA, *Biomaterials* 32(36) (2011) 9785–9795. doi:10.1016/j.biomaterials.2011.09.017.

139. Y. Chen, S.R. Bathula, J. Li, L. Huang, Multifunctional nanoparticles delivering small interfering rna and doxorubicin overcome drug resistance in cancer, *J. Biol. Chem.* 285(29) (2010) 22639–22650. doi:10.1074/jbc.M110.125906.

140. R. Arun, K.C.K. Ashok, V.V.N.S.S. Sravanthi, Cyclodextrins as drug carrier molecule: a review, *Sci. Pharm.* 76(4) (2008) 567–598. doi:10.3797/scipharm.0808-05.

141. M. Creixell, A.C. Bohorquez, M. Torres-Lugo, C. Rinaldi, EGFR-targeted magnetic nanoparticle heaters kill cancer cells without a perceptible temperature rise, *ACS Nano* 5(9) (2011) 7124–7129. doi:10.1021/nn201822b.

142. C.-J. Lai, R. Bao, X. Tao, J. Wang, R. Atoyan, H. Qu, D.-G. Wang, L. Yin, M. Samson, J. Forrester, B. Zifcak, G.-X. Xu, S. DellaRocca, H.-X. Zhai, X. Cai, W.E. Munger, M. Keegan, C.V. Pepicelli, C. Qian, CUDC-101, a multitargeted inhibitor of histone deacetylase, epidermal growth factor receptor, and human epidermal growth factor receptor 2, exerts potent anticancer activity. Therapeutics, targets, and chemical biology, *Cancer Res.* 70(9) (2010) 3647–3656. doi:10.1158/0008-5472.CAN-09-3360.

143. M. Garcia-Fuentes, D. Torres, M.J. Alonso, New surface-modified lipid nanoparticles as delivery vehicles for salmon calcitonin, *Int. J. Pharm.* 296(1–2) (2005) 122–132. doi:10.1016/j.ijpharm.2004.12.030.

144. S. Martins, S. Costa-Lima, T. Carneiro, A. Cordeiro-da-Silva, E.B. Souto, D.C. Ferreira, Solid lipid nanoparticles as intracellular drug transporters: an investigation of the uptake mechanism and pathway, *Int. J. Pharm.* 430(1–2) (2012) 216–227. doi:10.1016/j.ijpharm.2012.03.032.

145. J. Pardeike, A. Hommoss, R.H. Muller, Lipid nanoparticles (SLN, NLC) in cosmetic and pharmaceutical dermal products, *Int. J. Pharm.* 366(1–2) (2009) 170–184. doi:10.1016/j.ijpharm.2008.10.003.

146. R.K. Subedi, K.W. Kang, H.-K. Choi, Preparation and characterization of solid lipid nanoparticles loaded with doxorubicin, *Eur. J. Pharm. Sci.* 37(3–4) (2009) 508–513 doi:10.1016/j.ejps.2009.04.008.

147. Y. Barenholz, Doxil® — The first FDA-approved nanodrug: Lessons learned, *J. Control. Release* 160(2) (2012) 117–134. doi:10.1016/j.jconrel.2012.03.020.

148. Y. Chen, J.J. Wu, L. Huang, Nanoparticles targeted with ngr motif deliver c-myc siRNA and doxorubicin for anticancer therapy, *Mol. Ther.* 18(4) (2010) 828–834. doi:10.1038/mt.2009.291.

149. S.H. Kang, H.-J. Cho, G. Shim, S. Lee, S.-H. Kim, H.-G. Choi, C.-W. Kim, Y.-K. Oh, Cationic liposomal co-delivery of small interfering RNA and a MEK inhibitor for enhanced anticancer efficacy, *Pharm. Res.* 28 (2011) 3069–3078. doi:10.1007/s11095-011-0569-4.

150. G. Shim, S.-E. Han, Y.-H. Yu, S. Lee, H.Y. Lee, K. Kim, I.C. Kwon, T.G. Park, Y.B. Kim, Y.S. Choi, C.-W. Kim, Y.-K. Oh, Trilysinoyl oleylamide-based cationic liposomes for systemic co-delivery of siRNA and an anticancer drug, *J. Control. Release* 155(1) (2011) 60–66. doi:10.1016/j.jconrel.2010.10.017.

151. Y.H. Yu, E. Kim, D.E. Park, G. Shim, S. Lee, Y.B. Kim, C.-W. Kim, Y.-K. Oh, Cationic solid lipid nanoparticles for co-delivery of paclitaxel and siRNA, *Eur. J. Pharm. Biopharm.* 80(2) (2011) 268–273. doi:10.1016/j.ejpb.2011.11.002.

152. R. Koynova, L. Wang, R.C. MacDonald, Cationic phospholipids forming cubic phases: lipoplex structure and transfection efficiency, *Mol. Pharm.* 5(5) (2008) 739–744. doi:10.1021/mp800011e.

153. M. Saad, O.B. Garbuzenko, T. Minko, Co-delivery of siRNA and an anticancer drug for treatment of multidrug-resistant cancer, *Nanomedicine* 3(6) (2008) 761–776. doi:10.2217/17435889.3.6.761.

154. S.I. Kim, D. Shin, T.H. Choi, J.C. Lee, G.J. Cheon, K.Y. Kim, M. Park, M. Kim, Systemic and specific delivery of small interfering RNAs to the liver mediated by apolipoprotein A-I, *Mol. Ther.* 15 (2007) 1145–1152.

155. N. Yagi, I. Manabe, T. Tottori, A. Ishihara, F. Ogata, J.H. Kim, S. Nishimura, K. Fujiu, Y. Oishi, K. Itaka, Y. Kato, M. Yamauchi, R. Nagai, A nanoparticle system specifically designed to deliver short interfering RNA inhibits tumor growth in vivo, *Cancer Res.* 69 (2009) 6531–6538.

156. D.V. Morrissey, J.A. Lockridge, L. Shaw, K. Blanchard, K. Jensen, W. Breen, K. Hartsough, L. Machemer, S. Radka, V. Jadhav, N. Vaish, S. Zinnen, C. Vargeese, K. Bowman, C.S. Shaffer, L.B. Jeffs, A. Judge, I. MacLachlan, B. Polisky, Potent and persistent in vivo anti-HBV activity of chemically modified siRNAs, *Nat. Biotechnol.* 23 (2005) 1002–1007.

157. T.W. Geisbert, L.E. Hensley, E. Kagan, E.Z. Yu, J.B. Geisbert, K. Daddario-DiCaprio, E.A. Fritz, P.B. Jahrling, K. McClintock, J.R. Phelps, A.C. Lee, A. Judge, L.B. Jeffs, I. MacLachlan, Postexposure protection of guinea pigs against a lethal Ebola virus challenge is conferred by RNA interference, *J. Infect. Dis.* 193 (2006) 1650–1657.

158. T.S. Zimmermann, A.C. Lee, A. Akinc, B. Bramlage, D. Bumcrot, M.N. Fedoruk, J. Harborth, J.A. Heyes, L.B. Jeffs, M. John, A.D. Judge, K. Lam, K. McClintock, L.V. Nechev, L.R. Palmer, T. Racie, I. Rohl, S. Seiffert, S. Shanmugam, V. Sood, J. Soutschek, I. Toudjarska, A.J. Wheat, E. Yaworski, W. Zedalis, V. Koteliansky, M. Manoharan, H.P. Vornlocher, I. MacLachlan, RNAi-mediated gene silencing in non-human primates, *Nature* 441 (2006) 111–114.

159. C. Wolfrum, S. Shi, K.N. Jayaprakash, M. Jayaraman, G. Wang, R.K. Pandey, K.G. Rajeev, T. Nakayama, K. Charrise, E.M. Ndungo, T. Zimmermann, V. Koteliansky, M. Manoharan, M. Stoffel, Mechanisms and optimization of in vivo delivery of lipophilic siRNAs, *Nat. Biotechnol.* 25 (2007) 1149–1157.

160. S.A. Moschos, S.W. Jones, M.M. Perry, A.E. Williams, J.S. Erjefalt, J.J. Turner, P.J. Barnes, B.S. Sproat, M.J. Gait, M.A. Lindsay, Lung delivery studies using siRNA conjugated to TAT(48–60) and penetratin reveal peptide induced reduction in gene expression and induction of innate immunity, *Bioconjug. Chem.* 18(5) (2007) 1450–1459.

161. V.V. Ambardekar, H.Y. Han, M.L. Varney, S.V. Vinogradov, R.K. Singh, J.A. Vetro, The modification of siRNA with 3′ cholesterol to increase nuclease protection and suppression of native mRNA by select siRNA polyplexes, *Biomaterials* 32 (2011) 1404–1411.

162. Y. Oe, R.J. Christie, M. Naito, S.A. Low, S. Fukushima, K. Toh, Y. Miura, Y. Matsumoto, N. Nishiyama, K. Miyata, K. Kataoka, Actively-targeted polyion complex micelles stabilized by cholesterol and disulfide cross-linking for systemic delivery of siRNA to solid tumors, *Biomaterials* 35 (2014) 7887–7895.

163. S.E. Han, H. Kang, G.Y. Shim, M.S. Suh, S.J. Kim, J.S. Kim, Y.K. Oh, Novel cationic cholesterol derivative-based liposomes for serum-enhanced delivery of siRNA, *Int. J. Pharm.* 353 (2008) 260–269.

164. T. Kanazawa, K. Morisaki, S. Suzuki, Y. Takashima, Prolongation of life in rats with malignant glioma by intranasal siRNA/drug codelivery to the brain with cell penetrating peptide-modified micelles, *Mol. Pharm.* 11 (2014) 1471–1478.

165. M. Malhotra, C. Tomaro-Duchesneau, S. Saha, I. Kahouli, S. Prakash, Development and characterization of chitosan-PEG-TAT nanoparticles for the intracellular delivery of siRNA, *Int. J. Nanomed.* 8 (2013) 2041–2052.

166. L. Crombez, M.C. Morris, S. Dufort, G. Aldrian-Herrada, Q. Nguyen, G.McMaster, J.L. Coll, F. Heitz, G. Divita, Targeting cyclin B1 through peptide-based delivery of siRNA prevents tumour growth, *Nucleic Acids Res.* 37 (2009) 4559–4569.

167. M.C. Morris, E. Gros, G. Aldrian-Herrada, M. Choob, J. Archdeacon, F. Heitz, G. Divita, A non-covalent peptide-based carrier for in vivo delivery of DNA mimics, *Nucleic Acids Res.* 35 (2007) e49.

168. T. Ishihara, M. Goto, K. Kodera, H. Kanazawa, Y. Murakami, Y. Mizushima, M. Higaki, Intracellular delivery of siRNA by cell-penetrating peptides modified with cationic oligopeptides, *Drug Deliv.* 16 (2009) 153–159.

169. T.L. Cuellar, D. Barnes, C. Nelson, J. Tanguay, S.F. Yu, X. Wen, S.J. Scales, J. Gesch, D. Davis, A. van Brabant Smith, D. Leake, R. Vandlen, C.W. Siebel, Systematic evaluation of antibody-mediated siRNA delivery using an industrial platform of THIOMAB-siRNA conjugates, *Nucleic Acids Res.* 43 (2015) 1189–1203.

170. E. Song, P. Zhu, S.K. Lee, D. Chowdhury, S. Kussman, D.M. Dykxhoorn, Y. Feng, D. Palliser, D.B. Weiner, P. Shankar, W.A. Marasco, J. Lieberman, Antibody mediated in vivo delivery of small interfering RNAs via cell-surface receptors, *Nat. Biotechnol.* 23 (2005) 709–717.

171. Y.D. Yao, T.M. Sun, S.Y. Huang, S. Dou, L. Lin, J.N. Chen, J.B. Ruan, C.Q. Mao, F.Y. Yu, M.S. Zeng, J.Y. Zang, Q. Liu, F.X. Su, P. Zhang, J. Lieberman, J. Wang, E. Song, Targeted delivery of PLK1-siRNA by ScFv suppresses Her2+ breast cancer growth and metastasis, *Sci. Transl. Med.* 4(130) (2012) (130ra148). doi:10.1126/scitranslmed.3003601, www.ScienceTranslationalMedicine.org

172. C.F. Xia, Y. Zhang, Y. Zhang, R.J. Boado, W.M. Pardridge, Intravenous siRNA of brain cancer with receptor targeting and avidin-biotin technology, *Pharm. Res.* 24 (2007) 2309–2316.

173. S. Baeumer, N. Baeumer, N. Appel, L. Terheyden, J. Fremerey, S. Schelhaas, E. Wardelmann, F. Buchholz, W.E. Berdel, C. Muller-Tidow, Antibody-mediated delivery of anti-KRAS-siRNA in vivo overcomes therapy resistance in colon cancer, *Clin. Cancer Res.* 21(6) (2015) 1383–1394.

174. J.P. Dassie, X.Y. Liu, G.S. Thomas, R.M. Whitaker, K.W. Thiel, K.R. Stockdale, D.K. Meyerholz, A.P. McCaffrey, J.O. McNamara II, P.H. Giangrande, Systemic administration of optimized aptamer-siRNA chimeras promotes regression of PSMA expressing tumors, *Nat. Biotechnol.* 27 (2009) 839–849.

175. J.O. McNamara II, E.R. Andrechek, Y. Wang, K.D. Viles, R.E. Rempel, E. Gilboa, B.A. Sullenger, P.H. Giangrande, Cell type-specific delivery of siRNAs with aptamersiRNA chimeras, *Nat. Biotechnol.* 24 (2006) 1005–1015.

176. F. Pastor, D. Kolonias, P.H. Giangrande, E. Gilboa, Induction of tumour immunity by targeted inhibition of nonsense-mediated mRNA decay, *Nature* 465 (2010) 227–230.

177. U. Wullner, I. Neef, A. Eller, M. Kleines, M.K. Tur, S. Barth, Cell-specific induction of apoptosis by rationally designed bivalent aptamer-siRNA transcripts silencing eukaryotic elongation factor 2, *Curr. Cancer Drug Targets* 8 (2008) 554–565.

178. J. Zhou, K. Tiemann, P. Chomchan, J. Alluin, P. Swiderski, J. Burnett, X. Zhang, S. Forman, R. Chen, J. Rossi, Dual functional BAFF receptor aptamers inhibit ligand-induced proliferation and deliver siRNAs to NHL cells, *Nucleic Acids Res.* 41 (2013) 4266–4283.

179. K.W. Thiel, L.I. Hernandez, J.P. Dassie, W.H. Thiel, X. Liu, K.R. Stockdale, A.M. Rothman, F.J. Hernandez, J.O. McNamara II, P.H. Giangrande, Delivery of chemosensitizing siRNAs to HER2+-breast cancer cells using RNA aptamers, *Nucleic Acids Res.* 40 (2012) 6319–6337.

180. S.W. Choi, S.H. Lee, H. Mok, T.G. Park, Multifunctional siRNA delivery system: polyelectrolyte complex micelles of six-arm PEG conjugate of siRNA and cell penetrating peptide with crosslinked fusogenic peptide, *Biotechnol. Prog.* 26 (2010) 57–63.

181. D.J. Wong, S.A. Hurvitz, Recent advances in the development of anti-HER2 antibodies and antibody-drug conjugates, *Ann. Transl. Med.* 2 (2014) 122.

182. L. Cerchia, V. de Franciscis, Targeting cancer cells with nucleic acid aptamers, *Trends Biotechnol.* 28 (2010) 517–525.

183. P. Kumar, H.-S. Ban, S.-S. Kim et al., T cell-specific siRNA delivery suppresses HIV-1 infection in humanized mice, *Cell* 134(4) (2008) 577–586.

184. P. Guo, O. Coban, N.M. Snead et al., Engineering RNA for targeted siRNA delivery and medical application, *Adv. Drug Deliv. Rev.* 62(6) (2010) 650–666.

185. S. Abdelmawla, S. Guo, L. Zhang et al., Pharmacological characterization of chemically synthesized monomeric phi29 pRNA nanoparticles for systemic delivery, *Mol. Ther.* 19(7) (2011) 1312–1322.

186. D. Shu, Y. Shu, F. Haque, S. Abdelmawla, P. Guo, Thermodynamically stable RNA three-way junction for constructing multifunctional nanoparticles for delivery of therapeutics, *Nat. Nanotechnol.* 6(10) (2011) 658–667.

187. F. Haque, D. Shu, Y. Shu et al., Ultrastable synergistic tetravalent RNA nanoparticles for targeting to cancers, *Nano Today* 7(4) (2012) 245–257.

188. B.R. Meade, S.F. Dowdy, Exogenous siRNA delivery using peptide transduction domains/cell penetrating peptides, *Adv. Drug Deliv. Rev.* 59(2–3) (2007) 134–140.

189. Y.S. Cho, G.Y. Lee, H.K. Sajja et al., Targeted delivery of siRNA-generating DNA nanocassettes using multifunctional nanoparticles, *Small* 9 (11) (2013) 1964–1973. doi:10.1002/smll.201201973.

190. B.S. Nielsen, F. Rank, M. Illemann, L.R. Lund, K. Danø, Stromal cells associated with early invasive foci in human mammary ductal carcinoma in situ coexpress urokinase and urokinase receptor, *Int. J. Cancer* 120(10) (2007) 2086–2095.

191. F. Blasi, P. Carmeliet, uPAR: a versatile signalling orchestrator, *Nat. Rev. Mol. Cell Biol.* 3(12) (2002) 932–943.

192. Loutfy H. Madkour, *Reactive Oxygen Species (ROS), Nanoparticles, and Endoplasmic Reticulum (ER) Stress-Induced Cell Death Mechanisms.* Paperback ISBN: 9780128224816. Imprint: Academic Press Published Date: 1st August 2020. https://www.elsevier.com/books/reactive-oxygen-species-ros-nanoparticles-and-endoplasmic-reticulum-er-stress-induced-cell-death-mechanisms/madkour/978-0-12-822481-6.

193. Loutfy H. Madkour, *Nanoparticles Induce Oxidative and Endoplasmic Reticulum Antioxidant Therapeutic Defenses.* Copyright 2020 Publisher Springer International Publishing. Copyright Holder Springer Nature Switzerland AG eBook ISBN 978-3-030-37297-2 DOI 10.1007/978-3-030-37297-2 Hardcover ISBN 978-3-030-37296-5 Series ISSN 2194-0452 Edition Number 1. https://www.springer.com/gp/book/9783030372965?utm_campaign=3_pier05_buy_print&utm_content=en_08082017&utm_medium=referral&utm_source=google_books#otherversion=9783030372972.

194. Loutfy H. Madkour, *Nucleic Acids as Gene Anticancer Drug Delivery Therapy.* 1st Edition. Publishing house: Elsevier, (2020). Paperback ISBN: 9780128197776 Imprint: Academic Press Published Date: 2nd January 2020 Imprint: Academic Press Copyright: Paperback ISBN: 9780128197776 © Academic Press 2020 Published: 2nd January 2020 Imprint: Academic Press Paperback ISBN: 9780128197776. https://www.elsevier.com/books/nucleic-acids-as-gene-anticancer-drug-deliverytherapy/madkour/978-0-12–819777-6.

195. Loutfy H. Madkour, *Nanoelectronic Materials: Fundamentals and Applications (Advanced Structured Materials)* 1st ed. 2019 Edition: https://link.springer.com/book/10.1007%2F978-3-030-21621-4 Series Title Advanced Structured Materials Series Volume 116 Copyright 2019 Publisher Springer International Publishing Copyright Holder Springer Nature Switzerland AG. eBook ISBN 978-3-030-21621-4 DOI 10.1007/978-3-030-21621-4 Hardcover ISBN 978-3-030-21620-7 Series ISSN 1869-8433 Edition Number 1 Number of Pages XLIII, 783 Number of Illustrations 122 b/w illustrations, 494 illustrations in colour Topics. ISBN-10: 3030216209 ISBN-13: 978-3030216207 #117 in Nanotechnology (Books) #725 in Materials Science (Books) #187336 in Textbooks. https://books.google.com.eg/books/about/Nanoelectronic_Materials.html?id=YQXCxAEACAAJ&source=kp_book_description&redir_esc=y; https://www.springer.com/gp/book/9783030216207.

5 Small Interfering RNAs, MicroRNAs, and NPs in Gynecological Cancers

Gynecological cancers (GCs) are often diagnosed at advanced stages, limiting the efficacy of available therapeutic options. Modulation of tumor microenvironment by miRNAs can possibly explain some of their reported biological effects. miRNA signatures have been proposed as biomarkers for the early detection of GCs, even the various subtypes of individual GCs. miRNA signatures are also being pursued as predictors of response to therapies. However, siRNA therapeutics has to face important drawbacks in therapy including stability and successful siRNA delivery *in vivo*. In this regard, the development of effective siRNA delivery systems has helped to address these issues by opening novel therapeutic windows which have allowed building up important advances in nanomedicine. It is time to ponder over the knowledge gained so that more meaningful pre-clinical and translational studies can be designed to better realize the potential that miRNAs have to offer.

5.1 INTRODUCTION

Cancer has become one of the most complex diseases due to numerous genetic disorders and cellular abnormalities. Cancer disease continues to be a major health concern worldwide, being the second leading cause of death in the world. According to the World Health Organization (WHO), nearly ten million people are estimated to die of cancer by the year 2020. Cancer has been known as the number one cause of deaths in developed countries in the current century [1–3]. While remarkable efforts have been developed during the past few decades in the detection, prevention, and treatment [4,5], signaling pathway complexities that regulate cancer progression together with its tumor microenvironment heterogeneity and metastasis remain as serious obstacles to find efficient cancer treatments [6,7]. Nowadays, treatments based on single chemotherapeutic drugs generally face a lack of effectiveness in cancer therapy, whereas two or more combined therapeutic methods involving various mechanisms of action are needed to achieve certain effectiveness in cancer therapy.

The currently used therapies are non-selective, leading to side effects responsible for prolonged and expensive recovery, often followed by relapse at later time points. In this context, the selective targeting may provide a platform for the development of novel, more effective diagnostic tools and/or less harmful treatments [8]. Targeted therapies using monoclonal antibodies (mAb) against overexpressed receptors (e.g., Herceptin) have improved clinical outcomes [9]. Moreover, nanomaterials have also become an interesting alternative approach for the administration of drugs,

reducing the side effects (e.g., biodegradable nanoparticles loaded with docetaxel) [10]. The impact of these nanomedicines on human health may be enormous if the right combination of targeting molecules and drugs becomes available with defined chemical structures. This has been demonstrated with the explosion of the antibodies-drug conjugates field [11]. However, the control of the number and position of the drugs on the antibodies, as well as the design of auto-immolative linkers to help trigger drug release after internalization, is still far to be solved although this is an active field of development [12].

Recently, much attention has been paid to the potential application of RNA interference (RNAi) for cancer treatment [8,13]. RNAi is the term given to the ability of a double-stranded RNA (dsRNA) containing a homologous sequence to a specific gene leading to sequence-specific gene silencing. RNAi is an endogenous post-transcriptional regulation process that consists of small regulatory RNAs including microRNAs (miRNAs) or small interfering RNAs (siRNAs) which are able to silence target messenger RNAs (mRNAs) in a sequence-specific procedure [14]. After the discovery of RNAi in Caenorhabditis elegans [15,16] and subsequent demonstration of siRNA activity in mammalian cells, RNAi has received considerable attention as an effective therapy for multiple diseases like cancer and viral infections, particularly for those diseases with "undruggable" molecular targets [17,18].

Today, RNAi has become a powerful technology for gene function studies and has been recently used in therapeutic applications [18–20]. The main role of the RNAi in cells is the down-regulation of specific proteins (Figure 5.1). RNAi mechanism is triggered initially by the enzyme Dicer, which cleaves dsRNAs into short double-stranded siRNAs of 21–25 nt. The siRNA passenger strand is then unwound, and the siRNA guide strand is loaded into the RNA-induced silencing complex (RISC), leading to cleavage of target mRNAs by Argonaute 2 (Ago2) when the guide strand sequence is paired with an mRNA complementary sequence [21–23]. This important mechanism has allowed opening novel therapeutic approaches by designing oligonucleotide molecules by using mRNA transcripts sequences found in the existing human genomic data. Therefore, a careful sequence selection and synthesis of tailored siRNAs may have enormous repercussions in therapy as almost all genes might be down-regulated as well as splice variants, separate transcripts, or mutations might also be specifically targeted. As a consequence, this powerful approach might help circumvent the limitations exhibited by small molecule drugs in conventional cancer therapy treatments, leading to drug

DOI: 10.1201/9781003229674-5

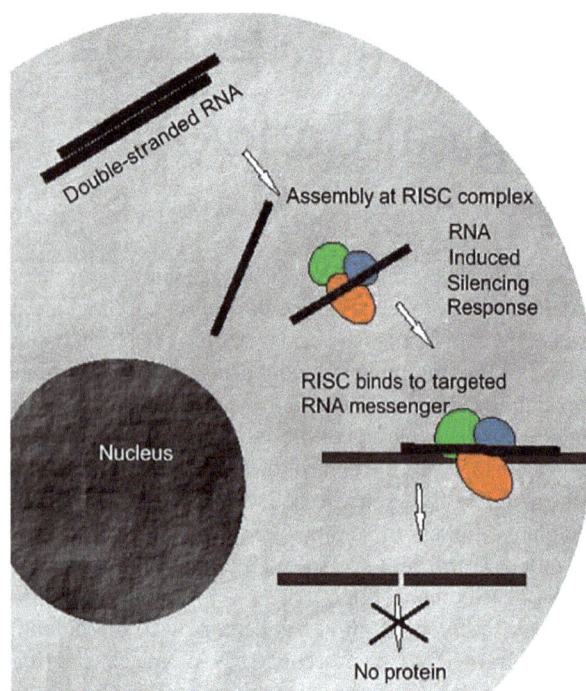

FIGURE 5.1 Mechanism of action of siRNA molecules. SiRNA duplexes are incorporated in the RNA-induced silencing complex (RISC). Then, siRNA are unwinded and the strand with lower thermodynamic stability at its 5′ end remains in the complex and guides it to the complementary mRNA. The target mRNA is then cleaved and protein expression is abolished or reduced.

development processes based on gene functionality [21]. Therefore, the development of this therapeutic strategy may have a high impact on modern medicine [20,24,25].

However, siRNA technology faces multiple obstacles regarding efficient delivery and effectiveness. To overcome this issue, siRNA intracellular delivery strategies should be nontoxic and stable at the site of action for succeeding therapeutic applications of RNAi [26–28]. Currently, different methods including mechanical (ultrasound), physical methods [29], electroporation [30], hydrodynamic tail vein injections in mice [31], and the use of a gene gun have been carried out for delivering siRNA *in vivo*. In addition, local administrations (e.g., intraperitoneal, intravenous, subcutaneous injections) and chemical methods based on synthesizing non-viral vehicles (e.g., polymers [32–34], cationic lipids [35,36], and peptides [37,38]) have also been successfully used among others. To demonstrate the potential of RNAi-based therapeutics, several proof-of-concept studies including bio-distribution, efficiency of delivery, and toxicity caused by cationic delivery vehicles have been carefully analyzed.

5.2 siRNA TECHNOLOGY IN CANCER THERAPY

siRNA has been investigated as an effective treatment for viral disease as well as cancer extensively with the aim of blocking multiple disease-causing genes [39]. RNAi was discovered for the first time in the nematode *Caenorhabditis*

elegans; however, this process has been also found in many different eukaryotes species, including vertebrates, plants, and insects. In mammalian cells, researchers reported that synthetic siRNAs were also able to promote RNAi and, therefore, silence the expression of altered proteins [15–17,40].

Numerous chemical modifications have been proposed in order to increase efficacy and potency in RNAi for *in vivo* use [41]. In this regard, rational chemical designs have allowed siRNA passenger strands to be more likely to modification than siRNA guide strands. These synthetic strategies have enabled to replace either non-bridging oxygen on the phosphate linkage with a sulfur atom, the 2′-hydroxyl group modification of the sugar ring with a methyl group ($2'\text{-OCH}_3$) and ethyl group ($2'\text{-OCH}_2\text{CH}_3$), among others [42–45]. In addition, other strategies have been developed to deliver siRNAs safely in the cytoplasm. While most naked siRNAs have been effective for a good number of tumor cells *in vitro*, these siRNAs have unfortunately failed when injected *in vivo* by systemic administrations [46].

Immunotherapy has gained increasing attention as a promising strategy for treating cancer by promoting the host immune system activation. This activation may occur by simply introducing cytokines, cancer vaccines, mAb, or using antigen-presenting cells through Toll-like receptors [47]. Dendritic cells (DCs) are the strongest antigen-exhibiting cells that have the capacity to stimulate naïve T cells and stimulate differentiation and growth of B cells. Furthermore, they include a system of leukocytes broadly distributed in all tissues. DC therapy may offer a novel and promising immunotherapeutic method for the prevention and treatment of advanced cancer as well as autoimmune disorders [48,49].

DC immunization has been broadly studied in clinical trials involving several types of malignancies like melanoma, prostate cancer, and renal cell carcinoma, among others [50–54]. The use of DC therapy has proved to be effective and a safe strategy in inducing antitumor immunity to patients containing advanced-stage cancer diseases [51,55]. Several models have been proposed with the aim of isolating DCs *in vitro*. For example, Zhang et al developed a method to favor DC differentiation through contact circulating monocytes with natural killer cell subsets in order to find optimal protocols for DC vaccination [56]. According to *in vivo* studies, DCs can promote T cell-mediated tumor eradication and controlled tumor-bearing hosts when *ex vivo* isolation has been implemented with tumor antigens. These perceptions have prompted clinical trials to explore both immunologic and clinical impacts of antigen-loaded DCs regulated as therapeutic vaccines to patients containing specific tumors. Some promising outcomes reported from clinical trials in patients with melanoma and malignant prostate tumors showed that immunotherapeutic strategies involving the development of antigen-presenting cells in DCs might demonstrate the effectiveness of this process to certain human tumors [50]. However, DC clinical effectiveness has not been as good as researchers expected in some specific cancers probably due to the heterogeneity and different methods to monocyte production as well as DC differentiation.

Interestingly, novel approaches have been implemented involving dendritic cell-based therapies and other therapies like RNAi in order to overcome these drawbacks and find a reliable vaccine for cancer therapy [57]. For example, Qian et al reported that siRNA may be combined to DC-based therapy in order to manipulate CD40 expression levels and therefore reduce the functional capability of DC to stimulate allogeneic T cells. In this regard, silencing of CD40 expression on DCs might be used for generating tolerance-promoting DCs with the aim of applying in autoimmunity and transplantation processes [58].

Recently, Liu et al prepared a specific cationic nanoparticle in order to deliver indoleamine 2, 3-dioxygenase (IDO) siRNA and tyrosine-related protein 2 (Trp2) to DCs [59]. The authors were able to inhibit IDO expression, trigger T-cell immune reaction and consequently favor the secretion of cytokines like IL-6, IFN-ϒ, and TNF-α as well as promote DC differentiation when compared to traditional control DC vaccines. Thus, *in vitro* and *in vivo* studies in the B16-F10 mouse model proved this approach to be effective in reducing melanoma tumor growth and therefore enhancing the immune response in mice.

5.3 siRNA-BASED GENE SILENCING

Great efforts have been made to understand how dsRNAs, siRNAs, and miRNAs are able to affect control expression in eukaryotic cells. As described previously, siRNA technology mediates, specifically, gene silencing at different levels like mRNA degradation, chromatin modification, and translational repression [60–64]. Remarkable findings were also found and confirmed that transcriptional gene silencing was conserved in mammalian cells when mediated by siRNAs [65]. Despite the advantages and interest showed by siRNA-based technology as an effective therapeutic approach, many obstacles like efficient cellular uptake, long-term stabilities, and off-target effects have been reported. These important issues have reduced siRNA effectiveness when used *in vitro* and/or injected in animal models as well.

While the enhancement of siRNA stability has been successfully solved by introducing chemical modifications at the level of sugar and phosphate groups, advances in efficient siRNA delivery systems to transport siRNAs safely into the cytoplasm of targeted cells is a vital element in cancer therapy [66,67]. For this purpose, viral vectors (e.g., lentivirus, retrovirus, and adenovirus) have become potential vectors for siRNA delivery due to their ability to encapsulate and deliver genetic materials into cells [68,69]. Despite such viral vectors having been shown highly transfection efficacies, their clinical usage is still limited due to possible risks of immune responses, mutation, and inflammation. To minimize such undesirable effects and exploit the potential of RNAi-based technology, a good number of synthetic non-viral vectors have been proposed to impart siRNA delivery safely and effectively [22,35].

5.4 OFF-TARGET EFFECTS AND STIMULATION OF IMMUNE RESPONSE

The specificity of action carried out by siRNA molecules depends upon the uniqueness of the selected sequences; however, many other factors may also have an impact on a lack of specificity [70]. Several types involving siRNA off-target effects have been described and thoroughly reviewed [71]. It is well known that mammalian immune cells tend to express a family of receptors so-called Toll-like receptors (TLRs) which also have the ability to recognize pathogens and molecules derived from microbes. In addition, some synthetic siRNA sequences as well as their non-viral vehicles have proved to promote the activation of immune system cells, producing inflammatory cytokines and Type I interferon *in vitro* and *in vivo* by activating TLR7 and TLR8 in a sequence-dependent manner [72].

Other significant off-target effect associated with siRNA delivery falls into the miRNA-like off-target silencing. miRNAs are small non-coding endogenous RNA molecules that have the ability to regulate gene expression of several genes in the same way as siRNAs do. This undesirable sequence-specific activity is mainly produced via siRNA base pairing with sequences located at the 3'-UTR regions of mRNAs. As a consequence, many transcripts might be affected dealing with multiple-site cleavage translational blocks [73,74].

Finally, the RNAi machinery saturation mediated by synthetic siRNAs is another source of off-target. Some data have shown that synthetic siRNAs when entering the RNAi pathway tend to compete with endogenous miRNAs for RISC. This process has been observed in certain model studies in which both transcript upregulation and target script down-regulation have been observed. Efforts to mitigate or reduce such off-target effects have been effectively studied by designing effective modified siRNAs [75–79].

5.5 DELIVERY SYSTEMS

5.5.1 LIPID-BASED NANOVECTORS FOR siRNA DELIVERY

Various kinds of systems have been employed for delivering siRNA, such as antibody conjugates, micelles, natural polysaccharides, peptides, synthetic cationic polymers, and microparticles among others. Nevertheless, some lipid-based formulations and other lipid-like materials such as liposomes, niosomes, and stable nucleic acid lipid particles (SNALPs) have proved to be effective drug delivery systems as promising strategies for *in vivo* siRNA delivery [80–85] (Figure 5.2).

5.5.2 LIPOSOMES AND LIPOPLEXES

As non-viral vectors, liposomes have become a powerful platform as a pharmaceutical carrier to facilitate the delivery of small molecule drugs and macromolecules [86]. Liposomes are made up of phospholipids which tend to form closed lipid bilayers in aqueous solvents dealing with

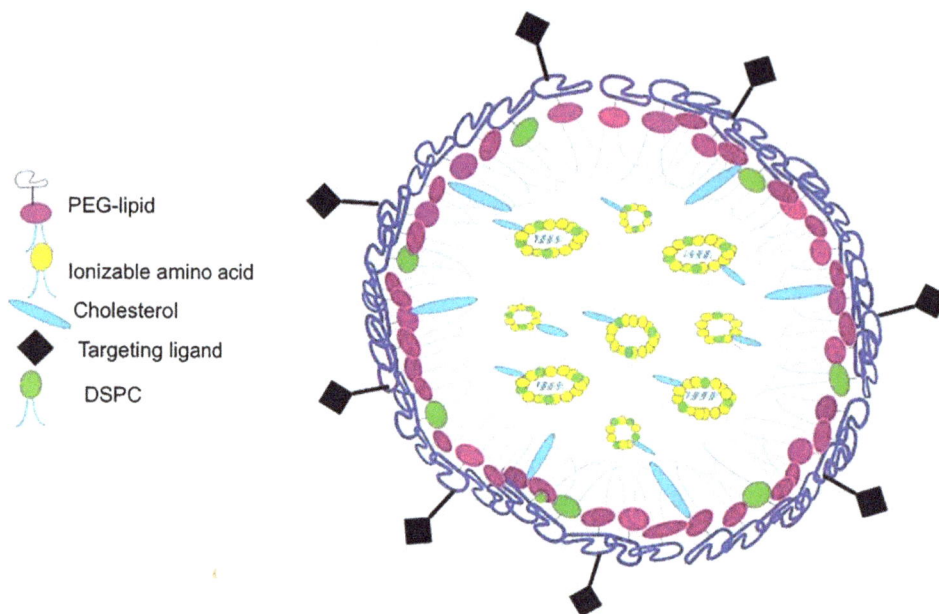

FIGURE 5.2 A schematic image of LNPs siRNA showing a nanostructured core.

particle formation of nanometric size. In addition to loading a good number of substances like active drugs, proteins, peptides, antibodies, and nucleic acids, liposomes have been also used in the transport of photosensitizers needed for promoting photo-dynamic therapy [87]. The second and third generation of liposomes have also been proposed by including certain ligands or loading polymers which have the ability to recognize specific receptors or enhance liposome stabilities, respectively [88]. These advances have allowed liposomes to be used in a good number of clinical applications and also be injected according to different administration routes.

Nucleic acids, in particular antisense oligonucleotides (ASOs), and siRNAs have been widely incorporated into liposomal nanocarriers (Table 5.1) [35,62].

This electrostatic combination has resulted in obtaining the corresponding lipoplexes, which have helped nucleic acids increase both their long-term stabilities and cellular internalization. Positive and negative charged together with neutral liposomes have been used as vehicles for transporting siRNA molecules efficiently [91] (Figure 5.3). In this regard, cationic lipids have attracted significant attention

as appropriate non-viral vehicles. This interest has allowed designing convenient synthetic strategies and characterizing a plethora of cationic lipids. Structurally, cationic lipids consist of three general components: (i) the lipid tail(s); (ii) the cationic head group, and (iii) the linkers and/or backbones that connect to both parts. Some studies have suggested a relationship between the efficiency and lipid structure; however, this involvement still remains a central goal in siRNA delivery [82].

While anionic liposomes are usually cleared from circulation, cationic liposomes (e.g., DC-Cholesterol, DOTAP, and AtuFECT01 among others) in combination with helper lipids (e.g., Cholesterol, DOPE, and DPhyPE) have proved efficient in siRNA delivery at optimized N/P ratios. However, reducing toxicity levels still remains crucial when forming these types of lipoplexes [92–94]. To solve these issues, neutral liposomes [e.g., 1,2-dioleoyl-sn-glycero-3-phosphatidyl-choline (DOPC)] have been prepared in order to reduce such toxicity and therefore increase biocompatibility although their entrapment efficiency might be compromised [95].

TABLE 5.1

Summary of siRNA-Loaded Encapsulated Liposomes Utilized for siRNA Delivery [89]

Liposome Components	Target Cells	Target Genes	References
DOPC	HeyA8, SKOV3ip1	EphA2	[13]
Egg PC, Chol, PEG-PE, DOTAP, R8	SK-MES-1	HDM2	[23]
Lipidoid, Chol, PEGlipids	Hepatocytes	Factor VII, ApoB	[23]
DOTAP, Chol, PEGlipids	HeLa	GFP	[23]
DLinDMA, DSPC, Chol, PEG-C-DMA	HepG2	HBV263, HBV1583	[32]
DOTAP, DOPE, PEGPE, Chol, Anti-EGFR	NCI-H322	Luciferase	[90]

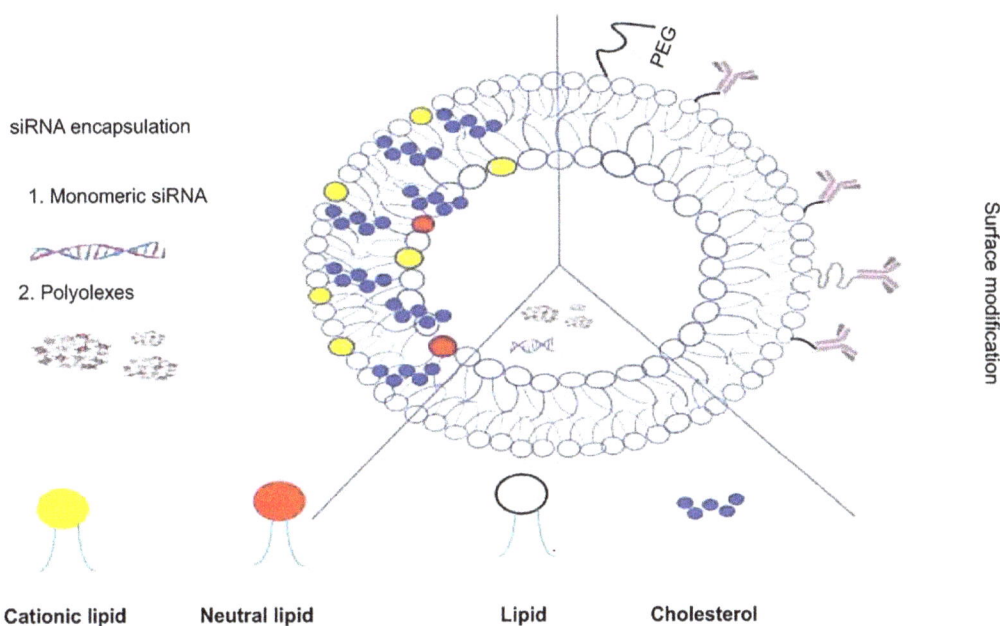

FIGURE 5.3   A schematic representations of several strategies for encapsulating siRNA in liposomes.

The use of neutral lipid-based formulations has enabled the successful siRNA delivery *in vivo* in mouse models, showing tumor growth inhibition and consequently the down-regulation of targeted genes [67]. Several siRNA-based treatments against ovarian cancer were suggested by Sood et al [96]. In this study, DOPC-encapsulated siRNA targeting the oncoprotein Ephrin Type-A receptor 2 was highly effective (65%) in reducing its expression after 48 h of being administered in a single dose in an orthotopic model. Interestingly, the authors found that this liposomal formulation when injected both intraperitoneal and intravenous reduced the ovarian tumor size in mice xenograft models with the same efficiency. In addition, treatments with DOPC-based liposomes were also studied in order to target interleukin-8, β-2 adrenergic receptor, and focal adhesion-kinase by mediating intraperitoneal delivery of siRNAs in an ovarian cancer mouse model [96].

In spite of obtaining powerful and effective nanovehicles based on formulating lipid molecules and siRNAs, liposomes and niosomes85 have been properly tuned in order to promote targeted delivery in specific organs and tissues. This strategy has enabled the preparation of unique lipid-based platforms bearing the arginine-glycine-aspartic acid (RGD) peptide [97] or decorated with an octa-arginine (R8) cell-penetrating peptide (CPPs) [98]. These two strategies have confirmed increased particle stability, biocompatibility, and good siRNA therapeutic response without affecting cellular viability remarkably.

5.5.3   STABLE NUCLEIC ACID LIPID PARTICLES (SNALPs)

SNALPs have become a promising delivery platform for siRNA molecules in different animal models. This formulation is made up of a lipid bilayer based on a mixture of fusogenic and cationic lipids, which enables endosomal release and therefore facilitates the siRNA cellular uptake. In addition, the SNALP surface is also coated during the formulation process with a PEG-lipid conjugate that provides hydrophilicity and a neutral layer with the aim of stabilizing these particles in the bloodstream when injected *in vivo* [35]. The first use of SNALPs was reported by Zimmermann et al. to silence the apolipoprotein B (Apo B) gene expression in non-human primates with a single dose (2.5 mg/kg) of siRNA [99]. Optimized formulations based on modifying SNALPs chemically increased their siRNA efficacy *in vivo* by reducing doses until 0.01 mg/kg when targeting a hepatic endogenous gene [82].

Other important applications of SNALPs have been reported and reviewed in the literature [100]. For example, McLachlan et al. formulated a siRNA targeting the polymerase gene *in vivo* in order to fully protect guinea pigs against Ebola virus [101]. More recently, SNALP technology has been successfully employed to favor the silencing of mTTR expression [102]. Clinical results confirmed the suitability and therapeutic effect of this siRNA–SNALP combination in humans, giving rise to the first RNAi therapeutic in the market [68,103].

5.6   POLYMERIC NANOPARTICLES

The past decades have witnessed the large development of polymeric nanosized materials as drug carriers, becoming some of the top-selling drugs [102,104]. Synthetic or naturally siRNA-occurring nanopolymers are colloidal solid materials, specially designed to be degraded *in vivo* without producing toxic components [105]. Several polymeric nanoparticles have been approved as drug carriers for human use [106]. Due to their excellent properties, a variety of polymers including cationic polymers such as polyethyl-enimine (PEI), polysaccharides such as cyclodextrin (CD) and chitosan have been studied for siRNA delivery [90,107]. As a general rule, polymer nanoparticles exhibit positively charged units to facilitate electrostatic binding of siRNA; however, the use of covalent strategies involving siRNA and polymers have been frequently prepared by using degradable linkers such as disulfide or thiol-maleimide bonds [108].

5.6.1 Cyclodextrin (CD) Nanoparticles

Cyclodextrins are naturally occurring oligosaccharides that are produced during the bacterial digestion of cellulose. They have been well studied and characterized as pharmaceutical excipients with a favorable toxicological profile [109–111] (Figure 5.4). CD-containing polycation nanoparticles are exciting polymer-based siRNA delivery systems, as they are able to self-assemble with siRNA dealing to shape colloidal particles of about 50 nm in diameter. In addition, their terminal imidazole groups help in the release and intracellular trafficking of nucleic acids. A complex system consisting of a siRNA, the human transferrin protein to engage transferrin receptors on the surface of the cancer cells, a CD-based polymer, and polyethylene glycol (PEG) has been described to increase the stability of nanoparticles in biological fluids [112,113].

An example of this system is CALAA-01, which is a targeted nanocomplex that includes an anti-R2 siRNA [114]. This targeted therapeutic system has been designed to inhibit tumor growth. The selected siRNA prevents the tumor from growing via RNAi to decrease expression of the M2 subunit of R2 (ribonucleotide reductase). This system was used in clinical studies in patients bearing solid tumors [115].

5.6.2 Chitosan and Inulin Nanoparticles

Chitosan and inulin are naturally occurring polysaccharides used for the preparation of siRNA formulations. Chitosan, which contains hydroxyl and amino groups, is widely used as a drug carrier due to its low cost, easy degradability, and biocompatibility. Chitosan has positive charges

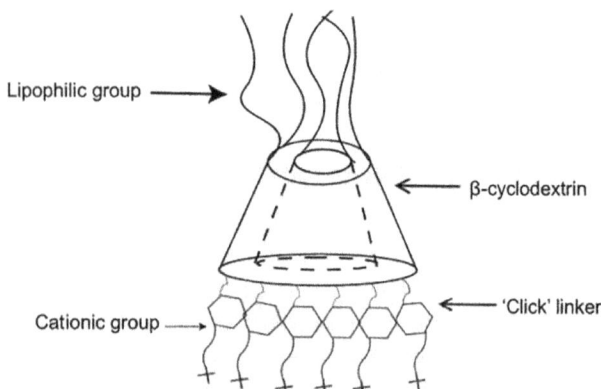

FIGURE 5.4 Schematic illustration of a Cyclodextrin structure.

under slightly acidic conditions, allowing the formation of nanoparticles or complexes by interaction with siRNA molecules [116,117]. Interestingly, optimized chitosan formulations containing folic acid as a targeting ligand resulted in increasing siRNA cellular uptake to tumor cells producing an enhancement in gene-silencing properties in HeLa and OV-3 cell lines [117]. Furthermore, grafting chitosan with PEG [118] and polyethylenenimine [119] enables it for *in vivo* use through intravenous or intraperitoneal administration [118,119]. Chitosan is frequently used in combination with other carriers such as poly(L-lactide) (PLLA) porous microparticle [120,121] or the triblock polymer poly(L-lactide)-poly(ethyleneglycol)-poly(L-lactide) (PLLA-PEG-PLLA) to increase storage stability and decrease immunogenicity [122]. These formulations, prepared by supercritical fluid technology [123], allowed the addition of multiple polymers as well as other chemotherapeutic drugs such as paclitaxel [122] and doxorubicin [121].

Another polysaccharide used recently in siRNA delivery is inulin. This polysaccharide, made up of fructose and glucose units, is usually processed with oligoamines such as ethylenediamine [124] or diethylenetriamine and imidazole [125,126] in order to generate cationic groups for siRNA binding and therefore favor endosomal escape.

5.6.3 Polyethylenimine (PEI)

Polyethylenimine (PEI) is one of the most-studied cationic polymers for the transfection of oligonucleotides, siRNA, and plasmid DNA [127]. It is accessible either in a branched or linear shape and has many molecular weights [128]. The high charge density of PEI is considered a good property for the complexation of siRNA and facilitates the endosomal escape by the proton sponge effect [127]. However, high-molecular-weight PEI has exhibited significant toxicity in many cell lines [128]. The use of PEI as a non-viral vehicle to deliver siRNAs was demonstrated to have an efficient antiviral effect in a guinea pig model of Ebola virus infection [129] and a murine model of influenza infection [130]. The first successful application of PEI delivery of siRNA in cancer was the inhibition of human EGF receptor 2 (HER2) in mouse models of ovarian cancer [131]. If provided the appropriate molecular weight polymer and structure to avoid toxicities, for systemic use, PEI appears to be a promising siRNA delivery system [132].

At present, research on PEI is directed towards the development of mixed polymers, especially with PEG [133] and polysaccharides such as chitosan [119] to reduce potential toxic effects and decrease the removal of nanoparticles by the reticuloendothelial system (RES). To direct PEI siRNA complexes to specific target cells, PEI has been modified with receptor-mediated ligands such as folic acid, mannose, N-acetylgalactosamine, and others [133].

5.6.4 Anionic Polymers

Poly-L-lactic-co-glycolic acid (PLGA) is a biocompatible, well-studied, and biodegradable polymer used for decades in pharmaceutical applications [134,135]. The PGLA polymer has the advantage of exhibiting lower toxicity when compared with cationic polymers and cationic lipids. On the other side, PLGA cannot form electrostatic complexes with siRNA as both are negatively charged. One way to overcome this issue is to use PLGA nanocapsules in order to encapsulate oligonucleotides bearing 5′-lipophilic molecules. These resulting polymer microspheres have provided sustained release of the modified siRNAs and antisense oligodeoxynucleotides within 24 h when administered subcutaneously [136]. Another interesting approach is to react polyamines or positively charged dendrimers with some of the carboxyl groups of PLGA in order to generate additional positive charges that can be used for electrostatic binding [135]. In addition, siRNAs may also be covalently linked to PLGA via intracellular cleavable disulfide linkers [137].

Hyaluronic acid (HA) is also an anionic polymer that plays a pivotal role as a ligand against the CD44 receptor, which is highly overexpressed in tumor cells. The combination of PLGA and HA has also been used to co-deliver paclitaxel together with a siRNA against focal adhesion kinase , which is overexpressed in breast, colon, and ovarian cancers [138]. The resulting PLGA nanoparticles were shown to possess a highly selective delivery of the paclitaxel and siRNA to CD44+ cells.

5.6.5 CATIONIC DENDRIMERS

Cationic dendrimers with extremely branched peripheral chain ends are well-defined artificial macromolecules. These can be synthesized by adding several layer branches. Each branched layer represents a superior generation molecule [134]. The precise core-shell nanostructures of dendrimers enable drug loading by surface adsorption, interior encapsulation, or chemical conjugation (Figure 5.5). The dendrimer surface can be functionalized to build a variety of functions for a good number of applications. Dendrimers have a well-defined chemical structure and size in comparison with alternative linear polymers with a spherical form. To deliver negatively charged plasmid DNA, siRNAs, and ASOs, dendrimers containing a high density of positive charges on the surface have been used [139,140]. Polycationic dendrimers including poly-propylenimine and poly-(amidoamine) (PAMAM) dendrimers have been investigated for siRNA delivery in past years. PAMAM-mediated siRNA delivery is usually found at nucleolus and even perinuclear locations. In a study designed for increasing the siRNA loading capacity, dendrimers were additionally improved with magnetofluorescent nanoworms to create "dendriworms" [141]. After adding the dendriworm-carrying siRNAs to human glioblastoma cells, the siRNA dendrimers quickly internalized into the cells and escaped into the cytosol. The delivered siRNAs were demonstrated to silence the expression of the targeted gene *in vivo* [142].

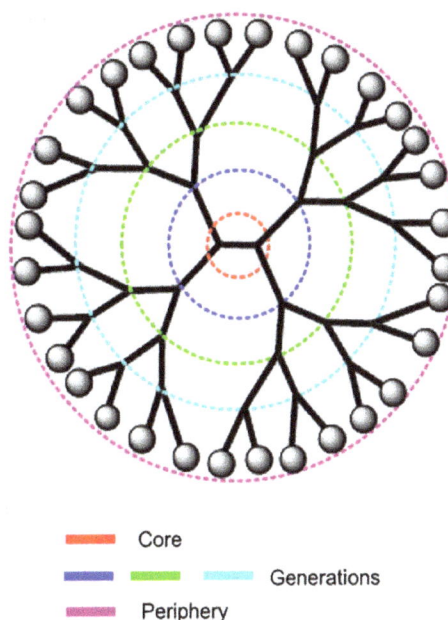

FIGURE 5.5 A schematic representation of a dendrimer showing the central core, the peripherical sites, and the consecutive generations.

5.7 CARBON NANOTUBES (CNTs)

Carbon nanotubes (CNTs) have been considered as potential nucleic acid and drug delivery vehicles within the nanomedicine field [143,144]. They can be either singlewalled CNTs (a single layer of graphene sheets) or multiwalled CNTs, which can be prepared using multiple layers. In addition, CNTs can be modified with additional functional groups and also offer a structural advantage due to their very large surface. This can be used for loading therapeutic drugs like proteins and nucleic acids. In order to form complexes with siRNA, positively charged functionalized single-walled CNTs (SWCNTs+) have been prepared. In a model study, siRNA designed to inhibit telomerase reverse transcriptase (TERT) was complexed with SWCNTs+ and incubated with tumor cells. The complexes TERT siRNA: SWCNTs+ were effective in delivering siRNA and knockdown the expression of TERT in a variety of tumor cells [145].

5.8 INORGANIC NANOPARTICLES (INPs)

In the past decades, inorganic nanoparticles (INPs) have emerged as alternative nanomaterials to traditional lipid formulations for siRNA delivery [146]. Specifically, magnetic nanoparticles and gold nanoparticles have been extensively studied for siRNA delivery and *in vivo* imaging because of their biocompatibility and reduced toxicity [146,147]. For example, mesoporous silica nanoparticles have been used as interesting vehicles for delivering siRNAs in cancer cells. Recently, Ngamcherdtrakul et al. successfully prepared 50 nm INPs decorated with PEI, PEG, and an antibody [148]. These authors were able to establish a lyophilization protocol for these modified INPs and, therefore, promote the formation of complexes with siRNAs. Interestingly, these siRNA nanoconstructs were stable, showed luciferase silencing inhibition, and were able to display antiproliferative effect *in vitro*. Other INPs like carbonate apatite have also been studied by Tiash et al. In this work, the authors used these NPs as vehicles for delivering siRNA, targeting GFR genes (egfr1 and erbb2) simultaneously in mouse models, showing the ability of these siRNA complexes to reduce tumor growth and reduce cell viability [149].

5.8.1 MAGNETIC NANOPARTICLES (MNPs)

Magnetic nanoparticles (MNPs) have been extensively employed as magnetic resonance imaging (MRI) contrast agents for tumor imaging and drug delivery as well. Iron oxide nanoparticles can be synthesized to obtain particles of small nanometric size with narrow and high magnetization values. In addition, MNPs have been shown to induce cancer-cell apoptosis by magnetic heating because of their excellent contrast signal in MRI [150]. In addition, MNPs can be coated with siRNAs as well as other chemotherapeutic agents in order to promote delivery to the tumor site by applying external magnetic fields. Some representative examples inducing cellular death by magnetic heating have been reported [151,152].

5.8.2 GOLD NANOPARTICLES (AuNPs)

Gold nanoparticles (AuNPs) have been used as effective nanomaterials for siRNA delivery applications for several reasons [147,153,154]. First, functional diversity can be easily obtained with the creation of multifunctional monolayers, and second, AuNPs can be prepared in a scalable fashion with low size disparity. AuNPs have been widely utilized for gene therapy targets in preclinical animal model and *in vitro* studies because of their low toxicity, rapid endosomal escape, high payload, efficient uptake, increased half-life, specific, efficient, extensive transcriptional activation of the innate immune response, and selective gene silencing and transfection [155]. AuNPs were effectively employed as a platform for the delivery of B-cell lymphoma 2 (Bcl-2)or vascular endothelial growth factor (VEGF) siRNAs to a human cervical carcinoma cell line or into a human glioma cell line, for silencing of enhanced green fluorescent protein and luciferase reporter genes [156,157].

5.9 LIMITATIONS TO THE siRNA THERAPEUTIC APPROACH

Table 5.2 summarizes some of the limitations described for siRNA delivery [158]. Degradation in serum of siRNA therapeutic molecules is one of the major limitations for the therapeutic use of these molecules. Double-stranded siRNA molecules are more stable than single-stranded ASOs. For this reason, unmodified siRNA in saline buffer has been described to be successful for human treatments. However, these cases have been mostly focused for the treatment of ocular diseases by local administration [159].

Most of the siRNA molecules used for therapeutic uses are partially modified since a large number of modifications may block RISC binding to siRNA and therefore prevent RNAi mechanism [166]. Frequently, these modifications are located near the 3' and 5'-ends of the passenger and guide strands, where it has been demonstrated that they have a strong impact in the following properties: (i) avoiding exonuclease degradation action [74,166]; (ii) increasing affinity to RISC [76]; (iii) preventing the passenger strand loading [76]; (iv) lowering innate immunostimulation response; [79] and (v) avoiding miRNA-like effects [75]. Another interesting siRNA chemical modification is the preparation of siRNA conjugates covalently [160], especially lipid conjugates such as cholesterol. Such lipid-siRNA conjugates have exhibited exonuclease resistance, promoted cellular uptake, and also increased serum circulation time by binding to serum proteins [161,163].

Carbohydrate-siRNA conjugates and, especially, N-acetyl-galactosamine (GalNAc)-siRNA conjugates have also being used for *in vivo* targeting to hepatocytes. A large impact on cellular uptake was observed with siRNAs

TABLE 5.2
Intracellular and Extracellular Limitations of RNAi

Limitation	Solution(s)	References
A. Intracellular		
mRNA targeting	Chemical modification of siRNA	[42]
Endosomal escape	Acid-responsive polymers/lipid complexation	[127]
	Conjugation or complexation with fusogenic peptides	[160]
B. Extracellular		
Targeting to specific cells	Vector modification with targeting ligands	[106]
Degradation in serum	Peptide/polymer/lipid complexation	[161]
	Chemical modification with PEG, etc.	[113,114]
	Nanoparticle encapsulation	[162]
Internalization	Peptide/polymer/lipid complexation for charge neutralization	[159]
	Conjugation or complexation with CPPs	[163]
	Ligand modification for receptor-mediated endocytosis	[164,165]

that were conjugated with triantennary GalNAc residues. Transfection experiments corroborated high specificity and gene silencing levels in the liver [167]. Peptide-siRNA conjugates, especially CPPs and fusogenic peptides [160] have been also described to potentiate cellular uptake and facilitate endosomal escape, being a good alternative for anticancer siRNA delivery.

Most of the clinical trials involving systemic delivery of siRNA molecules have used lipid formulations including liposomes, SNALPs, and other types of lipid formulations that contain cationic lipids to form complexes with siRNA molecules. One of the first human clinical trials for cancer treatment used two siRNA molecules formulated in lipid nanoparticles to treat liver metastasis of colon cancer [168]. These formulations were actively taken up by the liver but the treatment of cancer to other tissues was not demonstrated.

As shown in this chapter, the development of novel approaches based on nanomaterials is one of the most active areas of development for future medicines for cancer treatment. Polymeric nanoparticles are one of the most promising alternatives for the near future. The knowledge generated in the past decades for the delivery of chemotherapeutic agents using biocompatible nanopolymers will trigger the development of novel formulations that may include combinations of chemotherapeutic agents together with one or several siRNA molecules targeting overexpressed proteins for a more efficient and less toxic medicines. These nanomaterials as well as gold and superparamagnetic iron oxide nanoparticles (SPION) nanoparticles also allow the introduction of specific targeting molecules that will direct the accumulation of the therapeutic molecules near the tumors, increasing the passive accumulation of nanoparticles by the enhanced permeability and retention effect. The addition of acid-responsive polymers such as PEI and peptides may also increase the efficacy by facilitating endosomal escape. A limitation on the use of nanomaterials is the potential *in vivo* aggregation with serum proteins and

subsequent removal by the RES. This undesired effect may be prevented by the incorporation of PEG [137].

Finally, a novel approach with high potential is the use of DNA scaffolds for the delivery of siRNA [169]. For example, DNA dumbbell [170], DNA nanoribbons [171], and spherical nucleic acids (SNAs) [172] have been described as alternative systems which are biodegradable, non-toxic, and also nonimmunogenic. These DNA scaffolds have proved to be effective when they have incorporated targeting ligands, siRNA drugs as well as chemotherapeutic drugs with high precision [164,173].

5.10 siRNA IN CLINICAL TRIALS FOR CANCER THERAPY

Recently, RNAi-based treatment has been rapidly developed into clinical trials. In addition, it has been studied for treating diverse diseases, such as cancer, respiratory infection, age-related macular degeneration, glaucoma, and hypercholesterolemia, among others [165]. So far, at least 20 clinical trials have been initiated using siRNA- and miRNA-based therapeutics [162]. Although there are many ways to engage RNAi pathways, currently the majority of the clinical trials involve siRNA technology [115,174–176].

In a recent report from a phase I study on patients with refractory or relapsed solid cancer, Davis et al. provided the first clinical evidence that RNAi could be achieved by administering siRNA against the M2 subunit of ribonucleotide reductase (RRM2) [110].

Recently, the therapeutic potential of RNAi as a revolutionary modern class of medicine was demonstrated in cancer therapy for the treatment of inaccessible solid tumors via systemic administration by delivering Atu027 [177] and CALAA-01 [115] developed by Silence Therapeutics and Calando Pharmaceuticals Inc, respectively (Table 5.3). In 2008, CALAA-01 was employed for treating the first patient in a phase I clinical trial. In these studies, a siRNA

TABLE 5.3
Selection of Clinical Trials against Cancer Using siRNA Drugs

siRNA Drug	Formulation	Target	Disease	Phase	Sponsor	References
CALAA-01	Rondel® nanoparticles (CD)	M2 subunit of ribonucleotide reductase (RRM2)	Solid tumors	I	Calando pharmaceuticals	[115]
Atu027	siRNA with 2′-O-Me and cationic lipid	Protein Kinase N3 (PKN3)	Advanced solid tumors (metastatic pancreatic cancer	I	Silence therapeutics GmbH	[178]
ALN-RSV	Lipid nanoparticles	VEGF gene and KSP gene	Solid tumors (liver metastasis from colon cancer)	I	Alnylam pharmaceuticals	[179]
DCR-MYC	Lipid nanoparticles	Myc	Hepatocellular carcinoma	I	Dicerna pharmaceuticals	[180]
siRNAEphA2-DOPC	DOPC liposomes	Ephrin type-A receptor2 (EphA2) gene	Advanced cancers	I	M.D. Anderson Cancer center	[181]
siG12DLODER	LODER® (polymer)	KRAS (mutation G12D in KRAS oncogene)	Solid tumors (advanced pancreatic cancer)	II	Silenseed Ltd	[182]

2′-O-Me, 2′-O-methyl-RNA units; CD, cyclodextrins; DOPC, 1,2-dioleoyl-snglycero-3-phosphatidylcholine neutral liposomes; LODER®, LOcal Drug EluteR; VEGF, vascular endothelial growth factor.

nanoparticle targeting protein kinase N3 (PKN3) or RRM2 was administered intravenously for the treatment of solid tumors [115]. Recently Atu027, a siRNA targeting protein kinase N3 (PKN3), is being used in a clinical trial together with gemcitabine for the treatment of advanced or metastatic pancreatic cancer (clinicaltrials.gov Identifier: NCT01808638).

An interesting therapeutic approach has been shown by Tabernero et al. [178]. In this study, two different siRNAs targeting two genes (vascular endothelial growth factor, VEGF, and kinesin spindle protein, KSP) involved in angiogenesis were formulated in the same lipid formulation. The authors showed that siRNAs were able to promote mRNA cleavage and antitumor activity in humans. This lipid formulation (ALN-RSV) (Alnylam Pharmaceuticals) demonstrated complete regression of liver metastases and endometrial cancer in some cases.

A similar lipid formulation is being used for silencing Myc oncoprotein which is deregulated in over half of human malignancies. In a recent dose-escalation work, the clinical activity of DCR-MYC was evaluated in patients with advanced solid tumors, multiple myeloma, or lymphoma, showing good clinical and metabolic responses over various dose levels [179].

Recently, the use of 1,2-dioleoyl-sn-glycero-3-phosphatidylcholine liposomes for systemic siRNA delivery was evaluated in phase 1 clinical trial to inhibit the Ephrin type-A receptor2 (EphA2) gene [180]. The liposomal formulation was well tolerated, and clinical trials are ongoing.

In another approach, Silenseed has used the insertion of a specialized bio-polymeric "scaffold" containing the siRNA drug into the solid tumor core. The LODER® polymer matrix has been used in a clinical trial for silencing a mutated K-RAS oncogene relevant for pancreatic ductal adenocarcinoma [181].

Although there are not a large number of siRNAs in advanced clinical trials, RNAi is a noteworthy mechanism for advanced novel therapeutics because, in cancer cells, the functionality and expression of overexpressed damaging genes are significantly reduced by siRNAs. Nonetheless, once applying RNAi techniques *in vivo*, the most obstacle to achieving gene silencing is the delivery of therapeutic siRNA molecules [179]. Thus, the clinical application of siRNA therapy faces several challenges to achieve safe effective dosages in target cells and to maintain oligonucleotide stability in circulation.

The strategies for the observation of the distribution and therapeutic effects as well as techniques for enhancing cellular uptake are also essential [18,156]. First clinical trials have shown encouraging results. An interesting direction is the use of combinations of chemotherapeutic agents and siRNA as well as the combination of several siRNA, targeting overexpressed proteins involved in different metabolic routes such as oncogenes, control of the nucleotide pool, angiogenesis, telomeres, antiapoptotic genes, and so on. Finally, the use of exosomes derived from mesenchymal stromal cells will be evaluated in a clinical trial for the delivery KrasG12D siRNA in patients of pancreatic cancer with KrasG12D mutation (clinicaltrials.gov Identifier: NCT03608631). Exosomes are natural lipid particles secreted by cells that play a crucial role in protecting and transporting macromolecules such as endogenous microRNA and mRNA. These interesting properties have triggered the interest in the use of such exosomes as potential nanovehicles for internalization of therapeutic molecules.

5.11 GYNECOLOGICAL CANCERS (GCs)

Gynecological cancers (GCs) are the cancers that originate from, and affect, women's reproductive organs such as the cervix, ovary, uterus/endometrium, vagina, and vulva. GCs originate in different places within a woman's pelvis, the area between the hip bones and below the stomach. Each GC is unique, with its own signs and symptoms as well as risk factors. The risk for GCs increases with age. In the United States, almost 90,000 women are diagnosed with GCs every year, and more than 28,000 women die from these malignancies [183]. Among the different GCs, ovarian, cervical, and endometrial cancers are the most frequent and, thus, are considered major women's health issues. Although endometrial cancer (EC) is the most common GC among women, ovarian cancer (OC) is the most lethal type [184], and despite scientific advancements, mortality rates of GCs continue to rise [183]. Both early diagnosis and limited treatment options for advanced GCs are contributing factors to their high mortality, emphasizing the need for further advancements in these areas.

Recent years have witnessed a growing interest in the field of miRNAs (also referred to as miRs) because of their potential to regulate diverse biological processes [185]. miRNAs are small, non-coding RNA molecules, approximately 20–22 nucleotides in length. In general, miRNAs regulate the expression of genes by binding to the 3′-untranslated regions (3′-UTRs) of target messenger-RNAs (mRNAs) with partial or full complementarity, resulting in either translational repression or degradation of target mRNAs [185]. The human genome encodes several thousand miRNAs, and the knowledge about their identity and functions is constantly emerging. It is believed that miRNAs regulate the expression of more than one-third of all human genes [186]. In this chapter, we discuss the deregulation of miRNAs in GCs, their established or putative functions, and clinical and translational relevance. Considering the high incidence and mortality, we will mainly focus on ovarian, cervical, and endometrial cancers as the representative GCs.

5.12 DYSREGULATION OF miRNAs IN GYNECOLOGICAL CANCERS

Dysregulation of miRNAs in GCs has been reported in multiple studies, suggesting their pathobiological importance. Here, we discuss some of these reports on the differential expression of miRNAs in ovarian, cervical, and

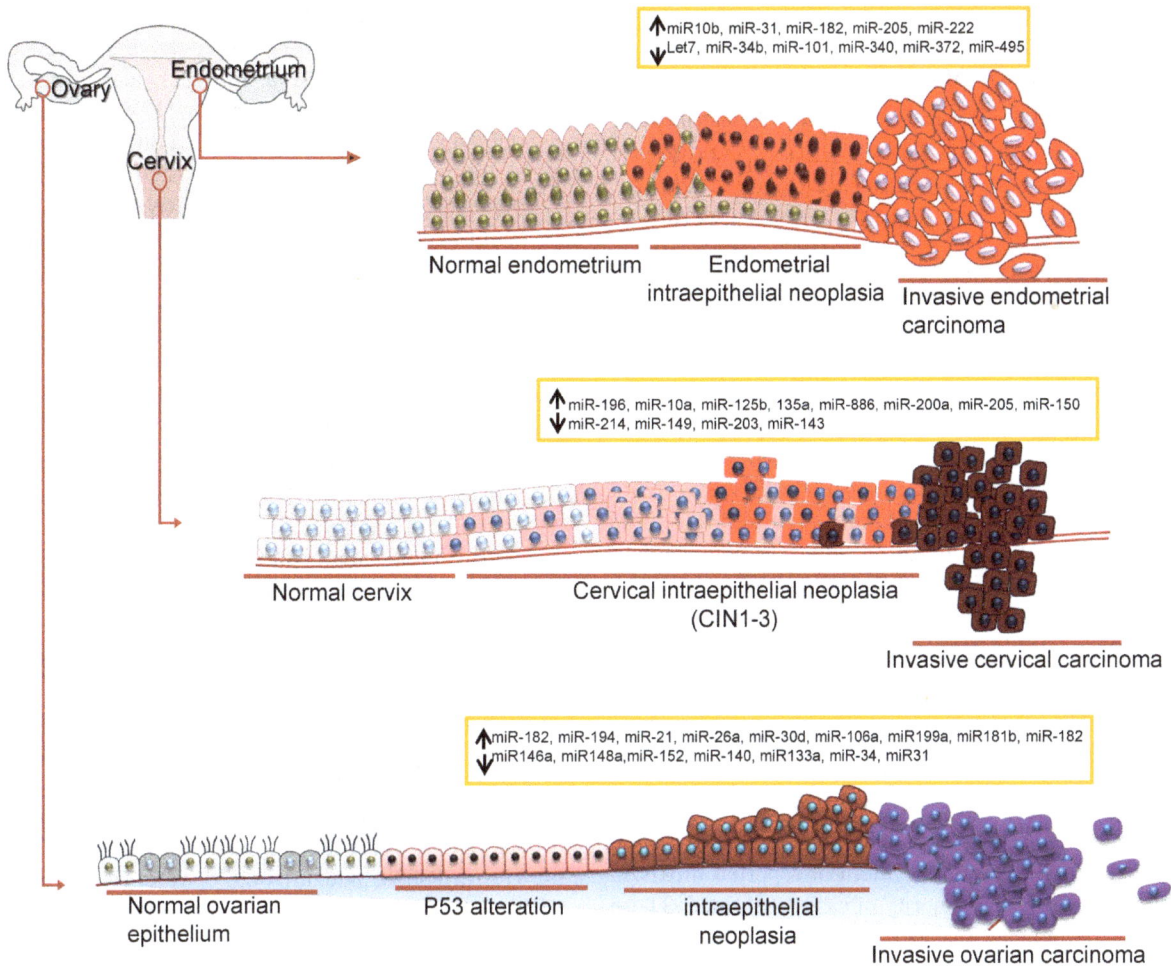

FIGURE 5.6 Role of miRNAs in the development and progression of gynecological malignancies. During the progression of gynecological cancers (ovarian cancers, cervical cancers, and endometrial cancers), miRNAs are highly dysregulated. Tumor-suppressor miRNAs are either lost or their expression down-regulated at the initiation stages, while oncogenic miRNAs get up-regulated, facilitating the progression of disease. The miRNAs identified in this figure are only representative and a comprehensive list is available in the individual tables.

endometrial cancers and highlight their significance in the development and progression of gynecological malignancies (Figure 5.6) [187].

5.12.1 OVARIAN CANCER

OC is the deadliest GC in the USA [188] (Table 5.4). Approximately 70% of the patients with OC are diagnosed with advanced disease [189], resulting in poor prognosis, even with aggressive and immediate treatments. Several studies have reported miRNA profiling from serum, plasma, and tissues of OC patients and have successfully identified distinct miRNA signatures. Zhang et al. were the first to demonstrate differential expression of miRNAs in OC [190]. Their study identified a copy number loss of the regions that harbor miR-15a and miR-16-1 in 23.9% of OC cases. Using deep sequencing of samples from normal and malignant ovarian tissues, Wyman et al. discovered six novel differentially expressed miRNAs (miR-2114*, miR-2115*, miR-2116*, miR-2114*, miR-449* and miR-548q)

[191]. In addition, their study also identified miRNAs that were differentially expressed in OC histologic subtypes. miR-449a was specific to serous, miR-499-5p/miR-375/ miR196a/miR-196b/miR-182 were specific to endometrioid, and miR-486-5p/miR-144/miR-30a/miR-199a-5p were specific to clear cell carcinoma [191]. Based on miRNA microarray data obtained from analysis on normal ovarian surface epithelium and ovarian tumors, Shahab and coworkers identified 42 miRNAs, out of which 33 were over-expressed and 9 miRNAs were down-regulated in OC [192]. In a recent study, small RNA sequencing was performed on normal tubal and high-grade serous OC samples, leading to the identification of differential expression of several miRNAs, of which 59 were known and 20 were novel [193]. Another recent study identified 1156 deregulated miRNAs in OC [194]. miR-1, miR-133a, and miR-451 were under-expressed while miR-141, miR-200a, miR-200c, and miR-3613 were significantly elevated in most of the OC patients. Resnick et al. investigated differentially expressed miRNAs in the serum of OC patients

TABLE 5.4

Gynecological Cancer Statistics

Gynecological Cancer	Estimated New Cases	Estimated Deaths
Ovarian cancer	22,440	14,080
Cervical cancer	12,820	4,210
Endometrial cancer	61,380	10,920

Estimates are rounded to the nearest ten, as reported in American Cancer Society's Cancer Facts & Figures 2017 [188].

and observed that miR-21, miR-29a, miR-92, miR-93, and miR-126 were significantly over-expressed, while miR-155, miR-127, and miR-99b were underexpressed [195]. From the plasma of patients with OC, a specific miRNA signature was detected. This included 19 down-regulated and three over-expressed miRNAs in OC patients, as compared to plasma of controls [193]. Moreover, six miRNAs, miR-126, miR-150, miR-17, miR-20a, miR-106b, and miR-92a, were efficient enough to distinguish benign plasma from that of the sample of OC patients. Nam et al., using miRNA microarray, identified several deregulated miRNAs [196]. In 17 out of 20 cases, miR-21 was most frequently up-regulated while miR-125b was down-regulated in 19 of 20 patients [196]. Their study further identified distinct miRNA signatures in OC cases, as compared with normal ovarian tissues. Further, the expression pattern of reported miRNAs was homogenous in the majority of cases examined. These studies clearly indicate that aberrant expression of miRNAs may have clinical relevance.

5.12.2 CERVICAL CANCER

Cervical cancer (CC) is another common gynecologic malignancy in the USA [188] (Table 5.4). Several factors, such as environmental, genetic, epigenetic, and viral (HPV) infection are believed to be the common etiological causes for cervical carcinogenesis. Growing evidence suggests that miRNAs exhibit a special expression pattern in CC patients, compared to normal women. Using hybridization arrays, Chen et al. examined the expression of 1450 miRNAs in cervical carcinoma vs. normal cervical tissue [197]. They identified 89 differentially expressed miRNAs; 62 miRNAs were more abundantly expressed; and 27 miRNAs exhibited downregulated expression. Furthermore, miRNAs with up-regulated expression in CC tissues were also readily detectable in serum. Some of the common miRNAs exhibiting higher levels in serum and tissue specimens were miR-1246, miR-20a, miR-2392, miR-3147, miR-3162–5p, and miR-4484 [197]. Lee et al. observed altered expression of 70 miRNAs in cervical carcinomas [198]. These included 68 over-expressed and two down-regulated miRNAs. Gocze et al. performed miRNA profiling of primary human CC samples and detected significantly high levels of miR-203, miR-27a, miR-196a, miR-34a, miR-155, miR-221,

and miR-21 in cervical carcinoma, irrespective of clinical grading and HPV status [199]. Moreover, overexpression of miR-34a, miR-196a, miR-27a, miR-221, and miR-21 was found to be the specific signature for HPV-positive cervical carcinomas. Wilting et al. identified differential expression of 106 miRNAs during the consecutive stages of CC development [200]. Twenty-seven miRNAs showed early transiently altered expression in high-grade precancerous lesions (CIN2–3) lesions only. Late altered expression of 46 miRNAs was seen in squamous-cell carcinomas and 33 miRNAs were continuously altered in both high-grade precancerous lesions and squamous-cell carcinomas.

Recently, Nagamitsu et al. examined the miRNA expression profile in serum specimens from CC patients by miRCURY LNA microRNA array [201]. Their data suggested that 6 of 1223 miRNAs were increased >3.0-folds in CC patients, as compared to healthy subjects. miR-1290 was identified to be significantly higher in 45 CC samples. Sharma and coworkers identified novel miRNA signatures in HPV-mediated cervical carcinogenesis in Indian women [202]. They identified 100 differentially expressed miRNAs in precancerous cervix (70 up-regulated and 30 down-regulated miRNAs) and 383 differentially expressed miRNAs in CC (350 upregulated and 33 down-regulated miRNAs). Further, 182 miRNAs were differentially expressed in HPV-16/18-positive vs. HPV-negative CC cell lines. Several novel miRNAs, namely miR-500, miR-505, miR-711, miR-888, and miR-892b were also discovered in pre-cancerous and CC cases in the Indian population [202]. Sequencing data by Jia et al. on serum specimens from CC patients vs. healthy controls revealed 12 miRNAs specific to CC, suggesting their use as a promising fingerprint for CC [203]. Li et al. performed a meta-analysis of 27 studies that consisted of 943 normal and 1132 cancer samples [204]. One hundred and ninety-five miRNAs were elevated, and 96 were found to be down-regulated in CC tissues, compared to normal cervical specimens [187]. Thus, miRNAs, being highly deregulated in CC, may play role in their pathobiology.

5.12.3 ENDOMETRIAL CANCER

EC is the most frequently diagnosed GC [188] (Table 5.4). A number of studies have looked at the miRNA profiles in EC using tumor tissues and other fluidic samples with a goal to identify disease-specific biomarkers. From serum samples of 46 patients with EC and 28 women without a history of cancer, miRNA profiling was performed using qRT-PCR, and miR-186, miR-222, and miR-223 were identified to be highly elevated [205]. Only miR-204 was expressed at low levels in EC patients. Similarly, another group identified 47 differentially expressed miRNAs in EC vs healthy individuals [206]. Of these, 26 miRNAs were down-regulated and 21, highly expressed. Eight miRNAs were selected and their expression examined in 58 type-IEC patients. miR-141, miR-200a, and miR-205 were up-regulated while miR-143 and miR-145 were found to be down-regulated.

For the identification of miRNA signature for endometrial adenocarcinoma, a study identified 112 novel miRNAs specific to endometrial adenocarcinoma, among which miR-182 and miR-183 were highly expressed [207]. In ten pairs of EC and adjacent non-cancer endometrium, miRNA expression profiling revealed the elevated level of 17 miRNAs and reduced levels of 6 miRNAs [208]. From tissue and plasma samples of 77 EC and 45 healthy controls, expression profiling of 866 human miRNAs was performed. Study revealed a distinct pattern of 21 miRNAs in EC specimens. The expression pattern of several miRNAs was found to be associated with International Federation of Gynecology and Obstetrics (FIGO) stage, grade, relapse, and nodal metastases. Furthermore, as compared to single miRNAs, the miRNA signatures from tissue and EC plasma specimens could efficiently classify EC with higher accuracy. MiR-92a/miR-205/miR-410 and miR-92a/miR-410 was the proposed miRNA signature for tumor tissue, and miR-9/miR-1228 and miR-9/miR-92 was identified to be the plasma-specific miRNA signature of EC [209]. Similar to this, another study reported that subtypes of EC exhibit a distinct miRNA pattern [210]. A specific miRNA signature could distinguish tumor from normal specimens, and miRNA profile differed between type I or II tumors. Working on a similar line, miRNA profiling of grade 1–2 EC suggested specific miRNAs to be an efficient tool for surgical staging in early-stage EC. Significantly low levels of miR-375, miR-184, miR-34c-5p, miR-34c-3p, and miR-34b-5p in the primary tumor of EC, with positive lymph nodes, were detected. Women with high miR-375 or reduced expression of miR-184 were more likely to have positive lymph nodes [211].

Altogether, these studies suggest that miRNAs are dysregulated in GCs. They impact the development and progression of GCs and could be helpful in the effective clinical management of the disease.

5.13 BIOLOGICAL SIGNIFICANCE OF miRNAs IN GYNECOLOGICAL CANCERS

miRNAs regulate a number of genes with diverse physiological roles. Consequently, the effects of miRNAs are apparent on many biological functions. Some of the better studied biological effects of miRNAs are on cell growth, proliferation, migration, invasion, and metastasis. These effects are discussed in the next few subsections.

5.13.1 CELL PROLIFERATION, SURVIVAL, AND STEMNESS

The effects of miRNAs on the proliferation and growth of cells representing GCs are very well studied. Such effects are often the very first biological effects investigated. Over the past several years, a number of publications have detailed the loss or gain of expression of miRNAs in OC, CC, and EC, with the resulting impact on growth, proliferation, and apoptosis. Due to the enormous number of such reports, a detailed discussion on all of these

miRNAs and their target genes is beyond the scope of this article. However, a comprehensive list is provided in [187]. While some miRNAs have been shown to correlate with increased cell proliferation and growth in CC [212–225], EC [226–232], and OC [233–240], others have been associated with reduced proliferation and/or induced apoptosis in CC [241–271], EC [272–280], and OC [281–327]. As evident, miRNAs have been reported to target a number of genes, mostly mutually exclusive, leading to their effects on cancer cell proliferation.

The miRNAs that induce proliferation of GCs often do so by either targeted inhibition of tumor suppressor genes or the activation of oncogenes. A few examples of such regulation are miRNA-mediated regulations of tumor suppressors p53 and PTEN. p53 is a very well-characterized tumor suppressor gene [328]. In an early report on the role of miRNAs in OC cells' proliferation, miR-34b and miR-34/c were reported to be significantly down-regulated (12-folds) as a consequence of p53 inactivation [329]. The two miRNAs, cooperatively, reduced proliferation as well as anchorage-independent cell growth, thus mediating p53 effects. miR-31 is another miRNA that is associated with the p53 pathway, particularly in serous OCs [330] and has anti-proliferative properties [309]. In a later study, miR-34a was also reported to be a negative regulator of OC proliferation, and its action was shown to be mediated through its regulation of AXL [331]. The p53 pathway has been shown to be affected by miRNAs in CC cells as well. TP53INP1 (tumor protein p53-induced nuclear protein 1), a p53 target gene, was shown responsible for the proliferation-inhibitory role of miR-17 [242]. PTEN is another classical tumor-suppressor [332]. It is a target of miR-21 [333,334], miR-130a [335], miR-222 [336] in CC cells; a target of miR-200 [337,338], miR-205 [230,339], miR-429 [338] in EC cells, and a target of miR-21 [340], miR-106a [341], miR-205 [342], miR-214 [343], and miR-630 [344] in OC. miR-21 induces OC cell proliferation through its targeting of PTEN [340] as well as PDCD4 [345]. PDCD4 has also been identified as a target of miR-21 in HeLa CC cells responsible for miR-21-induced cell proliferation [346].

miRNAs do not just regulate tumor suppressors. They affect oncogenic signals and signaling pathways as well. NF-kB signaling, for instance, is a target of miR-9 [347]. miR-9 is frequently down-regulated in OC, and its overexpression in OC cells can downregulate NF-kB, resulting in reduced proliferation. The NF-kB miRNA interactions are further supported by a study in serous OC cells, which observed shorter survival of OC patients with high expression of NF-kB [348]. NF-kB repressed miR-134 expression, resulting in increased expression of its target TAB1, and chemoresistance. In CC cells, NF-kB positively regulates miR-130a by binding to its promoter [335]. miR-130a inhibits PTEN, resulting in increased proliferation and growth of OC cells. A role of IKK-β in miRNA regulation of NF-kB has been demonstrated in CC cells. miR-429 represses its target IKK-b which leads to down-regulation of NF-kB, reduced proliferation and increased apoptosis [349]. A number of other pro-survival pathways are also affected by miRNAs. miR-491 induces apoptosis by targeting EGFR, which leads to inhibition of Akt and MAPK pathways [350]. This results in BIM accumulation and the inhibition of Bcl-xl. EGFR family is also targeted by tumor suppressor miRNAs, such as, miR-133a in CC [250], miR-125b in EC [275], and miR-133b in OC cells [293]. miR-15a and miR-16 regulate OC cell proliferation by targeting oncogenic Bmi-1 [351].

The "stemness" of distinct sub-populations of cancer cells is their ability to self-renew and maintain tumors by producing new cancer cells [352]. Such "cancer stem cells (CSCs)" are known to be involved in cancer metastasis and resistance to therapies. As such, a role of miRNAs in determining the stemness of GCs has also been evaluated. In a recent study [353], the OC cells with stem-cell-like properties were reported to express active STAT3 signaling with a mechanistic involvement of miR-92a in the regulation of wnt signaling antagonist DKK1. The miR-92a-STAT3-mediated stemness was shown to be important for chemoresistance. Wnt signaling is also targeted by miR-1207, an miRNA that promotes stemness in OC cells [354]. In another study on OC [355], miR-34a and miR-137 were observed to be important for stemness, as determined by their role in sphere formation and invasion. These suppressor miRNAs were down-regulated in OC, resulting in de-repression of their target Snail. Snail promoted invasion and sphere formation by inducing EMT. Low levels of miR-34a and miR-137 correlated with poor survival of OC patients [355].

miRNAs have been investigated for their effects on GC cells with expression of specific stem cells markers. In an early report on the topic [356], miR-200a was observed to be down-regulated in CD133/1-positive OC stem cells. ZEB2, the target of miR-200a, influenced invasion of CSCs by inhibiting e-cadherin. Later, another member of the miR-200 family, miR-200c, was shown to regulate stemness in OC [357]. miR-200c was reported to be downregulated in CD117/CD44-positive ovarian CSCs with resulting increased expression of ZEB1 and vimentin. Low levels of miR-200c correlated with increased colony formation and invasion *in vitro* and increased pulmonary metastases *in vivo*. A few other miRNAs have also been shown to negatively regulate GC stemness. miR-98 inhibits the stemness of ovarian CSCs by targeting EZH2 [358] while miR-134 inhibits ovarian CSCs (CD44/CD133-positive) by targeting RAB27A [359] and endometrial CSCs by targeting protein O-glucosyltrasferase 1 (POGLUT1) [360]. miR-136 has recently been reported to target Notch-3 oncogene and the OC stemness [361]. The effects of miR-136 are evident on CSC phenotype and paclitaxel resistance of OC cells, as over-expression of this miRNA re-sensitizes OC cells to paclitaxel. miR-106a has a distinct effect on GC stemness. In SKOV3 OC cells, over-expression of miR-106a was reported to result in increased CD24/CD133- positive stem cell populations [362]. These studies suggest a correlation between miRNA expression, CSC markers, and the resulting effects on CSC-mediated resistance to therapies and metastases. Evidently, a majority of such studies have

focused on ovarian cancer (OC), and it remains to be seen if miRNAs can similarly stemness of other gynecological malignancies like breast cancer (BrC) as well.

5.13.2 INVASION AND METASTASIS

Invasion of cancer cells into surrounding tissues and their metastases to distant organs account for a majority of cancer-associated deaths. Therefore, there has been a wide interest in understanding the ability of miRNAs to regulate the process of invasion and metastases, with possible implications in therapy. Studies have revealed the potential of different miRNAs to either inhibit or induce invasion and/or metastasis of different GCs [187]. For example, miR-126 inhibits invasion of EC cells [363]. miR-34a also inhibits invasion, but via differing mechanisms in different cancer cells. In EC cells, it suppresses L1CAM [364], while Notch signaling is its target in CC cells [365]. miR-218 has two different targets within CC cells, focal adhesion pathways [366] and survivin [367], which regulate to mediate effects on invasion. miR-183 targets MMP3 to inhibit invasion of CC cells [368], while miR-375 inhibits invasion by targeting transcription factor SP1 [369]. miR-205 [370] promotes invasion of EC cells and miR-346 promotes migration and invasion of CC cells by positively regulating AGO2 (argonaute 2) [371].

As discussed above, PTEN and PDCD4 play a role in miRNA-regulated cancer cell proliferation. miR-21-targeting of PTEN [340] and PDCD4 [345] also affects the invasive potential of OC cells. In addition, PTEN mediates miR-17 effects [372] while PDCD4 is implicated in miR-182-mediated invasion of ovarian carcinomas [373]. Other miRNAs that regulate invasion of GCs are miR-124 [374], miR-335 [375], miR-339 [376], miR-130b [377], and miR-181 [378]. miR-182 seems to be important for OC metastasis because its inhibition was shown to result in significantly reduced tumor burden, local invasion, and distant metastasis in an *in vivo* orthotopic model of serous ovarian carcinoma [379]. miR-22 is a potential metastasis-suppressing miRNA in OC cells with putative regulation of several pro-metastatic genes [380]. miR-204 is another metastasis-suppressor miRNA that plays a role in the regulation of OC metastasis through its target, brain-derived neurotrophic factor [381]. miR-138 also associates negatively with OC cells' invasion and metastasis [382]. Its suppressive action is believed to involve SOX4 (SRY-related high mobility group box 4) and HIF-1a (hypoxia-inducible factor-1 a). HIF-1a is also a target of miR-199a [383]. Expression of miR-373 inversely correlates with clinical stage and histological grade of epithelial OCs, and its target is the oncogenic Rab22a [384].

EMT is an important mechanism that plays a key role in invasion and metastasis of cancer cells. A number of miRNAs have been demonstrated to regulate EMT, thereby playing a role in the regulation of invasion and metastasis. miR-200 family, a known family of tumor suppressor miRNAs with well-characterized role in EMT of cancer cells [385], has been implicated in EMT of OC cells [386,387] as well as CC cells [388,389]. Another member of this family, miR-429, has also been shown to reverse EMT [390]. miR-200a's role in suppressing OC invasion has been attributed to its ability to target CD133/1-positive OC stem cells [356], while the ability of miR-200c to inhibit metastasis has been linked to down-regulation of mesenchymal markers vimentin/ZEB1 and up-regulation of epithelial marker E-cadherin in CD117 and CD44-positive OC stem cells [357].

EMT is also regulated by several other miRNAs, with implications on migration and invasion, in CC, EC, and OC cells [355,391–403]. miR-181a mediates TGF-β-mediated EMT in a smad7-dependent manner and its expression correlates with poor outcome and shorter time to recurrence in patients with epithelial OC [404]. In HeLa and SiHa CC cells, smad7 is a target of miR-519d, an oncogenic miRNA that promotes metastasis [405]. Tumor suppressor let-7a targets smad4 to suppress TGF-β-mediated proliferation of CC cells [406]. In EC cells, smad3 is targeted by miR-23a to modulate TGF-β-mediated EMT [407]. miR-29b [408] and miR-30d [409] inhibit TGF-β-mediated EMT. Through their targets, Id-1 (inhibitor of DNA binding 1) and snail, respectively, they modulate TGF-β-mediated EMT in OC cells.

5.13.3 Modulation of Tumor Microenvironment

A role of tumor microenvironment in GCs has been realized [410,411] and the exact mechanism is being explored. In a study that compared normal fibroblasts vs. cancer-associated fibroblasts (CAFs), an important component of TME, miR-148a was found to be significantly down-regulated in 15 of 16 patient-derived CAFs [412]. Consistent with the tumor-suppressive function of this miRNA, conditioned media from CAFs inhibited the migration of multiple EC cell lines. Wnt signaling was shown to be affected by this down-regulation of miR-148a. Since wnt signaling is known to be important for TME, especially the stromal compartment [413], deregulated miR-148 in CAFs provides a mechanism for the role of miRNAs in TME-guided tumorigenesis. Mitra et al. compared the miRNA profile of primary CAFs and adjacent normal fibroblasts in OC patients, and they also performed miRNA profiling in induced CAFs established from normal fibroblasts upon co-culture with tumor cells and normal fibroblasts [414]. They identified miR-214 and miR-31 to be down-regulated and miR-155 up-regulated in CAFs. Furthermore, re-expression of miR-214 and miR-31, and inhibition of miR-155, could revert the CAF phenotype to normal fibroblasts. This clearly indicates a direct role of miRNAs in reversible conversion of normal fibroblasts into CAFs.

In view of the low-oxygen hypoxic conditions in TME, HIF-1α's expression and role has been a subject of interest in TME [415]. Regulation of HIF-1α by miR-199a, with involvement of dynamin 2 and lysloxidase, is believed to play an important role in metastasis of OC cells under hypoxic condition in the TME [383]. Another target of hypoxia-responsive miR-199a is c-met [416]. Reduced levels of miR-199a in TME hypoxic conditions can lead to increased c-met, with resulting activation of Akt pathway and the increased proliferation and invasiveness. In

a 3-dimensional culture model of OC TME, an essential role of miR-193b has been demonstrated wherein miR-193b is down-regulated through a direct interaction of OC cells with the mesothelial cells in the microenvironment [417]. Suppression of miR-193b results in de-repression of its target urokinase-type plasminogen activator, a well-known tumor-associated protease that is involved in invasion and metastases of various human cancers [418]. This activation of uPA results in increased invasion of OC cells into the omentum in an *in vivo* mouse xenograft model as well the human omental pieces *ex vivo* [417].

As an indirect evidence of regulation of TME by miRNAs, hedgehog signaling is regulated by miR-506 in CC cells [419]. Hedgehog signaling is an important modulator of TME where it plays a critical role by creating a niche that favors cancer cell growth, chemoresistance, and metastasis [420]. Further, lysophosphatidic acid (LPA), a mitogenic lipid present within the ovarian TME, has been reported to induce the expression of miR-30c-2* [421]. Expression of this miRNA is also affected by epidermal growth factor and the platelet-derived growth factor. This miRNA, affected by tumor microenvironment, seems to counter cell growth by targeting oncogenic BCL9, suggesting a complex regulatory mechanism in cancer cells. Using a preclinical mouse model, it has been demonstrated that delivery of immunostimulatory miR-155 specifically to tumor-associated leukocytes can re-program immunological control of metastatic OCs [422]. Thus, there are multiple evidences in support of the role of miRNAs in TME.

5.13.4 Chemoresistance Mechanisms

Resistance to chemotherapies, i.e., chemoresistance, is another characteristic of cancer cells responsible for making this disease particularly lethal. There are reports on the role of miRNAs in determining response to chemotherapies in GCs [423] (Table 5.5). Cisplatin and paclitaxel are two drugs that have been studied in detail in GCs, with regards to a role of miRNAs in determining sensitivity and/or acquisition of resistance. The results vary from mere exploration of expression status in sensitive vs. resistant cells to more mechanistic explorations.

In addition, its role in cancer cell proliferation, invasion, and metastasis, PTEN plays a role in cancer drug resistance as well [451]. miR-93 was identified as a regulator of PTEN/Akt signaling pathway [431]. It directly targeted PTEN to regulate apoptosis and the sensitivity to cisplatin [431]. In a study that investigated miRNA profiles of sensitive vs. cisplatin-resistant OC cells SKOV3, miR-130a was observed to be up-regulated in the resistant cells [434]. miR-130a was, similarly, found elevated in cisplatin-resistant OC cells A2780 as well, compared to the parental cells [452]. Interestingly, PTEN was determined to be a target of this miRNA in both these studies [434,452]. In addition, miR-130a could inhibit MDR1 [434,452] and NRP1 (neuropilin 1) [453], which suggests that this miRNA can influence multidrug resistance.

TABLE 5.5

miRNAs Reported to Modulate Resistance of Gynecological Cancers to Therapy

miRNA	Gynecological Cancer	Role in Chemoresistance	References
Let-7a	Ovarian	Biomarker for response to paclitaxel	[424]
Let-7i	Ovarian	Reverses paclitaxel resistance	[425]
miR-9	Ovarian	Down-regulated in paclitaxel-resistant tumor samples	[426]
miR-21	Ovarian	Over-expressed in cisplatin-resistant cells	[427]
miR-29	Ovarian	Down-regulated in cisplatin resistant cells	[428]
miR-31	Ovarian	Down-regulated in paclitaxel resistant cells	[429]
		Over-expressed in cisplatin resistant cells	[430]
miR-93	Ovarian	Targets PTEN and regulates sensitivity to cisplatin	[431]
miR-106a	Ovarian	Expression correlates with paclitaxel resistance	[432]
miR-125b	Ovarian	Induces cisplatin resistance	[433]
miR-130a	Ovarian	Induces cisplatin and multidrug resistance	[434]
miR-130b	Ovarian	Negatively correlates with multidrug resistance	[435]
miR-145	Ovarian	Epigenetically silenced in paclitaxel-resistant cells	[436]
miR-152	Ovarian	Increases sensitivity to cisplatin	[437]
miR-155	Cervical	Reverses EMT and cisplatin resistance	[438]
miR-185	Ovarian	Increases sensitivity to cisplatin	[437]
miR-186	Ovarian	Negative regulator of EMT and resulting cisplatin resistance	[439]
miR-199b	Ovarian	Epigenetically silenced in cisplatin-resistant cells	[440]
miR-200s	Ovarian	Determines response to paclitaxel-based therapy	[441,442]
miR-214	Ovarian	Induces cisplatin resistance	[343]
miR-218	Cervical	Increases cisplatin sensitivity	[443,444]
miR-224	Cervical	Increases paclitaxel sensitivity	[445]
miR-375	Cervical	Up-regulated in paclitaxel resistant cells	[446,447]
miR-376c	Ovarian	Induces cisplatin resistance	[448]
miR-497	Ovarian	Hypermethylated in cisplatin resistant cells and tumors	[449]
miR-506	Ovarian	Determines sensitivity to cisplatin by inhibiting EMT	[450]
miR-591	Ovarian	Down-regulated in paclitaxel resistant cells	[432]

The phenomenon of EMT is known to play a role in acquired resistance to therapy. miR-186 was shown to affect EMT and the resulting cisplatin resistance of OC cells through its target Twist 1 [439]. miR-115 has been reported to reverse cisplatin resistance in CC cells by reversing EMT [438]. In addition to influencing EMT, as discussed in the preceding sub-section, miR-200 family can also determine the response to paclitaxel-based therapy, which suggests a possible role as biomarker of response to such therapy [441,454]. Restoration of miR-200c has been linked to enhanced sensitivity to paclitaxel [442]. Let-7a, another tumor suppressor miRNA that belongs to the let-7 family, has also been proposed as a potential biomarker for determining response to paclitaxel [424]. With the objective of delivering let-7i specifically to OC cells, let-7i was combined with MUC1 aptamer [425]. Once delivered, let-7i was observed to down-regulate cell cycle-associated factors, resulting in the reversal of paclitaxel resistance. miR-506 is another microRNA that negatively regulates EMT and the resulting chemoresistance of OC cells [450]. Because of its inverse connection with EMT, it was found to associate with favorable response to therapy and overall progression-free survival in an analysis that looked at two independent cohorts of epithelial OC patients with a combined sample size of 598 patients [450]. The results were confirmed *in*

vivo where miR-506 sensitized cells to cisplatin treatment. miR-25 has been shown to reverse EMT, leading to sensitization to cisplatin in HeLa and CaSki CC cells [455].

In a study that compared paclitaxel-sensitive and the derived paclitaxel-resistant KFr13 cells, miR-31 was found to be down-regulated in the resistant cells [429]. miR-31's over-expression resulted in reduced MET, which was proposed to be the mediator of miR-31 effects on paclitaxel sensitivity. Further proof of a role of miR-31 in OC cells' acquired resistance to chemotherapy was provided in a later study that observed elevated STMN1 (stathmin 1) levels in tissue samples from OC patients with resistance to taxanes, compared to samples from taxane-responsive patients [456].

Comparison of taxane-sensitive vs. resistant OC cells confirmed the increased STMN1 levels in resistant cells and also revealed regulation of STMN1 by miR-31. miRNA profiling of formalin-fixed paraffin-embedded OC patient samples helped list a number of up- and down-regulated miRNAs, among which miR-9 was shortlisted as a down-regulated miRNA with possible implications in the survival of OC patients [426].

Let-7e [457], miR-29 [428], miR-128 [458], miR-136 [459], miR-155 [460], miR-199a [461], miR-216b [462], miR-449a [463], miR-489 [464], miR-595 [465], miR-634 [466], and miR-770 [467] inversely correlate with cisplatin resistance in

OC, while miR-218 [443,444] increases sensitivity to cisplatin in CC cells. miR-21 [427,468], miR-125b [433], miR-214 [343], miR-224 [469], miR-376c [448], and miR-509 [470] induce cisplatin resistance in OC. A number of other miRNAs, such as miR-106a [432,471], miR-130b [472], miR-134 [473], miR-145 [436], miR-149 [474], miR-186 [475], miR-197 [476], miR-429 [477], miR-433 [478], miR-490 [479], and miR-591 [432] have been linked to paclitaxel and/or cisplatin resistance in OC. miR-125a [480], miR-224 [445], and miR-375 [446,447] expression has been linked with paclitaxel resistance in CC cells. Interestingly, although a reduced expression of miR-31 was observed to correlate with paclitaxel resistance [429], its over-expression was reported to drive cisplatin resistance [481].

5.14 CLINICAL SIGNIFICANCE OF miRNAs IN GYNECOLOGICAL CANCERS

The discovery of miRNAs and recent knowledge on their role in GC pathobiology has created substantial opportunities for translating the miRNA research into clinical settings. Furthermore, data from emerging studies clearly highlight the clinical significance of these miRNAs in the diagnosis and prognosis of gynecologic malignancies. In the sections below, we have described the implication of these miRNAs as potential diagnostic and prognostic biomarkers.

5.14.1 TOOLS FOR EARLY AND DIFFERENTIAL DIAGNOSIS

For the successful treatment of any cancer, early diagnosis is critical. Unfortunately, after several years of research, no major improvements have been made toward the early detection and screening of the GCs. The human epididymis protein 4 (HE4) is an important biomarker for gynecological malignancies [205,482], but its sensitivity in patients has been reported as a possible limiting factor [483]. CA125 is another biomarker for gynecological malignancies, but several factors hinder its implication to be used as a specific biomarker [484]. For example, higher levels of serum CA125 are also reported to be associated with pregnancy,

menstruation, and endometriosis [485]. Even though it has been documented that HE4 has better diagnostic performance than CA125 for early-stage diagnosis of EC [486], follow-up studies are highly warranted for identification of novel biomarkers that could serve as superior diagnostic biomarkers for this malignancy. Recently, miRNAs have gained significant attention as novel diagnostic markers.

miRNAs have the potential to screen/identify cancer patients from healthy individuals, suggesting that the inclusion of these miRNAs along with the current diagnostic markers in combination or alone may yield improved diagnosis and early detection of gynecologic malignancies (Table 5.6). In this direction, a recent study identified miR-222, miR-223, miR-186, and miR-204 to be the potent miRNAs for the diagnostics of EC [205]. This study also suggested a positive correlation between HE4 levels with miR-222 and miR-223 and a negative correlation with miR-204. Further, serum miR-204 and HE4 were shown to possess best diagnostic performance in the discrimination of patients with EC vs healthy controls. In the confirmed OC patients, Resnick et al. observed that the level of conventionally used biomarker CA125 was very low, but a specific miRNA subset, miR-21, miR-92, and miR-93, was highly elevated in OC patients, suggesting the implication of these miRNAs in disease diagnosis with high precision [195]. Earlier studies have reported the overexpression of miR-944 in several gynecological malignancies, while its clinical significance remained largely unknown [232]. Zuberi et al. observed that miR-200a, miR-200b, and miR-200c levels were significantly higher in OC, as compared to normal controls [487]. The area under curve of receiver operating characteristic (ROC) further suggested that miR-200a and miR-200c could be used as an efficient diagnostic tool. Based on ROC and logistic regression analyses, Zheng et al. proposed a diagnostic miRNA panel [488]. Let-7f and miR-205 together were found to provide high diagnostic accuracy for OC, particularly for stage-I tumors. The accuracy of detection was further improved when these two miRNAs were combined with CA-125. Moreover, Zheng and coworkers also reported significantly higher level of

TABLE 5.6
miRNAs with Potential Role as Diagnostic Markers in Gynecological Cancers

miRNA	Gynecological Cancer	Putative Diagnostic Role	References
Let-7f/miR-205	Ovarian	Accurate diagnosis of stage-I tumors	[488]
miR-21/miR-92/miR-93	Ovarian	Elevated in patients	[195]
miR-30a	Ovarian	Diagnostic marker for clear-cell carcinoma subtype	[489]
miR-92a/miR-205/miR-410	Endometrial	miRNA signature for diagnosis	[209]
miR-192/miR-194	Ovarian	Diagnostic markers for mucinous subtype	[489]
miR-196	Cervical	Elevated serum levels in patients	[490]
miR-200s	Ovarian	Differentially expressed in patients	[487]
miR-203	Cervical	Diagnostic marker	[491]
miR-204	Endometrial	Correlates negatively with diagnostic marker HE4	[205]
miR-222/miR-223	Endometrial	Correlate positively with diagnostic marker HE4	[205]
miR-483	Ovarian	Diagnostic marker for stage III and IV tumors	[488]

miR-483–5p in stage III and IV patients as compared to patients with stages I and II [488].

Calura et al. identified miRNAs that could be used as diagnostic markers [489]. These miRNAs could specifically discriminate clear cell and mucinous histotypes of OC—higher expression of miR-30a and miR-30a was specific to clear cell carcinoma while that of miR-192/194 was specific to mucinous histotype. Jia and coworkers identified a miRNA fingerprint for EC detection [492]. This fingerprint/panel included four serum miRNAs; miR-222, miR-223, miR-186, and miR-204. The AUC curve of this miRNA signature was remarkably higher than that of CA-125. In 104 EC tissue samples, Torres et al. identified several miRNAs to be altered [209]. miRNA signatures miR-92a/miR-205/miR-410 and miR-92a/miR-410 could efficiently classify tumor tissues with higher accuracy, as compared to single miRNAs. miRNA signatures from plasma, i.e., miR-9/miR-92a and miR-9/miR-1228, were able to classify the plasma samples of EC patients with high accuracy. Their study thus suggested that these miRNA signatures hold a great promise to be used as promising biomarkers for early detection of EC. A recent study by Coimbra and coworkers found that the expression levels miR-203 and of ∆Np63 mRNA positively correlate with each other in CC tissues and could serve as a promising tool for the screening of CC [491]. Liu et al. suggested the use of miR-196 as a diagnostic marker based on their observation that serum levels of miR-196a are elevated in CC patients as well as in cervical intraepithelial neoplasia [490]. Altogether, these reports underscore the potential of miRNAs to be used as valuable tools for discriminating GCs from normal cases and classifying the tumor stage and grade, either alone, or in combination with other biomarkers.

5.14.2 PREDICTIVE AND PROGNOSTIC BIOMARKERS

Recent studies have revealed that the levels of miRNAs are associated with the prognosis of gynecologic malignancies. He et al. compared the levels of miR-944 in 68 EC tissues vs. 20 normal endometrial specimens [232]. They identified miR-944 to be consistently up-regulated in EC tissues, and clinicopathological studies suggested high level of miR-944 association with FIGO stages and pathology classification of EC. Further, Kaplan–Meier analysis suggested that patients exhibiting high miR-944 have a shorter survival time. Zuberi et al. examined the association of miR-200a, miR-200b, and miR-200c with clinicopathological factors and progression of OC [487]. They identified an association of miR-200a and miR-200c with disease progression. miR-200a alone was associated with tumor stage and histology, while high level of miR-200c in patients was associated with lymph node metastasis [487].

Zhai et al. reported miR-194 to be remarkably decreased in EC, which correlated with the cancer stage [493]. The decreased expression of miR-194 also associated with poor prognosis. Zheng et al. performed a study on 300 patients with OC and found significantly reduced levels of let-7f

in OC patients, compared to healthy controls, suggesting low levels of let-7f to be predictive of poor prognosis [488]. Down-regulation of miR-497 in CC was reported by Luo et al. [494]. Their study identified a correlation of miR-497 levels with FIGO stage and lymph node metastases. Moreover, based on multivariate cox analysis, decreased miR-497 expression was demonstrated to associate with poor prognosis of CC. miR-181a-1 has been reported to be over-expressed in various malignancies, and its role in the carcinogenesis has also been documented. He et al. observed high expression of miR-181a in type I and type II EC [495]. Interestingly, the higher expression of miR-181a was seen in type II EC, rather than type I EC, suggesting that miR-181a could serve as a novel biomarker for EC. Shapira et al. [496] examined miRNA levels in the plasma samples of pre-surgery vs. follow-up OC patients. They identified a special signature of five different miRNAs in women with short overall survival, as compared to those exhibiting long overall survival. With the aim of identifying miRNAs in plasma for predicting response to treatment and outcome, Halvorsen and coworkers performed miRNA profiling in the plasma of OC patients with different histology, grade, and FIGO stages [497]. Of 754 unique miRNAs identified, decreased miR-1274a, miR-200b, and miR-141 levels were significantly associated with better survival. Low miR-1274a correlated with therapeutic outcome, while miR-200c was associated with prolonged progression-free survival when treated with bevacizumab, as compared to standard therapeutic regimen [497].

Torres et al. also identified a special miRNA signature in EC that associated with FIGO stage, grade, relapse, and nodal metastases [209]. Signatures consisting of miR-200a and miR-205 could predict the relapse with high accuracy. Moreover, miRNA signatures from tissues, i.e., miR-1228/miR-200c/miR-429 and miR-1228/miR-429 were independent prognostic markers of overall and progression-free survival, respectively. Wilczynski et al. observed that elevated miR-205 expression was associated with better overall survival, thus suggesting its potential clinical utility as a prognostic marker of EC [498]. Working on the similar line in advanced OC, Parikh et al. observed an association between high expression of miR-181a and shorter recurrence time [404]. Yang et al. suggested miR-320 as a potential biomarker of radiosensitivity in CC, based on their observation that this miRNA was considerably low in C33AR cells, a radio-resistant CC cell line [499]. Vecchione et al. identified a signature of 23 miRNAs associated with chemoresistance [500]. Further analysis demonstrated that miR-484, -642, and -217 could predict the chemoresistance of ovarian tumors. Nam et al. identified several miRNAs that could discriminate chemosensitive from chemoresistant cases and detected significant down-regulation of miR-199a and miR-7039 in the chemoresistant group. They also examined the usefulness of miRNAs for detecting chemoresistant disease and reported that the down-regulation of miR-199a could be an efficient marker for predicting chemoresistant disease [196]. Using the Kaplan–Meier analysis, a very recent study examined the correlation between serum levels of miR-425-5p and the overall survival of CC patients [501]. The results suggested a positive correlation of miR-425-5p with tumor stage and positive lymph node metastasis. High serum levels of miR-425-5p were suggested to predict poor survival, and cox proportional hazards risk analysis identified miR-425-5p to be an independent prognostic factor for CC.

A correlation between serum miR-196a levels and the tumor size, grade, lymph node metastasis, and FIGO stage was suggested by Liu and coworkers [490]. Based on multivariate analysis, authors reported that higher serum miR-196a levels in CC patients were an independent predictor for poor survival. miR-31 has also been reported to be an independent prognostic factor in CC [502]. Multivariate and cox regression analysis demonstrated that high expression of miR-31 associated with poorer overall survival. Moreover, its correlation with FIGO stages and node metastases was also reported. In a pilot study on the role of miRNAs in the prediction of the drug/treatment sensitivity, Benson and coworkers identified plasma miRNAs that can predict the outcomes of a carboplatin with decitabine in platinum-resistant recurrent OC patients [503]. They reported that a decreased circulating miR-148b-5p expression level was associated with longer progression-free survival, suggesting its potential as a novel biomarker of therapeutic response. Plasma samples were collected from 33 OC patients, and it was observed that patients with no miR-200b variation have longer progression-free survival. Also, patients with positive variation had higher risk of disease progression [503]. Together, these studies highlight the significance of miRNAs in the prognostic assessments of gynecological malignancies.

5.14.3 Next-Generation of Therapeutics

Results from preclinical studies suggest that miRNAs can be exploited as possible therapeutic weapons against GC. miRNA mimics, miRNA nanoformulations, miRNA masks, miRNA sponges, and adenovirus-mediated miRNA delivery systems are now being utilized to achieve the gain or loss of miRNA function. For example, MRX34, a liposomal miR-34 mimic, has been successfully tested as an miRNA-based anticancer drug in human phase I trial in patients with advanced hepatocellular carcinoma, thus highlighting the feasibility of translating miRNAs into cancer therapy in clinical settings [504]. miR-520d-3p has been identified as a tumor suppressor in OC [505]. Nano-liposomes loaded with miR-520d-3p and EphA2-siRNA exhibited potent antitumor effect and greater therapeutic efficacy *in vivo* than any of the single treatment. miR-34 family of miRNAs is frequently down-regulated in OC and often associated with metastatic disease [506]. Replacement therapy of miR-34 in the metastatic SKOV3 OC cells could inhibit the tumor cell proliferation and metastatic potential [331]. miR-182 overexpression is known to promote the aggressiveness of OC. Xu et al. examined the delivery of anti-miR-182 to an animal model mimicking human OC [379]. It was reported that anti-miR-182 treatment is potent enough to inhibit tumor growth and metastasis. Recently, Dwivedi et al. tested miR-15a and miR-16 nanoliposomes, either alone or in combination, in a pre-clinical chemoresistant orthotopic mouse model of OC [507]. Their results demonstrated that combination therapy of miR-15a and miR-16 without cisplatin yielded better therapeutic response as compared to cisplatin treatment. Thus, the advent of miR replacement therapy offers novel ammunition for the treatment of GC.

5.15 CONCLUSION AND FUTURE PERSPECTIVES

Cancer is accounted for one of the most prevalent diseases with high mortality rates in the world. It is considered one of the major challenges of medical treatment and health [508]. For instance, colorectal cancer with more than 1.2 million new cases causes 600 thousand deaths per year and is the fourth cause of deaths worldwide [509]. Nearly 50,000 people will die in the USA per year, and nearly 135,000 new cases will be diagnosed [510].

In addition to surgery and classical chemotherapeutic and radiation methods, there is a need for novel and less aggressive treatments. RNAi can be considered a promising alternative for cancer therapy as it is less toxic than classical chemotherapy. In addition, siRNAs have been studied for the treatment of various human diseases such as genetic disorders, ocular conditions, cardiovascular diseases, viral infections, and cancers. The ability to target virtually any gene(s) is one of the most attractive aspects of siRNA therapeutics when treatments involving protein-based drugs or small molecules cannot be properly used.

However, a major restriction within the therapeutic applications of siRNA is the low cellular uptake of unmodified siRNAs as they cannot penetrate the cells with high efficiency. For this reason, siRNA molecules need to be complexed or conjugated with an appropriate carrier system. In addition, their fast degradation in cellular cytoplasm and plasma lead to short half-lives. For this reason, numerous strategies involving the combination of biocompatible and versatile non-viral carriers with siRNAs containing modifications and optimized sequences have resulted in potential RNAi-based drugs as efficient medicines into the clinic.

Although a large number of excellent works [511–514] have been described, future studies are required to concentrate on the *in vivo* safety profiles of the nanoparticle-based delivery systems like polymers, cationic lipids, dendrimers, and inorganic nanoparticles, including undesirable cytotoxicity and immune stimulation. For the clinical usage of siRNA-based cancer therapeutics, the development of biocompatible, biodegradable, and safe biodegradable nanoparticle delivery systems is still necessary together with the development of simple and reproducible protocols for the production of batches for regulatory assessment and clinical trials.

Despite the progress in our understanding of the molecular basis of gynecologic malignancies, no major progress has been made in the improvement of patients' survival. For past several years, miRNAs have established themselves as molecules of interest, with possible implications in diagnosis as well as prognosis of GCs. Some interesting observations have led to promising role of miRNAs in therapy of multiple cancers of gynecological origin. Based on the available and emerging data, miRNAs can possibly impact future therapeutic strategies of carcinomas of cervical, endometrial, and ovarian origin. However, before this becomes a reality, our understanding of diverse functionality of miRNAs needs to mature further. miRNAs can target multiple genes, and a single gene can be targeted by multiple miRNAs. Thus, there is certain level of redundancy in miRNA-regulation of genes, which needs to be explored. Further, even after numerous reports on the topic, we do not fully understand the complex nature of miRNA-mediated regulation. As an example, miR-26a was first shown to promote OC proliferation through its suppression of ER-a [515]. Subsequently, it was shown to inhibit proliferation of OC cells through its regulation of CDC6 [516]. In CC model, miR-26a inhibits cell proliferation, migration, and invasion *in vitro* and also inhibits tumor growth *in vivo* in a xenograft model [517]. Similarly, miR-31/miR-214/miR-494 and miR-222 [518,519] have different reported roles in different GCs. Thus, there are conflicting reports on the functionality of a single miRNA within a specific GC as well as across different GCs. While this can possibly be explained by closely related yet distinct miRNA isotypes and the cell line-specific effects, an outcome of targeting of multiple target genes by the same miRNA, the phenomenon needs to be conclusively understood if the knowledge gained from these observations is to be translated into therapy. As a first step, it is critical to cross-validate the findings by independent teams of researchers before reaching conclusions with regards to the functionality of miRNAs. After a successful and definitive understanding of the role that miRNAs play in etiology of GC will come the question as to how miRNAs or the anti-miRs can be systemically delivered, as part of therapy. The strategies to manipulate miRNA levels in cancer patients need to be developed further because when the results from pre-clinical studies emerge, immediate translation to clinics should be possible for the benefit of millions of patients worldwide hoping for a cure and the end to sufferings.

REFERENCES

1. M. Ebrahimi, F. Moazzen, V. Marmari, et al. In silico analysis, cloning and expression of recombinant CD166 in E. coli BL21 (DE3) as a marker for detection and treatment of colorectal cancer, *J. Med. Microbiol. Diagnosis.* 06(01) (2017) 1–6. doi: 10.4172/2161-0703.1000249.
2. R.G.J. Vries, M. Huch, H. Clevers, Stem cells and cancer of the stomach and intestine, *Mol. Oncol.* 4(5) (2010) 373–384. doi: 10.1016/j. molonc.2010.05.001.
3. H. Dana, An overview of cancer stem cell, *J. Stem Cell Res Ther.* 1(4) (2017) 169–174. doi: 10.15406/jsrt.2016.01.00029.
4. X. Zhang, X. Li, Q. You, X. Zhang, Prodrug strategy for cancer cell-specific targeting: a recent overview, *Eur. J. Med. Chem.* 139 (2017) 542–563. doi: 10.1016/j. ejmech.2017.08.010.
5. S.H. Hassanpour, M. Dehghani, Review of cancer from perspective of molecular, *J. Cancer Res. Pract.* 4(4) (2017) 127–129. doi: 10.1016/j.jcrpr.2017.07.001.
6. M. Saraswathy, S. Gong, Recent developments in the co-delivery of siRNA and small molecule anticancer drugs for cancer treatment, *Mater Today* 17(6) (2014) 298–306. doi: 10.1016/j. mattod.2014.05.002.
7. T. Endoh, T. Ohtsuki, Cellular siRNA delivery using cell-penetrating peptides modified for endosomal escape, *Adv. Drug Delivery Rev.* 61(9) (2009) 704–709. doi: 10.1016/j. addr.2009.04.005.
8. R. Siegel, J. Ma, Z. Zou, A. Jemal, Cancer statistics, *CA Cancer J. Clin.* 64(1) (2014) 9–29. doi: 10.3322/caac.21208.
9. J.-P. Spano, D. Azria, A. Gonçalves, Patients' satisfaction in early breast cancer treatment: change in treatment over time and impact of HER2-targeted therapy, *Crit. Rev. Oncol. Hematol.* 94(3) (2015) 270–278. doi: 10.1016/j. critrevonc.2015.01.007.
10. C. Wee Gan, S. Chien, S.-S. Feng, Nanomedicine: enhancement of chemotherapeutical efficacy of docetaxel by using a biodegradable nanoparticle formulation, *Curr. Pharm. Des.* 16(21) (2010) 2308–2320. doi: 10.2174/138161210791920487.
11. S. Panowski, S. Bhakta, H. Raab, P. Polakis, J.R. Junutula, Sitespecific antibody drug conjugates for cancer therapy, *MAbs.* 6(1) (2013) 34–45. doi: 10.4161/mabs.27022.
12. M. Leal, P. Sapra, S.A. Hurvitz, et al., Antibody–drug conjugates: an emerging modality for the treatment of cancer, *Ann. N. Y. Acad Sci.* 1321(1) (2014) 41–54. doi: 10.1111/nyas.12499.
13. S. Jain, K. Pathak, A. Vaidya, Molecular therapy using siRNA: recent trends and advances of multi target inhibition of cancer growth, *Int. J. Biol. Macromol.* 116 (2018) 880–892. doi: 10.1016/j. ijbiomac.2018.05.077.
14. H. Mahmoodzad, M. Ardaneh, E. Zeinalinia, et al. Microrna a new gate in cancer and human disease: a review, *J. Biol. Sci.* 17(6) (2017) 247–254. doi: 10.3923/jbs.2017.247.254.
15. A. Fire, S. Xu, M.K. Montgomery, S.A. Kostas, S.E. Driver, C.C. Mello, Potent and specific genetic interference by double-stranded RNA in Caenorhabditis elegans, *Nature* 391 (1998) 806. doi: 10.1038/35888.
16. N.J. Caplen, S. Parrish, F. Imani, A. Fire, R.A. Morgan, Specific inhibition of gene expression by small double-stranded RNAs in invertebrate and vertebrate systems, *Proc. Natl. Acad. Sci.* 98(17) (2001) 9742–9747. doi: 10.1073/pnas.171251798.
17. S.M. Elbashir, J. Harborth, W. Lendeckel, A. Yalcin, K. Weber, T. Tuschl, Duplexes of 21-nucleotide RNAs mediate RNA interference in cultured mammalian cells, *Nature* 411(6836) (2001) 494–498. doi: 10.1038/35078107.
18. D.H. Kim, J.J. Rossi, Strategies for silencing human disease using RNA interference, *Nat. Rev. Genet.* 8(3) (2007) 173–184. doi: 10.1038/nrg2006.
19. H. Dana, G.M. Chalbatani, H. Mahmoodzadeh, et al. Molecular mechanisms and biological functions of siRNA, *Int. J. Biomed. Sci.* 13(2) (2017) 48–57.
20. J. Yang, Patisiran for the treatment of hereditary transthyretin-mediated amyloidosis, *Expert Rev. Clin. Pharmacol.* 12(2) (2019) 95–99. doi: 10.1080/17512433.2019.1567326.

21. C. Lorenzer, M. Dirin, A.M. Winkler, V. Baumann, J. Winkler, Going beyond the liver: progress and challenges of targeted delivery of siRNA therapeutics, *J. Control Release* 203 (2015) 1–15. doi: 10.1016/j.jconrel.2015.02.003.

22. C.A. Hong, Y.S. Nam, Functional nanostructures for effective delivery of small interfering RNA therapeutics, *Theranostics* 4(12) (2014) 1211–1232. doi: 10.7150/thno.8491.

23. S.-Y. Lee, S.J. Lee, Y.-K. Oh, et al. Stability and cellular uptake of polymerized siRNA (poly-siRNA)/polyethylenimine (PEI) complexes for efficient gene silencing, *J. Control Release* 141(3) (2009) 339–346. doi: 10.1016/j.jconrel.2009.10.007.

24. B. Sjouke, D.M.W. Balak, U. Beuers, V. Ratziu, E.S.G. Stroes, Is mipomersen ready for clinical implementation? A transatlantic dilemma, *Curr. Opin. Lipidol.* 24 (2013) 4. doi: 10.1097/MOL.0b013e328362dfd9.

25. J. Burnett, J. Rossi, RNA-based therapeutics: current progress and future prospects, *Chem. Biol.* 19(1) (2012) 60–71. doi: 10.1016/j.chembiol.2011.12.008.

26. S. Biswas, P.P. Deshpande, G. Navarro, N.S. Dodwadkar, V.P. Torchilin, Lipid modified triblock PAMAM-based nanocarriers for siRNA drug co-delivery, *Biomaterials* 34(4) (2013) 1289–1301. doi: 10.1016/j.biomaterials.2012.10.024.

27. K.A. Whitehead, R. Langer, D.G. Anderson, Knocking down barriers: advances in siRNA delivery, *Nat. Rev. Drug Discov.* 8(2) (2009) 129–138. doi: 10.1038/nrd2742.

28. G.R. Rettig, M.A. Behlke, Progress toward in vivo use of siRNAs-II, *Mol. Ther.* 20(3) (2012) 483–512. doi: 10.1038/mt.2011.263.

29. S. Tsunoda, O. Mazda, Y. Oda, et al. Sonoporation using microbubble BR14 promotes pDNA/siRNA transduction to murine heart, *Biochem. Biophys. Res. Commun.* 336(1) (2005) 118–127. doi: 10.1016/j.bbrc.2005.08.052.

30. T. Kishida, H. Asada, S. Gojo, et al. Sequence-specific gene silencing in murine muscle induced by electroporation-mediated transfer of short interfering RNA, *J. Gene Med.* 6(1) (2004) 105–110. doi: 10.1002/jgm.456.

31. D.V. Morrissey, K. Blanchard, L. Shaw, et al. Activity of stabilized short interfering RNA in a mouse model of hepatitis B virus replication, *Hepatology* 41(6) (2005) 1349–1356. doi: 10.1002/hep.20702.

32. S. Zhang, B. Zhao, H. Jiang, B. Wang, B. Ma, Cationic lipids and polymers mediated vectors for delivery of siRNA, *J. Control Release* 123(1) (2007) 1–10. doi: 10.1016/j.jconrel.2007.07.016.

33. W.J. Kim, S.W. Kim, Efficient siRNA delivery with non-viral polymeric vehicles, *Pharm. Res.* 26(3) (2009) 657–666. doi: 10.1007/s11095-008-9774-1.

34. D.J. Gary, N. Puri, Y.Y. Won, Polymer-based siRNA delivery: perspectives on the fundamental and phenomenological distinctions from polymer-based DNA delivery, *J. Control Release* 121(1–2) (2007) 64–73. doi: 10.1016/j.jconrel.2007.05.021.

35. Y.C. Tseng, S. Mozumdar, L. Huang, Lipid-based systemic delivery of siRNA, *Adv. Drug. Delivery Rev.* 61(9) (2009) 721–731. doi: 10.1016/j.addr.2009.03.003.

36. Z. Hassani, G.F. Lemkine, P. Erbacher, et al. Lipid-mediated siRNA delivery down-regulates exogenous gene expression in the mouse brain at picomolar levels, *J. Gene Med.* 7(2) (2005) 198–207. doi: 10.1002/jgm.659.

37. F. Simeoni, M.C. Morris, F. Heitz, G. Divita, Insight into the mechanism of the peptide-based gene delivery system MPG: implications for delivery of siRNA into mammalian cells, *Nucleic Acids Res.* 31(11) (2003) 2717–2724. doi: 10.1093/nar/gkg385.

38. F. Simeoni, M.C. Morris, F. Heitz, G. Divita, Peptide-based strategy for siRNA delivery into mammalian cells. In: G.G. Carmichael, N.J. Totowa (eds.) *RNA Silencing: Methods and Protocols*, vol. 309. Humana Press (2005), 251–260. doi: 10.1385/1-59259-935-4:251.

39. B. Farrow, B.M. Evers, T. Iwamura, C. Murillo, K.L. O'Connor, P. Rychahou, Inhibition of pancreatic cancer cell growth and induction of apoptosis with novel therapies directed against protein kinase A, *Surgery* 134(2) (2003) 197–205. doi: 10.1067/msy.2003.220.

40. D.S. Schwarz, G. Hutvágner, B. Haley, P.D. Zamore, Evidence that siRNAs function as guides, not primers, in the Drosophila and human RNAi pathways, *Mol. Cell* 10(3) (2002) 537–548. doi: 10.1016/S1097-2765(02)00651-2.

41. M.A. Behlke, Chemical modification of siRNAs for in vivo use, *Oligonucleotides* 18(4) (2008) 305–320. doi: 10.1089/oli.2008.0164.

42. Y. Chiu, T.M. Rana, siRNA function in RNAi: a chemical modification analysis, *RNA* 9 (2003) 1034–1048. doi: 10.1261/rna.5103703.2000.

43. A.H.S. Hall, J. Wan, E.E. Shaughnessy, B.R. Shaw, K.A. Alexander, RNA interference using boranophosphate siRNAs: structure-activity relationships, *Nucleic Acids Res.* 32(20) (2004) 5991–6000. doi: 10.1093/nar/gkh936.

44. T. Dowler, D. Bergeron, A.L. Tedeschi, L. Paquet, N. Ferrari, M.J. Damha, Improvements in siRNA properties mediated by 2′-deoxy-2′-fluoro-β-D-arabinonucleic acid (FANA), *Nucleic Acids Res.* 34(6) (2006) 1669–1675. doi: 10.1093/nar/gkl033.

45. J.K. Watts, G.F. Deleavey, M.J. Damha, Chemically modified siRNA: tools and applications, *Drug Discov. Today* 13(19–20) (2008) 842–855. doi: 10.1016/j.drudis.2008.05.007.

46. C. Xu, J. Wang, Delivery systems for siRNA drug development in cancer therapy, *Asian J. Pharm. Sci.* 10(1) (2015) 1–12. doi: 10.1016/j.ajps.2014.08.011.

47. S. Ghafouri-Fard, siRNA and cancer immunotherapy, *Immunotherapy* 4(9) (2012) 907–917. doi: 10.2217/imt.12.87.

48. R. Klippstein, D. Pozo, Nanotechnology-based manipulation of dendritic cells for enhanced immunotherapy strategies, *Nanomed. Nanotechnol. Biol. Med.* 6(4) (2010) 523–529. doi: 10.1016/j.nano.2010.01.001.

49. J. Banchereau, R.M. Steinman, Dendritic cells and the control of immunology, *Nature* 392 (1998) 245–252. doi: 10.1038/32588.

50. L. Fong, E.G. Engleman, Dendritic cells in cancer immunotherapy, *Pathology* (2000) 245–273. doi: 10.1146/annurev.immunol.21.120601.141040.

51. J. Constantino, C. Gomes, A. Falcão, B.M. Neves, M.T. Cruz, Dendritic cell-based immunotherapy: a basic review and recent advances, *Immunol. Res.* 65(4) (2017) 798–810. doi: 10.1007/s12026-017-8931-1.

52. N. Verra, D. De Jong, A. Bex, et al. Infiltration of activated dendritic cells and T cells in renal cell carcinoma following combined cytokine immunotherapy, *Eur. Urol.* 48(3) (2005) 527–533. doi: 10.1016/j.eururo.2005.03.031.

53. H. Van Poppel, S. Joniau, S.W. Van Gool, Vaccine therapy in patients with renal cell carcinoma, *Eur. Urol.* 55(6) (2009) 1333–1344. doi: 10.1016/j.eururo.2009.01.043.

54. A.M. Asemissen, P. Brossart, Vaccination strategies in patients with renal cell carcinoma, *Cancer Immunol. Immunother.* 58(7) (2009) 1169–1174. doi: 10.1007/s00262-009-0706-7.

55. S. Anguille, E.L. Smits, E. Lion, V.F. Van Tendeloo, Z.N. Berneman, Clinical use of dendritic cells for cancer therapy, *Lancet Oncol.* 15(7) (2014) 257–267. doi: 10.1016/S1470-2045(13)70585-0.

56. A.L. Zhang, U. Purath, I.H. Tarner, et al. Natural killer cells trigger differentiation of monocytes into dendritic cells, *Blood* 110(7) (2007) 2484–2493. doi: 10.1182/blood-2007-02-076364.

57. Z. Wang, D.D. Rao, N. Senzer, J. Nemunaitis, RNA interference and cancer therapy, *Pharm. Res.* (2011) 2983–2995. doi: 10.1007/s11095-011-0604-5.

58. M. Li, H. Qian, T.E. Ichim, et al. Induction of RNA interference in dendritic cells, *Immunol. Res.* 30(2) (2004) 215–230. doi: 10.1385/IR:30:2:215.

59. S. Liu, D. Liu, M. Ji, et al. An indoleamine 2, 3-dioxygenase siRNA nanoparticle-coated and Trp2-displayed recombinant yeast vaccine inhibits melanoma tumor growth in mice, *J. Control Release* 273 (2018) 1–12. doi: 10.1016/j.jconrel.2018.01.013.

60. W. Filipowicz, L. Jaskiewicz, F.A. Kolb, R.S. Pillai, Post-transcriptional gene silencing by siRNAs and miRNAs, *Curr. Opin. Struct. Biol.* 15 (2005) 331–341. doi: 10.1016/j.sbi.2005.05.006.

61. L. He, G.J. Hannon, MicroRNAs: small RNAs with a big role in gene regulation, *Nat. Rev. Genet.* 5(7) (2004) 522–531. doi: 10.1038/nrg1379.

62. D. Castanotto, J.J. Rossi, The promises and pitfalls of RNA-interference-based therapeutics, *Nature* 457(7228) (2009) 426–433. doi: 10.1038/nature07758.

63. K. Tatiparti, S. Sau, S. Kashaw, A. Iyer, siRNA delivery strategies: a comprehensive review of recent developments, *Nanomaterials* 7(4) (2017) 77. doi: 10.3390/nano7040077.

64. S. Massadeh, M. Al Aamery, Nano-materials for gene therapy: an efficient way in overcoming challenges of gene delivery, *J. Biosens. Bioelectron.* 7(1) (2016) 1–12. doi: 10.4172/2155-6210.1000195.

65. K.V. Morris, S.W.-L. Chan, S.E. Jacobsen, D.J. Looney, Small interfering RNA-induced transcriptional gene silencing in human cells, *Cell* 305(1) (2004) 1289–1293.

66. J. Li, S. Xue, Z.W. Mao, Nanoparticle delivery systems for siRNA-based therapeutics, *J. Mater. Chem. B* 4(41) (2016) 6620–6639. doi: 10.1039/c6tb01462c.

67. Y.K. Oh, T.G. Park, siRNA delivery systems for cancer treatment, *Adv. Drug Delivery Rev.* 61(10) (2009) 850–862. doi: 10.1016/j.addr.2009.04.018.

68. M. Chen, Q. Du, H.-Y. Zhang, C. Wahlestedt, Z. Liang, Vector-based siRNA delivery strategies for high-throughput screening of novel target genes, *J. RNAi Gene Silencing* 1(1) (2005) 5–11.

69. N.S. Lee, T. Dohjima, G. Bauer, et al. Expression of small interfering RNAs targeted against HIV-1 rev transcripts in human cells, *Nat. Biotechnol.* 20(5) (2002) 500–505. doi: 10.1038/nbt0502-500.

70. S. Moffatt, siRNA-based nanoparticles for cancer therapy: hurdles and hopes, *MOJ Proteomics Bioinf.* 4(6) (2017) 4–6. doi: 10.15406/mojpb.2016.04.00142.

71. A.L. Jackson, P.S. Linsley, Recognizing and avoiding siRNA off-target effects for target identification and therapeutic application, *Nat. Rev. Drug Discov.* 9(1) (2010) 57–67. doi: 10.1038/nrd3010.

72. J.T. Marques, B.R.G. Williams, Activation of the mammalian immune system by siRNAs, *Nat. Biotechnol.* 23 (2005) 1399. doi: 10.1038/nbt1161.

73. A. Alagia, R. Eritja, siRNA and RNAi optimization, *Wiley Interdisc. Rev. RNA* 7(3) (2016) 316–329. doi: 10.1002/wrna.1337.

74. J.B. Bramsen, M.M. Pakula, T.B. Hansen, et al. A screen of chemical modifications identifies position-specific modification by UNA to most potently reduce siRNA off-target effects, *Nucleic Acids Res.* 38(17) (2010) 5761–5773. doi: 10.1093/nar/gkq341.

75. S.R. Suter, A. Ball-Jones, M.M. Mumbleau, et al. Controlling miRNA-like off-target effects of an siRNA with nucleobase modifications, *Org. Biomol. Chem.* 15(47) (2017) 10029–10036. doi: 10.1039/c7ob02654d.

76. A. Alagia, A.F. Jorge, A. Aviñó, et al. Exploring PAZ/3′-overhang interaction to improve siRNA specificity. A combined experimental and modeling study, *Chem. Sci.* 9(8) (2018) 2074–2086. doi: 10.1039/c8sc00010g.

77. H.S. Kang, D. Lee, C.J. Li, et al. Asymmetric shorter-duplex siRNA structures trigger efficient gene silencing with reduced nonspecific effects, *Mol. Ther.* 17(4) (2009) 725–732. doi: 10.1038/mt.2008.298.

78. M. Sioud, Advances in RNA sensing by the immune system: separation of siRNA unwanted effects from RNA interference, *Methods Mol. Biol.* 629 (2010) 33–52. doi: 10.1007/978-1-60761-6573_3.

79. F. Eberle, M. Peter, C. Richert, et al. Modifications in small interfering RNA that separate immunostimulation from RNA interference, *J. Immunol.* 180(5) (2014) 3229–3237. doi: 10.4049/ jimmunol.180.5.3229.

80. Slobodkin G, Wilkinson L, Pence C, et al. Versatile cationic lipids for siRNA delivery, *J. Control Release* 158(2) (2011) 269–276. doi: 10.1016/j.jconrel.2011.11.006.

81. Y.Y.C. Tam, S. Chen, P.R. Cullis, Advances in lipid nanoparticles for siRNA delivery, *Pharmaceutics* 5(3) (2013) 498–507. doi: 10.3390/pharmaceutics5030498.

82. S.C. Semple, A. Akinc, J. Chen, et al. Rational design of cationic lipids for siRNA delivery, *Nat. Biotechnol.* 28 (2010) 172. doi: 10.1038/nbt.1602.

83. K.T. Love, K.P. Mahon, G. Christopher, et al. Correction for Love et al., Lipid-like materials for low-dose, in vivo gene silencing, *Proc. Natl. Acad. Sci.* 107(21) (2010) 9915. doi: 10.1073/pnas.1005136107.

84. M.T. Abrams, M.L. Koser, J. Seitzer, et al. Evaluation of efficacy, biodistribution, and inflammation for a potent siRNA nanoparticle: effect of dexamethasone co-treatment, *Mol. Ther.* 18(1) (2010) 171–180. doi: 10.1038/mt.2009.208.

85. S. Grijalvo, G. Puras, J. Zárate, et al. Cationic niosomes as non-viral vehicles for nucleic acids: challenges and opportunities in gene delivery, *Pharmaceutics* 11 (2019) 2. doi: 10.3390/pharmaceutics11020050.

86. B.S. Pattni, V.V. Chupin, V.P. Torchilin, New developments in liposomal drug delivery, *Chem. Rev.* 115(19) (2015) 10938–10966. doi: 10.1021/acs.chemrev.5b00046.

87. A. Derycke, Liposomes for photodynamic therapy, *Adv. Drug Delivery Rev.* 56(1) (2003) 17–30. doi: 10.1016/j.addr.2003.07.014.

88. T. Minko, R.I. Pakunlu, Y. Wang, J.J. Khandare, M. Saad, New generation of liposomal drugs for cancer, *Anticancer Agents Med. Chem.* 6(6) (2014) 537–552. doi: 10.2174/187152006778699095.

89. G.M. Chalbatani, H. Dana, E. Gharagouzloo, S. Grijalvo, R. Eritja, C.D. Logsdon, F. Memari, S.R. Miri, M.R. Rad, V. Marmari, Small interfering RNAs (siRNAs) in cancer therapy: a nano-based approach, *Int. J. Nanomed.* 14 (2019) 3111–3128.

90. R. Cheng, F. Feng, F. Meng, C. Deng, J. Feijen, Z. Zhong, Glutathione-responsive nano-vehicles as a promising platform for targeted intracellular drug and gene delivery, *J. Control Release* 152(1) (2011) 2–12. doi: 10.1016/j.jconrel.2011.01.030.

91. B. Ozpolat, A.K. Sood, G. Lopez-Berestein, Liposomal siRNA nanocarriers for cancer therapy, *Adv. Drug Delivery Rev.* 66 (2014) 110–116. doi: 10.1016/j.addr.2013.12.008.

92. A. Duchemin, B. Evrard, G. Piel, V. Sanna, A. Lechanteur, D. Mottet, Cationic liposomes carrying siRNA: impact of lipid composition on physicochemical properties, cytotoxicity and endosomal escape, *Nanomaterials* 8(5) (2018) 270. doi: 10.3390/nano8050270.

93. A. Santel, M. Aleku, O. Keil, et al. A novel siRNA-lipoplex technology for RNA interference in the mouse vascular endothelium, *Gene Ther.* 13(16) (2006) 1222–1234. doi: 10.1038/sj.gt.3302777.

94. M. Aleku, P. Schulz, O. Keil, et al. Atu027, a liposomal small interfering RNA formulation targeting protein kinase N3, inhibits cancer progression, *Cancer Res.* 68(23) (2008) 9788–9798. doi: 10.1158/0008-5472.CAN-08-2428.

95. S.Y. Wu, N.A.J. McMillan, Lipidic systems for in vivo siRNA delivery, *Aaps J.* 11(4) (2009) 639–652. doi: 10.1208/s12248-009-9140-1.

96. C.N. Landen, W.M. Merritt, L.S. Mangala, et al. Intraperitoneal delivery of liposomal siRNA for therapy of advanced ovarian cancer, *Cancer Biol. Ther.* 5(12) (2006) 1708–1713. doi: 10.4161/cbt.5.12.3468.

97. Y. Cheng, Y. Ji, RGD-modified polymer and liposome nanovehicles: recent research progress for drug delivery in cancer therapeutics, *Eur. J. Pharm. Sci.* 128 (2019) 8–17. doi: 10.1016/j.ejps.2018.11.023.

98. S.I. Mattern-Schain, R.K. Fisher, P.C. West, et al. Cell mimetic liposomal nanocarriers for tailored delivery of vascular therapeutics, *Chem. Phys. Lipids.* 218 (2019) 149–157. doi: 10.1016/j.chemphyslip.2018.12.009.

99. T.S. Zimmermann, A.C.H. Lee, A. Akinc, et al. RNAi-mediated gene silencing in non-human primates, *Nature* 441(1) (2006) 111–114. doi: 10.1038/nature04688.

100. W. Ho, X.Q. Zhang, X. Xu, Biomaterials in siRNA delivery: a comprehensive review, *Adv. Healthcare Mater.* 5(21) (2016) 2715–2731. doi: 10.1002/adhm.201600418.

101. V. Sood, A.N. Honko, I. McLachlan, et al. Postexposure protection of non-human primates against a lethal Ebola virus challenge with RNA interference: a proof-of-concept study, *Lancet* 375(9729) (2010) 1896–1905. doi: 10.1016/s0140-6736(10)60357-1.

102. R.R. Nikam, K.R. Gore, Journey of siRNA: clinical developments and targeted delivery, *Nucleic Acid Ther.* 28(4) (2018) 209–224. doi: 10.1089/nat.2017.0715.

103. P.J.C. Lin, Y.K. Tam, Chapter 9: Controlling protein expression by delivery of RNA therapeutics using lipid nanoparticles. In: M. Filice, J.B.T. Ruiz-Cabello (eds.) *Micro and Nano Technologies.* Elsevier: Amsterdam, the Netherlands (2019) 277–310. doi: 10.1016/B978-0-12-814470-1.00009-5.

104. J. Zhao, G. Weng, J. Li, J. Zhu, J. Zhao, Polyester-based nanoparticles for nucleic acid delivery, *Mater Sci. Eng. C.* 92 (2018) 983–994. doi: 10.1016/j.msec.2018.07.027.

105. D.B. Rozema, D.L. Lewis, D.H. Wakefield, et al. Dynamic PolyConjugates for targeted in vivo delivery of siRNA to hepatocytes, *Proc. Natl. Acad. Sci.* 104(32) (2007) 12982–12987. doi: 10.1073/pnas.0703778104.

106. E. Wagner, Polymers for sirna delivery: inspired by viruses to be targeted, dynamic, and precise, *Acc. Chem. Res.* 45(7) (2012) 1005–1013. doi: 10.1021/ar2002232.

107. R. Farra, F. Musiani, F. Perrone, et al. Polymer-mediated delivery of siRNAs to hepatocellular carcinoma: variables affecting specificity and effectiveness, *Molecules* 23(4) (2018). doi: 10.3390/molecules23040777.

108. R.G. Parmar, M. Poslusney, M. Busuek, et al. Novel endosomolytic poly(amido amine) polymer conjugates for systemic delivery of siRNA to hepatocytes in rodents and nonhuman primates, *Bioconjug. Chem.* 25(5) (2014) 896–906. doi: 10.1021/bc400527e.

109. R. Kanasty, J.R. Dorkin, A. Vegas, D. Anderson, Delivery materials for siRNA therapeutics, *Nat. Mater.* 12(11) (2013) 967–977. doi: 10.1038/nmat3765.

110. M.E. Davis, The first targeted delivery of siRNA in humans via a self-assembling, cyclodextrin polymer-based nanoparticle: from concept to clinic, *Mol. Pharm.* 6(3) (2009) 659–668. doi: 10.1021/mp900015y.

111. A.M. O'Mahony, B.M.D.C. Godinho, J. Ogier, et al. Click-modified cyclodextrins as nonviral vectors for neuronal siRNA delivery, *ACS Chem. Neurosci.* 3(10) (2012) 744–752. doi: 10.1021/cn3000372.

112. A. Díaz-Moscoso, L. Le Gourriérec, M. Gómez-García, et al. Polycationic amphiphilic cyclodextrins for gene delivery: synthesis and effect of structural modifications on plasmid DNA complex stability, cytotoxicity, and gene expression, *Chem. A Eur. J.* 15(46) (2009) 12871–12888. doi: 10.1002/chem.200901149.

113. E. Miele, G.P. Spinelli, E. Miele, et al. Nanoparticle-based delivery of small interfering RNA: challenges for cancer therapy, *Int. J. Nanomed.* 7 (2012) 3637–3657. doi: 10.2147/IJN. S23696.

114. G. Sica, Z. Chen, Z. Wang, et al. RRM2 regulates Bcl-2 in head and neck and lung cancers: a potential target for cancer therapy, *Clin. Cancer Res.* 19(13) (2013) 3416–3428. doi: 10.1158/1078-0432.ccr-13-0073.

115. M.E. Davis, D. Seligson, A. Tolcher, et al. Evidence of RNAi in humans from systemically administered siRNA via targeted nanoparticles, *Nature* 464(7291) (2010) 1067–1070. doi: 10.1038/nature08956.

116. M.B. Hovgaard, U.L. Rahbek, S.Z. Glud, et al. RNA interference in vitro and in vivo using a novel chitosan/siRNA nanoparticle system, *Mol. Ther.* 14(4) (2006) 476–484. doi: 10.1016/j.ymthe.2006.04.010.

117. K. Dai, F. Winnik, X. Qiu, et al. Low molecular weight chitosan conjugated with folate for siRNA delivery in vitro: optimization studies, *Int. J. Nanomed.* 7 (2012) 5833. doi: 10.2147/ijn.s35567.

118. S.C. De Smedt, B. Nysten, C.S. Le Duff, et al. Chitosan nanoparticles for siRNA delivery: optimizing formulation to increase stability and efficiency, *J. Control Release* 176 (2014) 54–63. doi: 10.1016/j.jconrel.2013.12.026.

119. Y.K. Kim, A. Minai-Tehrani, J.H. Lee, C.S. Cho, M.H. Cho, H.L. Jiang, Therapeutic efficiency of folated poly(ethylene glycol)-chitosangraft-polyethylenimine-Pdcd4 complexes in H-ras12V mice with liver cancer, *Int. J. Nanomed.* 8 (2013) 1489–1498. doi: 10.2147/IJN.S42949.

120. R.K. Kankala, X.F. Lin, H.F. Song, et al. Supercritical fluid-assisted decoration of nanoparticles on porous microcontainers for codelivery of therapeutics and inhalation therapy of diabetes, *ACS Biomater. Sci. Eng.* 4(12) (2018) 4225–4235. doi: 10.1021/acsbiomaterials.8b00992.

121. P.-Y. Xu, R.K. Kankala, Y.-J. Pan, H. Yuan, S.-B. Wang, A.-Z. Chen, Overcoming multidrug resistance through inhalable siRNA nanoparticles-decorated porous microparticles based on supercritical fluid technology, *Int. J. Nanomed.* 13 (2018) 4685–4698. doi: 10.2147/IJN.S169399.

122. S.-B. Wang, A.-Z. Chen, N. Tang, X.-Q. Su, Y.-Q. Kang, Preparation and antitumor effect evaluation of composite microparticles co-loaded with siRNA and paclitaxel by a supercritical process, *J. Mater. Chem B.* 3(31) (2015) 6439–6447. doi: 10.1039/c5tb00715a.

123. R.K. Kankala, B.-Q. Chen, C.-G. Liu, H.-X. Tang, S.-B. Wang, A.-Z. Chen, Solution-enhanced dispersion by supercritical fluids: an ecofriendly nanonization approach for processing biomaterials and pharmaceutical compounds, *Int J. Nanomed.* 13 (2018) 4227–4245. doi: 10.2147/IJN.S166124.

124. M. Licciardi, A. Li Volsi, C. Sardo, N. Mauro, G. Cavallaro, G. Giammona, Inulin-ethylenediamine coated SPIONs magnetoplexes: a promising tool for improving siRNA delivery, *Pharm. Res.* 32(11) (2015) 3674–3687. doi: 10.1007/s11095-015-1726-y.

125. C. Sardo, R. Farra, M. Licciardi, et al. Development of a simple, biocompatible and cost-effective inulin-diethylene-triamine based siRNA delivery system, *Eur. J. Pharm. Sci.* 75 (2015) 60–71. doi: 10.1016/j.ejps.2015.03.021.

126. C. Sardo, E.F. Craparo, B. Porsio, G. Giammona, G. Cavallaro, Improvements in rational design strategies of inulin derivative polycation for siRNA delivery, *Biomacromolecules* 17(7) (2016) 2352–2366. doi: 10.1021/acs.biomac.6b00281.

127. A. Aigner, Delivery systems for the direct application of siRNAs to induce RNA interference (RNAi) in vivo, *J. Biomed. Biotechnol.* 2006 (2006) 1–15. doi: 10.1155/JBB/2006/71659.

128. S. Akhtar, I.F. Benter, Review series nonviral delivery of synthetic siRNAs in vivo, *J. Clin. Invest.* 117(12) (2007) 3623–3632. doi: 10.1172/JCI33494.

129. A. Judge, E.A. Fritz, J.R. Phelps, et al. Postexposure protection of guinea pigs against a lethal ebola virus challenge is conferred by RNA interference, *J. Infect. Dis.* 193(12) (2006) 1650–1657. doi: 10.1086/504267.

130. A. Bai, J. Chen, L. Filip, T. Nguyen, Q. Ge, H.N. Eisen, Inhibition of influenza virus production in virus-infected mice by RNA interference, *Proc. Natl. Acad. Sci.* 101(23) (2004) 8676–8681. doi: 10.1073/pnas.0402486101.

131. B. Urban-Klein, S. Werth, S. Abuharbeid, F. Czubayko, A. Aigner, RNAi-mediated gene-targeting through systemic application of polyethylenimine (PEI)-complexed siRNA in vivo, *Gene Ther.* 12 (2004) 461. doi: 10.1038/sj.gt.3302425.

132. S. Akhtar, I. Benter, Toxicogenomics of non-viral drug delivery systems for RNAi: potential impact on siRNA-mediated gene silencing activity and specificity, *Adv. Drug Delivery Rev.* 59(2–3) (2007) 164–182. doi: 10.1016/j.addr.2007.03.010.

133. A.P. Pandey, K.K. Sawant, Polyethylenimine: a versatile, multifunctional non-viral vector for nucleic acid delivery, *Mater. Sci. Eng. C.* 68 (2016) 904–918. doi: 10.1016/j.msec.2016.07.066.

134. J. Wang, Z. Lu, M.G. Wientjes, J.L.S. Au, Delivery of siRNA therapeutics: barriers and carriers, *Aaps J.* 12(4) (2010) 492–503. doi: 10.1208/s12248-010-9210-4.

135. C. Fornaguera, S. Grijalvo, M. Galán, et al. Novel non-viral gene delivery systems composed of carbosilane dendron functionalized nanoparticles prepared from nano-emulsions as non-viral carriers for antisense oligonucleotides, *Int. J. Pharm.* 478(1) (2015) 113–123. doi: 10.1016/j.ijpharm.2014.11.031.

136. A. Khan, M. Benboubetra, P.Z. Sayyed, et al. Sustained polymeric delivery of gene silencing antisense ODNs, siRNA, DNAzymes and ribozymes: in vitro and in vivo studies, *J. Drug Target.* 12(6) (2004) 393–404. doi: 10.1080/10611860400003858.

137. S. Svenson, R.I. Case, R.O. Cole, et al. Tumor selective silencing using an RNAi-conjugated polymeric nano-pharmaceutical, *Mol. Pharm.* 13(3) (2016) 737–747. doi: 10.1021/acs.molpharmaceut.5b00608.

138. Y. Byeon, J.-W. Lee, W.S. Choi, et al. CD44-targeting PLGA nanoparticles incorporating paclitaxel and FAK siRNA overcome chemoresistance in epithelial ovarian cancer, *Cancer Res.* 78(21) (2018) 6247–6256. doi: 10.1158/0008-5472.CAN-17-3871.

139. J. Winkler, Nanomedicines based on recombinant fusion proteins for targeting therapeutic siRNA oligonucleotides, *Ther. Delivery* 2(7) (2011) 891–905. doi: 10.4155/tde.11.56.

140. T.L. Kaneshiro, Z.R. Lu, Targeted intracellular code-livery of chemotherapeutics and nucleic acid with a well-defined dendrimer-based nanoglobular carrier, *Biomaterials* 30(29) (2009) 5660–5666. doi: 10.1016/j.biomaterials.2009.06.026.

141. S. Bhatia, H. Zhu, A. Birjiniuk, et al. Functional delivery of siRNA in mice using dendriworms, *ACS Nano* 3(9) (2009) 2495–2504. doi: 10.1021/nn900201e.

142. J. Zhou, K.T. Shum, J.C. Burnett, J.J. Rossi, Nanoparticle-based delivery of RNAi therapeutics: progress and challenges, *Pharmaceuticals* 6(1) (2013) 85–107. doi: 10.3390/ph6010085.

143. W. Cheung, F. Pontoriero, O. Taratula, A.M. Chen, H. He, DNA and carbon nanotubes as medicine, *Adv Drug Delivery Rev.* 62(6) (2010) 633–649. doi: 10.1016/j.addr.2010.03.007.

144. D. Lynn Kirkpatrick, M. Weiss, A. Naumov, G. Bartholomeusz, R. Bruce Weisman, O. Gliko, Carbon nanotubes: solution for the therapeutic delivery of siRNA? *Materials (Basel)* 5(2) (2012) 278–301. doi: 10.3390/ma5020278.

145. Z. Zhang, X. Yang, Y. Zhang, et al. Delivery of telomerase reverse transcriptase small interfering RNA in complex with positively charged single-walled carbon nanotubes suppresses tumor growth, *Clin. Cancer Res.* 12(16) (2006) 4933–4939. doi: 10.1158/1078-0432.CCR-05-2831.

146. Y. Jiang, S. Huo, J. Hardie, X.-J. Liang, V.M. Rotello, Progress and perspective of inorganic nanoparticle-based siRNA delivery systems, *Expert Opin. Drug Delivery* 13(4) (2016) 547–559. doi: 10.1517/17425247.2016.1134486.

147. M.E. Gindy, R.K. Prud'homme, Multifunctional nanoparticles for imaging, delivery and targeting in cancer therapy, *Expert Opin. Drug Delivery* 6(8) (2009) 865–878. doi: 10.1517/17425240902932908.

148. T. Sangvanich, D. Bejan, S. Gu, W. Yantasee, M. Reda, W. Ngamcherdtrakul, Lyophilization and stability of antibody-conjugated mesoporous silica nanoparticle with cationic polymer and PEG for siRNA delivery, *Int. J. Nanomed.* 13 (2018) 4015–4027. doi: 10.2147/ijn.s164393.

149. S. Tiash, N.I.B. Kamaruzman, E.H. Chowdhury, Carbonate apatite nanoparticles carry siRNA(s) targeting growth factor receptor genes egfr1 and erbb2 to regress mouse breast tumor, *Drug Delivery* 2017;24 (1):1721–1730. doi: 10.1080/10717544.2017.1396385.

150. J. Courty, A. Latorre, A. Villanueva, et al. Efficient treatment of breast cancer xenografts with multifunctionalized iron oxide nanoparticles combining magnetic hyperthermia and anti-cancer drug delivery, *Breast Cancer Res.* 17(1) (2015) 1–17. doi: 10.1186/s13058-015-0576-1.

151. D. Cai, R. Long, Y. Liu, et al. Bacterial magnetosomes-based nanocarriers for co-delivery of cancer therapeutics in vitro, *Int. J. Nanomed.* 13 (2018) 8269–8279. doi: 10.2147/ijn.s180503.

152. Z. Wu, J. Shen, L.-M. Zhang, et al. Magnetic cationic amylose nanoparticles used to deliver survivin-small interfering RNA for gene therapy of hepatocellular carcinoma in vitro, *Nanomaterials* 7(5) (2017) 110. doi: 10.3390/nano7050110.

153. M. Roca, H. Aj, Probing cells with noble metal nanoparticle aggregates, *Nanomedicine* 3(4) (2008) 555–565. doi: 10.2217/17435889.3.4.555.

154. Z.P. Xu, Q.H. Zeng, G.Q. Lu, A.B. Yu, Inorganic nanoparticles as carriers for efficient cellular delivery, *Chem. Eng. Sci.* 61(3) (2006) 1027–1040. doi: 10.1016/j.ces.2005.06.019.

155. J.K.L. Wong, N. Habib, A.M. Seifalian, R. Mohseni, A.A. Hamidieh, R.E. MacLaren, Will nanotechnology bring new hope for gene delivery? *Trends Biotechnol.* 35(5) (2017) 434–451. doi: 10.1016/j. tibtech.2016.12.009.

156. R. Mendes, A.R. Fernandes, P.V. Baptista, Gold nanoparticle approach to the selective delivery of gene silencing in cancer-The case for combined delivery? *Genes (Basel).* 8(3) (2017) 94. doi: 10.3390/genes8030094.

157. W. Hou, P. Wei, L. Kong, R. Guo, S. Wang, X. Shi, Partially PEGylated dendrimer-entrapped gold nanoparticles: a promising nanoplatform for highly efficient DNA and siRNA delivery, *J. Mater. Chem. B.* 4(17) (2016) 2933–2943. doi: 10.1039/c6tb00710d.

158. T. Tokatlian, T. Segura, siRNA applications in nanomedicine, *Wiley Interdiscip. Rev. Nanomed. Nanobiotechnol.* 2(3) (2010) 305–315. doi: 10.1002/wnan.81.

159. J.M. Benitez-Del-Castillo, J. Moreno-Montañés, I. Jiménez-Alfaro, et al. Safety and efficacy clinical trials for SYL1001, a novel short interfering RNA for the treatment of dry eye disease, *Invest. Ophthalmol. Vis. Sci.* 57(14) (2016) 6447–6454. doi: 10.1167/iovs.16-20303.

160. S. Grijalvo, A. Alagia, A.F. Jorge, R. Eritja, Covalent strategies for targeting messenger and non-coding RNAs: an updated review on siRNA, miRNA and anti-miR conjugates, *Genes (Basel)* 9 (2018) 2. doi: 10.3390/genes9020074.

161. M. Manoharan, C. Andree, P. Amaya, et al. Identification of siRNA delivery enhancers by a chemical library screen, *Nucleic Acids Res.* 43(16) (2015) 7984–8001. doi: 10.1093/nar/gkv762.

162. C. Chakraborty, A.R. Sharma, G. Sharma, C.G.P. Doss, S.-S. Lee, Therapeutic miRNA and siRNA: moving from bench to clinic as next generation medicine, *Mol. Ther. Nucleic Acids* 8 (2017) 132–143. doi: 10.1016/j.omtn.2017.06.005.

163. J. Soutschek, A. Akinc, B. Bramlage, et al. Therapeutic silencing of an endogenous gene by systemic administration of modified siRNAs, *Nature* 432(7014) (2004) 173–178. doi: 10.1038/nature03121.

164. H. Li, L. Wang, C. Fan, H. Gu, Q. Hu, DNA nanotechnology-enabled drug delivery systems, *Chem. Rev.* (2018). doi: 10.1021/acs.chemrev.7b00663.

165. Z. Ni, P. Hui, Emerging pharmacologic therapies for wet age-related macular degeneration, *Ophthalmologica* 223(6) (2009) 401–410. doi: 10.1159/000228926.

166. J.C. Perales, V.E. Marquez, R. Eritja, S.M. Ocampo, M. Terrazas, Effect of north bicyclo3.1.0.hexane 2′-Deoxy-pseudosugars on RNA Interference: a novel class of siRNA modification, *ChemBioChem* 12(7) (2011) 1056–1065. doi: 10.1002/cbic.201000791.

167. J.K. Nair, J.L.S. Willoughby, A. Chan, et al. Multivalent N-Acetylgalactosamine-conjugated siRNA localizes in hepatocytes and elicits robust RNAi-mediated gene silencing, *J. Am. Chem. Soc.* 136(49) (2014) 16958–16961. doi: 10.1021/ja505986a.

168. R.E. Meyers, G.J. Weiss, V.A. Clausen, et al. First-in-humans trial of an RNA interference therapeutic targeting VEGF and KSP in cancer patients with liver involvement, *Cancer Discov.* 3(4) (2013) 406–417. doi: 10.1158/2159-8290.cd-12-0429.

169. J.S. Donahoe, M. Nahrendorf, R. Langer, et al. Molecularly self-assembled nucleic acid nanoparticles for targeted in vivo siRNA delivery, *Nat. Nanotechnol.* 7(6) (2012) 389–393. doi: 10.1038/nnano.2012.73.

170. C. Salvans, I. Brun-Heath, I. Ivani, et al. Rational design of novel N-alkyl-N capped biostable RNA nanostructures for efficient long-term inhibition of gene expression, *Nucleic Acids Res.* 44(9) (2016) 4354–4367. doi: 10.1093/nar/gkw169.

171. C. He, Y. Weizmann, W. Lin, D. Liu, T.R. Gannett, G. Chen, Enzymatic synthesis of periodic DNA nanoribbons for intracellular pH sensing and gene silencing, *J. Am. Chem. Soc.* 137(11) (2015) 3844–3851. doi: 10.1021/ja512665z.

172. W. Ruan, M. Zheng, Y. An, et al. DNA nanoclew templated spherical nucleic acids for siRNA delivery, *Chem. Commun.* 54(29) (2018) 3609–3612. doi: 10.1039/c7cc09257a.

173. A.F. Jorge, R. Eritja, Overview of DNA self-assembling: progresses in biomedical applications, *Pharmaceutics* 10 (2018) 4. doi: 10.3390/pharmaceutics10040268.

174. Y. Xin, M. Huang, W.W. Guo, Q. Huang, L. Zhang, G. Jiang, Nanobased delivery of RNAi in cancer therapy, *Mol. Cancer* 16(1) (2017) 1–9. doi: 10.1186/s12943-017-0683-y.

175. M.S. Shim, S. Wong, Y.J. Kwon, SiRNA as a conventional drug in the clinic? Challenges and current technologies, *Drug Discov. Today Technol.* 9(2) (2012) e167–e173. doi: 10.1016/j. ddtec.2012.01.003.

176. M. Ferrari, Vectoring siRNA therapeutics into the clinic, *Nat. Rev. Clin. Oncol.* 7 (2010) 485. doi: 10.1038/nrclinonc.2010.131.

177. A. Santel, J. Kaufmann, D. Strumberg, et al. First-in-human phase I Study of the liposomal RNA interference therapeutic Atu027 in patients with advanced solid tumors, *J. Clin. Oncol.* 32(36) (2014) 4141–4148. doi: 10.1200/jco.2013.55.0376.

178. J. Tabernero, G.I. Shapiro, P.M. LoRusso, et al. First-in-humans trial of an RNA interference therapeutic targeting VEGF and KSP in cancer patients with liver involvement, *Cancer Discov.* 3(4) (2013) 406–417. doi: 10.1158/2159-8290.CD-12-0429.

179. A.W. Tolcher, K.P. Papadopoulos, A. Patnaik, et al. Safety and activity of DCR-MYC, a first-in-class Dicer-substrate small interfering RNA (DsiRNA) targeting MYC, in a phase I study in patients with advanced solid tumors, *J. Clin. Oncol.* 33(15_suppl) (2015) 11006. doi: 10.1200/jco.2015.33.15_suppl.11006.

180. M.J. Wagner, A.K. Sood, G. Lopez-Berestein, et al. Preclinical mammalian safety studies of EPHARNA (DOPC Nanoliposomal EphA2-Targeted siRNA), *Mol. Cancer Ther.* 16(6) (2017) 1114–1123. doi: 10.1158/1535-7163.mct-16-0541.

181. T. Golan, E.Z. Khvalevsky, A. Hubert, et al. RNAi therapy targeting KRAS in combination with chemotherapy for locally advanced pancreatic cancer patients, *Oncotarget* 6(27) (2015) 24560–24570. doi: 10.18632/oncotarget.4183.

182. H. Mahmoodzadeh, F. Moazzen, N. Mehmandoost, et al. Cloning and expression of C2 and V Domains of ALCAM Protein in E. coli BL21 (DE3), *Clin. Microbiol. Open Access* 6(1) (2017) 1–6. doi: 10.4172/2327-5073.1000271.

183. A.B. Bourla, D. Zamarin, Immunotherapy: new strategies for the treatment of gynecologic malignancies, *Oncology (Williston Park)* 30 (2016) 59–69.
184. Y. Collins, K. Holcomb, E. Chapman-Davis, D. Khabele, J.H. Farley, Gynecologic cancer disparities: a report from the health disparities taskforce of the society of gynecologic oncology, *Gynecol. Oncol.* 133 (2014) 353e361.
185. S. Jonas, E. Izaurralde, Towards a molecular understanding of microRNAmediated gene silencing, *Nat. Rev. Genet.* 16 (2015) 421e433.
186. X. Zhong, G. Coukos, L. Zhang, miRNAs in human cancer, *Methods Mol. Biol.* 822 (2012) 295e306.
187. S.K. Srivastava, A. Ahmad, H. Zubair, O. Miree, S. Singh, R.P. Rocconi, J. Scalici, A.P. Singh, MicroRNAs in gynecological cancers: Small molecules with big implications, *Cancer Letters* 407 (2017) 123–138.
188. R.L. Siegel, K.D. Miller, A. Jemal, Cancer statistics, *CA: Cancer J. Clin.* 67 (2017) 7–30.
189. A. Dehal, J.J. Smith, G.M. Nash, Cytoreductive surgery and intraperitoneal chemotherapy: an evidence-based review e past, present and future, *J. Gastrointest. Oncol.* 7 (2016) 143–157.
190. L. Zhang, J. Huang, N. Yang, J. Greshock, M.S. Megraw, A. Giannakakis, et al., microRNAs exhibit high frequency genomic alterations in human cancer, *Proc. Natl. Acad. Sci. U. S. A.* 103 (2006) 9136–9141.
191. S.K. Wyman, R.K. Parkin, P.S. Mitchell, B.R. Fritz, K. O'Briant, A.K. Godwin, et al., Repertoire of microRNAs in epithelial ovarian cancer as determined by next generation sequencing of small RNA cDNA libraries, *PLoS One* 4 (2009) e5311.
192. S.W. Shahab, L.V. Matyunina, R. Mezencev, L.D. Walker, N.J. Bowen, B.B. Benigno, et al., Evidence for the complexity of microRNA-mediated regulation in ovarian cancer: a systems approach, *PLoS One* 6 (2011) e22508.
193. J. Brouwer, J. Kluiver, R.C. de Almeida, R. Modderman, M.M. Terpstra, K. Kok, et al., Small RNA sequencing reveals a comprehensive miRNA signature of BRCA1-associated high-grade serous ovarian cancer, *J. Clin. Pathol.* 69 (11) (2016) 979–985. doi: 10.1136/jclinpath-2016-203679
194. R.L. Wu, S. Ali, S. Bandyopadhyay, B. Alosh, K. Hayek, M.F. Daaboul, et al., Comparative analysis of differentially expressed miRNAs and their downstream mRNAs in ovarian cancer and its associated endometriosis, *J. Cancer Sci. Ther.* 7 (2015) 258–265.
195. K.E. Resnick, H. Alder, J.P. Hagan, D.L. Richardson, C.M. Croce, D.E. Cohn, The detection of differentially expressed microRNAs from the serum of ovarian cancer patients using a novel real-time PCR platform, *Gynecol. Oncol.* 112 (2009) 55–59.
196. E.J. Nam, H. Yoon, S.W. Kim, H. Kim, Y.T. Kim, J.H. Kim, et al., MicroRNA expression profiles in serous ovarian carcinoma, *Clin. Cancer Res.* 14 (2008) 2690–2695.
197. J. Chen, D. Yao, Y. Li, H. Chen, C. He, N. Ding, et al., Serum microRNA expression levels can predict lymph node metastasis in patients with early stage cervical squamous cell carcinoma, *Int. J. Mol. Med.* 32 (2013) 557–567.
198. J.W. Lee, C.H. Choi, J.J. Choi, Y.A. Park, S.J. Kim, S.Y. Hwang, et al., Altered MicroRNA expression in cervical carcinomas, *Clin. Cancer Res.* 14 (2008) 2535–2542.
199. K. Gocze, K. Gombos, K. Juhasz, K. Kovacs, B. Kajtar, M. Benczik, et al., Unique microRNA expression profiles in cervical cancer, *Anticancer Res.* 33 (2013) 2561–2567.
200. S.M. Wilting, P.J. Snijders, W. Verlaat, A. Jaspers, M.A. van de Wiel, W.N. van Wieringen, et al., Altered microRNA expression associated with chromosomal changes contributes to cervical carcinogenesis, *Oncogene* 32 (2013) 106–116.
201. Y. Nagamitsu, H. Nishi, T. Sasaki, Y. Takaesu, F. Terauchi, K. Isaka, Profiling analysis of circulating microRNA expression in cervical cancer, *Mol. Clin. Oncol.* 5 (2016) 189–194.
202. S. Sharma, S. Hussain, K. Soni, P. Singhal, R. Tripathi, V.G. Ramachandran, et al., Novel MicroRNA signatures in HPV-mediated cervical carcinogenesis in Indian women, *Tumour Biol. J. Int. Soc. Oncodevel. Biol. Med.* 37 (2016) 4585–4595.
203. W. Jia, Y. Wu, Q. Zhang, G.E. Gao, C. Zhang, Y. Xiang, Expression profile of circulating microRNAs as a promising fingerprint for cervical cancer diagnosis and monitoring, *Mol. Clin. Oncol.* 3 (2015) 851–858.
204. M.Y. Li, X.X. Hu, Meta-analysis of microRNA expression profiling studies in human cervical cancer, *Med. Oncol. (Northwood, Lond. Engl.)* 32 (2015) 510.
205. M. Montagnana, M. Benati, E. Danese, S. Giudici, M. Perfranceschi, O. Ruzzenenete, et al., Aberrant MicroRNA expression in patients with endometrial cancer, *Int. J. Gynecol. Cancer Off. J. Int. Gynecol. Cancer Soc.* 27 (2017) 459–466.
206. Y. Wang, S. Adila, X. Zhang, Y. Dong, W. Li, M. Zhou, et al., MicroRNA expression signature profile and its clinical significance in endometrioid carcinoma, *Zhonghua Bing Li Xue Za Zhi* 43 (2014) 88–94.
207. S. Jurcevic, B. Olsson, K. Klinga-Levan, MicroRNA expression in human endometrial adenocarcinoma, *Cancer Cell Int.* 14 (2014) 88.
208. W. Wu, Z. Lin, Z. Zhuang, X. Liang, Expression profile of mammalian microRNAs in endometrioid adenocarcinoma, *Eur. J. Cancer Prev.* 18 (2009) 50–55.
209. A. Torres, K. Torres, A. Pesci, M. Ceccaroni, T. Paszkowski, P. Cassandrini, et al., Diagnostic and prognostic significance of miRNA signatures in tissues and plasma of endometrioid endometrial carcinoma patients, *Int. J. Cancer* 132 (2013) 1633–1645.
210. E.S. Ratner, D. Tuck, C. Richter, S. Nallur, R.M. Patel, V. Schultz, et al., MicroRNA signatures differentiate uterine cancer tumor subtypes, *Gynecol. Oncol.* 118 (2010) 251–257.
211. G. Canlorbe, Z. Wang, E. Laas, S. Bendifallah, M. Castela, M. Lefevre, et al., Identification of microRNA expression profile related to lymph node status in women with early-stage grade 1–2 endometrial cancer, *Mod. Pathol. Off. J. U. S. Can. Acad. Pathol.* 29 (2016) 391–401.
212. M.J. Long, F.X. Wu, P. Li, M. Liu, X. Li, H. Tang, MicroRNA-10a targets CHL1 and promotes cell growth, migration and invasion in human cervical cancer cells, *Cancer Lett.* 324 (2012) 186–196.
213. X.M. Xu, X.B. Wang, M.M. Chen, T. Liu, Y.X. Li, W.H. Jia, et al., MicroRNA-19a and -19b regulate cervical carcinoma cell proliferation and invasion by targeting CUL5, *Cancer Lett.* 322 (2012) 148–158.
214. S. Zhao, D. Yao, J. Chen, N. Ding, F. Ren, MiR-20a promotes cervical cancer proliferation and metastasis in vitro and in vivo, *PLoS one* 10 (2015) e0120905.
215. Y. Sun, X. Yang, M. Liu, H. Tang, B4GALT3 up-regulation by miR-27a contributes to the oncogenic activity in human cervical cancer cells, *Cancer Lett.* 375 (2016) 284–292.

216. C. Zhou, L. Shen, L. Mao, B. Wang, Y. Li, H. Yu, miR-92a is upregulated in cervical cancer and promotes cell proliferation and invasion by targeting FBXW7, *Biochem. Biophys. Res. Commun.* 458 (2015) 63–69.

217. Z. Su, H. Yang, M. Zhao, Y. Wang, G. Deng, R. Chen, MicroRNA-92a promotes cell proliferation in cervical cancer via inhibiting p21 expression and promoting cell cycle progression, *Oncol. Res.* 25 (2017) 137–145.

218. Y. Xu, S. Zhao, M. Cui, Q. Wang, Down-regulation of microRNA-135b inhibited growth of cervical cancer cells by targeting FOXO1, *Int. J. Clin. Exp. Pathol.* 8 (2015) 10294–10304.

219. J. Li, L. Hu, C. Tian, F. Lu, J. Wu, L. Liu, microRNA-150 promotes cervical cancer cell growth and survival by targeting FOXO4, *BMC Mol. Biol.* 16 (2015) 24.

220. G. Lao, P. Liu, Q. Wu, W. Zhang, Y. Liu, L. Yang, et al., Mir-155 promotes cervical cancer cell proliferation through suppression of its target gene LKB1, *Tumour Biol. J. Int. Soc. Oncodev. Biol. Med.* 35 (2014) 11933–11938.

221. L. Yang, Y.L. Wang, S. Liu, P.P. Zhang, Z. Chen, M. Liu, et al., miR-181b promotes cell proliferation and reduces apoptosis by repressing the expression of adenylyl cyclase 9 (AC9) in cervical cancer cells, *FEBS Lett.* 588 (2014) 124–130.

222. J. Zhang, F. Zheng, G. Yu, Y. Yin, Q. Lu, miR-196a targets netrin 4 and regulates cell proliferation and migration of cervical cancer cells, *Biochem. Biophys. Res. Commun.* 440 (2013) 582–588.

223. H. Xie, Y. Zhao, S. Caramuta, C. Larsson, W.O. Lui, miR-205 expression promotes cell proliferation and migration of human cervical cancer cells, *PLoS One* 7 (2012) e46990.

224. Y.K. Yang, W.Y. Xi, R.X. Xi, J.Y. Li, Q. Li, Y.E. Gao, MicroRNA-494 promotes cervical cancer proliferation through the regulation of PTEN, *Oncol. Rep.* 33 (2015) 2393–2401.

225. H. Dang, P. Zheng, Y. Liu, X. Wu, X. Wu, MicroRNA-543 acts as a prognostic marker and promotes the cell proliferation in cervical cancer by BRCA1- interacting protein 1, *Tumour Biol. J. Int. Soc. Oncodevel. Biol. Med.* 39 (2017). doi: 10.1177/1010428317691187.

226. H. Chen, Y. Fan, W. Xu, J. Chen, C. Xu, X. Wei, et al., miR-10b inhibits apoptosis and promotes proliferation and invasion of endometrial cancer cells via targeting HOXB3, *Cancer Biother. Radiopharm.* 31 (2016) 225–231.

227. T. Mitamura, H. Watari, L. Wang, H. Kanno, M. Kitagawa, M.K. Hassan, et al., microRNA 31 functions as an endometrial cancer oncogene by suppressing Hippo tumor suppressor pathway, *Mol. Cancer* 13 (2014) 97.

228. Y. Guo, Y. Liao, C. Jia, J. Ren, J. Wang, T. Li, MicroRNA-182 promotes tumor cell growth by targeting transcription elongation factor A-like 7 in endometrial carcinoma, *Cell. Physiol. Biochem. Int. J. Exp. Cell. Physiol. Biochem. Pharmacol.* 32 (2013) 581–590.

229. E.J. Devor, B.M. Schickling, H.D. Reyes, A. Warrier, B. Lindsay, M.J. Goodheart, et al., Cullin-5, a ubiquitin ligase scaffold protein, is significantly underexpressed in endometrial adenocarcinomas and is a target of miR-182, *Oncol. Rep.* 35 (2016) 2461–2465.

230. G. Zhang, X. Hou, Y. Li, M. Zhao, MiR-205 inhibits cell apoptosis by targeting phosphatase and tensin homolog deleted on chromosome ten in endometrial cancer Ishikawa cells, *BMC Cancer* 14 (2014) 440.

231. B. Liu, Q. Che, H. Qiu, W. Bao, X. Chen, W. Lu, et al., Elevated MiR-222-3p promotes proliferation and invasion of endometrial carcinoma via targeting ERalpha, *PLoS One* 9 (2014) e87563.

232. Z. He, H. Xu, Y. Meng, Y. Kuang, miR-944 acts as a prognostic marker and promotes the tumor progression in endometrial cancer, *Biomed. Pharmacother.* 88 (2017) 902–910.

233. X. Fan, Y. Liu, J. Jiang, Z. Ma, H. Wu, T. Liu, et al., miR-20a promotes proliferation and invasion by targeting APP in human ovarian cancer cells, *Acta Biochim. Biophys. Sin.* 42 (2010) 318–324.

234. H. Zhang, Z. Zuo, X. Lu, L. Wang, H. Wang, Z. Zhu, MiR-25 regulates apoptosis by targeting Bim in human ovarian cancer, *Oncol. Rep.* 27 (2012) 594–598.

235. X. Yang, X. Zhong, J.L. Tanyi, J. Shen, C. Xu, P. Gao, et al., mir-30d regulates multiple genes in the autophagy pathway and impairs autophagy process in human cancer cells, *Biochem. Biophys. Res. Commun.* 431 (2013) 617–622.

236. T. Liang, L. Li, Y. Cheng, C. Ren, G. Zhang, MicroRNA-194 promotes the growth, migration, and invasion of ovarian carcinoma cells by targeting protein tyrosine phosphatase nonreceptor type 12, *OncoTargets Ther.* 9 (2016) 4307–4315.

237. L. Yang, Q.M. Wei, X.W. Zhang, Q. Sheng, X.T. Yan, MiR-376a promotion of proliferation and metastases in ovarian cancer: potential role as a biomarker, *Life Sci.* 173 (2017) 62–67.

238. X. Zhang, J. Liu, D. Zang, S. Wu, A. Liu, J. Zhu, et al., Upregulation of miR-572 transcriptionally suppresses SOCS1 and p21 and contributes to human ovarian cancer progression, *Oncotarget* 6 (2015) 15180–15193.

239. A.H. Wu, Y.L. Huang, L.Z. Zhang, G. Tian, Q.Z. Liao, S.L. Chen, MiR-572 prompted cell proliferation of human ovarian cancer cells by suppressing PPP2R2C expression, *Biomed. Pharmacother.* 77 (2016) 92–97.

240. X. Ying, Q. Li-ya, Z. Feng, W. Yin, L. Ji-hong, MiR-939 promotes the proliferation of human ovarian cancer cells by repressing APC2 expression, *Biomed. Pharmacother.* 71 (2015) 64–69.

241. S. Liu, P. Zhang, Z. Chen, M. Liu, X. Li, H. Tang, MicroRNA-7 downregulates XIAP expression to suppress cell growth and promote apoptosis in cervical cancer cells, *FEBS Lett.* 587 (2013) 2247–2253.

242. Q. Wei, Y.X. Li, M. Liu, X. Li, H. Tang, MiR-17-5p targets TP53INP1 and regulates cell proliferation and apoptosis of cervical cancer cells, *IUBMB Life* 64 (2012) 697–704.

243. J.H. Wang, L. Zhang, Y.W. Ma, J. Xiao, Y. Zhang, M. Liu, et al., microRNA-34upregulated retinoic acid-inducible gene-I promotes apoptosis and delays cell cycle transition in cervical cancer cells, *DNA Cell Biol.* 35 (2016) 267–279.

244. K.S. Chandrasekaran, A. Sathyanarayanan, D. Karunagaran, Downregulation of HMGB1 by miR-34a is sufficient to suppress proliferation, migration and invasion of human cervical and colorectal cancer cells, *Tumour Biol. J. Int. Soc. Oncodevel. Biol. Med.* 37 (2016) 13155–13166.

245. F. Huang, C. Lin, Y.H. Shi, G. Kuerban, MicroRNA-101 inhibits cell proliferation, invasion, and promotes apoptosis by regulating cyclooxygenase-2 in Hela cervical carcinoma cells, *Asian Pac. J. Cancer Prev.* 14 (2013) 5915–5920.

246. C. Zhou, G. Li, J. Zhou, N. Han, Z. Liu, J. Yin, miR-107 activates ATR/Chk1 pathway and suppress cervical cancer invasion by targeting MCL1, *PLoS One* 9 (2014) e111860.

247. Z. Fan, H. Cui, X. Xu, Z. Lin, X. Zhang, L. Kang, et al., MiR-125a suppresses tumor growth, invasion and metastasis in cervical cancer by targeting STAT3, *Oncotarget* 6 (2015) 25266–25280.

248. X. Qin, Y. Wan, S. Wang, M. Xue, MicroRNA-125a-5p modulates human cervical carcinoma proliferation and migration by targeting ABL2, *Drug Des. Devel. Ther.* 10 (2016) 71–79.

249. F. Cui, X. Li, X. Zhu, L. Huang, Y. Huang, C. Mao, et al., MiR-125b inhibits tumor growth and promotes apoptosis of cervical cancer cells by targeting phosphoinositide 3-kinase catalytic subunit delta, *Cell. Physiol. Biochem. Int. J. Exp. Cell. Physiol. Biochem. Pharmacol.* 30 (2012) 1310–1318.

250. X. Song, B. Shi, K. Huang, W. Zhang, miR-133a inhibits cervical cancer growth by targeting EGFR, *Oncol. Rep.* 34 (2015) 1573–1580.

251. B. Li, X.X. Yang, D. Wang, H.K. Ji, MicroRNA-138 inhibits proliferation of cervical cancer cells by targeting c-Met, *Eur. Rev. Med. Pharmacol. Sci.* 20 (2016) 1109–1114.

252. N. Zhou, D. Fei, S. Zong, M. Zhang, Y. Yue, MicroRNA-138 inhibits proliferation, migration and invasion through targeting hTERT in cervical cancer, *Oncol. Lett.* 12 (2016) 3633–3639.

253. B. Deng, Y. Zhang, S. Zhang, F. Wen, Y. Miao, K. Guo, MicroRNA-142-3p inhibits cell proliferation and invasion of cervical cancer cells by targeting FZD7, *Tumour Biol. J. Int. Soc. Oncodevel. Biol. Med.* 36 (2015) 8065–8073.

254. L. Liu, X. Yu, X. Guo, Z. Tian, M. Su, Y. Long, et al., miR-143 is downregulated in cervical cancer and promotes apoptosis and inhibits tumor formation by targeting Bcl-2, *Mol. Med. Rep.* 5 (2012) 753–760.

255. C. Luo, J. Qiu, MiR-181a inhibits cervical cancer development via downregulating GRP78, *Oncol. Res.* (2017).

256. N. Wang, H. Wei, D. Yin, Y. Lu, Y. Zhang, Q. Zhang, et al., MicroRNA-195 inhibits proliferation of cervical cancer cells by targeting cyclin D1a, *Tumour Biol. J. Int. Soc. Oncodevel. Biol. Med.* 37 (2016) 4711–4720.

257. X. Du, L.I. Lin, L. Zhang, J. Jiang, microRNA-195 inhibits the proliferation, migration and invasion of cervical cancer cells via the inhibition of CCND2 and MYB expression, *Oncol. Lett.* 10 (2015) 2639–2643.

258. Z. Li, H. Wang, Z. Wang, H. Cai, MiR-195 inhibits the proliferation of human cervical cancer cells by directly targeting cyclin D1, *Tumour Biol. J. Int. Soc. Oncodevel. Biol. Med.* 37 (2016) 6457–6463.

259. X. Zhu, K. Er, C. Mao, Q. Yan, H. Xu, Y. Zhang, et al., miR-203 suppresses tumor growth and angiogenesis by targeting VEGFA in cervical cancer, *Cell. Physiol. Biochem. Int. J. Exp. Cell. Physiol. Biochem. Pharmacol.* 32 (2013) 64–73.

260. R.Q. Peng, H.Y. Wan, H.F. Li, M. Liu, X. Li, H. Tang, MicroRNA-214 suppresses growth and invasiveness of cervical cancer cells by targeting UDP-N-acetylalpha-D-galactosamine: polypeptide N-acetylgalactosaminyltransferase 7, *J. Biol. Chem.* 287 (2012) 14301–14309.

261. L. Wu, H. Li, C.Y. Jia, W. Cheng, M. Yu, M. Peng, et al., MicroRNA-223 regulates FOXO1 expression and cell proliferation, *FEBS Lett.* 586 (2012) 1038–1043.

262. X. Wang, Y. Xia, microRNA-328 inhibits cervical cancer cell proliferation and tumorigenesis by targeting TCF7L2, *Biochem. Biophys. Res. Commun.* 475 (2016) 169–175.

263. T. Fujii, K. Shimada, A. Asano, Y. Tatsumi, N. Yamaguchi, M. Yamazaki, et al., MicroRNA-331-3p suppresses cervical cancer cell proliferation and E6/E7 expression by targeting NRP2, *Int. J. Mol. Sci.* 17 (8) (2016) 1351. doi:10.3390/ijms17081351.

264. X.R. Li, H.J. Chu, T. Lv, L. Wang, S.F. Kong, S.Z. Dai, miR-342–3p suppresses proliferation, migration and invasion by targeting FOXM1 in human cervical cancer, *FEBS Lett.* 588 (2014) 3298–3307.

265. C. Shi, Z. Zhang, MicroRNA-362 is downregulated in cervical cancer and inhibits cell proliferation, migration and invasion by directly targeting SIX1, *Oncol. Rep.* 37 (2017) 501–509.

266. R.Q. Tian, X.H. Wang, L.J. Hou, W.H. Jia, Q. Yang, Y.X. Li, et al., MicroRNA-372 is down-regulated and targets cyclin-dependent kinase 2 (CDK2) and cyclin A1 in human cervical cancer, which may contribute to tumorigenesis, *J. Biol. Chem.* 286 (2011) 25556–25563.

267. Y. Deng, Y. Xiong, Y. Liu, miR-376c inhibits cervical cancer cell proliferation and invasion by targeting BMI1, *Int. J. Exp. Pathol.* 97 (2016) 257–265.

268. X.J. Lai, X.Y. Cheng, L.D. Hu, microRNA 421 induces apoptosis of c-33a cervical cancer cells via down-regulation of Bcl-xL, *Genet. Mol. Res.* 15 (2016) gmr15048853. doi: http://dx.doi.org/10.4238/gmr15048853.

269. H. Ye, X. Yu, J. Xia, X. Tang, L. Tang, F. Chen, MiR-486-3p targeting ECM1 represses cell proliferation and metastasis in cervical cancer, *Biomed. Pharmacother.* 80 (2016) 109–114.

270. J. Cong, R. Liu, X. Wang, H. Jiang, Y. Zhang, MiR-634 decreases cell proliferation and induces apoptosis by targeting mTOR signaling pathway in cervical cancer cells, *Artif. Cells Nanomed. Biotechnol.* 44 (2016) 1694–1701.

271. X.F. Chen, Y. Liu, MicroRNA-744 inhibited cervical cancer growth and progression through apoptosis induction by regulating Bcl-2, *Biomed. Pharmacother.* 81 (2016) 379–387.

272. P. Liu, M. Qi, C. Ma, G. Lao, Y. Liu, Y. Liu, et al., Let7a inhibits the growth of endometrial carcinoma cells by targeting aurora-B, *FEBS Lett.* 587 (2013) 2523–2529.

273. E. Hiroki, F. Suzuki, J. Akahira, S. Nagase, K. Ito, J. Sugawara, et al., MicroRNA-34b functions as a potential tumor suppressor in endometrial serous adenocarcinoma, *Int. J. Cancer* 131 (2012) E395–E404.

274. Y. Konno, P. Dong, Y. Xiong, F. Suzuki, J. Lu, M. Cai, et al., MicroRNA-101 targets EZH2, MCL-1 and FOS to suppress proliferation, invasion and stem cell-like phenotype of aggressive endometrial cancer cells, *Oncotarget* 5 (2014) 6049–6062.

275. C. Shang, Y.M. Lu, L.R. Meng, MicroRNA-125b down-regulation mediates endometrial cancer invasion by targeting ERBB2, *Med. Sci. Monit. Int. Med. J. Exp. Clin. Res.* 18 (2012) r149–155.

276. W. Xie, W. Qin, Y. Kang, Z. Zhou, A. Qin, MicroRNA-340 inhibits tumor cell proliferation and induces apoptosis in endometrial carcinoma cell line RL 95-2, *Med. Sci. Monit. Int. Med. J. Exp. Clin. Res.* 22 (2016) 1540–1546.

277. B.L. Liu, K.X. Sun, Z.H. Zong, S. Chen, Y. Zhao, MicroRNA-372 inhibits endometrial carcinoma development by targeting the expression of the Ras homolog gene family member C (RhoC), *Oncotarget* 7 (2016) 6649–6664.

278. W. Ye, J. Xue, Q. Zhang, F. Li, W. Zhang, H. Chen, et al., MiR-449a functions as a tumor suppressor in endometrial cancer by targeting CDC25A, *Oncol. Rep.* 32 (2014) 1193–1199.

279. K.X. Sun, Y. Chen, S. Chen, B.L. Liu, M.X. Feng, Z.H. Zong, et al., The correlation between microRNA490–3p and TGFalpha in endometrial carcinoma tumorigenesis and progression, *Oncotarget* 7 (2016) 9236–9249.

280. Y.Y. Xu, J. Tian, Q. Hao, L.R. Yin, MicroRNA-495 down-regulates FOXC1 expression to suppress cell growth and migration in endometrial cancer, *Tumour Biol. J. Int. Soc. Oncodevel. Biol. Med.* 37 (2016) 239–251.

281. W. Li, Z. Liu, L. Chen, L. Zhou, Y. Yao, MicroRNA-23b is an independent prognostic marker and suppresses ovarian cancer progression by targeting runt-related transcription factor-2, *FEBS Lett.* 588 (2014) 1608–1615.

282. J. Yan, J.Y. Jiang, X.N. Meng, Y.L. Xiu, Z.H. Zong, MiR-23b targets cyclin G1 and suppresses ovarian cancer tumorigenesis and progression, *J. Exp. Clin. Cancer Res. CR* 35 (2016) 31.

283. J. Lin, L. Zhang, H. Huang, Y. Huang, L. Huang, J. Wang, et al., MiR-26b/KPNA2 axis inhibits epithelial ovarian carcinoma proliferation and metastasis through downregulating OCT4, *Oncotarget* 6 (2015) 23793–23806.

284. H. Jiang, L. Qu, Y. Wang, J. Cong, W. Wang, X. Yang, miR-99a promotes proliferation targeting FGFR3 in human epithelial ovarian cancer cells, *Biomed. Pharmacother.* 68 (2014) 163–169.

285. A. Semaan, A.M. Qazi, S. Seward, S. Chamala, C.S. Bryant, S. Kumar, et al., MicroRNA-101 inhibits growth of epithelial ovarian cancer by relieving chromatin-mediated transcriptional repression of p21(waf(1)/cip(1)), *Pharm. Res.* 28 (2011) 3079–3090.

286. H.B. Zheng, X.G. Zheng, B.P. Liu, miRNA-101 inhibits ovarian cancer cells proliferation and invasion by downregulating expression of SOCS-2, *Int. J. Clin. Exp. Med.* 8 (2015) 20263–20270.

287. J. Yang, G. Li, K. Zhang, MiR-125a regulates ovarian cancer proliferation and invasion by repressing GALNT14 expression, *Biomed. Pharmacother.* 80 (2016) 381–387.

288. Y. Guan, H. Yao, Z. Zheng, G. Qiu, K. Sun, MiR-125b targets BCL3 and suppresses ovarian cancer proliferation, *Int. J. Cancer* 128 (2011) 2274–2283.

289. M. Lee, E.J. Kim, M.J. Jeon, MicroRNAs 125a and 125b inhibit ovarian cancer cells through post-transcriptional inactivation of EIF4EBP1, *Oncotarget* 7 (2016) 8726–8742.

290. L. Bi, Q. Yang, J. Yuan, Q. Miao, L. Duan, F. Li, et al., MicroRNA-127-3p acts as a tumor suppressor in epithelial ovarian cancer by regulating the BAG5 gene, *Oncol. Rep.* 36 (2016) 2563–2570.

291. G. Tan, X. Cao, Q. Dai, B. Zhang, J. Huang, S. Xiong, et al., A novel role for microRNA-129-5p in inhibiting ovarian cancer cell proliferation and survival via direct suppression of transcriptional co-activators YAP and TAZ, *Oncotarget* 6 (2015) 8676–8686.

292. J. Guo, B. Xia, F. Meng, G. Lou, miR-133a suppresses ovarian cancer cell proliferation by directly targeting insulin-like growth factor 1 receptor, *Tumour Biol. J. Int. Soc. Oncodevel. Biol. Med.* 35 (2014) 1557–1564.

293. X. Liu, G. Li, MicroRNA-133b inhibits proliferation and invasion of ovarian cancer cells through Akt and Erk1/2 inactivation by targeting epidermal growth factor receptor, *Int. J. Clin. Exp. Pathol.* 8 (2015) 10605–10614.

294. W. Tang, Y. Jiang, X. Mu, L. Xu, W. Cheng, X. Wang, MiR-135a functions as a tumor suppressor in epithelial ovarian cancer and regulates HOXA10 expression, *Cell. Signal.* 26 (2014) 1420–1426.

295. J. Guo, B. Xia, F. Meng, G. Lou, miR-137 suppresses cell growth in ovarian cancer by targeting AEG-1, *Biochem. Biophys. Res. Commun.* 441 (2013) 357–363.

296. L. Zhang, Z. Li, F. Gai, Y. Wang, MicroRNA-137 suppresses tumor growth in epithelial ovarian cancer in vitro and in vivo, *Mol. Med. Rep.* 12 (2015) 3107–3114.

297. X. Li, W. Chen, W. Zeng, C. Wan, S. Duan, S. Jiang, microRNA-137 promotes apoptosis in ovarian cancer cells via the regulation of XIAP, *Br. J. Cancer* 116 (2017) 66–76.

298. H. Lan, W. Chen, G. He, S. Yang, miR-140-5p inhibits ovarian cancer growth partially by repression of PDGFRA, *Biomed. Pharmacother.* 75 (2015) 117–122.

299. L. Wang, J. He, H. Xu, L. Xu, N. Li, MiR-143 targets CTGF and exerts tumor suppressing functions in epithelial ovarian cancer, *Am. J. Transl. Res.* 8 (2016) 2716–2726.

300. Q. Xu, L.Z. Liu, X. Qian, Q. Chen, Y. Jiang, D. Li, et al., MiR-145 directly targets p70S6K1 in cancer cells to inhibit tumor growth and angiogenesis, *Nucleic Acids Res.* 40 (2012) 761–774.

301. H. Wu, Z. Xiao, K. Wang, W. Liu, Q. Hao, MiR-145 is downregulated in human ovarian cancer and modulates cell growth and invasion by targeting p70S6K1 and MUC1, *Biochem. Biophys. Res. Commun.* 441 (2013) 693–700.

302. X. Chen, C. Dong, P.T. Law, M.T. Chan, Z. Su, S. Wang, et al., MicroRNA-145 targets TRIM2 and exerts tumor-suppressing functions in epithelial ovarian cancer, *Gynecol. Oncol.* 139 (2015) 513–519.

303. Y. Cui, K. She, D. Tian, P. Zhang, X. Xin, miR-146a inhibits proliferation and enhances chemosensitivity in epithelial ovarian cancer via reduction of SOD2, *Oncol. Res.* 23 (2016) 275–282.

304. X. Zhou, F. Zhao, Z.N. Wang, Y.X. Song, H. Chang, Y. Chiang, et al., Altered expression of miR-152 and miR-148a in ovarian cancer is related to cell proliferation, *Oncol. Rep.* 27 (2012) 447–454.

305. S. Zhao, Z. Wen, S. Liu, Y. Liu, X. Li, Y. Ge, et al., MicroRNA-148a inhibits the proliferation and promotes the paclitaxel-induced apoptosis of ovarian cancer cells by targeting PDIA3, *Mol. Med. Rep.* 12 (2015) 3923–3929.

306. M. Zhao, Z. Su, S. Zhang, L. Zhuang, Y. Xie, X. Li, Suppressive role of microRNA-148a in cell proliferation and invasion in ovarian cancer through targeting transforming growth factor-beta-induced 2, *Oncol. Res.* 24 (2016) 353–360.

307. J.S. Imam, K. Buddavarapu, J.S. Lee-Chang, S. Ganapathy, C. Camosy, Y. Chen, et al., MicroRNA-185 suppresses tumor growth and progression by targeting the Six1 oncogene in human cancers, *Oncogene* 29 (2010) 4971–4979.

308. H. Nakano, Y. Yamada, T. Miyazawa, T. Yoshida, Gain-of-function microRNA screens identify miR-193a regulating proliferation and apoptosis in epithelial ovarian cancer cells, *Int. J. Oncol.* 42 (2013) 1875–1882.

309. F.F. Ibrahim, R. Jamal, S.E. Syafruddin, N.S. Ab Mutalib, S. Saidin, R.R. MdZin, et al., MicroRNA-200c and microRNA-31 regulate proliferation, colony formation, migration and invasion in serous ovarian cancer, *J. Ovarian Res.* 8 (2015) 56.

310. S. Li, Y. Li, Z. Wen, F. Kong, X. Guan, W. Liu, microRNA-206 overexpression inhibits cellular proliferation and invasion of estrogen receptor alphapositive ovarian cancer cells, *Mol. Med. Rep.* 9 (2014) 1703–1708.

311. B. Xia, S. Yang, T. Liu, G. Lou, miR-211 suppresses epithelial ovarian cancer proliferation and cell-cycle progression by targeting cyclin D1 and CDK6, *Mol. Cancer* 14 (2015) 57.

312. Q. Wu, X. Ren, Y. Zhang, X. Fu, Y. Li, Y. Peng, et al., MiR-221-3p targets ARF4 and inhibits the proliferation and migration of epithelial ovarian cancer cells, Biochem. *Biophys. Res. Commun.* 497(4) (2017) 1162–1170. doi: 10.1016/j.bbrc.2017.01.002.

313. T. Guo, W. Yu, S. Lv, C. Zhang, Y. Tian, MiR-302a inhibits the tumorigenicity of ovarian cancer cells by suppression of SDC1, *Int. J. Clin. Exp. Pathol.* 8 (2015) 4869–4880.

314. T. Ge, M. Yin, M. Yang, T. Liu, G. Lou, MicroRNA-302b suppresses human epithelial ovarian cancer cell growth by targeting RUNX1, *Cell. Physiol. Biochem. Int. J. Exp. Cell. Physiol. Biochem. Pharmacol.* 34 (2014) 2209–2220.

315. C. Wen, X. Liu, H. Ma, W. Zhang, H. Li, miR3383p suppresses tumor growth of ovarian epithelial carcinoma by targeting Runx2, *Int. J. Oncol.* 46 (2015) 2277–2285.

316. Y. Jin, M. Zhao, Q. Xie, H. Zhang, Q. Wang, Q. Ma, MicroRNA-338-3p functions as tumor suppressor in breast cancer by targeting SOX4, *Int. J. Oncol.* 47 (2015) 1594–1602.

317. J. Liu, Y. Dou, M. Sheng, Inhibition of microRNA-383 has tumor suppressive effect in human epithelial ovarian cancer through the action on caspase-2 gene, *Biomed. Pharmacother.* 83 (2016) 1286–1294.

318. R.L. Han, F.P. Wang, P.A. Zhang, X.Y. Zhou, Y. Li, miR-383 inhibits ovarian cancer cell proliferation, invasion and aerobic glycolysis by targeting LDHA, *Neoplasma* 64 (2) (2017) 244–252. doi: 10.4149/neo_2017_211.

319. Y. Lv, Y. Lei, Y. Hu, W. Ding, C. Zhang, C. Fang, miR-448 negatively regulates ovarian cancer cell growth and metastasis by targeting CXCL12, *Clin. Transl. Oncol. Off. Publ. Fed. Span. Oncol. Soc. Natl. Cancer Inst. Mexico* 17 (2015) 903–909.

320. S. Chen, X. Chen, Y.L. Xiu, K.X. Sun, Y. Zhao, MicroRNA-490–3P targets CDK1 and inhibits ovarian epithelial carcinoma tumorigenesis and progression, *Cancer Lett.* 362 (2015) 122–130.

321. J. Yuan, K. Wang, M. Xi, MiR-494 inhibits epithelial ovarian cancer growth by targeting c-Myc, *Med. Sci. Monit. Int. Med. J. Exp. Clin. Res.* 22 (2016) 617–624.

322. X. Zhao, Y. Zhou, Y.U. Chen, F. Yu, miR-494 inhibits ovarian cancer cell proliferation and promotes apoptosis by targeting FGFR2, *Oncol. Lett.* 11 (2016) 4245–4251.

323. Z. Lin, J. Zhao, X. Wang, X. Zhu, L. Gong, Overexpression of microRNA-497 suppresses cell proliferation and induces apoptosis through targeting paired box 2 in human ovarian cancer, *Oncol. Rep.* 36 (2016) 2101–2107.

324. R. Liu, F. Liu, L. Li, M. Sun, K. Chen, MiR-498 regulated FOXO3 expression and inhibited the proliferation of human ovarian cancer cells, *Biomed. Pharmacother.* 72 (2015) 52–57.

325. G. Liu, Y. Sun, P. Ji, X. Li, D. Cogdell, D. Yang, et al., MiR-506 suppresses proliferation and induces senescence by directly targeting the CDK4/6-FOXM1 axis in ovarian cancer, *J. Pathol.* 233 (2014) 308–318.

326. Y. Pang, H. Mao, L. Shen, Z. Zhao, R. Liu, P. Liu, MiR-519d represses ovarian cancer cell proliferation and enhances cisplatin-mediated cytotoxicity in vitro by targeting XIAP, *OncoTargets Ther.* 7 (2014) 587–597.

327. C. Shi, Z. Zhang, miR-761 inhibits tumor progression by targeting MSI1 in ovarian carcinoma, *Tumour Biol. J. Int. Soc. Oncodevel. Biol. Med.* 37 (2016) 5437–5443.

328. M.S. Greenblatt, W.P. Bennett, M. Hollstein, C.C. Harris, Mutations in the p53 tumor suppressor gene: clues to cancer etiology and molecular pathogenesis, *Cancer Res.* 54 (1994) 4855–4878.

329. D.C. Corney, A. Flesken-Nikitin, A.K. Godwin, W. Wang, A.Y. Nikitin, Micro- RNA-34b and MicroRNA-34c are targets of p53 and cooperate in control of cell proliferation and adhesion-independent growth, *Cancer Res.* 67 (2007) 8433–8438.

330. C.J. Creighton, M.D. Fountain, Z. Yu, A.K. Nagaraja, H. Zhu, M. Khan, et al., Molecular profiling uncovers a p53-associated role for microRNA-31 in inhibiting the proliferation of serous ovarian carcinomas and other cancers, *Cancer Res.* 70 (2010) 1906–1915.

331. R. Li, X. Shi, F. Ling, C. Wang, J. Liu, W. Wang, et al., MiR-34a suppresses ovarian cancer proliferation and motility by targeting AXL, *Tumour Biol. J. Int. Soc. Oncodevel. Biol. Med.* 36 (2015) 7277–7283.

332. M.S. Song, L. Salmena, P.P. Pandolfi, The functions and regulation of the PTEN tumour suppressor, *Nat. Rev. Mol. Cell Biol.* 13 (2012) 283–296.

333. J. Xu, W. Zhang, Q. Lv, D. Zhu, Overexpression of miR-21 promotes the proliferation and migration of cervical cancer cells via the inhibition of PTEN, *Oncol. Rep.* 33 (2015) 3108–3116.

334. O. Peralta-Zaragoza, J. Deas, A. Meneses-Acosta, O.G.F. De la, G. Fernandez-Tilapa, C. Gomez-Ceron, et al., Relevance of miR-21 in regulation of tumor suppressor gene PTEN in human cervical cancer cells, *BMC Cancer* 16 (2016) 215.

335. Y. Feng, S. Zhou, G. Li, C. Hu, W. Zou, H. Zhang, et al., Nuclear factor-kappaBdependent microRNA-130a upregulation promotes cervical cancer cell growth by targeting phosphatase and tensin homolog, *Arch. Biochem. Biophys.* 598 (2016) 57–65.

336. Y. Sun, B. Zhang, J. Cheng, Y. Wu, F. Xing, Y. Wang, et al., MicroRNA-222 promotes the proliferation and migration of cervical cancer cells, *Clin. Invest. Med. Med. Clin. Exp.* 37 (2014) E131.

337. R. Li, J.L. He, X.M. Chen, C.L. Long, D.H. Yang, Y.B. Ding, et al., MiR-200a is involved in proliferation and apoptosis in the human endometrial adenocarcinoma cell line HEC-1B by targeting the tumor suppressor PTEN, *Mol. Biol. Rep.* 41 (2014) 1977–1984.

338. K. Yoneyama, O. Ishibashi, R. Kawase, K. Kurose, T. Takeshita, miR-200a, miR-200b and miR-429 are oncomiRs that target the PTEN gene in endometrioid endometrial carcinoma, *Anticancer Res.* 35 (2015) 1401–1410.

339. W. Xin, X. Liu, J. Ding, J. Zhao, Y. Zhou, Q. Wu, et al., Long non-coding RNA derived miR-205-5p modulates human endometrial cancer by targeting PTEN, *Am. J. Transl. Res.* 7 (2015) 2433–2441.

340. Y. Lou, X. Yang, F. Wang, Z. Cui, Y. Huang, MicroRNA-21 promotes the cell proliferation, invasion and migration abilities in ovarian epithelial carcinomas through inhibiting the expression of PTEN protein, *Int. J. Mol. Med.* 26 (2010) 819–827.

341. L. Chen, F. Zhang, X.G. Sheng, S.Q. Zhang, Y.T. Chen, B.W. Liu, MicroRNA-106a regulates phosphatase and tensin homologue expression and promotes the proliferation and invasion of ovarian cancer cells, *Oncol. Rep.* 36 (2016) 2135–2141.

342. J. Li, K. Hu, G. Gong, D. Zhu, Y. Wang, H. Liu, et al., Upregulation of MiR-205 transcriptionally suppresses SMAD4 and PTEN and contributes to human ovarian cancer progression, *Sci. Rep.* 7 (2017) 41330.

343. H. Yang, W. Kong, L. He, J.J. Zhao, J.D. O'Donnell, J. Wang, et al., MicroRNA expression profiling in human ovarian cancer: miR-214 induces cell survival and cisplatin resistance by targeting PTEN, *Cancer Res.* 68 (2008) 425–433.

344. Y.T. Zou, J.Y. Gao, H.L. Wang, Y. Wang, H. Wang, P.L. Li, Downregulation of microRNA-630 inhibits cell proliferation and invasion and enhances chemosensitivity in human ovarian carcinoma, *Genet. Mol. Res.* 14 (2015) 8766–8777.

345. Y. Lou, Z. Cui, F. Wang, X. Yang, J. Qian, miR-21 downregulation promotes apoptosis and inhibits invasion and migration abilities of OVCAR3 cells, *Clin. Invest. Med. Med. Clin. Exp.* 34 (2011) E281.

346. Q. Yao, H. Xu, Q.Q. Zhang, H. Zhou, L.H. Qu, MicroRNA-21 promotes cell proliferation and down-regulates the expression of programmed cell death 4 (PDCD4) in HeLa cervical carcinoma cells, *Biochem. Biophys. Res. Commun.* 388 (2009) 539–542.

347. L.M. Guo, Y. Pu, Z. Han, T. Liu, Y.X. Li, M. Liu, et al., MicroRNA-9 inhibits ovarian cancer cell growth through regulation of NF-kappaB1, *FEBS J.* 276 (2009) 5537–5546.

348. T. Shuang, M. Wang, Y. Zhou, C. Shi, D. Wang, NF-kappaB1, c-Rel, and ELK1 inhibit miR-134 expression leading to TAB1 upregulation in paclitaxel resistant human ovarian cancer, *Oncotarget* 8 (2017) 24853–24868.

349. J.Y. Fan, Y.J. Fan, X.L. Wang, H. Xie, H.J. Gao, Y. Zhang, et al., miR-429 is involved in regulation of NF-kappaBactivity by targeting IKK beta and suppresses oncogenic activity in cervical cancer cells, *FEBS Lett.* 591 (2017) 118–128.

350. C. Denoyelle, B. Lambert, M. Meryet-Figuiere, N. Vigneron, E. Brotin, C. Lecerf, et al., miR-491–5p-induced apoptosis in ovarian carcinoma depends on the direct inhibition of both BCL-XL and EGFR leading to BIM activation, *Cell Death Dis.* 5 (2014)–1445.

351. R. Bhattacharya, M. Nicoloso, R. Arvizo, E. Wang, A. Cortez, S. Rossi, et al., MiR-15a and MiR-16 control Bmi-1 expression in ovarian cancer, *Cancer Res.* 69 (2009) 9090–9095.

352. H. Clevers, Cancer therapy: defining stemness, *Nature* 534 (2016) 2.

353. M.W. Chen, S.T. Yang, M.H. Chien, K.T. Hua, C.J. Wu, S.M. Hsiao, et al., The STAT3-miRNA-92-Wnt signaling pathway regulates spheroid formation and malignant progression in ovarian cancer, *Cancer Res.* 77 (2017) 1955–1967.

354. G. Wu, A. Liu, J. Zhu, F. Lei, S. Wu, X. Zhang, et al., MiR-1207 overexpression promotes cancer stem cell-like traits in ovarian cancer by activating the Wnt/beta-catenin signaling pathway, *Oncotarget* 6 (2015) 28882–28894.

355. P. Dong, Y. Xiong, H. Watari, S.J. Hanley, Y. Konno, K. Ihira, et al., MiR-137 and miR-34a directly target Snail and inhibit EMT, invasion and sphere-forming ability of ovarian cancer cells, *J. Exp. Clin. Cancer Res. CR* 35 (2016) 132.

356. Q. Wu, R. Guo, M. Lin, B. Zhou, Y. Wang, MicroRNA-200a inhibits CD133/1+ ovarian cancer stem cells migration and invasion by targeting E-cadherin repressor ZEB2, *Gynecol. Oncol.* 122 (2011) 149–154.

357. D. Chen, Y. Zhang, J. Wang, J. Chen, C. Yang, K. Cai, et al., MicroRNA-200c overexpression inhibits tumorigenicity and metastasis of CD117+CD44+ ovarian cancer stem cells by regulating epithelial-mesenchymal transition, *J. Ovarian Res.* 6 (2013) 50.

358. T. Liu, L. Hou, Y. Huang, EZH2-specific microRNA-98 inhibits human ovarian cancer stem cell proliferation via regulating the pRb-E2F pathway, *Tumour Biol. J. Int. Soc. Oncodevel. Biol. Med.* 35 (2014) 7239–7247.

359. C. Chang, T. Liu, Y. Huang, W. Qin, H. Yang, J. Chen, MicroRNA-134-3p is a novel potential inhibitor of human ovarian cancer stem cells by targeting RAB27A, *Gene* 605 (2017) 99–107.

360. Y. Gao, T. Liu, Y. Huang, MicroRNA-134 suppresses endometrial cancer stem cells by targeting POGLUT1 and Notch pathway proteins, *FEBS Lett.* 589 (2015) 207–214.

361. J.Y. Jeong, H. Kang, T.H. Kim, G. Kim, J.H. Heo, A.Y. Kwon, et al., MicroRNA-136 inhibits cancer stem cell activity and enhances the anti-tumor effect of paclitaxel against chemoresistant ovarian cancer cells by targeting Notch3, *Cancer Lett.* 386 (2017) 168–178.

362. Z. Liu, E. Gersbach, X. Zhang, X. Xu, R. Dong, P. Lee, et al., miR-106a represses the Rb tumor suppressor p130 to regulate cellular proliferation and differentiation in high-grade serous ovarian carcinoma, *Mol. Cancer Res.* 11 (2013) 1314–1325.

363. X. Zhao, D. Zhu, C. Lu, D. Yan, L. Li, Z. Chen, MicroRNA-126 inhibits the migration and invasion of endometrial cancer cells by targeting insulin receptor substrate 1, *Oncol. Lett.* 11 (2016) 1207–1212.

364. U. Schirmer, K. Doberstein, A.K. Rupp, N.P. Bretz, D. Wuttig, H. Kiefel, et al., Role of miR-34a as a suppressor of L1CAM in endometrial carcinoma, *Oncotarget* 5 (2014) 462–472.

365. R.T. Pang, C.O. Leung, T.M. Ye, W. Liu, P.C. Chiu, K.K. Lam, et al., MicroRNA-34a suppresses invasion through downregulation of Notch1 and Jagged1 in cervical carcinoma and choriocarcinoma cells, *Carcinogenesis* 31 (2010) 1037–1044.

366. N. Yamamoto, T. Kinoshita, N. Nohata, T. Itesako, H. Yoshino, H. Enokida, et al., Tumor suppressive microRNA-218 inhibits cancer cell migration and invasion by targeting focal adhesion pathways in cervical squamous cell carcinoma, *Int. J. Oncol.* 42 (2013) 1523–1532.

367. R. Kogo, C. How, N. Chaudary, J. Bruce, W. Shi, R.P. Hill, et al., The microRNA-218~Survivin axis regulates migration, invasion, and lymph node metastasis in cervical cancer, *Oncotarget* 6 (2015) 1090–1100.

368. D. Fan, Y. Wang, P. Qi, Y. Chen, P. Xu, X. Yang, et al., MicroRNA-183 functions as the tumor suppressor via inhibiting cellular invasion and metastasis by targeting MMP-9 in cervical cancer, *Gynecol. Oncol.* 141 (2016) 166–174.

369. F. Wang, Y. Li, J. Zhou, J. Xu, C. Peng, F. Ye, et al., miR-375 is down-regulated in squamous cervical cancer and inhibits cell migration and invasion via targeting transcription factor SP1, *Am. J. Pathol.* 179 (2011) 2580–2588.

370. N. Su, H. Qiu, Y. Chen, T. Yang, Q. Yan, X. Wan, miR-205 promotes tumor proliferation and invasion through targeting ESRRG in endometrial carcinoma, *Oncol. Rep.* 29 (2013) 2297e2302.

371. J. Guo, J. Lv, M. Liu, H. Tang, miR-346 up-regulates argonaute 2 (AGO2) protein expression to augment the activity of other MicroRNAs (miRNAs) and contributes to cervical cancer cell malignancy, *J. Biol. Chem.* 290 (2015) 30342–30350.

372. Y. Fang, C. Xu, Y. Fu, MicroRNA-17-5p induces drug resistance and invasion of ovarian carcinoma cells by targeting PTEN signaling, *J. Biol. Res. (Thessalonike, Greece)* 22 (2015) 12.

373. Y.Q. Wang, R.D. Guo, R.M. Guo, W. Sheng, L.R. Yin, MicroRNA-182 promotes cell growth, invasion, and chemoresistance by targeting programmed cell death 4 (PDCD4) in human ovarian carcinomas, *J. Cell. Biochem.* 114 (2013) 1464–1473.

374. H. Zhang, Q. Wang, Q. Zhao, W. Di, miR-124 inhibits the migration and invasion of ovarian cancer cells by targeting SphK1, *J. Ovarian. Res.* 6 (2013) 84.

375. J. Cao, J. Cai, D. Huang, Q. Han, Q. Yang, T. Li, et al., miR-335 represents an invasion suppressor gene in ovarian cancer by targeting Bcl-w, *Oncol. Rep.* 30 (2013) 701–706.

376. W. Shan, J. Li, Y. Bai, X. Lu, miR-339-5p inhibits migration and invasion in ovarian cancer cell lines by targeting NACC1 and BCL6, *Tumour Biol. J. Int. Soc. Oncodev. Biol. Med.* 37 (2016) 5203–5211.

377. D. Paudel, W. Zhou, Y. Ouyang, S. Dong, Q. Huang, R. Giri, et al., MicroRNA-130b functions as a tumor suppressor by regulating RUNX3 in epithelial ovarian cancer, *Gene* 586 (2016) 48–55.

378. Y. Xia, Y. Gao, MicroRNA-181b promotes ovarian cancer cell growth and invasion by targeting LATS2, *Biochem. Biophys. Res. Commun.* 447 (2014) 446–451.

379. X. Xu, B. Ayub, Z. Liu, V.A. Serna, W. Qiang, Y. Liu, et al., Anti-miR182 reduces ovarian cancer burden, invasion, and metastasis: an in vivo study in orthotopic xenografts of nude mice, *Mol. Cancer Ther.* 13 (2014) 1729–1739.

380. J. Li, S. Liang, H. Yu, J. Zhang, D. Ma, X. Lu, An inhibitory effect of miR-22 on cell migration and invasion in ovarian cancer, *Gynecol. Oncol.* 119 (2010) 543–548.

381. J.S. Imam, J.R. Plyler, H. Bansal, S. Prajapati, S. Bansal, J. Rebeles, et al., Genomic loss of tumor suppressor miRNA-204 promotes cancer cell migration and invasion by activating AKT/mTOR/Rac1 signaling and actin reorganization, *PLoS One* 7 (2012) e52397.

382. Y.M. Yeh, C.M. Chuang, K.C. Chao, L.H. Wang, MicroRNA-138 suppresses ovarian cancer cell invasion and metastasis by targeting SOX4 and HIF-1alpha, *Int. J. Cancer* 133 (2013) 867–878.

383. H.P. Joshi, I.V. Subramanian, E.K. Schnettler, G. Ghosh, R. Rupaimoole, C. Evans, et al., Dynamin 2 along with microRNA-199a reciprocally regulate hypoxia-inducible factors and ovarian cancer metastasis, *Proc. Natl. Acad. Sci. U. S. A.* 111 (2014) 5331–5336.

384. Y. Zhang, F.J. Zhao, L.L. Chen, L.Q. Wang, K.P. Nephew, Y.L. Wu, et al., MiR-373 targeting of the Rab22a oncogene suppresses tumor invasion and metastasis in ovarian cancer, *Oncotarget* 5 (2014) 12291–12303.

385. A. Ahmad, A. Aboukameel, D. Kong, Z. Wang, S. Sethi, W. Chen, et al., Phosphoglucose isomerase/autocrine motility factor mediates epithelial-mesenchymal transition regulated by miR-200 in breast cancer cells, *Cancer Res.* 71 (2011) 3400–3409.

386. S.M. Park, A.B. Gaur, E. Lengyel, M.E. Peter, The miR-200 family determines the epithelial phenotype of cancer cells by targeting the E-cadherin repressors ZEB1 and ZEB2, *Genes Dev.* 22 (2008) 894–907.

387. A. Bendoraite, E.C. Knouf, K.S. Garg, R.K. Parkin, E.M. Kroh, K.C. O'Briant, et al., Regulation of miR-200 family microRNAs and ZEB transcription factors in ovarian cancer: evidence supporting a mesothelial-to-epithelial transition, *Gynecol. Oncol.* 116 (2010) 117–125.

388. Y.X. Cheng, Q.F. Zhang, L. Hong, F. Pan, J.L. Huang, B.S. Li, et al., MicroRNA-200b suppresses cell invasion and metastasis by inhibiting the epithelial-mesenchymal transition in cervical carcinoma, *Mol. Med. Rep.* 13 (2016) 3155–3160.

389. Y.X. Cheng, G.T. Chen, C. Chen, Q.F. Zhang, F. Pan, M. Hu, et al., MicroRNA-200b inhibits epithelial-mesenchymal transition and migration of cervical cancer cells by directly targeting RhoE, *Mol. Med. Rep.* 13 (2016) 3139–3146.

390. J. Chen, L. Wang, L.V. Matyunina, C.G. Hill, J.F. McDonald, Overexpression of miR-429 induces mesenchymal-to-epithelial transition (MET) in metastatic ovarian cancer cells, *Gynecol. Oncol.* 121 (2011) 200–205.

391. H. Tan, Q. He, G. Gong, Y. Wang, J. Li, J. Wang, et al., miR-382 inhibits migration and invasion by targeting ROR1 through regulating EMT in ovarian cancer, *Int. J. Oncol.* 48 (2016) 181–190.

392. Z. Yang, X.L. Wang, R. Bai, W.Y. Liu, X. Li, M. Liu, et al., miR-23a promotes IKKalpha expression but suppresses ST7L expression to contribute to the malignancy of epithelial ovarian cancer cells, *Br. J. Cancer* 115 (2016) 731–740.

393. Y. Tang, Y. Wang, Q. Chen, N. Qiu, Y. Zhao, X. You, MiR-223 inhibited cell metastasis of human cervical cancer by modulating epithelial-mesenchymal transition, *Int. J. Clin. Exp. Pathol.* 8 (2015) 11224–11229.

394. P. Dong, M. Kaneuchi, H. Watari, J. Hamada, S. Sudo, J. Ju, et al., MicroRNA-194 inhibits epithelial to mesenchymal transition of endometrial cancer cells by targeting oncogene BMI-1, *Mol. Cancer* 10 (2011) 99.

395. B.L. Li, C. Lu, W. Lu, T.T. Yang, J. Qu, X. Hong, et al., miR-130b is an EMTrelated microRNA that targets DICER1 for aggression in endometrial cancer, *Med. Oncol. (Northwood, Lond. Engl.)* 30 (2013) 484.

396. P. Dong, M. Kaneuchi, H. Watari, S. Sudo, N. Sakuragi, MicroRNA-106b modulates epithelial-mesenchymal transition by targeting TWIST1 in invasive endometrial cancer cell lines, *Mol. Carcinog.* 53 (2014) 349–359.

397. C.N. Kent, I.K. Guttilla Reed, Regulation of epithelial-mesenchymal transition in endometrial cancer: connecting PI3K, estrogen signaling, and microRNAs, *Clin. Transl. Oncol. Off. Publ. Fed. Spanish Oncol. Soc. Natl. Cancer Inst. Mexico* 18 (2016) 1056–1061.

398. P. Dong, K. Ihira, Y. Xiong, H. Watari, S.J. Hanley, T. Yamada, et al., Reactivation of epigenetically silenced miR-124 reverses the epithelial-to-mesenchymal transition and inhibits invasion in endometrial cancer cells via the direct repression of IQGAP1 expression, *Oncotarget* 7 (2016) 20260–20270.

399. C. Jin, R. Liang, miR-205 promotes epithelial-mesenchymal transition by targeting AKT signaling in endometrial cancer cells, *J. Obstet. Gynaecol. Res.* 41 (2015) 1653–1660.

400. J. Yao, B. Deng, L. Zheng, L. Dou, Y. Guo, K. Guo, miR-27b is upregulated in cervical carcinogenesis and promotes cell growth and invasion by regulating CDH11 and epithelial-mesenchymal transition, *Oncol. Rep.* 35 (2016) 1645–1651.

401. Y. Wang, X. Dong, B. Hu, X.J. Wang, Q. Wang, W.L. Wang, The effects of Micro-429 on inhibition of cervical cancer cells through targeting ZEB1 and CRKL, *Biomed. Pharmacother.* 80 (2016) 311–321.

402. X. Zhang, D. Cai, L. Meng, B. Wang, MicroRNA-124 inhibits proliferation, invasion, migration and epithelial-mesenchymal transition of cervical carcinoma cells by targeting astrocyte-elevated gene-1, *Oncol. Rep.* 36 (2016) 2321–2328.

403. D. Xu, S. Liu, L. Zhang, L. Song, MiR-211 inhibits invasion and epithelial-to-mesenchymal transition (EMT) of cervical cancer cells via targeting MUC4, *Biochem. Biophys. Res. Commun.* 485 (2017) 556–562.

404. A. Parikh, C. Lee, P. Joseph, S. Marchini, A. Baccarini, V. Kolev, et al., micro-RNA-181a has a critical role in ovarian cancer progression through the regulation of the epithelial-mesenchymal transition, *Nat. Commun.* 5 (2014) 2977.

405. J.Y. Zhou, S.R. Zheng, J. Liu, R. Shi, H.L. Yu, M. Wei, MiR-519d facilitates the progression and metastasis of cervical cancer through direct targeting Smad7, *Cancer Cell Int.* 16 (2016) 21.

406. T. Wu, X. Chen, R. Peng, H. Liu, P. Yin, H. Peng, et al., Let7a suppresses cell proliferation via the TGFbeta/SMAD signaling pathway in cervical cancer, *Oncol. Rep.* 36 (2016) 3275–3282.

407. P. Liu, C. Wang, C. Ma, Q. Wu, W. Zhang, G. Lao, MicroRNA-23a regulates epithelial-to-mesenchymal transition in endometrial endometrioid adenocarcinoma by targeting SMAD3, *Cancer Cell Int.* 16 (2016) 67.

408. Y. Teng, L. Zhao, L. Zhang, W. Chen, X. Li, Id-1, a protein repressed by miR-29b, facilitates the TGFbeta1-induced epithelial-mesenchymal transition in human ovarian cancer cells, *Cell. Physiol. Biochem. Int. J. Exp. Cell. Physiol. Biochem. Pharmacol.* 33 (2014) 717–730.

409. Z. Ye, L. Zhao, J. Li, W. Chen, X. Li, miR-30d blocked transforming growth\factor beta1-induced epithelial-mesenchymal transition by targeting snail in ovarian cancer cells, *Int. J. Gynecol. Cancer Off. J. Int. Gynecol. Cancer Soc.* 25 (2015) 1574–1581.

410. J.M. Hansen, R.L. Coleman, A.K. Sood, Targeting the tumour microenvironment in ovarian cancer, *Eur. J. Cancer* 56 (2016) 131–143.

411. A.S. Felix, J. Weissfeld, R. Edwards, F. Linkov, Future directions in the field of endometrial cancer research: the need to investigate the tumor microenvironment, *Eur. J. Gynaecol. Oncol.* 31 (2010) 139–144.

412. O. Aprelikova, J. Palla, B. Hibler, X. Yu, Y.E. Greer, M. Yi, et al., Silencing of miR-148a in cancer-associated fibroblasts results in WNT10B-mediated stimulation of tumor cell motility, *Oncogene* 32 (2013) 3246–3253.

413. M.L. Macheda, S.A. Stacker, Importance of Wnt signaling in the tumor stroma microenvironment, *Curr. Cancer Drug Targets* 8 (2008) 454–465.

414. A.K. Mitra, M. Zillhardt, Y. Hua, P. Tiwari, A.E. Murmann, M.E. Peter, et al., MicroRNAs reprogram normal fibroblasts into cancer-associated fibroblasts in ovarian cancer, *Cancer Discov.* 2 (2012) 1100–1108.

415. E.L. LaGory, A.J. Giaccia, The ever-expanding role of HIF in tumour and stromal biology, *Nat. Cell Biol.* 18 (2016) 356–365.

416. Y. Kinose, K. Sawada, K. Nakamura, I. Sawada, A. Toda, E. Nakatsuka, et al., The hypoxia-related microRNA miR-199a-3p displays tumor suppressor functions in ovarian carcinoma, *Oncotarget* 6 (2015) 11342–11356.

417. A.K. Mitra, C.Y. Chiang, P. Tiwari, S. Tomar, K.M. Watters, M.E. Peter, et al., Microenvironment-induced downregulation of miR-193b drives ovarian cancer metastasis, *Oncogene* 34 (2015) 5923–5932.

418. K. Dass, A. Ahmad, A.S. Azmi, S.H. Sarkar, F.H. Sarkar, Evolving role of uPA/uPAR system in human cancers, *Cancer Treat. Rev.* 34 (2008) 122–136.

419. S.Y. Wen, Y. Lin, Y.Q. Yu, S.J. Cao, R. Zhang, X.M. Yang, et al., miR-506 acts as a tumor suppressor by directly targeting the hedgehog pathway transcription factor Gli3 in human cervical cancer, *Oncogene* 34 (2015) 717–725.

420. A. Hanna, L.A. Shevde, Hedgehog signaling: modulation of cancer properties and tumor mircroenvironment, *Mol. Cancer* 15 (2016) 24.

421. W. Jia, J.O. Eneh, S. Ratnaparkhe, M.K. Altman, M.M. Murph, MicroRNA-30c-2* expressed in ovarian cancer cells suppresses growth factor-induced cellular proliferation and downregulates the oncogene BCL9, *Mol. Cancer Res.* 9 (2011) 1732–1745.

422. J.R. Cubillos-Ruiz, L.F. Sempere, J.R. Conejo-Garcia, Good things come in small packages: therapeutic antitumor immunity induced by microRNA nanoparticles, *Oncoimmunology* 1 (2012) 968–970.

423. W.T. Chen, Y.J. Yang, Z.D. Zhang, Q. An, N. Li, W. Liu, et al., MiR-1307 promotes ovarian cancer cell chemoresistance by targeting the ING5 expression, *J. Ovarian Res.* 10 (2017) 1.

424. L. Lu, P. Schwartz, L. Scarampi, T. Rutherford, E.M. Canuto, H. Yu, et al., MicroRNA let-7a: a potential marker for selection of paclitaxel in ovarian cancer management, *Gynecol. Oncol.* 122 (2011) 366–371.

425. N. Liu, C. Zhou, J. Zhao, Y. Chen, Reversal of paclitaxel resistance in epithelial ovarian carcinoma cells by a MUC1 aptamer-let-7i chimera, *Cancer Invest.* 30 (2012) 577e582.

426. X. Li, Y. Lu, Y. Chen, W. Lu, X. Xie, MicroRNA profile of paclitaxel-resistant serous ovarian carcinoma based on formalin-fixed paraffin-embedded samples, *BMC Cancer* 13 (2013) 216.

427. J.K. Chan, K. Blansit, T. Kiet, A. Sherman, G. Wong, C. Earle, et al., The inhibition of miR-21 promotes apoptosis and chemosensitivity in ovarian cancer, *Gynecol. Oncol.* 132 (2014) 739–744.

428. P.N. Yu, M.D. Yan, H.C. Lai, R.L. Huang, Y.C. Chou, W.C. Lin, et al., Downregulation of miR-29 contributes to cisplatin resistance of ovarian cancer cells, *Int. J. Cancer* 134 (2014) 542–551.

429. T. Mitamura, H. Watari, L. Wang, H. Kanno, M.K. Hassan, M. Miyazaki, et al., Downregulation of miRNA-31 induces taxane resistance in ovarian cancer cells through increase of receptor tyrosine kinase MET, *Oncogenesis* 2 (2013) e40.

430. P. Samuel, R.C. Pink, D.P. Caley, J.M. Currie, S.A. Brooks, D.R. Carter, Overexpression of miR-31 or loss of KCNMA1 leads to increased cisplatin resistance in ovarian cancer cells, *Tumour Biol. J. Int. Soc. Oncodevel. Biol. Med.* 37 (2016) 2565–2573.

431. X. Fu, J. Tian, L. Zhang, Y. Chen, Q. Hao, Involvement of microRNA-93, a new regulator of PTEN/Akt signaling pathway, in regulation of chemotherapeutic drug cisplatin chemosensitivity in ovarian cancer cells, *FEBS Lett.* 586 (2012) 1279–1286.

432. J.H. Huh, T.H. Kim, K. Kim, J.A. Song, Y.J. Jung, J.Y. Jeong, et al., Dysregulation of miR-106a and miR-591 confers paclitaxel resistance to ovarian cancer, *Br. J. Cancer* 109 (2013) 452–461.

433. F. Kong, C. Sun, Z. Wang, L. Han, D. Weng, Y. Lu, et al., miR-125b confers resistance of ovarian cancer cells to cisplatin by targeting pro-apoptotic Bcl-2 antagonist killer 1, *J. Huazhong Univ. Sci. Technol. Med. Sci.* 31 (2011) 543–549.

434. L. Yang, N. Li, H. Wang, X. Jia, X. Wang, J. Luo, Altered microRNA expression in cisplatin-resistant ovarian cancer cells and upregulation of miR-130a associated with MDR1/P-glycoprotein-mediated drug resistance, *Oncol. Rep.* 28 (2012) 592–600.

435. C. Yang, J. Cai, Q. Wang, H. Tang, J. Cao, L. Wu, et al., Epigenetic silencing of miR-130b in ovarian cancer promotes the development of multidrug resistance by targeting colony-stimulating factor 1, *Gynecol. Oncol.* 124 (2012) 325–334.

436. X. Zhu, Y. Li, C. Xie, X. Yin, Y. Liu, Y. Cao, et al., miR-145 sensitizes ovarian cancer cells to paclitaxel by targeting Sp1 and Cdk6, *Int. J. Cancer* 135 (2014) 1286–1296.

437. Y. Xiang, N. Ma, D. Wang, Y. Zhang, J. Zhou, G. Wu, et al., MiR-152 and miR-185 co-contribute to ovarian cancer cells cisplatin sensitivity by targeting DNMT1 directly: a novel epigenetic therapy independent of decitabine, *Oncogene* 33 (2014) 378–386.

438. C. Lei, Y. Wang, Y. Huang, H. Yu, Y. Huang, L. Wu, et al., Up-regulated miR155 reverses the epithelial-mesenchymal transition induced by EGF and increases chemo-sensitivity to cisplatin in human Caski cervical cancer cells, *PLoS One* 7 (2012) e52310.

439. X. Zhu, H. Shen, X. Yin, L. Long, C. Xie, Y. Liu, et al., miR-186 regulation of Twist1 and ovarian cancer sensitivity to cisplatin, *Oncogene* 35 (2016) 323–332.

440. M.X. Liu, M.K. Siu, S.S. Liu, J.W. Yam, H.Y. Ngan, D.W. Chan, Epigenetic silencing of microRNA-199b-5p is associated with acquired chemoresistance via activation of JAG1-Notch1 signaling in ovarian cancer, *Oncotarget* 5 (2014) 944–958.

441. S. Leskela, L.J. Leandro-Garcia, M. Mendiola, J. Barriuso, L. Inglada-Perez, I. Munoz, et al., The miR-200 family controls beta-tubulin III expression and is associated with paclitaxel-based treatment response and progression-free survival in ovarian cancer patients, *Endocr. Relat. Cancer* 18 (2011) 85–95.

442. D.M. Cittelly, I. Dimitrova, E.N. Howe, D.R. Cochrane, A. Jean, N.S. Spoelstra, et al., Restoration of miR-200c to ovarian cancer reduces tumor burden and increases sensitivity to paclitaxel, *Mol. Cancer Ther.* 11 (2012) 2556–2565.

443. J. Li, Z. Ping, H. Ning, MiR-218 impairs tumor growth and increases chemosensitivity to cisplatin in cervical cancer, *Int. J. Mol. Sci.* 13 (2012) 16053–16064.

444. R. Dong, H. Qiu, G. Du, Y. Wang, J. Yu, C. Mao, Restoration of microRNA218 increases cellular chemosensitivity to cervical cancer by inhibiting cell-cycle progression, *Mol. Med. Rep.* 10 (2014) 3289–3295.

445. F. Lin, P. Wang, Y. Shen, X. Xie, Upregulation of microRNA-224 sensitizes human cervical cells SiHa to paclitaxel, *Eur. J. Gynaecol. Oncol.* 36 (2015) 432–436.

446. Y. Shen, P. Wang, Y. Li, F. Ye, F. Wang, X. Wan, et al., miR-375 is upregulated in acquired paclitaxel resistance in cervical cancer, *Br. J. Cancer* 109 (2013) 92–99.

447. Y. Shen, J. Zhou, Y. Li, F. Ye, X. Wan, W. Lu, et al., miR-375 mediated acquired chemo-resistance in cervical cancer by facilitating EMT, *PLoS One* 9 (2014) e109299.

448. G. Ye, G. Fu, S. Cui, S. Zhao, S. Bernaudo, Y. Bai, et al., MicroRNA 376c enhances ovarian cancer cell survival by targeting activin receptor-like kinase 7: implications for chemoresistance, *J. Cell Sci.* 124 (2011) 359–368.

449. S. Xu, G.B. Fu, Z. Tao, J. OuYang, F. Kong, B.H. Jiang, et al., MiR-497 decreases cisplatin resistance in ovarian cancer cells by targeting mTOR/P70S6K1, *Oncotarget* 6 (2015) 26457–26471.

450. G. Liu, D. Yang, R. Rupaimoole, C.V. Pecot, Y. Sun, L.S. Mangala, et al., Augmentation of response to chemotherapy by microRNA-506 through regulation of RAD51 in serous ovarian cancers, *J. Natl. Cancer Inst.* 107 (7) (2015) djv108. doi: 10.1093/jnci/djv108.

451. L.M. Dillon, T.W. Miller, Therapeutic targeting of cancers with loss of PTEN function, *Curr. Drug Targets* 15 (2014) 65–79.

452. N. Li, L. Yang, H. Wang, T. Yi, X. Jia, C. Chen, et al., MiR-130a and MiR-374a function as novel regulators of cisplatin resistance in human ovarian cancer A2780 cells, *PLoS One* 10 (2015) e0128886.

453. C. Chen, Y. Hu, L. Li, NRP1 is targeted by miR-130a and miR-130b, and is associated with multidrug resistance in epithelial ovarian cancer based on integrated gene network analysis, *Mol. Med. Rep.* 13 (2016) 188–196.

454. A. Brozovic, G.E. Duran, Y.C. Wang, E.B. Francisco, B.I. Sikic, The miR-200 family differentially regulates sensitivity to paclitaxel and carboplatin in human ovarian carcinoma OVCAR-3 and MES-OV cells, *Mol. Oncol.* 9 (2015) 1678–1693.

455. J. Song, Y. Li, miR-25-3p reverses epithelial-mesenchymal transition via targeting Sema4C in cisplatin-resistance cervical cancer cells, *Cancer Sci.* 108 (2017) 23–31.

456. M.K. Hassan, H. Watari, T. Mitamura, Z. Mohamed, S.F. El-Khamisy, Y. Ohba, et al., P18/Stathmin1 is regulated by miR-31 in ovarian cancer in response to taxane, *Oncoscience* 2 (2015) 294–308.

457. J. Cai, C. Yang, Q. Yang, H. Ding, J. Jia, J. Guo, et al., Deregulation of let-7e in epithelial ovarian cancer promotes the development of resistance to cisplatin, *Oncogenesis* 2 (2013) e75.

458. B. Li, H. Chen, N. Wu, W.J. Zhang, L.X. Shang, Deregulation of miR-128 in ovarian cancer promotes cisplatin resistance, *Int. J. Gynecol. Cancer Off. J. Int. Gynecol. Cancer Soc.* 24 (2014) 1381–1388.

459. H. Zhao, S. Liu, G. Wang, X. Wu, Y. Ding, G. Guo, et al., Expression of miR-136 is associated with the primary cisplatin resistance of human epithelial ovarian cancer, *Oncol. Rep.* 33 (2015) 591–598.

460. W. Chen, L. Huang, C. Hao, W. Zeng, X. Luo, X. Li, et al., MicroRNA-155 promotes apoptosis in SKOV3, A2780, and primary cultured ovarian cancer cells, *Tumour Biol. J. Int. Soc. Oncodevel. Biol. Med.* 37 (2016) 9289–9299.

461. Z. Wang, Z. Ting, Y. Li, G. Chen, Y. Lu, X. Hao, microRNA-199a is able to reverse cisplatin resistance in human ovarian cancer cells through the inhibition of mammalian target of rapamycin, *Oncol. Lett.* 6 (2013) 789–794.

462. Y. Liu, Z. Niu, X. Lin, Y. Tian, MiR-216b increases cisplatin sensitivity in ovarian cancer cells by targeting PARP1, *Cancer Gene Ther.* 24 (2017) 208–214.

463. Y. Zhou, Q. Chen, R. Qin, K. Zhang, H. Li, MicroRNA-449a reduces cell survival and enhances cisplatin-induced cytotoxicity via downregulation of NOTCH1 in ovarian cancer cells, *Tumour Biol. J. Int. Soc. Oncodevel. Biol. Med.* 35 (2014) 12369–12378.

464. H. Wu, Z. Xiao, H. Zhang, K. Wang, W. Liu, Q. Hao, MiR-489 modulates cisplatin resistance in human ovarian cancer cells by targeting Akt3, *Anticancer Drugs* 25 (2014) 799–809.

465. S. Tian, M. Zhang, X. Chen, Y. Liu, G. Lou, MicroRNA-595 sensitizes ovarian cancer cells to cisplatin by targeting-ABCB1, *Oncotarget* 7 (2016) 87091–87099.

466. M.T. van Jaarsveld, P.F. van Kuijk, A.W. Boersma, J. Helleman, I.W.F. van, R.H. Mathijssen, et al., miR-634 restores drug sensitivity in resistant ovarian cancer cells by targeting the Ras-MAPK pathway, *Mol. Cancer* 14 (2015) 196.

467. H. Zhao, X. Yu, Y. Ding, J. Zhao, G. Wang, X. Wu, et al., MiR-770-5p inhibits cisplatin chemoresistance in human ovarian cancer by targeting ERCC2, *Oncotarget* 7 (2016) 53254–53268.

468. I.M. Echevarria-Vargas, F. Valiyeva, P.E. Vivas-Mejia, Upregulation of miR-21 in cisplatin resistant ovarian cancer via JNK-1/c-Jun pathway, *PLoS One* 9 (2014) e97094.

469. H. Zhao, T. Bi, Z. Qu, J. Jiang, S. Cui, Y. Wang, Expression of miR-224-5p is associated with the original cisplatin resistance of ovarian papillary serous carcinoma, *Oncol. Rep.* 32 (2014) 1003–1012.

470. W. Chen, W. Zeng, X. Li, W. Xiong, M. Zhang, Y. Huang, et al., MicroRNA-509-3p increases the sensitivity of epithelial ovarian cancer cells to cisplatin-induced apoptosis, *Pharmacogenomics* 17 (2016) 187–197.

471. H. Li, H. Xu, H. Shen, H. Li, microRNA-106a modulates cisplatin sensitivity by targeting PDCD4 in human ovarian cancer cells, *Oncol. Lett.* 7 (2014) 183–188.

472. C. Zong, J. Wang, T.M. Shi, MicroRNA 130b enhances drug resistance in human ovarian cancer cells, *Tumour Biol. J. Int. Soc. Oncodevel. Biol. Med.* 35 (2014) 12151–12156.

473. T. Shuang, M. Wang, C. Shi, Y. Zhou, D. Wang, Down-regulated expression of miR-134 contributes to paclitaxel resistance in human ovarian cancer cells, *FEBS Lett.* 589 (2015) 3154–3164.

474. Y. Zhan, F. Xiang, R. Wu, J. Xu, Z. Ni, J. Jiang, et al., MiRNA-149 modulates chemosensitivity of ovarian cancer A2780 cells to paclitaxel by targeting MyD88, *J. Ovarian Res.* 8 (2015) 48.

475. K.X. Sun, J.W. Jiao, S. Chen, B.L. Liu, Y. Zhao, MicroRNA-186 induces sensitivity of ovarian cancer cells to paclitaxel and cisplatin by targeting ABCB1, *J. Ovarian Res.* 8 (2015) 80.

476. D. Zou, D. Wang, R. Li, Y. Tang, L. Yuan, X. Long, et al., MiR-197 induces Taxol resistance in human ovarian cancer cells by regulating NLK, *Tumour Biol. J. Int. Soc. Oncodevel. Biol. Med.* 36 (2015) 6725–6732.

477. L. Wang, R. Mezencev, M. Svajdler, B.B. Benigno, J.F. McDonald, Ectopic overexpression of miR-429 induces mesenchymal-to-epithelial transition (MET) and increased drug sensitivity in metastasizing ovarian cancer cells, *Gynecol. Oncol.* 134 (2014) 96–103.

478. K. Weiner-Gorzel, E. Dempsey, M. Milewska, A. McGoldrick, V. Toh, A. Walsh, et al., Overexpression of the microRNA miR-433 promotes resistance to paclitaxel through the induction of cellular senescence in ovarian cancer cells, *Cancer Med.* 4 (2015) 745–758.

479. S. Chen, X. Chen, Y.L. Xiu, K.X. Sun, Z.H. Zong, Y. Zhao, microRNA 490-3P enhances the drug-resistance of human ovarian cancer cells, *J. Ovarian Res.* 7 (2014) 84.

480. Z. Fan, H. Cui, H. Yu, Q. Ji, L. Kang, B. Han, et al., MiR-125a promotes paclitaxel sensitivity in cervical cancer through altering STAT3 expression, *Oncogenesis* 5 (2016) e197.

481. P. Samuel, R.C. Pink, D.P. Caley, J.M. Currie, S.A. Brooks, D.R. Carter, Overexpression of miR-31 or loss of KCNMA1 leads to increased cisplatin resistance in ovarian cancer cells, *Tumour Biol. J. Int. Soc. Oncodevel. Biol. Med.* 37 (2016) 2565–2573.

482. M. Montagnana, G. Lippi, O. Ruzzenente, V. Bresciani, E. Danese, S. Scevarolli, et al., The utility of serum human epididymis protein 4 (HE4) in patients with a pelvic mass, *J. Clin. Lab. Anal.* 23 (2009) 331–335.

483. Y. Bie, Z. Zhang, Diagnostic value of serum HE4 in endometrial cancer: a meta-analysis, *World J. Surg. Oncol.* 12 (2014) 169.

484. E.V. Hogdall, L. Christensen, S.K. Kjaer, J. Blaakaer, A. Kjaerbye-Thygesen, S. Gayther, et al., CA125 expression pattern, prognosis and correlation with serum CA125 in ovarian tumor patients. From the Danish "MALOVA" *Ovarian Cancer Study, Gynecol. Oncol.* 104 (2007) 508–515.

485. D. Badgwell, R.C. Bast Jr., Early detection of ovarian cancer, *Dis. Markers* 23 (2007) 397–410.

486. X. Liu, F. Zhao, L. Hu, Y. Sun, Value of detection of serum human epididymis secretory protein 4 and carbohydrate antigen 125 in diagnosis of early endometrial cancer of different pathological subtypes, *Onco. Targets Ther.* 8 (2015) 1239–1243.

487. M. Zuberi, R. Mir, J. Das, I. Ahmad, J. Javid, P. Yadav, et al., Expression of serum miR-200a, miR-200b, and miR-200c as candidate biomarkers in epithelial ovarian cancer and their association with clinicopathological features, *Clin. Transl. Oncol. Off. Publ. Fed. Span. Oncol. Soc. Natl. Cancer Inst. Mexico* 17 (2015) 779–787.

488. H. Zheng, L. Zhang, Y. Zhao, D. Yang, F. Song, Y. Wen, et al., Plasma miRNAs as diagnostic and prognostic biomarkers for ovarian cancer, *PLoS One* 8 (2013) e77853.

489. E. Calura, R. Fruscio, L. Paracchini, E. Bignotti, A. Ravaggi, P. Martini, et al., MiRNA landscape in stage I epithelial ovarian cancer defines the histotype specificities, *Clin. Cancer Res.* 19 (2013) 4114–4123.

490. P. Liu, F. Xin, C.F. Ma, Clinical significance of serum miR-196a in cervical intraepithelial neoplasia and cervical cancer, *Genet. Mol. Res.* 14 (2015) 17995–18002.

491. E.C. Coimbra, M.D.A. Conceiçao Gomes Leitao, M.R. Junior, T.H.D.E. Oliveira, J.D.A. Costa Silva Neto, A.C.D.E. Freitas, Expression profile of MicroRNA-203 and its DeltaNp63 target in cervical carcinogenesis: prospects for cervical cancer screening, *Anticancer Res.* 36 (2016) 3939–3946.

492. W. Jia, Y. Wu, Q. Zhang, G. Gao, C. Zhang, Y. Xiang, Identification of four serum microRNAs from a genome-wide serum microRNA expression profile as potential non-invasive biomarkers for endometrioid endometrial cancer, *Oncol. Lett.* 6 (2013) 261–267.

493. H. Zhai, M. Karaayvaz, P. Dong, N. Sakuragi, J. Ju, Prognostic significance of miR-194 in endometrial cancer, *Biomark. Res.* 1(12) (2013). doi: 10.1186/2050-7771-1-12.

494. M. Luo, D. Shen, X. Zhou, X. Chen, W. Wang, MicroRNA-497 is a potential prognostic marker in human cervical cancer and functions as a tumor suppressor by targeting the insulin-like growth factor 1 receptor, *Surgery* 153 (2013) 836–847.

495. S. He, S. Zeng, Z.W. Zhou, Z.X. He, S.F. Zhou, Hsa-microRNA-181a is a regulator of a number of cancer genes and a biomarker for endometrial carcinoma in patients: a bioinformatic and clinical study and the therapeutic implication, *Drug Des. Devel. Ther.* 9 (2015) 1103–1175.

496. I. Shapira, M. Oswald, J. Lovecchio, H. Khalili, A. Menzin, J. Whyte, et al., Circulating biomarkers for detection of ovarian cancer and predicting cancer outcomes, *Br. J. cancer* 110 (2014) 976–983.

497. A.R. Halvorsen, G. Kristensen, A. Embleton, C. Adusei, M.P. Barretina-Ginesta, P. Beale, et al., Evaluation of prognostic and predictive significance of circulating microRNAs in ovarian cancer patients, *Dis. Markers* 2017 (2017) 3098542.

498. M. Wilczynski, J. Danielska, M. Dzieniecka, B. Szymanska, M. Wojciechowski, A. Malinowski, Prognostic and clinical significance of miRNA-205 in endometrioid endometrial cancer, *PLoS One* 11 (2016) e0164687.

499. C.X. Yang, S.M. Zhang, J. Li, B. Yang, W. Ouyang, Z.J. Mei, et al., MicroRNA-320 regulates the radiosensitivity of cervical cancer cells C33AR by targeting beta-catenin, *Oncol. Lett.* 12 (2016) 4983–4990.

500. A. Vecchione, B. Belletti, F. Lovat, S. Volinia, G. Chiappetta, S. Giglio, et al., A microRNA signature defines chemoresistance in ovarian cancer through modulation of angiogenesis, *Proc. Natl. Acad. Sci. U. S. A.* 110 (2013) 9845–9850.

501. L. Sun, R. Jiang, J. Li, B. Wang, C. Ma, Y. Lv, et al., MicoRNA-425-5p is a potential prognostic biomarker for cervical cancer, *Ann. Clin. Biochem.* 54 (2017) 127–133.

502. N. Wang, Y. Zhou, L. Zheng, H. Li, MiR-31 is an independent prognostic factor and functions as an oncomir in cervical cancer via targeting ARID1A, *Gynecol. Oncol.* 134 (2014) 129–137.

503. E.A. Benson, T.C. Skaar, Y. Liu, K.P. Nephew, D. Matei, Carboplatin with decitabine therapy, in recurrent platinum resistant ovarian cancer, alters circulating miRNAs concentrations: a pilot study, *PLoS One* 10 (2015) e0141279.

504. M.S. Beg, A.J. Brenner, J. Sachdev, M. Borad, Y.K. Kang, J. Stoudemire, et al., Phase I study of MRX34, a liposomal miR-34a mimic, administered twice weekly in patients with advanced solid tumors, *Invest. New Drugs* 35 (2017) 180–188.

505. M. Nishimura, E.J. Jung, M.Y. Shah, C. Lu, R. Spizzo, M. Shimizu, et al., Therapeutic synergy between microRNA and siRNA in ovarian cancer treatment, *Cancer Discov.* 3 (2013) 1302–1315.

506. D.C. Corney, C.I. Hwang, A. Matoso, M. Vogt, A. Flesken-Nikitin, A.K. Godwin, et al., Frequent downregulation of miR-34 family in human ovarian cancers, *Clin. Cancer Res.* 16 (2010) 1119–1128.

507. S.K. Dwivedi, S.B. Mustafi, L.S. Mangala, D. Jiang, S. Pradeep, C. Rodriguez- Aguayo, et al., Therapeutic evaluation of microRNA-15a and microRNA-16 in ovarian cancer, *Oncotarget* 7 (2016) 15093–15104.

508. H. Mahmoodzadeh, F. Moazzen, N. Mehmandoost, et al. Cloning and expression of C2 and V domains of ALCAM Protein in E. coli BL21 (DE3), *Clin. Microbiol. Open Access* 6(1) (2017) 1–6. doi: 10.4172/2327-5073.1000271.

509. H. Dana, V. Marmari, A. Mazraeh, A. Ghamari, M.M. Forghanifard, Cloning and expression of the V-domain of the CD166 in prokaryotic host cell, *Int. J. Cancer Ther. Oncol.* 5(1) (2017). http://ijcto.org/index.php/IJCTO/article/view/ijcto51.10.

510. H. Dana, CD166 as a stem cell marker? A potential target for therapy colorectal cancer? *J. Stem Cell Res. Ther.* 1(6) (2017) 6–9. doi: 10.15406/jsrt.2016.01.00041.

511. Loutfy H. Madkour. *Reactive Oxygen Species (ROS), Nanoparticles, and Endoplasmic Reticulum (ER) Stress-Induced Cell Death Mechanisms* (2020). https://www.elsevier.com/books/reactive-oxygen-species-ros-nanoparticles-and-endoplasmic-reticulum-er-stress-induced-cell-death-mechanisms/madkour/978-0-12-822481-6.

512. Loutfy H. Madkour, *Nanoparticles Induce Oxidative and Endoplasmic Reticulum Antioxidant Therapeutic Defenses* (2020). https://www.springer.com/gp/book/9783030372965?utm_campaign=3_pier05_buy_print&utm_content=en_08082017&utm_medium=referral&utm_source=google_books#otherversion=9783030372972.

513. Loutfy H. Madkour, *Nucleic Acids as Gene Anticancer Drug Delivery Therapy* (1st edn) (2020). https://www.elsevier.com/books/nucleic-acids-as-gene-anticancer-drug-delivery therapy/madkour/978-0-12-819777-6.

514. Loutfy H. Madkour, *Nanoelectronic Materials: Fundamentals and Applications (Advanced Structured Materials)* (1st edn) (2019) https://link.springer.com/book/10.1007%2F978-3-030-21621-4, https://books.google.com.eg/books/about/Nanoelectronic_Materials.html?id=YQXCxAEACAAJ&source=kp_book_description&redir_esc=y, https://www.springer.com/gp/book/9783030216207.

515. W. Shen, M. Song, J. Liu, G. Qiu, T. Li, Y. Hu, et al., MiR-26a promotes ovarian cancer proliferation and tumorigenesis, *PLoS One* 9 (2014) e86871.

516. T.Y. Sun, H.J. Xie, H. He, Z. Li, L.F. Kong, miR-26a inhibits the proliferation of ovarian cancer cells via regulating CDC6 expression, *Am. J. Transl. Res.* 8 (2016) 1037–1046.

517. J. Dong, L. Sui, Q. Wang, M. Chen, H. Sun, MicroRNA-26a inhibits cell proliferation and invasion of cervical cancer cells by targeting protein tyrosine phosphatase type IVA 1, *Mol. Med. Rep.* 10 (2014) 1426–1432.

518. C. Sun, N. Li, B. Zhou, Z. Yang, D. Ding, D. Weng, et al., miR-222 is upregulated in epithelial ovarian cancer and promotes cell proliferation by downregulating P27kip1, *Oncol. Lett.* 6 (2013) 507–512.

519. X. Fu, Y. Li, A. Alvero, J. Li, Q. Wu, Q. Xiao, et al., MicroRNA-222-3p/GNAI2/AKT axis inhibits epithelial ovarian cancer cell growth and associates with good overall survival, *Oncotarget* 7 (2016) 80633–80654.

6 Nanoparticle–Based RNA (siRNA) Combination Therapy Toward Overcoming Drug Resistance in Cancer

6.1 SMALL INTERFERENCE RNA (siRNA)

RNA interference (RNAi) is a process by which RNA molecules, with sequences complementary to a gene's coding sequence, induce degradation of corresponding messenger RNAs (mRNAs), thus blocking the translation of the mRNA into protein [1,2]. RNAi is initiated by exposing cells to long dsRNA via transfection or endogenous expression. dsRNAs are processed into smaller fragments (usually 21–23 nucleotides) of small interfering RNAs (siRNA) [3], which form a complex with the RNA-induced silencing complexes [4]. Introduction of siRNA into mammalian cells leads to downregulation of target genes without triggering interferon responses [3]. Molecular therapy using siRNA has shown great potential for diseases caused by abnormal gene overexpression or mutation, such as various cancers, viral infections, and genetic disorders, as well as for pain management. In the last ten years, a tremendous effort has been made in biomedical therapeutic application of gene silencing in humans. Phase I studies of siRNA for the treatment of age-related macular degeneration and respiratory syncytial virus provided promising data with no sign of nonspecific toxicity [5,6]. However, there are many challenges to be overcome for siRNA cancer therapeutics, including safety, stability, and effective siRNA delivery.

The major barrier facing siRNA therapeutics is the efficiency of delivery to the desired cell type, tissue, or organ. siRNAs do not readily pass through the cell membrane due to their size and negative charge. Cationic liposome-based strategies are usually used for the cellular delivery of chemically synthesized or *in vitro* transcribed siRNA [7]. However, there are many problems with lipid-based delivery systems *in vivo*, such as rapid clearance by the liver and lack of target tissue specificity. Delivery systems can be categorized into physical methods, conjugation methods, and natural carrier (viruses and bacteria) and nonviral carrier methods [8]. DNA-based expression cassettes that express short hairpin RNA (shRNA) are usually delivered to target cells *ex vivo* by viruses and bacteria, and these modified cells are then reinfused back into the patient [9]. The popular adenovirus- and adeno-associated virus-derived vectors provide efficient delivery for shRNA expression [10]. However, there are problems with delivery using viral vectors, such as insertional mutagenesis and immunogenicity [11]. Nonviral gene delivery systems are highly attractive for gene therapy because they are safer and easier to produce than viral vectors.

Nanotechnology has made significant advances in the development of efficient siRNA delivery systems. Current nonviral delivery systems can be categorized as organic and inorganic [12]. Organic complexes include lipid complexes, conjugated polymers, and cationic polymers, whereas inorganic nanoparticles include magnetic nanoparticles, quantum dots, carbon nanotubes, and gold nanoparticles.

6.2 NOVEL COMBINATION THERAPY

The long-standing challenge in cancer drug resistance and the urgent need for novel combination therapy are highlighted in a recent perspective by Woodcock et al., who liken the complexity of cancer biology to webs of interconnected routes with multiple redundancies [13]. Very tellingly, this analogy points out the inadequacy of single-drug therapy, whose one-dimensional action mechanism often activates and strengthens the alternative pathways, prompting the emergence of chemoresistance mutations and tumor relapse. In an aim to increase treatment efficacy, combination chemotherapy has long been adopted as the standard of care against many cancer types. It is generally acknowledged that through the proper drug combination the treatment can promote synergistic actions, improve target selectivity, and deter the development of cancer drug resistance [14].

Despite being a clinical standard, current combination approach through the cocktail administration leaves plenty of room for improvements. While *in vitro* cellular studies have generated many leads for combinatorial regimens, their clinical results are often met with little improvement in efficacy and, at times, higher toxicity [15,16]. One major factor that separates *in vitro* success from impressive clinical outcomes is the varying pharmacokinetics among different drugs. Upon systemic administration, drugs undergo distinctive physiological fates and non-uniform distribution. Predicting and controlling the therapeutic mixtures that reach the diseased cells and tissues, therefore, become a major clinical challenge. The common approach based on maximum-tolerated dose fails to take into account the intricate pharmacologic interactions that are sensitive to both dosing and sequencing of combinatorial drugs. One strategy toward more effective combination therapies thus is devising a better scheme for precise and controlled delivery of multiple therapeutic agents.

DOI: 10.1201/9781003229674-6

Advances in nanotechnology have opened up unprecedented opportunities in controlled drug delivery and novel combination strategies. Nanoscale particles between 10 and 200 nm in diameter have shown more favorable pharmacokinetic profiles as compared to small-molecule drugs; these drug-loaded nanoparticles exhibit prolonged systemic circulation lifetime, sustained drug release kinetics, and better tumor accumulations through both passive and active mechanisms [17–20]. Recently, nanocarriers are gaining increasing attention for their ability to co-encapsulate multiple therapeutic agents and to synchronize their delivery to the diseased cells. Various nanoparticle platforms such as liposomes, polymeric micelles, dendrimers, and mesoporous silica particles have been used to carry broad classes of therapeutics including cytotoxic agents, chemosensitizers, small interference RNA (siRNA), and antiangiogenic agents. In this chapter, we will cover several nanoparticulate systems that have been used for co-encapsulation and co-delivery of multiple drugs. In this chapter, we discuss recent advances in nanoparticle-mediated siRNA delivery systems and the application of these systems in clinical trials for cancer therapy. Furthermore, we offer perspectives on future applications of siRNA therapeutics. We will then summarize nanoparticle-based combination strategies to overcome the experimental models of multidrug resistance (MDR) in cancer. Lastly, in light of the complexity in clinical cancer drug resistance, we will offer insights on emerging features in nanoparticle drug delivery that promise broader applicability and better design for combination therapy. These features include co-encapsulating hydrophobic and hydrophilic drugs, precise and ratiometric control over drug loading, and sequenced drug release.

6.3 NANOPARTICULATE SYSTEMS FOR COMBINATORIAL DRUG DELIVERY

Nanoparticulate systems such as liposomes, polymeric micelles, and polymer–drug conjugates have led to about two dozen clinically approved therapeutic products [18]. Herein, we highlight the nanocarriers that have been demonstrated to carry two or more types of therapeutic payloads. While these systems share the common aim in promoting synergism through controlled combinatorial drug delivery, each platform has its unique strength and characteristics. The different particle structures, materials, and preparation processes are emphasized here to provide design considerations toward developing combinatorial therapeutics.

6.3.1 LIPOSOMES

Liposomes are spherical vesicles consisting of amphiphilic phospholipid bilayers. Phosphatidylcholine and phosphatidylethanolamine are the common building blocks for liposomal preparation whereas cholesterol is a frequent additive that serves to modify the rigidity of the lipid membranes. Liposomes are typically prepared by rehydrating lipid films

to form multilamellar vesicles (MLV), which subsequently undergo mechanical extrusions to form unilamellar vesicles [21]. The resulting structure contains a lipid bilayer and an inner aqueous core, which are capable of carrying lipophilic and hydrophilic drugs, respectively.

Liposomal drug loading can be accomplished either through active extrusion or through passive diffusion. In the active extrusion approach, drugs are suspended along with the phospholipids in aqueous solution. The resulting mixture of MLV and drugs are then extruded through membrane with defined pore size to form drug-loaded liposomes. In the passive diffusion approach, liposomes are first prepared and then mixed with solubilized drugs. These drug molecules then enter the liposomes by diffusing through the lipid bilayers. Multidrug-loaded liposomes can be prepared using either of the loading schemes followed by filtration of unloaded drugs. For instance, in preparing CPX-351, a combinatorial liposome for leukemia treatment, cytarabine is hydrated and extruded with the lipid components yielding cytarabine-loaded liposomes. These liposomes are then incubated with daunorubicin to achieve dual-drug encapsulation [22]. Currently, liposomes are the only nanoparticle-based combinatorial drug delivery platform that has entered clinical trials.

6.3.2 POLYMERIC NANOPARTICLES

In contrast to liposomal vehicles that carry drug cargoes in their aqueous cavity, polymeric nanoparticles contain a solid, polymer-filled core that is better suited for water-insoluble drug payloads. The solid structure also gives polymeric nanoparticles higher stability, more sustained and controllable drug release profiles, and more uniform size distribution. Polymeric nanoparticles are typically prepared through the self-assembly of amphiphilic diblock copolymers. A variety of polymers have been used to prepare polymeric nanoparticles, including biodegradable synthetic polymers such as poly(lactic-co-glycolic acid) (PLGA) and polycaprolactone (PCL) and natural polymers such as polysaccharides and polypeptides [23–25]. In general, drug encapsulation into polymeric nanoparticles is achieved by mixing the drugs with the polymer solution. As the polymers self-assemble into particles, they physically entrap the drug compounds. Multiple hydrophobic therapeutic compounds have been loaded simultaneously through this physical entrapment approach. Other encapsulation schemes have taken advantage of the synthesis flexibility in the polymeric building blocks. Through drug–polymer conjugations and particle functionalization, more advanced combinatorial drug encapsulation schemes have been developed to extend compatibility to hydrophilic drugs [26–28], precisely controlled drug-loading ratios [29], and fine-tuned drug release sequence and kinetics [30,31].

6.3.3 POLYMER–DRUG CONJUGATES

Covalently attaching therapeutic agents to water-soluble polymers is another approach that improves the drugs' systemic circulation lifetime and reduces their exposure

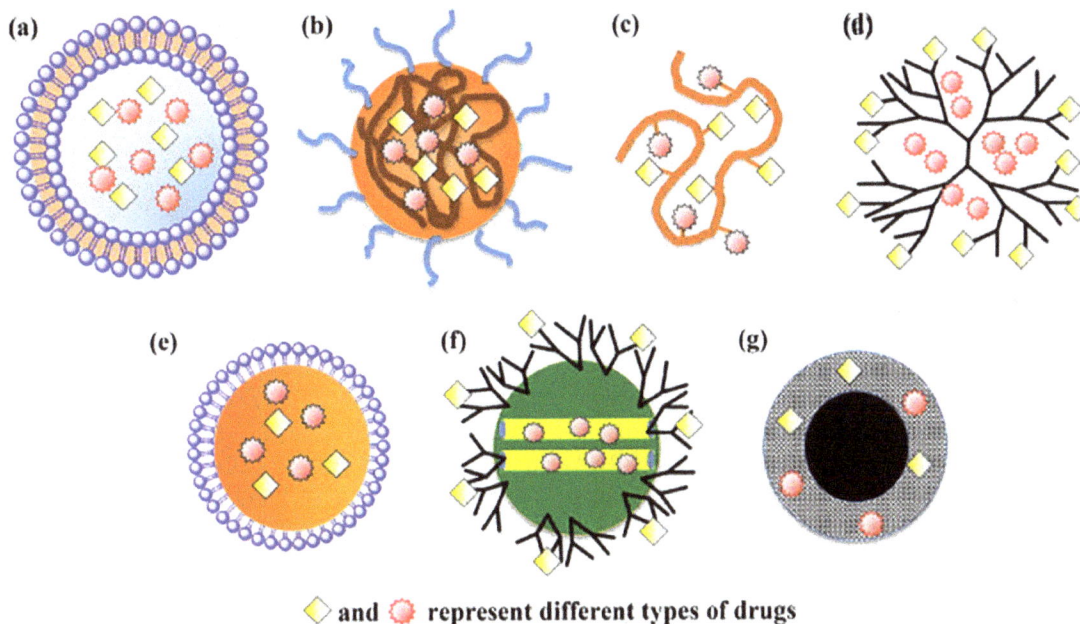

◇ and ◯ represent different types of drugs

FIGURE 6.1 Schematic illustration of nanoscale drug carriers used for combinatorial drug delivery: (a) liposome, (b) polymeric micelle, (c) polymer–drug conjugate, (d) dendrimer, (e) oil nanoemulsion, (f) mesoporous silica nanoparticle, and (g) iron oxide nanoparticle.

to normal tissues. Many low-molecular-weight anticancer drugs such as paclitaxel, doxorubicin (DOX), and camptothecin have shown improved pharmacokinetic profiles and clinical efficacy following polymer conjugation [32]. Polyethylene glycol, poly (L-glutamic acid), and N-(2-hydroxypropyl) methacrylamide (HPMA) are examples of polymers that have been accepted into clinical practice [33]. Owing to the multivalent functional groups on these polymers, recent research efforts have synthesized conjugates with a combination of drugs to the polymer chains and demonstrated cooperative efficacy [34,35]. Since drugs need to be detached from the polymer conjugates to take effects, it is possible to modify the drug release kinetics through the use of environment- or enzyme-sensitive linkers [34].

6.3.4 Dendrimers

Dendrimers are hyperbranched polymers that are characterized by a central inner core surrounded by layers of repeating units and an outermost layer of multivalent functional groups. The tree-like globular morphology initiates from the core and branches outward in a symmetrical fashion. While the outer functional groups can be coupled with charged polar molecules through electrostatic interactions, the hydrophobic pockets spanning the inside of dendrimers favor the encapsulation of uncharged, non-polar molecules [36]. Despite that dendrimers are in a relatively nascent stage as a drug delivery platform, their unique structural attribute has drawn interest for the concurrent delivery of hydrophobic and hydrophilic therapeutic agents [37].

6.3.5 Other Nanoparticles

Other nanoparticles that have been demonstrated to deliver therapeutic cargoes in combination include oil nanoemulsions [38], mesoporous silica nanoparticles [39], and iron oxide nanoparticles [40,41]. For the oil emulsion, hydrophobic drug mixture is homogenized along with the oil and loaded in the oil phase of the resulting nanoemulsions. In the case of the mesoporous nanoparticles and the iron oxide particles, the inorganic cores are functionalized with additional polymeric matrices to carry multiple drug payloads. A graphical illustration of the different multidrug-loaded nanoparticle platforms can be found in Figure 6.1.

6.4 LIPID-BASED NANOVECTORS FOR SYSTEMIC siRNA DELIVERY

6.4.1 Liposomes/Lipoplexes

Liposomes/lipoplexes have been extensively explored as nonviral vectors for plasmid and siRNA delivery [42]. Lipoplexes are complexes between cationic lipids and nucleic acids (mainly as plasmid DNA) [43]. Although neutral liposomes are more biocompatible than cationic lipids and have superior pharmacokinetics, they have low entrapment efficiency due to the lack of interaction between neutral lipids and anionic polynucleotides during formulation [44]. To increase entrapment efficiency, Landen Jr. et al. developed a method of formulating 1,2-dioleoylsn- glycero-3-phosphatidylcholine- (DOPC-) encapsulated siRNA liposomes that involves dissolving DOPC and siRNA in excess tertiary-butanol in the presence of the nonionic detergent Tween 20 [45]. DOPC-encapsulated siRNA targeting the oncoprotein EphA2 was highly effective in reducing EphA2 expression 48 h after administration of a single dose in an orthotopic model of ovarian carcinoma [45]. Treatment with DOPC-encapsulated siRNA via intravenous or intraperitoneal injections was highly effective in reducing both *in vivo* expression of target genes (e.g., EphA2, FAK, neuropilin-2, or IL-8) and tumor weight in mouse models of different human cancers [45–48]. In 2012, M.D. Anderson Cancer Center initiated a phase I dose-escalation trial for neutral liposome (DOPC) targeting of Eph2 in patients with advanced, recurrent cancer (http://www.clinicaltrials.gov/ct2/show/NCT01591356).

Cationic lipids, such as dioleoyl phosphatidylethanolamine and 1,2-dioleoyl-3-trimethylammonium-propane (DOTAP), form lipoplexes with negatively charged siRNA [44,49]. Cationic liposomes are routinely used for delivery of siRNA or plasmid DNA into mammalian cells *in vitro* [50]. However, surface interactions of cationic liposomes with the tumor cells produce an electrostatically derived binding site-barrier effect, inhibiting further association of the delivery systems with tumor spheroids [51]. In addition, although cationic liposomes efficiently take up siRNA, limited success has been achieved with these systems in *in vivo* gene silencing, probably due to their intracellular stability and resultant failure to release siRNA contents [49]. Finally, the effectiveness of cationic liposomes has been limited by their toxicity. The use of cationic liposomes *in vivo* elicited dose-dependent toxicity and pulmonary inflammation by promoting release of reactive oxygen intermediates [52–54]. This effect was more pronounced with the multivalent cationic liposomes than with the monovalent cationic lipids, such as DOTAP [53].

The coating of liposomes with hydrophilic molecules, such as polyethylene glycol (PEG), and reduced uptake by the reticuloendothelial system (RES) results in enhanced circulatory half-life [55]. In 2006, Santel et al. developed a novel liposomal siRNA formulation based on cationic lipids (siRNA-lipoplex/AtuPLEX), containing neutral fusogenic and PEG-modified lipid components, for improved pharmacokinetics and cellular uptake, and more efficient siRNA release [56,57]. Using this formulation to target endothelia-specific genes, such as CD31 (platelet endothelial cell adhesion molecule-1) or TIE-2, they demonstrated downregulation of the corresponding mRNAs and proteins in mice [57]. Atu027 is a lipoplexed siRNA molecule specifically targeting the expression of protein kinase N3, which has been identified as a downstream effector of the phosphoinositol-3-kinase signaling pathway [58]. Atu027 has been reported to inhibit lymph node metastasis in orthotopic prostate and pancreatic cancer mouse models and to inhibit hematogenous metastasis to the target organ lung in various mouse lung metastasis models [58,59]. Silence Therapeutics (London, UK) is performing a phase I trial of Atu027, which was well tolerated up to a dose of 0.180 mg/kg and was not associated with dose-dependent toxicities, in patients with colorectal cancer metastasized to the liver [60]. Dose escalation is

currently being investigated. Using liposomal encapsulation of siRNA nanoparticles, another delivery platform, tauRNAi, has been developed by Marina Biotech (Bothell, WA, USA). This drug is in the preclinical stage for hepatocellular carcinoma [61].

6.4.2 STABLE NUCLEIC ACID LIPID PARTICLES AND LIPIDOIDS

Solid lipid-based systems have been developed as alternatives to emulsions, liposomes, microparticles, and polymeric nanoparticles for systemic delivery of siRNA and include stable nucleic acid lipid particles (SNALPs) and cationic solid-lipid nanoparticles [62,63]. Jeffs et al. developed a new "spontaneous vesicle formation" method for the preparation of rapid and reproducible stabilized plasmid lipid particles for nonviral, systemic gene therapy [64]. Using this controlled, stepwise dilution method, Morrissey et al. developed SNALPs, which are PEG-conjugated lipid nanoparticles comprised of siRNA encapsulated inside a lipid bilayer of neutral lipids and PEG-lipid fusion regulators [62]. Stabilized siRNA targeting hepatitis B virus (HBV) RNA was incorporated into SNALPs and administered by intravenous injection into mice carrying replicating HBV, resulting in reduction of the level of HBV DNA. Furthermore, reductions were seen in serum HBV DNA for up to 6 weeks with weekly dosing. Zimmermann et al. have demonstrated that intravenous injection of ApoB-targeting siRNAs encapsulated in SNALPs resulted in significant dose-dependent silencing *ApoB*mRNA in the livers of both mice and nonhuman primates [65]. A single administration of 2.5 mg/kg SNALP-formulated siRNA was well tolerated and reduced *ApoB* mRNA expression in the liver by up to 90%, lasting for 11 days at the highest siRNA dose. SNALP-formulated siRNA targeting the essential cell-cycle proteins polo-like kinase 1 (PLK1) and kinesin spindle protein (KSP) showed potent antitumor efficacy in both hepatic and subcutaneous tumor models [66]. Tekmira Pharmaceuticals Corporation (Burnaby, BC, Canada) initiated a phase I trial of SNALP-encapsulated siRNA targeting PLK1 (TKM 080301) in December 2010 (http://www.clinicaltrials.gov/ct2/show/NCT01262235). This is a dose-escalation trial conducted at multiple clinical centers, designed to determine TKM 080301 safety, tolerability, and pharmacokinetics in adult patients with solid tumors or lymphomas that are refractory to standard therapy or for whom there is no standard therapy. Alnylam Pharmaceuticals (Cambridge, MA, USA) has developed SNALP-formulated siRNAs targeting vascular endothelial growth factor (VEGF) and KSP in ALN-VSP02, the first dual-targeted siRNA drug. In April 2009, a phase I dose-escalation trial was initiated (http://www.clinicaltrials.gov/ct2/show/NCT00882180). Interim data from pharmacodynamic measurements provided preliminary evidence of clinical activity for the treatment of advanced solid tumors with liver involvement. Additional results from the initial 28 patients in the first six-dose cohorts demonstrated that ALN-VSP02 was generally well tolerated at the highest dose (1.25 mg/kg) [67]. The study has not yet reached a maximum tolerated dose and the trial continues to enroll patients in a dose-escalating manner. In another phase I trial, several patients with stable disease have advanced to a multicenter, open label, extension study to collect long-term safety data (http://www.clinicaltrials.gov/ct2/show/NCT01158079).

Lipidoid nanoparticles are lipid-like delivery molecules comprised of cholesterol and PEG-modified lipids specific for delivery of specific siRNA [67]. To improve SNALP-mediated delivery, Akinc et al. developed a new chemical method to allow rapid synthesis of a large library of lipidoids and tested their efficacy in siRNA delivery [68]. The leading candidate, the 98N12-5 lipidoid-based siRNA formulation, showed 75%–90% reduction in ApoB or FVII factor expression in hepatocytes in nonhuman primates and mice [68,69]. This formulation facilitated gene silencing at orders-of-magnitude lower doses of siRNA than those required by the original SNALP formulation, resulting in reduced toxicity [70].

6.5 COMBINATORIAL NANOPARTICLES AGAINST MULTIDRUG RESISTANCE IN CANCER

Many combinatorial nanoparticle formulations have been successful in reversing MDR in *in vitro* and *in vivo* cancer models through co-delivering combinations of chemosensitizing agents and chemotherapy agents [71,72]. Among the many cellular mutations that diminish the effectiveness of anticancer drugs, the over-expression of multidrug transporters and the altered apoptosis are the two underlying mechanisms through which cancer cells acquire resistance to multiple structurally and mechanistically different drugs [13,73]. In transporter-dependent MDR, an upregulated level of transmembrane drug efflux pumps under the ATP-binding cassette (ABC) superfamily actively export drugs to reduce their effective intracellular concentration. These transporters act on a variety of anticancer drugs. For instance, Pglycoprotein (P-gp), an ATP-driven pump over-expressed in liver, ovarian, pancreatic, and gastrointestinal cancers [74–80], can readily pump out DOX, vinblastine, and paclitaxel. In apoptotic pathway-dependent MDR, pro-survival mutations such as the deregulation of BCL2 and nuclear factor kappa B (NF-κB) enable cancer cells to tolerate drug-inflicted injuries and significantly decrease their apoptotic response. To this date, a number of chemosensitizers have been developed to inhibit drug-efflux pumps and to restore the proper apoptotic signaling. In addition, the emergence of siRNA has made possible the silencing of MDR-related genes. Nanoparticles that combine these MDR modulators and cytotoxic drugs have the ability to sensitize drug resistant cancer cells to the chemotherapeutic payloads. Herein we highlight different combinatorial nanoparticle formulations against the effect of MDR in cancer.

6.5.1 COMBINATION OF EFFLUX PUMP INHIBITORS WITH CHEMOTHERAPEUTICS

Compared to small-molecule drugs which diffuse through cellular membrane and are susceptible to transmembrane multidrug transporter, nanoparticles carry a high dose of drug payloads that can overwhelm the drug efflux kinetics. In addition, since nanoparticles enter cells through endocytosis, they shuttle the drug cargoes away from the drug-pump-spanning cellular membrane [74–76]. Building upon these inherent advantages, therapeutic nanoparticles containing a combination of cytotoxic drugs and efflux pump inhibitors, such as cyclosporine, verapamil, and tariquidar, have further aided the suppression of MDR effect. These co-encapsulation strategies also address the poor pharmacokinetics and high systemic toxicity frequently associated with these chemosensitizers [81,82].

The first attempt to co-deliver chemosensitizer with chemotherapeutics in a single nanocarrier was a polyalkylcyanoacrylate nanoparticle system loaded with P-gp-inhibiting cyclosporin A (CyA) and DOX [83]. Against a DOX-resistant leukemia cell line (P388), Soma et al. showed that the co-encapsulation of CyA and DOX results in a nearly 2-fold increase in toxicity as compared to DOX-only nanoparticles. It should also be noted that the enhanced efficacy was not observed when free CyA was applied with the DOX-only nanoparticles. The finding suggests that nanoparticle-coordinated delivery of two bioactive agents is essential for their cooperative activity.

MDR reversion through the combination of P-gp modulators and cytotoxic drugs has also been achieved with oil nanoemulsions [38], polymeric micelles [84], and liposomes [38,85–87]. A summary of these combinatorial nanoparticles can be found in Table 6.1. Some of these nanoparticle formulations have shown improved efficacy against drug-resistant tumors *in vivo*. Liang et al., for instance, prepared a stealth liposomal formulation combining vincristine and quinacrine and tested it against a murine model bearing the MDR K562 human chronic myelogenous leukemia. The study showed superior efficacy by the combinatorial liposomal formulation as opposed to the cocktail administration of the free drugs. The quinacrine was found to restore the MDR cells' response to vincristine, as was confirmed by the increased activity of caspase 9 and 3 [87].

Surface functionalization of nanoparticles with cancer-targeting ligands has been proposed to prevent the MDR modulators from affecting normal tissues. Since multidrug-binding proteins play a key role in regulating the exchange of molecules at the intestinal lining and blood brain barrier [93,94], their molecular substrates and inhibitors can greatly affect physiological functions. Against healthy tissues, MDR modulators can disrupt cellular metabolisms and inflict injuries. Cardiotoxicity, nephrotoxicity, and neurotoxicity, for instance, are among the common side effects of these modulator compounds [95]. In an aim to reduce systemic exposure of drug-efflux-pump blockers, Wu et al. prepared a transferrin-conjugated liposome containing

TABLE 6.1

Selected Examples of Combinatorial Nanoparticle Formulations Containing Chemotherapeutics and Chemosensitizers

Nanocarrier Platform	Chemotherapeutic	Chemosensitizing Agent	Indication	Status[a]	References
Liposome	Topotecan	Amlodipine	Leukemia	*In vivo*	[86]
Liposome	Vincristine	Quinacrine	Leukemia	*In vivo*	[87]
Liposome	Paclitaxel	Tariquidar	Ovarian cancer	*In vitro*	[85]
Liposome (transferrin-conjugated)	Doxorubicin	Verapamil	Leukemia	*In vitro*	[84]
Liposome (cationic)	Doxorubicin	MRP-1 and BCL2 siRNA	Lung cancer	*In vitro*	[88]
Cationic core-shell nanoparticle	Paclitaxel siRNA	BCL2-siRNA	Breast cancer	*In vitro*	[89]
PLGA-PEG nanoparticle	Vincristine	Verapamil	Breast cancer	*In vitro*	[90]
PLGA-PEG-biotin nanoparticle	Paclitaxel	Tariquidar	Various cancer types	*In vivo*	[91]
PLA-PEG-biotin nanoparticle	Paclitaxel	P-gp siRNA	Various cancer types	*In vivo*	[92]
Polyalkylcyanoacrylate nanoparticle	Doxorubicin	Cyclosporine A	Various cancer types	*In vitro*	[83]
Oil nanoemulsion	Paclitaxel	Curcumin	Ovarian cancer	*In vitro*	[38]
Mesoporous silica nanoparticle	Doxorubicin	BCL2-siRNA	Ovarian cancer	*In vitro*	[39]

[a] *In vivo* refers to live animal-based tests and *in vitro* refers to cultured cell-based studies.

both DOX and verapamil. In addition to achieving MDR reversal, the ligand-functionalized formulation showed faster accumulation *in vitro* to a drug-resistant leukemia cell line (K562) and demonstrated higher degree of MDR reversal as compared to the non-functionalized liposomal combination [84]. In a different study, Patil et al., using a biotin-conjugated PLGA nanoparticle co-encapsulating paclitaxel and tariquidar, also showed that the nanoparticle functionalized with the breast-cancer-targeting moiety not only improves tumor reduction *in vivo* but also improves the overall survival of the inoculated mice as compared to the non-targeted formulations [91]. The targeted, concurrent delivery of chemosensitizers and chemotherapeutics promises a safer and more effective approach in treating MDR tumors.

6.5.2 Combinations of Pro-apoptotic Compounds with Chemotherapeutics

In response to MDR associated with the alterations of the apoptosis pathways, therapeutic nanoparticles have been co-encapsulated with compounds that repair the dysfunctional apoptotic signaling. One example of such pro-apoptotic compound is ceramide, which is produced by cells under environmental stress and serves as a key messenger in programmed cell death. Some MDR cancer cells hinder apoptosis initiation by over-expressing glucosyl-ceramide synthase that converts ceramide to its inactive, glycosylated form. To address the ceramide metabolism, a polymeric micelle formulation based on poly(ethylene oxide)-poly(epsilon caprolactone) (PEO-PCL) was prepared to co-deliver exogenous ceramide and paclitaxel [96]. Against a paclitaxel-resistant ovarian cancer cell line (SKOV-3TR), the combinatorial formulation was found to raise paclitaxel sensitivity of the MDR cells to the same level as non-MDR cells. Combination with ceramide showed a

100-fold increase in efficacy as compared to paclitaxel-only nanoparticles. Caspase activity study and western blotting results suggest that the co-delivery of ceramide encouraged programmed cell death in the MDR cells. In a more recent study, the combinatorial formulation of ceramide and paclitaxel was found to show improved efficacy against MDR tumors *in vivo* using a PLGA nanoparticle system [97]. The co-delivery system was shown to increase apoptotic activity and tumor reductions in murine models without significant liver toxicity or reduction in white blood cell count.

Other combinatorial nanoparticle formulations have been prepared to combat drug resistance caused by the over-expression of NF-κB. These nuclear factors have been implicated to the production of anti-apoptotic proteins as well as to paclitaxel resistance [98]. A chitosan-based nanoparticle system was prepared to co-deliver DOX with a NF-κB inhibitor, pyrrolidine dithiocarbamate (PDTC) [99]. In addition to combination therapy, the chitosan-based nanoparticle also employs active targeting and stimuli-responsive drug release kinetics to maximize DOX retention and sensitivity in the MDR cancer cells. Another example of NF-κB inhibitor, curcumin, which also blocks multidrug transporters, has also been co-delivered with chemotherapeutics in oil nanoemulsions and in PLGA nanoparticles [38,100]. A summary of combinatorial nanoparticles containing pro-apoptotic compounds and chemotherapeutics can be found in Table 6.1.

6.5.3 Combinations of MDR-Targeted siRNA with Chemotherapeutics

The advancement in siRNA technology and its application to cancer treatment promise highly specific therapeutic options that silence target genes [101]. MDR-targeted siRNA have been constructed to target the likes of MRP1 (a MDR-associated protein) and BCL2 (an anti-apoptotic protein) genes, but their therapeutic application is hindered by the rapid degradation of siRNA molecules in serum, lack of cellular target selectivity, and poor cellular uptake [102]. Several studies have used nanoparticles to deliver siRNA both *in vitro* and *in vivo* and showed enhanced gene transfection through nanoparticle-mediated cellular uptake [103–105]. Such enhancement can be attributed to the improvements in siRNA stability and pharmacokinetic profiles. In investigating the effect of nanoformulations on siRNA delivery, Gao et al. showed that unmodified siRNA are cleared from the blood circulation through plasma degradation and renal excretion within minutes of intravenous injection. In a pegylated liposomal formulation, however, the clearance was much slower, with 30% of the siRNA remaining in the blood after 30 min [106]. More recently, Paolo et al. also demonstrated that a ligand-functionalized liposomal formulation significantly improved the pharmacokinetics of siRNA, retaining ~20% of the siRNA content 24 h following the administration. The attachment of targeting ligands to these nanoparticles also offered the opportunity to address the off-targeting issue in siRNA delivery [107]. Even though siRNA as a therapeutic agent is still in the developmental stage, early success in nanoparticle-based siRNA transfection has led many to explore the feasibility of combining chemotherapeutics and siRNA using a variety of nanocarrier platforms (Table 6.1).

A poly ((N-methyldietheneamine sebacate)-co-((cholesteryl oxocarbonylamido ethyl) methyl bis(ethylene) ammonium bromide) sebacate) (P(MDS-co-CES)) nanoparticle formulation was among one of the earlier efforts in demonstrating the potential of combinatorial nanoparticle co-delivering chemotherapeutics and siRNA [89]. The cationic amphiphilic copolymer self-assembled into a core-shell structured nanoparticle with a positive surface charge. The negatively charged, BCL2-targeted siRNA readily formed a complex with the nanocarrier through electrostatic interaction. The resulting paclitaxel- and siRNA-loaded nanoparticle was successful in down-regulating the expression of BCL2 and more effective against a breast cancer cell line (MDA-MB-231) *in vitro* as compared to the individual agents and their cocktail mixture. Using another polymeric nanoparticle formulation, Patil et al. later demonstrated the *in vivo* application of paclitaxel-siRNA combination against a mouse model of drug-resistant tumor. An siRNA sequence aiming to knock down the expression of P-gp drug transporter was complexed to a PLGA-PEI (polyethyleneimine) copolymer [92]. It was found that the paclitaxel-siRNA nanoparticle resulted in significantly higher paclitaxel retention in the MDR cancer cells. A targeted formulation of the combinatorial nanoparticle showed observable reduction of the drug resistant tumor xenograft, which had little response to paclitaxel without the MDR gene silencing.

Liposomes, dendrimers, and silica nanoparticles are among the other nanoparticle formulations used to deliver combinations of siRNA and chemotherapy drugs. Saad et al. prepared a cationic liposome using positively charged 1,2-dioleoyl-3-trimethylammonium-propane for the co-delivery of MRP1 and BCL2 siRNA in combination with DOX [88]. The formulation suppressed MDR effects by silencing both the drug efflux activity and anti-apoptotic signaling. Generation 3 dendrimers with silsesquioxane cubic core and poly(L-lysine) have been prepared to deliver siRNA-DOX mixture [108]. The dendrimer system, which is also conjugated to an RGD-based tumor-targeting peptide, showed excellent gene silencing and growth inhibition in glioblastoma cells (U87). Inorganic nanoparticles can also be complexed with siRNA upon functionalization with a positively charged outer shell. Mesoporous silica nanoparticles, for instance, have been used to co-deliver MDR-targeted siRNA and DOX, following surface coating with PEI [109] and with amine-terminated dendrimers [39]. Both of these formulations showed resensitization of MDR cancer cells to DOX *in vitro*.

6.6 COMBINATION STRATEGIES AGAINST CLINICAL CANCER DRUG RESISTANCE

While the upregulation of multidrug transporters and altered apoptosis pathways remain the major targets of interest in experimental MDR cancer models, clinical occurrence of cancer drug resistance is usually caused by more complicated and less defined mechanisms. Combinatorial nanoparticles containing multiple cytotoxic drugs with different mechanisms of action are, therefore, commonly adopted in an aim to target the multi-faceted nature of clinical cancer drug resistance. In this section, we highlight the developments that lead to more sophisticated combinatorial nanoparticle designs and enable higher level of tuning in the drug combinations. Selected examples of combinatorial nanoparticles containing multiple cytotoxic drugs can be found in Table 6.2.

6.6.1 COMBINATORIAL NANOPARTICLES CO-ENCAPSULATING HYDROPHOBIC AND HYDROPHILIC DRUGS

Most nanoparticle-based drug combinations are comprised of drug compounds with similar water solubility. Liposomal drug combinations, for instance, typically contain hydrophilic drugs owing to liposome's aqueous core whereas polymeric nanoparticle formulations preferentially carry water-insoluble drugs in their hydrophobic core [113]. The difficulty in co-encapsulating hydrophobic and hydrophilic drugs imposes a major limitation on the possible therapy combinations. To broaden the applicability of combinatorial nanoparticles, Zhang et al. conducted a pioneering work in co-encapsulating hydrophobic and hydrophilic drugs on a polymeric nanoparticle platform [28]. In the study, RNA aptamers were conjugated to the surface of PLGA-PEG polymeric micelles loaded with hydrophobic anticancer drug, docetaxel. The aptamers serve as targeting moieties to prostate cancer cells and at the same time carry the hydrophilic DOX through intercalation. The resulting nanoparticle

TABLE 6.2

Selected Examples of Combinatorial Nanoparticle Formulations Containing Multiple Cytotoxic Drugs

Nanocarrier Platform	Drug Combinations	Indication	Significance	Status	References
Liposome (CPX-351)	5:1 cytarabine and daunorubicin	Acute myeloid leukemia	Ratiometric drug loading with synergistic ratio maintained *in vivo*	Phase II	[110]
Liposome (CPX-1)	1:1 irinotecan and floxuridine	Colorectal cancer	Ratiometric drug loading with synergistic ratio maintained *in vivo*	Phase II	[111,112]
PLGA-PEG nanoparticle (aptamer-conjugated)	Cisplatin and docetaxel	Prostate cancer	Hydrophobic and hydrophilic drugs are co-encapsulated with differential drug release	*In vitro*	[27]
PLGA-PEG nanoparticle (aptamer-conjugated)	Doxorubicin and docetaxel	Prostate cancer	Hydrophobic and hydrophilic drugs are co-encapsulated	*In vitro*	[28]
Lipid-polymer hybrid nanoparticle	Doxorubicin and camptothecin	Pancreatic cancer	Adjustable ratiometric drug loading	*In vitro*	[29]
Lipid-coated PLGA nanocell	Combretastatin and doxorubicin	Lung carcinoma and melanoma	Temporally sequenced drug release achieves higher efficacy	*In vivo*	[30]
PLGA-PEG nanoparticle	Combretaastatin and paclitaxel	Lung carcinoma and melanoma	Temporally sequenced drug release achieves higher efficacy	*In vivo*	[31]
HPMA-Gem-Dox	Gemcitabine and doxorubicin	Prostate cancer and various cancer types	Enzyme-labile drug linkers enables differential drug release	*In vivo*	[34]

formulation was able to concurrently deliver DOX and hydrophobic docetaxel to the targeted cancer cells.

Chemical modifications have also been employed to improve drug molecules' compatibility with carrier platforms. Kolishetti et al., for example, conjugated hydrophilic cisplatin to a polylactide (PLA) derivative and co-encapsulated the resulting prodrug with docetaxel in PLGA nanoparticles [27]. The conjugated cisplatin drug detaches from the hydrophobic PLA chain and releases from the polymeric core upon intracellular reduction. The combinatorial nanoparticle formulation of the two mechanistically distinct anticancer drugs showed higher toxicity in prostate cancer than single-drug-loaded nanoparticles. Applying the same principle in modifying drugs' solubility profiles, Aryal et al., chemically modified hydrophilic gemcitabine to enable its co-encapsulation with paclitaxel in a lipid-coated PLGA nanoparticle system [26]. But, instead of modifying the hydrophilic compound with a hydrophobic polymer derivative, Aryal et al. covalently joined gemcitabine to the hydrophobic drug with a hydrolyzable linker. This approach yielded a water-insoluble drug–drug conjugate that enabled the uniform loading of the two drug species. The conjugate was readily hydrolyzed in mildly acidic condition and the dual-drug-load nanoparticle showed strong toxicity against a human pancreatic cancer cell line (XPA3).

6.6.2 COMBINATORIAL NANOPARTICLES WITH PRECISE RATIOMETRIC DRUG LOADING

Drug-to-drug ratio has been found to govern the efficacy of combination treatments. Multiple studies suggest that the degree of synergism and antagonism of a combination therapy is highly dependent on the relative concentrations between the combined drugs [114,115]. By unifying the pharmacokinetics of their cargoes, combinatorial

nanoparticles open the avenue to co-delivering multiple drugs at a predetermined ratio that maximizes the combination efficacy. Currently, dual-drug liposomes with precise molar ratios have been prepared, and their superiority over traditional combination therapy are highlighted by the clinical trials of CPX-351, a 5:1 cytarabine and daunorubicin formulation for acute leukemia treatment [22,116,117], and CPX-1, a 1:1 irinotecan and floxuridine formulation for colorectal cancer treatment [111]. These liposomes demonstrate the ability to maintain the synergistic drug ratios *in vivo* and are more effective than the cocktail administration of the free drugs. In preparing these fixed-ratio, dual-drug liposomes, the empty liposomal carriers are incubated with individual drug solution. Incubation conditions such as liposome-to-drug ratio, solvent, temperature, and incubation time are carefully monitored to encapsulate the desirable concentration of drugs [118].

In polymeric nanoparticles, drug co-encapsulation through noncovalent physical entrapment leads to batch-to-batch variability in drug concentrations. In response to this issue, Aryal et al. devised a strategy to enable consistent and controllable ratiometric drug loading by covalently attaching drugs to polymer chains with uniform length and structure [29]. The polymer conjugation provides a predominant hydrophobicity to overwhelm the drugs' intrinsic solubility. As a proof-of-concept, DOX and camptothecin (CPT) were used to synthesize polymer conjugates with uniform molecular weight. The lipid-coated polymeric nanoparticles prepared from different mixtures of the two drug–polymer conjugates showed consistent size distribution. More importantly, the final loading yield of DOX and CPT follows the same molar ratio as the drug–polymer conjugates used during the nanoparticle preparation. The study demonstrated that the combinatorial nanoparticles were more potent than the cocktail mixture of the single-drug-loaded nanoparticles. The drug–polymer conjugation approach could be applied to other drug types and paves the road to the facile assembly of ratiometrically controlled multidrug-loaded nanoparticles.

6.6.3 COMBINATORIAL NANOPARTICLES WITH TEMPORALLY SEQUENCED DRUG RELEASE

The effect of temporally sequenced drug release is most clearly found in a lipid-coated PLGA nanoparticle system developed by Sengupta et al. that combines an antiangiogenic factor, combretastatin, with DOX [30]. In this formulation, the antiangiogenic agent is loaded in the lipid coatings and has much faster release kinetics than the polymer-conjugated DOX. The system takes advantage of the physiology of tumors, whose rapid, uninhibited growth relies on the nutrients supplied by newly formed blood vessels. Once the nanoparticles reach the tumor target, the fast-released combretastatin shuts off the surrounding vessels, enclosing the DOX-encapsulated nanoparticles within the tumor. As compared to a liposomal formulation of combretastatin and DOX, which lacks the sequenced drug release, the lipid-coated PLGA nanoparticle showed superior efficacy and lower systemic toxicity in murine models bearing Lewis lung carcinoma and B16/F10 melanoma. The same treatment philosophy was also applied in a PEG–PLA formulation in which combretastatin was physically entrapped and paclitaxel was covalently attached to the polymeric core. This therapeutic strategy that quarantines and kills tumors from the inside out presents a unique advantage of nanoparticle-based combination therapy [31].

Combinatorial nanoparticles with temporally sequenced drug release also promise better-tailored treatments that optimally deliver the biochemical agents at the appropriate cellular stage. For drug combinations with different action mechanisms, sequencing is particularly important to the drugs' cooperative effect. Many chemotherapeutics are most potent in specific cell cycles, and, therefore, improper sequencing could lead to unintended cell cycle arrest and diminish response to the subsequent drug [119]. Currently, several combinatorial nanoparticle formulations have shown differential drug release kinetics among their drug cargoes [27,28,34]. While further investigations are warranted to examine the effect of sequenced drug release on the cellular level, these nanoparticle designs could open the door to more precise multimodal targeting against molecular pathways of cancer cells.

6.7 GOLD NANOPARTICLES RADIOSENSITIZATION EFFECT IN RADIATION THERAPY OF CANCER

In the recent years, application of nanoparticles in diagnosis and treatment of cancer has been the issue of extensive research. Among these studies some have focused on the dose enhancement effect of gold nanoparticles (GNPs) in radiation therapy of cancer. On the other hand, some studies indicated energy dependency of dose enhancement effect, and the others have studied the GNP size effect in association with photon energy. However, in some aspects of GNP-based radiotherapy, the results of recent studies do not seem very conclusive in spite of relative agreement on the basic physical interaction of photoelectric between GNPs and low-energy photons. The main idea behind the GNP dose enhancement in some studies is not able to explain the results especially in recent investigation on cell lines and animal models radiation therapy using GNPs.

Nanoparticles are defined as microscopic particles between 1 and 100 nm, but definitions including particles of up to 1 µM have also been reported [120]. In cancer treatment they have provided better penetration ability for substances used for therapy and diagnosis with lower risk compared to conventional drugs [121,122]. Nanoparticle distribution is influenced by different parameters, like size and their ability to use cancerous cells features for own inactivation [123]. Radiation therapy with ionizing radiations including X-rays, gamma rays, and high energy particles is employed extensively for treatment of almost all types of solid tumors. Unfortunately, ionizing radiations do not discriminate between cancerous and normal cells. Thus, normal tissue damage is still the dose-limiting factor that diminishes tumor-cell eradication in radiation therapy. Application of tumor-specific nanoparticles in radiation therapy has aimed to improve the radiation therapy outcomes by inducing more toxicity for tumors and less for normal tissues. Among various nanoparticles, preclinical studies have reported gold nanoparticles' (GNPs) radiosensitization effect in conjunction with different photon beams [124–128]. Although Monte Carlo simulations of GNPs have demonstrated physical dose enhancement of about 60% for low-energy photons of ^{192}Ir brachytherapy sources and also X-rays in kilovoltage range [129], the biological study of Jain et al. found comparable sensitization effect at kilovoltage and megavoltage X-ray energies [130]. It was suggested that physical dose enhancement based on increased X-ray absorption could not be the main mechanism of sensitization. However, it should be noted that the used GNP dimensions have been different in these studies. In other words, in the MC study GNPs with diameter of 100 nm were used, while in the biological study, the diameter of 1.9 nm were used.

In the pioneering study of Hainfeld et al., a GNP with the diameter of 1.9 nm was injected intravenously into mammary tumor-bearing mice in combination with 250 kVp X-ray [125]. Results showed a 86% 1-year survival for new method compared to 20% for X-rays alone. Another study was conducted by Chang et al. on melanoma tumor-bearing mice using 13 nm GNP in conjunction with a single dose of 25 Gy of 6 MeV electron beam [124]. It resulted in significant reduction in tumor volume compared to a control group. Additionally, the number of apoptotic cells in GNP plus irradiation animals was two times higher than irradiation alone.

It is believed that interactions of X-rays and GNP result in the release of photoelectrons from high Z gold atoms as well as generation of auger electrons. The range of these electrons is very short with relative to photons, and a pronounced energy is deposited in cells containing GNP or in direct proximity to gold atoms.

The controversial results concerning GNP radiosensitization could be originated from the differences in performed investigations in terms of key parameters including GNP shape, size, concentration and type of cell lines, and radiation energy and type. To address the problem, the affecting parameters in GNP X-ray radiosensitization were comprehensively evaluated by Burn et al. The most efficient factors were found to be large-sized GNP, high molar concentration and 50 KeV photons with possible dose enhancement factor of 6 [123].

In the present sections, the principles behind the GNP radiosensitization will be discussed, and the results of the related studies will be reviewed. In the present sections the results of the available reports and articles [131] were analyzed and compared, and the final status of the GNP-RT was discussed.

6.8 INTERACTION OF X-RAY AND GAMMA RADIATIONS WITH GNPs

Before clinical application of GNP-based radiation therapy, it is a requisite to comprehend the GNP interactions on the cellular level and its molecular partners in biochemical reactions for further optimizations. On the other hand, the X-ray interaction with high-Z GNP and subsequent mechanisms which lead to dose enhancement should be explained for further applications.

The irradiation stability and cytotoxicity of GNPs for radiotherapy purposes was evaluated by Zhang et al. They found no obvious instability and size variation in spherical GNPs with the diameter of 15 nm following gamma radiation of 2000–10,000 Rontgen. Cytotoxicity results showed that the extremely high concentration of GNP could cause a sharp drop off in K562 cell viability, while the low concentration did not affect the cell viability [132].

Based on the energies of ionizing photons, different types of interactions occur between photons and GNPs. The photoelectric effect is the predominant process for photons with energy from 10 to 500 keV. The result of this process is the production of electrons, characteristic X-ray of gold atoms or auger electrons. In photoelectric interaction between photons and GNPs, a vacancy in a K, L, or M shell following photoelectric absorption results in a de-excitation of the atomic system, either by characteristic X-ray or Auger-electron emission. The relative probability of these de-excitation processes is given by the fluorescence yield. Fluorescence yield is strongly dependent on atomic number (Z), being small for light atoms and large for heavy atoms such as gold.

For photons above 500 keV, the Compton scattering and excitation are observed. The Compton scattering will result in atom re-excitation and production of Compton electrons which leads to subsequent photoelectric effect. There are certain selection rules which prohibit photon emission entirely after atom excitation and phonon emission occurs. In phonon emission, the excitation energy flows into the host lattice as low grade heat. This is referred to as a quenching process. The high energy excitation in gold induces lots of phonons and less photons, because the dominant transition of GNPs is photon–phonon transition processing [128,132].

For photon energies higher than 1.02 MeV, pair production process dominates and results in positron and electron pairs. For all of these interactions, except Compton scattering, the cross section of photon interactions depends strongly on Z, when the photoelectric and pair production effect probabilities are proportional to Z^3 and Z^2 of atoms. Consequently, it is expected that the interaction of X-and γ ray with gold atoms deliver considerable energy GNPs, which are transformed to energetic, free electrons and thermal energy.

6.9 MONTE CARLO MODELING OF GNP DOSE ENHANCEMENT EFFECT

Using the GEANT4MCcode a ^{192}Ir brachytherapy source, BEBIG was simulated and benchmarked against the available published dosimetric data for model validation [129]. Two geometries, including parallel beam geometry and 4π beam geometry, were used for MC simulations. The parallel beams were used to resemble the external beam irradiations using two parallel beams. The GNP with a diameter of 100 nm was uniformly distributed into a nanoparticle region with a grid of 450 nm. Moreover, dose enhancement by a volume of gold–water mixture with the same concentration was also simulated. For two parallel beams with 380 keV photons, the maximum dose enhancement of 28% and 36% were seen for gold nanoparticle and gold–water mixture which lead to 16.2% overestimation for gold–water mixture. However, it should be noted that as photons pass through the nanoparticle region, the dose values fall below those for non-gold case. Additionally, it gets more pronounced for lower energies that have been used in majority of previous studies on GNP dose enhancement effect. Also, the self-absorption of the high atomic region could be a problem in creating a uniform dose distribution for treatments using GNPs. According to the MC simulation for GNPs dose enhancement, the GNPs effect comes mainly from higher photoelectric interactions which are inversely proportional to the photon energy (αE^{-3}). As we know from basic radiation physics, the photoelectric interaction coefficient is significantly raised in energies just above gold's K-edge binding energy, i.e. 80.7 keV. In the study of Zhang et al., they explained the enhancement effect by the fact that as the energy of photoelectrons was about 300 for 380 keV photon, the range of photo electrons was about 85 μm, much longer than the gold diameter of 100 nm. Consequently, the photoelectrons had the chance to deposit their energy in the water surrounding the nanoparticles.

In the study of Cho, the MC method was used to evaluate the dose enhancement effect of GNP-based radiation therapy by 140 kVp X-rays, 4 and 6 MV photon beams, and ^{192}Ir gamma rays [133]. The dose enhancement ratio of 2 was obtained for the 140 kVp X-ray case with gold concentration of 7 mgAu/g tumor assuming no gold outside the tumor. The tumor dose enhancement ratio for the 4 and 6 MV photon beams ranged from about 1% to 7%, depending on the amount of gold within the tumor and photon beam qualities. For the ^{192}Ir case, the dose enhancement ratio of 5%–31%, depending on radial distance and gold concentration, was reported.

In another study by Cho et al. [134] the feasibility of gold nanoparticle-aided radiation therapy (GNRT) using low-energy photons was studied by MC calculations. Brachytherapy sources of 50 kVp X-rays, ^{125}I and ^{169}Yb were used to calculate macroscopic dose enhancement factors (MDEF), defined as the ratio of the average dose in the tumor region with and without the presence of gold nanoparticles during the irradiation of the tumor. A significant tumor dose enhancement of more than 40% was found, using 50 kVp X-rays, ^{125}I, and ^{169}Yb sources and gold nanoparticles. For a tumor loaded with 18 mgAu/g, the respective MDEFs of 116%, 92%, and 108% were reported for ^{125}I, 50 kVp, and ^{169}Yb at the distance of 1.0 cm from the center of the source. Whereas, for the concentration of 7 mg Au/g, it decreased to 68%, 57%, and 44%, respectively, for the same sources. They concluded that GNRT using the clinically used brachytherapy sources is feasible and could be exploited for brachytherapy with low-energy photons, especially with a high dose rate ^{169}Yb source.

6.10 GNP SENSITIZATION IN CELL LINE AND ANIMAL MODELS

In the first study by Hainfeld, GNPs were employed to enhance radiotherapy toxicity for cancerous cells in mice [125]. Mice with subcutaneous breast cancers were divided into three groups. The first one received GNP injection prior to 250 kVp X-ray radiotherapy. The second group received radiation only, and the last group received GNPs only. The 1-year survival rates were found to be 86% for the GNP and radiation group versus 20% for the radiation alone and 0% for the gold alone groups. The increased radiosensitivity was attributed to high-Z radioenhancement by GNPs.

In the study by Chang et al., the increased apoptotic and dose-enhancing effects of GNP in combination with single dose clinical electron beams on tumor-bearing mice were reported [124]. Murine B16F10 melanoma cells lines were cultured and then also transplanted into mice leg. The cell lines and tumor-bearing mice were irradiated with a single dose of 25 Gy using 6 MV electron beam in combination with GNPs. Moreover, the accumulation of GNPs in cell lines and mice were detected and quantized. The cell survival results showed that GNP radiosensitized B16F10 melanoma cells in the colony formation assay meaningfully,

with P value of 0.02. For tumor-bearing mice it was revealed that the tumor growth was retarded more considerably comparing to the control and radiation only group ($P < 0.05$). Additionally, the extent of apoptosis was found (almost two times) higher for the GNP plus radiation group relative to the radiation alone group. They suggested the application of GNP-based radiation therapy with electrons for melanoma treatments. Chang et al. [124] used GNP with an average size of 13 nm to benefit from higher sensitization effect, according to the previous study of Chithrani et al. [135].

In the study of Burn et al., DNA plasmid solution combined with GNP was irradiated to investigate the response of this key molecule for GNP radiation therapy. GNPs with diameters of 8.1, 20.2, 37.5, 74, and 92 and photon effective energies from 15 to 70 keV were used [123]. With a GNP: DNA ratio of 1:5 and 49 keV effective energy, a linear relationship was observed for enhancement factor in terms of loss of supercoiled DNA and GNP diameter. For diameters from 8 to 92 nm, the enhancement factor raised to 3 for the largest GNP diameter in their study.

Zhang et al. studied the enhancement in radiation sensitivity in prostate cancer by gold nanoparticles [127]. Human prostate carcinoma DU-145 cells were exposed to 200 kVp X-rays and 15 nM TGS–GNPs, or 15nM Glucose–GNPs, or GNPs plus irradiation. The cytotoxicity induced by GNPs, irradiation, or GNPs plus irradiation was measured using a standard colorimetric MTT assay. The results indicated that either TGS–GNPs or X-ray induced an inhibition of cell growth by ~14% or 16% individually. However, a combination of TGS–GNPs and X-ray produced an inhibition of cell growth of 30.57%, while the combination of Glucose–GNPs plus X-ray induced an inhibition of cell growth by 46%.

In the *in vitro* study of Kong et al., two functional molecules of GNPs, including cysteamine (AET) and thioglucose (Glu), were synthesized and cell uptake and radiation cytotoxicity enhancement in a breast-cancer cell line (MCF-7) versus a nonmalignant breast-cell line (MCF-10A) were studied. Transmission electron microscopy (TEM) results showed that cancer cells take up functional Glu-GNPs significantly more than naked GNPs. The results showed that these functional GNPs have little or no toxicity to these cells. Different radiations such as 200 kVp X-rays and gamma-rays were applied to radiation therapy of the cells, with and without functional GNPs. The results showed that the radiotherapy in association with GNPs killed significantly more breast-cancer cells compared to those without GNP [136].

6.11 IMPACT OF RADIATION ENERGY

The beam energy is one of the major factors influencing the radiation therapy effectiveness. In radiation therapy of tumors loaded with high-Z elements, the physical concepts of photoelectric interaction has been employed for photon energy selection. In other words, it is physically obvious that the possibility of photoelectric interaction is raised when the photon energy is just above the k-edge of high-Z elements. Additionally, the release of photoelectrons and Auger electrons leads to a great energy deposition in the vicinity of nanoparticles. However, this pure physical concept was not completely realized in practice. Biston et al. used a combination of synchrotron irradiation and cis-diamminedichloroplatinum (II) on rat F98 glioma cells below and above the K-edge of platinum (78.4 keV). Surprisingly, the results were identical for both cases. The suggested reason for such a strange event was that for an incident photon with the energy of K-edge, all the energy is spent to eject K-electron and the photoelectron would not receive enough energy to result in excessive damage to surrounding material.

Another influencing factor which should be taken into account to explain the observed discrepancies is absorption differences between high-Z element and surrounding medium. In Figure 6.2, the variation of relative mass energy absorption coefficient of gold to water is presented. The data was derived from National Institute of Standards and Technology (NIST). As can be seen, the maximum value locates around 40–50 keV, which means that the highest achievable enhancement factor with GNPs could be realized with the photon energy of 40–50 keV. The finding of Burn et al. was in accordance with the theoretical assumption on optimum energy of photons suggested for radiation therapy with GNPs. On the other hand, the application of low energy photons for radiation therapy is associated with the problem of high skin dose and rapid drop off of absorbed dose with depth. In the MeV energies used for the current radiation therapy, the ratio of absorption between gold and water becomes theoretically negligible, as can be seen in Figure 6.2. However, as other studies have shown, the enhancement effect can be seen also with MeV range of photons. In higher energies, the photon interaction with matter produces Compton electrons with a spectrum of energy which have higher absorption coefficient with GNPs

compared to the surrounding biological matter. It can be suggested that some refinement in photon energies and more studies on sensitizing effect of GNPs with higher energy photon may help to overcome the keV range photon problems in radiation therapy with GNPs. Another approach to avoid higher dose to skin with low energy photons is to use GNPs with newly developed miniature X-ray sources which can be inserted into the body and located beside or inside the tumor using laparoscopic and endoscopic techniques [123].

6.12 BIOMEDICAL APPLICATIONS OF GRAPHENE OXIDE (GO)

Graphene oxide (GO) have received considerable attention with respect to their utilization in biomedical applications. However, GO-related safety issues concerning human vasculature are very limited. In these sections, we report for the first time the differential size-related biological effects of GOs on endothelial cells (ECs). Notably, subnanometer- and nanometer-sized GOs induce apoptotic death in ECs via autophagy activation. A molecular mechanism for the GO-induced autophagic cell death through the PLCb3/IP3/Ca^{2+}/JNK signaling axis has been proposed [137]. The findings could provide a better understanding of the GO size-dependent cytotoxicity in vasculature and facilitate the future development of safer biomedical applications of GOs.

GO induces apoptotic cell death in endothelial cells by activating autophagy via calcium-dependent phosphorylation of c-Jun N-terminal kinases. Despite the rapid expansion of the biomedical applications of graphene oxide (GO), safety issues related to GO, particularly with regard to its effects on vascular endothelial cells (ECs), have been poorly evaluated. To explore possible GO-mediated vasculature cytotoxicity and determine lateral GO size relevance, four types of GO have been constructed: micrometer-sized GO (MGO; 1089.9 ± 135.3 nm), submicrometer-sized GO (SGO; 390.2 ± 51.4 nm), nanometer-sized GO (NGO;

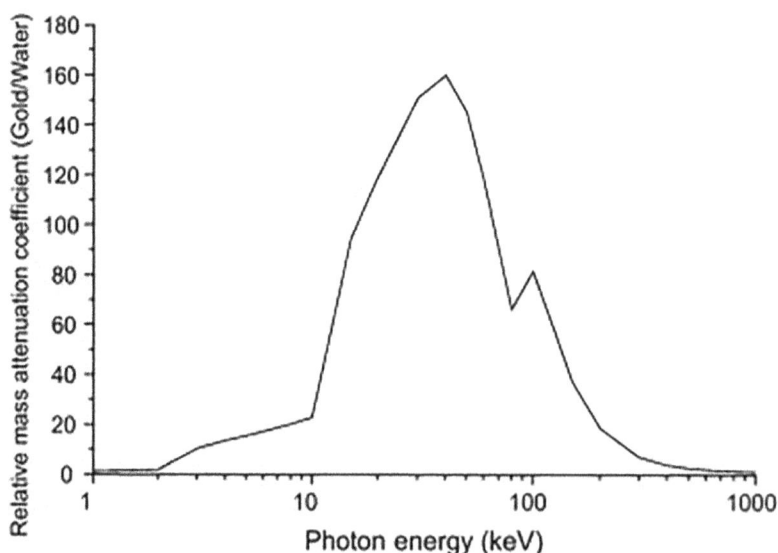

FIGURE 6.2 The variation of relative mass attenuation coefficient of gold to water with photon energy.

65.5 ± 16.3 nm), and graphene quantum dots (GQDs). All types but GQD showed a significant decrease in cellular viability in a dose-dependent manner. Notably, SGO or NGO, but not MGO, potently induced apoptosis while causing no detectable necrosis. Subsequently, SGO or NGO markedly induced autophagy through a process dependent on the c-Jun Nterminal kinase (JNK)-mediated phosphorylation of B-cell lymphoma 2 (Bcl-2), leading to the dissociation of Beclin-1 from the Beclin-1–Bcl-2 complex. Autophagy suppression attenuated the SGO- or NGO-induced apoptotic cell death of ECs, suggesting that SGO- or NGO-induced cytotoxicity is associated with autophagy. Moreover, SGO or NGO significantly induced increased intracellular calcium ion (Ca^{2+}) levels. Intracellular Ca^{2+} chelation with BAPTA-AM significantly attenuated microtubule-associated protein 1A/1B-light chain 3-II accumulation and JNK phosphorylation, resulting in reduced autophagy. Furthermore, it has been found that SGO or NGO induced Ca^{2+} release from the endoplasmic reticulum through the PLC b3/IP3/IP3R signaling axis.

Graphene comprises a two-dimensional, single-atom-thick sheet made of planar sp2-hybridized carbon atoms, with a large surface area on both sides of the planar axis [138]. Graphene is part of a much broader graphene family of nanomaterials (GFNs) that include single-layer graphene, few-layer graphene (2–10 graphene layers), graphene oxide (GO; normally a single layer), reduced GO (normally a single layer), and graphite [139]. In recent years, graphene and its derivatives have received considerable attention with respect to their utilization in biomedical applications such as biosensing [140], drug delivery [141,142], diagnosis [143], bio-imaging, and tissue engineering [144,145]. Such applications are possible because the extremely high specific surface areas of graphene or GO can interact with various biomolecules and colloidal dispersions of individualized graphene sheets or GO can be easily engineered without metallic impurities [146]. In the field of biomedical applications, GO is becoming the favored form of GFN because of its better solubility/dispersibility in water and under physiological conditions than native graphene [139,147,148]. Therefore, the biomedical applications of GO are expected to rapidly expand in the near future. Despite this interest, however, GO-related safety issues concerning human health have not yet been fully evaluated, and more exhaustive nanotoxicological and human safety studies are urgently required.

Recently, several studies were conducted to assess the *in vitro* and *in vivo* toxic effects of GO, but contradictory results were obtained; some studies clearly showed no particular risks, whereas others indicated that GO contributes to health hazards [149–152]. The toxicities and biological responses of GO may depend on intrinsic factors such as lateral size, stiffness, hydrophobicity, surface functionalization, dose administered, and purity [139,153,154]. Among these, lateral size has been reported to differentially regulate cellular responses, and these experimental data provide invaluable clues for the appropriate design and engineering

of GO with the intent to target cells or subcellular organelles. Yue et al. demonstrated that at different lateral sizes (350 nm and 2 μm), GO exhibited different initial cell interaction processes and intracellular compartmentalization in phagocytic cell lines. In addition, cellular responses such as inflammatory cytokine release are dependent on the sizes of GO nanosheets [152]. However, the effect of GO lateral size on cellular responses is poorly understood and must be urgently addressed.

Other studies have shown that GO may induce size- and dose-dependent cytotoxicities in various cell lines, although some results are contradictory with regard to the type of cell, conditions of cell culture, chemical nature of cell surface membranes, and expression of genes in each cell line [149,150]. Currently, the mechanisms of GO-induced cytotoxicity in various cell lines have not been fully elucidated. However, the depletion of mitochondrial membrane potential, which increases the generation of intracellular reactive oxygen species and triggers apoptosis through the activation of the mitochondrial pathway, is considered to be the most important mechanism underlying GO-induced cytotoxicity [155,156]. In addition, recent studies suggested that autophagy is another critical mechanism of GO-induced cytotoxicity; notably, Chen et al. reported the induction of autophagy and toll-like receptor (TLR) signaling, leading to inflammatory responses, in murine macrophage-like RAW264.7 cells after incubation with GO nanosheets [149].

Autophagy is considered to be a cytoprotective process involved in the normal turnover of long-lived proteins and whole organelles to maintain a healthy cellular status [157]. However, recent data strongly demonstrate that autophagy is intimately linked to apoptosis or necrosis and serves both pro-survival and pro-death functions. Autophagy regulation requires an orchestrated interplay between many signaling molecules, including mammalian target of rapamycin (mTOR) kinase, which has the most potent impact on autophagy [158,159]. Once activated, mTOR inhibits autophagy via the phosphorylation of autophagy-related proteins. AMP activated protein kinase (AMPK) activation can lead to autophagy by negatively regulating mTOR [160,161]. The tumor suppressor protein p53 can trigger autophagy by phosphorylating AMPK and further inhibiting the mTOR signaling pathway [160]. Beclin-1 also plays a critical role in autophagosome formation and crosstalk between autophagy and apoptosis [161]. The BH3 domain-mediated binding of Beclin-1 to B-cell lymphoma 2 (Bcl-2) and B-cell lymphoma-extra large (Bcl-XL) inhibits autophagy. However, the c-Jun N-terminal kinase (JNK) 1- or extracellular signal-regulated kinase (ERK)-mediated phosphorylation of Bcl-2 or death-associated protein kinase-mediated phosphorylation of Beclin-1 induces the dissociation of the Beclin-1–Bcl-2/Bcl-XL complex, thus inhibiting autophagy [161–165]. Intracellular calcium ions (Ca^{2+}) can regulate the activation of JNK and the apoptotic signaling pathway [166].

Future biomedical applications of GO nanosheets will require frequent, systemic intravascular administration as GO nanosheet trafficking and systemic translocation are conducted by blood cells in circulation. GO nanosheets should also interact with or traverse the endothelial cell (EC) linings of blood vessels to function in target cells or tissues. Moreover, because blood vessels are critical for maintaining homeostasis in the human body, ECs should be protected from potential damage. Therefore, safety studies involving human primary blood components and ECs should be performed prior to expanding the human use of GO nanosheets. Several studies have reported that GO and its derivatives adversely affect erythrocytes and platelets as well as dendritic cells and monocytes/macrophages [150,151,167,168]. However, the current understanding of GO-mediated cytotoxicity in ECs is limited and warrants further detailed investigation.

The study [137] aimed to evaluate the effects of different-sized GOs on EC cytotoxicity and to elucidate the mechanism(s) underlying GO-mediated cellular damage. We demonstrate for the first time that submicro- and nano-sized GOs induced apoptotic cell death by triggering autophagy in ECs. Calcium-dependent JNK activation, leading to the phosphorylation of Bcl-2 and subsequent dissociation of Beclin-1 from the Beclin-1–Bcl-2 complex, may establish the mechanism of GO-induced autophagy in ECs. The results [137] elucidate the mechanism underlying the size-dependent cytotoxicity of GOs in the vasculature and may facilitate the development of a safer biomedical application of GOs.

6.12.1 CHARACTERIZATION OF GOs

With the exception of graphene quantum dots (GQDs), GOs were prepared [137] at different sizes using a modified version of the methods reported by Hummer, with additional sonication [169]. The size of GOs except GQD was determined by measuring the hydrodynamic diameter of GOs dispersed in aqueous solution. The average size of freshly prepared GOs was 1089.9 ± 135.3 nm; this was further decreased to 390.2 ± 51.4 nm and 65.5 ± 16.3 nm after sonication for 5 and 180 min, respectively. These GOs were referred to as micrometer-sized GO (MGO), submicrometer-sized GO (SGO), and nanometer-sized GO (NGO), respectively. GQDs were prepared by refluxing GO with nitric acid to yield particles ~5 nm in size (similar to the reported size of GQDs produced by Shen et al. [170]) as determined by transmission electron microscopy (TEM); these particles also exhibited distinctive blue fluorescence specific to GQDs. The atomic force microscopic image analyses of four different sized GOs revealed distinctively that they are thin sheet-shaped and single-layered GOs with ~1.0 nm thickness. GOs featured negative zeta-potential values of -22.35 ± 0.71 mV, -35.20 ± 0.81 mV, -31.08 ± 0.49 mV, and -34.35 ± 0.64 mV for GQD, NGO, SGO, and MGO, respectively (Figure 6.3).

These characteristics of GOs suggest hydrophilicity and good dispersion in an aqueous solution, which may be advantageous for the utilization of GOs in biomedical applications such as bioimaging, drug delivery, and phototherapy. Furthermore, the chemical composition of GOs with various size was analyzed by XPS. The C1 s XPS-spectra of GOs except GQD showed the significant peaks at 284.1, 285.5, and 287.0 eV corresponding to C–C = C, C–O, and C = O, respectively, indicating that NGO, SGO, and MGO were partially oxidized. In the spectrum of GQD, the peaks at 286.4 and 289.3 eV corresponding to C–O and C = O, respectively, were significant, indicating that GQD was highly oxidized due to secondary oxidation.

6.12.2 INDUCTION OF APOPTOSIS BY GOs IN ENDOTHELIAL CELLS (ECs)

To determine the biological activities of GOs with different sizes on primary human umbilical vein ECs (HUVECs), cells were treated with different concentrations (5, 10, or 25 µg/mL) of MGO, SGO, NGO, or GQD for 24 h, after which cellular viability was determined. MGO, SGO, and NGO, but not GQD, induced significant decreases in cellular viability in a dose-dependent manner (Figure 6.4a). To clarify whether these GO-mediated decreases in cellular viability resulted from the induction of apoptosis or necrosis, HUVECs were treated with GOs as indicated, stained with fluorescein isothiocyanate (FITC)-conjugated annexin V and propidium iodide (PI), and subjected to flow cytometric analysis. SGO or NGO markedly induced apoptosis in ECs, whereas MGO induced necrosis rather than apoptosis in a dose-dependent manner (Figure 6.4b). In SGO- or NGO treated ECs, caspase-3/7 activation was substantially increased as assessed by the pro-caspase-3 cleavage and caspase-3/7 activity assays (Figure 6.4c). Moreover, pretreatment with z-VAD-fmk, a pan-caspase inhibitor, markedly blocked the SGO- or NGO-mediated decreases in cellular viability and increased caspase-3/7 activity (Figure 6.4d and e), but had no effect on cellular viability in MGO-treated ECs (Figure 6.4d), indicating that SGO or NGO induces apoptotic cell death in ECs.

Increasing evidence has shown that autophagy and apoptosis can act cooperatively, antagonistically, or synergistically to regulate cell fates, depending on the specific cellular context [160,171,172]. To explore whether SGO- or NGO-induced apoptotic cell death in ECs resulted from an interplay between autophagy and apoptosis, we evaluated the effects of GOs on the induction of autophagy in HUVECs. The conversion of microtubule-associated protein 1A/1B-light chain 3 (LC3)-I to LC3-II, a hallmark of autophagy, was markedly increased in ECs treated with SGO or NGO in a dose-dependent manner, but not in cells treated with MGO or GQDs (Figure 6.5a). Autophagy induction was further supported by the following findings: when green fluorescent protein (GFP)–LC3 fusion proteins were expressed in ECs, markedly increased numbers of

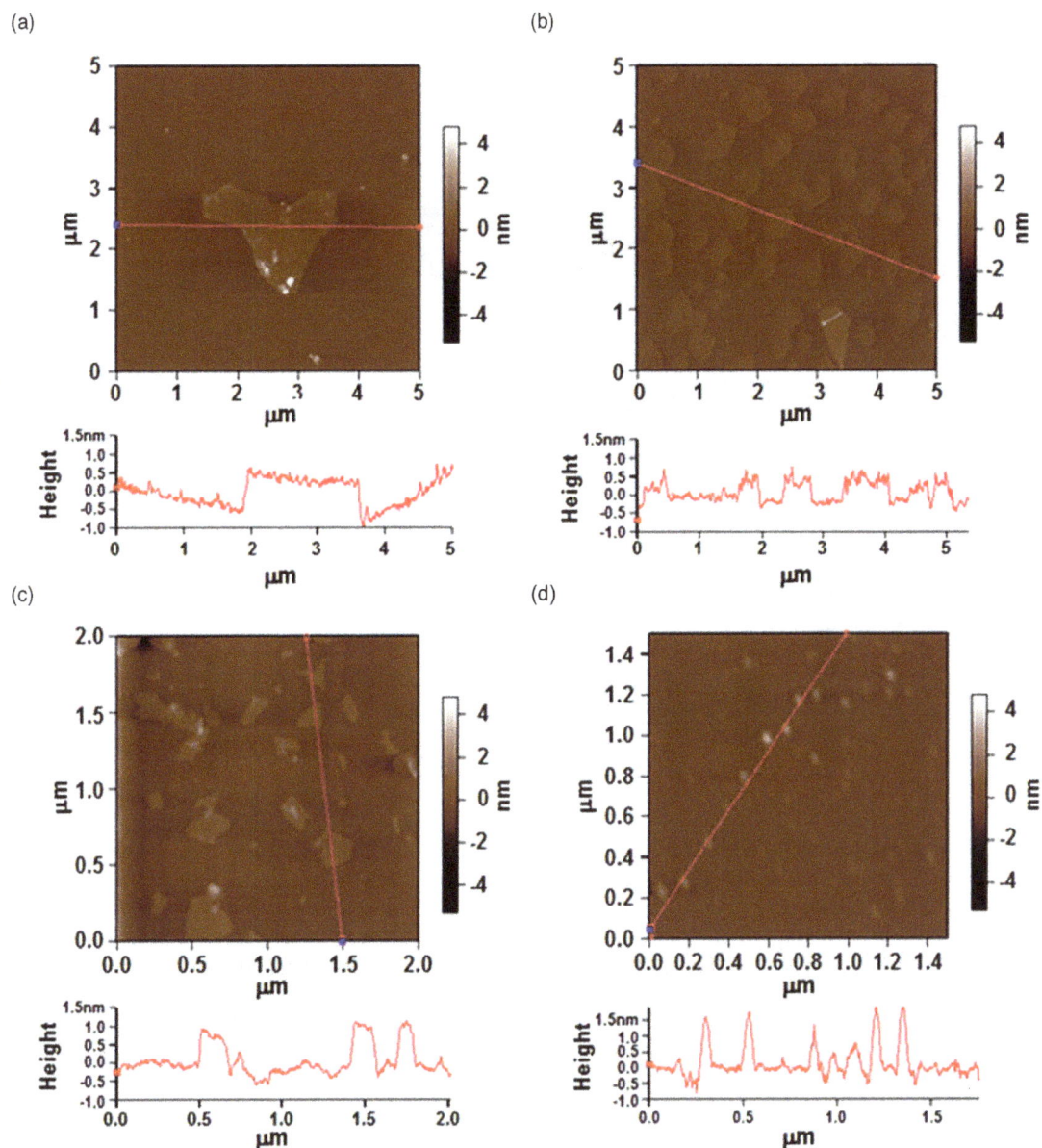

FIGURE 6.3 Atomic force microscopy images and line profiles of four different forms of graphene oxide. (a) Micrometer-sized graphene oxide (GO; MGO), (b) submicrometer-sized GO (SGO), (c) nanometer-sized (NGO), and (d) graphene quantum dots (GQDs).

cytoplasmic punctae, due to GFP–LC3 accumulation in autophagosomes, were observed in SGO- or NGO-treated ECs; in contrast, a ubiquitous, diffuse pattern of cytosolic green fluorescence was observed in control and MGO or GQD-treated ECs (Figure 6.5b).

Although increased numbers of autophagosomes, indicated by the accumulation of LC3-II or increased numbers of GFP-LC3 punctae, suggest the induction of autophagy, this phenomenon is not always indicative of autophagy induction and may represent either enhanced autophagosome generation or a block in both autophagolysomal maturation and the autophagy pathway completion.

Therefore, additional experimental methods are needed to distinguish between the induction of autophagy and inhibition of downstream steps such as the impairment of lysosomal function and/or fusion of autophagosomes with lysosomes [173]. In this context, we performed turnover assays for LC3 and other autophagy substrates, such as p62, to determine whether the overall autophagic flux had been induced. As shown in Figure 6.5c, ECs treated with SGO or NGO in the presence of bafilomycin A1 (Baf A1), a lysosomal inhibitor, exhibited marked increases in LC3-II accumulation, indicating that increased amounts of LC3 in autophagosomes had already been delivered to lysosomes for degradation. In addition, the total cellular expression levels of p62 decreased in a time-dependent manner (Figure 6.5d) in SGO- or NGO-treated ECs, indicating an increase in autophagic activity because p62 is selectively incorporated into the autophagosome through direct binding to LC3 and is efficiently degraded by autophagy [174].

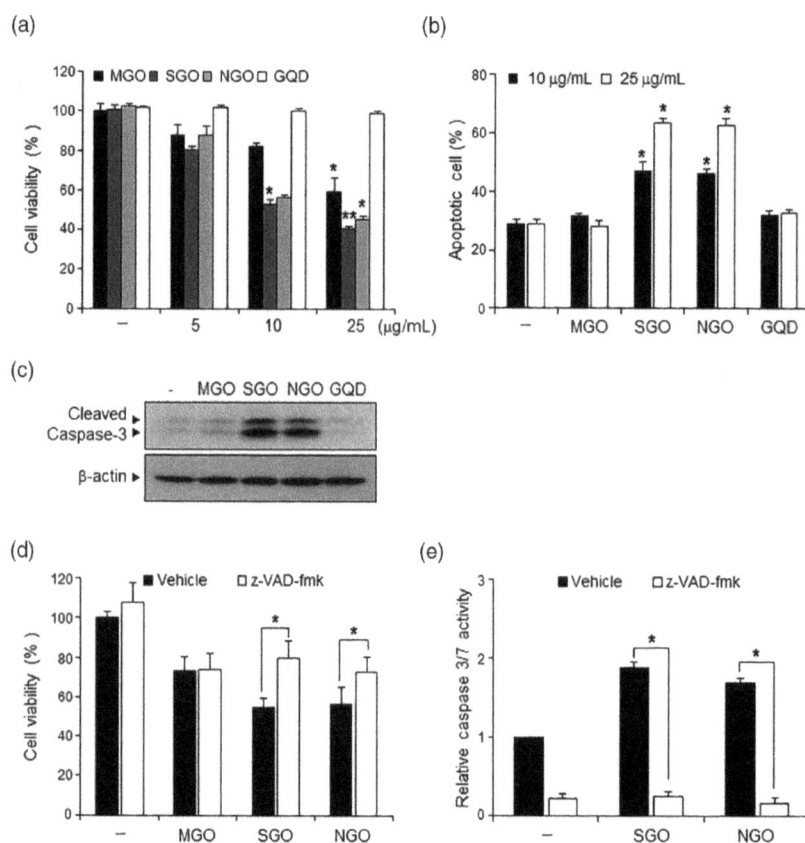

FIGURE 6.4 Graphene oxide-mediated induction of apoptosis in endothelial cells. (a) Assessment of endothelial cell (EC) viability following treatment with GOs. Human umbilical vein ECs (HUVECs) were treated with the indicated concentrations of GOs for 24 h and analyzed using the WST-1 assay. Quantitative data are reported as means ± standard deviations (SD). *$p < 0.005$ or **$p < 0.001$ versus untreated controls. (b) Representative bar graph of the percentages of apoptotic cells (early apoptotic cell: annexin-V+/PI_, late apoptotic cell: annexin-V+/PI+) quantified by flow cytometric analysis. Quantitative data are reported as means ± SD. *$p < 0.005$ versus untreated controls. (c) Western blot analysis of caspase-3 activation in HUVECs following treatment with 25 μg/mL GOs for 24 h. (d and e) Effect of a pan-caspase inhibitor, z-VAD-fmk, on GO-induced apoptotic cell death. HUVECs were pretreated with 100-μM z-VAD-fmk or vehicle for 30 min and subsequently treated with GOs at 25 μg/mL for 24 h. (d) Cell viability was determined using the WST-1 assay. Quantitative data are reported as means ± SD. *$p < 0.005$ versus vehicle control. (e) Relative caspase.

6.12.3 INHIBITION OF AUTOPHAGY ATTENUATES SGO- OR NGO-INDUCED APOPTOTIC CELL DEATH

Next, to examine the role of autophagy in SGO- and NGO-induced apoptotic cell death, HUVECs were treated with SGO or NGO after transfection with LC3-specific small interfering RNA (siRNA). LC3-specific siRNA treatment blocked SGO- or NGO-induced autophagy as determined by the reduced LC3-II accumulation in those cells (Figure 6.6a). This impaired SGO- or NGO-induced autophagy following transfection with LC3-specific siRNA resulted in a significant inhibition of pro-caspase-3 cleavage and caspase-3/7 enzymatic activity (Figure 6.6b and c) and consequent apoptotic cell death as assessed using terminal deoxynucleotidyl transferase-mediated deoxy uridine triphosphate nick end labeling (TUNEL) and trypan blue exclusion assays and in comparison with ECs transfected with control siRNA (Figure 6.6d). Taken together, these results clearly suggest that SGO or NGO promote apoptotic cell death through autophagy induction in ECs.

Recently, cytoplasmic p53 was reported to regulate apoptosis and block autophagy through the inhibition of the AMPK/mTOR-signaling pathway, although the relationship between autophagy and p53 remains complicated [160]. The levels of p53 in GO-treated HUVECs to evaluate the potential involvement of p53 in GO-mediated autophagy induction have been examined next. A marked decrease in p53 protein expression was observed in SGO- or NGO-treated ECs, whereas no significant differences were observed in MGO or GQD-treated ECs (Figure 6.7a), suggesting that a decrease in p53 triggers AMPK activation, thus inhibiting mTOR signaling and inducing autophagy. Unexpectedly, no significant change in AMPK phosphorylation was observed in SGO- or NGO-treated HUVECs, despite the decreased p53 levels in those cells (Figure 6.7b). In addition, treatment with the proteasome inhibitor MG132, in an attempt to recover p53 protein levels, did not affect the GO-mediated induction of autophagy (Figure 6.7b). Collectively, these results indicate that SGO or NGO induce autophagy in a ROS- or AMPK-independent manner.

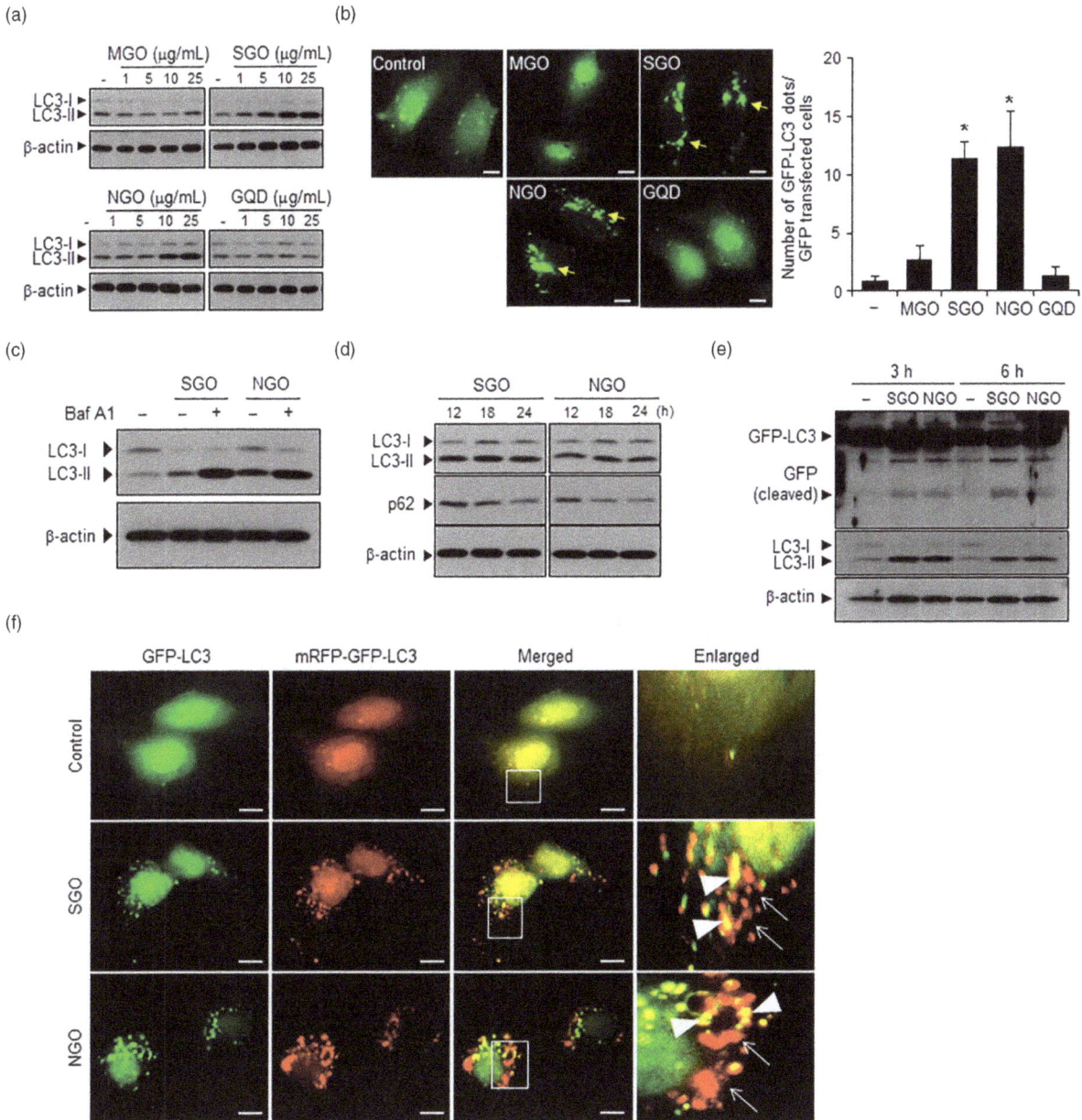

FIGURE 6.5 Induction of autophagy in SGO- or NGO-treated ECs. (a) Western blot analysis of microtubule-associated protein 1A/1B-light chain 3 (LC3)-I to LC3-II conversion in HUVECs treated with GOs at the indicated concentrations for 24 h. (b) Representative images of green fluorescent protein (GFP)–LC3 punctae in HUVECs after treatment with GOs at 25 μg/mL for 12 h (left panel). Scale bar = 10 μm. Bar graph indicates the number of GFP–LC3 dots per transfected cells (right panel). Quantitative data are reported as means ± standard deviations. *$p < 0.005$ versus untreated control. (c) Effect of a lysosomal inhibitor, Bafilomycin A1 (Baf A1), on SGO- or NGO-induced autophagy in HUVECs. HUVECs were pretreated with 10 nM Baf A1 for 30 min and subsequently treated with SGO or NGO for 5 h. LC3-I to LC3-II conversion was detected by Western blot analysis. (d) Western blot analysis of the LC3-I to LC3-II conversion and p62 protein levels in HUVECs treated with 25 μg/mL GOs for the indicated times. (e) Western blot analysis of cleaved GFP fragments from GFP–LC3. HUVECs transiently transfected with a GFP–LC3 plasmid were treated with 25 μg/mL GOs for the indicated times and subjected to Western blotting with an antibody specific for GFP. (f) Representative images of mRFP–GFP–LC3 punctae. Colocalization of GFP and red fluorescent protein (RFP), indicated by yellow dots in the overlapped GFP and RFP images, is visible in autophagosomes (arrowhead), whereas only RFP fluorescence, indicated by red punctae, is observed in autolysosomes (arrow). Scale bar = 10 μm.

Next, it has been determined the effects of GOs on the activation of mitogen-activated protein kinase (MAPK) signaling in ECs. As shown in Figure 6.7c, treatment with SGO or NGO markedly induced the phosphorylation of p38 MAPK and JNKs but not ERKs, whereas MGO had no marked effects on MAPK signaling pathways. The effects of SGO and NGO on autophagy induction in the presence of specific MAPK signaling pathway inhibitors have been

(a)

(b)

(c)

(d)

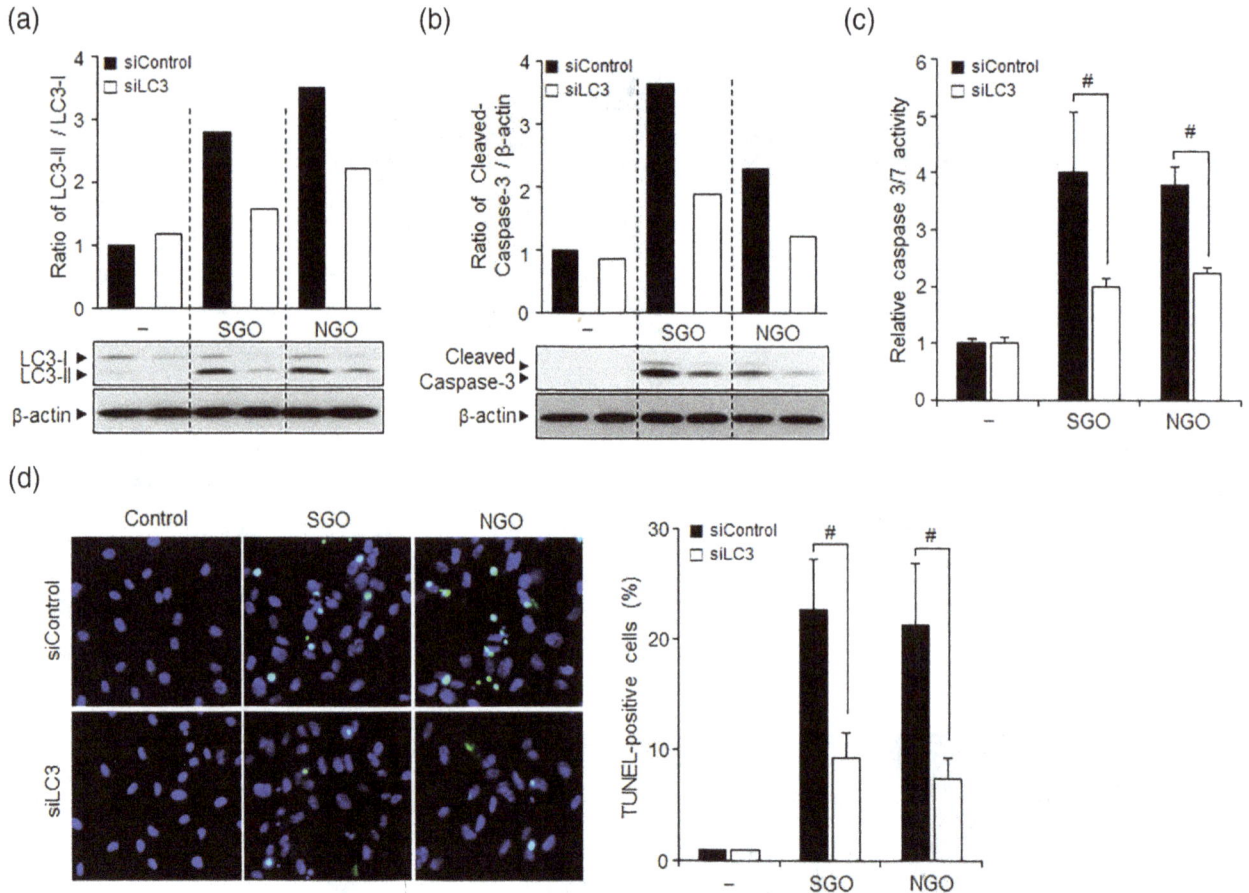

FIGURE 6.6 Inhibition of autophagy attenuates the SGO- or NGO-induced apoptotic cell death. (a) Western blot analysis of LC3-I to LC3-II conversion in HUVECs transfected with LC3-targeted or control siRNA. After 48 h, control or LC3 siRNA-transfected HUVECs were treated with 25 μg/mL SGO or NGO for 5 h. Relative LC3-II to LC3-I ratios are indicated in the graph. Data were quantified using Image J software. (b) Western blot analysis of caspase-3 activation in control or LC3 siRNA-transfected HUVECs with 25 μg/mL SGO or NGO for 24 h. Cleaved caspase-3 band densities were analyzed using Image J software and normalized against b-actin expression. (c) Relative caspase-3/7 activity in control siRNA- or LC3 siRNA-transfected HUVECs. Quantitative data are reported as means ± SD. #$p < 0.01$ versus control siRNA. (d) Terminal deoxynucleotidyl transferase mediated deoxy uridine triphosphate nick end labeling (TUNEL) assay findings were analyzed using fluorescent microscopy (left panel, magnification; ×100). Blue fluorescence indicates DAPI nuclear staining; green fluorescence indicates TUNEL-positive nuclear staining. Bar graph shows the percentages of cells containing fragmented DNA (right panel). Quantitative data are reported as means ± SD. #$p < 0.01$ versus control siRNA.

tested. SGO- or NGO-mediated LC3-II accumulation was significantly attenuated by treatment with the JNK inhibitor SP600125, but not the p38 inhibitor SB203580 (Figure 6.7d). Similarly, the transfection of ECs with JNK-specific siRNA after treatment with SGO or NGO significantly inhibited the accumulation of LC3-II (Figure 6.7e), indicating that SGO- or NGO-induced autophagy is mediated by JNK signaling pathway activation.

Next, The signaling pathways that play critical roles in SGO- or NGO-mediated autophagy induction in ECs have been scrutinized. The core molecular machinery involved in autophagosome formation and the signaling pathways that stimulate autophagy have been studied in detail. Among these, reactive oxygen species (ROS) are considered to be among the most potent regulators of autophagy. Whereas the total Bcl-2 protein level was not affected by GO treatment (Figure 6.8a), GO treatment also affected the interaction between Beclin-1 and Bcl-2 in ECs as assessed using

an immunoprecipitation assay (Figure 6.8b). Similarly, significant decreases in Bcl-2 and Beclin-1 co-localization signals were observed in SGO- and NGO treated ECs relative to controls. An immunofluorescence double co-localization experiment (Figure 6.8c) revealed that these decreases were due to the dissociation of Beclin-1 from the complex, thus suggesting that JNK regulates SGO- or NGO-mediated autophagic activity in ECs through Bcl-2 phosphorylation, leading to the dissociation of Beclin-1 from the Beclin-1–Bcl-2 complex.

To further clarify the role of Beclin-1 in SGO- or NGO-mediated autophagy induction and apoptotic cell death, HUVECs were treated with Beclin-1-specific siRNA, and the effects of SGO and NGO treatment on autophagy and/or apoptosis were examined in these cells. Compared to control ECs, Beclin-1 knockdown reduced LC3-II accumulation after treatment with SGO or NGO (Figure 6.9a). The inhibition of autophagy in ECs in response to Beclin-1 depletion

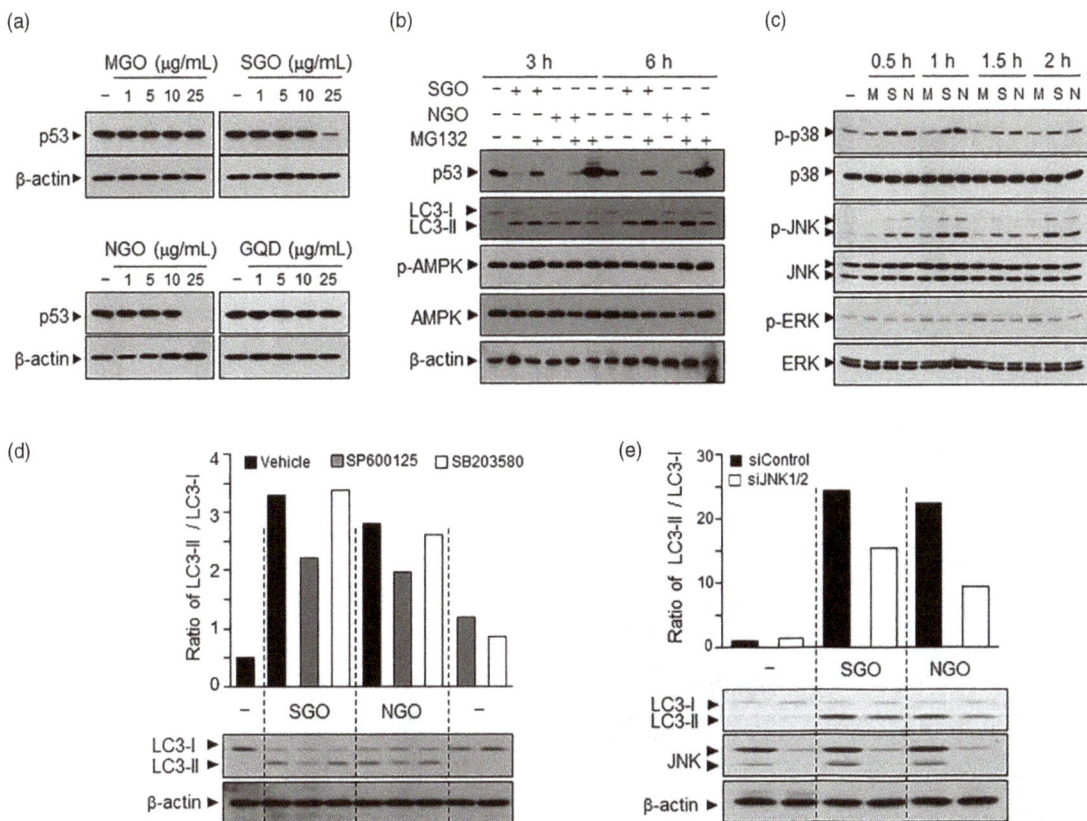

FIGURE 6.7 SGO- and NGO-induced autophagy depends on JNK signaling pathway activation. (a and c) Western blot analysis of p53 protein levels and p38, c-Jun N-terminal kinase (JNK), and extracellular-signal-regulated kinase (ERK) phosphorylation. HUVECs were treated with GOs at the indicated concentrations for 24 h or for the indicated times with 25 µg/mL GOs (M, MGO; S, SGO; and N, NGO). (b) Western blot analysis of p53 protein levels, AMPK phosphorylation, and LC3-I to LC3-II conversion. HUVECs were pre-treated with 10-mM MG132 (proteasome inhibitor) for 30 min and subsequently treated with SGO or NGO for the indicated times. (d and e) Western blot analysis of the LC3-I to LC3-II conversion following treatment with JNK inhibitor (SP600125) or JNK1/2 siRNA. Relative LC3-II to LC3-I ratios are indicated in the graphs. Data were quantified using the Image J software.

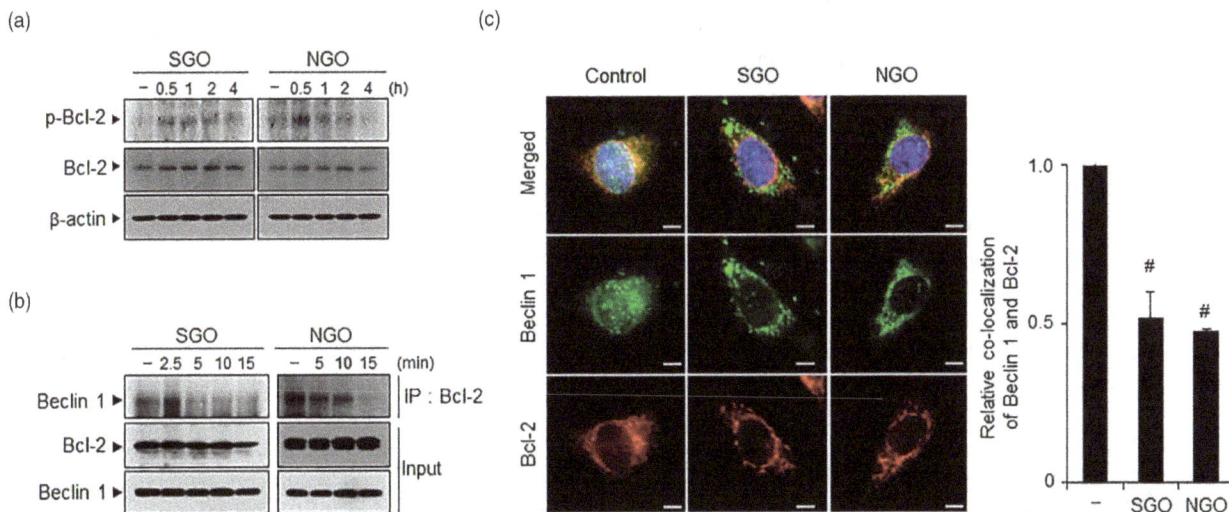

FIGURE 6.8 JNK induces autophagy in ECs through B-cell lymphoma 2 phosphorylation, leading to the dissociation of Beclin-1 from the Beclin-1–Bcl-2 complex. (a) Western blot analysis of B-cell lymphoma 2 (Bcl-2) phosphorylation. HUVECs were treated with SGO or NGO at 25 µg/mL for the indicated times. (b) Coimmunoprecipitation of Beclin-1 and Bcl-2 from HUVECs treated with SGO or NGO for the indicated times. (c) Representative fluorescence image of Beclin-1 (Green) and Bcl-2 (Red) colocalization in HUVECs treated with 25 µg/mL SGO or NGO for 30 min (left panel). Bar graph of the percentage of Bcl-2 spots that colocalized with Beclin-1 (right panel). Quantitative data are reported as means ± SD. #$p < 0.01$ versus untreated control. Scale bar = 10 µm.

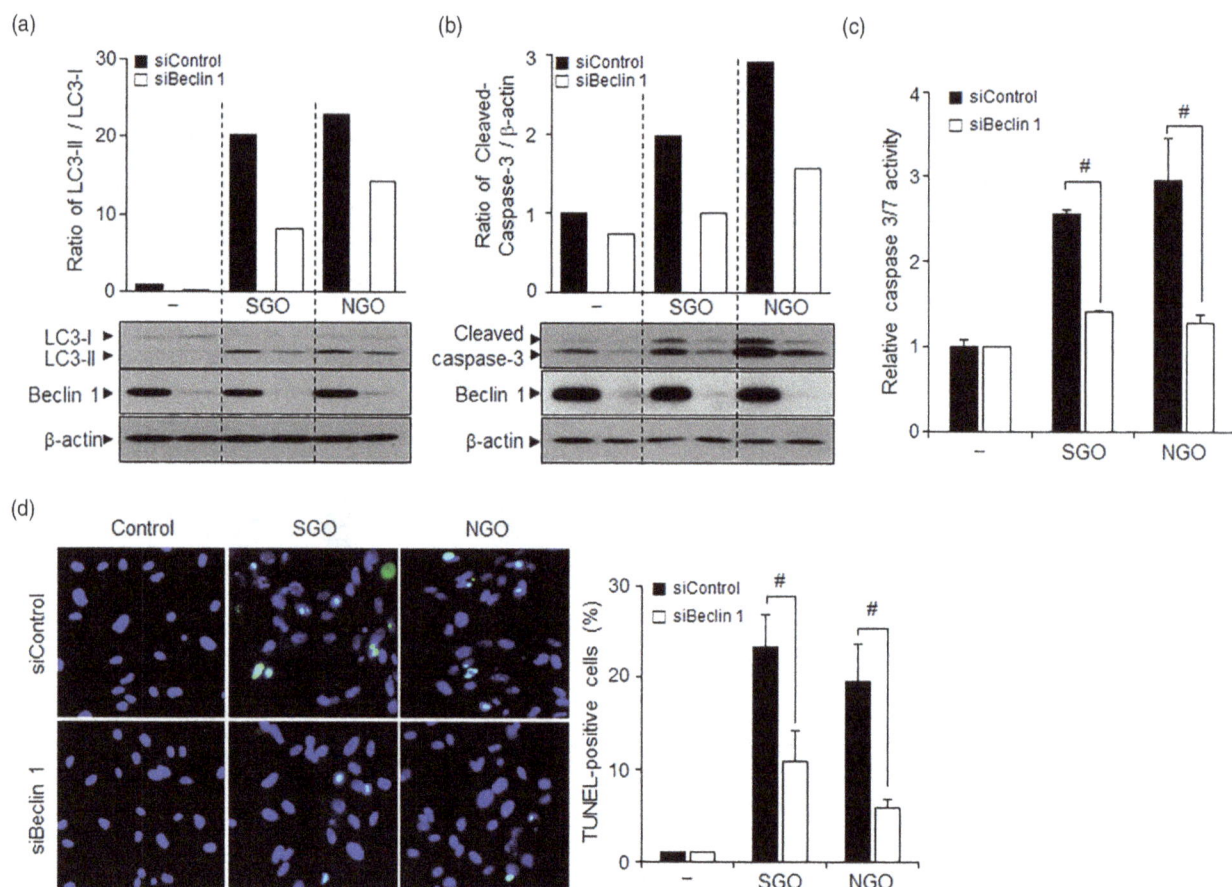

FIGURE 6.9 The role of Beclin-1 in SGO- or NGO-mediated induction of autophagy and apoptotic cell death. (a and b) Western blot analysis of the LC3-I to LC3-II conversion and caspase-3 activation in control siRNA- or Beclin-1 siRNA-transfected HUVECs. HUVECs were transfected with control siRNA or Beclin-1 siRNA; after 48 h, cells were treated with 25 µg/mL of SGO or NGO for 5 h (a) or 24 h (b). Relative LC3-II to LC3-I ratios and relative levels of cleaved caspase-3 are indicated in the graphs. Data were quantified using Image J software. Cleaved caspase-3 band densities were normalized against b-actin. (c) Relative caspase-3/7 activity in control siRNA- or Beclin-1 siRNA-transfected HUVECs. Quantitative data are reported as means ± SD. #$p < 0.01$ versus control siRNA. (d) TUNEL assay detection via fluorescent microscopy. Blue fluorescence indicates 4,6-diamidino-2-phenylindole (DAPI) nuclear staining; green fluorescence indicates TUNEL-positive nuclear staining (left panel). Percentage of cells that contain fragmented DNA (right panel, magnification; ×100). Quantitative data are reported as means ± SD. #$p < 0.01$ versus control siRNA.

also led to a decrease in SGO- or NGO-mediated apoptosis as determined via pro-caspase-3 cleavage, caspase-3/7 activity assays, TUNEL staining, and trypan blue exclusion assays (Figure 6.9b–d). All these results strongly suggest that JNK plays an essential regulatory role in the SGO- or NGO-mediated induction of autophagy and apoptosis through the phosphorylation of Bcl-2, resulting in the dissociation of Beclin-1 from the Beclin-1–Bcl-2 complex and the subsequent induction of Beclin-1-mediated autophagy.

6.12.4 SGO or NGO Increases Intracellular Ca²⁺ Levels by Activating Calcium Channels, and Elevated Intracellular Ca²⁺ Activate Subsequent Downstream Intracellular Events Related to GO-Mediated Autophagy

Ca²⁺ has long been known to play an important role in numerous cellular processes, including cell death regulation,

and therefore, the cytosolic Ca²⁺ concentration should be tightly regulated. Notably, the endoplasmic reticulum (ER) and mitochondria serve as primary Ca²⁺ storage organelles [166,175]. As Ca²⁺ is a key signaling molecule upstream of MAPKs, we hypothesized that SGO or NGO induces JNK phosphorylation and consequent autophagy activation in ECs by increasing intracellular Ca²⁺ levels. An apparent increase in Ca²⁺ levels was observed in SGO- or NGO treated ECs, whereas no significant changes were found in MGO- or GQD-treated ECs (Figure 6.10a).

To further determine the role of intracellular Ca²⁺ in SGO- or NGO-mediated autophagy activation, HUVECs were preincubated with BAPTA-AM, a highly selective cell-permeant chelator of intracellular Ca²⁺, for 30min before treatment with SGO or NGO; LC3-II accumulation and JNK phosphorylation were subsequently measured. As shown in Figure 6.10b and c, the chelation of intracellular Ca²⁺ with BAPTA-AM apparently suppressed JNK phosphorylation and LC3-II accumulation. The inositol

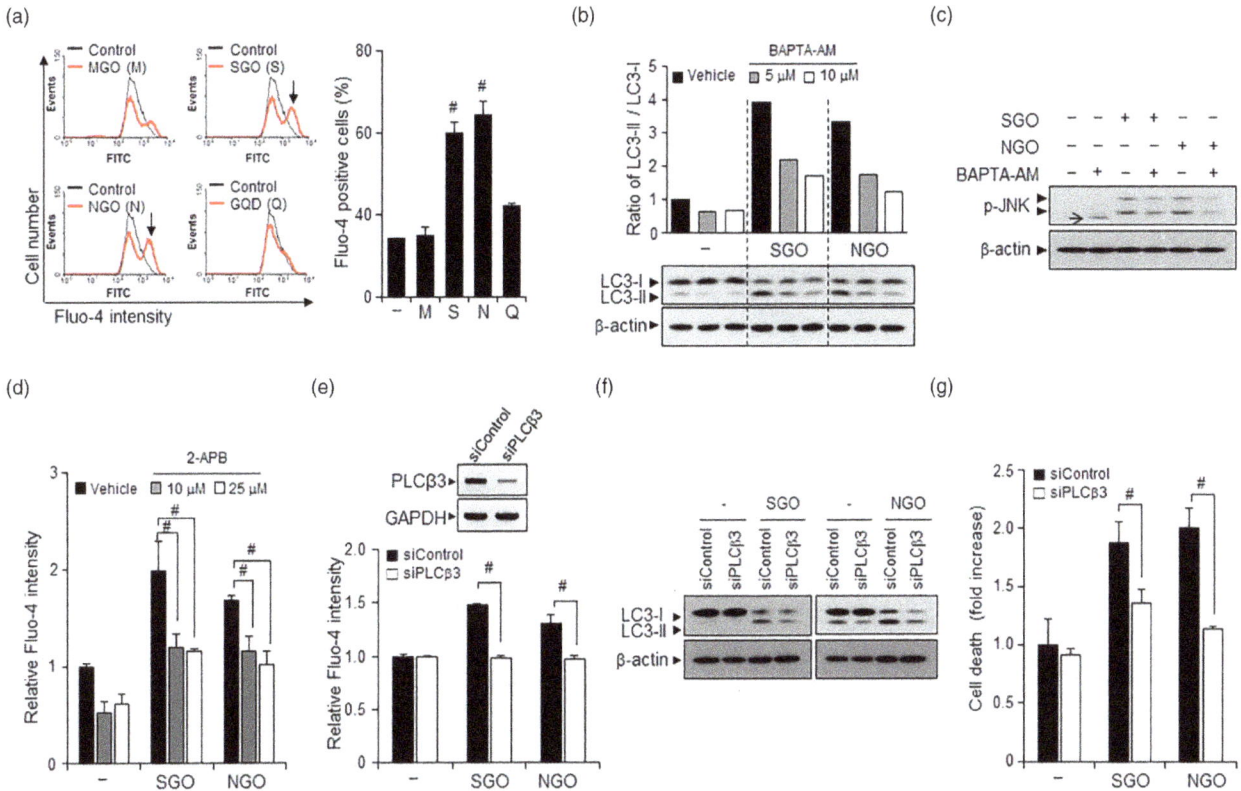

FIGURE 6.10 SGO and NGO induce autophagy through the PLCb3/IP3/Ca^{2+}/JNK signaling axis. (a) Histogram data from flow cytometric experiments reveal increased fluo4-NM fluorescence intensity in HUVECs treated with 25 μg/mL GOs (left panel). The bar graph indicates the percentages of fluo4-NM positive cells (right panel). Quantitative data are reported as means ± SD. #$p < 0.01$ versus untreated control. (b and c) Western blot analysis of LC3-I to LC3-II conversion and JNK phosphorylation in SGO- or NGO-treated HUVECs in the presence or absence of BAPTA-AM. HUVECs were pretreated with BAPTA-AM for 30 min, followed by an additional incubation with 25 μg/mL SGO or NGO for 3 h (b) or 30 min (c). Relative LC3-II to LC3-I ratios are indicated in the graphs. Data were quantified using Image J software. The arrow indicates a nonspecific band. (d) HUVECs were pretreated with 2-APB for 30 min, followed by additional 30-min incubation with 25 μg/mL SGO or NGO, followed by the quantitative estimation of changes in the mean fluorescence intensity of fluo4-NM. Quantitative data are reported as means ± SD. #$p < 0.01$ versus vehicle control. (e and f) HUVECs were transfected with control siRNA or PLCb3 siRNA for 48 h. (e) Reverse transcription polymerase chain reaction (RT-PCR) analysis of phospholipase C (PLC) b3 mRNA levels (upper panel). Quantitative estimates of changes in the mean fluorescence intensity of fluo4-NM in control siRNA- or PLC b3 siRNA-transfected HUVECs (lower panel). Quantitative data are reported as means ± SD. #$p < 0.01$ versus control siRNA (f) Western blot analysis of LC3-I to LC3-II conversion in control siRNA- or PLCb3 siRNA-transfected HUVECs following treatment with SGO or NGO. (g) Determination of cell death in control siRNA- or PLCb3 siRNA-transfected HUVECs following treatment with SGO or NGO. Quantitative data are reported as means ± SD. #$p < 0.01$ versus control siRNA.

1,4,5-trisphosphate receptor (IP3R), a Ca^{2+} channel, is activated by IP3 binding and regulates Ca^{2+} levels in the cytosol. The inhibition of IP3R with 2-aminoethoxydiphenyl borate (2-APB) apparently attenuated the SGO- and NGO-induced elevation of intracellular Ca^{2+} levels, whereas extracellular Ca^{2+} removal using ethylene glycol tetraacetic acid (EGTA) had no significant effects, indicating that the increased intracellular Ca^{2+} levels observed following SGO or NGO treatment is released from internal ER pools to the cytosol (Figure 6.10d).

Thus, in the above sections of this study [137], experimental data regarding the differential size-related biological effects of GOs on ECs have been presented. Additionally, it has been demonstrated for the first time that GOs induce apoptotic death in ECs via autophagy activation. As presented in Figure 6.11, SGOs or NGOs induce autophagic cell death

through the PLCb3/IP3/Ca^{2+}/JNK signaling axis. Although further investigations are required before the current findings can be clinically applied, these data will provide a better understanding of the mechanism underlying GO size-dependent cytotoxicity in vasculature and facilitate the future development of safer biomedical applications of GOs.

6.13 CONCLUSION AND OUTLOOK

Multidrug-loaded nanoparticles present a powerful and versatile platform for anticancer drug delivery. The synthesis flexibility of nanoparticle platforms has enabled unprecedented control in delivering a wide range of therapeutics. Various strategies based on combinatorial nanoparticles opened up many promising options toward addressing cancer drug resistance. Specific chemosensitizing agents,

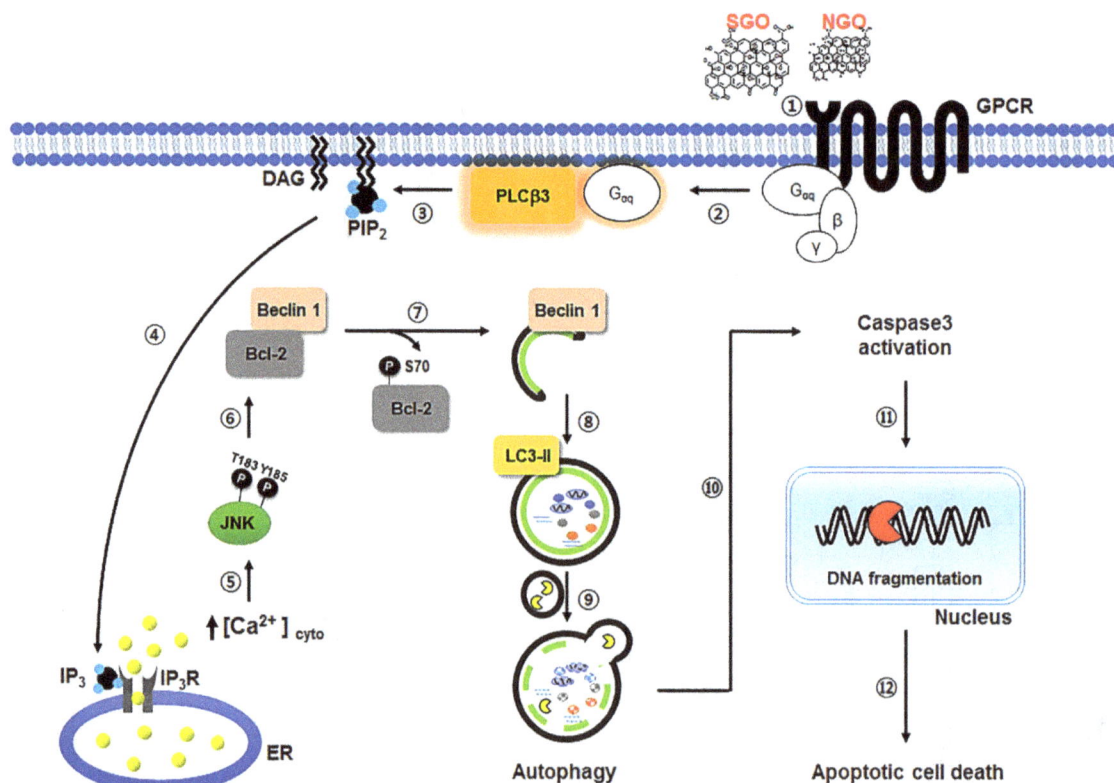

FIGURE 6.11 Overview of GO-induced apoptotic cell death pathway in ECs. SGO and NGO bind to the cell membrane, leading to G protein-coupled receptor (GPCR) stimulation. Following the activation of GPCR, the Gaq subunit induces PLC β3 activation, which hydrolyzes phosphatidylinositol-4,5-bisphosphate (PIP_2) to diacylglycerol (DAG) and inositol 1,4,5-trisphosphate (IP_3). Subsequently, IP_3 binds the IP_3 receptor (IP_3R) on the endoplasmic reticulum (ER) to induce Ca^{2+} efflux from ER. Subsequently, the increased intracellular Ca^{+2} level induced JNK phosphorylation, followed by Bcl-2 phosphorylation at serine 70 (S70) and dissociation of the Bcl-2–Beclin-1 complex. Following the dissociation of Beclin-1 from Bcl-2, activated Beclin-1 induces autophagy via LC3. As a result, autophagy induced by SGO or NGO induces apoptotic cell death via caspase-3 activation and DNA fragmentation.

for instance, have been used in combination with chemotherapeutics to suppress MDR with defined mechanisms. In clinical cancer treatment, drugs with different modes of action can be combined in a precisely controlled manner to maximize therapeutic efficacy and to minimize the likelihood of drug resistance development. Enabling uniform and concurrent delivery of drug combinations, maintaining the synergistic drug ratios, and controlling drug exposure sequence are the major advantages of nanoparticle-based combination therapy over the traditional cocktail administration. While batch-to-batch inconsistency and manufacturability are among the key challenges in many combinatorial nanoparticles, we believe that ongoing efforts on the advancement of combinatorial nanoparticles will lead to the ideal combination therapy sought after by physicians and oncologists.

Various nanoparticle-based delivery systems [176–179] such as cationic lipids, polymers, dendrimers, and inorganic nanoparticles have been demonstrated to provide effective and efficient siRNA delivery *in vitro* and *in vivo*. Future studies must focus on the *in vivo* safety profiles of the various delivery systems, including undesirable immune stimulation

and cytotoxicity. It is critical to develop safe, biocompatible, and biodegradable nanoparticle delivery systems for the clinical application of RNAi-based cancer therapeutics.

Since RNAi was discovered, various nonviral vector delivery systems for siRNA delivery have been explored extensively. Although significant advances have been made in the development of efficient *in vivo* siRNA delivery, there are still many challenges and barriers that must be overcome to achieve the ideal formulation in terms of selectivity, efficacy, and safety. Only a few nanoparticle-based siRNA delivery systems have been approved by the FDA and are in clinical trials for cancer therapy. Delivery systems can improve specificity of cancer-cell targeting, prevent nonspecific delivery of siRNA, and may also protect the siRNA during transport. Nanoparticles conjugated to the targeting ligand for effective siRNA delivery increase the chance of binding the tumor surface receptor; however, the process also increases the overall size of the nanoparticle.

The concept of using GNPs for radiation therapy has been studied by several experimental and MC simulation investigations during last years. Although the enhancement of radiation dose in tumors loaded with high-Z materials have been attempted for several decades, the emergence of new gold nanoparticles with biocompatible characteristics has motivated scientists to investigate their applications in conjunction with radiation therapy. The results of all aforementioned studies are agreed in that GNPs can enhance the dose deposition phenomenon in GNP loaded tumors. But there are controversial results about the impact of photon energy and GNP size in recently published articles. To optimize the technique of GNP-based radiation therapy for clinical application, some studies should be carried out to address the effect of photon energy and GNP size separately. Also, more biological experiments on cell lines and animal models are required to clarify the observed differences in dose enhancement effect concerning the magnitude of enhancement effect and impact of cell type in GNP-based radiation therapy.

REFERENCES

1. G.J. Hannon, RNA interference, *Nature* 418(6894) (2002) 244–251.
2. P.A. Sharp, RNAi and double-strand RNA, *Genes Dev.* 13(2) (1999) 139–141.
3. S.M. Elbashir, J. Harborth, W. Lendeckel, A. Yalcin, K. Weber, T. Tuschl, Duplexes of 21-nucleotide RNAs mediate RNA interference in cultured mammalian cells, *Nature* 411(6836) (2001) 494–498.
4. E. Bernstein, A.A. Caudy, S.M. Hammond, G.J. Hannon, Role for a bidentate ribonuclease in the initiation step of RNA interference, *Nature* 409(6818) (2001) 363–366.
5. E. Check, Acrucial test, *Nat. Med.* 11(3) (2005) 243–244.
6. J. DeVincenzo, J.E. Cehelsky, R. Alvarez et al., Evaluation of the safety, tolerability and pharmacokinetics of ALN-RSV01, a novel RNAi antiviral therapeutic directed against respiratory syncytial virus (RSV), *Antiviral Res.* 77(3) (2008) 225–231.
7. L. Aagaard, J.J. Rossi, RNAi therapeutics: principles, prospects and challenges, *Adv. Drug Delivery Rev.* 59(2–3) (2007) 75–86.
8. X. Yuan, S. Naguib, Z. Wu, Recent advances of siRNA delivery by nanoparticles, *Expert Opin. Drug Delivery* 8(4) (2011) 521–536.
9. J.C. Burnett, J.J. Rossi, K. Tiemann, Current progress of siRNA/shRNA therapeutics in clinical trials, *Biotechnol. J.* 6(9) (2011) 1130–1146.
10. Y.P. Liu, B. Berkhout, MiRNA cassettes in viral vectors: problems and solutions, *Biochimica et Biophysica Acta* 1809(11–12) (2011) 732–745.
11. P.L. Sinn, S.L. Sauter, P.B. McCray Jr., Gene therapy progress and prospects: development of improved lentiviral and retroviral vectors-design, biosafety, and production, *Gene Ther.* 12(14) (2005) 1089–1098.
12. Y. Wang, Z. Li, Y. Han, L.H. Liang, A. Ji, Nanoparticle based delivery system for application of siRNA in vivo, *Curr. Drug Metab.* 11(2) (2010) 182–196.
13. J. Woodcock, J.P. Griffin, R.E. Behrman, Development of novel combination therapies, *N. Engl. J. Med.* 364 (2011) 985–987.
14. V.T. DeVita Jr, R.C. Young, G.P. Canellos, Combination versus single agent chemotherapy: a review of the basis for selection of drug treatment of cancer, *Cancer* 35 (1975) 98–110.
15. C. Delbaldo, S. Michiels, N. Syz, J.C. Soria, T. Le Chevalier, J.P. Pignon, Benefits of adding a drug to a single-agent or a 2-agent chemotherapy regimen in advanced non-small-cell lung cancer: a meta-analysis, *J. Am. Med. Assoc.* 292 (2004) 470–484.
16. M. Di Maio, P. Chiodini, V. Georgoulias, D. Hatzidaki, K. Takeda, F.M. Wachters, et al. Meta-analysis of single-agent chemotherapy compared with combination chemotherapy as second-line treatment of advanced non-small-cell lung cancer, *J. Clin. Oncol.* 27 (2009) 1836–1843.
17. A.Z. Wang, F. Gu, L. Zhang, J.M. Chan, A. Radovic-Moreno, M.R. Shaikh, et al. Biofunctionalized targeted nanoparticles for therapeutic applications, *Expert Opin. Biol. Ther.* 8 (2008) 1063–1070.
18. L. Zhang, F.X. Gu, J.M. Chan, A.Z. Wang, R.S. Langer, O.C. Farokhzad, Nanoparticles in medicine: therapeutic applications and developments, *Clin. Pharmacol. Ther.* 83 (2008) 761–769.
19. C.M. Hu, S. Kaushal, H.S. Tran Cao, S. Aryal, M. Sartor, S. Esener, et al. Half-antibody functionalized lipid-polymer hybrid nanoparticles for targeted drug delivery to carcinoembryonic antigen presenting pancreatic cancer cells, *Mol. Pharm.* 7 (2010) 914–920.
20. C.M. Hu, L. Zhang, Therapeutic nanoparticles to combat cancer drug resistance, *Curr Drug Metab* 10 (2009) 836–841.
21. A.D. Bangham, M.M. Standish, J.C. Watkins, Diffusion of univalent ions across the lamellae of swollen phospholipids, *J. Mol. Biol.* 13 (1965) 238–252.
22. W.F. Bayne, L.D. Mayer, C.E. Swenson, Pharmacokinetics of CPX-351 (cytarabine/daunorubicin HCl) liposome injection in the mouse, *J. Pharm. Sci.* 98 (2009) 2540–2548.
23. Y. Takakura, M. Hashida, Macromolecular drug carrier systems in cancer chemotherapy: macromolecular prodrugs, *Crit. Rev. Oncol. Hematol.* 18 (1995) 207–231.
24. F. Kratz, U. Beyer, M.T. Schutte, Drug–polymer conjugates containing acid cleavable bonds, *Crit. Rev. Ther. Drug Carrier Syst.* 16 (1999) 245–288.
25. L. Liu, K. Xu, H. Wang, P.K. Tan, W. Fan, S.S. Venkatraman, et al. Self-assembled cationic peptide nanoparticles as an efficient antimicrobial agent, *Nat. Nanotechnol.* 4 (2009) 457–463.
26. S. Aryal, C.M. Hu, L. Zhang, Combinatorial drug conjugation enables nanoparticle dual-drug delivery, *Small* 6 (2010) 1442–1448.
27. N. Kolishetti, S. Dhar, P.M. Valencia, L.Q. Lin, R. Karnik, S.J. Lippard, et al. Engineering of self-assembled nanoparticle platform for precisely controlled combination drug therapy, *Proc. Natl. Acad. Sci. U. S. A.* 107 (2010) 17939–17944.
28. L. Zhang, A.F. Radovic-Moreno, F. Alexis, F.X. Gu, P.A. Basto, V. Bagalkot, et al. Codelivery of hydrophobic and hydrophilic drugs from nanoparticle-aptamer bioconjugates, *ChemMedChem* 2 (2007) 1268–1271.
29. S. Aryal, C.M. Hu, L. Zhang, Polymeric nanoparticles with precise ratiometric control over drug loading for combination therapy, *Mol. Pharm.* 8 (2011) 1401–1407.
30. S. Sengupta, D. Eavarone, I. Capila, G. Zhao, N. Watson, T. Kiziltepe, et al. Temporal targeting of tumour cells and neovasculature with a nanoscale delivery system, *Nature* 436 (2005) 568–572.
31. Z. Wang, P.C. Ho, A nanocapsular combinatorial sequential drug delivery system for antiangiogenesis and anticancer activities, *Biomaterials* 31 (2010) 7115–7123.

32. C. Li, S. Wallace, Polymer–drug conjugates: recent development in clinical oncology, *Adv. Drug Delivery Rev.* 60 (2008) 886–898.

33. F. Greco, M.J. Vicent, Polymer–drug conjugates: current status and future trends, *Front Biosci.* 13 (2008) 2744–2756.

34. T. Lammers, V. Subr, K. Ulbrich, P. Peschke, P.E. Huber, W.E. Hennink, et al. Simultaneous delivery of doxorubicin and gemcitabine to tumors in vivo using prototypic polymeric drug carriers. *Biomaterials* 30 (2009) 3466–3475.

35. H. Krakovicova, T. Etrych, K. Ulbrich, HPMA-based polymer conjugates with drug combination. *Eur. J. Pharm. Sci.* 37 (2009) 405–412.

36. L. Zhao, Y. Cheng, J. Hu, Q. Wu, T. Xu, Host-guest chemistry of dendrimer-drug complexes. 3. Competitive binding of multiple drugs by a single dendrimer for combination therapy, *J. Phys. Chem. B* 113 (2009) 14172–14179.

37. R.K. Tekade, T. Dutta, V. Gajbhiye, N.K. Jain, Exploring dendrimer towards dual drug delivery: pH responsive simultaneous drug-release kinetics, *J. Microencapsul.* 26 (2009) 287–296.

38. S. Ganta, M. Amiji, Coadminstration of paclitaxel and curcumin in nanoemulsion formulations to overcome multidrug resistance in tumor cells, *Mol. Pharm.* 6 (2009) 928–939.

39. A.M. Chen, M. Zhang, D. Wei, D. Stueber, O. Taratula, T. Minko, et al. Co-delivery of doxorubicin and Bcl-2 siRNA by mesoporous silica nanoparticles enhances the efficacy of chemotherapy in multidrug-resistant cancer cells, *Small* 5 (2009) 2673–2677.

40. F. Dilnawaz, A. Singh, C. Mohanty, S.K. Sahoo, Dual drug loaded superparamagnetic iron oxide nanoparticles for targeted cancer therapy, *Biomaterials* 31 (2010) 3694–3706.

41. A. Singh, F. Dilnawaz, S. Mewar, U. Sharma, N.R. Jagannathan, S.K. Sahoo, Composite polymeric magnetic nanoparticles for co-delivery of hydrophobic and hydrophilic anticancer drugs and MRI imaging for cancer therapy, *ACS Appl. Mater. Interfaces* 3 (2011) 842–856.

42. D.B. Fenske, P.R. Cullis, Liposomal nanomedicines, *Expert Opin. Drug Delivery*, 5(1) (2008) 25–44.

43. A. Elouahabi, J.-M. Ruysschaert, Formation and intracellular trafficking of lipoplexes and polyplexes, *Mol. Ther.* 11(3) (2005) 336–347.

44. S.Y. Wu, N.A.J. McMillan, Lipidic systems for in vivo siRNA delivery, *AAPS J.* 11(4) (2009) 639–652.

45. C.N. Landen Jr., A. Chavez-Reyes, C. Bucana et al., Therapeutic EphA2 gene targeting in vivo using neutral liposomal small interfering RNA delivery, *Cancer Res.* 65(15) (2005) 6910–6918.

46. J. Halder, A.A. Kamat, C.N. Landen Jr. et al., Focal adhesion kinase targeting using in vivo short interfering RNA delivery in neutral liposomes for ovarian carcinoma therapy, *Clin. Cancer Res.* 12(16) (2006) 4916–4924.

47. M.J. Gray, G. Van Buren, N.A. Dallas et al., Therapeutic targeting of neuropilin-2 on colorectal carcinoma cells implanted in the murine liver, *J. Nat. Cancer Inst.* 100(2) (2008) 109–120.

48. W.M. Merritt, Y.G. Lin, W.A. Spannuth et al., Effect of interleukin-8 gene silencing with liposome-encapsulated small interfering RNA on ovarian cancer cell growth, *J. Nat. Cancer Inst.* 100(5) (2008) 359–372.

49. B. Ozpolat, A.K. Sood, G. Lopez-Berestein, Nanomedicine based approaches for the delivery of siRNA in cancer, *J. Internal Med.* 267(1) (2010) 44–53.

50. S. Taetz, A. Bochot, C. Surace et al., Hyaluronic acid-modified DOTAP/DOPE liposomes for the targeted delivery of antitelomerase siRNA to CD44-expressing lung cancer cells, *Oligonucleotides* 19(2) (2009) 103–116.

51. K. Kostarelos, D. Emfietzoglou, A. Papakostas, W.-H. Yang, A. Ballangrud, G. Sgouros, Binding and interstitial penetration of liposomes within avascular tumor spheroids, *Int. J. Cancer* 112(4) (2004) 713–721.

52. S. Dokka, D. Toledo, X. Shi, V. Castranova, Y. Rojanasakul, Oxygen radical-mediated pulmonary toxicity induced by some cationic liposomes, *Pharm. Res.* 17(5) (2000) 521–525.

53. S. Spagnou, A.D. Miller, M. Keller, Lipidic carriers of siRNA: differences in the formulation, cellular uptake, and delivery with plasmid DNA, *Biochemistry*, 43(42) (2004) 13348–13356.

54. H. Lv, S. Zhang, B. Wang, S. Cui, J. Yan, Toxicity of cationic lipids and cationic polymers in gene delivery, *J. Controlled Release* 114(1) (2006) 100–109.

55. M. Uner, G. Yener, Importance of solid lipid nanoparticles (SLN) in various administration routes and future perspectives, *Int. J. Nanomed.* 2(3) (2007) 289–300.

56. A. Santel, M. Aleku, O. Keil et al., RNA interference in the mouse vascular endothelium by systemic administration of siRNA-lipoplexes for cancer therapy, *GeneTherapy* 13(18) (2006) 1360–1370.

57. A. Santel, M. Aleku, O. Keil et al., Anovel siRNA-lipoplex technology for RNA interference in the mouse vascular endothelium, *GeneTherapy*, 13(16) (2006) 1222–1234.

58. M. Aleku, P. Schulz, O. Keil et al., Atu027, a liposomal small interfering RNA formulation targeting protein kinase N3, inhibits cancer progression, *Cancer Res.* 68(23) (2008) 9788–9798.

59. A. Santel, M. Aleku, N. Roder et al., Atu027 prevents pulmonary metastasis in experimental and spontaneous mouse metastasis models, *Clin. Cancer Res.* 16(22) (2010) 5469–5480.

60. D. Strumberg, B. Schultheis, U. Traugott et al., Phase I clinical development of Atu027, a siRNA formulation targeting PKN3 in patients with advanced solid tumors, *Int. J. Clin. Pharmacol. Ther.* 50(1) (2012) 76–78.

61. V. Brower, RNA interference advances to early-stage clinical trials, *J. Nat. Cancer Inst.* 102(19) (2010) 1459–1461.

62. D.V. Morrissey, J.A. Lockridge, L. Shaw et al., Potent and persistent in vivo anti-HBV activity of chemically modified siRNAs, *Nat. Biotechnol.* 23(8) (2005) 1002–1007.

63. J. Jin, K.H. Bae, H. Yang et al., In vivo specific delivery of c-Met siRNA to glioblastoma using cationic solid lipid nanoparticles, *Bioconjugate Chem.* 22(12) (2011) 2568–2572.

64. L.B. Jeffs, L.R. Palmer, E.G. Ambegia, C. Giesbrecht, S. Ewanick, I. MacLachlan, Ascalable, extrusion-free method for efficient liposomal encapsulation of plasmidDNA, *Pharm. Res.* 22(3) (2005) 362–372.

65. T.S. Zimmermann, A.C.H. Lee, A. Akinc et al., RNAi-mediated gene silencing in non-human primates, *Nature* 441(7089) (2006) 111–114.

66. A.D. Judge, M. Robbins, I. Tavakoli et al., Confirming the RNAi-mediated mechanism of action of siRNA-based cancer therapeutics in mice, *J. Clin. Invest.* 119(3) (2009) 661–673.

67. H. Shen, T. Sun, M. Ferrari, Nanovector delivery of siRNA for cancer therapy, *Cancer Gene Ther.* 19(6), (2012) 367–373.

68. A. Akinc, A. Zumbuehl, M. Goldberg et al., A combinatorial library of lipid-like materials for delivery of RNAi therapeutics, *Nat. Biotechnol.* 26(5) (2008) 561–569.

69. A. Akinc, M. Goldberg, J. Qin et al., Development of lipidoid-siRNA formulations for systemic delivery to the liver, *Mol. Ther.* 17(5) (2009) 872–879.

70. K.T. Love, K.P. Mahon, C.G. Levins et al., Lipid-like materials for low-dose, in vivo gene silencing, *Proc. Nat. Acad. Sci. U. S. A.* 107(5) (2010) 1864–1869.

71. A. Shapira, Y.D. Livney, H.J. Broxterman, Y.G. Assaraf, Nanomedicine for targeted cancer therapy: towards the overcoming of drug resistance, *Drug Resist Updat.* 14 (2011) 150–163.

72. G.N. Chiu, M.Y. Wong, L.U. Ling, I.M. Shaikh, K.B. Tan, A. Chaudhury, et al. Lipid-based nanoparticulate systems for the delivery of anti-cancer drug cocktails: implications on pharmacokinetics and drug toxicities, *Curr. Drug Metab.* 10 (2009) 861–874.

73. M.M. Gottesman, Mechanisms of cancer drug resistance, *Annu. Rev. Med.* 53 (2002) 615–627.

74. M. Koval, K. Preiter, C. Adles, P.D. Stahl, T.H. Steinberg, Size of IgG-opsonized particles determines macrophage response during internalization, *Exp. Cell Res.* 242 (1998) 265–273.

75. J. Huwyler, A. Cerletti, G. Fricker, A.N. Eberle, J. Drewe, By-passing of P-glycoprotein using immunoliposomes. *J. Drug Target* 10 (2002) 73–79.

76. J. Rejman, V. Oberle, I.S. Zuhorn, D. Hoekstra, Size-dependent internalization of particles via the pathways of clathrin- and caveolae-mediated endocytosis, *Biochem. J.* 377 (2004) 159–169.

77. M. Bebawy, M. Chetty, Gender differences in p-glycoprotein expression and function: effects on drug disposition and outcome, *Curr. Drug Metab.* 10 (2009) 322–328.

78. D.M. Bradshaw, R.J. Arceci, Clinical relevance of transmembrane drug efflux as a mechanism of multidrug resistance. *J. Clin. Oncol.* 16 (1998) 3674–3690.

79. M. Hennessy, J.P. Spiers, A primer on the mechanics of P-glycoprotein the multidrug transporter, *Pharmacol. Res.* 55 (2007) 1–15.

80. H. Yuan, X. Li, J. Wu, J. Li, X. Qu, W. Xu, et al. Strategies to overcome or circumvent P-glycoprotein mediated multidrug resistance, *Curr. Med. Chem.* 15 (2008) 470–476.

81. R. Advani, G.A. Fisher, B.L. Lum, J. Hausdorff, J. Halsey, M. Litchman, et al. A phase I trial of doxorubicin, paclitaxel, and valspodar (PSC 833), a modulator of multidrug resistance, *Clin. Cancer Res.* 7 (2001) 1221–1229.

82. P.M. Fracasso, M.F. Brady, D.H. Moore, J.L. Walker, P.G. Rose, L. Letvak, et al. Phase II study of paclitaxel and valspodar (PSC 833) in refractory ovarian carcinoma: a gynecologic oncology group study, *J. Clin. Oncol.* 19 (2001) 2975–2982.

83. C.E. Soma, C. Dubernet, D. Bentolila, S. Benita, P. Couvreur, Reversion of multidrug resistance by co-encapsulation of doxorubicin and cyclosporin A in polyalkylcyanoacrylate nanoparticles, *Biomaterials* 21 (2000) 1–7.

84. J. Wu, Y. Lu, A. Lee, X. Pan, X. Yang, X. Zhao, et al. Reversal of multidrug resistance by transferrin-conjugated liposomes co-encapsulating doxorubicin and verapamil, *J. Pharm. Pharm. Sci.* 10 (2007) 350–357.

85. N.R. Patel, A. Rathi, D. Mongayt, V.P. Torchilin, Reversal of multidrug resistance by co-delivery of tariquidar (XR9576) and paclitaxel using long-circulating liposomes, *Int. J. Pharm.* 416 (2011) 296–299.

86. X. Li, W.L. Lu, G.W. Liang, G.R. Ruan, H.Y. Hong, C. Long, et al. Effect of stealthy liposomal topotecan plus amlodipine on the multidrug-resistant leukaemia cells in vitro and xenograft in mice. *Eur. J. Clin. Invest.* 36 (2006) 409–418.

87. G.W. Liang, W.L. Lu, J.W. Wu, J.H. Zhao, H.Y. Hong, C. Long, et al. Enhanced therapeutic effects on the multi-drug resistant human leukemia cells in vitro and xenograft in mice using the stealthy liposomal vincristine plus quinacrine, *Fundam. Clin. Pharmacol.* 22 (2008) 429–437.

88. M. Saad, O.B. Garbuzenko, T. Minko, Co-delivery of siRNA and an anticancer drug for treatment of multidrug-resistant cancer, *Nanomedicine (Lond)* 3 (2008) 761–776.

89. Y. Wang, S. Gao, W.H. Ye, H.S. Yoon, Y.Y. Yang, Co-delivery of drugs and DNA from cationic core-shell nanoparticles self-assembled from a biodegradable copolymer, *Nat. Mater.* 5 (2006) 791–796.

90. X.R. Song, Z. Cai, Y. Zheng, G. He, F.Y. Cui, D.Q. Gong, et al. Reversion of multidrug resistance by co-encapsulation of vincristine and verapamil in PLGA nanoparticles, *Eur. J. Pharm. Sci.* 37 (2009) 300–305.

91. Y. Patil, T. Sadhukha, L. Ma, J. Panyam, Nanoparticle-mediated simultaneous and targeted delivery of paclitaxel and tariquidar overcomes tumor drug resistance, *J. Control Release* 136 (2009) 21–29.

92. Y.B. Patil, S.K. Swaminathan, T. Sadhukha, L. Ma, J. Panyam, The use of nanoparticle- mediated targeted gene silencing and drug delivery to overcome tumor drug resistance, *Biomaterials* 31 (2010) 358–365.

93. R. Bendayan, G. Lee, M. Bendayan, Functional expression and localization of P-glycoprotein at the blood brain barrier. *Microsc. Res. Tech.* 57 (2002) 365–380.

94. X. Cao, L.X. Yu, C. Barbaciru, C.P. Landowski, H.C. Shin, S. Gibbs, et al. Permeability dominates in vivo intestinal absorption of P-gp substrate with high solubility and high permeability, *Mol. Pharm.* 2 (2005) 329–340.

95. R. Rezzani, Cyclosporine A and adverse effects on organs: histochemical studies, *Prog. Histochem. Cytochem.* 39 (2004) 85–128.

96. L.E. van Vlerken, Z. Duan, M.V. Seiden, M.M. Amiji, Modulation of intracellular ceramide using polymeric nanoparticles to overcome multidrug resistance in cancer. *Cancer Res.* 67 (2007) 4843–4850.

97. L.E. van Vlerken, Z. Duan, M.V. Seiden, M.M. Amiji, Augmentation of therapeutic efficacy in drug-resistant tumor models using ceramide coadministration in temporal-controlled polymer-blend nanoparticle delivery systems, *AAPS J.* 12 (2010) 171–180.

98. N.M. Patel, S. Nozaki, N.H. Shortle, P. Bhat-Nakshatri, T.R. Newton, S. Rice, et al. Paclitaxel sensitivity of breast cancer cells with constitutively active NFkappaB is enhanced by IkappaBalpha super-repressor and parthenolide, *Oncogene* 19 (2000) 4159–4169.

99. L. Fan, F. Li, H. Zhang, Y. Wang, C. Cheng, X. Li, et al. Co-delivery of PDTC and doxorubicin by multifunctional micellar nanoparticles to achieve active targeted drug delivery and overcome multidrug resistance, *Biomaterials* 31 (2010) 5634–5642.

100. R. Misra, S.K. Sahoo, Coformulation of doxorubicin and curcumin in poly(D, Llactide-co-glycolide) nanoparticles suppresses the development of multidrug resistance in K562 cells, *Mol. Pharm.* 8 (2011) 852–866.

101. A. de Fougerolles, H.P. Vornlocher, J. Maraganore, J. Lieberman, Interfering with disease: a progress report on siRNA-based therapeutics, *Nat. Rev. Drug Discov.* 6 (2007) 443–453.

102. M. Bartsch, A.H. Weeke-Klimp, D.K. Meijer, G.L. Scherphof, J.A. Kamps, Cell-specific targeting of lipid-based carriers for ODN and DNA, *J. Liposome Res.* 15 (2005) 59–92.

103. K. Nakamura, A.S. Abu Lila, M. Matsunaga, Y. Doi, T. Ishida, H. Kiwada, A double modulation strategy in cancer treatment with a chemotherapeutic agent and siRNA. *Mol. Ther.* 19 (2011) 2040–2047.

104. P.L. Felgner, T.R. Gadek, M. Holm, R. Roman, H.W. Chan, M. Wenz, et al. Lipofection: a highly efficient, lipid-mediated DNA-transfection procedure, *Proc. Natl. Acad. Sci. U. S. A.* 84 (1987) 7413–7417.

105. P.L. Felgner, G.M. Ringold, Cationic liposome-mediated transfection, *Nature* 337 (1989) 387–388.

106. S. Gao, F. Dagnaes-Hansen, E.J. Nielsen, J. Wengel, F. Besenbacher, K.A. Howard, et al. The effect of chemical modification and nanoparticle formulation on stability and biodistribution of siRNA in mice, *Mol. Ther.* 17 (2009) 1225–1233.

107. D. Di Paolo, C. Brignole, F. Pastorino, R. Carosio, A. Zorzoli, M. Rossi, et al. Neuroblastoma-targeted nanoparticles entrapping siRNA specifically knockdown ALK, *Mol. Ther.* 19 (2011) 1131–1140.

108. T.L. Kaneshiro, Z.R. Lu, Targeted intracellular codelivery of chemotherapeutics and nucleic acid with a well-defined dendrimer-based nanoglobular carrier, *Biomaterials* 30 (2009) 5660–5666.

109. H. Meng, M. Liong, T. Xia, Z. Li, Z. Ji, J.I. Zink, et al. Engineered design of mesoporous silica nanoparticles to deliver doxorubicin and P-glycoprotein siRNA to overcome drug resistance in a cancer cell line. *ACS Nano* 4 (2010) 4539–4550.

110. P. Tardi, S. Johnstone, N. Harasym, S. Xie, T. Harasym, N. Zisman, et al. In vivo maintenance of synergistic cytarabine:daunorubicin ratios greatly enhances therapeutic efficacy, *Leuk .Res.* 33 (2009) 129–139.

111. G. Batist, K.A. Gelmon, K.N. Chi, W.H. Miller Jr, S.K. Chia, L.D. Mayer, et al. Safety, pharmacokinetics, and efficacy of CPX-1 liposome injection in patients with advanced solid tumors, *Clin. Cancer Res.* 15 (2009) 692–700.

112. T.O. Harasym, P.G. Tardi, N.L. Harasym, P. Harvie, S.A. Johnstone, L.D. Mayer, Increased preclinical efficacy of irinotecan and floxuridine coencapsulated inside liposomes is associated with tumor delivery of synergistic drug ratios, *Oncol. Res.* 16 (2007) 361–374.

113. H.C. Shin, A.W. Alani, H. Cho, Y. Bae, J.M. Kolesar, G.S. Kwon, A 3-in-1 polymeric micelle nanocontainer for poorly water-soluble drugs, *Mol. Pharm.* 8 (2011) 1257–1265.

114. V. Pavillard, D. Kherfellah, S. Richard, J. Robert, D. Montaudon, Effects of the combination of camptothecin and doxorubicin or etoposide on rat glioma cells and camptothecin-resistant variants, *Br. J. Cancer* 85 (2001) 1077–1083.

115. M. Raitanen, V. Rantanen, J. Kulmala, H. Helenius, R. Grenman, S. Grenman, Supraadditive effect with concurrent paclitaxel and cisplatin in vulvar squamous cell carcinoma in vitro, *Int. J. Cancer* 100 (2002) 238–243.

116. W.S. Lim, P.G. Tardi, N. Dos Santos, X. Xie, M. Fan, B.D. Liboiron, et al. Leukemia selective uptake and cytotoxicity of CPX-351, a synergistic fixed-ratio cytarabine: daunorubicin formulation, in bone marrow xenografts, *Leuk. Res.* 34 (2010) 1214–1223.

117. E.J. Feldman, J.E. Lancet, J.E. Kolitz, E.K. Ritchie, G.J. Roboz, A.F. List, et al. First-in-man study of CPX-351: a liposomal carrier containing cytarabine and daunorubicin in a fixed 5:1 molar ratio for the treatment of relapsed and refractory acute myeloid leukemia, *J. Clin. Oncol.* 29 (2011) 979–985.

118. P.G. Tardi, N. Dos Santos, T.O. Harasym, S.A. Johnstone, N. Zisman, A.W. Tsang, et al. Drug ratio-dependent antitumor activity of irinotecan and cisplatin combinations in vitro and in vivo, *Mol. Cancer Ther.* 8 (2009) 2266–2275.

119. M.A. Shah, G.K. Schwartz, Cell cycle-mediated drug resistance: an emerging concept in cancer therapy, *Clin. Cancer Res.* 7 (2001) 2168–2181.

120. N.P. Praetorius, T.K. Mandal, Engineered nanoparticles in cancer therapy. *Recent Pat Drug Delivery Formul.* 1 (2007) 37–51.

121. P. Mukherjee, R. Bhattacharya, N. Bone, Y.K. Lee, C.R. Patra, S. Wang, et al. Potential therapeutic application of gold nanoparticles in B-chronic lymphocytic leukemia (BCLL): enhancing apoptosis. *J. Nanobiotechnol.* 5 (2007) 4.

122. E. Porcel, S. Liehn, H. Remita, N. Usami, K. Kobayashi, Y. Furusawa, et al. Platinum nanoparticles: a promising material for future cancer therapy? *Nanotechnology* 21 (2010) 85–103.

123. E. Burn, L. Sanche, C. Sicard-Roselli, Parameters governing gold nanoparticle X-ray radiosensitization of DNA in solution, *Colloids Surf B: Biointerfaces* 72 (2009) 128–134.

124. M.Y. Chang, A.L. Shiau, Y.H. Chen, C.J. Chang, H.H. Chen, C.L. Wu, Increased apoptotic potential and dose-enhancing effect of gold nanoparticles in combination with single-dose clinical electron beams on tumor-bearing mice, *Cancer Sci.* 99 (2008) 1479–1484.

125. J.F. Hainfeld, D.N. Slatkin, H.M. Smilowitz, The use of gold nanoparticles to enhance radiotherapy in mice, *Phys. Med. Biol.* 49 (2004) N309–15.

126. J.F. Hainfeld, F.A. Dilmanian, Z. Zhong, D.N. Slatkin, J.A. Kalef-Ezra, Smilowitz HM. Gold nanoparticles enhance the radiation therapy of a murine squamous cell carcinoma, *Phys. Med. Biol.* 55 (2010) 3045–3059.

127. X. Zhang, J.Z. Xing, J. Chen, L. Ko, J. Amanie, S. Gulavita, et al. Enhanced radiation sensitivity in prostate cancer by gold-nanoparticles, *Clin. Invest. Med.* 31 (2008) E160–7.

128. Y. Zheng, D.J. Hunting, P. Ayotte, L. Sanche, Radiosensitization of DNA by gold nanoparticles irradiated with high-energy electrons, *Radiat. Res.* 169 (2008) 19–27.

129. S.X. Zhang, J. Gao, T.A. Buchholz, Z. Wang, M.R. Salehpour, R.A. Drezek, et al. Quantifying tumor-selective radiation dose enhancements using gold nanoparticles: a monte carlo simulation study, *Biomed. Microdev.* 11 (2009) 925–933.

130. S. Jain, J. Coulter, K. Butterworth, A. Hounsell, F. Currel, K. Price, et al. Gold nanoparticles as sensitizers for radiation therapy at clinically relevant megavoltage X-ray energies (2010). http://www.asco.org/ASCOv2/Meetings/ Abstracts?&vmview=abstdetail view&confID=73&abstrac tID=30431.

131. A. Mesbahi, A review on gold nanoparticles radiosensitization effect in radiation therapy of cancer, *Rep. Pract. Oncol. Radiothe.* 15 (2010) 176–180.

132. X.D. Zhang, M.L. Guo, H.Y. Wu, Y.M. Sun, Y.Q. Ding, X. Feng, et al. Irradiation stability and cytotoxicity of gold nanoparticles for radiotherapy, *Int. J. Nanomed.* 4 (2009) 165–173.

133. S.H. Cho, Estimation of tumour dose enhancement due to gold nanoparticles during typical radiation treatments: a preliminary Monte Carlo study, *Phys. Med. Biol.* 50 (2005) N163–73.

134. S.H. Cho, B.L. Jones, S. Krishnan, The dosimetric feasibility of gold nanoparticle-aided radiation therapy (GNRT) via brachytherapy using low-energy gamma-/X-ray sources, *Phys. Med. Biol.* 54 (2009) 4889–4905.

135. B.D. Chithrani, A.A. Ghazani, W.C. Chan, Determining the size and shape dependence of gold nanoparticle uptake into mammalian cells, *Nano Lett.* 6 (2006) 662–668.

136. T. Kong, J. Zeng, X. Wang, X. Yang, J. Yang, S. McQuarrie, et al. Enhancement of radiation cytotoxicity in breast-cancer cells by localized attachment of gold nanoparticles, *Small* 4 (2008) 1537–1543.

137. M.-H. Lim, I.C. Jeung, J. Jeong, S.-J. Yoon, S.-H. Lee, J. Park, Y.-S. Kang, H. Lee, Y.-J. Park, H.G. Lee, S.-J. Lee, B.S. Han, N.W. Song, S.C. Lee, J.-S. Kim, K.-H. Bae, J.-K. Min. Graphene oxide induces apoptotic cell death in endothelial cells by activating autophagy via calcium-dependent phosphorylation of c-Jun N-terminal kinases, *Acta. Biomater.* 46 (2016) 191–203.

138. A.K. Geim, Graphene: status and prospects, *Science* 324 (2009) 1530–1534.

139. V.C. Sanchez, A. Jachak, R.H. Hurt, A.B. Kane, Biological interactions of graphene-family nanomaterials: an interdisciplinary review, *Chem. Res. Toxicol.* 25 (2012) 15–34.

140. Y. Wang, Y. Shao, D.W. Matson, J. Li, Y. Lin, Nitrogen-doped graphene and its application in electrochemical biosensing, *ACS Nano* 4 (2010) 1790–1798.

141. H. Bao, Y. Pan, Y. Ping, N.G. Sahoo, T. Wu, L. Li, J. Li, L.H. Gan, Chitosanfunctionalized graphene oxide as a nanocarrier for drug and gene delivery, *Small* 7 (2011) 1569–1578.

142. X. Fan, G. Jiao, W. Zhao, P. Jin, X. Li, Magnetic Fe_3O_4-graphene composites as targeted drug nanocarriers for pH-activated release, *Nanoscale* 5 (2013) 1143–1152.

143. L. Feng, L. Wu, X. Qu, New horizons for diagnostics and therapeutic applications of graphene and graphene oxide, *Adv. Mater.* 25 (2013) 168–186.

144. S.H. Ku, M. Lee, C.B. Park, Carbon-based nanomaterials for tissue engineering, *Adv. Healthcare Mater.* 2 (2013) 244–260.

145. G. Lalwani, A.M. Henslee, B. Farshid, L. Lin, F.K. Kasper, Y.X. Qin, A.G. Mikos, B. Sitharaman, Two-dimensional nanostructure-reinforced biodegradable polymeric nanocomposites for bone tissue engineering, *Biomacromolecules* 14 (2013) 900–909.

146. C.J. Shih, S. Lin, R. Sharma, M.S. Strano, D. Blankschtein, Understanding the pH-dependent behavior of graphene oxide aqueous solutions: a comparative experimental and molecular dynamics simulation study, *Langmuir* 28 (2012) 235–241.

147. C. Bussy, H. Ali-Boucetta, K. Kostarelos, Safety considerations for graphene: lessons learnt from carbon nanotubes, *Acc. Chem. Res.* 46 (2013) 692–701.

148. C. Chung, Y.K. Kim, D. Shin, S.R. Ryoo, B.H. Hong, D.H. Min, Biomedical applications of graphene and graphene oxide, *Acc. Chem. Res.* 46 (2013) 2211–2224.

149. G.Y. Chen, H.J. Yang, C.H. Lu, Y.C. Chao, S.M. Hwang, C.L. Chen, K.W. Lo, L.Y. Sung, W.Y. Luo, H.Y. Tuan, Y.C. Hu, Simultaneous induction of autophagy and toll-like receptor signaling pathways by graphene oxide, *Biomaterials* 33 (2012) 6559–6569.

150. K.H. Liao, Y.S. Lin, C.W. Macosko, C.L. Haynes, Cytotoxicity of graphene oxide and graphene in human erythrocytes and skin fibroblasts, *ACS Appl. Mater. Interfaces* 3 (2011) 2607–2615.

151. G. Qu, S. Liu, S. Zhang, L. Wang, X. Wang, B. Sun, N. Yin, X. Gao, T. Xia, J.J. Chen, G.B. Jiang, Graphene oxide induces toll-like receptor 4 (TLR4)-dependent necrosis in macrophages, *ACS Nano* 7 (2013) 5732–5745.

152. H. Yue, W. Wei, Z. Yue, B. Wang, N. Luo, Y. Gao, D. Ma, G. Ma, Z. Su, The role of the lateral dimension of graphene oxide in the regulation of cellular responses, *Biomaterials* 33 (2012) 4013–4021.

153. W. Hu, C. Peng, M. Lv, X. Li, Y. Zhang, N. Chen, C. Fan, Q. Huang, Protein coronamediated mitigation of cytotoxicity of graphene oxide, *ACS Nano* 5 (2011) 3693–3700.

154. Y. Zhang, S.F. Ali, E. Dervishi, Y. Xu, Z. Li, D. Casciano, A.S. Biris, Cytotoxicity effects of graphene and single-wall carbon nanotubes in neural phaeochromocytoma-derived PC12 cells, *ACS Nano* 4 (2010) 3181–3186.

155. N. Chatterjee, H.J. Eom, J. Choi, A systems toxicology approach to the surface functionality control of graphene-cell interactions, *Biomaterials* 35 (2014) 1109–1127.

156. M.C. Duch, G.R. Budinger, Y.T. Liang, S. Soberanes, D. Urich, S.E. Chiarella, L.A. Campochiaro, A. Gonzalez, N.S. Chandel, M.C. Hersam, G.M. Mutlu, Minimizing oxidation and stable nanoscale dispersion improves the biocompatibility of graphene in the lung, *Nano Lett.* 11 (2011) 5201–5207.

157. S.C. Nussenzweig, S. Verma, T. Finkel, The role of autophagy in vascular biology, *Circ. Res.* 116 (2015) 480–488.

158. C. He, D.J. Klionsky, Regulation mechanisms and signaling pathways of autophagy, *Annu. Rev. Genet.* 43 (2009) 67–93.

159. B. Ravikumar, C. Vacher, Z. Berger, J.E. Davies, S. Luo, L.G. Oroz, F. Scaravilli, D.F. Easton, R. Duden, C.J. O'kane, D.C. Rubinsztein, Inhibition of mTOR induces autophagy and reduces toxicity of polyglutamine expansions in fly and mouse models of Huntington disease, *Nat. Genet.* 36 (2004) 585–595.

160. K. Jing, K.S. Song, S. Shin, N. Kim, S. Jeong, H.R. Oh, J.H. Park, K.S. Seo, J.Y. Heo, J. Han, J.I. Park, C. Han, T. Wu, G.R. Kweon, S.K. Park, W.H. Yoon, B.D. Hwang, K. Lim, Docosahexaenoic acid induces autophagy through p53/AMPK/Mtor signaling and promotes apoptosis in human cancer cells harboring wild-type p53, *Autophagy* 7 (2011) 1348–1358.

161. G. Marino, M. Niso-Santano, E.H. Baehrecke, G. Kroemer, Self-consumption: the interplay of autophagy and apoptosis, *Nat. Rev. Mol. Cell Biol.* 15 (2014) 81–94.

162. Y. Liu, Y. Yang, Y.C. Ye, Q.F. Shi, K. Chai, S. Tashiro, S. Onodera, T. Ikejima, Activation of ERK-p53 and ERK-mediated phosphorylation of Bcl-2 are involved in autophagic cell death induced by the c-Met inhibitor SU11274 in human lung cancer A549 cells, *J. Pharmacol. Sci.* 118 (2012) 423–432.

163. A.J. Meijer, P. Codogno, Signalling and autophagy regulation in health, aging and disease, *Mol. Aspects Med.* 27 (2006) 411–425.

164. Y. Wei, S. Pattingre, S. Sinha, M. Bassik, B. Levine, JNK1-mediated phosphorylation of Bcl-2 regulates starvation-induced autophagy, *Mol. Cell* 30 (2008) 678–688.

165. E. Zalckvar, H. Berissi, L. Mizrachy, Y. Idelchuk, I. Koren, M. Eisenstein, H. Sabanay, R. Pinkas-Kramarski, A. Kimchi, DAP-kinase-mediated phosphorylation on the BH3 domain of beclin 1 promotes dissociation of beclin 1 from Bcl-XL and induction of autophagy, *EMBORep.* 10 (2009) 285–292.

166. J. Kim, R.P. Sharma, Calcium-mediated activation of c-Jun NH2-terminal kinase (JNK) and apoptosis in response to cadmium in murine macrophages, *Toxicol. Sci.* 81 (2004) 518–527.

167. S.K. Singh, M.K. Singh, M.K. Nayak, S. Kumari, S. Shrivastava, J.J. Grácio, D. Dash, Thrombus inducing property of atomically thin graphene oxide sheets, *ACS Nano* 5 (2011) 4987–4996.

168. W. Wang, Z. Li, J. Duan, C. Wang, Y. Fang, X.D. Yang, In vitro enhancement of dendritic cell-mediated anti-glioma immune response by graphene oxide, *Nanoscale Res. Lett.* 9 (2014) 311.

169. W.S. Hummers, R.E. Offeman, Preparation of graphitic oxide, *J. Am. Chem. Soc.* 80 (1958) 1339.

170. J. Shen, Y. Zhu, Y. Yang, J. Zong, J. Zhang, C. Li, One-pot hydrothermal synthesis of graphene quantum dots surface-passivated by polyethylene glycol and their photoelectric conversion under near-infrared light, *New J. Chem.* 36 (2012) 97–101.

171. S. Hussain, F. Al-Nsour, A.B. Rice, J. Marshburn, B. Yingling, Z. Ji, J.I. Zink, N.J. Walker, S. Garantziotis, Cerium dioxide nanoparticles induce apoptosis and autophagy in human peripheral blood monocytes, *ACS Nano* 6 (2012) 5820–5829.

172. L. Jia, R.R. Dourmashkin, P.D. Allen, A.B. Gray, A.C. Newland, S.M. Kelsey, Inhibition of autophagy abrogates tumour necrosis factor alpha induced apoptosis in human T-lymphoblastic leukaemic cells, *Br. J. Haematol.* 98 (1997) 673–685.

173. N. Mizushima, T. Yoshimori, B. Levine, Methods in mammalian autophagy research, *Cell* 140 (2010) 313–326.

174. G. Bjørkøy, T. Lamark, A. Brech, H. Outzen, M. Perander, A. Øvervatn, H. Stenmark, T. Johansen, P62/SQSTM1 forms protein aggregates degraded by autophagy and has a protective effect on huntingtin-induced cell death, *J. Cell Biol.* 171 (2005) 603–614.

175. S. Orrenius, B. Zhivotovsky, P. Nicotera, Regulation of cell death: the calcium apoptosis link, *Nat. Rev. Mol. Cell Biol.* 4 (2003) 552–565.

176. Loutfy H. Madkour, *Reactive Oxygen Species (ROS), Nanoparticles, and Endoplasmic Reticulum (ER) Stress-Induced Cell Death Mechanisms.* (2020). https://www.elsevier.com/books/reactive-oxygen-species-ros-nanoparticles-and-endoplasmic-reticulum-er-stress-induced-cell-death-mechanisms/madkour/978-0-12-822481-6.

177. Loutfy H. Madkour, *Nanoparticles Induce Oxidative and Endoplasmic Reticulum Antioxidant Therapeutic Defenses.* 1st Edition, Springer Nature, Switzerland AG (2020). https://www.springer.com/gp/book/9783030372965?utm_campaign=3_pier05_buy_print&utm_content=en_08082017&utm_medium=referral&utm_source=google_books#otherversion=9783030372972.

178. Loutfy H. Madkour, *Nucleic Acids as Gene Anticancer Drug Delivery Therapy.* 1st Edition. Elsevier, Amsterdam, Netherlands (2020). https://www.elsevier.com/books/nucleic-acids-as-gene-anticancer-drug-deliverytherapy/madkour/978-0-12-819777-6.

179. Loutfy H. Madkour, *Nanoelectronic Materials: Fundamentals and Applications.* Advanced Structured Materials Series, Volume 116, 1st Edition, Springer Nature, Switzerland AG (2019). https://link.springer.com/book/10.1007%2F978-3-030-21621-4; https://books.google.com.eg/books/about/Nanoelectronic_Materials.html?id=YQXCxAEACAAJ&source=kp_book_description&redir_esc=y; and https://www.springer.com/gp/book/9783030216207.

7 Advantages and Limitations of RNAi Delivery for Cancer Biological Therapeutics Imaging

Advantages and limitations of RNAi for cancer biological therapeutics imaging

In the development of RNAi-based therapeutics, imaging methods can provide a visible and quantitative way to investigate the therapeutic effect at anatomical, cellular, and molecular level; to noninvasively trace the distribution; and to study the biological processes in preclinical and clinical stages. Their abilities are important not only for therapeutic optimization and evaluation but also for shortening of the time of drug development to market. Typically, imaging-functionalized RNAi therapeutics delivery that combines nanovehicles and imaging techniques to study and improve their biodistribution and accumulation in tumor site has been progressively integrated into anticancer drug discovery and development processes.

7.1 INTRODUCTION

Since it was discovered that double-stranded RNA (dsRNA) can induce RNA interference (RNAi) in Caenorhabditis elegans [1], the capability of RNAi that can suppress the expression of target genes with high specificity and efficacy has been confirmed with small RNA sequences (siRNA/miRNA) [2]. Since then, much effort has been directed to develop RNAi therapeutics into clinic as a potential disruptive tool for new conservative and personalized treatment of a broad range of diseases [3], including viral infection [4], eye disorder [5], inflammatory disease [6], cardiovascular disease [7], genetic disorder [8], and cancer [9–11].

Currently, both naked siRNAs and nanoparticle-mediated delivery of RNA fragments have been investigated for cancer therapy. The administration route for naked siRNA is critically reliant on its accessibility to the target sites inside the body. Most of the naked siRNA fragments have been administered topically, which has the advantages of high bioavailability in target organs and low adverse reactions compared to systemic administration. The systemic administration of siRNA fragments requires them to reach the right organs or tissues after dispersing in the body and passing through the biological barriers, which is virtually impossible for naked small RNAs. The systemic delivery of siRNAs or other small therapeutic RNAs to target sites is impeded by many factors including nuclease degradation and rapid systemic elimination of "naked" small RNAs in biological systems [12]; intrinsic negative charge nature on the surface of small RNAs makes them very difficult

to transfer into cells that too also with negatively charged surface of bilayer phospholipid membrane [13]. Therefore, a variety of delivery systems have been engineered to address above issues and deliver small RNAs specifically to target sites, including tumors and inflammatory foci, for instance, lipid nanoparticles made with cationic lipids; lipidol and other lipid materials [14–17]; polymeric nanoparticles made with polyethylenimine (PEI); dendrimers; membrane-disruptive and cyclodextrin-containing polymers [18–20]; membrane-disruptive peptides [21,22]; aptamer-siRNA chimeras [23]; single-chain fragmented antibodies [24]; supramolecular assemblies [25–27]; inorganic nanoparticles, including multishell nanoparticles, mesoporous nanoparticles, and carbon-based nanomaterials [28]; and so on [29–33]. However, the entrapment of nano-sized carriers in the reticuloendothelial system (RES), the vascular endothelial resistance in tissues, the barriers of extracellular matrix, and the intracellular release from endosomal uptake [34,35] are the major challenges for the systemic delivery of RNAi therapeutics. In addition, the siRNA-based therapeutics encounter safety concerns owing to unexpected adverse effects, including off-target effects, innate immune responses, proinflammatory cytokine induction, and spleen toxicity, which were found in the early studies of those candidates [8,36–38].

There are three major aspects of scientific challenges in developing RNAi therapeutics for cancer therapy (Figure 7.1): (i) target gene selection for RNAi and gene vector development for either systemic or local administration; (ii) product screening and preclinical evaluation including the relative efficacy, biodistribution, pharmacokinetics, and toxicity; and (iii) clinical study of the efficacy, safety, pharmacokinetics, and optimal dose. It has been proven that noninvasive imaging methods and biomarker detection could speed up the development of RNAi therapeutics [39–41]. Developing powerful imaging techniques and methods is important for providing valuable information by visualizing, characterizing, and quantifying the biological processes of RNAi therapeutics and monitoring their therapeutic effects and factors that are crucial for the optimization of RNAi cancer therapeutics.

Generally, in vivo imaging of RNAi refers to the utilization of a variety of imaging modalities, including bioluminescence imaging (BLI) [42], photoluminescence imaging [43,44], magnetic resonance imaging (MRI) [45], positron emission tomography (PET) [46], single-photon emission

DOI: 10.1201/9781003229674-7

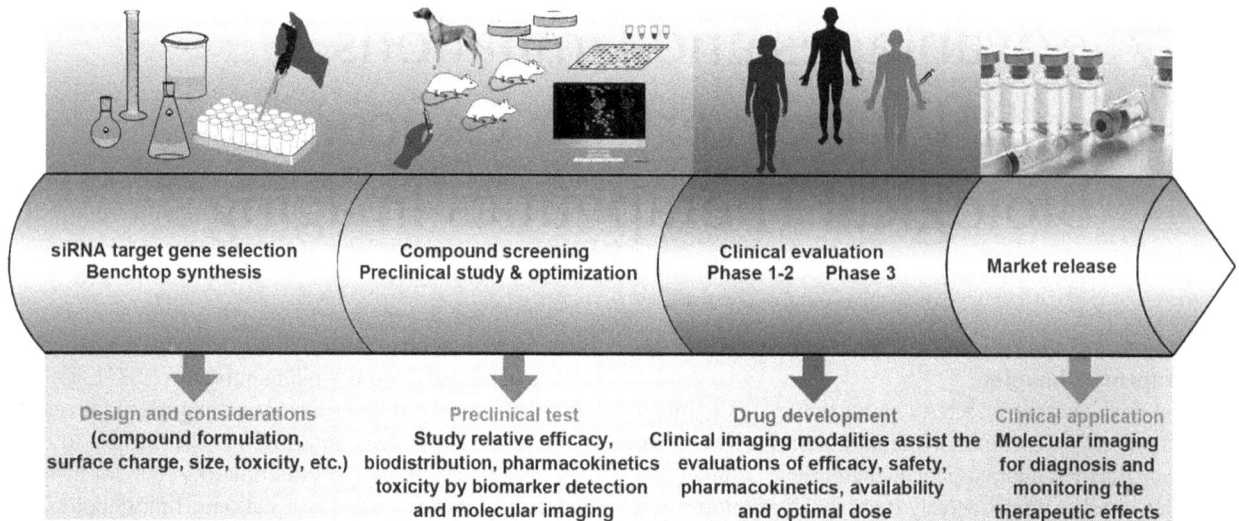

FIGURE 7.1 The workflow of developing RNAi therapeutics and translating them for clinical applications. There are mainly four steps for this, including targeting gene selection, compound screening, clinical evaluation, and market release. Imaging methods could assist the development of RNAi therapeutics at every step in the RNAi therapeutics development processes, including marking for gene selection, tracing the small RNA sequences for pharmacokinetics study, evaluating the gene-silencing efficacy, and diagnosing tumors and monitoring the therapeutic effects.

computed tomography (SPECT) [47], and ultrasound [48], to quantitatively and/or qualitatively visualize the *in vivo* behavior of the RNAi therapeutics. Many imaging modalities have been applied for RNAi researches. The therapeutic genes have been directly or indirectly marked with a variety of imaging contrast agents to make them detectable in biological systems with clinically relevant imaging equipment. These probe-labeled systems with target delivery function hold high promise for studying the pharmacological properties of RNAi therapeutics in clinical translation. This chapter highlights the current status of RNAi-based cancer therapeutics in clinical trials with discussion of selected cases. Before addressing the current progresses of applying various imaging techniques in RNAi therapeutics development, we will discuss the biological barriers and challenges for developing RNAi therapeutics and emphasize the design considerations of non-viral gene delivery vehicles for targeting tumors. Finally, the perspective of applying various imaging techniques for developing RNAi cancer therapeutics is described in more detail.

7.2 RNAi CANCER THERAPEUTICS IN CLINICAL TRIALS

The significant advantages of RNAi strategy are its high specificity together with infinite choice of genes that can be applied for cancer therapy. The RNAi therapeutics could interfere with angiogenesis, metastasis, chemoresistance of tumors, and the proliferation of cancer cells [49,50]. The intrinsic features of RNAi therapeutics make RNAi a novel strategy for cancer treatment. Therefore, a myriad of RNAi therapeutics is under investigation for this purpose. Recently, around 10 types of RNAi-based cancer

therapeutics have entered the early stage of clinical trial (Table 7.1), demonstrating potential capability of RNAi with specific gene-silencing efficacy for cancer treatment. Although the ongoing clinical trials provide encouraging results for future commercial success, many obstacles still remain ahead for applying RNAi therapeutics in humans. Here, we highlight the current status of two selected cases in clinical evaluation.

The siRNA-loaded lipid nanoparticles (Atu027) have been applied clinically to suppress the expression of protein kinase N3 (PKN3) [63]. PKN3 is an effector of PI3K pathway related to the modulation of cell growth, differentiation, survival, motility, and adhesion as well as immune cell and glucose transport function. Chronic activation of PI3K pathway could prevent various human cancers and inhibit the growth of malignant cells [64]. Although numerous signaling molecules can be considered as therapeutic candidates to mediate the PI3K pathway, their upstream inhibition could trigger signal cascades with undesirable signal regulation of normal cells associated with various side effects. For this reason, PKN3 is considered to be a proper effector to adjust the growth of metastatic cancer cells with activated PI3K [65]. The results from animal studies indicate that Atu027 could effectively knock down the expression of PKN3 gene in the vascular endothelium to inhibit tumor growth and metastasis [63]. In clinical study of Atu027, no interferon response or activation of cytokines was observed, which may be due to liposomal encapsulation of siRNA with enhanced safety while avoiding triggering side reactions during circulation [66]. Thus, Atu027 was well tolerated, and no dose-dependent toxicity was observed. Recent study of using Atu027 to treat advanced solid tumors has found that up to 41% of patients exhibited

TABLE 7.1

Current Clinical Status of RNAi Therapeutics for Cancer Treatment

Indications	Name	Delivery Route	Target	Delivery System	Development Phase	References
Advanced solid tumors	siRNA-EphA2-DOPC	Intravenous injection	EphA2	Lipid-based nanoparticles	Preclinical	[51]
Metastatic tumors or cannot be removed by surgery	APN401	Intravenous injection	E3 ubiquitin ligase Cbl-b	*Ex vivo* transfection	Preclinical	[52]
Metastatic melanoma, absence of CNS metastases	iPsiRNA	Intradermal injection	LMP2, LMP7, MECL1	*Ex vivo* transfection	Phase I, completed	[53]
Advanced solid tumors	Atu027	Intravenous infusion	PKN3	Lipid-based nanoparticles	Phase I, completed	[54]
Pancreatic ductal adenocarcinoma; Pancreatic cancer	siG12D LODER	Intratumoral implantation	KRASG12D	LODER polymer	Phase I, completed	[55]
Primary or secondary liver cancer	TKM-080,301	Hepatic intra-arterial injection	PLK1	Lipid-based nanoparticles	Phase I, completed	[56]
METAVIR F3–4	ND-L02-s0201	Intravenous injection	HSP47	Lipid-based nanoparticles	Phase I, recruiting	[57]
Solid tumors; multiple myeloma; non-Hodgkin's lymphoma	DCR-MYC	Intravenous infusion	MYC	Lipid-based nanoparticles	Phase I, recruiting	[58]
Cancer; solid tumor	CALAA-01	Intravenous injection	RRM2	cyclodextrin-containing polymer	Phase I, terminated	[59]
Neuroendocrine tumors; adrenocortical carcinoma	TKM 080301	Intravenous infusion	PLK1	Lipid-based nanoparticles	Phase I/II, recruiting	[60]
Solid tumors	ALN-VSP02	Intravenous injection	KSP, VEGF	Lipid-based nanoparticles	Phase I, completed	[61,62]

no further progression of tumors after eight weeks of treatment [67]. Since Atu027 targets tumor stroma instead of tumor cells, it is expected that this treatment will be effective for all type of vascularized metastatic cancers.

Another clinical trial product that targets kinesin spindle protein (KSP) and vascular endothelial growth factor (VEGF) for treating solid tumors is ALN-VSP02. KSP is a type of motor protein that plays a central role in the proper separation of emerging spindle poles during mitosis, and it is upregulated in many types of cancer cells. Therefore, KSP is another attractive target for cancer therapy by RNAi therapeutics, as silencing its expression will lead to cell cycle arrest at mitosis through the formation of an abnormal mitotic spindle and finally inducing apoptosis [68]. VEGF, which is involved in angiogenesis and lymphangiogenesis, is overexpressed in numerous cancer types [69,70]. Blocking the expression of VEGF is expected to inhibit angiogenesis and suppress tumor growth [71]. The dually targeted RNAi drug (ALN-VSP02) is in clinical trial, aimed for treating solid tumors (Figure 7.2a). In the first in-human study, the clinical activity, safety, and pharmacokinetics of ALN-VSP02 were evaluated, demonstrating good systemic tolerance and acceptable toxicity with biweekly intravenous administration. The results also demonstrated that the expression levels of both target genes were decreased in multiple patients, including one patient with complete regression of liver metastases from

endometrial cancer (Figure 7.2b and c) [11]. Although ALN-VSP02 has achieved some success in clinical trials, some interesting results should be noticed. The infusion-related reactions (IRR) of ALNVSP02 seem to be complement-mediated, not cytokine-induced. Additionally, it was found that ALN-VSP02 could cause spleen toxicity with prolonged dosing. The patient with endometrial cancer had a more than 50% decrease in blood flow (Ktrans) and a 90% reduction in spleen size [11]. Based on the above observations, some improvements are suggested for future development of stable nucleic acid lipid particle (SNALP)-based cancer siRNA therapeutics to improve the safety. It includes using more efficacious and less immunogenic lipid components and reducing the size of SNALP-based drug delivery systems to be small enough to improve the circulation time and benefit the accumulation in solid tumors through the enhanced permeability and retention (EPR) effect. Finally, the biodegradability of SNALP should be optimized to reduce the spleen toxicity, which was induced by lipid accumulation along the endosomal–lysosomal pathway.

To date, owing to the low stability, poor systemic distribution, possible side reactions, and low bioavailability of naked siRNA, most siRNA-based therapeutics in clinical trials are formulated by encapsulation within lipid-based particles. These early trials hold great potential for cancer therapy, especially allowing RNAi to be precisely tailored in each case. However, many challenges still need to be

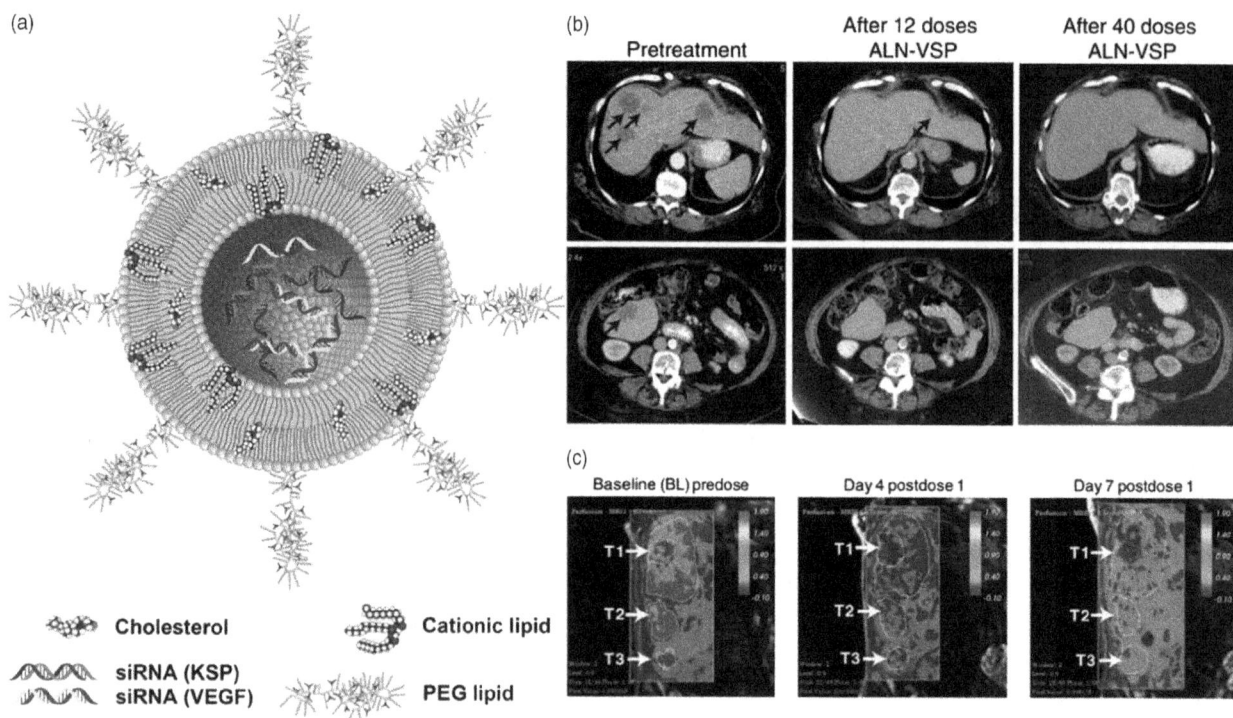

FIGURE 7.2 (a) Schematic structure of ALN-VSP formulation: The siRNA lipid nanoparticle is composed of cationic or ionizable lipid with cholesterol and encapsulated with two different siRNAs to target KSP and VEGF genes. The nanoparticles are stabilized by surface binding of PEGylated lipids. (b) CT images demonstrated a complete response of ALN-VSP in an endometrial cancer patient with multiple liver metastatic tumors (black arrows). (c) Dynamic contrast-enhanced MRI (DCE-MRI) images from another patient with three metastatic pancreatic neuroendocrine tumors in the right lobe of the liver (white arrows). A significant change of tumor blood flow was observed during the treatment at 0.7 mg/kg (indicated in red). (Adapted with permission from Ref. [11].)

solved for personalized cancer therapy by RNAi to become a reality. First, RNAi delivery systems with high efficiency and low toxicity are needed for early (Phase I) clinical trial. Then, an adequate knockdown of target genes needs to be achieved in later trials of Phase I to Phase II. Besides, possible off-target effects in normal tissues should be avoided for safety consideration (Phase II). The positive or negative correlation of target knockdown with tumor regression should be analyzed during Phase II to verify the feasibility for Phase III study. Finally, for future clinical applications, the distribution, metabolism, and degradation of siRNA loaded nanocarriers need to be extensively studied.

7.3 BIOLOGICAL BARRIERS FOR RNAi CANCER THERAPEUTICS

Although several siRNA-based therapeutics have been evaluated in early phase clinical studies, there are various biological barriers that need to be conquered for successful clinical translation, such as efficient delivery of RNAi therapeutics to tumors after reaching the circulation, overcoming the vascular barrier, cellular uptake, and endosomal escape (Figure 7.3). Because many target sites are not accessible or not convenient for local administration, the systemic administration of RNAi therapeutics is essential. To fully exploit the therapeutic potential of RNAi

therapeutics, developing effective and biocompatible gene delivery systems that could specifically target cancer cells in the body is a key factor. Generally, gene vehicles with diameter ranging from 10 to 100 nm are suitable for systemic administration. These gene vectors are needed to be stable enough and well dispersed in blood. Besides, gene vectors decorated with targeting moieties could facilitate specific cellular uptake by cancer cells, a strategy that is important to evade the innate immune stimulation in the body [72]. In such cases, noninvasive imaging tools can be utilized to study the pharmacokinetic properties of RNAi therapeutics and monitor their effects in a visible way. In order to accelerate the screening process, imaging techniques with adequate spatial resolution and sensitivity for small animals should be used for determining the temporal and spatial biodistribution of the developed compounds. This may help reduce irrational costs and allow the selection of the most promising candidates during the early stage of drug development [73].

7.3.1 ADMINISTRATION BARRIER

Administration through oral route is obviously the most convenient approach for patients. However, it is currently challenging for treating cancers through the oral administration of RNAi therapeutics due to difficulties in accessing

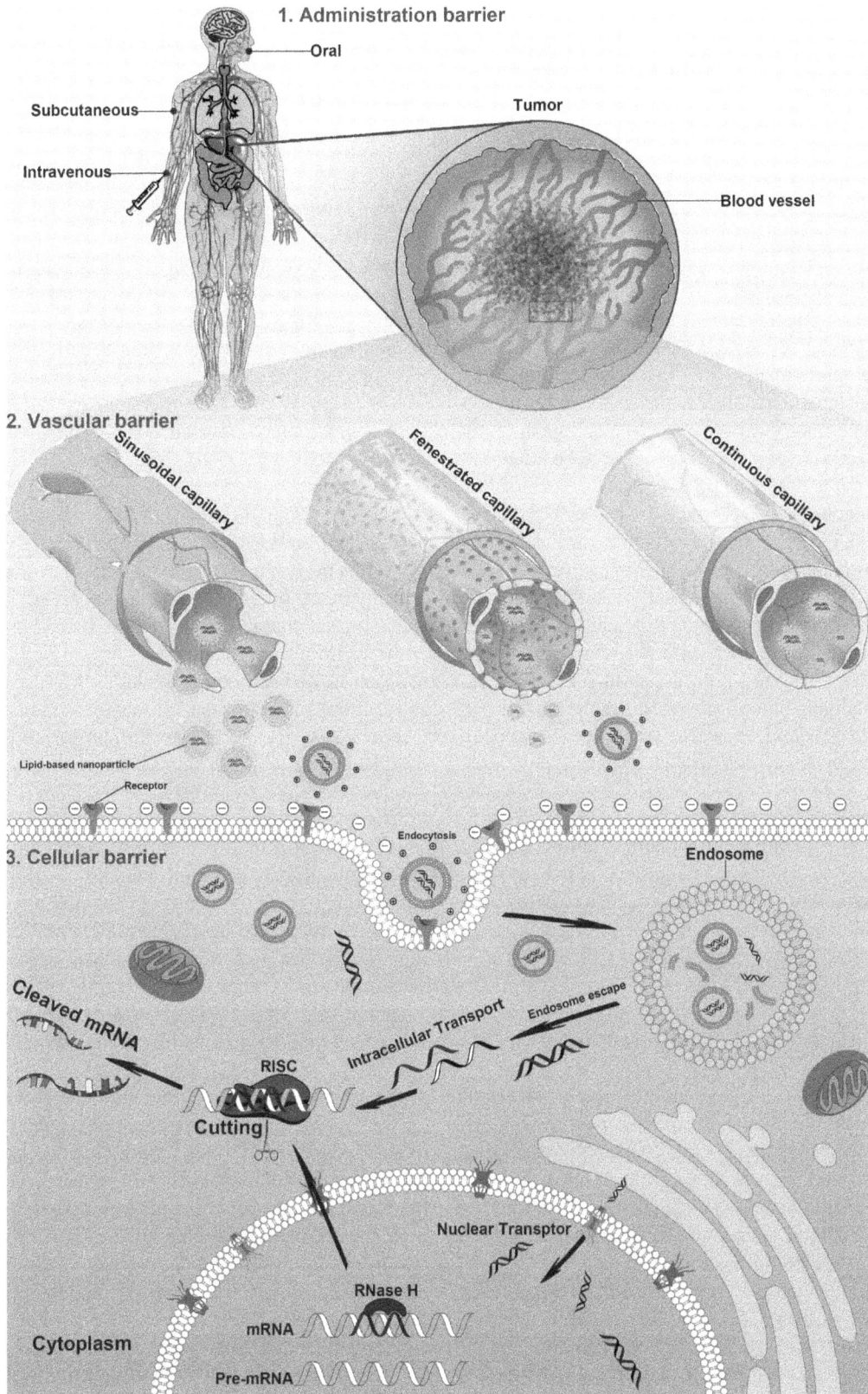

FIGURE 7.3 Schematic illustration of nanocarrier-mediated delivery of RNAi therapeutics: the biological barriers for gene silencing in cancer treatment include reaching the circulation, crossing the vascular barrier, cellular uptake, and endosomal escape. Following systemic administration in patients, the RNAi therapeutics could be transported to the blood vessels in tumor tissues. The gene vectors could escape from the sinusoidal and fenestrated capillaries and retain in the tumor regions. The gene vectors could be taken by cancer cells through endocytosis or ligand- mediated intracellular transport and then transferred into the cytoplasm to silence target genes for cancer therapy.

tumor sites, including poor intestinal stability and insufficient permeability across intestinal epithelium into circulation [34]. Subcutaneous administration is another route for the systemic delivery of RNAi therapeutics. The drugs can reach the circulation directly from the interstitial space of subcutaneous connective tissue to the capillaries by traversing through the vascular barrier or through lymphatic drainage. Compared to intravenous administration, the sustained entry of drugs into circulation through subcutaneous route can achieve almost complete absorption without first-pass effect in the liver. A clinical example of RNAi therapeutics using subcutaneous administration to treat transthyretin-mediated amyloidosis is ALN-TTRsc, which could achieve approximately 90% knockdown of the transthyretin gene expression in liver in a phase-I study [74]. For the subcutaneous administration of RNAi therapeutics, the lipophilicity and size of gene vectors have to be taken into account to avoid endocytosis by phagocytic cells in subcutis and lymph node drainage, which subsequently influence the potency of RNAi therapeutics. For further details on designing desirable properties of siRNA delivery system, please refer to the following reviews [17,19,75–79]. The most direct way for RNAi therapeutics to reach blood circulation is intravenous or infusion injection. Currently, several RNAi products for systemic administration have entered clinical evaluation for cancer treatment (Table 7.1). In order to identify and validate gene vector candidates for specific administration route of siRNA delivery during preclinical stage, *in vitro* and *in vivo* optical imaging can be assisted as a fast and inexpensive method for compound screening by visualizing and evaluating the biocompatibility, stability, absorption, and distribution in live subjects in a real-time manner, as well as biological interactions at subcellular level.

7.3.2 VASCULAR BARRIER

Passing through the endothelium of vasculature is a key step for RNAi therapeutics. Depending on the vascular permeability of target organs or tissues, a certain half-life of RNAi therapeutics in plasma is required. A successful gene silencing in the liver primarily benefits from the discontinuous sinusoidal capillaries, as the large openings in the endothelium can greatly access the leaked RNAi nanocarriers from the vasculature. Such pores in sinusoidal capillaries are wide openings for both passive and active passages of RNAi nanocarriers up to 100 nm in size from bloodstream to hepatocytes in liver. Tumor capillaries are discontinuous, with considerable variation of cell composition, the basement membrane, and pericyte coverage. Kobayashi et al. suggested that four important factors should be considered when passive targeting is involved [80]: (i) internal and external blood flow of tumor, (ii) tumor vascular permeability, (iii) structural barriers enforced by extracellular matrix and tumor cells, and (4) intratumoral interstitial pressure. These factors can certainly influence the accumulation of

certain sized nanoparticles or molecules in tumor tissue by EPR effect [81]. In order to take advantage of the EPR effect in tumor tissues, or receptor mediated transcytotic pathway through vascular endothelium [34], longer half-life for RNAi therapeutics is necessary. In contrast to sinusoidal or tumor capillaries, the fenestrated capillaries have much smaller pores (60–80 nm in diameter) in endothelium covered with continuous basal lamina, which can prevent the diffusion of large-scale nanoparticles. They are mainly located in the endocrine glands, intestines, pancreas, and glomeruli of kidneys. The tightness, shape of the pores, continuous basal lamina, and extracellular matrix should be considered for designing non-hepatic tissues-targeted RNAi-based formulations and delivery strategies.

The stability of RNAi therapeutics in blood circulation is of primary importance for arriving tumor tissues. A major challenge is to evade the phagocytic uptake by mononuclear phagocyte system (MPS) in the bloodstream [82]. The formulation size, surface electrostatic nature, and stability can certainly affect the uptake by MPS. It is more likely to interact with MPS and other components in the bloodstream if they possess large size and excessive net charge [83]. Thus, the formulations are generally of minimum net charge through modification with hydrophilic and neutral molecules to increase the stability. Introducing poly(ethylene glycol) (PEG) shell to the surface of RNAi vectors is a general approach for stabilization. However, the high stability achieved by PEGylation can reduce uptake by target cells [84]. This can be solved by attaching targeting moieties to RNAi therapeutics [85]. The vascular endothelium is negatively charged because the heparin sulfate proteoglycans are on the cell surface and in the extracellular matrix. Additionally, tumor vascularity is controlled by oxygen supply and some metabolites [86]. It has been observed that increasing the tumor vascularity could result in more efficient delivery of RNAi agents to solid tumors [87]. It was reported that nanoparticles with smaller size and increased lipophilicity could lead to higher level of accumulation in tumor tissues [88]. To evaluate the delivery efficiency and *in vivo* behavior of the potential RNAi therapeutics, quantitative functional, and molecular imaging can be integrated to provide valuable information concerning pharmacokinetics and biodistribution properties in animal models, such as quantitative visualization of compound absorption and distribution in tissues and organs, as well as elimination time after the administration, and the amount of compounds reaching target tissues. Usually, the quantitative imaging assessment can be performed in a real-time, whole-body, and noninvasive way by selecting appropriate imaging techniques. In this method, the compound is often labeled with specific imaging probes corresponding to the imaging modality for further applications. A great benefit of this approach is that the animals can be imaged repeatedly for longitudinal studies, which minimizes the number of animals needed for a given experiment [89].

7.3.3 CELLULAR BARRIER

Cellular uptake is critical for successful delivery of RNAi therapeutics into the cytoplasm for gene silencing. Basically, cell membrane is comprised of hydrophobic phospholipid bilayer embedded with various functional proteins. The innate negatively charged cell surface provides an external biological barrier to naked siRNA molecules. The small cationic peptides, cationic lipids, and polymers have often been applied to facilitate the cellular uptake of siRNA molecules via endocytosis [90]. However, for targeted delivery of RNAi therapeutics into cancer cells, the receptor-mediated endocytosis is mostly preferred, and various ligands have been used for targeted delivery of RNAi therapeutics, including folate [91], transferrin [92], and aptamers [93]. Those ligands could specifically interact with receptors overexpressed on the surface of cancer cells to promote cellular uptake. Pros and cons of using various targeting ligands for siRNA therapeutics have been reviewed elsewhere [94]. Once entering into target cells, the success in approaching RNA induced silencing complex (RISC) in cytoplasm is largely dependent on endosomal escape. It has been suggested that endosomal escape should occur before late endosomes fuse with lysosomes, which contains certain digestive enzymes [95]. For cationic polymers, which could enhance endosomolysis via absorbing protons and preventing the acidification of the endosomes, the elevated influx of the protons to endosomes increases osmotic pressure that causes lysosome swelling and rupture, eventually releasing the gene vectors to cytoplasm [96,97]. Similarly, ionizable lipids with neutral charge in bloodstream can become positively charged in endosomes, subsequently leading to disruption of the endosome membrane [17]. Elucidating the mechanism of endosomal escape pathways can help develop new strategies for gene delivery without relying on acidification. For investigations of cellular uptake and intracellular trafficking, molecular/cellular imaging is an essential tool to demonstrate the ligand-receptor interaction, subcellular translocation, and mechanism of potential RNAi therapeutics. Fluorescent probes and radioactive isotope-labeled drug candidates are commonly used for whole-body and subcellular tracking to provide quantitative and qualitative information of biological processes occurring at cellular and molecular levels.

7.3.4 IMMUNE RESPONSE AND SAFETY

The key issue in the application of RNAi therapeutic is the safety without any undesirable side effects. Unwanted silencing of target genes in normal organs or tissues is called "off-target silencing" [38,98]. The siRNAs longer than 30 bp can induce the interferon pathway [36]. Such induction of interferon reaction is caused by the innate immune system because the human body recognizes long dsRNA as virus particles and triggers the innate immune system to overcome the infection. Several investigations showed that even low concentration of siRNAs can induce natural immunity by activating interferon expression [99]. It is suggested that the main mechanisms of immune response caused by some siRNAs are the stimulated production of proinflammatory cytokines through TLR-8 on monocytes and TLR-7 on dendritic cells in a sequence-dependent manner [36,100]. In order to overcome this problem, the therapeutic siRNAs should be less than 21–23 bp [36]. Chemical modifications including 2′-O-methylation are also performed to avoid immune activation of siRNAs. Hence, immunostimulatory effects of potential siRNA-based therapeutics must be evaluated in animals prior to the clinical trial until the exact mechanism of sequence-dependent siRNA-induced immune response is fully understood [101].

In addition to siRNA-induced immune activation, the formulation of siRNA-based nanoparticles also plays an important role in safety profile for systemic delivery. Presently, the collective results of siRNA SNALP-based nanoparticles (ALN-VSP), cationic liposome/lipoplexes (Atu027), and cyclodextrin-based polymers (CALAA-01) have shown RNAi efficacy and dose tolerability in early clinical development. Based on these valuable outcomes and lessons learned, several additional key investigations are suggested here. (i) The quality control assay for RNAi products must be performed to prevent structure alteration during the practical use. (ii) A better understanding of proinflammatory cytokine response is needed for developing more potent siRNA-based nanoparticles with less acute immunostimulatory events. The side effects could be reflected in the change of pathological states or pathological indicators, such as inflammation, enzyme levels, and other biological factors. (iii) Imaging techniques could be applied to study the safety of RNAi therapeutics. Once the safety evaluation of a potential RNAi therapeutic has been established in early trial, molecular imaging can assist in the establishment of biological activity at appropriate dosage range with acceptable toxicities associated with the detection, diagnosis, evaluation, treatment, and management of cancer.

7.4 IMAGING MODALITIES IN THE RNAi CANCER THERAPEUTICS DEVELOPMENT PROCESS

Noninvasive imaging techniques are important tools to visualize and quantify the biological processes of RNAi therapeutics at cellular or tissue levels in a real-time way. Imaging-guided delivery of RNAi therapeutics can trace the pathway of RNAi therapeutics inside the body, provide pathological information of tumors, evaluate the tumor targeted delivery, and provide further information about the pharmacokinetics of the RNAi therapeutics.

7.4.1 OPTICAL IMAGING

Optical imaging, mainly including fluorescence imaging and bioluminescence imaging (BLI), provides the most convenient way for preclinical study of RNAi knockdown due to their advantages including abundant choices of optical dyes, easy labeling, noninvasiveness, multi-channel imaging function, and whole-body real-time readout. Besides, the excellent sensitivity and inexpensive use of optical imaging (with maximum penetration depth of few centimeters [102,103]) make it a promising modality for real-time monitoring of siRNA delivery in small animals.

For fluorescence imaging, the animals are illuminated by a light at an appropriate wavelength to excite the fluorescent agents *in situ*, and then, the emitted light from fluorescent agents is filtered and detected by a charge-coupled device (CCD) camera maintained at low temperature (Figure 7.4a) [104]. Since both the excitation and emission lights used are low-energy photons, it is considerably safer than other imaging systems that involve ionizing radiation. However, the use of relatively low energy light results in limited tissue penetration due to the light absorption by tissue components, which makes it virtually impossible for deep tissue imaging in large animals or human subjects. Moreover, there are other intrinsic limitations for consideration, for example, the light scattering phenomenon during the light propagation in tissues can result in a blurry fluorescence image [105]. For *in vivo* optical imaging, autofluorescence is an undesired background signal emitted by natural fluorophores in tissues, which can overlay with fluorescent signal from optical probes, and consequently reduce the signal-to-noise ratio [105]. Near-infrared fluorescent (NIRF) agents are generally applied for labeling siRNA therapeutics, as NIRF emits light in the range of 650–900 nm with deep tissue penetration by minimizing the tissue absorption, scattering, and autofluorescence [106]. For instance, VEGF siRNAs labeled with cyanines dye (Cy5.5) were conjugated to PEG through disulfides to form micelles through the interaction with PEI [107]. With Cy5.5, the VEGF siRNA-loaded micelles could be traced for delivering siRNA into prostate cancer cells (PC3), and the accumulation of Cy5.5-labeled siRNA, siRNA/PEI mixture, and micelles could be detected in tumors, and the main organs also could be monitored after administration to PC-3 tumor-bearing mice. The fluorescent dyes could also be utilized to study the intracellular pathway of RNAi therapeutics. By image-based analysis of lipid nanoparticles (LNPs) incorporating A647-labeled siRNA, it was observed that the LNPs could enter cancer cells through clathrin-mediated endocytosis and macropinocytosis, while the efficiency of siRNA escape from endosome to cytosol was low (1%–2%) and the endosome escape only occurred when the LNPs were located in the compartment sharing early and late endosomal characteristics [108]. In addition, fluorescence imaging could provide multi-channel imaging functions by labeling RNAi therapeutics with multiple dyes. For instance, the Cy3 and Cy5-labeled siRNAs were covalently linked to PEG to form nanocarrier-like loop, which could generate signals for dual imaging of the products inside cancer cells based on the fluorescence resonance energy transfer (FRET) of the fluorophore pair

[109]. Furthermore, the RNAi therapeutics in blood circulation, leakage from blood to tumor tissues as well as distribution in tumor tissues can be monitored in a real-time manner with intravital confocal laser scanning microscopy (IVRTCLSM). For instance, the Cy5-siRNAincorporated polymeric micelles and naked siRNA (Cy5-siRNA) could be traced in blood circulation to study their pharmacokinetics *in vivo*, to investigate their entry from blood to tumor tissues, as well as their distribution in tumor tissues by utilizing IVRTCLSM (Figure 7.4b–d) [110–112].

Besides organic fluorescent dyes, other nanomaterials, such as quantum dots (QDs) [113], carbon dots (C-dots) [114], and up-converting nanoparticles (UCNPs) [115], are also used for optical imaging as well as for siRNA delivery due to their high signal intensity and photostability. Specifically, tumor-specific, multifunctional siRNA-loaded QDs were prepared to induce downregulation of the expression of epidermal growth factor receptor variant III (EGFRvIII), which plays an important role in interfering with the proliferation of various types of cancer cells, while the uptake of siRNA-QDs was monitored by fluorescence imaging [116]. Compared to QDs, the C-dots show advantages of better biocompatibility, lower cost, and easier preparation and are considered as a potential alternative to QDs [117]. The C-dots surface coated with alkyl–PEI2k could effectively deliver siRNA and transfect against firefly luciferase (fLuc) with inhibited expression of luciferase gene in 4 T1-luc cells, while maintaining their biocompatibility and fluorescence properties [118]. The UCNPs have gained increasing attention in recent years as a new generation of biological luminescent nanoprobes for cell labeling and optical imaging. It offers many advantages, such as deep penetration, low background autofluorescence, and high resistance to photo-bleaching, thus providing a promising optical imaging way for monitoring the siRNA transfection [119,120].

In contrast to fluorescence imaging, BLI does not require an external light illumination on the living subjects because the bioluminescence is produced by oxidation reaction of luciferin with catalytic assistance of luciferase enzyme in the body. Various luciferase genes can be introduced into biological systems via transfection techniques and expressed with corresponding luciferase enzymes (Figure 7.5a). In this technique, there is no interference from autofluorescence and endogenous bioluminescence. Thus, BLI can provide a higher signal sensitivity and better signal-to-noise ratio than fluorescence imaging. By exposing RNAi therapeutics to cancer cells or injecting to tumor-bearing animals, the expression of bioluminescent reporters and fluorescent proteins, such as luciferases, the green fluorescent protein (GFP), and red fluorescent protein (RFP) [121], could be tested to evaluate the gene-silencing efficacy of those products. This could be helpful in forecasting their interfering ability for screening the most effective siRNA therapeutics and the best formulations before further test in human. In one study, Kay's group demonstrated the feasibility of monitoring siRNA delivery and assessing

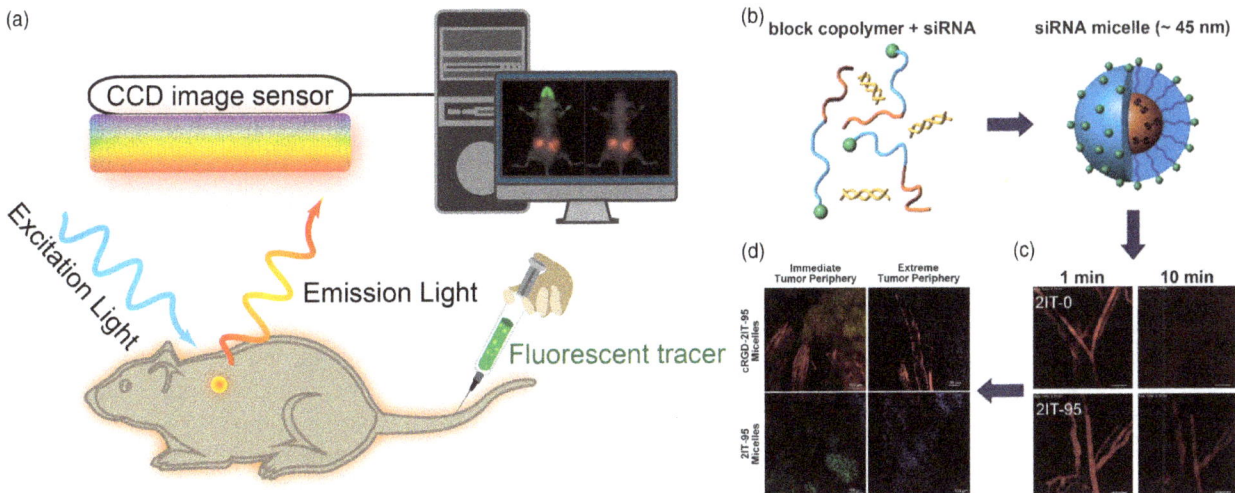

FIGURE 7.4 Optical fluorescence imaging. (a) A schematic illustration of the basic principle of *in vivo* fluorescence imaging. First, a fluorescently labeled RNAi therapeutics is injected into mouse body, and the subject is illuminated by an excitation light at specific wavelength, resulting an excitation of fluorescent molecules and subsequent emission light of different wavelength. The emitted light is filtered and then detected by CCD image sensor. The fluorescence signals and animal photo are finally converted to a single detailed image. The figures on right show using fluorescence imaging to trace polymeric micelles incorporated with dye-labeled siRNA in the mice body. (b) Schematic illustration of polymeric micelle structure formed by self-assembly of block copolymers with fluorescent dye-labeled siRNA. (c) Ear-lobe dermis snap-shots of blood circulation of two types of micelles after intravenous injection for 1 and 10 min. (d) Micro distribution of micelles incorporated with Cy5-labeled siRNA at 24 h post-injection. (red: siRNA; green: tumor cell nuclei; purple: other cell nuclei). (Adapted with permission from Ref. [110].)

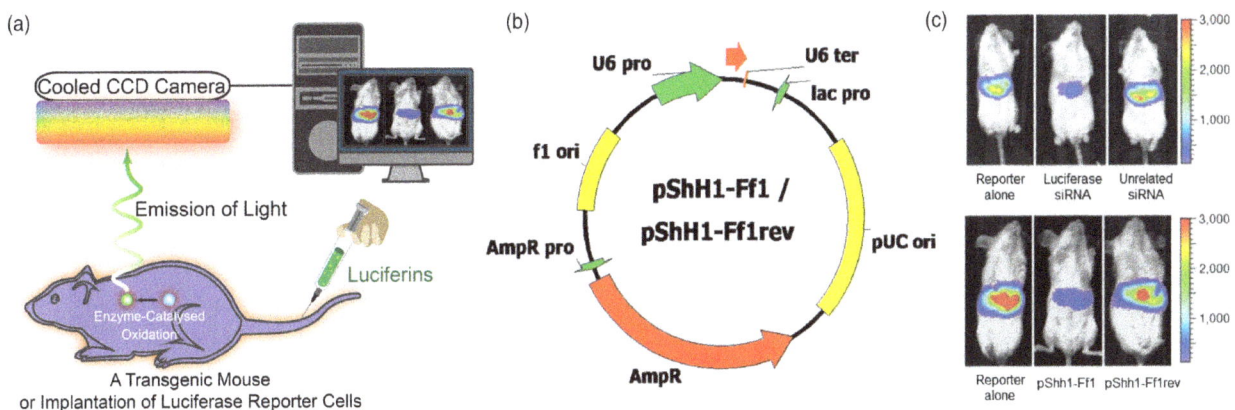

FIGURE 7.5 Optical bioluminescence imaging. (a) A schematic illustration of the basic principle of *in vivo* bioluminescence imaging. In this case, mouse with luciferase (Luc)-labeled cancer cells that express luciferase is required. After injecting the enzyme substrate luciferin into the mouse body, the bioluminescence light is generated when the luciferin molecules interact with luciferase via enzyme-catalyzed oxidation. Finally, the emitted light is detected by a cooled CCD camera and the image is produced by computer. (b) The plasmids used for transfection into mouse liver. (c) Representative images (upper image) of mice co-transfected with luciferase plasmid pGL3-control without siRNA, with luciferase siRNA or with unrelated siRNA. The results indicate that the luciferase expression was specifically suppressed by siRNA-mediated inhibition in adult mice, but the unrelated siRNAs had no effect. Another result from (c) (lower image) shows the gene silencing of luciferase expression by functional shRNAs (pShh1-Ff1). These outcomes demonstrated that the plasmid-encoded shRNAs can induce an effective and specific RNAi response *in vivo*. (Adapted with permission from Ref. [122].)

silencing effect by *in vivo* BLI (Figure 7.5b and c) [122]. In another study, by co-injection of luciferase plasmid and synthetic luciferase siRNA, the silencing effect in a variety of organs was monitored through BLI [123].Moreover, BLI was applied to assess the silencing of the activity of P-glycoprotein (Pgp), a multidrug resistance (MDR1) gene product overexpressed in multidrug-resistant cancer cells by using short hairpin RNA interference (shRNAi) [124]. The shRNAi-mediated downregulation of Pgp activity at cellular level or in animal models could be directly traced by BLI of Renilla luciferase (rLuc) reporter through its substrate, coelenterazine, which is also a known substrate for

Pgp transportation. Furthermore, the *in vivo* gene-silencing activity of luciferase siRNAs incorporated in calcium phosphate (CaP) nanoparticles was tested in a fLuc-expressing human cervical cancer cell line (HeLa-Luc). These nanoparticles were tested in transgenic mice (FVB/NJc1 female mice) with spontaneous pancreatic tumors by measuring the bioluminescence intensity with IVIS® after intraperitoneal injection of luciferin [125]. Recently, the kinetics of siRNA-mediated gene silencing combined with BLI was studied for the assessment of the best approach for gene silencing [126], for simulating/predicting the effective siRNA dose based on luciferase knockdown *in vitro*, and for studying the kinetics of luciferase knockdown by RNAi therapeutics in subcutaneous tumors and their effects.

GFP and its derivatives have also been widely utilized for imaging *in vitro* gene silencing of siRNA in numerous studies [127,128]. For instance, silica-gold nanoshells were covalently decorated with epilayer of poly(L-lysine) peptide (PLL) on the surface to load single-stranded antisense DNA oligonucleotides or double-stranded short-interfering RNA (siRNA) molecules with NIR laser irradiation-triggered release of gene segments and endosomal escape [128]. The gene-silencing efficacy was evaluated by measuring the downregulation of GFP in human lung cancer H1299 GFP/RFP cell line. Cancer cells and tumor-bearing animals were used to study the gene-silencing effects for screening the RNAi products and serve as a real-time tool to investigate the efficacy of siRNA delivery in preclinical studies. Understandably, the application of these technologies in humans is limited because of need of reporter gene transfection.

7.4.2 PET and SPECT

PET and SPECT are nuclear imaging techniques that use radioactive tracers and detect gamma rays to provide information of molecular signatures at molecular level within living subjects (Figure 7.6). Both imaging systems could afford excellent penetration depth in tissues and high sensitivity for whole-body imaging. For PET imaging, the specifically radiolabeled imaging agents are required for targeting and visualizing organs or tissues of interest. Imaging of radioactive tracer is achieved by detecting the high-energy photons (gamma ray) emitted from the radioactive isotopes during the spontaneous radioactive decay. More specifically, the nucleus of specific radioactive isotope undergoes a beta plus (β^+) decay due to its unstable nuclear system, while an excessive proton is converted into a neutron, a positron, and an electron neutrino [129]. Based on electron-positron annihilation, the collision between electron and positron produces two gamma ray photons traveling at opposite directions at approximately 180° from each other [130,131]. The gamma ray has ten times higher energy than X-ray, and large number of emitted paired photons from radioactive isotopes detected by gamma cameras provide angular and radial distance information from regional interest [131]. These features enable high signal sensitivity and reconstruction of quantitative tomographic images.

Owing to their highly quantitative and sensitive nature, radionuclide imaging techniques have been utilized for analyzing the pharmacokinetics and biodistribution of RNAi therapeutics [132]. Relatively short half-lived isotopes such as ^{18}F ($t_{1/2}$ =109.8 min) and ^{64}Cu ($t_{1/2}$ =12.7 h) are frequently used as radioactive tracers to label siRNA molecules or

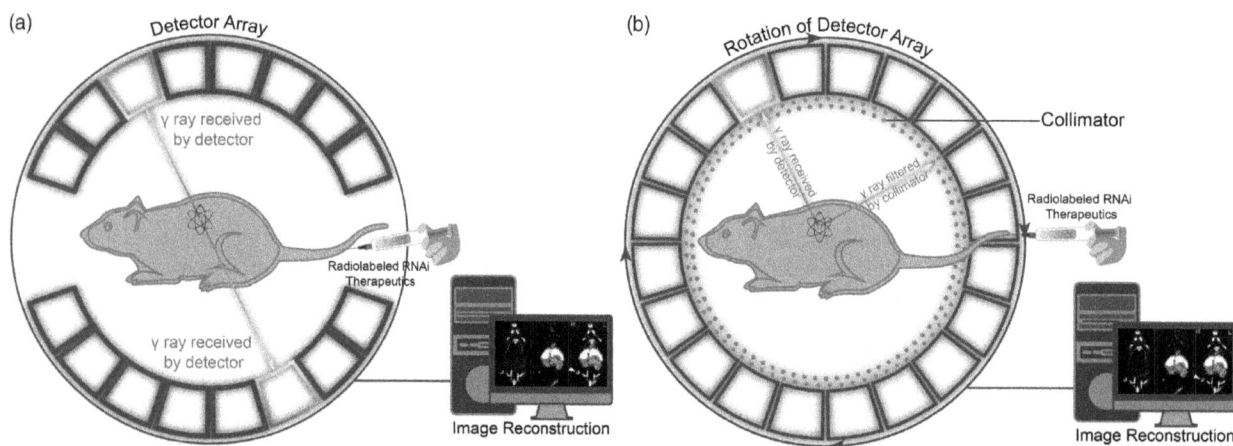

FIGURE 7.6 Positron emission tomography (PET) and single-photon emission computed tomography (SPECT). (a) A schematic illustration of the basic principles of *in vivo* PET imaging. In this technique, the radioactive isotope-labeled RNAi therapeutics is injected into animals. Positrons are emitted from the isotopes associating with electrons, which cause annihilation and subsequent production of two gamma (γ) rays. The two high-energy γ rays are traveling at 180° from each other. Then the γ rays are received by detector array with electrical signals and finally converted into tomographic images. (b) Another schematic illustration of the basic principle of *in vivo* SPECT imaging. First, the radioactive isotopes-labeled RNAi therapeutics is administered into the mouse to emit γ rays. The γ rays produced by isotopes in SPECT do not travel in opposite directions, instead, are collected by detector array that rotates around animals, while any diagonally incident γ rays are filtered by collimator. The γ rays received by detector array are converted and reconstructed into tomographic images.

drug delivery systems for PET imaging. In one recent study, core/shell-structured hollow gold nanospheres (HAuNS) were developed as a targeted NIR light-inducible delivery system for nuclear factor kappa-light-chain-enhancer of activated B cells (NF-κB) targeting siRNA [133]. By conjugating 1,4,7,10-tetraazacyclododecane-1,4,7,10- tetraacetic acid (DOTA) derivatives to the surface of nanospheres and labeling with ^{64}Cu, the HAuNS were applied for micro-PET/computed tomography (CT) imaging. The PET/CT images indicated that targeted HAuNS showed higher accumulation in tumors than nontargeted nanocarriers in HeLa cervical cancer bearing nude mice after intravenous injection (Figure 7.7). ^{18}F-labeled siRNA has also been investigated using PET to measure the pharmacokinetics and biodistribution of siRNA delivery systems [121]. For example, Oku et al. used Nsuccinimidyl 4–^{18}F-fluorobenzoate (^{18}F-SFB) to label siRNA for real time analysis of siRNA delivery [134]. PET images revealed that naked ^{18}F-labeled siRNA was cleared quite rapidly from the blood stream and excreted from the kidneys. However, the cationic liposome/^{18}F-labeled siRNA complexes tended to accumulate in the lung. There is an urgent need to develop facile and efficient ^{18}F-labeling methods for PET imaging of RNAi because most traditional ^{18}F-labeling strategies are time-consuming with low yield.

Single-photon emission computed tomography (SPECT) is similar to PET by utilizing radioactive materials that decay through the emission of single gamma rays (Figure 7.6). By comparison, SPECT scans are significantly less expensive than PET since the cyclotron is not required to generate short half-life radioisotopes [135]. SPECT uses isotopes with longer half-lives or from generator elution, such as ^{111}In ($t_{1/2} = 2.8$ days), ^{99m}Tc ($t_{1/2} = 6$h), ^{123}I ($t_{1/2} = 13.3$h), and ^{131}I ($t_{1/2} = 8$days), to provide information about localized function in internal organs with view of the distribution of radionuclides. However, as the emission of gamma rays cannot provide sufficient spatial information

for tomographic reconstruction, a special instrumental design for data acquisition is required, and the sensitivity of SPECT can be over one order of magnitude lower than PET [135]. In a recent study, siRNA was modified with hydrazinonicotinamide (HYNIC), a chelator for technetium-99 m (^{99m}Tc), to monitor siRNA at cellular level by gamma counting and microautoradiography [136]. Besides, the delivery process and biodistribution in tumor-bearing mice were assessed by whole-body imaging. Merkel et al. also employed SPECT to monitor the biodistribution and pharmacokinetics of siRNA labeled with a gamma emitter (e.g., $^{111}In/^{99m}Tc$) [137]. In the real-time perfusion investigation, rapid accumulation of gamma emitter-labeled siRNA in the liver and kidneys could be observed, followed by an increasing signal in the bladder. Quantification of scintillation counts in the regions of interest (ROI) revealed that the half-life of siRNA complexes in the blood pool is less than three min, suggesting a very rapid excretion into the bladder. Once the siRNA is labeled with radioactive probes, it can be used in noninvasive perfusion, kinetics, and biodistribution evaluation. This offers the advantage of real-time live imaging and investigation at various time points in the same animal to reduce the number of animals needed compared to conventional methods.

7.4.3 MRI

MRI is an important versatile technique that provides noninvasive imaging based on the principle of nuclear magnetic resonance (NMR), by using strong magnetic field and radiofrequency (RF) pulses to generate RF signal (relying on intrinsic physiological feature) for visualization (Figure 7.8a). Specifically, an atom nucleus consists of a number of protons and neutrons, each of which has a constant spin and produces angular momentum, which consequently leads to a net angular momentum in the nucleus. If there is an equal number of protons and neutrons

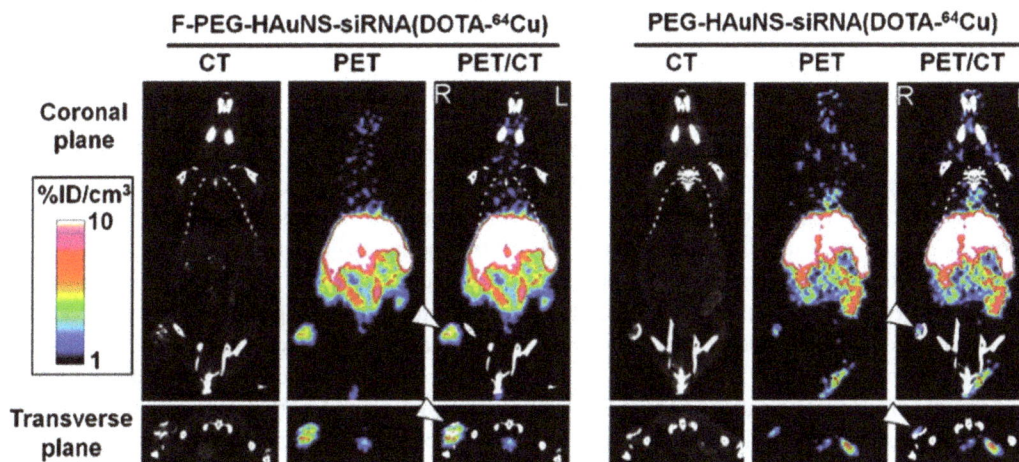

FIGURE 7.7 Micro-PET/CT images of nude mice bearing with HeLa cervical tumor xenografts in the right rear leg at 6h after intravenous injection of folic acid (F-PEG-HAuNS-siRNA (DOTA-^{64}Cu) or PEG-HAuNS-siRNA (DOTA-^{64}Cu). Tumors were marked by arrowheads. (Adapted with permission from Ref. [133].)

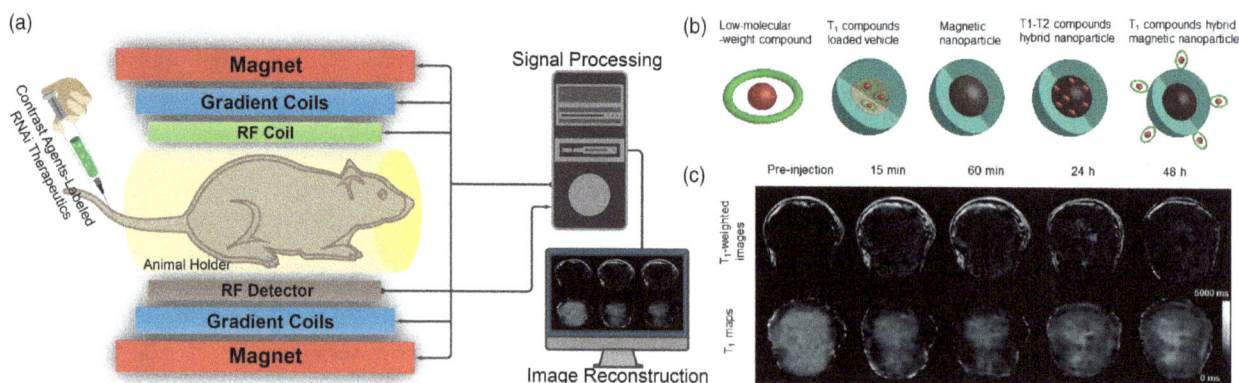

FIGURE 7.8 Magnetic resonance imaging (MRI). (a) A schematic illustration of the basic principle of *in vivo* MR imaging. In general, an MRI scanner consists of three types of coils: the first coil provides a strong homogenous magnetic field, the second coil generates the varying strength of magnetic field in X, Y, and Z directions to encode the spatial position of MR signal and the third coil produces the radio frequency to alter the magnetic dipoles of protons in the subject, generating MR signals to be detected and reconstructed into MR image by computer. MR contrast agents can be labeled onto RNAi therapeutics to track their distribution *in vivo* through T_1 and T_2 signal enhancement. (b) Typical contrast agents for MRI, including low molecular-weight paramagnetic compound, T_1 CA-loaded vehicle, magnetic nanoparticle, T_1-T_2 compounds hybrid nanoparticle, and T_1 compounds hybrid magnetic nanoparticle. (c) Representative T_1-weighted MR images (top) and quantitative T_1 maps (down) of a tumor (400 mm^3) before and after intravenous injection of siRNA-incorporated nanoplex at the dose of 300 mg/kg. (Adapted with permission from Ref. [142].)

in nucleus, net angular momentum is zero. If there is an unequal number of protons and neutrons, then the nucleus gives a specific net spin angular momentum. In the latter circumstances, the nuclear Larmor precession is gained when an external magnetic field is present, and the resonant absorption of RF pulses by nucleus will occur when the frequency of RF pulses equals to the Larmor precession rate. Finally, the RF signal is generated after the removal of external magnetic field [138]. In this regard, the ^{1}H nucleus is particularly useful for MRI since it is abundant in aqueous physiological environment and is magnetically active to give a large magnetic moment to generate RF. However, the RF signal can only be detected from an excess of nuclei with spins aligned either parallel or anti-parallel direction, an equal number of nuclei spins pointing in opposite direction cannot generate detectable MR signals [129]. Therefore, MRI is limited by low sensitivity with long signal acquisition time. Nonetheless, MRI has a number of unique advantages including high spatial resolution, deep tissue penetration, and excellent soft tissue contrast. MRI has been widely used in the clinic to study the anatomy as well as function of tissues. In addition to the development of high field scanners, the design of contrast agents (CAs) plays an important role to improve the image quality by enhancing the contrast of diseased regions while sparing normal tissues. Generally, the CAs could be classified as T_1 and T_2 CAs due to their magnetic properties and relaxation mechanisms (Figure 7.8b).

Superparamagnetic iron oxide nanoparticles (SPIONs) have the ability to decrease the spin–spin relaxation time for T_2-weighted imaging of specific tissues. There are several types of SPIONs approved as contrast agents for MRI in the clinic [139]. Recently, Mok et al. designed and synthesized a pH-sensitive siRNA-loaded nanovector based on SPIONs.

The SPIONs were modified with PEI, a commonly used gene transfection macromolecule, through acid-cleavable citraconic anhydride bonds and coated with anti-GFP siRNA and tumor-specific ligand, chlorotoxin (CTX) [140]. The nanovectors exhibited excellent magnetic property for MRI with a significantly higher r_2 (673 mM^{-1}s^{-1}) than the commercially available T_2 contrast agents (e.g., Feridex). More interestingly, the nanovectors did not elicit obvious cytotoxicity at pH 7.4, but exhibited significant cytotoxicity at pH 6.2 as a result of acidic environment-elicited cytotoxicity, which may be caused by the protonation of the primary amine at low pH. Meanwhile, the gene-silencing effect under acidic pH condition was significantly higher than that under physiological pH condition, because the surface of nanoparticles was nearly 3 times more negatively charged at pH 7.4 than that at pH 6.2. In another study, the formulation of polyethylene glycol-graft-polyethylenimine (PEG-g-PEI)-coated SPIONs were prepared, which was further modified with neuroblastoma cell specific disialoganglioside GD2 single-chain antibody fragment [141]. The nanocarriers could deliver Bcl-2 siRNA to cancer cells and knock down the expression of Bcl-2 mRNA. In addition, effective delivery of siRNA was confirmed through the *in vitro* and *in vivo* MR imaging studies.

Besides T_2 CAs, paramagnetic compounds, such as gadolinium and manganese-based compounds, which are widely applied as T_1 contrast agents, can elevate the relaxation potential by reducing the T_1 relaxation time. Recently, a type of nanoplex that self-assembled from fluorescein isothiocyanate (FITC)-labeled siRNA-chk duplexes and rhodamine labeled PEI, in which the PEI segments was linked to poly-L-lysine (PLL) with dual-labeling of Cy5.5 and Gd-DOTA, while the PLL-end was combined with prodrug enzyme bacterial cytosine deaminase (bCD) that can convert the nontoxic prodrug 5-fluorocytosine (5-FC) to cytotoxic 5-fluorouracil (5-FU), for imaging-guided RNAi cancer therapy [142]. The nanoplex labeled with different types of CAs could make it possible for MR and optical imaging of the delivery of siRNA and the function of prodrug enzyme in breast tumors for image-guided and molecular-targeted cancer therapy. For instance, the high-resolution T_1-weighted MR images and quantitative T_1 map of tumor region were obtained by MRI, and the contrast in tumor region was enhanced after the administration of nanoplex (Figure 7.8c) with T_1 value change as a result of the accumulation and diffusion of the nanoplex, demonstrating successful delivery of siRNA into tumor tissues, also confirmed by optical imaging. The delivered siRNA could down-regulate the activity of aggressive enzyme of choline kinase-α (Chk-α) in breast cancer cells, while the bCD could convert 5-FC to 5-FU, which procedure could be noninvasively monitored by ^{1}HMR spectroscopic imaging and ^{19}F MR spectroscopy. In another study, hollow manganese oxide nanoparticles (HMONs) were exploited as a theranostic nanoplatform for simultaneous cancer-targeted siRNA delivery and MR imaging [143]. In this study, HMON nanoparticles were coupled with 3,4-dihydroxy-Lphenylalanine conjugated branched PEI (PEI-DOPA) through the strong affinity between DOPA and metal oxides and further modified with Herceptin, a therapeutic monoclonal antibody to target Her-2 expressing cancer cells selectively. Although SPIONs have already been widely used as T_2 MRI contrast agents, they still have some drawbacks, such as magnetic susceptibility artifacts and negative contrast, which limit their clinical applications [144]. The development of T_1–T_2 dual-modal contrast agents has attracted considerable interest because they can provide the contrast for T_1-weighted imaging with high tissue resolution and for T_2-weighted imaging with high feasibility of lesions detection. Recently, Wang et al. reported a low-molecular-weight polyethylenimine (stPEI)-wrapped

and gadolinium-embedded iron oxide (GdIO) nanoclusters (GdIO–stPEI) for T_1–T_2 dual-modal MRI visible siRNA delivery, which exhibited high relaxivities for MRI measurements and suppressed expression of luciferase proteins for dual type of MR imaging-guided siRNA delivery [145].

7.4.4 Ultrasound

Ultrasound is a clinically widely equipped imaging modality for evaluating the structure, function, and blood flow of organs, which could provide images with high spatial and temporal resolution at low cost (Figure 7.9a). Ultrasound scanners can emit sound waves with frequencies between 1 and 20 MHz and receive feedback waves reflected by tissues based on density difference to build images for diagnosis [146], which could provide images in a real-time manner without processing delay after acquisition compared with other imaging modalities [40]. In principle, the signal reflected from tissues is insufficient for precise diagnosis because of artifacts from normal tissues. Thus, ultrasound contrast agents are essential to increase the imaging accuracy. Some contrast agents have been developed to enhance positive signal for ultrasound imaging [147–149], such as microbubbles [150–152], nanodroplets [153–156], nanobubbles [157,158], and liposomes [159,160] (Figure 7.9b). These are usually constructed with shell of proteins, polymers, lipids, or surfactants to maintain stability in the bloodstream as well as escaping from RES, while loading air or biologically inert heavy gas such as nitrogen, perfluorocarbons, and sulfur hexafluoride to generate echogenicity (Figure 7.9b) [161]. Besides, solid nanoparticles with cavities that can trap gas [162], and nanoparticles constructed with gas-generating materials have also been applied to enhance the contrast for ultrasound imaging [163].

Ultrasound demonstrates potential advantages in the development of RNAi therapeutics. First, when the ultrasound probe arrives at the tumor vasculature, with low

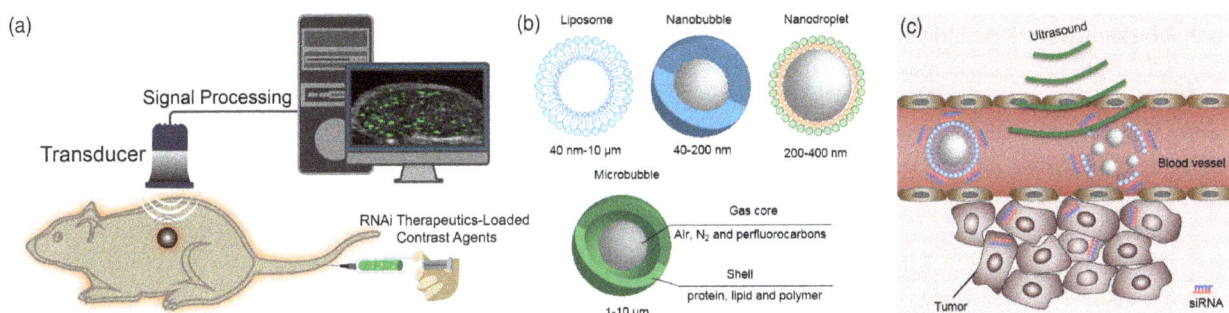

FIGURE 7.9 Ultrasound imaging. (a) A schematic illustration of the basic principle of *in vivo* ultrasound imaging. First, the ultrasound contrast agent that encapsulates RNAi therapeutics is injected into animals, then high-frequency sound waves are sent and penetrated into the subjects, while the time intervals of subsequent reflection of sound waves is recorded by a transducer. The detected signals are converted and constructed into images. A coupling medium is usually used between the contact surface of transducer and subject for sound wave transmission. (b) Typical contrast agents for ultrasound, such as liposome, nanobubble, nanodroplet, and microbubble. (c) Ultrasound-triggered destruction of siRNA-incorporated microbubbles. Ultrasound could disrupt the contrast agents with high acoustic pressure to release RNAi agents when delivered to the blood vessels of the tumor region. Then the released RNAi agents enter into tumor cells to silence target gene.

acoustic pressure (<100 kPa), it could be used to diagnose tumors for imaging-guided delivery of RNAi therapeutics and monitoring the therapeutic effects. Besides, by applying high acoustic pressure (100 kPa to several MPa), ultrasound could be applied to disrupt the probes to release cargos (drugs or RNAs) in target positions and change the permeability of cell membrane with more siRNA delivered intracellularly for gene silencing [151]. As a result, ultrasound can enhance therapeutic effect of RNAi therapeutics (Figure 7.9c) [148,164]. The siRNA molecules can be attached to the surface of microbubbles or trapped in the bilayer of liposomes, or siRNA-loaded nanoparticles can be incorporated into ultrasound probes. For instance, epidermal growth factor receptor (EGFR)-directed siRNA (EGFR-siRNA) could be efficiently attached to microbubbles with around 7 mg siRNA per 10^9 microbubbles and safely protect siRNA from RNase digestion [165]. The EGFR-siRNA-loaded microbubbles reduced the EGFR expression of murine squamous carcinoma cells *in vitro*, and the ultrasound triggered destruction of microbubbles released EGFR-siRNA specifically in the tumor region to effectively delay tumor growth, while the tumor volume was monitored by ultrasound.

However, microbubbles are limited to vascular compartment with poor tumor tissue penetration because of its large size and relatively poor stability. Therefore, ultrasound probes with much smaller size, such as nanobubbles, nanoparticles, and nanoscale liposomes, with better tumor tissue penetration properties have been fabricated for ultrasound diagnosis and ultrasound-mediated siRNA delivery with better tumor accumulation [156,166]. For instance, the ultrasound-sensitive siRNA nanobubbles made from positively charged liposomes with gas core and decorated with negatively charged siRNAs on the surface could effectively accumulate in the tumor tissues through EPR effect, demonstrating high potency for tumor imaging and targeted delivery of siRNA for RNAi therapy [167]. Moreover, high cellular affinity ligands have been introduced to the surface of ultrasound nanoprobes, for example, aptamer-decorated nanobubbles have been developed to specifically target the CCRF-CEM cells (T-cells, human acute lymphoblastic leukemia) for ultrasound imaging [158]. Other bioactive compounds, such as anticancer drugs and plasmid DNA, could also be co-loaded into probes for ultrasound imaging and combination therapy of tumors [159].

7.4.5 MULTIMODALITY IMAGING

Although each imaging modality has its unique advantages, it is also endowed with its intrinsic limitations, making it difficult to obtain accurate and reliable information on all aspects of structure and function about the target organs by a single imaging modality [168]. Table 7.2 summarizes some general features of classical imaging modalities including optical imaging, radionuclide imaging, MRI, and ultrasound imaging. To cope with the shortcomings of each modality, multimodality imaging combines different

imaging techniques and imaging probes and can provide some complementary information about RNAi therapeutics. However, in context of developing multimodality probes, it should be noted that challenges are involved especially for applications in living subjects. Since the multimodality probes are primarily nanoparticle based, such as organic dye-labeled iron oxides, gadolinium chelates functionalized QDs, magnetic microbubbles, radiolabeled C-dots, etc., the major problems may be associated with insufficient concentration of probes at target sites due to the undesired uptake by mononuclear phagocyte system (MPS). Other concerns include slow clearance time, long-term retention in tissues and organs, as well as the long-term toxicity. These issues are highly related to the physicochemical properties (e.g., chemical component, size distribution, final hydrodynamic diameter, shape, surface charge) of nanoprobes [169]. In addition, different modalities differ in their imaging sensitivity by large magnitude [170]. Thus, the combination of two different probes needs to be carefully designed with proper ratio [171]. Therefore, in order to reach the full potential of multimodality imaging, the participations of multidisciplinary scientists with solid background in nanotechnology, material science, pharmacology, pharmaceutical chemistry, clinical medicine, biomedical engineering, and instrumental techniques are essential in the early development stages [172,173].

A typical example of a multimodality probe-siRNA delivery system for *in vivo* imaging of RNAi has been reported by Medarova et al. [174]. In this study, a dual-purpose probe was developed, which was composed of iron oxide core and Cy5.5 dye on the surface. The probe was further modified with cell membrane translocation peptides to facilitate intracellular delivery of siRNA (Figure 7.10a). The successful delivery of GFP siRNA duplex to tumors was assessed by MRI and optical imaging of tumor-bearing animals after intravenous injection of the probes (Figure 7.10b and c). In another study, both commercial MRI contrast agents (Magnevist/Feridex) and Alexa-647 dye-labeled siRNA for targeting cyclooxygenase-2 (COX-2), an important therapeutic target in cancer, were encapsulated in PEGylated polycationic liposomes. The liposomes were used to assess the delivery and silencing effects of siRNA *in vivo* [175]. It was found that Feridex-loaded liposomes demonstrated better performance than that of Magnevist, which was further tested *in vivo*. Both MRI and optical imaging confirmed successful delivery of siRNA to MDA-MB-231 tumor.

Recently, PET/CT combined with BLI was also employed to monitor the whole-body biodistribution of RNAi therapeutics and assess their silencing effects of the expression of luciferase *in vivo* [176]. The nanoparticles were prepared with cyclodextrin-containing polycations and anti-Luc siRNAs with their 5′-end conjugated with 1,4,7,10-tetraazacyclododecane-1,4,7,10-tetraaceticacid (DOTA) for ^{64}Cu labeling. Micro-PET/CT was carried out to determine the distribution and tumor accumulation of siRNA-containing nanoparticles. No obvious difference in

TABLE 7.2
Features of Different Modalities for Structural, Functional, and Molecular Imaging of RNAi

Modality	Penetration depth	Sensitivity (Mol/L)	Spatial resolution	Physical medium	Imaging probes and amount of use	Advantages	Disadvantages
Optical FI	<1 cm	$\sim 10^{-9}$–10^{-12}	2–3 mm	Visible or NIR light	Organic dyes; QDs; C-dots; UCNPs — Microgram–milligram	High sensitivity; real-time imaging; nonionizing radiation; relatively inexpensive; short acquisition time; multiplexing capability	Low spatial resolution at greater depth; limited penetration depth; autofluorescence
Optical BLI	<2 cm	$\sim 10^{-15}$–10^{-17}	3–5 mm	Visible light	GFP; RFP — Microgram–milligram	High sensitivity; real-time imaging; no ionizing radiation; relatively inexpensive; short acquisition time; user friendly; multiplexing capability	Low spatial resolution at greater depth; Limited penetration depth; genetic reporter systems required
PET	Limitless	$\sim 10^{-11}$–10^{-12}	1–2 mm	High-energy γ-rays	Radiolabeled tracers — Nanograms	Excellent sensitivity; limitless penetration depth; quantitative data	High cost of cyclotron; Ionizing radiation; limited spatial resolution
SPECT	Limitless	10^{-10}–10^{-11}	1–2 mm	Low-energy γ-rays	Radiolabeled tracers — Nanogram	Excellent sensitivity; limitless penetration depth; no need of cyclotron; multiplexing capability	Relatively expensive; ionizing radiation; limited spatial resolution; semi-quantitative
MRI	Limitless	10^{-3}–10^{-5}	~1 mm	Radio wav	Gadolinium chelates; Iron oxides; Other magnetic nanoparticles — Microgram–milligram	Excellent spatial resolution; limitless penetration depth; quantitative data; no ionizing radiation	Relatively expensive; relatively low sensitivity and poor contrast; long acquisition time
US	Millimeters–centimeters (frequency dependent)	—	0.01–2 mm	Ultrasound waves	Microbubbles — Microgram–milligram	Relatively inexpensive; no ionizing radiation; quantitative data; no ionizing radiation; short acquisition time; high sensitivity with microbubbles	Limited penetration depth; poor low contrast; strong boundary effect; limited to imaging soft tissue only

BLI, bioluminescence imaging; FI, fluorescence imaging; US, ultrasound; NIR, near-infrared fluorescence; GFP, green fluorescent protein; RFP, red fluorescent protein; QDs, quantum dots; C-dots, Carbon nanodots; UCNPs, upconvertion nanoparticles.

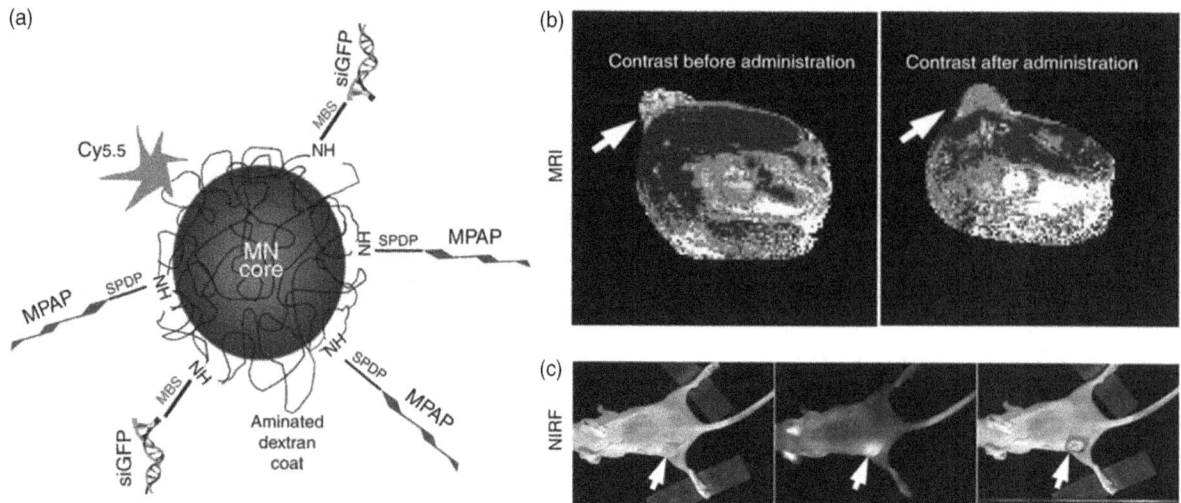

FIGURE 7.10 Multimodality *in vivo* imaging of RNAi by using MRI and optical imaging. (a) Schematic illustration of the multifunctional nanocarriers with core of magnetic nanoparticles, and surface conjugated with Cy5.5, GFP siRNA (siGFP), and membrane translocation peptides (MPAP). (b) *In vivo* MR imaging of mice bearing with subcutaneous LS174T human colorectal adenocarcinoma tumors (arrows) before and after the administration of the multifunctional nanocarriers, indicating significant drop of T2-weighted contrast enhancement in tumor regions after injection of the contrast agents. (c) A high-intensity NIRF signal in the tumor confirmed the successful delivery of the nanocarriers, while the left mouse with white light, middle one with NIRF, and right one with color-coded overlay. (Adapted with permission from Ref. [174].)

distribution between the targeted nanoparticles and non-targeted ones was observed. Meanwhile, the BLI revealed that the targeted nanoparticles had better RNAi effects one day after injection, demonstrating the importance of multimodal imaging. Thus, the combination of PET/CT and BLI is important to simultaneously monitor both the gene delivery and silencing effects of RNAi, which is critical for the design of RNAi therapeutics for clinical translation.

7.5 THERANOSTIC NANOMEDICINES

Theranostic nanomedicines contain both a diagnostic agent and one or more therapeutic drugs within one integrated system, enabling noninvasive diagnosis, therapy, and real-time monitoring of the therapeutic response at the same time [132,168,177,178]. Among various imaging techniques, computed tomography (CT) is one of the most commonly used non-invasive clinical imaging modalities because of its wide availability, high spatial resolution, unlimited depth, and accurate anatomical information with reconstructed three dimensional imaging [179–181]. Iodixanol (Visipaque) is a small iodinated molecule, clinically used as a CT contrast agent that has a low osmolality and great tolerability [182]. However, like all low molecular weight iodinated CT contrast agents, iodixanol has drawbacks like non-specific distribution and rapid renal clearance following i.v. injection [183]. In recent years, nanosized CT contrast agents have attracted great interest as they have several advantages over small molecular contrast agents such as prolonged circulation time, site-specific accumulation, and use for theranostics [184–187]. Some recent work showed systems with great promise of nanosized CT

contrast agents such as iodinated hyaluronic acid oligomer-based nano-assembled systems, theranostic self-assembly structures of gold nanoparticles, and multifunctional dendrimer-entrapped gold nanoparticles for simultaneous tumor imaging and therapy [188–190].

Among various types of nanoscale drug delivery systems, nanogels have attracted increasing attention since they have a large surface area for multivalent bioconjugation and a crosslinked three-dimensional network structure that offers great colloidal stability [191–193]. To achieve rapid release of the payload at the target site, pH, redox potential, and enzyme-responsive nanogels have been designed [194–201]. Nanogels based on hyaluronic acid (HA) have recently appeared as a unique system because HA is a hydrophilic natural material with excellent biocompatibility and intrinsic targeting ability toward CD44-overexpressing tumor cells [200,202–205]. HA nanoparticles have been used for efficient delivery of chemotherapeutics, proteins, as well as siRNA *in vitro* and *in vivo* [206–209].

We report on bioresponsive and fluorescent hyaluronic acid-iodixanol nanogels (HAI-NGs) for targeted CT imaging and chemotherapy of MCF-7 human breast tumor (Scheme 7.1). HAI-NGs were obtained from hyaluronic acid-cystamine-tetrazole (HA-Cys-Tet) and reductively degradable polyiodixanol-methacrylate (SS-PI-MA) via nanoprecipitation and a photo-click crosslinking reaction. HAI-NGs were designed with the following unique features: (i) both HA and iodixanol have excellent biocompatibility and are currently used in the clinic; (ii) the "tetrazole-ene" photo-click crosslinking reaction is highly selective, which prevents cross-reaction with most drugs and furthermore endows nanogels with bright green fluorescence [210,211];

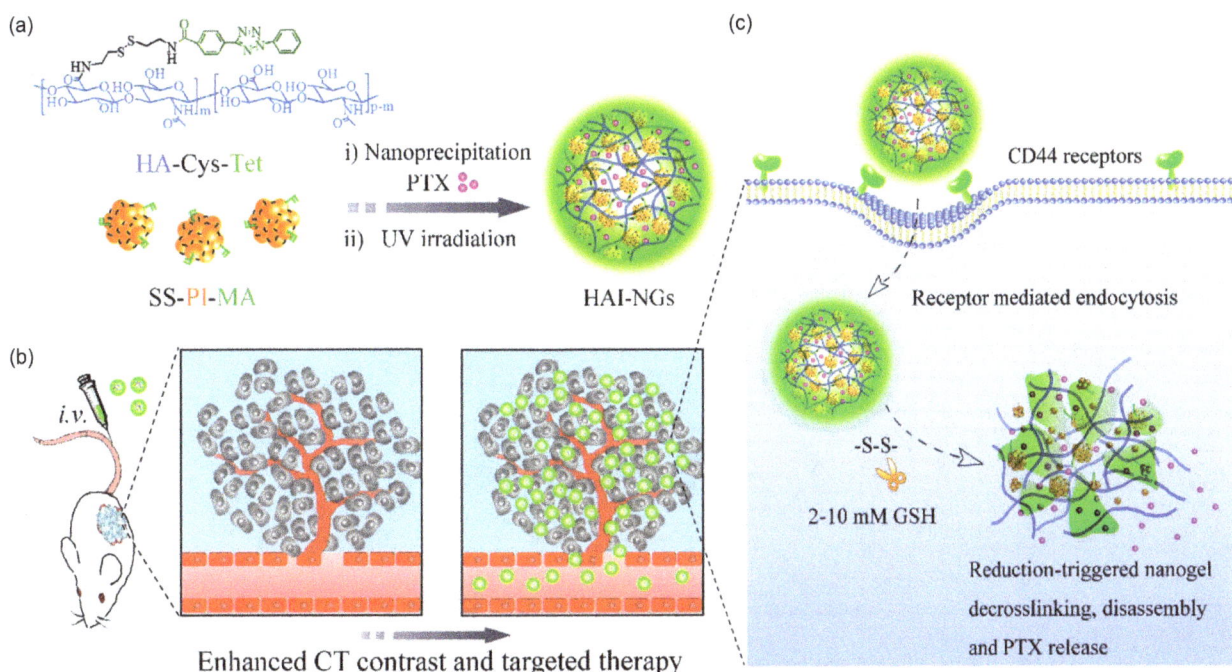

SCHEME 7.1 Illustration of bioresponsive and fluorescent hyaluronic acid-iodixanol nanogels for targeted X-ray computed tomography imaging and chemotherapy of breast tumors. (a) PTX-loaded HAI-NGs are prepared via nanoprecipitation followed by crosslinking via UV irradiation; (b) PTX-loaded HAI-NGs actively target and accumulate at MCF-7 tumors, resulting in enhanced CT contrast and targeted therapy; (c) PTX-loaded HAI-NGs are selectively internalized into the MCF-7 breast tumor cells via CD44 receptor-mediated endocytosis, nanogels are decrosslinked and disassembled in response to GSH in the cytosol, and PTX is quickly released into the cells.

(iii) HA can actively target CD44 receptors which are overexpressed on various malignant tumor cells and stem cells [212–215]; (iv) HAI-NGs can be used for targeted CT imaging *in vivo*; and (v) the reduction-sensitivity of HAI-NGs allows fast intracellular release of payloads like PTX to achieve efficient and targeted chemotherapy. Tetrazole (Tet) and cystamine diisocyanate (CDI) were synthesized according to previous reports [210,216]. Herein, the stability of HAI-NGs and the reduction-triggered PTX release from PTX loaded HAI-NGs were investigated. Furthermore, the targetability of HAI-NGs and antitumor activity of PTX loaded HAI-NGs toward MCF-7 cells, the pharmacokinetics and biodistribution, NIR and CT imaging, as well as therapeutic effects in MCF-7 human breast tumor xenografts in mice were evaluated.

7.6 PREPARATION OF NANOGELS AND TRIGGERED DRUG RELEASE

Hyaluronic acid-iodixanol nanogels (HAI-NGs) were readily obtained via nanoprecipitaion and photo-click crosslinking reaction from HACys-Tet and SS-PI-MA. Figure 7.11a shows that HAI-NGs had a small size of about 90 nm with a low polydispersity (PDI) of 0.11. TEM confirmed that HAI-NGs had a homogenous size distribution and spherical morphology (Figure 7.11b). Notably, HAI-NGs emitted bright green fluorescence under UV light (Figure 7.11c inset), which derives from pyrazoline cycloadducts produced by the "tetrazole-alkene" photo-click reaction [210,217].

Fluorescence spectroscopy displayed that HAI-NGs had a strong emission at ca. 485 nm (Figure 7.11c). The strong fluorescence of HAI-NGs can be used to monitor their *in vitro* and *in vivo* fate. HAI-NGs displayed excellent stability against extensive dilution as well as 10% serum. However, in the presence of 10 mM glutathione (GSH), HAI-NGs rapidly swelled and agglomerated, supporting their fast redox responsivity (Figure 7.11d).

In contrast, nearly complete PTX release was observed in the presence of 10 mM GSH under otherwise the same conditions, probably due to GSH triggered disulfide bond cleavage and de-crosslinking of the nanogels, corroborating that drug release can be accelerated in an intracellular reductive environment. Nanogels typically have a low loading and fast leakage of small molecule drugs [218]. Paclitaxel (PTX) could be easily loaded into HAI-NGs during nanoprecipitation. The high PTX loading and inhibited drug leakage of HAI-NGs is likely due to existence of strong π-π interactions between PTX and pyrazoline groups and iodixanol moieties in the nanogels [219].

7.7 CELLULAR UPTAKE AND CYTOTOXICITY OF PTX-LOADED HAI-NGs

Given their strong fluorescence, the cellular uptake of HAI-NGs into CD44 receptor overexpressing MCF-7 breast cancer cells could be conveniently traced by confocal laser scanning microscopy (CLSM). Notably, nanogel fluorescence was clearly observed in MCF-7 cells after 1 h

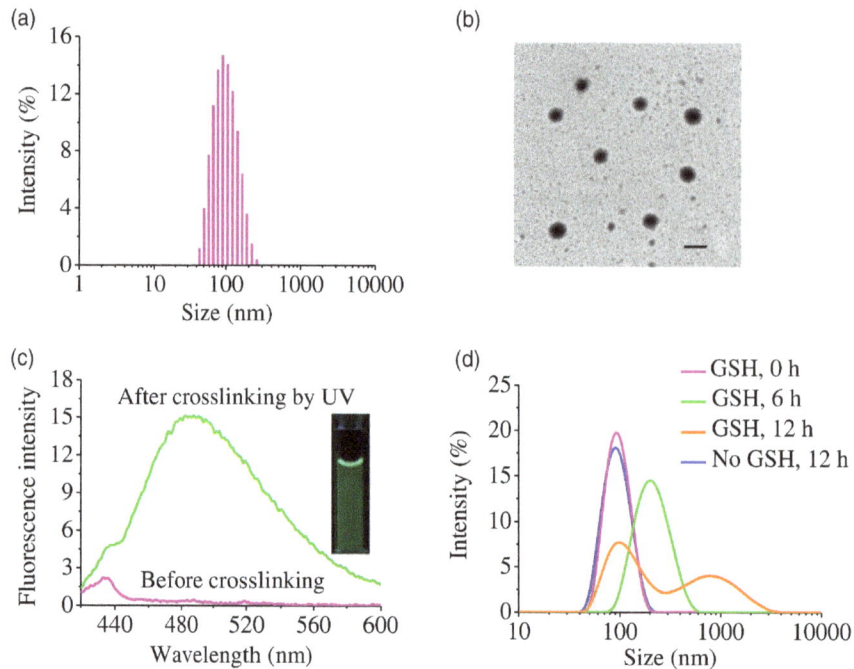

FIGURE 7.11 (a) Intensity size distribution of HAI-NGs determined by DLS. (b) TEM image of HAI-NGs (scale bar: 100 nm). (c) Fluorescent spectrum of HAI-NGs before and after crosslinking by UV irradiation. The insert shows a photograph of HAI-NGs under UV light. (d) Triggered destabilization of HAI-NGs in 10 mM GSH.

incubation, and the fluorescence became stronger at a prolonged incubation time of 2 or 4 h (Figure 7.12) [220]. The cellular uptake of nanogels was greatly inhibited and only weak nanogel fluorescence was discerned in the cell membrane of MCF-7 cells pre-incubated for 4 h with free HA, demonstrating that HAI-NGs are internalized by MCF-7 cells via a receptor-mediated mechanism. The application of using the fluorescence intensity of HAI-NGs via a CD44-mediated mechanism for both, L929 murine fibroblastic cells and MCF-7 cells. It was found that the fluorescence intensity of HAI-NGs in MCF-7 cells was much stronger than that in L929 cells, owing to a low expression of CD44 as negative controls in L929 murine fibroblastic cells.

MTT assays showed that blank HAI-NGs were practically non-toxic to MCF-7 cells (N93% cell viability) even at a high nanogel concentration of 1 mg/mL (Figure 7.13a), indicating that HAI-NGs possess excellent biocompatibility. In contrast, PTX-loaded HAI-NGs exhibited significant and dose dependent cytotoxicity against MCF-7 cells (Figure 7.13b). The half-maximal inhibitory concentration (IC_{50}) of PTX-loaded HAI-NGs was determined to be 0.52 μg/mL, comparable to that of free PTX (0.35 μg/mL), corroborating their efficient cellular internalization and rapid intracellular PTX release. The pre-treatment of MCF-7 cells with free HA for 4 h largely reduced the cytotoxic effect of PTX-loaded HAI-NGs, in line with the above CLSM observations that cellular uptake is inhibited by free HA.

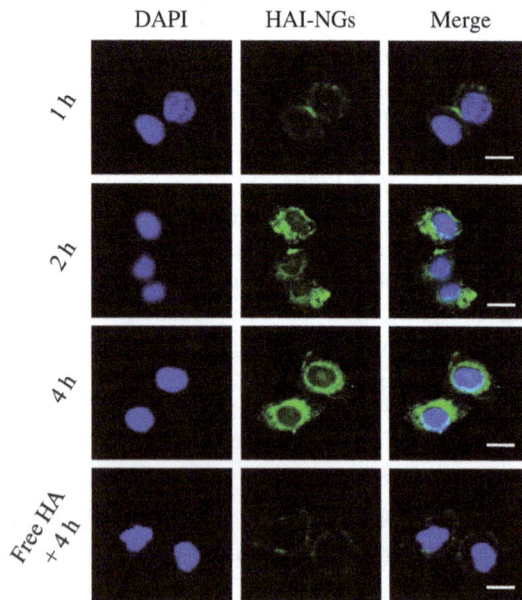

FIGURE 7.12 CLSM images of MCF-7 cells following 1 h, 2 h and 4 h incubation with HAI-NGs. Cells pre-treated with free HA (5 mg/mL) for 4 h before adding nanogels were used as a control. The scale bars correspond to 20 μm in all the images.

7.8 *IN VIVO* PHARMACOKINETICS, NEAR INFRARED IMAGING, AND BIODISTRIBUTION OF NANOGELS

To investigate the *in vivo* pharmacokinetics, PTX-loaded HAI-NGs were i.v. injected into BALB/c nude mice at 5 mg PTX/kg and the plasma levels of PTX at different time

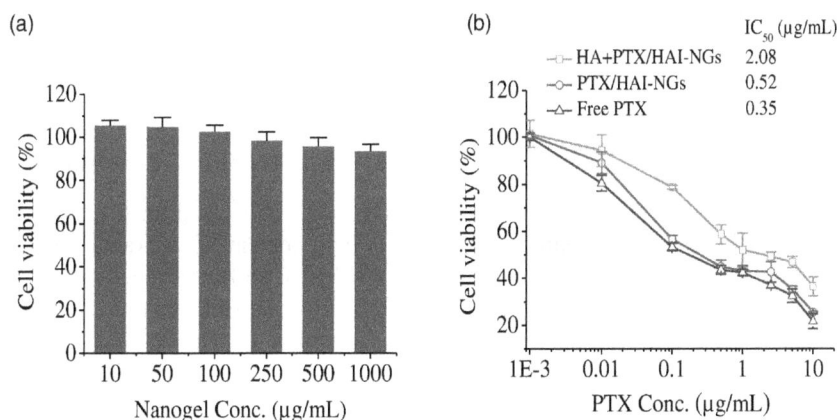

FIGURE 7.13 MTT assays of blank HAI-NGs and PTX/HAI-NGs in MCF-7 cells. (a) Viability of MCF-7 cells following 48h incubation with blank HAI-NGs; and (b) *In vitro* antitumor activity of PTX/HAI-NGs against MCF-7 cells. The cells were incubated with PTX/HAI-NGs for 4h, the medium was removed and replenished with fresh culture medium, and the cells were cultured for an additional 44h. The inhibition experiment was performed by pre-treating cells for 4h with free HA (5mg/mL) prior to incubation with PTX/HAI-NGs. Data are presented as mean±SD (n=4).

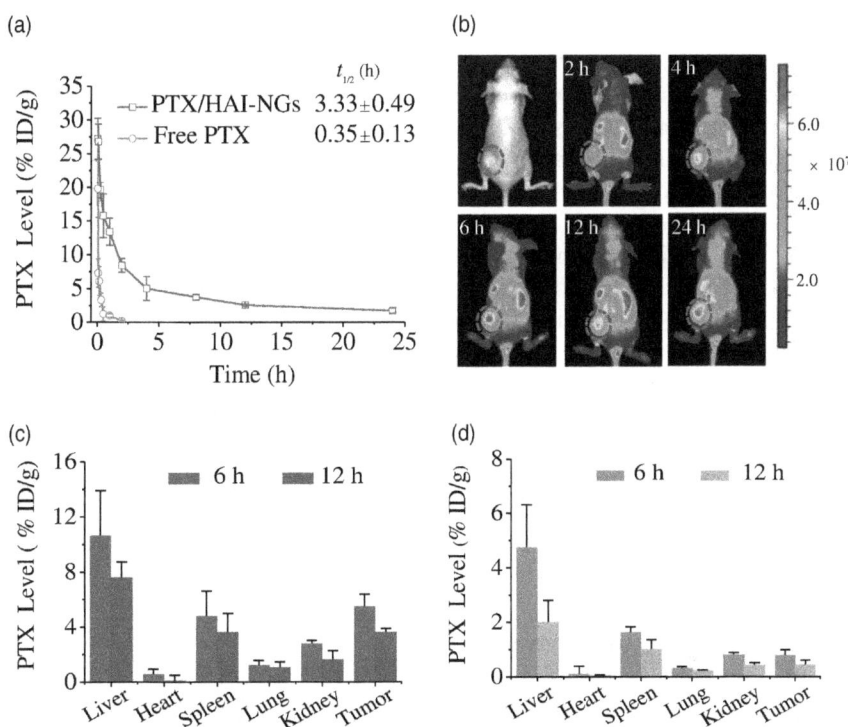

FIGURE 7.14 *In vivo* pharmacokinetics, NIR imaging and biodistribution studies. (a) *In vivo* pharmacokinetics of PTX/HAI-NGs and free PTX in mice. PTX level is expressed as % injected dose per gram of tissue (%ID/g). Data are presented as mean±SD (n=3); (b) *in vivo* fluorescence images of MCF-7 human breast tumor bearing nude mice at different time points following tail vein injection of Cy5-loaded nanogels. Circled areas indicate the locations of the tumor. PTX level, expressed as % injected dose per gram of tissue (%ID/g), in the tumor and different organs after 6 or 12h post injection of PTX/HAI-NGs (c) or free PTX (d). Data are presented as mean±SD (n=3).

points were determined by HPLC. Figure 7.14a displays that PTX-loaded HAI-NGs had a prolonged circulation time with an elimination half-life of 3.3h. [220] indicating that nanogels are stable in the circulation and drug leakage is low as a result of strong π-π interactions between PTX and pyrazoline group and iodixanol moieties in the nanogels [219]. In comparison, free PTX was rapidly eliminated

from the blood circulation, with an extremely short half-life time of 0.35h.

To visualize their tumor accumulation *in vivo*, a near infrared dye Cy5was loaded into HAI-NGs, and the serum Cy5 release was evaluated. It has been found that Cy5 release from HAI-NGs was slow, and within 24h, only 4.1% was released. Therefore, it is envisaged that Cy5 loaded HAI-NGs are also relatively stable in the circulation. Figure 7.14b shows real-time images of Cy5-loaded HAI-NGs in MCF-7 tumor-bearing mice. Notably, tumor accumulation of nanogels was clearly observed at 2 h post injection and reached a maximum at 6 h. This high tumor-targeting efficiency of nanogels is likely due to their small size, high stability, and active targeting effect. Interestingly, the fluorescence at the tumor site at 24 h again became stronger compared with that at 12 h, probably because the Cy5 fluorescence is partly self-quenched when loaded into the HAI-NGs due to the homo Förster resonance energy transfer (homo-FRET) effect [221]. When Cy5 molecules are partly released from the disassembled HAI-NGs in the reductive environment, the fluorescence of Cy5 in the tumor area may increase again. It is also noticed that besides in the tumor site, strong fluorescence was also observed in the liver and spleen, probably because after *i.v.* injection, nanogels are also captured by the RES system (mainly liver and spleen). As CD44 receptors are also expressed on liver and spleen cells, uptake of part of the nanogels by these organs may be inevitable".

To profile the *in vivo* biodistribution of PTX-loaded HAI-NGs in MCF-7 tumor-bearing mice, PTX levels in the tumor and different organs at 6 and 12 h post injection were quantitatively determined by HPLC. Notably, PTX-loaded nanogels exhibited a high tumor accumulation with 5.5% ID/g at 6 h (Figure 7.14c). The tumor PTX accumulation remained high (3.6% ID/g) at 12 h post injection. In comparison, free PTX displayed 7-and 15-fold lower tumor accumulation than PTX-loaded HAI-NGs at 6 and 12 h post injection, respectively (Figure 7.14d versus Figure 7.14c). The PTX level expressed in %ID for the tissues after injection with PTX/HAI-NGs also showed a relatively high retention of PTX in tumor tissue besides the high level in liver tissue and lower levels in the spleen. The levels after the administration of free PTX were investigated [220]. The pharmacokinetics, NIR imaging and biodistribution studies all point out that PTX-loaded HAI-NGs have a prolonged circulation time and significantly enhance PTX accumulation in the MCF-7 tumor.

7.9 ENHANCED CT IMAGING BY HAI-NGs

HAI-NGs can be used for CT imaging due to the presence of a high content of iodixanol. Figure 7.15a shows clearly that HAI-NGs effectively enhanced the CT contrast *in vitro*. The corresponding Hounsfield units (HU) values exhibited a linear correlation with HAI-NGs concentrations, suggesting that HAI-NGs can be used for quantitative CT studies. The application of HAI-NGs for *in vivo* CT diagnosis has been then evaluated. Interestingly, 5 min after intratumoral (i.t.) injection of 50 μL of HAI-NGs at an HAI-NGs concentration of 15 mg/mL (i.e. 60 mg iodine equiv./kg) into MCF-7 tumor-bearing nude mice, remarkably enhanced contrast was observed at the tumor site in the three-dimensional reconstructed images, with a marked increase of HU value from 37.2 to 182.8 (Figure 7.15b). It has been further investigated whether HAI-NGs can be applied for targeted CT imaging of CD44 overexpressed tumors.

The results showed that enhanced contrast was discerned in the MCF-7 tumor from both axial and coronal CT images, with HU values increasing from 37.0 to 82.6, at 7 h following intravenous injection of HAI-NGs into MCF-7 tumor bearing nude mice (Figure 7.16). The enhanced tumor contrast further confirms that HAI-NGs can target to and accumulate in the MCF-7 tumor. Notably, the high contrast signal at the tumor site lasted for a long time, which is advantageous for clinical diagnosis. In sharp contrast, little enhancement of HU value was observed at the tumor site for iodixanol (small molecule contrast agent) at the same iodine dose. Iodixanol was rapidly cleared from the body to the bladder. It is clear, therefore, that HAINGs are superior to iodixanol in targeted CT imaging of CD44 positive tumors.

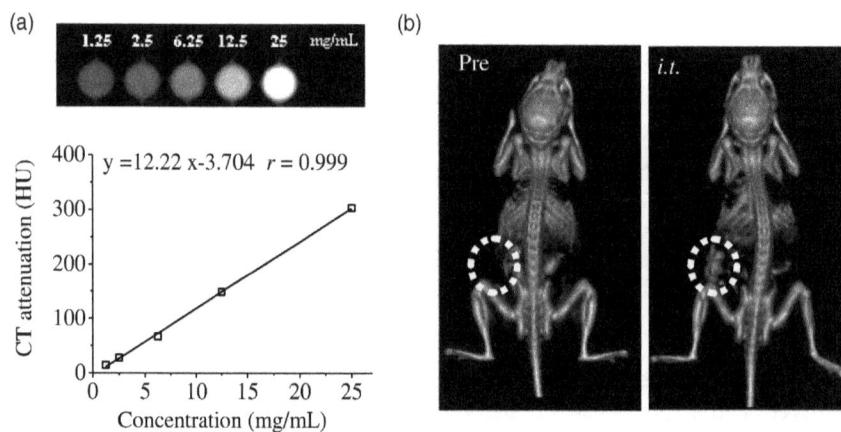

FIGURE 7.15   (a) HU measurements of HAI-NGs. The plot showed a linear correlation of CT calculated solution attenuation measured in Hounsfield units (HU) to HAI-NGs at varying concentrations from 1.25 to 25 mg/mL. (b) Three-dimensional reconstructed CT images of the MCF-7 tumor bearing mice following intratumoral (i.t.) injection of 50 μL of HAI-NGs at a concentration of 15 mg/mL (60 mg iodine equiv./kg). Circled areas indicate the location of the tumor.

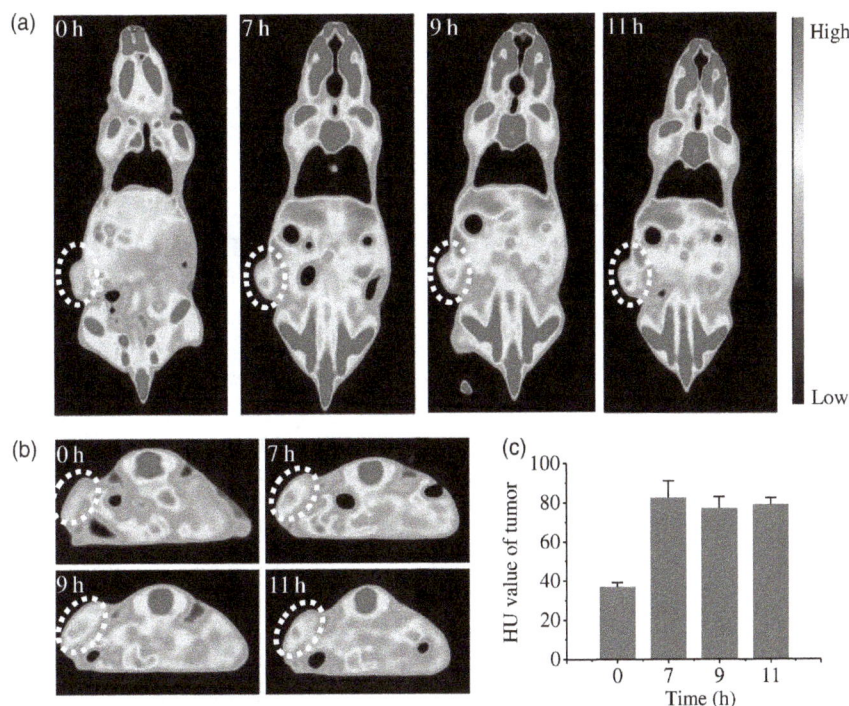

FIGURE 7.16 Axial CT images (a), coronal CT images (b) and HU value (c) of MCF-7 tumor bearing mice at 0 h, 7 h, 9 h and 11 h following tail vein injection of HAI-NGs at a concentration of 15 mg/mL (60 mg iodine equiv./kg). Circled areas indicate the position of the tumor.

7.10 *IN VIVO* TUMOR PENETRATION AND THERAPEUTIC EFFICACY OF PTX-LOADED HAINGs

In the process of tumor-targeted drug delivery, a series of biological barriers may influence the final therapeutic efficacy, among which are interstitial hindrance and tumor penetration [222,223]. The strong intrinsic fluorescence of HAI-NGs was utilized to track their distribution. The blood vessels and cell nuclei were stained by CD31 antibody and DAPI, respectively. Figure 7.17 reveals that HAI-NGs were located in the blood vessels at 2 h post *i.v.* injection. At a prolonged time of 6 h post injection, HAI-NGs extravagated from blood vessels to the interstitial space, displaying green

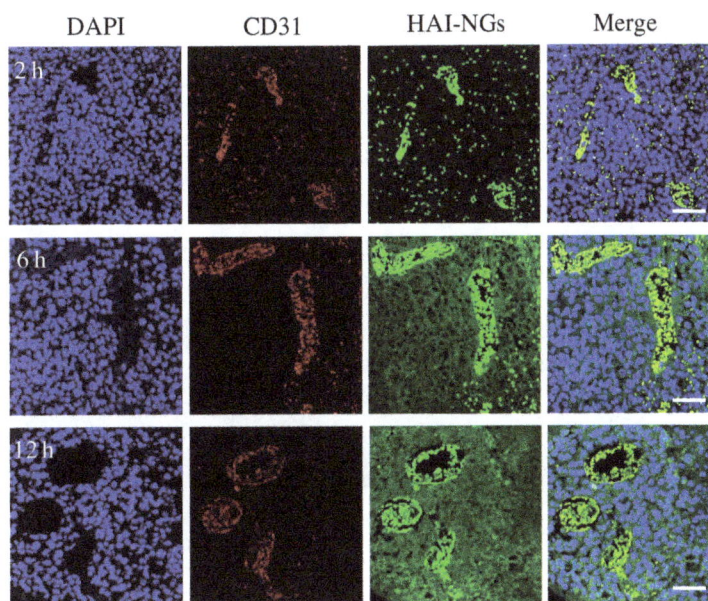

FIGURE 7.17 Tumor penetration of HAI-NGs observed by confocal microscopy. Tumor sections were obtained from MCF-7 tumor bearing mice following 2, 6 and 12 h tail vein injection of HAINGs (10 mg/mL). The nuclei were stained with DAPI (blue) and blood vessels were stained with CD31 (red). HAI-NGs have an intrinsic green fluorescence. The scale bar represents 50 μm.

fluorescence throughout the whole tumor. At 12 h post injection, HAI-NGs penetrated further deep into the tumor and were actively endocytosed by tumor cells, presenting bright green fluorescence around the cell nuclei. The above phenomena suggest that the HAI-NGs possess good tumor-penetration ability.

The antitumor efficacy of PTX-loaded HAI-NGs was evaluated in MCF-7 tumor-bearing mice at a dose of 5 mg PTX equiv./kg. The results [220] showed that PTX-loaded HAI-NGs exhibited effective inhibition of tumor growth, which was significantly better than that of free PTX (Figure 7.18a). The photographs of tumor blocks excised on day 24 further confirmed that mice treated with PTX-loaded HAI-NGs had the smallest tumor size (Figure 7.18b). Both PTX-loaded HAI-NGs and free PTX caused no change

of mice body weight (Figure 7.18c). Importantly, survival curves showed that PTX-loaded HAI-NGs effectively prolonged the survival time of the MCF-7 breast tumor bearing mice with all mice surviving over an experimental period of 65 d (Figure 7.18d). In contrast, mice treated with free PTX and PBS had a median survival time of 40 and 28 d, respectively. The histological analyses by H&E staining displayed that PTX-loaded HAI-NGs induced widespread necrosis of tumor tissue with little damage to the healthy organs including heart, liver, and kidney (Figure 7.18e), supporting that PTX-loaded HAI-NGs cause low systemic side effects. In comparison, hepatocellular necrosis (red arrows) was observed for free PTX treated mice, similar to previous reports [224,225]. It is evident that PTX-loaded HAI-NGs have low systemic toxicity and mediate efficient

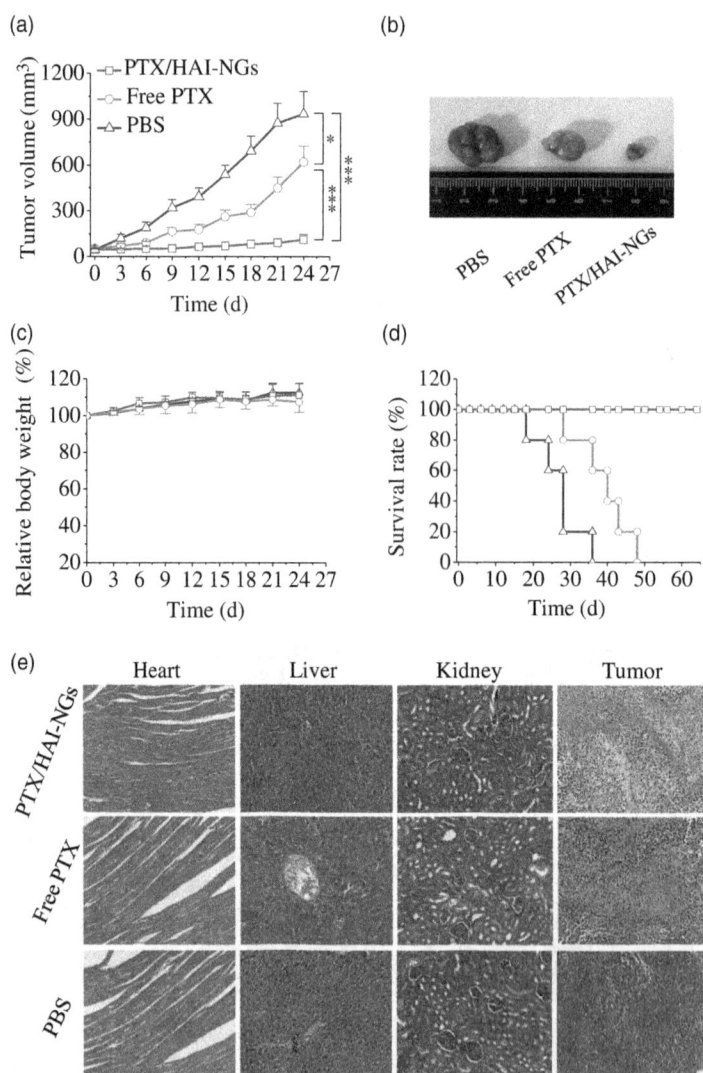

FIGURE 7.18 In *vivo* antitumor efficacy of PTX/HAI-NGs in MCF-7 tumor bearing nude mice. Free PTX and PBS were used as controls. The drug was given on day 0, 3, 6, 9, 12 (drug dosage: 5 mg PTX equiv./kg). (a) Tumor volume changes in time. Data are presented as mean ±SD (n=6). (b) Photographs of tumor blocks collected from different treatment groups on day 24. (c) Body weight changes of nude mice following different treatments within 24 days. (d) Survival rates of mice in different treatment groups within 60 d. Data are presented as means ±SD (n=5). * p<0.05, *** p<0.001. (e) H&E stained heart, liver, kidney and tumor sections excised from MCF-7 human breast tumor-bearing mice following 24 d treatment with PTX/HAINGs, free PTX or PBS. The images were obtained by a Leica microscope at 200× magnification. Red arrows indicate hepatocellular necrosis.

and targeted delivery of PTX to human breast tumors *in vivo*, resulting in effective suppression of tumor growth and markedly prolonged survival time.

7.11 CONCLUSIONS AND PERSPECTIVES

This chapter summarized the application of various imaging modalities for qualitative and quantitative assessments of RNAi therapeutics to promote their applications in cancer therapy and translate them into clinical applications. Overall, a variety of RNAi therapeutics has been developed and some of them are under clinical evaluation. Diverse imaging techniques have been applied to study the mechanism of gene transfection, route of delivery, systemic distribution in the body, gene-silencing effect, and therapeutic outcomes.

RNAi has demonstrated great potential for treating a wide range of diseases, especially for multidrug-resistant cancer treatment, which are difficult to be treated by conventional methods of chemotherapy and radiotherapy. Despite the positive progresses in translating some RNAi formulations into clinical trial for cancer therapy, several issues are required to be borne in mind for effective translation of RNAi therapeutics from bench to bedside: (i) How to optimize the parameters/conditions to accumulate sufficient amount of RNAi therapeutics in tumor tissues and translocate them into cancer cells; (ii) How to select the proper target to maximize the therapeutic effects of siRNA; and (iii) How to develop new effective gene carriers with high stability during circulation as well as controlled release function of payload nucleic acids inside cancer cells with high gene transfection effects. Finally, the ideal RNAi formulations should satisfy the requirement of specific delivery of RNAi agents to tumors and efficiently transfer into cancer cells to silence target genes at high performance for tumor suppression, while avoiding potential toxicity, side effects, and off-target silencing.

The advances in noninvasive imaging techniques [226–229] provide new approaches to visualize and quantify RNAi in cancer therapy and further understand the mechanism of RNAi intracellular and in the body. So far, several imaging modalities, such as optical imaging, MRI, ultrasound, and SPECT/PET, have been applied to assess the delivery of siRNA, to determine the biodistribution, and to monitor the therapeutic effects, leading to a significant contribution to the progresses of RNAi therapeutics, especially in the preclinical studies [230,231]. It is very important to establish proper evaluation models/systems with the aid of molecular imaging in preclinical studies and translate the animal results as important references for clinical trial in human. As each imaging modality has its intrinsic advantages and limitations, there is a trend to combine different imaging modalities for better tracing the fate of siRNA, the delivery vehicles, and the therapeutic effects, which is expected to maximize the potential of cancer therapy with RNAi therapeutics and help overcome the barriers that block the road to clinical translation.

The rational design of molecular imaging probes is essential to accurately monitor the biological processes of RNAi therapeutics and fully realize their potency in cancer therapy. Molecular imaging probes for RNAi-based cancer therapeutics, consisting of a variety of functional nanomaterials including lipids, metals, carbons, polymers, and biologics-based nanoparticles, should be relatively safe for clinical use with low toxicity and biodegradability in the body. Further development of new imaging contrast agents, which can increase the signal intensity for more reliable image analysis with cancer cell specific targeting ability, would optimize the diagnostic selectivity and provide more detailed and accurate pathological information about the biological processes of RNAi therapeutics in cancer treatment. Furthermore, the technical advances in imaging devices would enable proper patient selection and rapid translation of RNAi therapeutics into clinic.

We have demonstrated for the first time that bioresponsive and fluorescent hyaluronic acid-iodixanol nanogels (HAI-NGs) mediate targeted X-ray computed tomography (CT) imaging and chemotherapy of MCF-7 human breast tumor *in vivo*. Notably, HAI-NGs have integrated multiple functions including excellent biocompatibility, bright green fluorescence, high stability, superior targetability to CD44 overexpressing cells and fast glutathione-responsive drug release. The *in vivo* studies clearly show that PTX-loaded HAI-NGs have a prolonged circulation time, high tumor accumulation, and enhanced tumor penetration in MCF-7 breast tumor-bearing nude mice, resulting in effective tumor-growth inhibition, markedly improved survival rate, and reduced systemic toxicity as compared to free PTX. Furthermore, HAI-NGs via either intratumoral or intravenous injection lead to significantly enhanced CT imaging of MCF-7 breast tumors in nude mice as compared to iodoxanol. HAI-NGs provide a highly versatile and targeted theranostic nanoplatform that elegantly combines CT imaging with targeted chemotherapy toward CD44 overexpressing tumors.

REFERENCES

1. A. Fire, S. Xu, M.K. Montgomery, S.A. Kostas, S.E. Driver, C.C. Mello, Potent and specific genetic interference by double-stranded RNA in Caenorhabditis elegans, *Nature* 391 (1998) 806–811.
2. S.M. Elbashir, J. Harborth, W. Lendeckel, A. Yalcin, K. Weber, T. Tuschl, Duplexes of 21-nucleotide RNAs mediate RNA interference in cultured mammalian cells, *Nature* 411 (2001) 494–498.
3. S.L. Ginn, I.E. Alexander, M.L. Edelstein, M.R. Abedi, J. Wixon, Gene therapy clinical trials worldwide to 2012—an update, *J. Gene Med.* 15 (2013) 65–77.
4. E.P. Thi, C.E. Mire, R. Ursic-Bedoya, J.B. Geisbert, A.C.H. Lee, K.N. Agans, M. Robbins, D.J. Deer, K.A. Fenton, I. MacLachlan, T.W. Geisbert, Marburg virus infection in nonhuman primates: therapeutic treatment by lipid-encapsulated siRNA, *Sci. Transl. Med.* 6 (2014) 250ra116.

5. P.K. Kaiser, R.C. Symons, S.M. Shah, E.J. Quinlan, H. Tabandeh, D.V. Do, G. Reisen, J.A. Lockridge, B. Short, R. Guerciolini, Q.D. Nguyen, RNAi-based treatment for neovascular age-related macular degeneration by Sirna-027, *Am. J. Ophthalmol.* 150 (2010) 33–39, e32.

6. R.M. O'Connell, D.S. Rao, A.A. Chaudhuri, D. Baltimore, Physiological and pathological roles for microRNAs in the immune system, *Nat. Rev. Immunol.* 10 (2010) 111–122.

7. E. van Rooij, E.N. Olson, MicroRNA therapeutics for cardiovascular disease: opportunities and obstacles, *Nat. Rev. Drug Discov.* 11 (2012) 860–872.

8. T. Coelho, D. Adams, A. Silva, P. Lozeron, P.N. Hawkins, T. Mant, J. Perez, J. Chiesa, S. Warrington, E. Tranter, M. Munisamy, R. Falzone, J. Harrop, J. Cehelsky, B.R. Bettencourt, M. Geissler, J.S. Butler, A. Sehgal, R.E. Meyers, Q. Chen, T. Borland, R.M. Hutabarat, V.A. Clausen, R. Alvarez, K. Fitzgerald, C. Gamba-Vitalo, S.V. Nochur, A.K. Vaishnaw, D.W. Sah, J.A. Gollob, O.B. Suhr, Safety and efficacy of RNAi therapy for transthyretin amyloidosis, *N. Engl. J. Med.* 369 (2013) 819–829.

9. M.E. Davis, J.E. Zuckerman, C.H. Choi, D. Seligson, A. Tolcher, C.A. Alabi, Y. Yen, J.D. Heidel, A. Ribas, Evidence of RNAi in humans from systemically administered siRNA via targeted nanoparticles, *Nature* 464 (2010) 1067–1070.

10. H. Shen, T. Sun, M. Ferrari, Nanovector delivery of siRNA for cancer therapy, *Cancer Gene Ther.* 19 (2012) 367–373.

11. J. Tabernero, G.I. Shapiro, P.M. LoRusso, A. Cervantes, G.K. Schwartz, G.J. Weiss, L. Paz-Ares, D.C. Cho, J.R. Infante, M. Alsina, M.M. Gounder, R. Falzone, J. Harrop, A.C. White, I. Toudjarska, D. Bumcrot, R.E. Meyers, G. Hinkle, N. Svrzikapa, R.M. Hutabarat, V.A. Clausen, J. Cehelsky, S.V. Nochur, C. Gamba-Vitalo, A.K. Vaishnaw, D.W. Sah, J.A. Gollob, H.A. Burris 3rd, First-in-humans trial of an RNA interference therapeutic targeting VEGF and KSP in cancer patients with liver involvement, *Cancer Discov.* 3 (2013) 406–417.

12. F. Alexis, E. Pridgen, L.K.Molnar, O.C. Farokhzad, Factors affecting the clearance and biodistribution of polymeric nanoparticles, *Mol. Pharm.* 5 (2008) 505–515.

13. K.A. Whitehead, R. Langer, D.G. Anderson, Knocking down barriers: advances in siRNA delivery, *Nat. Rev. Drug Discov.* 8 (2009) 129–138.

14. W. Li, F.C. Szoka Jr., Lipid-based nanoparticles for nucleic acid delivery, *Pharm. Res.* 24 (2007) 438–449.

15. M.A. Mintzer, E.E. Simanek, Nonviral vectors for gene delivery, *Chem. Rev.* 109 (2009) 259–302.

16. A. Akinc, A. Zumbuehl, M. Goldberg, E.S. Leshchiner, V. Busini, N. Hossain, S.A. Bacallado, D.N. Nguyen, J. Fuller, R. Alvarez, A. Borodovsky, T. Borland, R. Constien, A. de Fougerolles, J.R. Dorkin, K. Narayanannair Jayaprakash, M. Jayaraman, M. John, V. Koteliansky, M. Manoharan, L. Nechev, J. Qin, T. Racie, D. Raitcheva, K.G. Rajeev, D.W. Sah, J. Soutschek, I. Toudjarska, H.P. Vornlocher, T.S. Zimmermann, R. Langer, D.G. Anderson, A combinatorial library of lipid-like materials for delivery of RNAi therapeutics, *Nat. Biotechnol.* 26 (2008) 561–569.

17. S.C. Semple, A. Akinc, J. Chen, A.P. Sandhu, B.L. Mui, C.K. Cho, D.W. Sah, D. Stebbing, E.J. Crosley, E. Yaworski, I.M. Hafez, J.R. Dorkin, J. Qin, K. Lam, K.G. Rajeev, K.F. Wong, L.B. Jeffs, L. Nechev, M.L. Eisenhardt, M. Jayaraman, M. Kazem, M.A. Maier, M. Srinivasulu, M.J. Weinstein, Q. Chen, R. Alvarez, S.A. Barros, S. De, S.K. Klimuk, T. Borland, V. Kosovrasti, W.L. Cantley, Y.K. Tam, M. Manoharan, M.A. Ciufolini, M.A. Tracy, A. de Fougerolles, I. MacLachlan, P.R. Cullis, T.D. Madden, M.J. Hope, Rational design of cationic lipids for siRNA delivery, *Nat. Biotechnol.* 28 (2010) 172–176.

18. C.C. Lee, J.A. MacKay, J.M. Frechet, F.C. Szoka, Designing dendrimers for biological applications, *Nat. Biotechnol.* 23 (2005) 1517–1526.

19. D.W. Pack, A.S. Hoffman, S. Pun, P.S. Stayton, Design and development of polymers for gene delivery, *Nat. Rev. Drug Discov.* 4 (2005) 581–593.

20. M. Thomas, A.M. Klibanov, Non-viral gene therapy: polycation-mediated DNA delivery, *Appl. Microbiol. Biotechnol.* 62 (2003) 27–34.

21. R.H. Mo, J.L. Zaro, W.C. Shen, Comparison of cationic and amphipathic cell penetrating peptides for siRNA delivery and efficacy, *Mol. Pharm.* 9 (2012) 299–309.

22. M.E. Martin, K.G. Rice, Peptide-guided gene delivery, *AAPS J.* 9 (2007) E18–E29.

23. J.P. Dassie, X.Y. Liu, G.S. Thomas, R.M. Whitaker, K.W. Thiel, K.R. Stockdale, D.K. Meyerholz, A.P. McCaffrey, J.O. McNamara 2nd, P.H. Giangrande, Systemic administration of optimized aptamer-siRNA chimeras promotes regression of PSMA expressing tumors, *Nat. Biotechnol.* 27 (2009) 839–849.

24. Y.D. Yao, T.M. Sun, S.Y. Huang, S. Dou, L. Lin, J.N. Chen, J.B. Ruan, C.Q. Mao, F.Y. Yu, M.S. Zeng, J.Y. Zang, Q. Liu, F.X. Su, P. Zhang, J. Lieberman, J. Wang, E. Song, Targeted delivery of PLK1-siRNA by ScFv suppresses Her2+ breast cancer growth and metastasis, *Sci. Transl. Med.* 4 (2012) 130ra148.

25. K.Y. Choi, O.F. Silvestre, X. Huang, N. Hida, G. Liu, D.N. Ho, S. Lee, S.W. Lee, J.I. Hong, X. Chen, A nanoparticle formula for delivering siRNA or miRNAs to tumor cells in cell culture and *in vivo, Nat. Protoc.* 9 (2014) 1900–1915.

26. K.Y. Choi, O.F. Silvestre, X. Huang, K.H. Min, G.P. Howard, N. Hida, A.J. Jin, N. Carvajal, S.W. Lee, J.I. Hong, X. Chen, Versatile RNA interference nanoplatform for systemic delivery of RNAs, *ACS Nano* 8 (2014) 4559–4570.

27. G. Liu, K.Y. Choi, A. Bhirde, M. Swierczewska, J. Yin, S.W. Lee, J.H. Park, J.I. Hong, J. Xie, G. Niu, D.O. Kiesewetter, S. Lee, X. Chen, Sticky nanoparticles: a platform for siRNA delivery by a bis(zinc(II) dipicolylamine)-functionalized, self-assembled nanoconjugate, *Angew. Chem. Int. Ed.* 51 (2012) 445–449.

28. V. Sokolova, M. Epple, Inorganic nanoparticles as carriers of nucleic acids into cells, *Angew. Chem. Int. Ed. Engl.* 47 (2008) 1382–1395.

29. K.A. Afonin, M. Viard, A.Y. Koyfman, A.N. Martins, W.K. Kasprzak, M. Panigaj, R. Desai, A. Santhanam, W.W. Grabow, L. Jaeger, E. Heldman, J. Reiser, W. Chiu, E.O. Freed, B.A. Shapiro, Multifunctional RNA nanoparticles, *Nano Lett.* 14 (2014) 5662–5671.

30. D.X. Cui, C.L. Zhang, B. Liu, Y. Shu, T. Du, D. Shu, K. Wang, F.P. Dai, Y.L. Liu, C. Li, F. Pan, Y.M. Yang, J. Ni, H. Li, B. Brand-Saberi, P.X. Guo, Regression of gastric cancer by systemic injection of RNA nanoparticles carrying both ligand and siRNA, *Sci. Rep.* 5 (2015) e10726.

31. H. Lee, A.K.R. Lytton-Jean, Y. Chen, K.T. Love, A.I. Park, E.D. Karagiannis, A. Sehgal, W. Querbes, C.S. Zurenko, M. Jayaraman, C.G. Peng, K. Charisse, A. Borodovsky, M. Manoharan, J.S. Donahoe, J. Truelove, M. Nahrendorf, R. Langer, D.G. Anderson, Molecularly self-assembled nucleic acid nanoparticles for targeted *in vivo* siRNA delivery, *Nat. Nanotechnol.* 7 (2012) 389–393.

32. P. Rychahou, F. Haque, Y. Shu, Y. Zaytseva, H.L. Weiss, E.Y. Lee, W. Mustain, J. Valentino, P. Guo, B.M. Evers, Delivery of RNA nanoparticles into colorectal cancer metastases following systemic administration, *ACS Nano* 9 (2015) 1108–1116.

33. D. Shu, H. Li, Y. Shu, G. Xiong, W.E. Carson 3rd, F. Haque, R. Xu, P. Guo, Systemic delivery of anti-miRNA for suppression of triple negative breast cancer utilizing RNA nanotechnology, *ACS Nano* 9 (2015) 9731–9740.

34. D. Haussecker, Current issues of RNAi therapeutics delivery and development, *J. Control. Release* 195 (2014) 49–54.

35. J. Wang, Z. Lu, M.G. Wientjes, J.L.S. Au, Delivery of siRNA therapeutics: barriers and carriers, *AAPS J.* 12 (2010) 492–503.

36. V. Hornung, M. Guenthner-Biller, C. Bourquin, A. Ablasser, M. Schlee, S. Uematsu, A. Noronha, M. Manoharan, S. Akira, A. de Fougerolles, S. Endres, G. Hartmann, Sequence-specific potent induction of IFN-alpha by short interfering RNA in plasmacytoid dendritic cells through TLR7, *Nat. Med.* 11 (2005) 263–270.

37. A.D. Judge, V. Sood, J.R. Shaw, D. Fang, K. McClintock, I. MacLachlan, Sequence dependent stimulation of the mammalian innate immune response by synthetic siRNA, *Nat. Biotechnol.* 23 (2005) 457–462.

38. A.L. Jackson, J. Burchard, J. Schelter, B.N. Chau, M. Cleary, L. Lim, P.S. Linsley, Widespread siRNA "off-target" transcript silencing mediated by seed region sequence complementarity, *RNA* 12 (2006) 1179–1187.

39. H. Hong, Y. Zhang, W.B. Cai, *In vivo* imaging of RNA Interference, *J. Nucl. Med.* 51 (2010) 169–172.

40. J.K. Willmann, N. van Bruggen, L.M. Dinkelborg, S.S. Gambhir, Molecular imaging in drug development, *Nat. Rev. Drug Discov.* 7 (2008) 591–607.

41. S.Y. Wu, G. Lopez-Berestein, G.A. Calin, A.K. Sood, RNAi therapies: drugging the undruggable, *Sci. Transl. Med.* 6 (2014) 240–247.

42. C.H. Contag, M.H. Bachmann, Advances in *in vivo* bioluminescence imaging of gene expression, *Annu. Rev. Biomed. Eng.* 4 (2002) 235–260.

43. F. Wang, X. Song, X. Li, J. Xin, S. Wang, W. Yang, J. Wang, K. Wu, X. Chen, J. Liang, J. Tian, F. Cao, Noninvasive visualization of microRNA-16 in the chemoresistance of gastric cancer using a dual reporter gene imaging system, *PLoS One* 8 (2013) e61792.

44. X. Huang, S. Lee, X. Chen, Design of "smart" probes for optical imaging of apoptosis, *Am. J. Nucl. Med. Mol Imaging* 1 (2011) 3–17.

45. D.E. Sosnovik, R. Weissleder, Emerging concepts in molecular MRI, *Curr. Opin. Biotechnol.* 18 (2007) 4–10.

46. M.M. Alauddin, Positron emission tomography (PET) imaging with (18)F-based radiotracers, *Am. J. Nucl. Med. Mol Imaging.* 2 (2012) 55–76.

47. P. Bhargava, G. He, A. Samarghandi, E.S. Delpassand, Pictorial review of SPECT/CT imaging applications in clinical nuclear medicine, *Am. J. Nucl. Med. Mol. Imaging* 2 (2012) 221–231.

48. P.A. Dayton, J.J. Rychak, Molecular ultrasound imaging using microbubble contrast agents, *Front. Biosci.* 12 (2007) 5124–5142.

49. S.I. Pai, Y.Y. Lin, B. Macaes, A. Meneshian, C.F. Hung, T.C. Wu, Prospects of RNA interference therapy for cancer, *Gene Ther.* 13 (2006) 464–477.

50. D.D. Rao, Z.H. Wang, N. Senzer, J. Nemunaitis, RNA Interference and personalized cancer therapy, *Discov. Med.* 81 (2013) 101–110.

51. M.D.A.C. Center, EphA2 Gene Targeting Using Neutral Liposomal Small Interfering RNA Delivery (IND# 72924): A Phase I Clinical Trial, https://clinicaltrials.gov/ct2/show/NCT01591356? term=NCT015913562012.

52. C.C.C.o.W.F. University, A Phase 1, Open-Label, Dose-Ranging Study to Assess the Safety and Immunologic Activity of APN401, https://clinicaltrials.gov/ct2/show/NCT021662552014.

53. S. Pruitt, Phase I Study of Active Immunotherapy of Metastatic Melanoma with Mature Autologous Dendritic Cells Transfected with Tumor Antigen RNA and Small Inhibitory RNAs to Alter Proteasomal Antigen Processing, https://clinicaltrials.gov/ct2/show/NCT006725422008.

54. S.T. GmbH, A Prospective, Open-label, Single Center, Dose Finding Phase I-Study with Atu027 (an siRNA Formulation) in Subjects with Advanced Solid Cancer, https://clinicaltrials.gov/ct2/show/NCT009385742009.

55. S. Ltd, Phase I—Escalating Dose Study of siG12D LODER (Local Drug EluteR) in Patients With Locally Advanced Adenocarcinoma of the Pancreas, and a Single Dose Study of siG12D LODER (Local Drug EluteR) in Patients With Non-operable Adenocarcinoma of the Pancreas, https://clinicaltrials.gov/ct2/show/NCT011887852010.

56. N.C.I. (NCI), A Phase 1 Dose Escalation Study of Hepatic Intra-Arterial Administration of TKM 080301 (Lipid Nanoparticles Containing siRNA Against the PLK1 Gene Product) in Patients with Colorectal, Pancreas, Gastric, Breast, Ovarian and Esophageal Cancers with Hepatic, https://clinicaltrials.gov/ct2/show/NCT014370072011.

57. N.D. Corporation, A Phase 1b/2, Open Label, Randomized, Repeat Dose, Dose Escalation Study to Evaluate the Safety, Tolerability, Biological Activity, and Pharmacokinetics of ND-L02-s0201 Injection, a Vitamin A-coupled Lipid Nanoparticle Containing siRNA Against HSP47, in Subjects with Moderate to Extensive Hepatic Fibrosis (METAVIR F3–4), https://clinicaltrials.gov/ct2/show/NCT022274592014.

58. I. Dicerna Pharmaceuticals, Phase I, Multicenter, Cohort Dose Escalation Trial to Determine the Safety, Tolerance, and Maximum Tolerated Dose of DCR-MYC, a Lipid Nanoparticle (LNP)-Formulated Small Inhibitory RNA (siRNA) Oligonucleotide Targeting MYC, in Patients with Refractory Locally Advanced or Metastatic Solid Tumor Malignancies, Multiple Myeloma, or Lymphoma, https://clinicaltrials.gov/ct2/show/NCT021105632014.

59. C. Pharmaceuticals, A Phase I, Dose-Escalating Study of the Safety of Intravenous CALAA-01 in Adults with Solid Tumors Refractory to Standard-of-Care Therapies, https://clinicaltrials.gov/ct2/show/NCT006890652008.

60. T.P. Corporation, A Phase 1/2 Dose Escalation Study to Determine the Safety, Pharmacokinetics, and Pharmacodynamics of Intravenous TKM-080301 in Patients with Advanced Solid Tumors, https://clinicaltrials.gov/ct2/show/NCT012622352010.

61. A. Pharmaceuticals, A Multi-Center, Open Label, Phase 1 Dose-Escalation Trial to Evaluate the Safety, Tolerability, Pharmacokinetics and Pharmacodynamics of Intravenous ALN-VSP02 in Patients with Advanced Solid Tumors with Liver Involvement, https://clinicaltrials.gov/ct2/show/NCT008821802009.

62. A. Pharmaceuticals, A Multi-center, Open-Label, Extension Study of ALN-VSP02 in Cancer Patients Who Have Responded to ALN-VSP02 Treatment, https://clinicaltrials.gov/ct2/show/NCT011580792009.

63. M. Aleku, P. Schulz, O. Keil, A. Santel, U. Schaeper, B. Dieckhoff, O. Janke, J. Endruschat, B. Durieux, N. Roder, K. Loffler, C. Lange, M. Fechtner, K. Mopert, G. Fisch, S. Dames, W. Arnold, K. Jochims, K. Giese, B. Wiedenmann, A. Scholz, J. Kaufmann, Atu027, a liposomal small interfering RNA formulation targeting protein kinase N3, inhibits cancer progression, *Cancer Res.* 68 (2008) 9788–9798.

64. A. Santel, M. Aleku, N. Roder, K. Mopert, B. Durieux, O. Janke, O. Keil, J. Endruschat, S. Dames, C. Lange, M. Eisermann, K. Loffler, M. Fechtner, G. Fisch, C. Vank, U. Schaeper, K. Giese, J. Kaufmann, Atu027 prevents pulmonary metastasis in experimental and spontaneous mouse metastasis models, *Clin. Cancer Res.* 16 (2010) 5469–5480.

65. F. Leenders, K. Mopert, A. Schmiedeknecht, A. Santel, F. Czauderna, M. Aleku, S. Penschuck, S. Dames, M. Sternberger, T. Rohl, A. Wellmann, W. Arnold, K. Giese, J. Kaufmann, A. Klippel, PKN3 is required for malignant prostate cell growth downstream of activated PI 3-kinase, *EMBO J.* 23 (2004) 3303–3313.

66. D. Strumberg, B. Schultheis, U. Traugott, C. Vank, A. Santel, O. Keil, K. Giese, J. Kaufmann, J. Drevs, Phase I clinical development of Atu027, a siRNA formulation targeting PKN3 in patients with advanced solid tumors, *Int. J. Clin. Pharmacol. Ther.* 50 (2012) 76–78.

67. B. Schultheis, D. Strumberg, A. Santel, C. Vank, F. Gebhardt, O. Keil, C. Lange, K. Giese, J. Kaufmann, M. Khan, J. Drevs, First-in-human phase I study of the liposomal RNA Interference therapeutic Atu027 in patients with advanced solid tumors, *J. Clin. Oncol.* 32 (2014) 4141–4148.

68. A. Blangy, H.A. Lane, P. d'Herin, M. Harper, M. Kress, E.A. Nigg, Phosphorylation by p34cdc2 regulates spindle association of human Eg5, a kinesin-related motor essential for bipolar spindle formation *in vivo*, *Cell* 83 (1995) 1159–1169.

69. J. Itakura, T. Ishiwata, B. Shen, M. Kornmann, M. Korc, Concomitant overexpression of vascular endothelial growth factor and its receptors in pancreatic cancer, *Int. J. Cancer* 85 (2000) 27–34.

70. C.A. Boocock, D.S. Charnockjones, A.M. Sharkey, J. Mclaren, P.J. Barker, K.A.Wright, P.R. Twentyman, S.K. Smith, Expression of vascular endothelial growth-factor and its receptors Flt and Kdr in ovarian-carcinoma, *J. Natl. Cancer Inst.* 87 (1995) 506–516.

71. N. Ferrara, H.P. Gerber, J. LeCouter, The biology of VEGF and its receptors, *Nat. Med.* 9 (2003) 669–676.

72. M.S. Duxbury, H. Ito, M.J. Zinner, S.W. Ashley, E.E. Whang, RNA interference targeting the M2 subunit of ribonucleotide reductase enhances pancreatic adenocarcinoma chemosensitivity to gemcitabine, *Oncogene* 23 (2004) 1539–1548.

73. Y.X. Wang, C.K. Ng, The impact of quantitative imaging in medicine and surgery: charting our course for the future, *Quant. Imaging. Med. Surg.* 1 (2011) 1–3.

74. V.K. Tracy Zimmermann, J. Harrop, A. Chan, J. Chiesa, G. Peters, R. Falzone, J. Cehelsky, S. Nochur, A. Vaishnaw, J. Gollob, Phase I First-in-Human Trial of ALN-TTRsc, a Novel RNA Interference Therapeutic for the Treatment of Familial Amyloidotic Cardiomyopathy (FAC), http://www.alnylam.com/web/wp-content/uploads/2013/09/ALN-TTRsc-PhI-HFSA-Poster-Sep2013.pdf2013.

75. K. Buyens, S.C. De Smedt, K. Braeckmans, J. Demeester, L. Peeters, L.A. van Grunsven, X.D. du Jeu, R. Sawant, V. Torchilin, K. Farkasova, M. Ogris, N.N. Sanders, Liposome based systems for systemic siRNA delivery: stability in blood sets the requirements for optimal carrier design, *J. Control. Release* 158 (2012) 362–370.

76. R. Kanasty, J.R. Dorkin, A. Vegas, D. Anderson, Delivery materials for siRNA therapeutics, *Nat. Mater.* 12 (2013) 967–977.

77. Y.K. Oh, T.G. Park, siRNA delivery systems for cancer treatment, *Adv. Drug Deliv. Rev.* 61 (2009) 850–862.

78. H. Yin, R.L. Kanasty, A.A. Eltoukhy, A.J. Vegas, J.R. Dorkin, D.G. Anderson, Non-viral vectors for gene-based therapy, *Nat. Rev. Genet.* 15 (2014) 541–555.

79. P. Zhang, Y. Chen, Y. Zeng, C. Shen, R. Li, Z. Guo, S. Li, Q. Zheng, C. Chu, Z.Wang, Z. Zheng, R. Tian, S. Ge, X. Zhang, N.S. Xia, G. Liu, X. Chen, Virus-mimetic nanovesicles as a versatile antigen-delivery system, *Proc. Natl. Acad. Sci. U. S. A.* 112 (2015) E6129–E6138.

80. H. Kobayashi, R.Watanabe, P.L. Choyke, Improving conventional enhanced permeability and retention (EPR) effects; what Is the appropriate Target? *Theranostics.* 4 (2014) 81–89.

81. Y. Matsumura, H. Maeda, A new concept for macromolecular therapeutics in cancer- chemotherapy—mechanism of tumoritropic accumulation of proteins and the antitumor agent Smancs, *Cancer Res.* 46 (1986) 6387–6392.

82. S.M. Moghimi, A.C. Hunter, J.C. Murray, Long-circulating and target-specific nanoparticles: theory to practice, *Pharmacol. Rev.* 53 (2001) 283–318.

83. K.J. Cho, X. Wang, S.M. Nie, Z. Chen, D.M. Shin, Therapeutic nanoparticles for drug delivery in cancer, *Clin. Cancer Res.* 14 (2008) 1310–1316.

84. L.E. van Vlerken, T.K. Vyas, M.M. Amiji, Poly(ethylene glycol)-modified nanocarriers for tumor-targeted and intracellular delivery, *Pharm. Res.* 24 (2007) 1405–1414.

85. I. Maclachlan, P. Cullis, Diffusible-PEG-lipid stabilized plasmid lipid particles, *Adv. Genet.* 53 (2005) 157–188 53pa. doi:10.1016/S0065-2660(05)53006-2

86. P. Vaupel, F. Kallinowski, P. Okunieff, Blood-flow, oxygen and nutrient supply, and metabolic microenvironment of human-tumors—a review, *Cancer Res.* 49 (1989) 6449–6465.

87. L. Li, R. Wang, D. Wilcox, X. Zhao, J. Song, X. Lin, W.M. Kohlbrenner, S.W. Fesik, Y. Shen, Tumor vasculature is a key determinant for the efficiency of nanoparticle mediated siRNA delivery, *Gene Ther.* 19 (2012) 775–780.

88. K. Huang, H. Ma, J. Liu, S. Huo, A. Kumar, T. Wei, X. Zhang, S. Jin, Y. Gan, P.C. Wang, S. He, X. Zhang, X.J. Liang, Size-dependent localization and penetration of ultrasmall gold nanoparticles in cancer cells, multicellular spheroids, and tumors *in vivo*, *ACS Nano* 6 (2012) 4483–4493.

89. L. Cunha, K. Szigeti, D. Mathe, L.F. Metello, The role of molecular imaging in modern drug development, *Drug Discov. Today* 19 (2014) 936–948.

90. B.R. Meade, S.F. Dowdy, Exogenous siRNA delivery using peptide transduction domains/ cell penetrating peptides, *Adv. Drug Deliv. Rev.* 59 (2007) 134–140.

91. D.B. Rozema, D.L. Lewis, D.H. Wakefield, S.C. Wong, J.J. Klein, P.L. Roesch, S.L. Bertin, T.W. Reppen, Q. Chu, A.V. Blokhin, J.E. Hagstrom, J.A. Wolff, Dynamic polyconjugates for targeted *in vivo* delivery of siRNA to hepatocytes, *Proc. Natl. Acad. Sci. U. S. A.* 104 (2007) 12982–12987.

92. A.L. Cardoso, S. Simoes, L.P. de Almeida, J. Pelisek, C. Culmsee, E. Wagner, M.C. Pedroso de Lima, siRNA delivery by a transferrin-associated lipid-based vector: a non-viral strategy to mediate gene silencing, *J. Gene Med.* 9 (2007) 170–183.

93. T.C. Chu, K.Y. Twu, A.D. Ellington, M. Levy, Aptamer mediated siRNA delivery, *Nucleic Acids Res.* 34 (2006) e73.

94. C. Lorenzer, M. Dirin, A.M. Winkler, V. Baumann, J. Winkler, Going beyond the liver: progress and challenges of targeted delivery of siRNA therapeutics, *J. Control. Release* 203 (2015) 1–15.

95. J. Gruenberg, F.G. van der Goot, Mechanisms of pathogen entry through the endosomal compartments, *Nat. Rev. Mol. Cell Biol.* 7 (2006) 495–504.

96. N.D. Sonawane, F.C. Szoka Jr., A.S. Verkman, Chloride accumulation and swelling in endosomes enhances DNA transfer by polyamine-DNA polyplexes, *J. Biol. Chem.* 278 (2003) 44826–44831.

97. O. Boussif, F. Lezoualc'h, M.A. Zanta, M.D. Mergny, D. Scherman, B. Demeneix, J.P. Behr, A versatile vector for gene and oligonucleotide transfer into cells in culture and *in vivo*: polyethylenimine, *Proc. Natl. Acad. Sci. U. S. A.* 92 (1995) 7297–7301.

98. S. Qiu, C.M. Adema, T. Lane, A computational study of off-target effects of RNA interference, *Nucleic Acids Res.* 33 (2005) 1834–1847.

99. A. Goodchild, N. Nopper, A. King, T. Doan, M. Tanudji, G.M. Arndt, M. Poidinger, L.P. Rivory, T. Passioura, Sequence determinants of innate immune activation by short interfering RNAs, *BMC Immunol.* 10 (2009) 40.

100. A.D. Judge, V. Sood, J.R. Shaw, D. Fang, K. McClintock, I. MacLachlan, Sequence dependent stimulation of the mammalian innate immune response by synthetic siRNA, *Nat. Biotechnol.* 23 (2005) 457–462.

101. M. Sioud, Does the understanding of immune activation by RNA predict the design of safe siRNAs? *Front. Biosci.* 13 (2008) 4379–4392.

102. E.M. Sevick-Muraca, J.P. Houston, M. Gurfinkel, Fluorescence-enhanced, near infrared diagnostic imaging with contrast agents, *Curr. Opin. Chem. Biol.* 6 (2002) 642–650.

103. J.V. Frangioni, *In vivo* near-infrared fluorescence imaging, *Curr. Opin. Chem. Biol.* 7 (2003) 626–634.

104. P. Zanzonico, Noninvasive imaging for supporting basic research, Small Animal Imaging: Basics and Practical Guide 2011, pp. 3–16.

105. F. Leblond, S.C. Davis, P.A. Valdés, B.W. Pogue, Pre-clinical whole-body fluorescence imaging: review of instruments, methods and applications, *J. Photochem. Photobiol., B* 98 (2010) 77–94.

106. Z. Guo, S. Park, J. Yoon, I. Shin, Recent progress in the development of near-infrared fluorescent probes for bioimaging applications, *Chem. Soc. Rev.* 43 (2014) 16–29.

107. S.H. Kim, J.H. Jeong, S.H. Lee, S.W. Kim, T.G. Park, Local and systemic delivery of VEGF siRNA using polyelectrolyte complex micelles for effective treatment of cancer, *J. Control. Release* 129 (2008) 107–116.

108. J. Gilleron, W. Querbes, A. Zeigerer, A. Borodovsky, G. Marsico, U. Schubert, K. Manygoats, S. Seifert, C. Andree, M. Stoter, H. Epstein-Barash, L. Zhang, V. Koteliansky, K. Fitzgerald, E. Fava, M. Bickle, Y. Kalaidzidis, A. Akinc, M. Maier, M. Zerial, Image-based analysis of lipid nanoparticle-mediated siRNA delivery, intracellular trafficking and endosomal escape, *Nat. Biotechnol.* 31 (2013) 638–646.

109. E. Chang, M.Q. Zhu, R. Drezek, Novel siRNA-based molecular beacons for dual imaging and therapy, *Biotechnol. J.* 2 (2007) 422–425.

110. R.J. Christie, Y. Matsumoto, K. Miyata, T. Nomoto, S. Fukushima, K. Osada, J. Halnaut, F. Pittella, H.J. Kim, N. Nishiyama, K. Kataoka, Targeted polymeric micelles for siRNA treatment of experimental cancer by intravenous injection, *ACS Nano* 6 (2012) 5174–5189.

111. R.J. Christie, K. Miyata, Y. Matsumoto, T. Nomoto, D. Menasco, T.C. Lai, M. Pennisi, K. Osada, S. Fukushima, N. Nishiyama, Y. Yamasaki, K. Kataoka, Effect of polymer structure on micelles formed between siRNA and cationic block copolymer comprising thiols and amidines, *Biomacromolecules* 12 (2011) 3174–3185.

112. Y. Oe, R.J. Christie, M. Naito, S.A. Low, S. Fukushima, K. Toh, Y. Miura, Y. Matsumoto, N. Nishiyama, K. Miyata, K. Kataoka, Actively-targeted polyion complex micelles stabilized by cholesterol and disulfide cross-linking for systemic delivery of siRNA to solid tumors, *Biomaterials* 35 (2014) 7887–7895.

113. A.A. Chen, A.M. Derfus, S.R. Khetani, S.N. Bhatia, Quantum dots to monitor RNAi delivery and improve gene silencing, *Nucleic Acids Res.* 33 (2005) e190.

114. J. Wang, P. Zhang, C. Huang, G. Liu, K.C. Leung, Y.X. Wang, High performance photoluminescent carbon dots for In Vitro and *In vivo* bioimaging: effect of nitrogen doping ratios, *Langmuir* 31 (2015) 8063–8073.

115. S. Jiang, Y. Zhang, K.M. Lim, E.K.W. Sim, L. Ye, NIR-to-visible upconversion nanoparticles for fluorescent labeling and targeted delivery of siRNA, *Nanotechnology* 20 (2009) e155101.

116. J. Jung, A. Solanki, K.A. Memoli, K. Kamei, H. Kim, M.A. Drahl, L.J. Williams, H.R. Tseng, K. Lee, Selective inhibition of human brain tumor cells through multifunctional quantum-dot-based siRNA delivery, *Angew. Chem. Int. Ed.* 49 (2010) 103–107.

117. J. Wang, G. Liu, K.C. Leung, R. Loffroy, P.X. Lu, Y.X. Wang, Opportunities and challenges of fluorescent carbon dots in translational optical imaging, *Curr. Pharm. Des.* 21 (2015) 5401–5416.

118. L. Wang, X. Wang, A. Bhirde, J. Cao, Y. Zeng, X. Huang, Y. Sun, G. Liu, X. Chen, Carbon- dot-based two-photon visible nanocarriers for safe and highly efficient delivery of siRNA and DNA, *Adv. Healthc. Mater.* 3 (2014) 1203–1209.

119. D.K. Chatterjee, M.K Gnanasammandhan, Y. Zhang, Small upconverting fluorescent nanoparticles for biomedical applications, *Small* 6 (2010) 2781–2795.

120. L. Wang, J. Liu, Y. Dai, Q. Yang, Y. Zhang, P. Yang, Z. Cheng, H. Lian, C. Li, Z. Hou, P. Ma, J. Lin, Efficient gene delivery and multimodal imaging by lanthanide-based upconversion nanoparticles, *Langmuir* 30 (2014) 13042–13051.

121. T.R. Nayak, L.K. Krasteva, W. Cai, Multimodality imaging of RNA Interference, *Curr. Med. Chem.* 20 (2013) 3664–3675.

122. A.P. McCaffrey, L. Meuse, T.T. Pham, D.S. Conklin, G.J. Hannon, M.A. Kay, RNA interference in adult mice, *Nature* 418 (2002) 38–39.

123. D.L. Lewis, J.E. Hagstrom, A.G. Loomis, J.A. Wolff, H. Herweijer, Efficient delivery of siRNA for inhibition of gene expression in postnatal mice, *Nat. Genet.* 32 (2002) 107–108.

124. A. Pichler, N. Zelcer, J.L. Prior, A.J. Kuil, D. Piwnica-Worms, *In vivo* RNA interference-mediated ablation of MDR1 P-glycoprotein, *Clin. Cancer Res.* 11 (2005) 4487–4494.

125. F. Pittella, H. Cabral, Y. Maeda, P. Mi, S. Watanabe, H. Takemoto, H.J. Kim, N. Nishiyama, K. Miyata, K. Kataoka, Systemic siRNA delivery to a spontaneous pancreatic tumor model in transgenic mice by PEGylated calcium phosphate hybrid micelles, *J. Control. Release* 178 (2014) 18–24.

126. D.W. Bartlett, M.E. Davis, Insights into the kinetics of siRNA-mediated gene silencing from live-cell and live-animal bioluminescent imaging, *Nucleic Acids Res.* 34 (2006) 322–333.

127. S.H. Kim, H. Mok, J.H. Jeong, S.W. Kim, T.G. Park, Comparative evaluation of target specific GFP gene silencing efficiencies for antisense ODN, synthetic siRNA, and siRNA plasmid complexed with PEI-PEG-FOL conjugate, *Bioconjug. Chem.* 17 (2006) 241–244.

128. R. Huschka, A. Barhoumi, Q. Liu, J.A. Roth, L. Ji, N.J. Halas, Gene silencing by gold nanoshell-mediated delivery and laser-triggered release of antisense oligonucleotide and siRNA, *ACS Nano* 6 (2012) 7681–7691.

129. M.L. James, S.S. Gambhir, A molecular imaging primer: modalities, imaging agents, and applications, *Physiol. Rev.* 92 (2012) 897–965.

130. M.E. Phelps, Positron emission tomography provides molecular imaging of biological processes, *Proc. Natl. Acad. Sci. U. S. A.* 97 (2000) 9226–9233.

131. S.I. Ziegler, Positron emission tomography: principles, technology, and recent developments, *Nucl. Phys. A.* 752 (2005) 679c–687c.

132. T. Lammers, S. Aime, W.E. Hennink, G. Storm, F. Kiessling, Theranostic nanomedicine, *Acc. Chem. Res.* 44 (2011) 1029–1038.

133. W. Lu, G. Zhang, R. Zhang, L.G. Flores 2nd, Q. Huang, J.G. Gelovani, C. Li, Tumor sitespecific silencing of NF-kappaB p65 by targeted hollow gold nanosphere-mediated photothermal transfection, *Cancer Res.* 70 (2010) 3177–3188.

134. K. Hatanaka, T. Asai, H. Koide, E. Kenjo, T. Tsuzuku, N. Harada, H. Tsukada, N. Oku, Development of double-stranded siRNA labeling method using positron emitter and its *in vivo* trafficking analyzed by positron emission tomography, *Bioconjug. Chem.* 21 (2010) 756–763.

135. F.M. Lu, Z. Yuan, PET/SPECT molecular imaging in clinical neuroscience: recent advances in the investigation of CNS diseases, *Quant. Imaging. Med. Surg.* 5 (2015) 433–447.

136. N. Liu, H. Ding, J.L. Vanderheyden, Z. Zhu, Y. Zhang, Radiolabeling small RNA with technetium-99 m for visualizing cellular delivery and mouse biodistribution, *Nucl. Med. Biol.* 34 (2007) 399–404.

137. O.M. Merkel, D. Librizzi, A. Pfestroff, T. Schurrat, M. Behe, T. Kissel, *In vivo* SPECT and real-time gamma camera imaging of biodistribution and pharmacokinetics of siRNA delivery using an optimized radiolabeling and purification procedure, *Bioconjug. Chem.* 20 (2009) 174–182.

138. W. Faulkner, Basic Principles of MRIOutSource 1996.

139. Y.X. Wang, Superparamagnetic iron oxide based MRI contrast agents: current status of clinical application, *Quant. Imaging. Med. Surg.* 1 (2011) 35–40.

140. H. Mok, O. Veiseh, C. Fang, F.M. Kievit, F.Y. Wang, J.O. Park, M. Zhang, pH-sensitive siRNA nanovector for targeted gene silencing and cytotoxic effect in cancer cells, *Mol. Pharm.* 7 (2010) 1930–1939.

141. M. Shen, F. Gong, P. Pang, K. Zhu, X. Meng, C. Wu, J. Wang, H. Shan, X. Shuai, An MRI-visible non-viral vector for targeted Bcl-2 siRNA delivery to neuroblastoma, *Int. J. Nanomedicine* 7 (2012) 3319–3332.

142. C. Li, M.F. Penet, F. Wildes, T. Takagi, Z.H. Chen, P.T. Winnard, D. Artemov, Z.M. Bhujwalla, Nanoplex delivery of siRNA and prodrug enzyme for multimodality image-guided molecular pathway targeted cancer therapy, *ACS Nano* 4 (2010) 6707–6716.

143. K.H. Bae, K. Lee, C. Kim, T.G. Park, Surface functionalized hollow manganese oxide nanoparticles for cancer targeted siRNA delivery and magnetic resonance imaging, *Biomaterials* 32 (2011) 176–184.

144. Z. Zhou, D. Huang, J. Bao, Q. Chen, G. Liu, Z. Chen, X. Chen, J. Gao, A synergistically enhanced T(1)–T(2) dual-modal contrast agent, *Adv. Mater.* 24 (2012) 6223–6228.

145. X. Wang, Z. Zhou, Z. Wang, Y. Xue, Y. Zeng, J. Gao, L. Zhu, X. Zhang, G. Liu, X. Chen, Gadolinium embedded iron oxide nanoclusters as T1–T2 dual-modal MRI-visible vectors for safe and efficient siRNA delivery, *Nanoscale* 5 (2013) 8098–8104.

146. H.D. Liang, M.J.K. Blomley, The role of ultrasound in molecular imaging, *Br. J. Radiol.* 76 (2003) S140–S150.

147. M.S. Shim, Y.J. Kwon, Stimuli-responsive polymers and nanomaterials for gene delivery and imaging applications, *Adv. Drug Deliv. Rev.* 64 (2012) 1046–1059.

148. E. Unger, T. Porter, J. Lindner, P. Grayburn, Cardiovascular drug delivery with ultrasound and microbubbles, *Adv. Drug Deliv. Rev.* 72 (2014) 110–126.

149. K.H. Martin, P.A. Dayton, Current status and prospects for microbubbles in ultrasound theranostics, *Wiley Interdiscip. Rev. Nanomed. Nanobiotechnol.* 5 (2013) 329–345.

150. S. Florinas, J. Kim, K. Nam, M.M. Janat-Amsbury, S.W. Kim, Ultrasound-assisted siRNA delivery via arginine-grafted bioreducible polymer and microbubbles targeting VEGF for ovarian cancer treatment, *J. Control. Release* 183 (2014) 1–8.

151. R.E. Vandenbroucke, I. Lentacker, J. Demeester, S.C. De Smedt, N.N. Sanders, Ultrasound assisted siRNA delivery using PEG-siPlex loaded microbubbles, *J. Control. Release* 126 (2008) 265–273.

152. Y. Liu, H. Miyoshi, M. Nakamura, Encapsulated ultrasound microbubbles: therapeutic application in drug/gene delivery, *J. Control. Release* 114 (2006) 89–99.

153. C.C. Chen, P.S. Sheeran, S.Y. Wu, O.O. Olumolade, P.A. Dayton, E.E. Konofagou, Targeted drug delivery with focused ultrasound-induced blood–brain barrier opening using acoustically-activated nanodroplets, *J. Control. Release* 172 (2013) 795–804.

154. X. Cheng, H. Li, Y. Chen, B. Luo, X. Liu, W. Liu, H. Xu, X. Yang, Ultrasound-triggered phase transition sensitive magnetic fluorescent nanodroplets as a multimodal imaging contrast agent in rat and mouse model, *PLoS One* 8 (2013), e85003.

155. P.A. Dayton, S. Zhao, S.H. Bloch, P. Schumann, K. Penrose, T.O. Matsunaga, R. Zutshi, A. Doinikov, K.W. Ferrara, Application of ultrasound to selectively localize nanodroplets for targeted imaging and therapy, *Mol. Imaging* 5 (2006) 160–174.

156. J. Jian, C. Liu, Y. Gong, L. Su, B. Zhang, Z. Wang, D. Wang, Y. Zhou, F. Xu, P. Li, Y. Zheng, L. Song, X. Zhou, India ink incorporated multifunctional phase-transition nanodroplets for photoacoustic/ultrasound dual-modality imaging and photoacoustic effect based tumor therapy, *Theranostics* 4 (2014) 1026–1038.

157. S. Horie, Y. Watanabe, M. Ono, S. Mori, T. Kodama, Evaluation of antitumor effects following tumor necrosis factor-alpha gene delivery using nanobubbles and ultrasound, *Cancer Sci.* 102 (2011) 2082–2089.

158. C.H. Wang, Y.F. Huang, C.K. Yeh, Aptamer-conjugated nanobubbles for targeted ultrasound molecular imaging, *Langmuir* 27 (2011) 6971–6976.

159. T. Yin, P. Wang, J. Li, Y. Wang, B. Zheng, R. Zheng, D. Cheng, X. Shuai, Tumor penetrating codelivery of siRNA and paclitaxel with ultrasound-responsive nanobubbles hetero-assembled from polymeric micelles and liposomes, *Biomaterials* 35 (2014) 5932–5943.

160. Z. Chen, K. Liang, J. Liu, M. Xie, X. Wang, Q. Lu, J. Zhang, L. Fang, Enhancement of survivin gene downregulation and cell apoptosis by a novel combination: liposome microbubbles and ultrasound exposure, *Med. Oncol.* 26 (2009) 491–500.

161. J. Castle, M. Butts, A. Healey, K. Kent, M. Marino, S.B. Feinstein, Ultrasound mediated targeted drug delivery: recent success and remaining challenges, *Am. J. Physiol. Heart Circ. Physiol.* 304 (2013) H350–H357.

162. O.F. Kaneko, J.K. Willmann, Ultrasound for molecular imaging and therapy in cancer, *Quant. Imaging. Med. Surg.* 2 (2012) 87–97.

163. S. Son, H.S. Min, D.G. You, B.S. Kim, I.C. Kwon, Echogenic nanoparticles for ultrasound technologies: evolution from diagnostic imaging modality to multimodal theranostic agent, *Nano Today* 9 (2014) 525–540.

164. V. Sboros, Response of contrast agents to ultrasound, *Adv. Drug Deliv. Rev.* 60 (2008) 1117–1136.

165. A.R. Carson, C.F. McTiernan, L. Lavery, M. Grata, X. Leng, J. Wang, X. Chen, F.S. Villanueva, Ultrasound-targeted microbubble destruction to deliver siRNA cancer therapy, *Cancer Res.* 72 (2012) 6191–6199.

166. Q.-L. Zhou, Z.-Y. Chen, Y.-X. Wang, F. Yang, Y. Lin, Y.-Y. Liao, Ultrasound-mediated local drug and gene delivery using nanocarriers, *Biomed. Res. Int.* (2014) e963891.

167. T. Yin, P. Wang, J. Li, R. Zheng, B. Zheng, D. Cheng, R. Li, J. Lai, X. Shuai, Ultrasound sensitive siRNA-loaded nanobubbles formed by hetero-assembly of polymeric micelles and liposomes and their therapeutic effect in gliomas, *Biomaterials* 34 (2013) 4532–4543.

168. D.E. Lee, H. Koo, I.C. Sun, J.H. Ryu, K. Kim, I.C. Kwon, Multifunctional nanoparticles for multimodal imaging and theragnosis, *Chem. Soc. Rev.* 41 (2012) 2656–2672.

169. H.S. Choi, J.V. Frangioni, Nanoparticles for biomedical imaging: fundamentals of clinical translation, *Mol. Imaging* 9 (2010) 291–310.

170. A.Y. Louie, Multimodality imaging probes: design and challenges, *Chem. Rev.* 110 (2010) 3146–3195.

171. O.C. Boerman, W.J.G. Oyen, Multimodality probes: amphibian cars for molecular imaging, *J. Nucl. Med.* 49 (2008) 1213–1214.

172. J.M. Idee, S. Louguet, S. Ballet, C. Corot, Theranostics and contrast-agents for medical imaging: a pharmaceutical company viewpoint, *Quant. Imaging. Med. Surg.* 3 (2013) 292–297.

173. Y.X. Wang, Physical scientists research biomedicine: a call for caution, *Chin. J. Cancer Res.* 27 (2015) 94–95.

174. Z. Medarova, W. Pham, C. Farrar, V. Petkova, A. Moore, *In vivo* imaging of siRNA delivery and silencing in tumors, *Nat. Med.* 13 (2007) 372–377.

175. M. Mikhaylova, I. Stasinopoulos, Y. Kato, D. Artemov, Z.M. Bhujwalla, Imaging of cationic multifunctional liposome-mediated delivery of COX-2 siRNA, *Cancer Gene Ther.* 16 (2009) 217–226.

176. D.W. Bartlett, H. Su, I.J. Hildebrandt, W.A. Weber, M.E. Davis, Impact of tumor specific targeting on the biodistribution and efficacy of siRNA nanoparticles measured by multimodality *in vivo* imaging, *Proc. Natl. Acad. Sci. U. S. A.* 104 (2007) 15549–15554.

177. X. Ma, Y. Zhao, X.-J. Liang, Theranostic nanoparticles engineered for clinic and pharmaceutics, *Acc. Chem. Res.* 44 (2011) 1114–1122.

178. J.H. Ryu, H. Koo, I.-C. Sun, S.H. Yuk, K. Choi, K. Kim, I.C. Kwon, Tumor targeting multifunctional nanoparticles for theragnosis: new paradigm for cancer therapy, *Adv. Drug Deliv. Rev.* 64 (2012) 1447–1458.

179. N. Lee, S.H. Choi, T. Hyeon, Nano-sized CT contrast agents, *Adv. Mater.* 25 (2013) 2641–2660.

180. F. Hallouard, N. Anton, P. Choquet, A. Constantinesco, T. Vandamme, Iodinated blood pool contrast media for preclinical X-ray imaging applications–a review, *Biomaterials* 31 (2010) 6249–6268.

181. Y. Liu, K. Ai, L. Lu, Nanoparticulate X-ray computed tomography contrast agents: from design validation to *in vivo* applications, *Acc. Chem. Res.* 45 (2012) 1817–1827.

182. H. Lusic, M.W. Grinstaff, X-ray-computed tomography contrast agents, *Chem. Rev.* 113 (2012) 1641–1666.

183. E. Jin, Z.-R. Lu, Biodegradable iodinated polydisulfides as contrast agents for CT angiography, *Biomaterials* 35 (2014) 5822–5829.

184. K.Y. Choi, G. Liu, S. Lee, X. Chen, Theranostic nanoplatforms for simultaneous cancer imaging and therapy: current approaches and future perspectives, *Nanoscale* 4 (2012) 330–342.

185. N. Anton, T.F. Vandamme, Nanotechnology for computed tomography: a real potential recently disclosed, *Pharm. Res.* 31 (2014) 20–34.

186. D.P. Cormode, P.C. Naha, Z.A. Fayad, Nanoparticle contrast agents for computed tomography: a focus on micelles, *Contrast Media Mol. Imaging* 9 (2014) 37–52.

187. X. Li, N. Anton, G. Zuber, T. Vandamme, Contrast agents for preclinical targeted X-ray imaging, *Adv. Drug Deliv. Rev.* 76 (2014) 116–133.

188. J.-Y. Lee, S.-J. Chung, H.-J. Cho, D.-D. Kim, Iodinated hyaluronic acid oligomer-based nanoassemblies for tumor-targeted drug delivery and cancer imaging, *Biomaterials* 85 (2016) 218–231.

189. H. Deng, Y. Zhong, M. Du, Q. Liu, Z. Fan, F. Dai, X. Zhang, Theranostic self-assembly structure of gold nanoparticles for NIR photothermal therapy and X-ray computed tomography imaging, *Theranostics* 4 (2014) 904–918.

190. J. Zhu, L. Zheng, S. Wen, Y. Tang, M. Shen, G. Zhang, X. Shi, Targeted cancer theranostics using alpha-tocopheryl succinate-conjugated multifunctional dendrimer-entrapped gold nanoparticles, *Biomaterials* 35 (2014) 7635–7646.

191. Y. Jiang, J. Chen, C. Deng, E.J. Suuronen, Z. Zhong, Click hydrogels, microgels and nanogels: emerging platforms for drug delivery and tissue engineering, *Biomaterials* 35 (2014) 4969–4985.

192. A.V. Kabanov, S.V. Vinogradov, Nanogels as pharmaceutical carriers: finite networks of infinite capabilities, *Angew. Chem. Int. Ed.* 48 (2009) 5418–5429.

193. X. Zhang, S. Malhotra, M. Molina, R. Haag, Micro-and nanogels with labile crosslinks from synthesis to biomedical applications, *Chem. Soc. Rev.* 44 (2015) 1948–1973.

194. W. Chen, K. Achazi, B. Schade, R. Haag, Charge-conversional and reduction-sensitive poly (vinyl alcohol) nanogels for enhanced cell uptake and efficient intracellular doxorubicin release, *J. Control. Release* 205 (2015) 15–24.

195. N. Morimoto, S. Hirano, H. Takahashi, S. Loethen, D.H. Thompson, K. Akiyoshi, Selfassembled pH-sensitive cholesteryl pullulan nanogel as a protein delivery vehicle, *Biomacromolecules* 14 (2013) 56–63.

196. L. Jiang, Q. Zhou, K. Mu, H. Xie, Y. Zhu, W. Zhu, Y. Zhao, H. Xu, X. Yang, pH/temperature sensitive magnetic nanogels conjugated with Cy5.5-labled lactoferrin for MR and fluorescence imaging of glioma in rats, *Biomaterials* 34 (2013) 7418–7428.

197. D. Steinhilber, M. Witting, X. Zhang, M. Staegemann, F. Paulus, W. Friess, S. Küchler, R. Haag, Surfactant free preparation of biodegradable dendritic polyglycerol nanogels by inverse nanoprecipitation for encapsulation and release of pharmaceutical biomacromolecules, *J. Control. Release* 169 (2013) 289–295.

198. H. Yang, Q. Wang, W. Chen, Y. Zhao, T. Yong, L. Gan, H. Xu, X. Yang, Hydrophilicity/ hydrophobicity reversable and redox-sensitive nanogels for anticancer drug delivery, *Mol. Pharm.* 12 (2015) 1636–1647.

199. X. Zhang, K. Achazi, D. Steinhilber, F. Kratz, J. Dernedde, R. Haag, A facile approach for dual-responsive prodrug nanogels based on dendritic polyglycerols with minimal leaching, *J. Control. Release* 174 (2014) 209–216.

200. C. Yang, X. Wang, X. Yao, Y. Zhang, W. Wu, X. Jiang, Hyaluronic acid nanogels with enzyme-sensitive cross-linking group for drug delivery, *J. Control. Release* 205 (2015) 206–217.

201. W. Chen, M. Zheng, F. Meng, R. Cheng, C. Deng, J. Feijen, Z. Zhong, In situ forming reduction-sensitive degradable nanogels for facile loading and triggered intracellular release of proteins, *Biomacromolecules* 14 (2013) 1214–1222.

202. X. Wei, T.H. Senanayake, G. Warren, S.V. Vinogradov, Hyaluronic acid-based nanogel-drug conjugates with enhanced anticancer activity designed for the targeting of CD44-positive and drug-resistant tumors, *Bioconjug. Chem.* 24 (2013) 658–668.

203. T.F. Stefanello, A. Szarpak-Jankowska, F. Appaix, B. Louage, L. Hamard, B.G. De Geest, B. van der Sanden, C.V. Nakamura, R. Auzély-Velty, Thermoresponsive hyaluronic acid nanogels as hydrophobic drug carrier to macrophages, *Acta Biomater.* 10 (2014) 4750–4758.

204. K. Liang, S. Ng, F. Lee, J. Lim, J.E. Chung, S.S. Lee, M. Kurisawa, Targeted intracellular protein delivery based on hyaluronic acid-green tea catechin nanogels, *Acta Biomater.* 33 (2016) 142–152.

205. J.J. Water, Y. Kim, M.J. Maltesen, H. Franzyk, C. Foged, H.M. Nielsen, Hyaluronic acidbased nanogels produced by microfluidics-facilitated self-assembly improves the safety profile of the cationic host defense peptide novicidin, *Pharm. Res.* 32 (2015) 2727–2735.

206. K. Park, M.-Y. Lee, K.S. Kim, S.K. Hahn, Target specific tumor treatment by VEGF siRNA complexed with reducible polyethyleneimine-hyaluronic acid conjugate, *Biomaterials* 31 (2010) 5258–5265.

207. Y. Zhong, J. Zhang, R. Cheng, C. Deng, F. Meng, F. Xie, Z. Zhong, Reversibly crosslinked hyaluronic acid nanoparticles for active targeting and intelligent delivery of doxorubicin to drug resistant CD44+ human breast tumor xenografts, *J. Control. Release* 205 (2015) 144–154.

208. E.J. Oh, K. Park, K.S. Kim, J. Kim, J.-A. Yang, J.-H. Kong, M.Y. Lee, A.S. Hoffman, S.K. Hahn, Target specific and long-acting delivery of protein, peptide, and nucleotide therapeutics using hyaluronic acid derivatives, *J. Control. Release* 141 (2010) 2–12.

209. J.K. Park, J.H. Shim, K.S. Kang, J. Yeom, H.S. Jung, J.Y. Kim, K.H. Lee, T.H. Kim, S.Y. Kim, D.W. Cho, Solid free-form fabrication of tissue-engineering scaffolds with a poly (lactic-co-glycolic acid) grafted hyaluronic acid conjugate encapsulating an intact bone morphogenetic protein-2/poly (ethylene glycol) complex, *Adv. Funct. Mater.* 21 (2011) 2906–2912.

210. Y. Fan, C. Deng, R. Cheng, F. Meng, Z. Zhong, In situ forming hydrogels via catalyst free and bioorthogonal "tetrazole-alkene" photo-click chemistry, *Biomacromolecules* 14 (2013) 2814–2821.

211. W. Song, Y. Wang, J. Qu, Q. Lin, Selective functionalization of a genetically encoded alkene-containing protein via "photoclick chemistry" in bacterial cells, *J. Am. Chem. Soc.* 130 (2008) 9654–9655.

212. S. Ganesh, A.K. Iyer, F. Gattacceca, D.V. Morrissey, M.M. Amiji, *In vivo* biodistribution of siRNA and cisplatin administered using CD44-targeted hyaluronic acid nanoparticles, *J. Control. Release* 172 (2013) 699–706.

213. J. Li, M. Huo, J. Wang, J. Zhou, J.M. Mohammad, Y. Zhang, Q. Zhu, A.Y. Waddad, Q. Zhang, Redox-sensitive micelles self-assembled from amphiphilic hyaluronic acid deoxycholic acid conjugates for targeted intracellular delivery of paclitaxel, *Biomaterials* 33 (2012) 2310–2320.

214. H.-j. Yao, Y.-g. Zhang, L. Sun, Y. Liu, The effect of hyaluronic acid functionalized carbon nanotubes loaded with salinomycin on gastric cancer stem cells, *Biomaterials* 35 (2014) 9208–9223.

215. P. Kesharwani, S. Banerjee, S. Padhye, F.H. Sarkar, A.K. Iyer, Hyaluronic acid engineered nanomicelles loaded with 3,4-difluorobenzylidene curcumin for targeted killing of CD44+ stem-like pancreatic cancer cells, *Biomacromolecules* 16 (2015) 3042–3053.

216. X. Wang, J. Zhang, R. Cheng, F. Meng, C. Deng, Z. Zhong, Facile synthesis of reductively degradable biopolymers using cystamine diisocyanate as a coupling agent, *Biomacromolecules* 17 (2016) 882–890.

217. Z. Yu, L.Y. Ho, Q. Lin, Rapid, photoactivatable turn-on fluorescent probes based on an intramolecular photoclick reaction, *J. Am. Chem. Soc.* 133 (2011) 11912–11915.

218. J. Peng, T. Qi, J. Liao, M. Fan, F. Luo, H. Li, Z. Qian, Synthesis and characterization of novel dual-responsive nanogels and their application as drug delivery systems, *Nanoscale* 4 (2012) 2694–2704.

219. Y. Shi, M.J. van Steenbergen, E.A. Teunissen, L.S. Novo, S. Gradmann, M. Baldus, C.F. van Nostrum, W.E. Hennink, π–π stacking increases the stability and loading capacity of thermosensitive polymeric micelles for chemotherapeutic drugs, *Biomacromolecules* 14 (2013) 1826–1837.

220. Y. Zhu, X. Wang, J. Chen, J. Zhang, F. Meng, C. Deng, R. Cheng, J. Feijen, Z. Zhong. Bioresponsive and fluorescent hyaluronic acid-iodixanol nanogels for targeted X-ray computed tomography imaging and chemotherapy of breast tumors. *J. Control. Release* 244 (2016) 229–239.

221. H. Kobayashi, P.L. Choyke, Target-cancer-cell-specific activatable fluorescence imaging probes: rational design and *in vivo* applications, *Acc. Chem. Res.* 44 (2010) 83–90.

222. V.P. Chauhan, R.K. Jain, Strategies for advancing cancer nanomedicine, *Nat. Mater.* 12 (2013) 958–962.

223. R.K. Jain, T. Stylianopoulos, Delivering nanomedicine to solid tumors, *Nat. Rev. Clin. Oncol.* 7 (2010) 653–664.

224. L. Liang, S.-W. Lin, W. Dai, J.-K. Lu, T.-Y. Yang, Y. Xiang, Y. Zhang, R.-T. Li, Q. Zhang, Novel cathepsin B-sensitive paclitaxel conjugate: higher water solubility, better efficacy and lower toxicity, *J. Control. Release* 160 (2012) 618–629.

225. Y. Zou, Y. Song, W. Yang, F. Meng, H. Liu, Z. Zhong, Galactose-installed photocrosslinked pH-sensitive degradable micelles for active targeting chemotherapy of hepatocellular carcinoma in mice, *J. Control. Release* 193 (2014) 154–161.

226. Loutfy H. Madkour, *Reactive Oxygen Species (ROS), Nanoparticles, and Endoplasmic Reticulum (ER) Stress-Induced Cell Death Mechanisms.* Paperback ISBN: 9780128224816. Imprint: Academic Press Published Date: 1st August 2020. https://www.elsevier.com/books/reactive-oxygen-species-ros-nanoparticles-and-endoplasmic-reticulum-er-stress-induced-cell-death-mechanisms/madkour/978-0-12-822481-6.

227. Loutfy H. Madkour, *Nanoparticles Induce Oxidative and Endoplasmic Reticulum Antioxidant Therapeutic Defenses.* Copyright 2020 Publisher Springer International Publishing. Copyright Holder Springer Nature Switzerland AG eBook ISBN 978-3-030-37297-2 DOI 10.1007/978-3-030-37297-2 Hardcover ISBN 978-3-030-37296-5 Series ISSN 2194-0452 Edition Number 1. https://www.springer.com/gp/book/9783030372965?utm_campaign=3_pier05_buy_print&utm_content=en_08082017&utm_medium=referral&utm_source=google_books#otherversion=9783030372972.

228. Loutfy H. Madkour, *Nucleic Acids as Gene Anticancer Drug Delivery Therapy.* 1st Edition. Publishing house: Elsevier, (2020). Paperback ISBN: 9780128197776 Imprint: Academic Press Published Date: 2nd January 2020 Imprint: Academic Press Copyright: Paperback ISBN: 9780128197776 © Academic Press 2020 Published: 2nd January 2020 Imprint: Academic Press Paperback ISBN: 9780128197776. https://www.elsevier.com/books/nucleic-acids-as-gene-anticancer-drug-deliverytherapy/madkour/978-0-12–819777-6.

229. Loutfy H. Madkour, *Nanoelectronic Materials: Fundamentals and Applications (Advanced Structured Materials)* 1st ed. 2019 Edition: https://link.springer.com/book/10.1007%2F978-3-030-21621-4 Series Title Advanced Structured Materials Series Volume 116 Copyright 2019 Publisher Springer International Publishing Copyright Holder Springer Nature Switzerland AG. eBook ISBN 978-3-030-21621-4 DOI 10.1007/978-3-030-21621-4 Hardcover ISBN 978-3-030-21620-7 Series ISSN 1869-8433 Edition Number 1 Number of Pages XLIII, 783 Number of Illustrations 122 b/w illustrations, 494 illustrations in colour Topics. ISBN-10: 3030216209 ISBN-13: 978-3030216207 #117 in Nanotechnology (Books) #725 in Materials Science (Books) #187336 in Textbooks. https://books.google.com.eg/books/about/Nanoelectronic_Materials.html?id=YQXCxAEACAAJ&source=kp_book_description&redir_esc=y; https://www.springer.com/gp/book/9783030216207.

230. Y.X.J. Wang, Y. Choi, Z.Y. Chen, S. Laurent, S.L. Gibbs, Molecular imaging: from bench to clinic, *Biomed. Res. Int.* 2014 (2014) 357258.

231. J. Wang, P. Mi, G. Lin, Y. Xiáng, J. Wáng, G. Liu, X. Chen, Imaging-guided delivery of RNAi for anticancer treatment, *Adv. Drug Deliv. Rev.* 104 (2016) 44–60.

8 Recent Development of Silica Nanoparticles as Delivery Biomedical Applications for Cancer Imaging and Therapy

8.1 NANOTECHNOLOGY IN CANCER DIAGNOSIS AND THERAPY

In the last two decades, applications of nanotechnology in cancer diagnosis and therapy have attracted significant attention [1–4]. A number of functional nanomaterials have been developed and evaluated for drug delivery [5,6], diagnostic sensors [7], imaging agents [8], and labeling probes [9]. Nanomaterials can be organic or inorganic [10,11], with a size from 1 nm to a few hundred nanometers [12,13], and surface charges from negative to positive or natural [14]. Gold nanoparticles [15], quantum dots [16], carbon nanotubes [17], magnetic nanoparticles [18], liposomes [19], and silica-based nanoparticles (SiNPs) [20] have been developed for imaging as well as drug and gene delivery. Furthermore, multifunctional nanomaterials with two or more different functions have been designed for cancer imaging and therapy both *in vitro* and *in vivo* [21–23].

Among these nanomaterials, SiNPs have gained special attention for tumor imaging and therapy due to their easy synthesis, uniform morphology, adjustable pore volume, controllable diameter, modifiable surface potential, easy functionalization, and significant biocompatibility [24–27]. There are two main types of SiNPs developed for tumor imaging and therapy: mesoporous silica nanoparticles (MSNs) [27] and core/shell silica nanoparticles (C/S-SiNPs) [26]. MSNs were successfully used for drug delivery and gene delivery because of their unique mesopores and nanochannels, which can render a high payload of the drug [28] and easy stimuli-controllable release [29]. C/S-SiNPs are useful for imaging agent delivery because imaging agents, such as fluorophores, quantum dots (QDs), and gold nanoparticles, can be easily doped into the nanoparticles. The shell structures can protect imaging agents inside the nanoparticles, and the signal from imaging agents gives the precise location of nanoparticles and tumor tissue [30]. SiNPs can accumulate in tumor tissues through passive targeting and active targeting [31,32]. More importantly, both MSNs and C/S-SiNPs

have shown a significant biocompatibility both *in vitro* and *in vivo* [33,34], a great property for tumor diagnosis and therapy in humans.

In this chapter, we will briefly discuss the synthetic methods and important characteristics of relatively well-studied SiNPs. Due to the importance of early cancer diagnosis, the applications of SiNPs in *in vitro* and *in vivo* imaging will be discussed as well. By varying imaging agents in SiNPs, the end products can be used in different imaging models, such as magnetic resonance imaging (MRI), fluorescence imaging, positron emission tomography (PET), and X-ray computed tomography (X-ray CT) imaging. Then, the applications of SiNPs in drug and gene delivery for tumor therapy will be summarized. Photosensitizers, photothermal agents, and chemotherapeutic agents can be successfully delivered to tumor cells and tissues by SiNPs. The loading and releasing mechanisms of drugs in MSNs and the applications of multifunctional nanomaterials bearing imaging and therapeutic features will be discussed. The different types of SiNPs for tumor imaging and therapy *in vitro* and *in vivo* coupled with their characteristics are summarized in Table 8.1.

8.2 CHARACTERISTICS OF SILICA NANOPARTICLES

8.2.1 PARTICLE SIZE

As a delivery vector, the particle size and pore dimension of SiNPs are crucial parameters and affected drug loading efficiency, pathway of cell uptake, biodistribution *in vivo*, and targeting efficiency in cancer diagnosis and therapy [52,53]. Through a reverse microemulsion method, monodispersed C/S-SiNPs can be easily constructed with a controllable size. For instance, Tan et al. investigated how the amount of ammonium hydroxide, surfactant, tetraethyl orthosilicate (TEOS), H_2O, and reaction time affects the size of SiNPs [54]. They found that the size of the dye-doped SiNPs was reverse proportional to the concentration of ammonium hydroxide and water to surfactant molar ratio, but direct

DOI: 10.1201/9781003229674-8

TABLE 8.1

The SiNPs for Tumor Imaging and Therapy *In Vitro* and *In Vivo*

Type	Diameter (nm)	Surface modification	Targets	Targeting pathway	Imaging mode	Therapeutic mode	Ref.
Core/shell SiNPs	20	Monoclonal antibodies	Cells	Active	Fluorescence (rhodamine B)		[35]
	30	Folic acid	Cells	Active	Fluorescence (DBF[a])		[36]
		Aptamer	Cells	Active	Fluorescence (FITC[b], RuBpy[c], TMR[d], and Cy5)		[37]
	31	RGD[e]	Cells	Active	Fluorescenc[c] (QDs[f]) and MRI (Gd)		[38]
	25	–NH$_2$	Cells	Cell uptake	Fluorescence (rhodamine 6G)	Antisense oligonucleotides	[39]
	105±6.8	–PO$_4^{3-}$	Xenografts		Fluorescence (MB[g])	PDT[h] (MB)	[40]
	25–42	–NH$_2$ and PEG[i]	Xenografts	Passive	Fluorescence (IR820)	PDT (PpIX[j])	[41]
	120		Xenografts	Cell uptake	Fluorescence (QDs)		[42]
		Folic acid	Cells and xenografts	Active	Dark-field scattering and CT/X-ray imaging (AuNR)	PTT[k] (AuNR[l])	[43]
MSNs	150		Cells	Cell uptake		Chemo (DOX[m]) and PTT (Pd@Ag)	[3]
	50	TAT peptide	Cells	Active	Fluorescence (DOX)	Chemo (DOX)	[44]
	110–130	Polyethylenimine	Cells	Cell uptake	Fluorescence (FITC)	siRNA and DNA	[13]
	~220		Cells	Cell uptake	Fluorescence (FITC)	Chemo (DOX)	[28]
	~110	RGD	Cells	Active	Fluorescence (FITC)	Chemo (CPT[n])	[45]
	245	Galactose	Cells	Active	Fluorescence (FITC)	Chemo (CPT) and PDT (porphyrin)	[46]
	200		Cells	Cell uptake	Fluorescence (DOX)	siRNA and Chemo (DOX)	[47]
	100–130	Folic acid	Xenografts	Active	Fluorescence (FITC)	Chemo (CPT)	[48]
	<100	PEG	Xenografts	Passive	MRI (Fe$_3$O$_4$)		[49]
	70±6	PEG	Xenografts	Passive	MRI (Fe$_3$O$_4$)	Chemo (DOX)	[50]
	100–130	Folic acid	Xenografts	Active		Chemo (CPT)	[32]
Silica nanorattle	125	PEG	Xenografts	Passive		Chemo (Dtxl[o])	[51]

a   4,4′-(1E, 1′E)-2,2′-(9,9-didecyl-9H-fluorene-2,7-diyl)bis(ethene-2,1-diyl)bis(N, N-dibutylaniline).

b   Fluorescein isothiocyanate.

c   Tris(bipyridine)ruthenium(II) chloride.

d   Tetramethylrhodamine.

e   Arg-Gly-Asp.

f   Quantum dots.

g   Methylene blue.

h   Photodynamic therapy.

i   Polyethylene glycol.

j   Protoporphyrin IX.

k   Photothermal therapy.

l   Gold nanorod.

m   Doxorubicin.

n   Camptothecin.

o   Docetaxel.

proportional to the amount of TEOS and reaction time [54]. In order to continuously control the size of the C/S-SiNPs in a more defined range, Zhao et al. developed a method by systematically varying the organic solvents used in a reverse microemulsion method [55]. Organic solvent may affect the surface area occupied by surfactant molecules, while the diameter of water droplet can increase with the length of the organic molecule. Eventually, through hydrolysis of TEOS on the surface of the droplet, the size of nanoparticles may change by varying the organic molecule.

C/S-SiNPs with a tunable size range from 10 to 100 nm were developed by simply varying the types of organic solvents.

Varying the amount of ammonium hydroxide was also useful for synthesizing MSNs with different sizes. Mou et al. synthesized MSNs with sizes from 30 to 280 nm using this strategy [52]. It was also found that the uptake of MSNs by cells was size-dependent and 50 nm was the preferable diameter for cell uptake. Pan et al. developed a tunable particle size of MSNs from 25 to 105 nm, and size effect on nuclear targeting was investigated [44]. They found that only MSNs of 50 nm or smaller can effectively target nucleus with the help of a TAT peptide. Using the Stöber method, large nanoparticles from 60 to 880 nm were synthesized by the Rosenzweig group by changing the amount of ammonium hydroxide [56]. The toxicity of SiNPs was also associated with their diameters. Hoet et al. developed a method to obtain amorphous spherical SiNPs of different sizes that ranged from 13.8 to 335.0 nm and investigated their cytotoxicity to human endothelial cells. It was found that the smaller the particles, the higher the toxicity to cells [57].

8.2.2 Surface Modification

The surface of SiNPs is usually negatively charged without further modification because of the presence of the hydroxyl group after hydrolysis of TEOS. However, it is convenient to modify the SiNPs' surface through the silane chemistry. Polyethylene glycol (PEG), amine, carboxyl, and phosphate groups could be easily conjugated to hydroxyl SiNPs by hydrolysis of the corresponding silanes. For example, He et al. synthesized three types of SiNPs with different surface charges, including OH-SiNPs, COOH-SiNPs, and PEG-SiNPs, and found that the biodistribution and excretion of the SiNPs were dependent on surface modifications. Neutrally charged SiNPs (PEG-SiNPs) exhibited relatively longer blood circulation and lower uptake by the reticuloendothelial system (RES) organs than the other two [33]. As a result, these PEG-modified SiNPs showed better passive targeting effects to the tumor site when they were used for the delivery of drugs and imaging agents [51,58].

Furthermore, as an effective delivery vector, active targeting is another strategy for better targeting efficiency. After surface modification with different functional groups, targeting molecules, including antibodies [59], peptides [45,60], folic acid [61], and aptamers [62], can be easily conjugated to the surface of SiNPs for active targeting tumor tissues [63]. For example, Lu et al. modified SiNPs with folic acids through EDC-NHS conjugation [32]. Tan et al. reported modification of COOH-SiNPs with aptamers through EDC-NHS conjugation reaction and used the aptamer-modified dye-doped SiNPs for the detection of cancer cells [31]. By using these strategies, the surface of SiNPs is easily modified with recognizing molecules to enhance the ability of the SiNPs to recognize cancer markers. Thus, the efficiency of SiNPs for cancer imaging and therapy is improved.

8.3 IMAGING APPLICATIONS OF SILICA NANOPARTICLES

With tunable particle sizes, easy surface modification, and good biocompatibility, SiNPs have been widely used for imaging of cancer cells or tissues both in vitro and in vivo. Imaging agents can be doped into or modified on the surface of SiNPs. In the next section, we will review the latest progress in SiNPs-mediated tumor imaging with fluorescence and MRI techniques.

8.3.1 Fluorescence Imaging

Fluorescence technology possesses high resolution compared to other imaging strategies, and the sensitivity of the fluorescence detection on cancer cells is promising [64,65]. Traditionally, fluorescent dyes suffer from the disadvantages of low brightness, photobleaching, and non-specific targeting [66]. However, fluorescent SiNPs may overcome these shortcomings and provide highly sensitive and selective tumor imaging. By doping thousands of fluorescent dye molecules into one SiNP, the brightness of SiNP was much higher than a single dye molecule [67]. For example, Herr et al. compared the fluorescence intensity between dye and dye-doped SiNPs [31]. Their results showed that an aptamer-modified dye-doped SiNP was brighter and more stable in fluorescence imaging than a dye-aptamer alone. Flow cytometry demonstrated that the signal from the SiNPs-aptamer was 100 times higher than that of the dye-aptamer. Therefore, these dye-doped SiNPs with high fluorescence intensity may be useful for creating highly sensitive biosensors [67]. Another important advantage of dye-doped SiNPs compared to free dye molecules is that silica matrix can protect the dye from photobleaching, allowing long-duration imaging of tumor cells and tissues [68]. As shown in Figure 8.1, with continual irradiation under a confocal microscope, the fluorescence of cells stained by pure FITC quenched almost completely within 20 min [69]. However, 60% of fluorescence in the FITC-doped SiNPs was retained for imaging after 20 min, and 30% of the fluorescence intensity was retained even after 1-h irradiation. This indicates that fluorescent SiNPs may have better photostability than free dyes and thus were more powerful as fluorescent markers for long-time imaging of living cells and tissues.

Moreover, the facileness to modify SiNPs makes the modification of targeting ligands convenient and effective. Targeting ligands, such as aptamers [70,71], antibodies [35,72], peptides [73], and folic acid [36,74], can be attached on SiNPs. Aptamer is a short fragment of DNA or RNA, which can selectively bind to certain targets, including ions, small biomolecules, peptides, and cells [75]. In 2011, Tan et al. developed an aptamer-conjugated nanoparticle for fluorescence imaging and extraction of tumor cells [37]. In this chapter, silica-coated magnetic and fluorophore-doped SiNPs modified with aptamers were used to recognize and

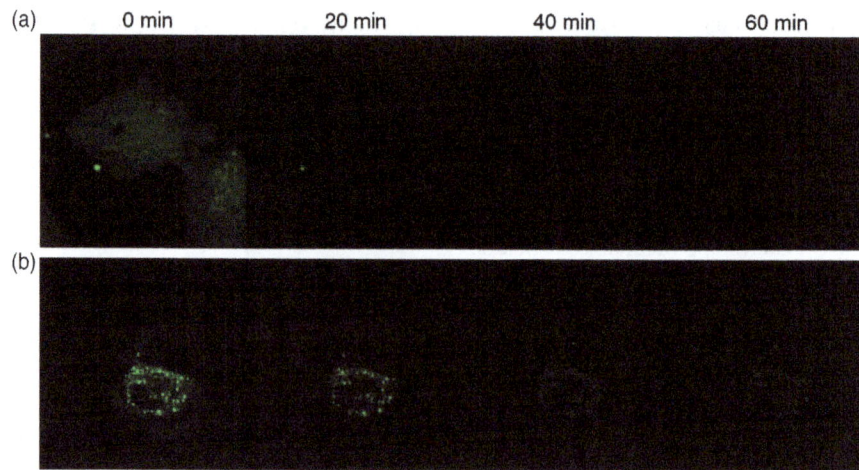

FIGURE 8.1 Confocal micrographs of continued irradiation of cells leading to photobleaching over a 1-h timescale. (A) FITC-loaded HUVEC cells. (B) 30 nm fluorescent silica-loaded cells. The cells are incubated with 100 μg/mL of nanomaterials for 3 h and are washed and subjected to continued irradiation for a period of 1 h. Images are taken every 20 min, and the photobleaching of pure FITC and FITC-loaded nanomaterials is studied. (Reprinted from Veeranarayanan et al. [69] with permission by the SpringerLink.)

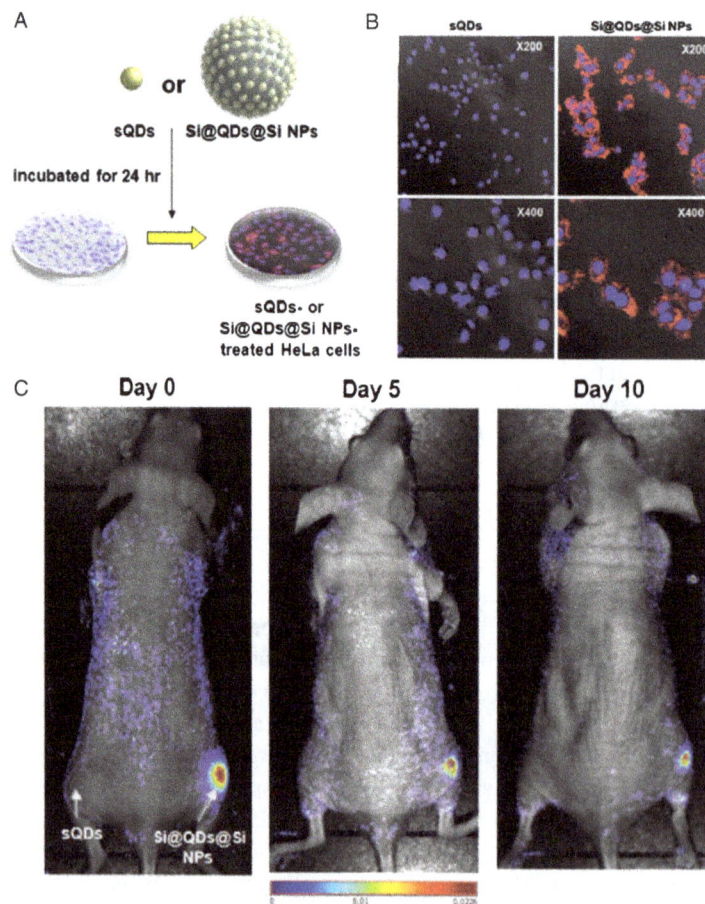

FIGURE 8.2 Cellular uptake *in vivo* test of single QDs and Si@QDs@Si NPs. (A) Illustration of sQD or Si@QDs@Si-NP labeling to HeLa cells. (B) Fluorescence images of sQD- and Si@QDs@Si-NP-uptaken cells (red color: QD, blue color: DAPI). (C) Maestro *in vivo* fluorescence image of sQD-labeled (left leg) and Si@QDs@Si-NP-labeled (right leg) cell-transplanted mouse. (Reprinted from Jun et al. [82] with permission by Wiley-VCH.)

isolate cancer cells from mixed cell populations using an external magnetic field.

The excellent optical characteristics of the dye-doped SiNPs ensure their usage as fluorescence agents for both tumor cells *in vitro* and *in vivo* imaging. Furthermore, the high biocompatibility and controllable size of SiNPs make *in vivo* tumor imaging possible [48,76]. The feasibility of SiNPs for *in vivo* imaging has been confirmed by many research groups. For instance, He et al. developed methylene blue-encapsulated phosphonate-terminated silica nanoparticles (MB-encapsulated PSiNPs) for *in vivo* imaging [30]. They found that the MB-encapsulated PSiNPs could be used as an effective NIR fluorescence imaging agent in mice using three different injection routes.

For *in vivo* imaging, there are two different pathways to target tumors with nanoparticles. The first one is passive targeting by enhanced permeability and retention (EPR) effect. In this case, certain sizes of particles would accumulate at the tumor sites rather than normal tissues because the newly formed blood vessels of tumor tissues were abnormal [40]. The small nanoparticles, such as gold nanoparticles [77], gold nanoclusters [78], quantum dots [79], and unconventional nanoparticles [80,81], have been used to prove this theory for tumor targeting *in vivo*. The second pathway is active targeting by modifying target ligands on the surface of nanoparticles. In 2010, Lu et al. investigated the biodistribution of fluorescent SiNPs in mice with xenograft tumors [48]. They found that both fluorescent mesoporous silica nanoparticles (FMSNs) and folic acid-modified fluorescent mesoporous silica nanoparticles (F-FMSNs) could preferentially accumulate in tumor tissues after injecting to mice through the tail vein injection. The tissue section of different organs also confirmed the results from the *in vivo* fluorescence imaging. In these two different types of nanoparticles, FMSNs targeted tumor through EPR effect, while the F-FMSNs targeted tumor through the folate receptor on the surface of tumor cells. Meanwhile, Qian et al. reported PEG-modified NIR SiNPs for mouse tumor imaging due to its deep penetration ability and low autofluorescence in NIR region [76]. The NIR SiNPs accumulated in the tumor tissues through EPR effects; also, these NIR SiNPs exhibited bright and stable NIR fluorescence that could be used for long-term *in vivo* imaging. It was noteworthy that SiNPs could be cleared from the mice through the hepatobiliary excretion, indicating their relatively low toxicity and perhaps high applicability in humans.

In order to enhance the performance of fluorescence imaging, other fluorescent nanomaterials have been coupled to SiNPs for cancer imaging. For instance, quantum dots, which possess brighter fluorescence, narrower photoluminescence spectra, and better photostability than traditional dyes, were embedded into SiNPs for tumor fluorescence imaging. In 2012, Jun et al. reported an ultrasensitive QDs-embedded SiNP for tumor fluorescence imaging (Figure 8.2A) [82]. Compared to a single QD, the QDs-embedded SiNPs showed brighter fluorescence intensity and increased uptake by HeLa cells (Figure 8.2B). For *in vivo* fluorescence

cell tracking, single QD-labeled- or QDs-embedded SiNPs labeled-HeLa cells were injected into mice for long-term fluorescence imaging, and the results showed that even after 10 days, the QDs-embedded SiNPs emitted strong fluorescence for *in vivo* imaging (Figure 8.2C). Therefore, the QDs-embedded SiNPs may have the potential for long-term fluorescence imaging *in vivo*.

8.3.2 MAGNETIC RESONANCE IMAGING (MRI)

Compared to fluorescence imaging, MRI has better penetration ability in tissues. As a result, MRI is routinely used as a primary diagnostic method for cancer in hospitals. However, most of the currently used MRI contrast agents are small molecules such as gadolinium chelates, which cannot provide a high contrast image for early diagnosis of cancer because of its low sensitivity and poor selectivity. By applying SiNPs, thousands of MRI agents like gadolinium chelates may be loaded into one nanoparticle. This high loading efficiency in SiNPs enhances the sensitivity of the MRI agent. Taylor et al. synthesized a highly efficient MSN-based MRI contrast agent for *in vitro* and *in vivo* MRI [41]. This MSN-based MRI contrast agent was an ideal platform for MRI benefitting from its large payload of Gd centers and enhanced water accessibility of the Gd chelates. This is the key parameter for the design of highly efficient MRI contrast agents. Lin et al. modified the Gd chelates onto SiNPs using layer-by-layer self-assembly coupled with doping a fluorescence contrast agent during the synthesis [42]. With the modification of a targeting peptide, the K7RGD-SiNPs had the ability to detect certain tumor cells using MRI and fluorescence imaging. Also, Gd chelates could be coated onto SiNPs through lipid coating [83]. Coupled with quantum dots doping in the same SiNPs, the imaging nanocomposite had the abilities of fluorescence imaging and MRI for tumor cells.

In addition, superparamagnetic iron oxide (SPIO) nanoparticles are another type of useful MRI contrast agents for tumor imaging *in vitro* and *in vivo*. In 2008, Kim et al. doped single magnetic iron oxide nanoparticle in MSNs (Fe_3O_4@$mSiO_2$), followed by doping the fluorescent dye in the silica shell to form multifunctional nanoparticles for tumor imaging and therapy (Figure 8.3A) [84]. PEG modification on SiNPs increased the biocompatibility and targeting efficiency to tumor sites through EPR effects. After intravenous injection of the Fe_3O_4@$mSiO_2$ into the mice implanted with MCF-7 cells, researchers took the T2-weighted MRI and observed that the T2 signal intensity in the tumor site decreased, indicating the accumulation of Fe_3O_4@$mSiO_2$ in the tumor site (Figure 8.3B). Meanwhile, the fluorescence of the Fe_3O_4@$mSiO_2$ in the tumor site was captured to verify the results from the T2-weighted MRI. Furthermore, the nanoparticles coupled with MRI agents and drugs were developed for simultaneous tumor imaging and therapy. For instance, Liong et al. enclosed multiple magnetites in the core of SiNPs and then doped fluorescent dye or drug in SiNPs to form a multifunctional delivery

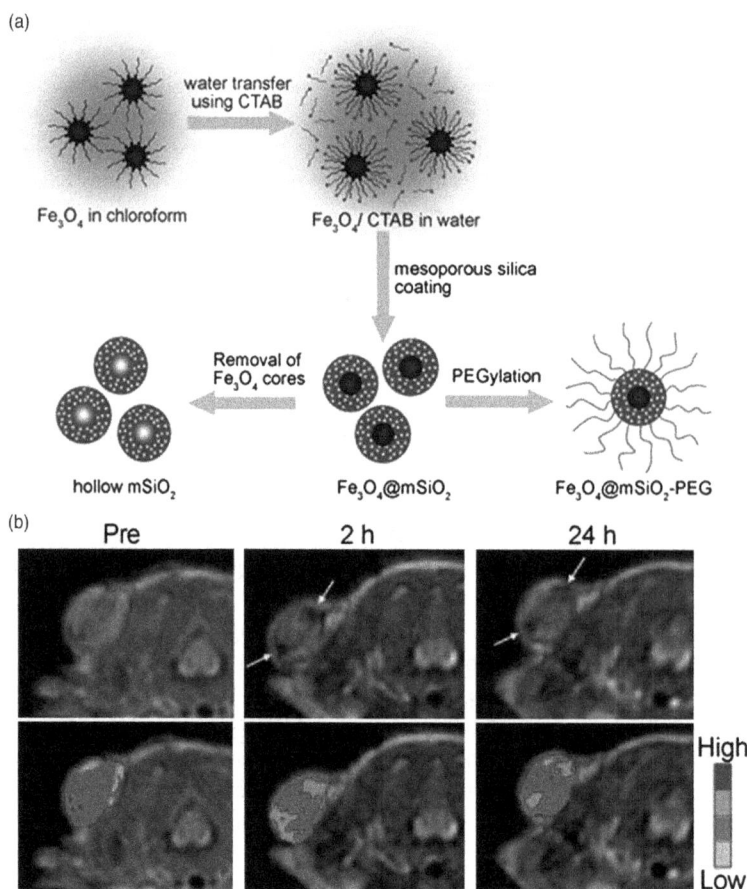

FIGURE 8.3 (A) Schematic illustration of the synthetic procedure for magnetite nanocrystal/mesoporous silica core/shell NPs. (B) Fluorescence images of subcutaneously injected MCF-7 cells labeled with Fe_3O_4@$mSiO_2(R)$ (10 μg Fem/L) and control MCF-7 cells without labeling into each dorsal shoulder of a nude mouse. (Reprinted from Kim et al. [84] with permission by Wiley-VCH.)

vehicle for tumor imaging and therapy. With the modification of folic acids on the surface of SiNPs, these multifunctional SiNPs showed the potential for active targeting tumor sites for diagnosis and therapy [38]. Lee et al. developed a novel silica nanovector for tumor MRI, fluorescence imaging, and drug delivery. The fluorescent dyes were doped into SiNPs, whereas multiple iron oxide nanoparticles were decorated on the surface of the SiNPs [49]. In addition to tumor imaging, iron oxide nanoparticles-embedded SiNPs were widely used for MRI of stem cells *in vitro* and *in vivo* by varying the targeting ligands [50,85].

8.4 DRUG AND GENE DELIVERY USING SILICA NANOPARTICLES

8.4.1 DRUG DELIVERY

SiNPs have been widely used for tumor therapy *in vitro* and *in vivo* because of their unique properties, such as large surface area and pore volume, easy functionalization, great biocompatibility, high stability, and controllable particle sizes. In the following section, we will discuss applications of SiNPs for drug delivery into tumor cells or tissues.

8.4.2 CHEMOTHERAPEUTIC AGENTS

Chemotherapy is a mainstream treatment of cancer. However, there are some limitations of existing chemotherapeutics, such as hydrophobicity, low targeting efficiency, side toxic effects, and unsatisfactory therapeutic efficacy. To overcome these limitations, biocompatible SiNPs have been employed as nanovehicles for tumor targeting imaging and therapy. Camptothecin (CPT) and its derivatives are one of the most promising anticancer drugs; however, their hydrophobic property limits their clinical applications. In order to transfer CPT efficiently into tumor tissues without modification of the molecule, Lu et al. reported a method for loading CPT in MSNs (MSNs/CPT) and delivering it to cancer cells to induce apoptosis [86]. Furthermore, they investigated anticancer effects of the MSNs/CPT *in vivo* [48]. Folic acid was modified onto MSNs for active targeting cancer cells (Figure 8.4A). As shown in Figure 8.4B, folic acid-modified MSNs/CPT resulted in a higher therapeutic efficiency to SK-BR-3 cells than that to MCF-7 cells because of the high-level expression of folate receptor on SK-BR-3 cells. In contrast, the MSNs/CPT without folic acid modification demonstrated similar cytotoxicity to these two human cancer cells. This indicated that the folic

(a)

Folic Acid

(b)

(c)

(d)

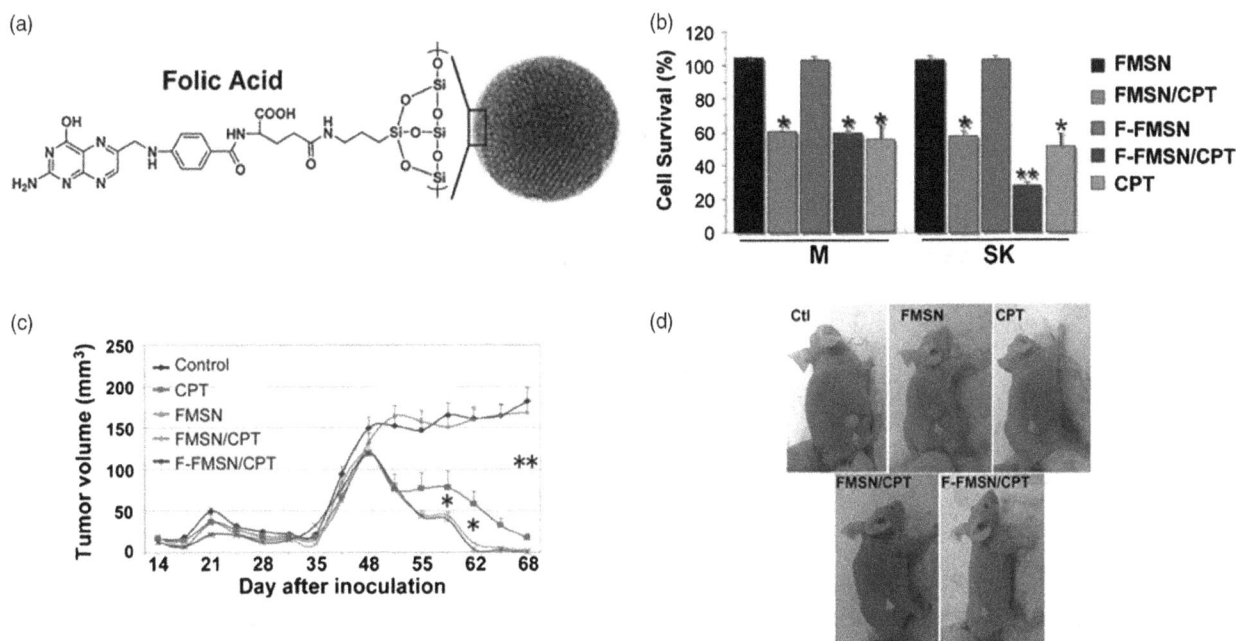

FIGURE 8.4 (A) Schematic illustration of FMSNs modified with folic acid-targeting ligands on the surface. (B) Cell proliferation assay with FMSNs and F-FMSNs in MCF10F (M) and SK-BR-3(SK) cells. The cells were treated for 48 h with 20 µg/mL of nanoparticles only (FMSN), CPT-loaded nanoparticles (FMSN/CPT), CPT-loaded F-FMSNs, or the same concentration of CPT dissolved in DMSO. The cells were then washed and stained with 10% WST-8 solution from the cell-counting kit (Dojindo Co.) for 2 h. The absorbances were measured at 450 nm with a plate reader. The percentages of each sample relative to control cells are presented as mean values ± SD. (C) The average tumor volumes are shown as means ± SD. $*=P<0.05$; $**=P<0.01$. (D) Representative images of mice from different groups. Red arrows indicate the location of subcutaneous tumors. (Reprinted from Lu et al. [48] with permission by Wiley-VCH.)

acid-mediated active targeting to folate receptor-positive tumor cells by MSNs showed efficacy in tumor treatment. Having achieved the exciting results from cancer cell treatment of MSNs/CPT, researchers investigated the *in vivo* tumor-suppressing effect of MSNs/CPT. As shown in Figure 8.4C and D, nude mice with xenografts of human breast cancer cell MCF-7 received different therapeutic agents. The MSNs/CPT and folic acid-modified MSNs/CPT showed faster tumor-shrinking effects in mice than those of the CPT alone group, and no obvious subcutaneous tumors were found in these two testing groups at the end points. In contrast, saline solution and MSNs did not inhibit the tumor growth in nude mice. In the work of Tsai et al., a non-cytotoxic anionic surfactant was coupled to the control releasing of a hydrophobic drug, resveratrol, loaded in the MSNs to kill HeLa cells [87]. The amount of resveratrol-loaded MSNs uptaken by tumor cells increased by almost fourfold compared to calcined MSNs due to the targeting delivery of surfactant. In another work, TAT peptide-modified MSNs were used for the delivery of doxorubicin (DOX) to nuclei of cancer cells [44]. With the modification of a TAT peptide on the surface of these MSNs, it was found that 50 nm or smaller TAT-MSNs can efficiently target the nucleus of HeLa cells. DOX in TAT-MSNs was released into the nucleus to kill cancer cells with enhanced efficiencies compared to MSNs. In addition, other targeting ligands such as aptamer have also been used for drug delivery using SiNPs [88].

In order to control the release of drugs loaded in SiNPs, stimuli-responsive released systems based on SiNPs were developed. MSNs have size-tunable pores, which allow adjusting the loading of different drug molecules and triggering the drug release from MSNs. Therefore, we will focus on the applications of stimuli-responsive release MSNs. These MSNs-based stimuli-responsive systems were originally developed by Lin's group [89]. The principle of these systems is shown in Figure 8.5 [25]. Drugs were loaded into MSNs through diffusion and chemical binding. Then, a gatekeeper, such as nanoparticles, organic molecules, and supermolecular assemblies, was used to regulate the encapsulation and release of drugs by certain stimulus conditions in tumor cells and tissues. Through this controllable loading and releasing manners in MSNs, the treatment efficacy for cancer increased markedly.

Using a self-complementary duplex DNA as the gatekeeper to control the release of drugs in certain regions, Chen et al. developed MSNs-based drug delivery system (DDS) for cancer therapy [90]. The drugs were trapped within the porous channels of MSNs, and then, the self-complementary duplex DNA was modified on the surface of MSNs to regulate the release of drugs. When the duplex DNA was denatured by heating or hydrolyzed by endonucleases in cancer cells, drugs in MSNs were released to kill cancer cells. Singh et al. coated MSNs with a shell of polymer, which was then triggered by the temperature and proteases presented in tumor cells [29]. Afterward, DOX

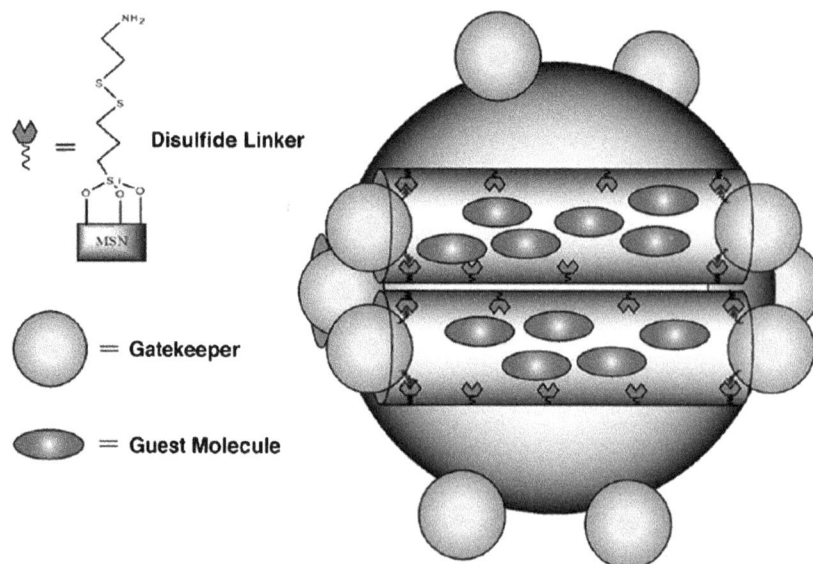

FIGURE 8.5 Representation of MSNs loaded with guest molecules and end-capped with a general gatekeeper. (Reprinted from Slowing et al. [25] with permission by Elsevier.)

that was doped in the core and shell was released into tumor cells to induce apoptosis. pH can also be used as another triggering factor for drug release from MSNs for tumor therapy. Meng et al. developed β-cyclodextrin (β-CD)-coated MSNs for DOX delivery into cancer cells [91]. The β-CD-based nanovalves were responsive to the endosomal acidification conditions in cancer cell lines. Upon the triggering by the acid condition, the DOX in the MSNs could be released into nuclei of cancer cells. Furthermore, Gao et al. investigated the effect of pore sizes and pH for drug release rates in MSNs-based DDSs [28]. With increasing pore sizes, drug release rates also increased. In addition, acid conditions could trigger the release of the drug into tumor cells.

Nanoparticles were another kind of gatekeeper for the controllable MSNs-based DDS. Quantum dots [89], gold nanoparticles [92], and iron oxide nanoparticles [49] have been investigated for controllable drug release systems. Utilizing stimuli-responsive DDSs based on MSNs, drugs for cancer therapy could be efficiently and specifically delivered to cancer cells and tissues *in vitro* and *in vivo*. Therefore, more effective therapy and fewer side effects of the chemotherapeutic drugs could be obtained by the stimuli-responsive MSNs.

8.4.3 Photodynamic Therapy Agents

Photodynamic therapy (PDT) of cancers is a relatively new treatment compared to chemotherapy. Photosensitizer, oxygen, and irradiation constitute necessary factors for PDT. Upon the irradiation of light, photosensitizers absorb photons and transfer the energy to surrounding oxygen to generate singlet oxygen that can irreversibly oxidize molecules, such as proteins and nucleic acids of tumor cells, resulting in cell killing.

Several photosensitizers have been developed for PDT. However, there are some limitations for clinical applications of these photosensitizers, such as hydrophobic property, low target efficiency to tumor sites, instability in biological environments, and side effects to normal cells. In order to overcome these limitations, SiNPs were used to deliver the photosensitizers to tumor cells with high targeting efficiency and low side effects. In 2003, Roy et al. entrapped a hydrophobic photosensitizer, 2-devinyl-2-(1-hexyloxyethyl) pyropheophorbide (HPPH), in SiNPs for tumor therapy [93]. With the irradiation of visible light, irreversible destruction of tumor cells was induced by singlet oxygen generated by the photodynamic process. To increase the penetration depth of light, Kim et al. used a two photo-absorbing fluorescent dye co-encapsulating with HPPH in SiNPs to form a photodynamic therapy system to effectively kill tumor cells [94]. In these two examples, the photosensitizers were encapsulated in the SiNPs through a physical process.

Drug leakage during systemic circulation is one of the disadvantages of these systems. Ohulchanskyy et al. covalently incorporated a photosensitizer to SiNPs and investigated singlet oxygen generation efficiency upon photo-irradiation [95]. Tumor cells incubated with these SiNPs demonstrated low survival rates than those of the control group. Zhang et al. described a versatile photosensitizer delivery system based on SiNPs for tumor therapy [96]. In their design, an upconverting nanoparticle was doped in SiNPs, and the photosensitizers were encapsulated within the silica shell. The surface of the silica shell was modified with antibodies that were specific for antigens of tumor cells. Upon the NIR irradiation, the upconverting nanoparticles absorbed the NIR light and transferred the energy to photosensitizers in the shell to generate singlet oxygen, leading to oxidative damage to tumor cells nearby the nanoparticles. An *in vivo*

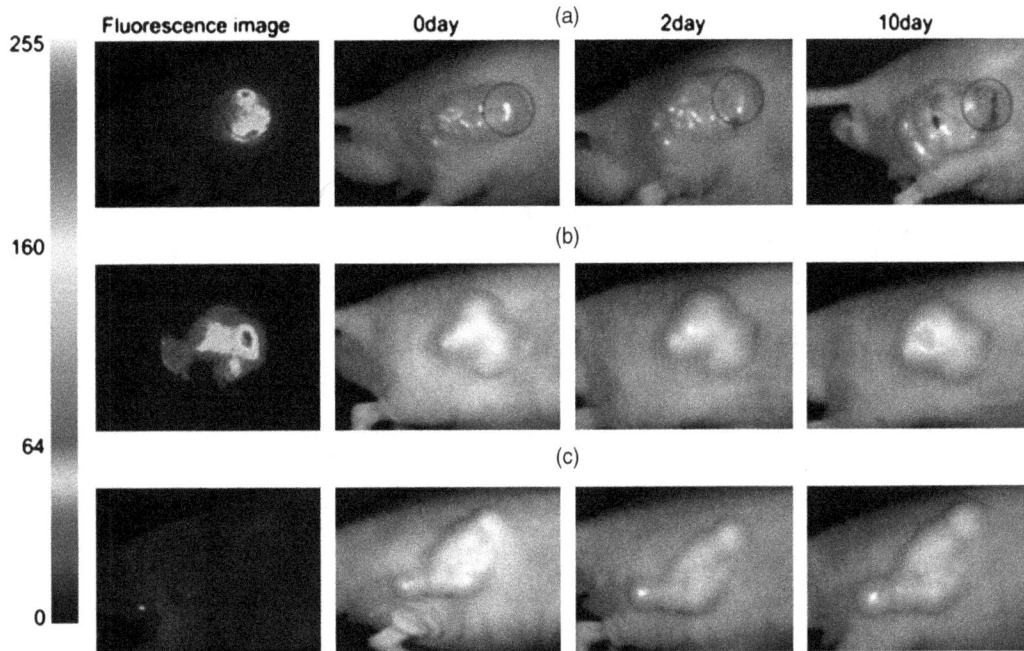

FIGURE 8.6 *In vivo* imaging and PDT of subcutaneous-HeLa-tumor-xenografted mice after different treatments: (A) 100 mL 44 mg/mL MB-encapsulated PSiNPs injection and 5-min light exposure with power intensity of 500 mw/cm², the red circle indicates the region injected the MB-encapsulated PSiNPs and with light exposure; (B) 100 mL 44 mg/mL MB-encapsulated PSiNPs injection; and (C) 5-min light exposure with power intensity of 500 mw/cm². (Reprinted from He et al. [30] with permission by Elsevier.)

PDT based on SiNPs was investigated by He et al. in 2009 [30]. Methylene blue (MB), a NIR photosensitizer, was doped in phosphate-modified SiNPs. It showed that these MB-SiNPs not only caused the death of tumor cells *in vitro*, but also induced damage on mouse tumor tissues due to the NIR irradiation (Figure 8.6). Meanwhile, fluorescence *in vivo* imaging was obtained by the fluorescence emission of MB in the SiNPs. Also, Gary-Bobo et al. combined a chemotherapeutic agent and photosensitizer into SiNPs for both chemotherapy and PDT to further enhance tumor killing [97]. Zhu et al. encapsulated the photosensitizers in small MSNs with a high loading capacity [98]. The resulting delivery system increased the amount of photosensitizers in cancer cells by two orders of magnitude, and the therapy efficiency was enhanced by more than fourfolds.

8.4.4 GENE THERAPY USING SiNPs-BASED VECTORS

The development of gene therapy technologies has generated great interest in cancer treatments about two decades ago. However, cancer gene therapy lacks specific delivery systems for carrying therapeutic genes to target tumor cells. Since He et al. reported that SiNPs could protect DNA from the cleavage by nucleases in 2003, these nanomaterials might have the potential for gene delivery to tumor cells [99]. Antisense oligonucleotide-loaded SiNPs were also developed for targeting HeLa cells by the same group [46]. It was found that these nanoparticles efficiently inhibited the proliferation and survival of HeLa cells. Xia et al. applied DNA- or siRNA-attached and polyethylenimine (PEI)-modified MSNs for gene therapy [11]. To improve

this technology, a GFP-containing siRNA was used as a model for siRNA delivery to kill tumor cells. Flow cytometry (Figure 8.7A) and fluorescence confocal microscopy (Figure 8.7B) were used to evaluate the transfection efficiency of the siRNA-loaded MSNs. The results showed that the MSNs coated with 10 kD PEI had the best transfection efficiency in transducing the GFP-siRNA into tumor cells. The fluorescence intensity of GFP in these cells was the lowest compared to the control groups due to the death of targeted cells. Meanwhile, a GFP-expressing plasmid was also delivered by MSNs into tumor cells to test the feasibility of the SiNPs for DNA delivery.

Overexpression of drug efflux transporters is one of the issues for cancer therapy. For example, P-glycoprotein (Pgp) is one of the well-known multiple drug resistance proteins. For efficient treatment of tumor cells with chemotherapeutics, siRNA used to silence the expression of Pgp was a new approach for the drug-resistant tumor cells. Meng et al. designed MSNs to deliver DOX and Pgp for tumor therapy [100]. This group found that the fluorescence intensity of DOX in tumor cells increased dramatically when the Pgp siRNA was co-delivered with DOX using MSNs, indicating that the Pgp expression was silenced by a Pgp siRNA on the MSNs. By staining with Annexin V/SYTOX, an apoptotic indicator, the tumor cells treated with the siRNA and DOX co-delivered MSNs showed significantly increased apoptosis compared to those treated with free DOX or DOX delivered by non-siRNA MSNs. Pgp is a pump-resistant protein for multidrug resistance, while for the nonpump resistance of multidrug resistance, activation of cellular antiapoptotic defense triggered by Bcl-2 protein is the main mechanism.

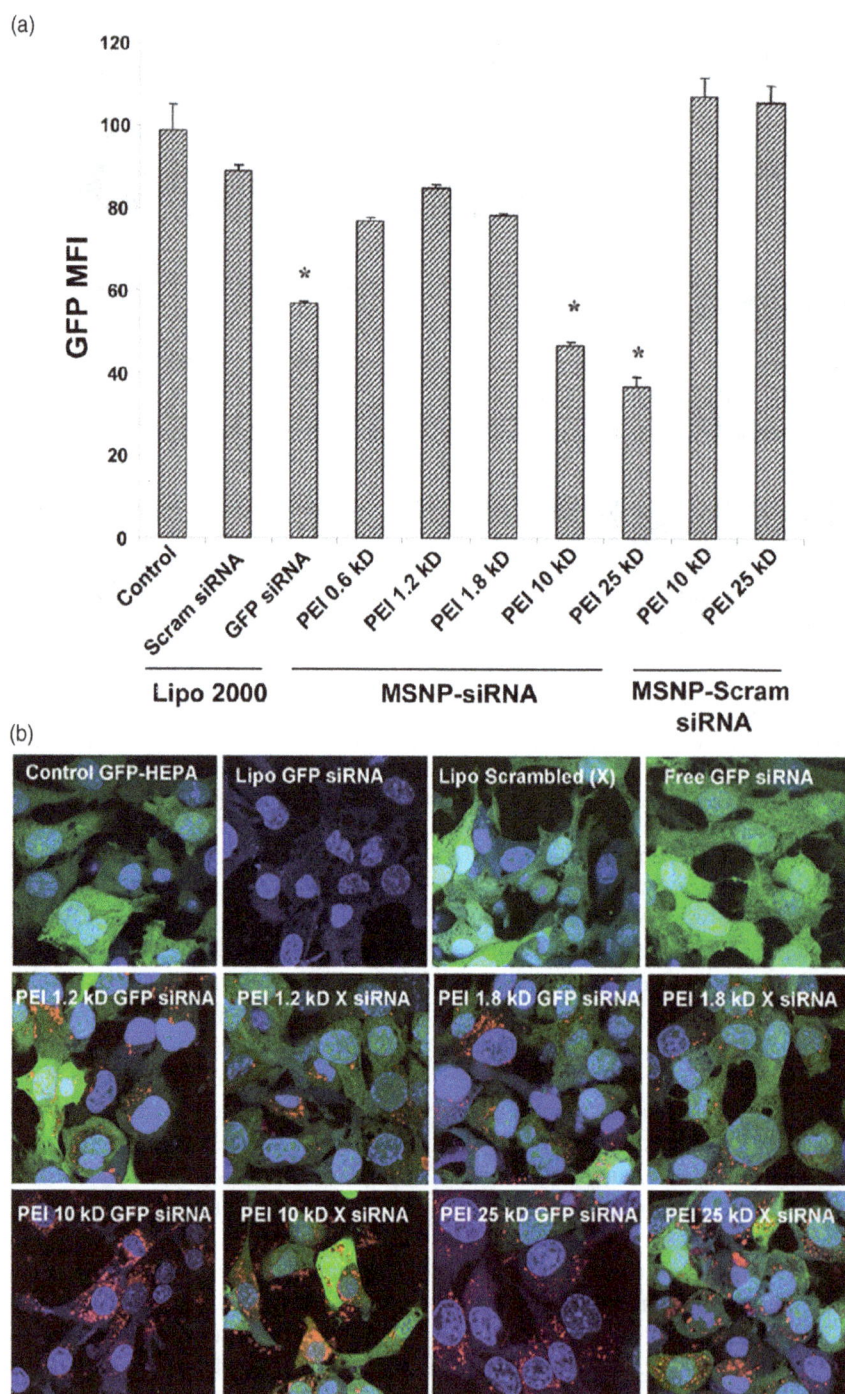

FIGURE 8.7 GFP knockdown by siRNA in stable transfected GFP-HEPA cells. HEPA-1 cells with stable GFP expression were used for siRNA knockdown assays. MSNP coated with different size PEI polymers was used to transfect GFP-specific or scrambled siRNA and the results compared with Lipofectamine 2000 as transfection agent. (A) GFP knockdown was assessed by flow cytometry in which GFP MFI was normalized to the value of control untransduced cells (100%). (B) Confocal pictures were taken showing GFP knockdown in GFP-HEPA cells. TEX 615-labeled siRNA was used to show the cellular localization of the nucleic acid bound particles (red dots). X, scrambled siRNA. The experiment was reproduced three times. (Reprinted from Gordon et al. [13] with permission by the American Chemical Society.)

To deliver a Bcl-2 siRNA into tumor cells, Chen et al. loaded Bcl-2 siRNA and DOX in MSNs to enhance chemotherapy [101]. DOX and Bcl-2 siRNA were loaded in the pore channel of MSNs (Figure 8.8). When the particles were taken up by tumor cells, the gatekeeper, G2 PAMAM, was opened by the acid pH in the endosome. Subsequently, DOX was released into cells to induce apoptosis, and Bcl-2 siRNA was released to silence Bcl-2 protein to increase apoptosis. Owing to the Bcl-2 siRNA-directed delivery, the chemotherapeutic efficacy of DOX was enhanced in tumor cells.

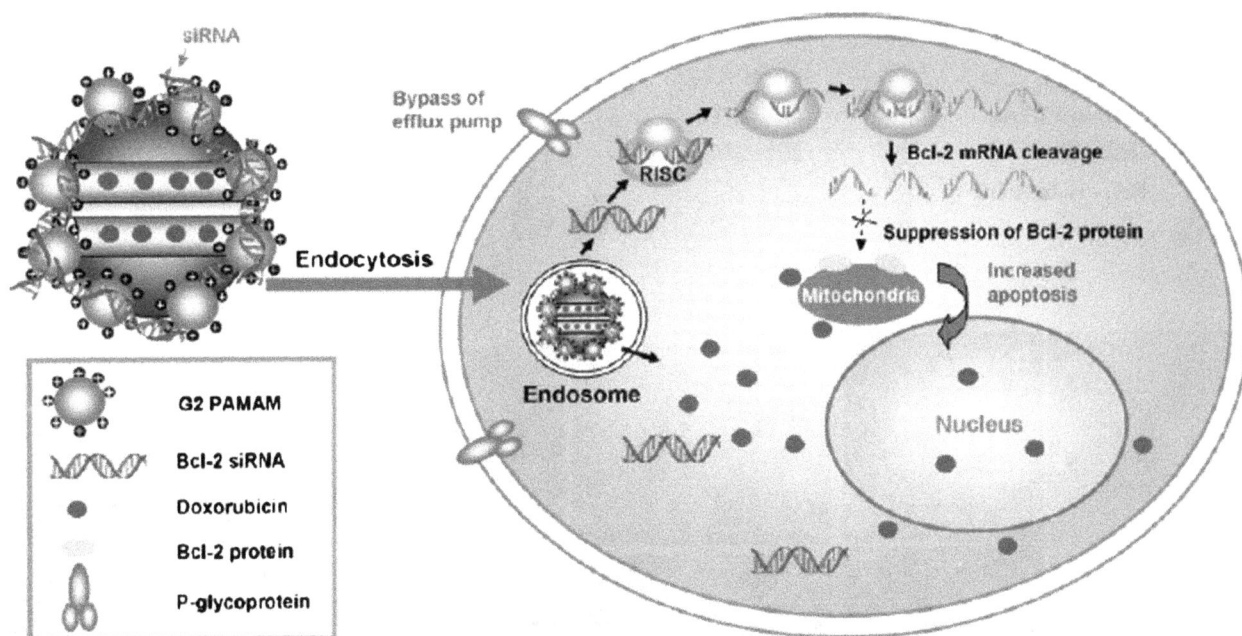

FIGURE 8.8 Schematic diagram of a co-delivery system based on MSNs to deliver Dox and Bcl-2-targeted siRNA simultaneously to A2780/AD human ovarian cancer cells for enhanced chemotherapy efficacy. (Reprinted from Chen et al. [101] with permission by Wiley-VCH.)

8.5 MULTIFUNCTIONAL SILICA NANOPARTICLES

To increase the therapy efficiency, not only is the therapy process important, but also diagnosis, especially at early stages, is crucial for patient survival. Theranostics has emerged as an interdisciplinary field by integrating imaging and therapy. Therefore, the development of novel multifunctional platforms for both imaging and therapy is one of the challenges in cancer treatments [39]. The success of SiNPs in the delivery of imaging agents and drugs attests to the potential of SiNPs for theranostics of tumor using multifunctional nanomaterial entities [102]. The capability of these multifunctional nanomaterials in imaging provides high-quality images for guiding therapeutic agents [47]. During and after the therapy, the images could be used for monitoring the effects of therapy. These properties may improve drug delivery efficacy and survival rates and minimize side effects of drugs to normal tissues.

There are at least three different models for multifunctional SiNPs including multimodel imaging, multimodel therapy, and multimodel theranostics. For the multimodel imaging system, the designed SiNPs possess different kinds of imaging strategies, such as optical imaging, MRI, PET, CT, and ultrasonic. This multimodel imaging system can greatly increase the diagnosis accuracy and sensitivity [47,103]. For example, Huang et al. developed a multifunctional MSN that incubated fluorescence imaging, MRI and PET for tumor imaging and probe localization [43]. The multimodel therapy system contains the SiNPs that incubated different therapeutic strategies. For example, chemotherapy, gene therapy, thermotherapy, PDT, and photothermal therapy (PTT) can be combined for the multimodel therapy of tumor [104,105]. The multimodel therapy system can enhance the therapeutic efficiency. Furthermore, the most important multifunctional SiNPs possess multimodel imaging abilities and multimodel therapeutic abilities for tumor diagnosis and therapy [106–109], which are illustrated as follows.

Liong et al. proposed the use of multifunctional MSNs for imaging, targeting, and drug delivery to tumors [38]. The iron oxide nanocrystal doped in MSNs and fluorescein on the silica shell provided the feasibility of MRI and fluorescence imaging for tumors. Folic acid was used to target tumor cells and tissues due to the high expression of folate receptor on tumor cells. A drug was loaded in the pore channel of MSNs for killing tumor cells. Meanwhile, the iron oxide nanocrystal could be used for magnetic manipulation to modulate the platform to a desired location. Therefore, the multifunctional MSNs boasted five functions together for tumor imaging and therapy. Chen et al. developed similar multifunctional SiNPs for simultaneous cell imaging and drug delivery [110]. Iron oxide nanocrystal or gold nanoparticles were doped in SiNPs and then co-loaded with a chemotherapeutic agent. *In vitro* and *in vivo* MRI and therapeutic functionalities of the platform were shown to be promising for tumor imaging and therapy in mice.

In 2011, Huang et al. constructed silica-modified gold nanorods for X-ray/CT imaging and photothermal therapy for tumor [111]. As shown in Figure 8.9A, gold nanorods were encapsulated in the silica nanoshell, which was modified with folic acids for active targeting tumor cells. Upon the irradiation of light, the tumor cells that underwent apoptosis were increased as stained by PI (Figure 8.9B).

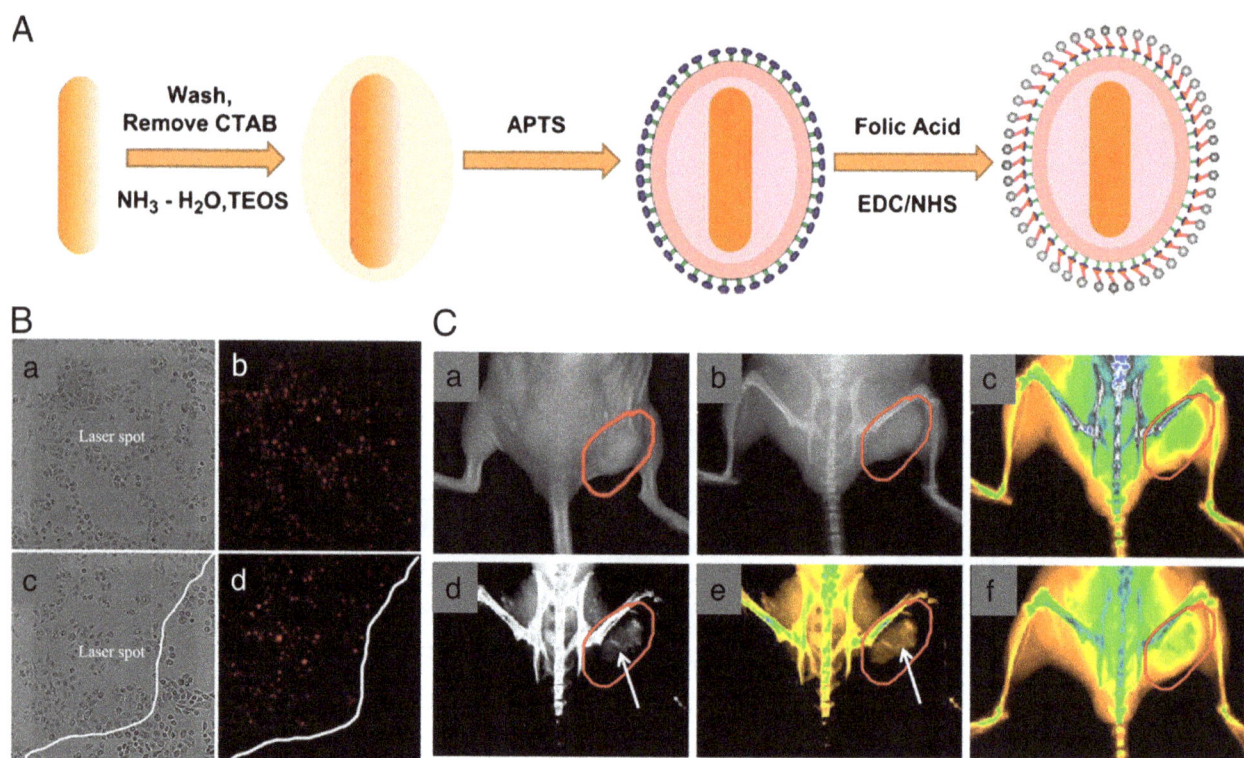

FIGURE 8.9   (A) Synthetic procedure of GNR-SiO$_2$-FA. (B) Photothermal therapy effects on GC803 cells incubated with 12.5 mM of GNR-SiO$_2$-FA for 24 h at 37°C in the dark prior to irradiation for 3 min with 808 nm laser. (a and b) MGC803 cells on the laser spot center, (d and d) GC803 cells on the boundary of laser spot. (a and c) Bright field, (b and d) fluorescence field. (C) Real-time *in vivo* X-ray images after intravenous injection of GNR-SiO$_2$-FA in nude mice at different time points. (a) The photograph of the tumor tissue; (b) the X-ray image at 0 h; (c) the X-ray image at 0 h (in color); (d) the X-ray image at 12 h; (e) the X-ray image at 12 h (in color); and (f) the X-ray image at 24 h (in color). (Reprinted from Huang et al. [111] with permission by Elsevier.)

Furthermore, *in vivo* X-ray imaging showed that tumor tissue displayed a sharp contrast compared to normal tissues (Figure 8.9C). To explore the thermal effect of gold nanoparticles, Huschka et al. investigated the thermal effect of gold nanoshell and gold nanorod for DNA release, which might be useful for tumor targeting gene delivery and therapy [112]. With a similar design, Zhang et al. developed mesoporous silica-coated gold nanorods (Au@SiO$_2$) for cancer treatment [113]. The Au@SiO$_2$ was monitored using two-photon imaging. Doxorubicin was also doped into the nanocomposite, which could be released by the low power density laser for chemotherapy. Meanwhile, with high power density laser, the gold nanorods induced photothermal effect could be used for the hyperthermia. Similarly, He et al. developed MB-doped SiNPs for simultaneous fluorescent imaging and PDT of tumor cells *in vitro* and tissues *in vivo* [30]. Zhao et al. doped upconversion nanoparticles into SiNPs, which were then coupled with photosensitizer for NIR imaging and PDT [114]. Interestingly, this nanomaterial also demonstrated good MR contrast in tumor cells and thereby could be used for MRI. In a recent review, Bardhan et al. summarized the design and synthesis of nanoshell-based theranostic agents using enhanced near-infrared fluorescence or MRI-guided photothermal ablation in both cellular models and animal models [115].

Collectively, the goals of theranostics may be achieved by combining imaging agents and therapeutic agents into appropriate SiNPs for tumor imaging and therapy. More importantly, these multifunctional nanoparticles may provide combined imaging strategies, such as fluorescence and MRI, fluorescence and X-ray imaging, fluorescence and Raman imaging, and MRI and X-ray imaging, for precise guidance of drug selection and monitoring the efficacy during tumor therapy.

8.6   BIOCOMPATIBILITY OF SILICA NANOPARTICLES

With the development of SiNPs for cancer diagnosis and therapy, the safety issues have been gradually recognized and need serious and full further investigation. The biocompatibility of SiNPs at different levels, including cells, tissues, and animals, was demonstrated by several groups. Because of the chemical inert of silica, the SiNPs showed great biocompatibility at different levels. However, the physiochemical properties, such as size, surface charge, and modification, can all play important roles in the toxicity and pharmacokinetics of SiNPs in the cells and animals. Meanwhile, because of the various synthesis methods and treated bio-matrixes, it is hard to draw a general conclusion about the toxicity of the SiNPs on cells and animals.

Herein, we briefly reviewed the recent developments of the investigations of the *in vitro* and *in vivo* toxicity of SiNPs regarding the size and surface modification of the nanoparticles.

The toxicity of SiNPs was affected by several factors, including the cell lines, concentrations, particle sizes, surface charges, particle shapes, and structures of the SiNPs. Mou et al. investigated the cellular uptake amount of different sized MSNs using HeLa cells [52]. They found that the MSNs of 50 nm diameter showed the highest uptake efficiency. Jin et al. synthesized different sized core/shell SiNPs and investigated their cytotoxicity [55]. It was found that the smaller SiNPs (23±3 nm) showed higher cytotoxicity than that of the larger SiNPs (85±5 nm). At the animal level, He et al. investigated the biodistribution and urinary excretion of MSNs with different particle sizes from 80 to 360 nm [116]. They found that the accumulation of MSNs in the liver and spleen and the excretion efficiency increased with the increase of particle size from 80, 120, to 200 nm after intravenous injection. However, within 1 month, neither MSNs nor PEGylated MSNs showed toxicity to the treated mice.

The surface modification of SiNPs was another factor that could affect the toxicity on the cells. The SiNPs with cationic charge surface had strong interaction with the cell membrane because of the electrostatic interaction, which would induce more immune response and cytotoxicity compared with the neutral and anion SiNPs. For the unmodified SiNPs, the surface was covered with silanol groups, which induced a negative charge of the SiNPs. However, other functional groups, such as amino group, carboxyl group, phosphonate group, and PEG, were easily modified on the surface of the SiNPs with the silanol chemistry. Among these groups, PEG was by far the best way to increase the dispersity and increase the biocompatibility of the SiNPs. With the modification of PEG, the blood half-life in small animals would significantly increase, and the accumulation in RES tissues would greatly decrease, which was enhancing the tumor targeting efficiency and biocompatibility. With PEGylation, the endocytosis of the SiNPs may be diminished, which could reduce the hemolytic activity and cytotoxicity [117,118]. After intravenous injection of different modified SiNPs, He et al. found that all the SiNPs accumulated in the liver and spleen with the increase of time [33]. However, the PEGylated SiNPs showed longer blood circulation times and lower uptake by the RES tissues than those of the hydroxyl modified SiNPs and carboxyl modified SiNPs. Meanwhile, all the SiNPs were partly excreted through the renal excretion route, which was confirmed by the fluorescence in the bladder and urine, and TEM images of SiNPs in the urine. The excretion process might greatly reduce the long-term toxicity of SiNPs *in vivo*.

8.7 MESOPOROUS SILICA NANOPARTICLES (MSNPs)

In the following sections, lipid-, protein-, and poly(NIPAM)-coated MSNPs are reviewed from the preparation, properties, and their potential application. We also introduce the

preparative methods including physical adsorption, covalent binding, and self-assembly on the MSNs' surfaces. Furthermore, the interaction between the aimed cells and these molecular-modified MSNs is discussed. We also demonstrate their typical applications, such as photodynamic therapy, bioimaging, controlled release, and selective recognition in biomedical field.

After the discovery of highly ordered mesoporous silica materials by the Mobil Corporation in 1992 [119,120], the preparation of mesoporous silica-based materials has become highly attractive due to their potential applications in the fields of catalysis, lasers, sensors, and environmental application [121–125]. In the past decade, more and more mesoporous silica-based composite materials were designed to apply in biomedical fields [24,27,126,127] since they were first reported as DDSs [128]. Several features result in mesoporous silica materials as good carriers in biomedical application. Firstly, they have the ordered pore network and homogeneous size for the drug loading; secondly, high pore volume and surface area will host the required amount of drug molecules; most importantly, a silanol-containing functionalized surface allows them to be modified easily to control over drug loading and release. Mesoporous silica materials made by the original procedures are mainly mesoporous silica sheets with disorganized morphologies. For increasing their biocompatibility, significant research efforts have been made toward the smaller size and monodispersity. In 2001, Cai et al. firstly obtained MCM-41 typed MSNs with 100 nm by using a dilute surfactant solution [129]. Later, various MSNs with well-defined and controllable particle morphology were developed by Lin's and other research groups in pursuit of biocompatible materials used in controlled release and DDSs [130–132]. These mesoporous silica materials with nanosizes are more valuable in biological application. Nano-sized particles are particularly interesting in medical and biological fields. They are often used as cell markers, gene transfection reagents, or MRI contrast agents to realize the maximization of cellular uptake [133,134]. Several studies have been done on their biocompatibility, cytotoxicity [135–137], blood compatibility [118,138,139], biodegradability [140,141], biodistribution, and excretion [116,142–144]. The downsides of MSNs, we think they are rigid and exhibit a little aggregation after modification. Furthermore, despite the MSNs' degradability has been reported, they still need more than days for degradation thoroughly.

Up to date, there are many reports on MSNs-based nanomaterials used in biomedical field. Some popular systems, such as cap systems, have been recently attracted great attention. Inorganic nanoparticles [145–147] or large molecules (cyclodextrins or rotaxanes) [91,148–150] have been used as the cap of the pores on the surface of MSNs. These caps are able to release entrapped guest molecules inside MSNs by using diverse physical and chemical stimuli. Some relevant review articles have been also reported [27,126,132]. Here, we will mainly introduce the lipid-, protein-, or poly(N-isopropylacrylamide) (poly(NIPAM))-modified MSNs used in biomedical field based on the recent works. These molecules are soft and biocompatible with the unique property, chemical conformation, and their own functions [151]. Our group has taken these species to assemble many different biomimetic systems as micro-/nanomaterials toward the biological applications [131,152–161].

Herein, we briefly summarize the abovementioned molecules coated MSN nanocomposites from preparation, property to potential applications. In the preparation section, layer-by-layer assembly, covalent linkage, and electrostatic interaction are described, respectively. Subsequently, biocompatibility, autofluorescence, and stimuli responsibility of these nanocomposites are introduced in detail. It demonstrates that these assembled molecules coated MSNs are suitable for the photodynamic therapy, cell imaging, controlled release, or selective recognition.

8.8 PREPARATION AND PROPERTIES OF THE FUNCTIONAL MOLECULES COATED MSNs

8.8.1 MSNs

Up to now, the preparation and characterization of MSNs are already recognized. Typically, they are prepared using a base-catalyzed solgel method reported by Cai and Lin's group, respectively [129,162]. As shown in Figure 8.10A,

the porous structure consists of a series of parallel channels with an average pore diameter of 3 nm that are packed in a 2D hexagonal geometry. These characteristics can also be proved by powder X-ray diffraction. The ordered porous structures enable MSNs to become good drug carriers due to their high surface areas (900–1500 cm^2/g) and large pore volumes (0.5–1.5 cm^3/g). Furthermore, Slowing et al. also reported that MCM-41 typed MSNs with the sizes ranging from 20 to 500 nm and with pore sizes ranging from 2 to 6 nm could be synthesized according to the modified methods [163]. MSN materials with various particle morphologies, such as spheres, ellipsoids, and rods, could also be prepared (Figure 8.10B–D) [164]. Zhang et al. also prepared different helical morphological MSN particles by the co-condensation of TEOS and hydrophobic organoalkoxysilane such as 3-mercaptopropyltrimethoxysilane (MPTS), using achiral surfactants as templates [130]. They synthesized the surfactant-extracted samples by using surfactants (either C16TAB or C18TAB) as a template. The morphology and pitch of helical mesostructured silica can be controlled by simply varying the amount of added organoalkoxysilane MPTS.

The size and porosity are important for their different biomedical applications. When MSN is used as drug carriers, the adsorption of molecules in MSN is determined by size

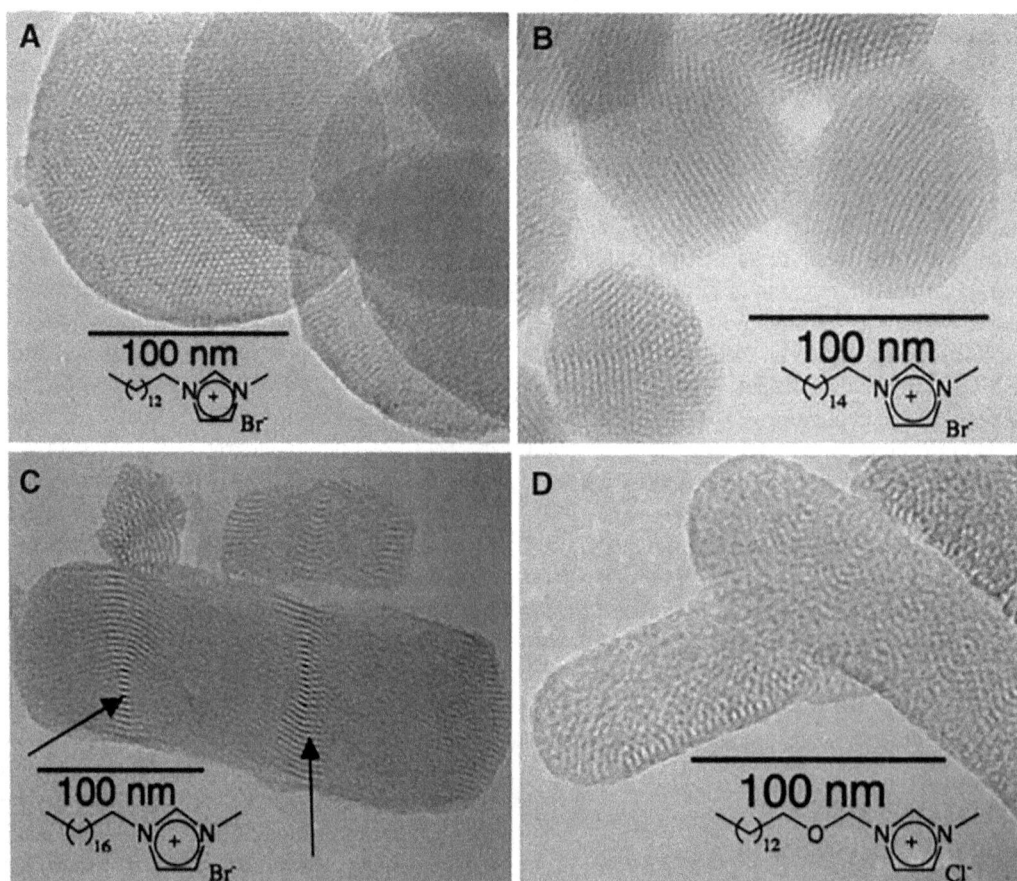

FIGURE 8.10 TEM images of MSNs with different morphology prepared by Trewyn et al. (A) spheres, (B) ellipsoids, (C) rods, and (D) tubes. (Reprinted with permission from Ref. [164] [Copyright 2004 American Chemical Society].)

of inner pores. The mesopore diameters can be tuned from 2 to 6nm, which make MSNs to host different sized drug molecules. The pore size also controls the drug release rate, which has been researched systemically by M. Vallet-Regi et al. [165]. The diameter of MSNs can also affect the interaction between MSNs and cells. Zhao et al. reported interaction of different sized MSNs with human red blood cell (RBC) membranes [166]. They found that small MSNs (ca. 100nm) were adsorbed to the surface of RBCs without disturbing the membrane while large MSNs (ca. 600nm) to RBCs induced a strong local membrane deformation leading to eventual hemolysis. They believe that size of MSNs is decisive in attractive interaction between MSNs and RBCs and the bending of the cell membrane. Only small MCM-41-type MSN materials (100–200nm) may be considered as potentially safe candidates for intravascular drug delivery. In the following introduction, we will mainly consider ca. 100nm sized spherical MSNs as MSNs except were mentioned especially.

8.8.2 LIPID-COATED MSNs

Supported lipid bilayers that mimic a cell membrane are well popular model systems for fundamental research and also are critical for the development of new types of biosensors, biodevices, and functional materials. On the supported surfaces, lipid bilayer not only can improve the biocompatibility of nanocomposites, but also can be used as a means to attach more biological functionality for them. For instance, due to the amphiphilic character of lipids, on the one hand, hydrophilic compounds can be adsorbed on bilayer surface via hydrophilic interactions, and on the other hand, hydrophobic molecules can be inserted in the bilayer hydrocarbon chain region via hydrophobic effects. Therefore, various micro-/nanomaterials, such as microcapsules [167–169], colloidal particles [170], nanotubes [155,171], and nanopatterns [172,173], were used as supported surface of lipid bilayers for more biofunctions.

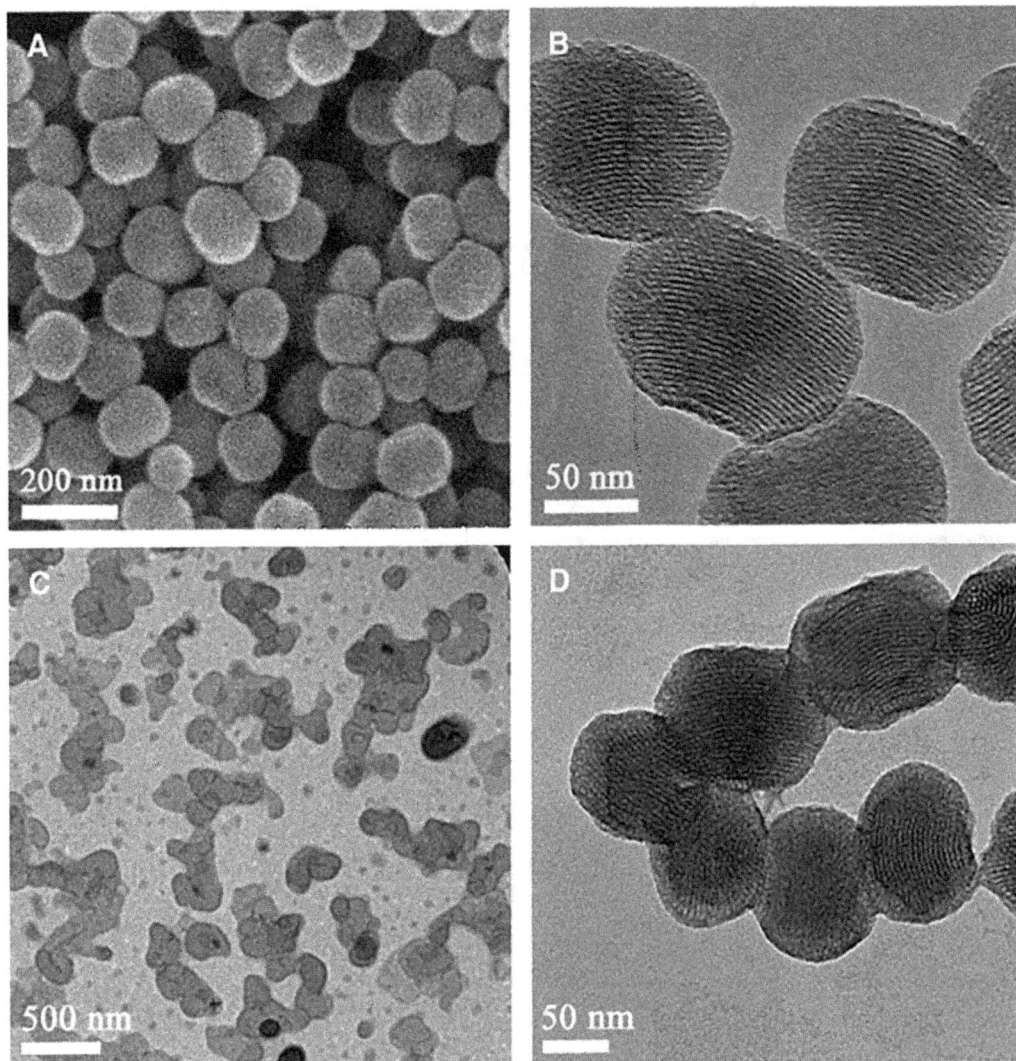

FIGURE 8.11 SEM (A) and TEM (B) of MSN after calcination; TEM (C) of vesicles of lipid mixture; TEM (D) of lipid-MSN-HB. The samples of C and D were stained with 1% phosphotungstic acid. (Reprinted with permission from Ref. [135] [Copyright 2010 Royal Society of Chemistry].)

Predictably, lipid bilayer-modified MSNs will not only improve their biocompatibility and biofunctions, but also maintain the properties of MSNs as ideal nanocarrier systems. Therefore, it has been prepared lipid-coated MSNs as photosensitive drug carriers in our recent work [135]. After being calcined, MSNs were dispersed into hypocrellin B (HB, a kind of photosensitive drug) solution for adsorption. Then, vesicles consisting of mixed phospholipids were coated on the surfaces of MSNs. TEMs (Figure 8.11B and D) showed the differences before and after coating phospholipid vesicles.

For further investigation, confocal laser scanning microscopy (CLSM) was used to observe the nanocomposites (Figure 8.12). From the results, phospholipid mixture can be adsorbed on the surface of MSNs through the higher fluidity of the lipid vesicles, and a subsequent easier fusion with the support [174,175]. The adsorption depends weakly on electrostatic attraction. As drug carriers, lipid-coated MSNs also make hydrophobic drug dispersing in water

very well. As we anticipate, the lipid layers can improve the cell compatibility of MSN materials. The result from flow cytometry measurement proves that lipid-coated MSNs can be more readily identified and internalized by cancer cells than bare MSNs.

Similarly, taking advantage of the amphiphilic character of lipid bilayer, we have assembled the thrombin-binding aptamer (TBA), anticancer drug docetaxel, as well as a hydrophilic PEG into the lipids bilayer and then coated them on the surfaces of MSNs [176]. Such assembled complexes can be used to suppress tumor cell proliferation and release anticancer drug into cell after cell uptake.

8.8.3 Protein-Coated MSNs

Protein is another native biomolecule that is often used for constructing biomaterials. As we know, for fragile protein, it is difficult to keep them stable during the entire process of assembling biomaterials. Up to now, various methods

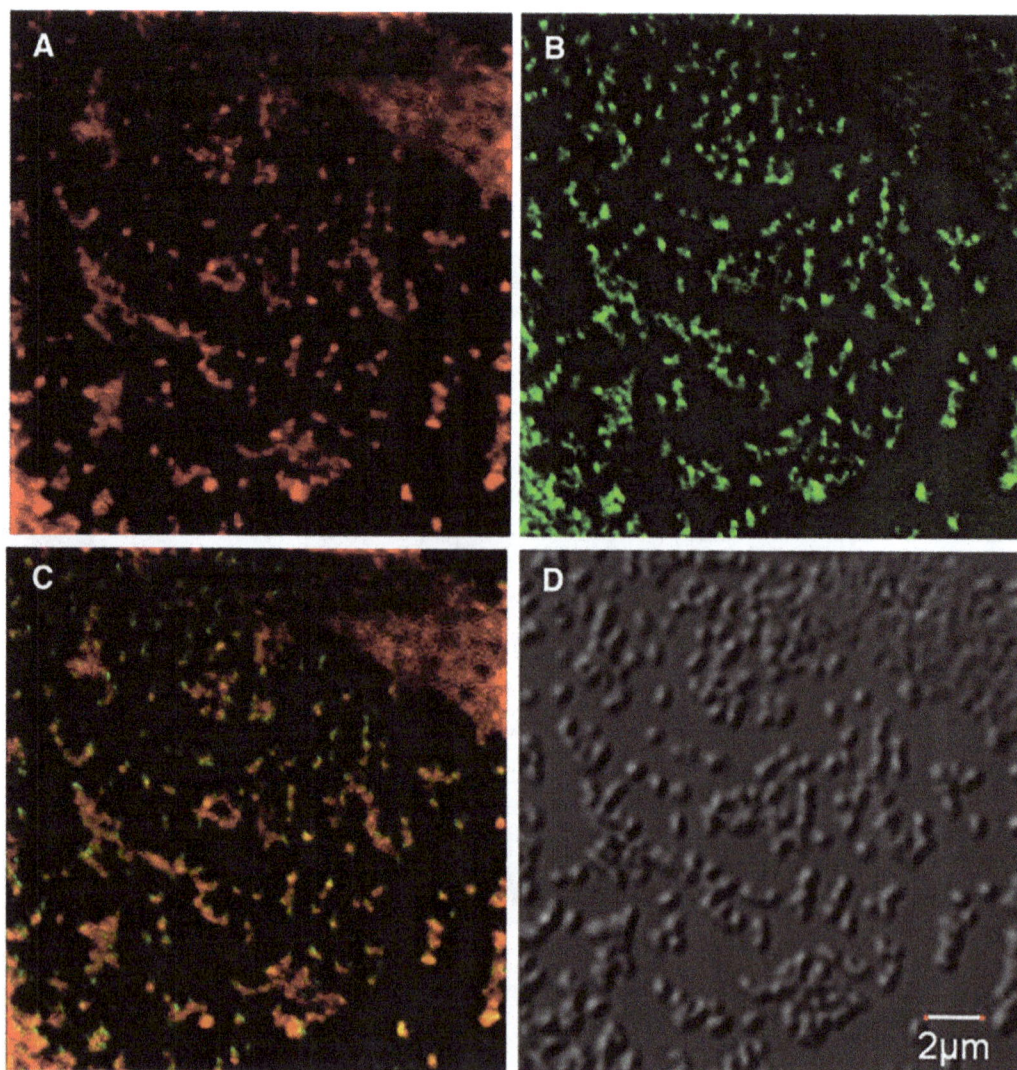

FIGURE 8.12 CLSM of lipid-MSN-HB particles in solution. The corresponding images of the HB (red) (A); NBD-PC in lipid mixture (green) (B); the overlapped image (C); and the pseudo-bright field image (d). Reprinted with permission from Ref. [135] (Copyright 2010 Royal Society of Chemistry).

have been used to construct stable protein films including the Langmuir–Blodgett (LB) technique, the solgel method, physical adsorption, and covalent cross-linking strategies [177–180]. In covalent cross-linking strategy, glutaraldehyde (GA) is a common protein-immobilized agent [181]. In the previous work, it has been made use of GA as a covalent cross-linker to fabricated hemoglobin and glucose oxidase (GOD) microcapsules via the layer-by-layer (LbL) assembly technique [182,183]. Recently, we used this strategy for coating protein, hemoglobin, and GOD, on the surface of MSNs with GA via the LbL method. The thickness of protein can be controlled by the number of assembly layers (Figure 8.13).

As we know, GOD catalyzes the oxidation and hydrolysis of β-D-glucose into gluconic acid and H_2O_2. In the presence of hemoglobin, H_2O_2 can react with the fluorogenic reagent Amplex Red to produce fluorescent compound resorufin. Therefore, when Amplex Red and β-D-glucose were added into an MSN@protein dispersed solution, we can detect the enzymatic activity and glucose sensitivity of coupled proteins through the adsorption/emission peak of resorufin at ~570/585 nm. The results also proved the hypothesis through real-time monitoring of glucose catalysis at different concentrations within MSN@protein using fluorescence spectrofluorometer (Figure 8.14). More interestingly, the MSN@protein particles presented the feature of autofluorescence without any external fluorochromes. The protein layers were constructed on the surface of MSNs via Schiff's base reaction between GA and protein. The autofluorescence can be attributed to the n−π* transition of C=N bonds in the Schiff's bases formed during the cross-linking reaction between the amino groups of proteins and the aldehyde groups of GA [184,185] since we have proved that the mixture of hemoglobin and GOD cannot present autofluorescence without the cross-linker GA under the same conditions.

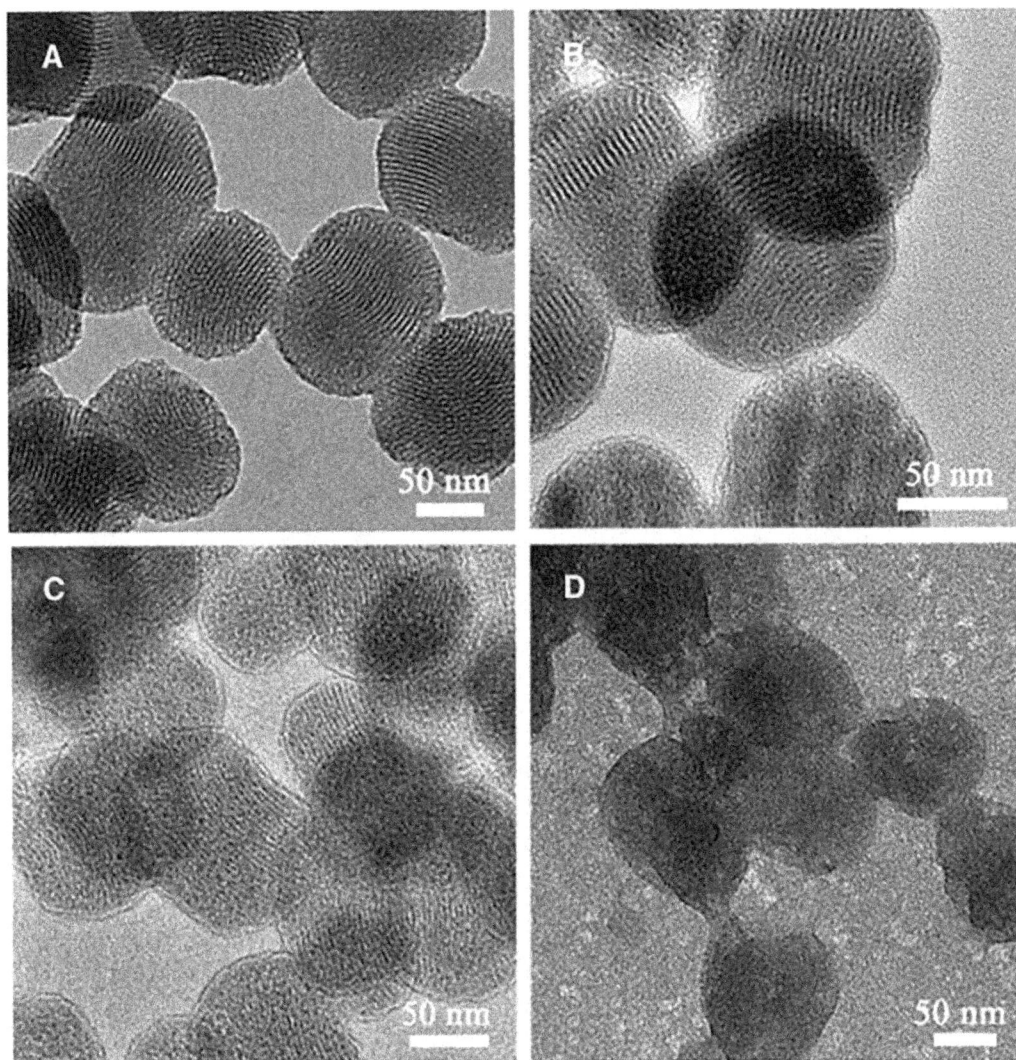

FIGURE 8.13   TEM images of protein-coated MSNs by different assembly layer numbers. (A) MSN; (B) MSN@(hemoglobin/GOD); (C) MSN@(hemoglobin/GOD)$_2$; and (D) MSN@(hemoglobin/GOD)$_3$. (Reprinted with permission from Ref. [136] [Copyright 2011 Royal Society of Chemistry].)

(a)

(b)

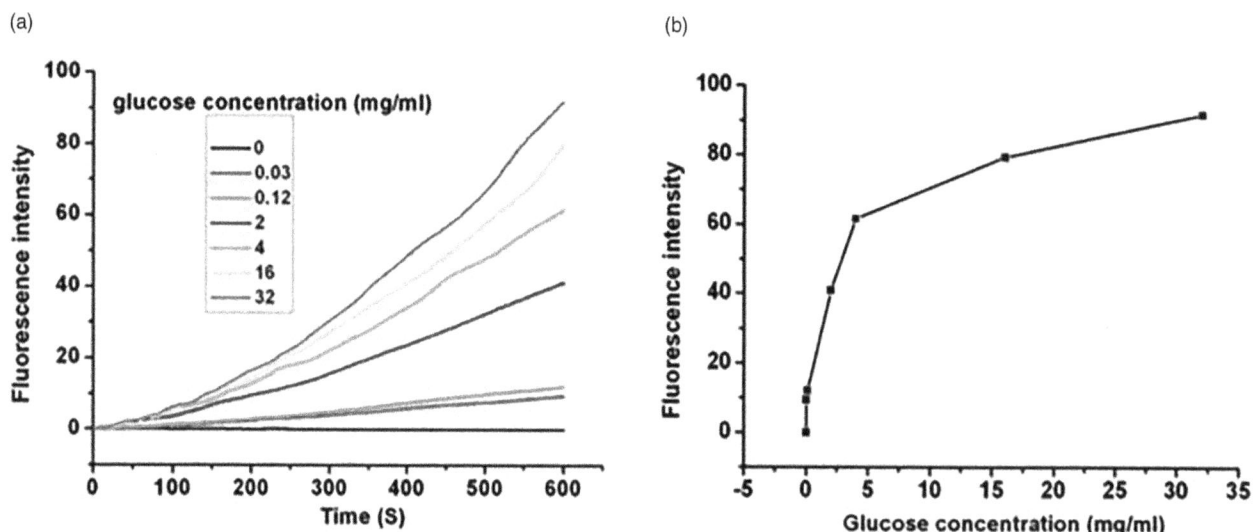

FIGURE 8.14 (A) Real-time monitoring of glucose catalysis at different concentrations within MSN@protein to analyze glucose consumption with respect to time using fluorescence spectrofluorometer. (B) Fluorescence intensity increased with the concentration of glucose at 585 nm after 10 min for glucose consumption. (Reprinted with permission from Ref. [136] [Copyright 2011 Royal Society of Chemistry].)

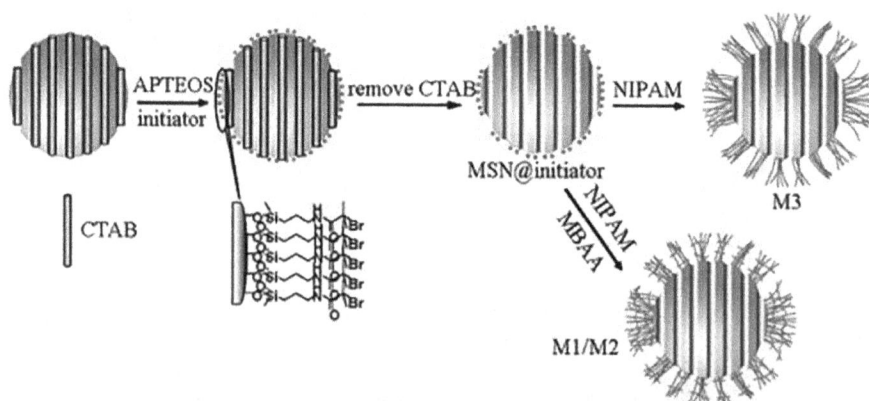

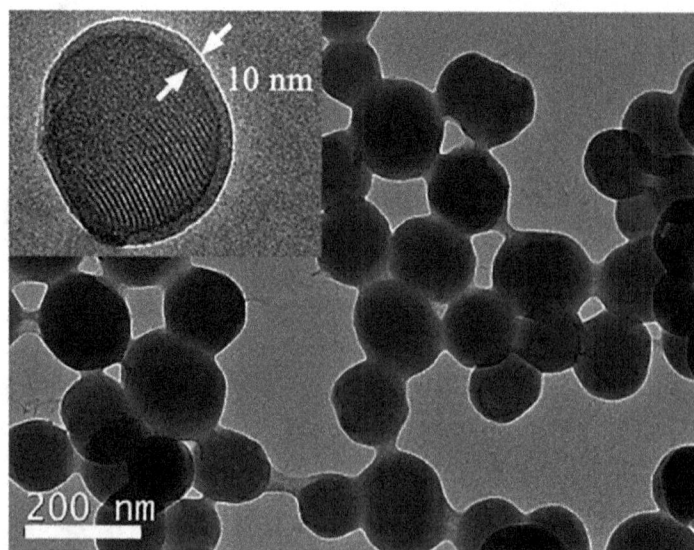

FIGURE 8.15 A schematic illustration of the surface functionalization for MSN and the fabrication of MSN@poly(NIPAM) and TEM of MSN@poly(NIPAM) through the "grafting from" method. (Reprinted with permission from Ref. [131] [Copyright 2008 Royal Society of Chemistry].)

8.8.4 Poly(NIPAM)-Coated MSNs

Poly(NIPAM) is well known as thermosensitive polymer, which will undergo phase transition when temperature is changed. Its lower critical solution temperature (LCST) at about 32°C is close to physiological temperature [186–188]. Several groups have reported that poly(NIPAM) does not present any sign of acute toxicity for some cell lines [189]. Therefore, poly(NIPAM) has often been designed as smart biosensors used as a drug delivery material, cell attachment/detachment matrix, and hemostatic agent [190–193]. "Grafting to" and "grafting from" are two typical methods to attach poly(NIPAM) onto substrate by chemical covalent interaction. "Grafting to" method means that end-functionalized polymer chains are attached directly to an appropriate substrate, while in "grafting from" approach, an initiator is modified on the surface of aimed materials. Then, the initiator-modified materials can initiate the polymerization of monomers through living/controlled polymerization, such as the surface-initiated atom transfer radical polymerization (ATRP).

For instance, You et al. grafted poly(NIPAM) to the surface of the preformed, thiol-functionalized MSN nanoparticles by the "grafting to" method [194]. At the same time, we reported MSN@poly(NIPAM) core/shell structured nanomaterials by ATRP and the "grafting from" method [131]. The synthetic process and typical sample are shown in Figure 8.15. The synthesized composite nanomaterial has both a mesoporous silica core and a thermosensitive poly(NIPAM) shell. The ATRP technique can incorporate more condensed polymers onto the substrate surfaces compared to the "grafting to" method. Polymer layers on the particle surface are more uniform with controllable thickness, while the inner channels remained. The measured

LCST of MSN@poly(NIPAM) material is about 32°C, which is consistent with pure poly(NIPAM) in water.

8.9 POTENTIAL APPLICATIONS AND OUTLOOKS

As mentioned above, such functional molecular/MSN nanocomposites provide new type of intelligent materials with core/shell structures. The soft organic layer endows MSNs with a novel functionality, while polyporous inorganic core makes nanocomposite more stable and also adsorbs more drugs when being used as drug carriers. Therefore, these organic–inorganic nanomaterials can be looked as novel nanotanks or nanocarriers in biomedical field. The application of such nanocomposites might be a favorable resolution to some novel challenges in controlled drug delivery in intelligent therapeutic system, molecular recognition, bioimaging, and so on.

8.9.1 In Photodynamic Therapy

Photodynamic therapy (PDT) is an effective and selective means of suppressing diseased tissues without altering the surrounding healthy tissue. It is based on the systemic or topical administration of a photosensitive drug, which is also known as a photosensitizer (PS) [195,196]. Light-activated PS can generate reactive oxygen species, which can irreversibly damage the treated tissues [197]. However, most PS molecules are hydrophobic and can aggregate easily in aqueous media, where PS aggregation will result in a decrease of their quantum yield and damage to healthy cells [198]. MSNs may be ideal PS carriers for PDT because they are hydrophilic and monodispersed. Nano-sized particles

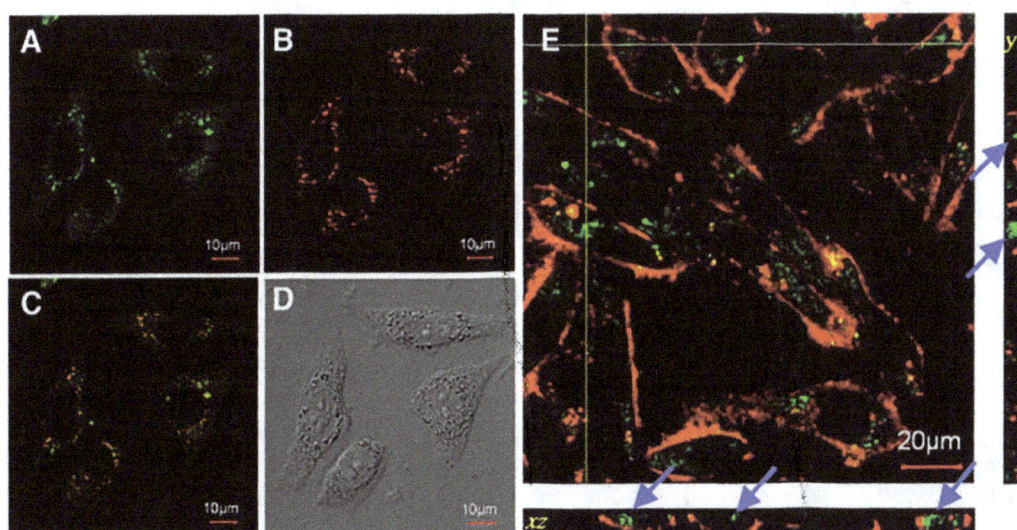

FIGURE 8.16 CLSM of MCF-7 cells and lipid-MSN-HB suspensions after 12 h of co-culturing. The corresponding images show the NBD-PC in lipid mixture (green) (A) and the HB (red) (B) taken up by the cells; the overlapped image (C) and the pseudo-bright field image (D). (E) MCF-7 cells after incubation in lipid-MSN in the presence of the FM4-64. The main image shows the area of xy section, while the white and yellow lines indicate the area of the xz and yz sections, respectively. The image shows the lipid-MSN particles surrounded by cell membrane (red). (Reprinted with permission from Ref. [135] [Copyright 2010 Royal Society of Chemistry].)

can also penetrate deep into tissues and be taken up efficiently by cancer cells. Especially for MSNs, they possess ordered porous structures and molecular oxygen can diffuse through the pores and interact with the PS loaded into the MSN carriers. The photogenerated reactive oxygen can diffuse out of the particle to generate the cytotoxic effect.

To take one example, lipid-coated MSNs have been used as photosensitive drug (HB) carriers for photodynamic experiment *in vitro* [135]. With the lipid modification, the carriers can be internalized more easily by MCF-7 cells (human breast carcinoma cells) through an endocytic mechanism (Figure 8.16). These intracellular HB-loaded lipid-MSNs show biocompatibility under darkness and high cytotoxicity after irradiation, which provides the possibility of controlled delivery and release of drugs. The results indicate that MSN-based materials can be used as good photosensitizer carriers in photodynamic therapy. There will be further opportunity to use these materials for photodetection.

8.9.2 In Cell Imaging

As we introduced before, nano-sized particles were particularly significant when they were used as cell markers to realize the maximization of cellular uptake. In our several work about biomolecules-modified MSNs, most composite MSNs presented good cell biocompatibility [131,135,136,174]. They could be readily attached onto the cell surface or internalized into the cells according to the uptake mechanism. For example, GA cross-linked protein (hemoglobin/GOD)-coated MSNs present autofluorescent

properties, which make them become good carrier candidate to be used in biological tracing. Furthermore, these protein-coated MSNs were found to be either adsorbed or embedded into HeLa cell membranes (Figure 8.17A–D). When another cell line (ESF cells) was selected, we found that MSN@protein also presented to be cell membrane friendly (Figure 8.17E–H). As is well known, cell membranes consist of lipid bilayers and membrane proteins. In this work, the system of MSN@protein might be more favorable to the structure of the cell membrane and internalized by the cell membrane. These unique features make this nanocomposite a good material as cell marker for cell imaging.

8.9.3 In Controlled Release

A facile functionalized surface of MSNs combined with the ATRP method provides a new strategy to construct stimuli-responsive polymer/MSN nanocomposites for controlled release. Recently, Yu and Sun et al. prepared pH-sensitive poly(N, N-dimethylaminoethyl methacrylate)-coated MSNs through the ATRP method for pH-responsive controlled release [199,200]. Another instance, poly(NIPAM)-coated MSNs reported by us can also be used in thermosensitive controlled release system [131]. In detail, a fluorescent molecule, FITC, was used as model guest molecule to test the encapsulation ability of the MSN@poly(NIPAM) particles. FITC can be entrapped by the stretched polymer chains at 20°C and be locked inside MSN at 40°C. After that, FITC will release again slowly from MSN@poly(NIPAM) at 20°C, but not at 40°C (Figure 8.18). The polymer chains on

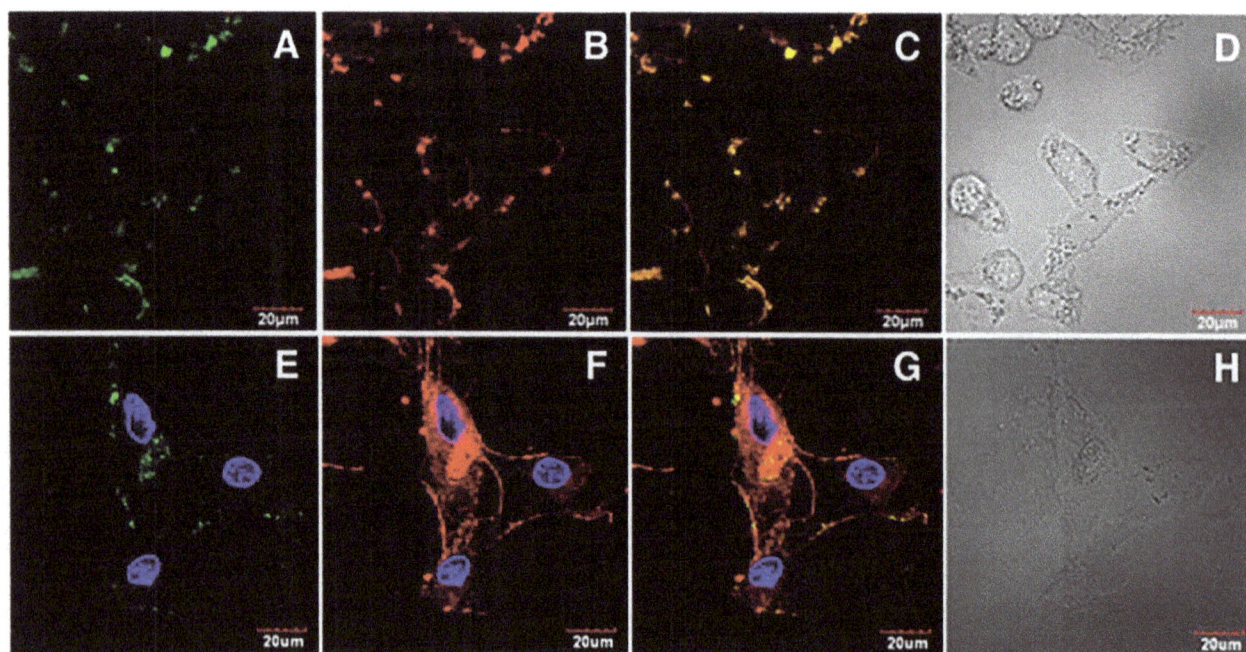

FIGURE 8.17 CLSM images of HeLa cells (A–D) and ESF cells (E–H) stained with FM 4-64 and MSN@protein suspensions after 12 h of co-culturing. The corresponding images of the MSN@protein nanoparticles (green) (A, E); FM 4-64 labeled cell membranes (red) (B, F); the overlapped image (C, G); and the pseudo-bright field image (D, H). (E–G, blue fluorescence comes from cell nucleus marker, Hoechst 33342). (Reprinted with permission from Ref. [136] [Copyright 2011 Royal Society of Chemistry].)

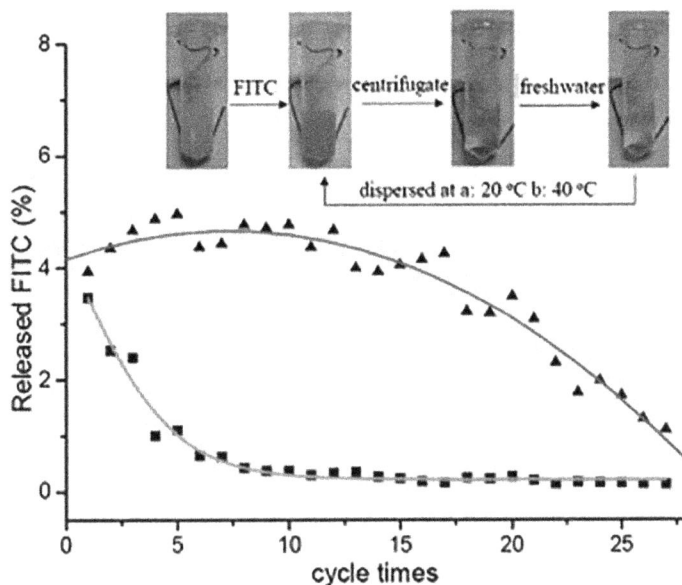

FIGURE 8.18 FITC release from MSN@poly(NIPAM) at different cycle times, which was recorded by UV absorbance at 480 nm. The freshwater was replaced, and FITC-loaded MSN@poly(NIPAM) particles were redispersed at 20°C (▲) or 40°C (■) for 15 min. The inset image illustrates the whole process. (Reprinted with permission from Ref. [131] [Copyright 2008 Royal Society of Chemistry].)

the surface of MSN will be stretched below LCST, which let guest molecule go into pores freely. However, the chains will collapse and block guest molecule from being released when raising the temperature above LCST. This process is reversible, which proves that the systems can be used in DDSs. What's more, the composite materials can be internalized into MCF-7 cells easily, which make it a promising material for application in drug carriers.

8.9.4 IN SELECTIVE RECOGNITION

Recent attention has been devoted to the design of nanodevices with highly efficient ligands that selectively recognize tumor-associated or tumor-specific antigens [201]. Nucleic acid ligand (aptamer) is a novel class of targeting molecules for therapeutic and diagnostic applications [202]. For example, 15-mer thrombin-binding aptamer (TBA) is such targeting molecules, which can inhibit the enzymatic function of thrombin [203–205]. The significant neoplastic biological effect of thrombin involves clotting-dependent mechanism and protease-activated receptor-1 (PAR-1)-related signaling; this leads to several tumor functions, specifically proliferation and angiogenesis [206–209]. In this work, it has been used TBA-tethered lipid-coated MSN composite as an extra and intracellular anticancer nanocarrier [176]. The composites comprise MSN as support core, mixed lipid layers with the incorporation of thrombin-binding aptamer and anticancer drug docetaxel as well as a hydrophilic PEG shell. Two approaches are involved in the whole tumor cell proliferation suppression process. Firstly, TBAA15 recombined on the bioconjugate selectively recognizes thrombin and inhibits its proteolytic capacity in the extracellular surroundings, which results in interference of signal transduction pathways activated by the interaction of thrombin and

PAR-1. Furthermore, incorporated docetaxel releases into cytoplasm where it triggered higher cellular cytotoxicity. The hybrid system constructed will be extended for combined anticancer treatment related to PAR-1 overexpressed.

8.10 CONCLUSIONS

In conclusion, the applications of SiNPs [210,211] in *in vitro* and *in vivo* tumor imaging demonstrated the potential for further developing the SiNPs into clinically useful reagents. Fluorescence imaging and MRI are currently the main strategies for the applications of SiNPs in cancer imaging. X-ray/CT may also be used along with SiNPs as imaging agents. As biocompatible nanomaterials, SiNPs can be used for drug delivery [212–215], especially for chemotherapeutic agents, photosensitizers, and photothermal agents. Stimuli-responsive MSNs for drug delivery and release have improved therapeutic efficacy and decreased side effects. Furthermore, the multifunctional SiNPs that combined imaging and therapy functionalization provided the most promising tool for tumor diagnostics and treatment.

However, there are some challenges that need to be resolved before successful applications of SiNPs in clinics. First of all, the delivery efficiency to the targeting tumor cells and tissues should be improved. Even several targeting ligands, including antibodies, aptamers, and peptides, have been tested for the active targeting for tumor diagnosis and therapy; most of them have great absorption in the liver and spleen. This might induce side effects to normal tissues and organs. Therefore, the excellent targeting efficiency to tumor is of great promise. Secondly, multifunctional SiNPs are in the early stage for tumor diagnosis and therapy. With different functions, the multifunctional SiNPs can accurately detect/arrive tumor sites and then kill the tumor cells.

Importantly, the therapy efficiency can also be monitored. By carefully designing of the multifunctional SiNPs, it will be of significance to accomplish all the necessary functions in one SiNP composite. Thirdly, the biocompatibility and toxicity of the SiNPs to normal tissues of rodents and primates need extensive investigation. Several investigations in SiNP toxicity have been recently carried out by different groups; however, it is premature to make a general conclusion on the toxicity of the SiNPs in biosystems. Much research needs to be done before the realization of the great potential of novel SiNPs in biomedical applications. For example, a systemic investigation for the toxicity *in vitro* and *in vivo* should be performed in small animals and primates. We look forward to witnessing more promising discoveries for tumor diagnosis and therapy using novel silica nanomaterials.

We have provided a brief overview of the immobilization of the functional molecules on the MSNs' surfaces by layer-by-layer methods, covalent linkage, or electrostatic interaction. The composite nanomaterials create various possibilities where both sophisticated functions of the molecules shells and mechanical stability of MSN cores are fulfilled. It is clear from the introduced work that functional molecules coated MSNs are stable and biocompatible. Moreover, such nanocomposites display much potential applications in biomedical field, such as photodynamic therapy, cell imaging, and selective recognition. These strategies might be universal methods for constructing hybrid organic–inorganic nanomaterials, which can be widely applied in biomedical field.

REFERENCES

1. Y. Zhao, B.G. Trewyn, I.I. Slowing, V.S.Y. Lin, Mesoporous silica nanoparticle-based double drug delivery system for glucose-responsive controlled release of insulin and cyclic AMP, *J. Am. Chem. Soc.* 131 (2009) 8398–8400.
2. Y.B. Patil, S.K. Swaminathan, T. Sadhukha, L. Ma, J. Panyam, The use of nanoparticle-mediated targeted gene silencing and drug delivery to overcome tumor drug resistance, *Biomaterials* 31 (2010) 358–365.
3. W. Fang, J. Yang, J. Gong, N. Zheng, Photo- and pH-triggered release of anticancer drugs from mesoporous silica-coated Pd@Ag nanoparticles, *Adv. Funct. Mater.* 22 (2012) 842–848.
4. Y. Klichko, M. Liong, E. Choi, S. Angelos, A.E. Nel, J.F. Stoddart, et al., Mesostructured silica for optical functionality, nanomachines, and drug delivery, *J. Am. Ceram. Soc.* 92 (2009) S2–S10.
5. J.H. Kim, Y.-W. Noh, M.B. Heo, M.Y. Cho, Y.T. Lim, Multifunctional hybrid nanoconjugates for efficient in vivo delivery of immunomodulating oligonucleotides and enhanced antitumor immunity, *Angew. Chem. Int. Ed.* 51 (2012) 9670–9673.
6. V. Bagalkot, X. Gao, siRNA-aptamer chimeras on nanoparticles: preserving targeting functionality for effective gene silencing, *ACS Nano.* 5 (2011) 8131–8139.
7. N.P. Sardesai, J.C. Barron, J.F. Rusling, Carbon nanotube microwell array for sensitive electrochemiluminescent detection of cancer biomarker proteins, *Anal. Chem.* 83 (2011) 6698–6703.
8. T. Chen, M.I. Shukoor, R. Wang, Z. Zhao, Q. Yuan, S. Bamrungsap, et al., Smart multifunctional nanostructure for targeted cancer chemotherapy and magnetic resonance imaging, *ACS Nano.* 5 (2011) 7866–7873.
9. Y. Gao, C. Yang, X. Liu, R. Ma, D. Kong, L. Shi, A multifunctional nanocarrier based on nanogated mesoporous silica for enhanced tumorspecific uptake and intracellular delivery, *Macromol. Biosci.* 12 (2012) 251–259.
10. S. Unezaki, K. Maruyama, J.-I. Hosoda, I. Nagae, Y. Koyanagi, M. Nakata, et al., Direct measurement of the extravasation of polyethyleneglycolcoated liposomes into solid tumor tissue by in vivo fluorescence microscopy, *Int. J. Pharm.* 144 (1996) 11–17.
11. T. Xia, M. Kovochich, M. Liong, H. Meng, S. Kabehie, S. George, et al., Polyethyleneimine coating enhances the cellular uptake of mesoporous silica nanoparticles and allows safe delivery of siRNA and DNA constructs, *ACS Nano.* 3 (2009) 3273–3286.
12. X. Wu, X. He, K. Wang, C. Xie, B. Zhou, Z. Qing, Ultrasmall near-infrared gold nanoclusters for tumor fluorescence imaging in vivo, *Nanoscale* 2 (2010) 2244–2249.
13. S. Gordon, E. Teichmann, K. Young, K. Finnie, T. Rades, S. Hook, In vitro and in vivo investigation of thermosensitive chitosan hydrogels containing silica nanoparticles for vaccine delivery, *Eur. J. Pharm. Sci.* 41 (2010) 360–368.
14. X. Gao, Y. Cui, R.M. Levenson, L.W. Chung, S. Nie, In vivo cancer targeting and imaging with semiconductor quantum dots, *Nat. Biotechnol.* 22 (2004) 969–976.
15. Y.C. Cheng, A. Samia, J.D. Meyers, I. Panagopoulos, B. Fei, C. Burda, Highly efficient drug delivery with gold nanoparticle vectors for in vivo photodynamic therapy of cancer, *J. Am. Chem. Soc.* 130 (2008) 10643–10647.
16. X. Michalet, F.F. Pinaud, L.A. Bentolila, J.M. Tsay, S. Doose, J.J. Li, et al., Quantum dots for live cells, in vivo imaging, and diagnostics, *Science* 307 (2005) 538–544.
17. H.K. Moon, S.H. Lee, H.C. Choi, In vivo near-infrared mediated tumor destruction by photothermal effect of carbon nanotubes, *ACS Nano.* 3 (2009) 3707–3713.
18. M. Lewin, N. Carlesso, C.H. Tung, X.W. Tang, D. Cory, D.T. Scadden, et al., Tat peptide-derivatized magnetic nanoparticles allow in vivo tracking and recovery of progenitor cells, *Nat. Biotechnol.* 18 (2000) 410–414.
19. Z. Cao, R. Tong, A. Mishra, W. Xu, G.C.L. Wong, J. Cheng, et al., Reversible cell-specific drug delivery with aptamer-functionalized liposomes, *Angew. Chem. Int. Ed.* 48 (2009) 6494–6498.
20. S.H. Wu, Y. Hung, C.Y.Mou, Mesoporous silica nanoparticles as nanocarriers, *Chem. Commun.* 47 (2011) 9972–9985.
21. B. Sumer, J. Gao, Theranostic nanomedicine for cancer, *Nanomedicine* 3 (2008) 137–140.
22. A. Louie, Multimodality imaging probes: design and challenges, *Chem. Rev.* 110 (2010) 3146–3195.
23. J.M. Rosenholm, C. Sahlgren, M. Linden, Multifunctional mesoporous silica nanoparticles for combined therapeutic, diagnostic and targeted action in cancer treatment, *Curr. Drug Targets* 12 (2011) 1166–1186.
24. B.G. Trewyn, S. Giri, I.I. Slowing, V.S.Y. Lin, Mesoporous silica nanoparticle based controlled release, drug delivery, and biosensor systems, *Chem. Commun.* 31 (2007) 3236–3245.
25. I.I. Slowing, J.L. Vivero-Escoto, C.-W. Wu, V.S.Y. Lin, Mesoporous silica nanoparticles as controlled release drug delivery and gene transfection carriers, *Adv. Drug. Deliv. Rev.* 60 (2008) 1278–1288.

26. S.W. Bae, W. Tan, J.I. Hong, Fluorescent dye-doped silica nanoparticles: new tools for bioapplications, *Chem. Commun.* 48 (2012) 2270–2282.

27. Z. Li, J.C. Barnes, A. Bosoy, J.F. Stoddart, J.I. Zink, Mesoporous silica nanoparticles in biomedical applications, *Chem. Soc. Rev.* 41 (2012) 2590–2605.

28. Y. Gao, Y. Chen, X. Ji, X. He, Q. Yin, Z. Zhang, et al., Controlled intracellular release of doxorubicin in multidrug-resistant cancer cells by tuning the shell-pore sizes of mesoporous silica nanoparticles, *ACS Nano.* 5 (2011) 9788–9798.

29. N. Singh, A. Karambelkar, L. Gu, K. Lin, J.S. Miller, C.S. Chen, et al., Bioresponsive mesoporous silica nanoparticles for triggered drug release, *J. Am. Chem. Soc.* 133 (2011) 19582–19585.

30. X. He, X. Wu, K. Wang, B. Shi, L. Hai, Methylene blue-encapsulated phosphonate-terminated silica nanoparticles for simultaneous in vivo imaging and photodynamic therapy, *Biomaterials* 30 (2009) 5601–5609.

31. J.K. Herr, J.E. Smith, C.D. Medley, D. Shangguan, W. Tan, Aptamerconjugated nanoparticles for selective collection and detection of cancer cells, *Anal. Chem.* 78 (2006) 2918–2924.

32. J. Lu, Z. Li, J.I. Zink, F. Tamanoi, In vivo tumor suppression efficacy of mesoporous silica nanoparticles-based drug-delivery system: enhanced efficacy by folate modification, *Nanomedicine* 8 (2012) 212–220.

33. X. He, H. Nie, K. Wang, W. Tan, X. Wu, P. Zhang, In vivo study of biodistribution and urinary excretion of surface-modified silica nanoparticles, *Anal. Chem.* 80 (2008) 9597–9603.

34. T. Liu, L. Li, X. Teng, X. Huang, H. Liu, D. Chen, et al., Single and repeated dose toxicity of mesoporous hollow silica nanoparticles in intravenously exposed mice, *Biomaterials* 32 (2011) 1657–1668.

35. R. Kumar, I. Roy, T.Y. Ohulchanskyy, L.N. Goswami, A.C. Bonoiu, E.J. Bergey, et al., Covalently dye-linked, surface-controlled, and bioconjugated organically modified silica nanoparticles as targeted probes for optical imaging, *ACS Nano.* 2 (2008) 449–456.

36. X. Wang, S. Yao, H.Y. Ahn, Y. Zhang, M.V. Bondar, J.A. Torres, et al., Folate receptor targeting silica nanoparticle probe for two-photon fluorescence bioimaging, *Biomed. Opt. Expr.* 1 (2010) 453–462.

37. C.D. Medley, S. Bamrungsap, W. Tan, J.E. Smith, Aptamer-conjugated nanoparticles for cancer cell detection, *Anal. Chem.* 83 (2011) 727–734.

38. M. Liong, J. Lu, M. Kovochich, T. Xia, S.G. Ruehm, A.E. Nel, et al., Multifunctional inorganic nanoparticles for imaging, targeting, and drug delivery, *ACS Nano.* 2 (2008) 889–896.

39. W.X. Mai, H. Meng, Mesoporous silica nanoparticles: a multifunctional nano therapeutic system, *Integr. Biol.* 5 (2013) 19–28.

40. Y. Matsumura, H. Maeda, A new concept for macromolecular therapeutics in cancer chemotherapy: mechanism of tumoritropic accumulation of proteins and the antitumor agent smancs, *Cancer Res.* 46 (1986) 6387–6392.

41. K.M.L. Taylor, J.S. Kim, W.J. Rieter, H. An, W. Lin, W. Lin, Mesoporous silica nanospheres as highly efficient MRI contrast agents, *J. Am. Chem. Soc.* 130 (2008) 2154–2155.

42. J.S. Kim, W.J. Rieter, K.M.L. Taylor, H. An, W. Lin, W. Lin, Self-assembled hybrid nanoparticles for cancer-specific multimodal imaging, *J. Am. Chem. Soc.* 129 (2007) 8962–8963.

43. X. Huang, F. Zhang, H. Wang, G. Niu, K.Y. Choi, M. Swierczewska, et al., Mesenchymal stem cell-based cell engineering with multifunctional mesoporous silica nanoparticles for tumor delivery, *Biomaterials* 34 (2013) 1772–1780.

44. L. Pan, Q. He, J. Liu, Y. Chen, M. Ma, L. Zhang, et al., Nuclear-targeted drug delivery of TAT peptide-conjugated monodisperse mesoporous silica nanoparticles, *J. Am. Chem. Soc.* 134 (2012) 5722–5725.

45. D.P. Ferris, J. Lu, C. Gothard, R. Yanes, C.R. Thomas, J.C. Olsen, et al., Synthesis of biomolecule-modified mesoporous silica nanoparticles for targeted hydrophobic drug delivery to cancer cells, *Small* 7 (2011) 1816–1826.

46. J. Peng, X. He, K. Wang, W. Tan, H. Li, X. Xing, et al., An antisense oligonucleotide carrier based on amino silica nanoparticles for antisense inhibition of cancer cells, *Nanomedicine* 2 (2006) 113–120.

47. R. Joshi, V. Feldmann, W. Koestner, C. Detje, S. Gottschalk, H.A. Mayer, et al., Multifunctional silica nanoparticles for optical and magnetic resonance imaging, *Biol. Chem.* 394 (2013) 125–135.

48. J. Lu, M. Liong, Z. Li, J.I. Zink, F. Tamanoi, Biocompatibility, biodistribution, and drug-delivery efficiency of mesoporous silica nanoparticles for cancer therapy in animals, *Small* 6 (2010) 1794–1805.

49. J.E. Lee, N. Lee, H. Kim, J. Kim, S.H. Choi, J.H. Kim, et al., Uniform mesoporous dye-doped silica nanoparticles decorated with multiple magnetite nanocrystals for simultaneous enhanced magnetic resonance imaging, fluorescence imaging, and drug delivery, *J. Am. Chem. Soc.* 132 (2009) 552–557.

50. H.M. Liu, S.H. Wu, Lu CW, Yao M, Hsiao JK, Hung Y, et al., Mesoporous silica nanoparticles improve magnetic labeling efficiency in human stem cells, *Small* 4 (2008) 619–626.

51. L. Li, F. Tang, H. Liu, T. Liu, N. Hao, D. Chen, et al., In vivo delivery of silica nanorattle encapsulated docetaxel for liver cancer therapy with low toxicity and high efficacy, *ACS Nano.* 4 (2010) 6874–6882.

52. F. Lu, S.-H. Wu, Y. Hung, C.-Y. Mou, Size effect on cell uptake in wellsuspended, uniform mesoporous silica nanoparticles, *Small* 5 (2009) 1408–1413.

53. F. Tang, L. Li, D. Chen, Mesoporous silica nanoparticles: synthesis, biocompatibility and drug delivery, *Adv. Mater.* 24 (2012) 1504–1534.

54. R.P. Bagwe, C. Yang, L.R. Hilliard, W. Tan, Optimization of dye-doped silica nanoparticles prepared using a reverse microemulsion method, *Langmuir* 20 (2004) 8336–8342.

55. Y. Jin, S. Lohstreter, D.T. Pierce, J. Parisien, M. Wu, C. Hall, et al., Silica nanoparticles with continuously tunable sizes: synthesis and size effects on cellular contrast imaging, *Chem. Mater.* 20 (2008) 4411–4419.

56. L.M. Rossi, L. Shi, F.H. Quina, Z. Rosenzweig, Stober synthesis of monodispersed luminescent silica nanoparticles for bioanalytical assays, *Langmuir* 21 (2005) 4277–4280.

57. D. Napierska, L.C.J. Thomassen, V. Rabolli, D. Lison, L. Gonzalez, M. Kirsch-Volders, et al., Size-dependent cytotoxicity of monodisperse silica nanoparticles in human endothelial cells, *Small* 5 (2009) 846–853.

58. V. Torchilin, Tumor delivery of macromolecular drugs based on the EPR effect, *Adv. Drug Deliv. Rev.* 63 (2011) 131–135.

59. N.S. Wilson, B. Yang, A. Yang, S. Loeser, S. Marsters, D. Lawrence, et al., An Fcgamma receptor-dependent mechanism drives antibody-mediated target-receptor signaling in cancer cells, *Cancer Cell* 19 (2011) 101–113.

60. B.R. Smith, Z. Cheng, A. De, A.L. Koh, R. Sinclair, S.S. Gambhir, Real-time intravital imaging of RGD-quantum dot binding to luminal endothelium in mouse tumor neovasculature, *Nano Lett.* 8 (2008) 2599–2606.

61. F. Porta, G.E.M. Lamers, J. Morrhayim, A. Chatzopoulou, M. Schaaf, H. den Dulk, et al., Folic acid-modified mesoporous silica nanoparticles for cellular and nuclear targeted drug delivery, *Adv. Healthcare Mater.* 2 (2012) 281–286.

62. S. Dhar, N. Kolishetti, S.J. Lippard, O.C. Farokhzad, Targeted delivery of a cisplatin prodrug for safer and more effective prostate cancer therapy in vivo, *Proc. Natl. Acad. Sci.* 108 (2011) 1850–1855.

63. L. Wang, W. Zhao, W. Tan, Bioconjugated silica nanoparticles: development and applications, *Nano Res.* 1 (2008) 99–115.

64. M.A. Calfon, A. Rosenthal, G. Mallas, A. Mauskapf, R.N. Nudelman, V. Ntziachristos, et al., In vivo near infrared fluorescence (NIRF) intravascular molecular imaging of inflammatory plaque, a multimodal approach to imaging of atherosclerosis, *J. Vis. Exp.* 54 (2011) e2257.

65. J. Condeelis, R. Weissleder, In vivo imaging in cancer, *Cold Spring Harb. Perspect. Biol.* 2 (2010) a003848.

66. V.A. Oleinikov, Semiconductor fluorescent nanocrystals (quantum dots) in biological biochips, *Bioorg. Khim.* 37 (2011) 171–189.

67. X. Zhao, R. Tapec-Dytioco, W. Tan, Ultrasensitive DNA detection using highly fluorescent bioconjugated nanoparticles, *J. Am. Chem. Soc.* 125: (2003) 11474–11475.

68. S. Santra, P. Zhang, K. Wang, R. Tapec, W. Tan, Conjugation of biomolecules with luminophore-doped silica nanoparticles for photostable biomarkers, *Anal. Chem.* 73 (2001) 4988–4993.

69. S. Veeranarayanan, A. Cheruvathoor Poulose, S. Mohamed, A. Aravind, Y. Nagaoka, Y. Yoshida, et al., FITC labeled silica nanoparticles as efficient cell tags: uptake and photostability study in endothelial cells, *J. Fluoresc.* 22 (2012) 537–548.

70. C.-L. Zhu, C.-H. Lu, Song X-Y, Yang H-H, Wang X-R. Bioresponsive controlled release using mesoporous silica nanoparticles capped with aptamer-based molecular gate, *J. Am. Chem. Soc.* 133 (2011) 1278–1281.

71. X. He, Y. Zhao, D. He, K. Wang, F. Xu, J. Tang, ATP-responsive controlled release system using aptamer-functionalized mesoporous silica nanoparticles, *Langmuir* 28 (2012) 12909–12915.

72. C.-P. Tsai, C.-Y. Chen, Y. Hung, F.-H. Chang, C.-Y. Mou, Monoclonal antibody-functionalized mesoporous silica nanoparticles (MSN) for selective targeting breast cancer cells, *J. Mater. Chem.* 19 (2009) 5737–5743.

73. P. Wu, X. He, K. Wang, W. Tan, D. Ma, W. Yang, et al., Imaging breast cancer cells and tissues using peptide-labeled fluorescent silica nanoparticles, *J. Nanosci. Nanotechnol.* 8 (2008) 2483–2487.

74. V. Lebret, L. Raehm, J.O. Durand, M. Smaihi, M.H. Werts, M. Blanchard-Desce, et al., Folic acid-targeted mesoporous silica nanoparticles for two-photon fluorescence, *J. Biomed. Nanotechnol.* 6 (2010) 176–180.

75. A.B. Iliuk, L. Hu, W.A. Tao, Aptamer in bioanalytical applications, *Anal. Chem.* 83 (2011) 4440–4452.

76. J. Qian, D. Wang, F. Cai, Q. Zhan, Y. Wang, S. He, Photosensitizer encapsulated organically modified silica nanoparticles for direct two photon photodynamic therapy and in vivo functional imaging, *Biomaterials* 33 (2012) 4851–4860.

77. R. Shukla, N. Chanda, A. Zambre, A. Upendran, K. Katti, R.R. Kulkarni, et al., Laminin receptor specific therapeutic gold nanoparticles (198AuNP-EGCg) show efficacy in treating prostate cancer, *Proc. Natl. Acad. Sci.* 109 (2012) 12426–12431.

78. X. Huang, Y. Luo, Z. Li, B. Li, H. Zhang, L. Li, et al., Biolabeling hematopoietic system cells using near-infrared fluorescent gold nanoclusters, *J. Phys. Chem. C* 115 (2011) 16753–16763.

79. G. Hong, J.T. Robinson, Y. Zhang, S. Diao, A.L. Antaris, Q. Wang, et al., In vivo fluorescence imaging with Ag2S quantum dots in the second near infrared region, *Angew. Chem. Int. Ed.* 124 (2012) 9956–9959.

80. L.Q. Xiong, Z.G. Chen, M.X. Yu, F.Y. Li, C. Liu, C.H. Huang, Synthesis, characterization, and in vivo targeted imaging of amine-functionalized rare-earth up-converting nanophosphors, *Biomaterials* 30 (2009) 5592–5600.

81. L. Xiong, Z. Chen, Q. Tian, T. Cao, C. Xu, F. Li, High contrast upconversion luminescence targeted imaging in vivo using peptide-labeled nanophosphors, *Anal. Chem.* 81 (2009) 8687–8694.

82. B.-H. Jun, D.W. Hwang, H.S. Jung, J. Jang, H. Kim, H. Kang, et al., Ultrasensitive, biocompatible, quantum-dot-embedded silica nanoparticles for bioimaging, *Adv. Funct. Mater.* 22 (2012) 1843–1849.

83. R. Koole, M.M. van Schooneveld, J. Hilhorst, K. Castermans, D.P. Cormode, G.J. Strijkers, et al., Paramagnetic lipid-coated silica nanoparticles with a fluorescent quantum dot core: a new contrast agent platform for multimodality imaging, *Bioconjug. Chem.* 19 (2008) 2471–2479.

84. J. Kim, H.S. Kim, N. Lee, T. Kim, H. Kim, T. Yu, et al., Multifunctional uniform nanoparticles composed of a magnetite nanocrystal core and a mesoporous silica shell for magnetic resonance and fluorescence imaging and for drug delivery, *Angew. Chem. Int. Ed.* 47 (2008) 8438–84341.

85. C.W. Lu, Y. Hung, J.K. Hsiao, M. Yao, T.H. Chung, Y.S. Lin, et al., Bifunctional magnetic silica nanoparticles for highly efficient human stem cell labeling, *Nano Lett.* 7 (2007) 149–154.

86. J. Lu, M. Liong, J.I. Zink, F. Tamanoi, Mesoporous silica nanoparticles as a delivery system for hydrophobic anticancer drugs, *Small* 3 (2007) 1341–1346.

87. C.H. Tsai, J.L. Vivero-Escoto, I.I. Slowing, I.J. Fang, B.G. Trewyn, V.S. Lin, Surfactant-assisted controlled release of hydrophobic drugs using anionic surfactant templated mesoporous silica nanoparticles, *Biomaterials* 32 (2011) 6234–6244.

88. X. He, L. Hai, J. Su, K. Wang, X. Wu, One-pot synthesis of sustainedreleased doxorubicin silica nanoparticles for aptamer targeted delivery to tumor cells, *Nanoscale* 3 (2011) 2936–2942.

89. C.Y. Lai, B.G. Trewyn, D.M. Jeftinija, K. Jeftinija, S. Xu, S. Jeftinija, et al., A mesoporous silica nanosphere-based carrier system with chemically removable CdS nanoparticle caps for stimuli-responsive controlled release of neurotransmitters and drug molecules, *J. Am. Chem. Soc.* 125 (2003) 4451–4459.

90. C. Chen, J. Geng, F. Pu, X. Yang, J. Ren, X. Qu, Polyvalent nucleic acid/mesoporous silica nanoparticle conjugates: dual stimuli-responsive vehicles for intracellular drug delivery, *Angew. Chem. Int. Ed.* 50 (2011) 882–886.

91. H. Meng, M. Xue, T. Xia, Y.-L. Zhao, F. Tamanoi, J.F. Stoddart, et al., Autonomous in vitro anticancer drug release from mesoporous silica nanoparticles by pH-sensitive nanovalves, *J Am. Chem. Soc.* 132 (2010) 12690–12697.

92. R. Liu, Y. Zhang, X. Zhao, A. Agarwal, L.J. Mueller, P. Feng, pH Responsive nanogated ensemble based on gold-capped mesoporous silica through an acid-labile acetal linker, *J. Am. Chem. Soc.* 132 (2010) 1500–1501.

93. I. Roy, T.Y. Ohulchanskyy, H.E. Pudavar, E.J. Bergey, A.R. Oseroff, J. Morgan, et al., Ceramic-based nanoparticles entrapping water-insoluble photosensitizing anticancer drugs: a novel drug-carrier system for photodynamic therapy, *J. Am. Chem. Soc.* 125 (2003) 7860–7865.

94. S. Kim, T.Y. Ohulchanskyy, H.E. Pudavar, R.K. Pandey, P.N. Prasad, Organically modified silica nanoparticles co-encapsulating photosensitizing drug and aggregation-enhanced two-photon absorbing fluorescent dye aggregates for two-photon photodynamic therapy, *J. Am. Chem. Soc.* 129 (2007) 2669–2675.

95. T.Y. Ohulchanskyy, I. Roy, L.N. Goswami, Y. Chen, E.J. Bergey, R.K. Pandey, et al., Organically modified silica nanoparticles with covalently incorporated photosensitizer for photodynamic therapy of cancer, *Nano Lett.* 7 (2007) 2835–2842.

96. P. Zhang, W. Steelant, M. Kumar, M. Scholfield, Versatile photosensitizers for photodynamic therapy at infrared excitation, *J. Am. Chem. Soc.* 129 (2007) 4526–4527.

97. M. Gary-Bobo, O. Hocine, D. Brevet, M. Maynadier, L. Raehm, S. Richeter, et al., Cancer therapy improvement with mesoporous silica nanoparticles combining targeting, drug delivery and PDT, *Int. J. Pharm.* 423 (2012) 509–515.

98. J. Zhu, H. Wang, L. Liao, L. Zhao, L. Zhou, M. Yu, et al., Small mesoporous silica nanoparticles as carriers for enhanced photodynamic therapy, *Chem. Asian J.* 6: (2011) 2332–2338.

99. X.X. He, K. Wang, W. Tan, B. Liu, X. Lin, C. He, et al., Bioconjugated nanoparticles for DNA protection from cleavage, *J. Am. Chem. Soc.* 125 (2003) 7168–7169.

100. H. Meng, M. Liong, T. Xia, Z. Li, Z. Ji, J.I. Zink, et al., Engineered design of mesoporous silica nanoparticles to deliver doxorubicin and P-glycoprotein siRNA to overcome drug resistance in a cancer cell line, *ACS Nano.* 4 (2010) 4539–4550.

101. A.M. Chen, M. Zhang, D. Wei, D. Stueber, O. Taratula, T. Minko, et al., Co-delivery of doxorubicin and Bcl-2 siRNA by mesoporous silica nanoparticles enhances the efficacy of chemotherapy in multidrug-resistant cancer cells, *Small* 5 (2009) 2673–2677.

102. Q. Zhang, F. Liu, K.T. Nguyen, X. Ma, X. Wang, B. Xing, et al., Multifunctional mesoporous silica nanoparticles for cancer-targeted and controlled drug delivery, *Adv. Funct. Mater.* 22 (2012) 5144–5156.

103. N. Lee, H.R. Cho, M.H. Oh, S.H. Lee, K. Kim, B.H. Kim, et al., Multifunctional Fe_3O_4/TaO(x) core/shell nanoparticles for simultaneous magnetic resonance imaging and X-ray computed tomography, *J. Am. Chem. Soc.* 134 (2012) 10309–10312.

104. H. Meng, W.X. Mai, H. Zhang, M. Xue, T. Xia, S. Lin, et al., Co-delivery of an optimal drug/siRNA combination using mesoporous silica nanoparticles to overcome drug resistance in breast cancer in vitro and in vivo, *ACS Nano.* 7 (2013) 994–1005.

105. J.M. Rosenholm, C. Sahlgren, M. Linden, Towards multifunctional, targeted drug delivery systems using mesoporous silica nanoparticles – opportunities & challenges, *Nanoscale* 2 (2010) 1870–1883.

106. H. Benachour, A. Seve, T. Bastogne, C. Frochot, R. Vanderesse, J. Jasniewski, et al., Multifunctional peptide-conjugated hybrid silica nanoparticles for photodynamic therapy and MRI, *Theranostics* 2 (2012) 889–904.

107. A. Mignot, C. Truillet, F. Lux, L. Sancey, C. Louis, F. Denat, et al., Atop-down synthesis route to ultrasmall multifunctional Gd-based silica nanoparticles for theranostic applications, *Chem. Asian J.* 19 (2013) 6122–6136.

108. N.-T. Chen, S.-H. Cheng, J.S. Souris, C.-T. Chen, C.-Y. Mou, L.-W. Lo, Theranostic applications of mesoporous silica nanoparticles and their organic/inorganic hybrids, *J. Mater. Chem. B* 1 (2013) 3128–3135.

109. X. Wang, H. Chen, Y. Zheng, M. Ma, Y. Chen, K. Zhang, et al., Aunanoparticle coated mesoporous silica nanocapsule-based multifunctional platform for ultrasound mediated imaging, cytoclasis and tumor ablation, *Biomaterials* 34 (2013) 2057–2068.

110. Y. Chen, H. Chen, D. Zeng, Y. Tian, F. Chen, J. Feng, et al., Core/shell structured hollow mesoporous nanocapsules: a potential platform for simultaneous cell imaging and anticancer drug delivery, *ACS Nano.* 4 (2010) 6001–6013.

111. P. Huang, L. Bao, C. Zhang, J. Lin, T. Luo, D. Yang, et al., Folic acid-conjugated silica-modified gold nanorods for X-ray/CT imaging-guided dual-mode radiation and photothermal therapy, *Biomaterials* 32 (2011) 9796–9809.

112. R. Huschka, J. Zuloaga, M.W. Knight, L.V. Brown, P. Nordlander, N.J. Halas, Light-induced release of DNA from gold nanoparticles: nanoshells and nanorods, *J. Am. Chem. Soc.* 133 (2011) 12247–12255.

113. Z. Zhang, L. Wang, J. Wang, X. Jiang, X. Li, Z. Hu, et al., Mesoporous silica-coated gold nanorods as a light-mediated multifunctional theranostic platform for cancer treatment, *Adv. Mater.* 24 (2012) 1418–1423.

114. Z. Zhao, Y. Han, C. Lin, D. Hu, F. Wang, X. Chen, et al., Multifunctional core–shell upconverting nanoparticles for imaging and photodynamic therapy of liver cancer cells, *Chem. Asian J.* 7 (2012) 830–837.

115. R. Bardhan, S. Lal, A. Joshi, N.J. Halas, Theranostic nanoshells: from probe design to imaging and treatment of cancer, *Acc. Chem. Res.* 44 (2011) 936–946.

116. Q. He, Z. Zhang, F. Gao, Y. Li, J. Shi, In vivo biodistribution and urinary excretion of mesoporous silica nanoparticles: effects of particle size and PEGylation, *Small* 7 (2011) 271–280.

117. Z. Tao, B.B. Toms, J. Goodisman, T. Asefa, Mesoporosity and functional group dependent endocytosis and cytotoxicity of silica nanomaterials, *Chem. Res. Toxicol.* 22 (2009) 1869–1880.

118. Q. He, J. Zhang, J. Shi, Z. Zhu, L. Zhang, W. Bu, et al., The effect of PEGylation of mesoporous silica nanoparticles on nonspecific binding of serum proteins and cellular responses, *Biomaterials* 31 (2010) 1085–1092.

119. J.S. Beck, J.C. Vartuli, W.J. Roth, M.E. Leonowicz, C.T. Kresge, K.D. Schmitt, et al., *J. Am. Chem. Soc.* 114 (1992) 10834–10843.

120. C.T. Kresge, M.E. Leonowicz, W.J. Roth, J.C. Vartuli, J.S. Beck, *Nature* 359 (1992) 710–712.

121. Y. Wan, D. Zhao, *Chem. Rev.* 107 (2007) 2821–2860.

122. J. Shi, *Chem. Rev.* 113 (2013) 2139–2181.

123. A. Stein, *Adv. Mater.* 15 (2003) 763–775.

124. M.E. Davis, *Nature* 417 (2002) 813–821.

125. A. Sayari, *Chem. Mater.* 8 (1996) 1840–1852.

126. P. Yang, S. Gai, J. Lin, *Chem. Soc. Rev.* 41 (2012) 3679–3698.

127. S. Wang, *Micropor. Mesopor. Mat.* 117 (2009) 1–9.

128. M. Vallet-Regi, A. Rámila, R.P. del Real, J. Pérez-Pariente, *Chem. Mater.* 13 (2000) 308–311.

129. Q. Cai, Z.-S. Luo, W.-Q. Pang, Y.-W. Fan, X.-H. Chen, F.-Z. Cui, *Chem. Mater.* 13 (2001) 258–263.

130. L. Zhang, S. Qiao, Y. Jin, L. Cheng, Z. Yan, G.Q. Lu, *Adv. Funct. Mater.* 18 (2008) 3834–3842.

131. Y. Yang, X. Yan, Y. Cui, Q. He, D. Li, A. Wang, et al., *J. Mater. Chem.* 18 (2008) 5731–5737.

132. B.G. Trewyn, I.I. Slowing, S. Giri, H.-T. Chen, V.S.Y. Lin, *Acc. Chem. Res.* 40 (2007) 846–853.

133. Y.-w. Jun, J.-w. Seo, J. Cheon, *Acc. Chem. Res.* 41 (2008) 179–189.

134. Y.-S. Lin, C.-P. Tsai, H.-Y. Huang, C.-T. Kuo, Y. Hung, D.-M. Huang, et al., *Chem. Mater.* 17 (2005) 4570–4573.

135. Y. Yang, W. Song, A. Wang, P. Zhu, J. Fei, J. Li, *Phys. Chem. Chem. Phys.* 12 (2010):4418–4422.

136. Y. Yang, Y. Jia, L. Gao, J.B. Fei, L.R. Dai, J. Zhao, et al., *Chem. Commun.* 47 (2011) 12167–12169.

137. S. Gai, P. Yang, D. Wang, C. Li, X. Li, et al., *J. Mater. Chem.* 21 (2011) 16420–16426.

138. I.I. Slowing, C.-W. Wu, J.L. Vivero-Escoto, V.S.Y. Lin, *Small* 5 (2009) 57–62.

139. Y.-S. Lin, C.L. Haynes, *J. Am. Chem. Soc.* 132 (2010) 4834–4842.

140. Q. He, J. Shi, M. Zhu, Y. Chen, F. Chen, *Micropor. Mesopor. Mat.* 131 (2010) 314–320.

141. V. Cauda, A. Schlossbauer, T. Bein, *Micropor. Mesopor. Mat.* 132 (2010) 60–71.

142. J. Lu, M. Liong, Z. Li, J.I. Zink, F. Tamanoi, *Small* 6 (2010) 1794–1805.

143. S.P. Hudson, R.F. Padera, R. Langer, D.S. Kohane, *Biomaterials* 29 (2008) 4045–4055.

144. J.S. Souris, C.-H. Lee, S.-H. Cheng, C.-T. Chen, C.-S. Yang, J.-a.A. Ho, et al., *Biomaterials* 31 (2010) 5564–5574.

145. C.-Y. Lai, B.G. Trewyn, D.M. Jeftinija, K. Jeftinija, S. Xu, S. Jeftinija, et al., *J. Am. Chem. Soc.* 125 (2003) 4451–4459.

146. S. Giri, B.G. Trewyn, M.P. Stellmaker, V.S.Y. Lin, *Angew. Chem. Int. Ed.* 44 (2005) 5038–5044.

147. F. Torney, B.G. Trewyn, V.S.Y. Lin, K. Wang, *Nat Nanotechnol* 2 (2007) 295–300.

148. K. Patel, S. Angelos, W.R. Dichtel, A. Coskun, Y.W. Yang, J.I. Zink, et al., *J. Am. Chem. Soc.* 130 (2008) 2382–2383.

149. H. Kim, S. Kim, C. Park, H. Lee, H.J. Park, C. Kim, *Adv. Mater.* 22 (2010) 4280–4283.

150. L. Du, S. Liao, H.A. Khatib, J.F. Stoddart, J.I. Zink, *J. Am. Chem. Soc.* 131 (2009) 15136–15142.

151. S. Scanlon, A. Aggeli, *Nano Today* 3 (2008) 22–30.

152. Q. He, J. Li, *Adv. Colloid Interface Sci.* 131 (2007) 91–98.

153. Q. He, Y. Cui, J. Li, *Chem. Soc. Rev.* 38 (2009) 2292–2303.

154. J. Li, H. Möhwald, Z. An, G. Lu, *Soft Matter* 1 (2005) 259–264.

155. Q. He, Y. Tian, H. Möhwald, J. Li, *Soft Matter* 5 (2009) 300–303.

156. W. Song, H. Möhwald, J. Li, *Biomaterials* 31 (2010) 1287–1292.

157. X. Yan, P. Zhu, J. Li, *Chem. Soc. Rev.* 39 (2010) 1877–1890.

158. Y. Cui, C. Tao, Y. Tian, Q. He, J. Li, *Langmuir* 22 (2006) 8205–8208.

159. Y. Cui, C. Tao, S. Zheng, Q. He, S. Ai, J. Li, *Macromol. Rapid Commun.* 26 (2005) 1552–1556.

160. D. Li, Y. Cui, K. Wang, Q. He, X. Yan, J. Li, *Adv. Funct. Mater.* 17 (2007) 3134–3140.

161. D. Li, Q. He, Y. Cui, K. Wang, X. Zhang, J. Li, *Chem. Eur. J.* 13 (2007) 2224–2229.

162. S. Huh, J.W. Wiench, J.-C. Yoo, M. Pruski, V.S.Y. Lin, *Chem. Mater.* 15 (2003) 4247–4256.

163. I. Slowing, B.G. Trewyn, S. Giri, V.S.Y. Lin, *Adv. Funct. Mater.* 17 (2007) 1225–1236.

164. B.G. Trewyn, C.M. Whitman, V.S.Y. Lin, *Nano Lett.* 4: (2004) 2139–2143.

165. M. Vallet-Regi, F. Balas, D. Arcos, *Angew. Chem. Int. Ed.* 46 (2007) 7548–7558.

166. Y. Zhao, X. Sun, G. Zhang, B.G. Trewyn, I.I. Slowing, V.S.Y. Lin, *ACS Nano.* 5 (2011) 1366–1375.

167. W. Qi, A. Wang, Y. Yang, M. Du, M.N. Bouchu, P. Boullanger, et al., *J. Mater. Chem.* 20 (2010) 2121–2127.

168. Z. An, H. Möhwald, J. Li, *Biomacromolecules* 7 (2006) 580–585.

169. Z. An, G. Lu, H. Möhwald, J. Li, *Chem. Eur. J.* 10 (2004) 5848–5852.

170. A.-L. Troutier, C. Ladavière, *Adv. Colloid Interface Sci.* 133 (2007) 1–21.

171. G. Lu, S. Ai, J. Li, *Langmuir* 21 (2005) 1679–1682.

172. X. Zhang, Q. He, Y. Cui, L. Duan, J. Li, *Biochem. Biophys. Res. Commun.* 349 (2006) 920–924.

173. X. Zhang, Q. He, X. Yan, P. Boullanger, J. Li, *Biochem. Biophys. Res. Commun.* 358 (2007) 424–428.

174. R. Rapuano, A.M. Carmona-Ribeiro, *J. Colloid Interface Sci.* 226 (2000) 299–307.

175. R. Rapuano, A.M. Carmona-Ribeiro, *J. Colloid Interface Sci.* 193 (1997) 104–111.

176. Gao L, Cui Y, He Q, Yang Y, Fei JB, Li JB. *Chem. Eur. J.* 17 (2011) 13170–13174.

177. Q. Wang, Z. Yang, Y. Gao, W. Ge, L. Wang, B. Xu, *Soft Matter* 4 (2008) 550–553.

178. K. Uto, K. Yamamoto, N. Kishimoto, M. Muraoka, T. Aoyagi, I. Yamashita, *J. Mater. Chem.* 18 (2008):3876–3884.

179. W. Qi, L. Duan, J. Li, *Soft Matter* 7 (2011) 1571–1576.

180. I. Hwang, K. Baek, M. Jung, Y. Kim, K.M. Park, D.-W. Lee, et al., *J. Am. Chem. Soc.* 129 (2007) 4170–4171.

181. A. Jayakrishnan, S.R. Jameela, *Biomaterials* 17 (1996) 471–484.

182. W. Qi, X. Yan, J. Fei, A. Wang, Y. Cui, J. Li, *Biomaterials* 30 (2009) 2799–2806.

183. L. Duan, Q. He, X. Yan, Y. Cui, K. Wang, J. Li, *Biochem. Biophys. Res. Commun.* 354 (2007) 357–362.

184. Y. Jia, J. Fei, Y. Cui, Y. Yang, L. Gao, J. Li, *Chem. Commun.* 47 (2011) 1175–1177.

185. W. Wei, L.Y. Wang, L. Yuan, Q. Wei, X.D. Yang, Z.G. Su, et al., *Adv. Funct. Mater.* 17 (2007) 3153–3158.

186. Y. Okada, F. Tanaka, *Macromolecules* 38 (2005) 4465–4471.

187. M. Karg, T. Hellweg, *Curr Opin Colloid Interface Sci.* 14 (2009) 438–450.

188. D. Li, Q. He, J. Li, *Adv. Colloid Interface Sci.* 149 (2009) 28–38.

189. D. Dubé, M. Francis, J.C. Leroux, F.M. Winnik, *Bioconjug. Chem.* 13 (2002) 685–692.

190. L. Dong, A.S. Hoffman, *J. Control Release* 15 (1991) 141–152.

191. S. Ohya, Y. Nakayama, T. Matsuda, *Biomacromolecules* 2 (2001) 856–863.

192. H.E. Canavan, X. Cheng, D.J. Graham, B.D. Ratner, D.G. Castner, *Langmuir* 21 (2005) 1949–1955.

193. T. Matsuda, M.J. Moghaddam, *Mater. Sci. Eng. C* 1 (1993) 37–43.

194. Y.-Z. You, K.K. Kalebaila, S.L. Brock, D. Oupický, *Chem. Mater.* 20 (2008) 3354–3359.

195. Y.N. Konan, R. Gurny, E. Allémann, *J. Photochem. Photobiol. B* 66: (2002) 89–106.

196. D.K. Chatterjee, L.S. Fong, Y. Zhang, *Adv. Drug Deliv. Rev.* 60 (2008):1627–1637.

197. T.J. Dougherty, C.J. Gomer, B.W. Henderson, G. Jori, D. Kessel, M. Korbelik, et al., *J. Natl. Cancer Inst.* 90 (1998) 889–905.

198. S. Wang, R. Gao, F. Zhou, M. Selke. *J. Mater. Chem.* 14 (2004) 487–493.

199. F. Yu, X. Tang, M. Pei, *Micropor. Mesopor. Mat.* 173 (2013) 64–69.

200. J.T. Sun, C.Y. Hong, C.Y. Pan, *J. Phys. Chem. C* 114 (2010) 12481–12486.

201. D. Peer, J.M. Karp, S. Hong, O.C. Farokhzad, R. Margalit, R. Langer, *Nat. Nanotechnol.* 2 (2007) 751–760.

202. J. Liu, Z. Cao, Y. Lu, *Chem. Rev.* 109 (2009) 1948–1998.

203. I. Smirnov, R.H. Shafer, *Biochemistry* 39 (2000) 1462–1468.

204. K.Y. Wang, S.H. Krawczyk, N. Bischofberger, S. Swaminathan, P.H. Bolton, *Biochemistry* 32 (1993) 11285–11292.

205. R.F. Macaya, P. Schultze, F.W. Smith, J.A. Roe, J. Feigon, *Proc. Natl. Acad. Sci. U. S. A.* 90 (1993) 3745–3749.

206. J.S. Palumbo, K.W. Kombrinck, A.F. Drew, T.S. Grimes, J.H. Kiser, J.L. Degen, et al., *Blood* 96 (2000) 3302–3309.

207. L. Hu, M. Lee, W. Campbell, R. Perez-Soler, S. Karpatkin, *Blood* 104 (2004) 2746–2751.

208. A. Russo, U.J.K. Soh, M.M. Paing, P. Arora, J. Trejo, *Proc. Natl. Acad. Sci. U. S. A.* 106 (2009) 6393–6397.

209. P. Arora, T.K. Ricks, J. Trejo, *J. Cell. Sci.* 120: (2007) 921–928.

210. X. Wu, M. Wu, J.X. Zhao, Recent development of silica nanoparticles as delivery vectors for cancer imaging and therapy, *Nanomed. Nanotechnol. Biol. Med.* 10 (2014) 297–312.

211. Y. Yang, J. Li, Lipid, protein and poly(NIPAM) coated mesoporous silica nanoparticles for biomedical applications, *Adv. Colloid Interface Sci.* 207 (2014) 155–163.

212. Loutfy H. Madkour, *Reactive Oxygen Species (ROS), Nanoparticles, and Endoplasmic Reticulum (ER) Stress-Induced Cell Death Mechanisms* (2020). Paperback ISBN: 9780128224816 Imprint: Academic Press. Published Date: 1st August 2020. https://www.elsevier.com/books/reactive-oxygen-species-ros-nanoparticles-and-endoplasmic-reticulum-er-stress-induced-cell-death-mechanisms/madkour/978-0-12-822481-6

213. Loutfy H. Madkour, *Nanoparticles Induce Oxidative and Endoplasmic Reticulum Antioxidant Therapeutic Defenses* (2020). Copyright 2020 Publisher Springer International Publishing Copyright Holder Springer Nature Switzerland AG eBook ISBN 978-3-030-37297-2. doi:10.1007/978-3-030-37297-2. Hardcover ISBN 978-3-030-37296-5. Series ISSN 2194-0452. Edition Number 1. https://www.springer.com/gp/book/9783030372965?utm_campaign=3_pier05_buy_print&utm_content=en_08082017&utm_medium=referral&utm_source=google_books#otherversion=9783030372972

214. Loutfy H. Madkour, *Nucleic Acids as Gene Anticancer Drug Delivery Therapy.* 1st Edition. Publishing House: Elsevier (2020). Paperback ISBN: 9780128197776. Imprint: Academic Press Published Date: 2nd January 2020 Imprint: Academic Press Copyright: Paperback ISBN: 9780128197776. © Academic Press 2020 Published: 2nd January 2020. Imprint: Academic Press Paperback ISBN: 9780128197776. https://www.elsevier.com/books/nucleic-acids-as-gene-anticancer-drug-delivery therapy/madkour/978-0-12-819777-6

215. Loutfy H. Madkour, *Nanoelectronic Materials: Fundamentals and Applications (Advanced Structured Materials)* 1st Edition. 2019 Edition. https://link.springer.com/book/10.1007%2F978-3-030-21621-4. Series Title: Advanced Structured Materials Series Volume 116. Copyright 2019 Publisher. Springer International Publishing Copyright Holder Springer Nature Switzerland AG. eBook ISBN 978-3-030-21621-4. doi:10.1007/978-3-030-21621-4. Hardcover ISBN 978-3-030-21620-7. Series ISSN 1869-8433. Edition Number 1. Number of Pages XLIII, 783 Number of Illustrations 122 b/w illustrations, 494 illustrations in colour Topics. ISBN-10: 3030216209. ISBN-13: 978-3030216207 #117 in Nanotechnology (Books) #725 in Materials Science (Books) #187336 in Textbooks. https://books.google.com.eg/books/about/Nanoelectronic_Materials.html?id=YQXCxAEACAAJ&source=kp_book_description&redir_esc=y

9 Application of Carbon Nanotubes in Cancer Vaccines as Drug Delivery Tools

9.1 INTRODUCTION

Cancer vaccines are one such intervention. Like traditional vaccines against infectious disease, cancer vaccines are comprised of cancer cell-derived antigens formulated in such a fashion as to provoke a potent immune response [1]. Typically, the antigenic payload of these vaccines is either mutated proteins arising as a direct result or as a by-product of tumorigenesis (so-called neoantigens), proteins which are overexpressed in tumors or proteins which are the result of aberrant expression of embryonic genes in tumors [2–4]. The antitumor immune responses elicited by the cancer vaccine are aimed to systemically target the cancer cells throughout the whole body; hence, cancer immunotherapy can be used to treat metastatic tumors [5]. Moreover, immunization with cancer vaccines can induce persistent T cell memory-specific against the tumor cells, providing long-lived protection and prolonged patient survival [6].

Unfortunately, while in preclinical models cancer vaccines have proven efficacious there has been limited progress in the development of human cancer vaccines, with a number of high profile candidates failing to meet their end points in clinical trials [7]. This is, in part, due to the failure to overcome tumor-induced immunosuppression [8,9]. However, there has been a surge of renewed interest in the field since the advent of checkpoint blockade and increased understanding of the immunosuppressive tumor microenvironment [10].

It is likely that a successful cancer vaccine will be composed of three components: the antigen, the adjuvant, and the delivery vehicle. This regime may or may not be supplemented with a checkpoint inhibitor. Speculating further it may be proposed that cancer vaccines will require novel formulations distinct from formulations previously used for infectious disease (such as alum absorbed antigen) as cancer immunity will primarily be driven by cell-mediated cytotoxic responses rather than antibody (Ab)-mediated humoral responses [11]. This chapter discusses one such formulation: carbon nanotubes (CNTs) in the context of cancer vaccines.

The use of CNTs as polyvalent tools for cancer treatment is progressing at a very fast pace. The most promising approach is the targeted delivery of drugs, designed to selectively direct the therapeutic treatment toward the tumors. CNTs may offer several advantages to overcome one of the main limitations of most existing anticancer therapies, namely the lack of selectivity. Herein, an account of the existing literature on CNT-based nanomedicine for cancer treatment is given. The most significant results obtained so far in the field of drug delivery are presented for many anticancer chemotherapeutics (doxorubicin, methotrexate (MTX), taxanes, platinum analogues, camptothecin, and gemcitabine), but also for immunotherapeutic and nucleic acids. Moreover, the alternative anticancer therapies based on thermal ablation and radiotherapy are discussed.

Despite significant advances, anticancer therapy strategies still suffer from severe drawbacks. One of the main limitations of most treatments is the lack of selectivity for the tumor tissues, resulting in severe side effects for patients that limit their compliance.

Another major problem related to anti-neoplastic chemotherapy is multidrug resistance (MDR) [12]. This phenomenon can often be ascribed to the activity of P-glycoprotein (P-gp), an efflux pump, able to recognize the drug and transport it out of the cells once it has been internalized, thus preventing it from exerting its cytotoxic action [13]. Importantly, P-gp-mediated MDR is often characteristic of residual tumor cells, limiting the efficacy of various chemotherapeutic agents.

Nanotechnology can help to overcome such limitations, by targeting cancer cells, either in non-specific, passive ways or via specific targeting ligand–receptor interactions. The passive targeting is mediated by the so-called enhanced permeability and retention (EPR) effect (Figure 9.1a–d) [14,15].

Cancer tissue is usually characterized by rapid and abrupt angiogenesis processes, resulting in leaky and defective blood vessels with large fenestrations, due to extensive endothelial cell disorganization. Also, the smooth muscle layer is frequently absent or abnormal in the vascular wall, leading to passive dilatation of vessels. The consequence is the enhanced extravasation of macromolecules in the tumor tissue, in contrast to low-molecular-weight molecules that undergo rapid renal clearance. Moreover, slower venous return and poor lymphatic drainage can lead to retention of accumulated macromolecules in the tumor. For these reasons, drug delivery using nanoscale systems would be more effective compared to the free drug. Moreover, this effect can be further enhanced by attaching targeting ligands to the nanocarriers such as antibodies or other targeting agents, able to recognize specific tumor markers.

DOI: 10.1201/9781003229674-9

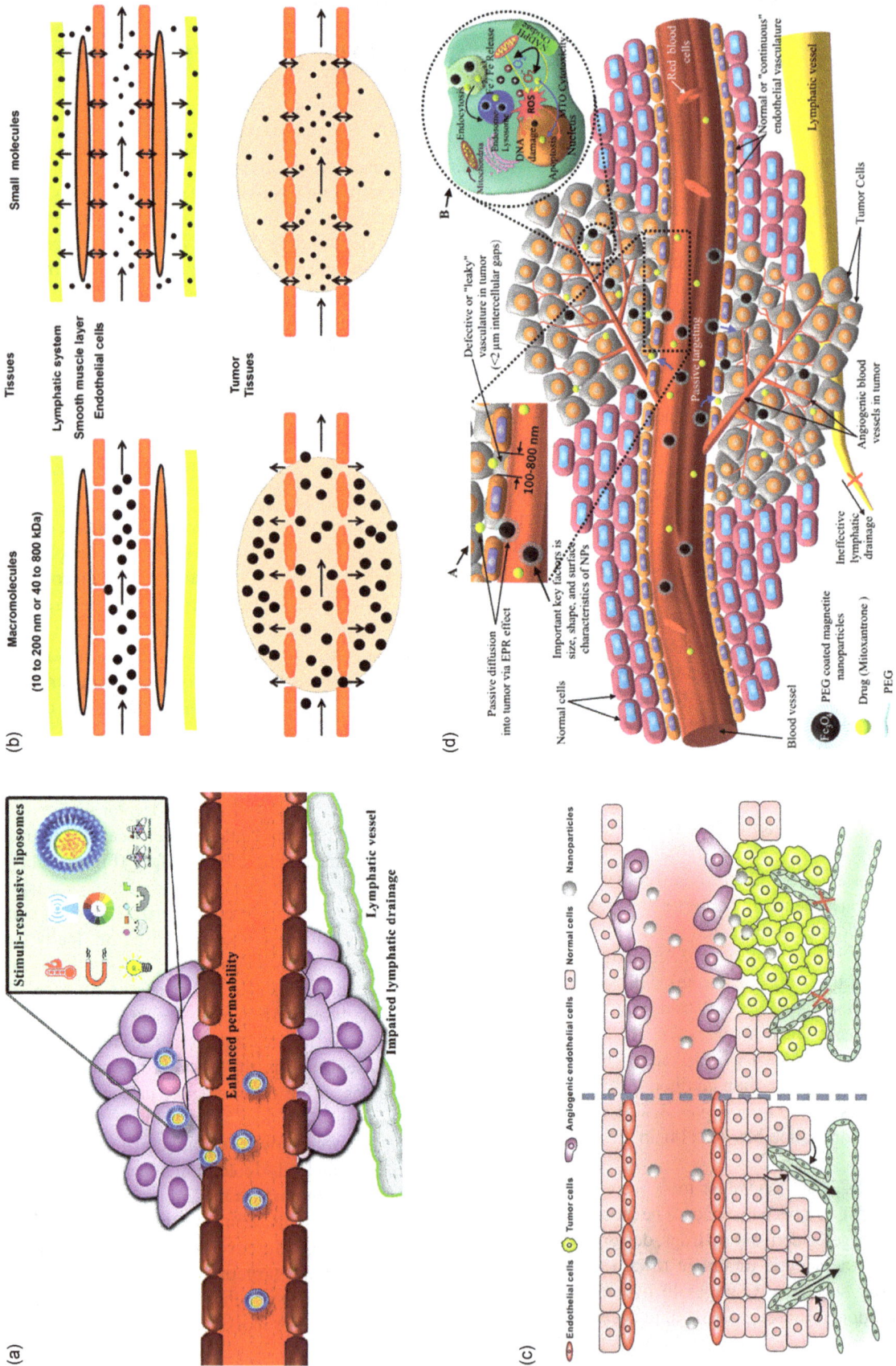

FIGURE 9.1 (a–c) Schematic representation of the passive targeting (enhanced permeability and retention (EPR) effect) of magnetic nanoparticles and anticancer drugs. (d) (A) Nanoparticles reach tumor cells selectively through the leaky vasculature surrounding the tumors, (B) Mechanisms of ROS induced by magnetite nanoparticles. First, NPs are internalized into the cell by endocytosis with subsequent formation of endocytotic vesicles; after that, the ions of magnetite are released from vesicles into the cell.

At the same time, the delivery of a drug through a carrier could involve different metabolic and cellular pathways, thus offering a way to elude MDR [16,17].

CNTs are among the most interesting nanovectors currently under investigation. Functionalized CNTs have shown great promise as novel delivery systems based on their ability to cross biological barriers. In fact, even though the specific mechanism of internalization (endocytosis or needle-like penetration) is still not fully elucidated, it is generally recognized that CNTs are able to enter cells, independent of cell type and functional groups at their surface [18,19]. In addition, their high surface area provides multiple attachment sites for molecules, allowing for polyvalent derivatization. Moreover, multiple *in vitro* and *in vivo* studies by different groups have shown, so far, that many types of chemically functionalized CNTs are biocompatible with the biological milieu, highlighting how the *in vivo* behavior of this material could be modulated by the degree and type of functionalization, both critical aspects that need to be accurately controlled [20–26].

Generally, in cancer treatment, most modalities currently used clinically aim at the elimination of cancer cells. In that context, different types of severely cytotoxic agents (e.g., small molecules, radiation) are utilized as "biologically active." Since considerable interest lately has surrounded the determination of the safety profile of CNT, particularly in terms of unintentional environmental exposure, a clear distinction in purpose needs to be comprehended. In cancer therapy, it is important to differentiate between the intended cytotoxicity from the therapeutic modality designed and the redundant possible toxicity from the carrier system itself, in this case the nanotube vector. While the former is required to achieve therapy, the latter needs to be minimized to avoid complications from therapy and side effects. There is emerging understanding that the physicochemical characteristics of CNTs play a critical role in their ensuing toxicological profile [27,28]. For instance, the length [27] and diameter [28] of the CNTs have been shown to be key players impacting their inflammogenic character. Shorter and thicker CNTs have been shown to be safer than their longer and thinner counterparts. Although such studies have only been performed with non-chemically functionalized (pristine) CNTs that are not explored therapeutically, it can begin to learn lessons and determine design parameters to be implemented in the development of CNT constructs for cancer therapy. Moreover, it is also becoming apparent that chemically functionalized CNTs and those suspensions exhibiting best aqueous dispersibility and stability in physiological environments can allow development in biomedical applications [22,29–31]. Another important factor considered to improve the overall safety profile of intentionally administered CNTs concerns their long-term tissue accumulation. Design of biodegradable CNTs, given the recent findings about their degradation *in vitro* [32] and *in vivo* [33], has become imperative. All the above suggest that, as with any other material developed with pharmacological intent (e.g., liposomes, polymeric micelles, dendrimers),

knowledge of the critical parameters and understanding of their biological implications are unavoidable steps to allow the utilization of CNTs in cancer therapy.

In this chapter, we analyze the most significant results reported so far in the field of drug delivery for cancer treatment. Conjugation of CNTs with many anticancer chemotherapeutics (doxorubicin, MTX, taxanes, platinum analogues, camptothecin, and gemcitabine), along with immunotherapeutic and nucleic acids, is considered. Moreover, alternative anticancer therapies based on thermal ablation and radiotherapy are also discussed [34].

Due to the advances in synthetic chemistry over the last few years, different biological nanomaterials [35] have been developed, which can be used for a variety of biological therapies, such as drug delivery, cancer diagnosis, treatment, and imaging. This group of nanomaterials includes quantum dots [36], dendrimers, CNTs, gold and silver nanoparticles, liposomes [37], and micelles [38,39].

9.2 CARBON NANOTUBES

CNTs are well-ordered, hollow, carbon graphitic nanomaterial with a range of properties. Some of these are a high aspect ratio, high surface area, and ultralightweight [40]. Typically, CNTs are classified as single-walled carbon nanotube (SWCNT) or multiwalled carbon nanotube (MWCNT). SWCNTs consist of a single cylindrical carbon layer with a diameter in the range of 0.4–2 nm [41], depending on the temperature at which they have been synthesized. It has been observed that a higher growth temperature gives a larger diameter. In contrast, MWCNTs are usually made from several cylindrical carbon layers with diameters in the range of 1–3 nm for the inner tubes and 2–100 nm for the outer tubes [42].

CNTs have attracted tremendous attention due to their unique properties as one of the most promising nanomaterials for a variety of biomedical applications [40]. In comparison with other nanomaterials, CNTs appear to be more dynamic in their biological application. For example, the main application of quantum dots is cancer cell imaging alone, while CNTs have the potential to be used not only in imaging but also for drug delivery and thermal ablation [43]. Application of CNTs for the delivery of drugs to their site of action has become one of the main areas of interest for different research groups. This is mainly because of the characteristics of these materials, including their unique chemical, physical, and biological properties, nanoneedle shape, hollow monolithic structure, and their ability to obtain the desired functional groups on their outer layers [40]. The shape of the CNT would allow these materials to enter the cell via different methods, such as passive diffusion across the lipid bilayer, or endocytosis, whereby the CNT attaches to the surface of the cell and is subsequently engulfed by the cell membrane [40,44]. The hollow monolithic structure of CNTs and their ability to bind desired functional groups make CNTs promising drug carriers. They can be functionalized to be more water-soluble and serum-stable, with low toxicity at the cellular level [40,45].

There has been great interest in the mechanism of cellular uptake of CNTs in the literature, and different methods have been investigated to elucidate this concept. Labeling CNTs with fluorescent materials, such as quantum dots, enables researchers to track the movement of CNTs [46]. Additionally, the detection of CNTs by nonlabeling methods such as transmission electronic microscopy or atomic force microscopy has also been undertaken [40,47]. The advantage of using atomic force microscopy is that it can operate in liquid form, allowing for measurement under near physiological conditions [44]. Figure 9.2 illustrates the presence of CNTs inside the cell with the aid of transmission electron microscopy [48]. Labeling CNTs with fluorescent agents and adding CNT-fluorescent agents to the cells have shown that CNTs are easily internalized into the nucleus [49,50]. Kam et al. reacted streptavidin-fluorescein isothiocyanate with CNTs and added this complex to HeLa cells. Their observation by confocal microscopy showed the presence of streptavidin-CNT inside the cells [51].

The method of attaching biological molecules to CNTs can vary. Drugs and biological molecules can either attach to the surface through functional groups or be loaded inside the CNTs. These methods are also called wrapping or filling modes of binding, respectively [52]. Another consideration while functionalizing CNTs is to improve their hydrophilicity. This can be achieved by reacting CNTs with strong acid, resulting in the formation of a carboxylic group on their surface, which increases their dispersibility in aqueous solutions. Alternatively, hydrophilic materials can be covalently or noncovalently attached to the surface of CNTs

[48,53]. Polyethylene glycol (PEG) coating can improve the hydrophilicity, biocompatibility, and immunogenicity of CNTs [38,54]. The aim of this chapter is to consider the biomedical applications of CNTs in drug delivery and targeting of cancer cells for thermal ablation. Furthermore, we seek to address issues related to possible toxic effects of CNTs.

In terms of the structure of the two types of CNTs, it has been proposed that the basic carbon arrangement of SWCNTs is different from that of MWCNTs. The structure of SWCNTs is organized according to armchair, zig-zag, chiral, or helical arrangements. On the other hand, the structure of MWCNTs can be divided into two types according to the arrangements of the graphite sheets. One is a "Russian-doll"-like structure where the graphite sheets are arranged in concentric layers and the other is a parchment-like model where the single sheet of graphite is rolled around itself [55].

CNTs can be synthesized by heating carbon black and graphite in a controlled flame environment. The major problem using this method is the irregularity in shape, size, mechanical strength, quality, and purity of the CNTs obtained [45]. To avoid these problems, techniques such as electric arc discharge, laser ablation, or catalytic decomposition of hydrocarbons have been suggested. Depending on the type of synthesis, different types of CNTs with different properties can be synthesized [41,56]. The appropriate fabrication technique can be utilized according to the intended application of the CNTs. For example, if CNTs are required for electric transport, SWCNTs should be used rather than MWCNTs. This is because SWCNTs can be either semi-conducting or metallic whereas MWCNTs are semiconducting [41]. In drug delivery, SWCNTs are known to be more efficient than MWCNTs. This is due to the one-dimensional structure of the SWCNT and efficient drug-loading capacity because of its ultrahigh surface area [57]. It has been shown that a SWCNT–anticancer drug complex has a much longer blood circulation time than the anticancer drug on its own, which can lead to more prolonged and sustained uptake of the drug by tumor cells via the EPR effect [58]. Various reports have suggested that once the functionalized SWCNT releases the drug into a specific area, it is gradually excreted from the body via the biliary pathway and finally in the feces [59]. This suggests that SWCNTs are suitable candidates for drug delivery and a promising nanoplatform for future cancer therapeutics.

SWCNTs can also be used for imaging. Single-molecule fluorescence spectroscopy and Raman spectroscopy techniques can be used to analyze the fluorescence and structural properties of SWCNTs. Results show that, unlike most single molecules or semiconductor nanoparticles, there are no spectral or intensity fluctuations for SWCNTs. Fluorescence spectra from individual nanotubes with identical structures have different emission energies and line widths that likely arise from defects in the local environment [60].

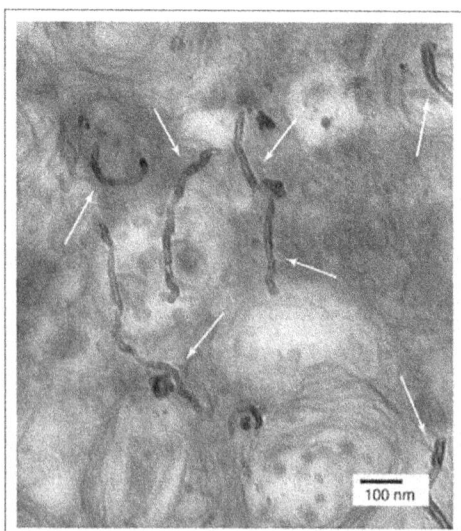

FIGURE 9.2 Transmission electronic microscopic imaging showing HeLa cells treated with functionalized multiwalled carbon nanotubes. As the white arrows illustrate, the functionalized carbon nanotubes were distributed into the cytoplasm. (Reprinted from Ref. [48]. Copyright 2005, with permission from Elsevier.)

MWCNTs are known to be more useful than SWCNTs for thermal treatment of cancer [61]. This is due to the fact that the MWCNTs release substantial vibrational energy after exposure to near-infrared light. The release of this energy within a tissue produces localized heating, which can be exploited to destroy cancer cells. Because MWCNTs have more available electrons per particle and also contain more metallic tubes than SWCNTs, they tend to absorb near-infrared radiation (NIR) at a faster rate.

9.3 CARBON NANOTUBES (CNTs) AS NANOCARRIERS

CNTs are synthetic allotropes of carbon. Allotropy is described as the chemical elements' ability to exist in more than one form. Three allotropic forms have been identified for carbon. The natural carbon allotropes include diamond, graphite (several layers of graphene), and amorphous carbon (non-crystalline form of carbon) [62]. The synthetic carbon allotropes that have been discovered include fullerene (sphere of carbon atoms) [63], graphene (single layer of graphite) [64], and CNT (cylinder consisting of rolled graphene layer(s)) (Figure 9.3) [65]. Morphologically, CNTs can be described as cylinders that are nanometers wide and nanometers to micrometers long, consisting of graphene rolled up in the form of single or multiple concentric layer(s) that are referred to as SWCNT or MWCNT, respectively [66].

9.3.1 SPHERES VS TUBES VS SHEETS AS NANOCARRIERS

In terms of carbonaceous nanomaterials, two carriers have been widely employed, namely CNT and the carbon nanosheet graphene oxide (GO). Unlike most other materials, there has been minimal work assessing the spherical form of carbon: fullerenes, as a carrier [67]. Therefore, it

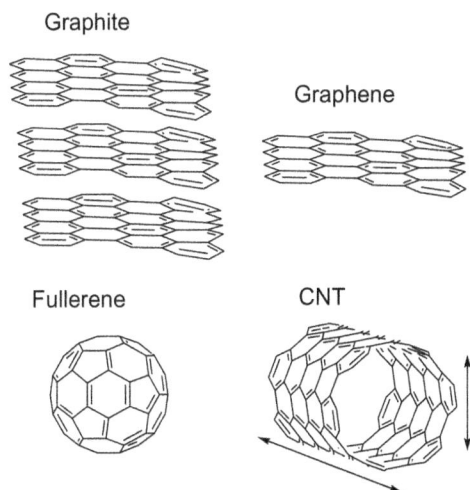

FIGURE 9.3 Different allotropes of carbon.

is difficult to attribute the observed effects to morphology or material composition when comparing CNT to other carriers. However, morphology-dependent behavior can be observed in other systems. For instance, Trewyn et al. compared the cellular uptake of silica nanoparticles that were either tube-shaped (100 nm wide and 600 nm long) or spherical-shaped (115 nm in diameter) of comparable surface charges [68]. The tube-shaped silica nanoparticles demonstrated higher uptake by CHO cells or fibroblast cells, *in vitro*, compared to the spherical ones. Similarly, Huang et al. have reported that internalization of rod-shaped silica nanoparticles (100 nm wide and 450 nm long) by the epithelial A375 line *in vitro* was higher compared to the spherical nanoparticles (100 nm in diameter) [69]. Whether the carrier's morphology-dependent cellular uptake affects the biological response induced by the loaded cargo demands future investigations. In light of these findings and hypotheses, comparative studies need to be carried out to investigate the cellular uptake and immunogenicity of CNTs versus spherical nanoparticles, ideally fullerenes but also the extensively studied poly(lactic-co-glycolic acid) (PLGA) nanoparticles and liposomes. The findings of such studies will undoubtedly contribute to the nanovaccinology field and further searches for nanocarriers with optimal morphological properties capable of efficient vaccine delivery.

The other commonly used carbon allotrope is the carbon nanosheet, GO [70–73]. The use of GO, as a cancer vaccine carrier, has been assessed by several groups. Yue et al. demonstrated that a subcutaneous injection of GO-OVA in C57BL/6 mice showed significantly elevated OVA-specific CTL response in comparison with OVA alone [74]. Furthermore, in a thymoma model, immunization of the aforementioned mice with GO-OVA was more efficient than OVA alone in limiting the growth of E.G7-OVA lymphoma cells. Testing the ability to induce protective antitumor immunity, Sinha et al. have reported that compared to C57BL/6 mice immunized with OVA alone, mice vaccinated with dextran-functionalized GO-OVA showed smaller tumor sizes after challenging with subcutaneous injection of OVA-expressing melanoma B16 cells [75]. These findings presented GO as a competent vaccine nanocarrier. Both CNTs and GO possess attractive properties of being able to incorporate the biomolecules of interest via simple surface adsorption. However, the proficiency of these carbon nanosheets (GO) compared to the CNTs in delivering vaccines remains in question. Zhang et al. have demonstrated that radiolabeled oxidized MWNTs were taken up in higher amounts compared to radiolabeled GO, by HeLa cells *in vitro* [76]. The degree of cellular uptake is a key, but is not the only, factor determining the intensity of elicited immune response. Proper comparative assessment of CNTs and GO uptake by the APCs and the subsequent impact on the induced immune response will assist future researches on further developing carbon nanocarriers suitable for vaccine delivery.

9.3.2 MECHANISMS OF CNTS' CELLULAR UPTAKE

Pristine (unmodified) CNTs are hydrophobic in nature and are thus characterized by their low dispersibility and high tendency to form aggregates in aqueous media. CNT bundle formation is attributed to the noncovalent interactions between the nanotubes such as the π-π stacking that occur between the aromatic rings of adjacent nanotubes. Thereby, it was essential to find chemical approaches that can improve (Cryptococcus neoformans) [77]. The functionalized MWNTs' internalization by these prokaryotic cells (which normally lack the ability to carry out active processes such as endocytosis) highlighted the MWNTs' utilization of mechanisms other than endocytosis for cell entry. In addition, it was shown that Jurkat leukemic T cell incubation with the functionalized MWNTs at 4°C in the presence of sodium azide did not inhibit the cellular uptake of MWNTs, which confirmed the involvement of passive cellular uptake mechanism. The contradicting mechanisms of CNTs' cellular uptake reported by different authors could be attributed to the properties of the CNTs used in these studies such as the CNTs' degree of individualization

and dispersibility in the cell culture media, which is highly dependent on the CNTs' functionalization density.

Mu et al. have studied the uptake of functionalized MWNTs by HEK293 epithelial cells using TEM [78]. In this study, single MWNTs were imaged penetrating the cell membrane, while MWNTs' bundles were found intracellular surrounded by endosomal membrane. Single MWNTs released from the MWNTs' bundle entrapped in endosomes were also imaged while penetrating the endosomal membrane, to enter the cytosol.

Collectively, from these studies, it could be concluded that CNTs can access the intracellular compartments via more than one mechanism of cell entry. This could be attributed to the length to width ratio of the CNTs that allows the, nanoneedle-shaped, CNTs to passively penetrate the cell membrane utilizing the hypothesized and experimentally demonstrated nanosyringe mechanism, in addition to the active endocytosis mechanism. The role of uptake cannot be understated as the ultimate goal of cancer vaccines is to induce tumor-specific cytotoxic and memory CD8+ T cell responses, capable of eradicating the established

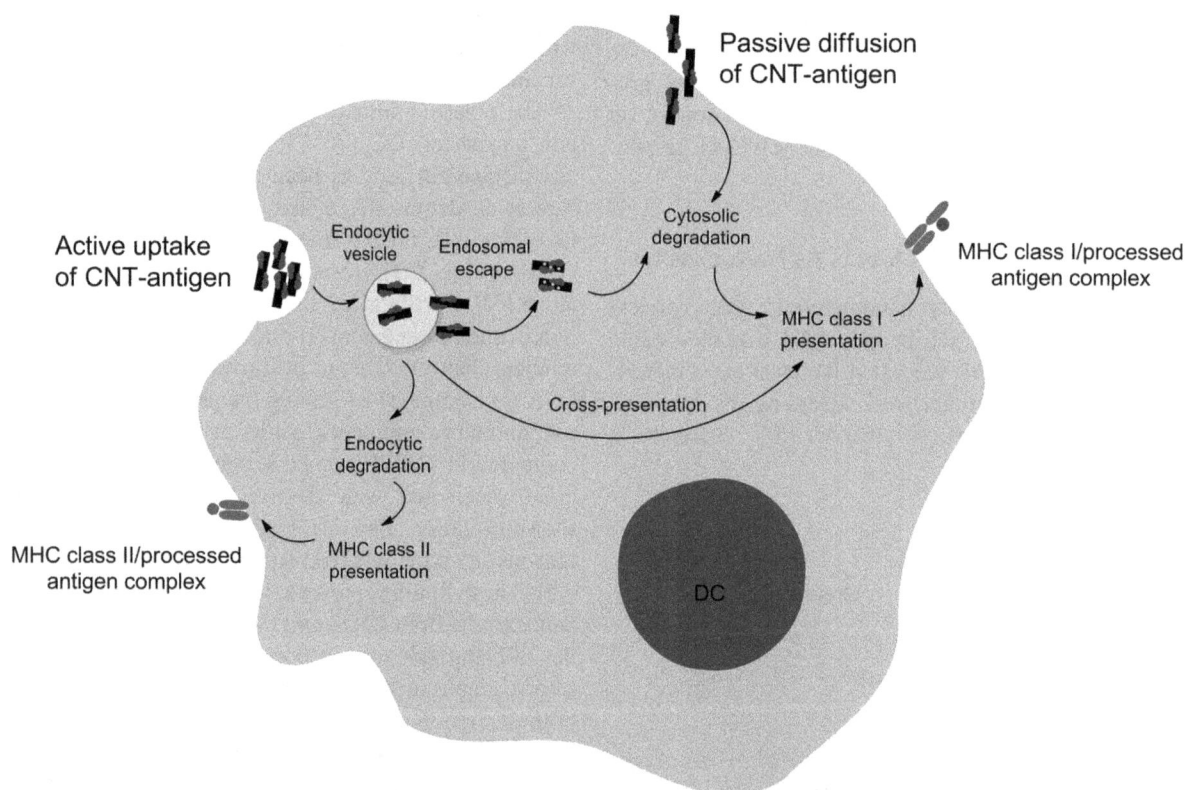

FIGURE 9.4 Proposed pathways for MHC presentation of CNTs-delivered antigens. CNTs could deliver the incorporated antigen to the cytosol of the DCs, via two proposed routes, where degradation by proteasome and subsequent MHC class I presentation occur. The ability of CNT-antigen conjugates to passively diffuse through the cell membrane could directly deliver the loaded antigen to the cytosol. Alternatively, following the active uptake of CNT-antigen conjugates by DCs and the subsequent endosomal escape, the incorporated antigen could gain entry into the cytosol. In addition, overcoming the need for endosomal escape, antigenic fragments yielded from antigens processed in the endosomes by endosomal proteases could be loaded onto the MHC class I molecules recycled from the plasma membrane. Furthermore, professional cross-priming DCs could translocate endocytosed antigenic cargo to the MHC class I pathway via the utilization of cross-presentation mechanism. Lysosomal degradation of CNTs-delivered antigens that fail to escape the endosomes could be followed by MHC class II presentation.

tumors and providing long-term protection, respectively [7]. Promoting antigen translocation to the DC's cytosol, where proteasomal processing occurs, could enhance antigen cross-presentation and, subsequently, the induction of antigen-specific CD8+ T cell response [79]. The fact that CNTs can passively diffuse through the cell membrane and reach the cytosol or leak through the endosomes into the cytosol following internalization via endocytosis could suggest that CNTs are qualified, as delivery vector, to translocate their loaded antigen to the cytosolic compartments (Figure 9.4) [49,77,78]. The CNTs' ability to penetrate the cell membrane might be assigned to their nanoneedle-like structure, which arises from their high aspect ratio (length to width ratio) [80]. Nevertheless, endosomal membrane disruption associated with CNTs' endosomal escape could induce cell damage [81,82]. Membrane disruption could activate NLRP3 inflammasome and consequently induce pyroptotic cell death [81,82] and is a concern that should not be overlooked on designing a CNT-based vaccine delivery system.

9.3.3 CNTs' Biocompatibility In Vitro

9.3.3.1 Effect of CNTs' Chemical Functionalization

Residual transition metal catalysts such as iron, cobalt, or nickel contained in the pristine CNTs can catalyze the intracellular formation of free radicals and oxidative stress leading to cytotoxic effects. For instance, treating HEK293 human kidney embryo cells with pristine SWNTs induced cell apoptosis and reduced cell proliferation [83]; additionally, incubating Calu-3 human epithelial cells with pristine MWNTs significantly reduced cell viability [84]. However, chemically functionalized CNTs have shown better biocompatibility profiles compared to the pristine material. This could be attributed to the fact that exposing pristine CNTs to chemical reactions followed by successive washing in organic solvents with the aid of bath sonication helps

in removing metal catalysts adsorbed onto the CNTs' wall. In addition, chemical reactions, such as bath sonication-assisted acid oxidation, that generate surface defects onto the CNTs help in removing trapped metal catalysts [85].

It could be suggested that [1] although chemical functionalization can improve the CNTs' purity and biocompatibility, the associated increase in CNTs' individualization increased their cellular uptake, thus the possibility of causing cytotoxic effects with increased dosage. In a similar fashion, Li et al. have demonstrated that as the positivity of chemically functionalized MWNTs was increased (by manipulating the surface chemistry), the cellular uptake by THP-1 cells (monocytic cell line) and BEAS-2B cells (bronchial epithelial cell line) was enhanced causing production of proinflammatory cytokines [86].

9.3.3.2 Biocompatibility with Immune Cells

Cytotoxic effects of CNTs on immune cells have been investigated in various studies. Using TEM imaging, it was demonstrated that carboxylate SWNTs formed less intracellular aggregates following incubation with human monocyte-derived macrophages and exerted lower effects on the cell viability than pristine SWNTs [87]. Treating murine RAW 264.7 macrophages with pristine SWNTs (26 wt% of iron) led to significant depletion of glutathione (oxidative stress biomarker) compared to treatment with carboxylate SWNTs (0.23 wt% of iron) [88]. The higher iron content of pristine SWNT than carboxylate SWNTs also led to significant increase in the formation of intracellular reactive oxygen species following incubation with rat NR8383 macrophages [89]. The length of the CNT could also determine the CNTs' biocompatibility. LPS-primed, human primary macrophages treated with long pristine MWNT (~13 μm). Figure 9.5 shows higher production of the NLRP3 inflammasome-mediated inflammatory cytokine IL-1β than shorter pristine MWNTs (1–10 μm)-treated macrophages [82,90].

Wang et al. have shown that treating human monocyte-derived DCs with carboxylate-MWNTs at 10–100 μg/mL for 48 h was not associated with a significant decrease in cell viability [91]. In addition, the carboxylate-MWNT treatment did not increase the DCs' expression of the CD80 or CD86 co-stimulatory molecules that suggested lack of MWNTs' adjuvanticity. However, cytokine production by MWNTs-treated DCs was not evaluated in this study. Dumortier et al. have demonstrated that culturing mice-derived B or T lymphocytes in the presence of SWNTs functionalized using 1,3-dipolar cycloaddition reaction did not induce cell death, provoke cell proliferation, or stimulate IFN-γ production [92]. Nevertheless, SWNTs functionalized via acid-oxidation and amide coupling reactions that exhibited lower aqueous dispersibility stimulated the production of TNF-α and IL-6 by macrophages in vitro. Although this study highlighted the effect of SWNTs' surface chemistry, and consequently the aqueous dispersibility, on the cytokine production by immune cells in vitro, it would be also useful to investigate the effect of different sized SWNTs.

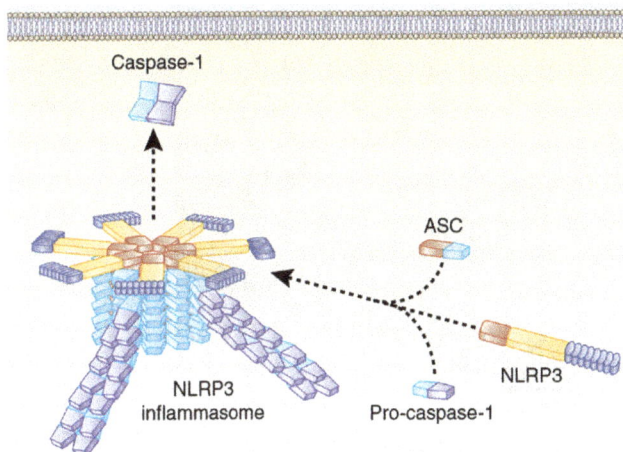

FIGURE 9.5 Inflammasome structure.

Pescatori et al. have also reported that incubating carboxylated or amine-functionalized MWNTs with Jurkat T cell line or THP-1 monocytic cell line did not induce cell apoptosis [93]. The uptake of the functionalized MWNTs by the THP-1 monocytic cells, but not the Jurkat T cells, increased the production of IL-6 and TNF-α proinflammatory cytokines. On the other hand, Medepalli et al. have found that DNA-functionalized SWNTs did not alter the cell phenotypes or activation markers' expression following the incubation with human blood-derived monocytes or lymphocytes [94]. Such discrepancy could be attributed to the CNTs' functionalization density, the used doses, and incubation time. These studies, therefore, suggested that the increased purity of functionalized CNTs could be accompanied by improved cytocompatibility. However, functionalized CNTs could still exert dose-dependent cytotoxic effects.

9.4 CNT FUNCTIONALIZATION TECHNIQUES

Despite the advantages of CNTs, there are limitations to their biomedical use. Purification of CNTs is still tedious. CNTs that are commercially available are severely contaminated with metal catalysts and amorphous carbons and are known to be generally insoluble and not biocompatible. In order to make these materials less toxic and more biocompatible, a number of procedures have been designed to attach appropriate molecules to the CNT surface, known as functionalization [95]. Generally, CNTs can be either covalently or noncovalently functionalized with different chemical groups [96]. In terms of CNT reactivity with functional groups, researchers have divided CNTs into two zones, i.e., the tips and the side walls. It has been shown that CNT tips have a higher affinity for binding functional groups than do the side walls [95].

9.4.1 NONCOVALENT FUNCTIONALIZATION

Noncovalent functionalization involves van der Waals interactions, π–π interactions, and hydrophobic interactions of biocompatible functional groups with the surface of the CNT. One of the main advantages of this type of bonding

is the minimal damage caused to the CNT surface. It has been suggested that noncovalent attachment preserves the aromatic structure and thus the electronic characteristics of CNTs. On the other hand, because noncovalent bonding provides a weak force between the functional group and the CNT, it is not suitable for targeted drug delivery applications [97].

9.4.2 COVALENT FUNCTIONALIZATION

Covalent binding of biocompatible groups to the surface of the CNT is another method of functionalization. Using this method, the surface of the CNT can be modified by different techniques, creating a suitable platform on the surface of these materials, enabling covalent attachment of biocompatible groups to the surface of CNTs. Oxidation of CNTs using strong acids is a method commonly used for generating covalent functionalization [41]. Briefly, concentrated nitric acid, concentrated sulfuric acid, and CNTs are sonicated and heated. This process allows for side-wall covalent functionalization, and carboxylic acid groups would be attached, rendering CNTs water-soluble. Figure 9.6 [39] shows a transmission electron microscopic CNT image before and after oxidization using a combination of nitric acid and sulfuric acid. These modifications would provide a suitable platform for the covalent attachment of biocompatible functional groups to the surface of the CNT, and the presence of a carboxylic group can improve CNT biocompatibility. It has been shown that a highly negative charge, developed as a result of the carboxylic group on the surface of the CNT, increases the hydrophilicity of these materials [41,42]. Oxidized CNTs can then be further coated with PEG, a hydrophilic substance with the ability to make CNTs more biostable [54]. Covalent binding of a functional group to the CNT can produce a stable functionalized CNT, making it more suitable for use as a vehicle for drug delivery. However, the side wall of the CNT is damaged during this process, resulting in alteration of other properties of the CNT [97,98]. Hence, CNTs functionalized by covalent bonding should not be used in some applications, including imaging [99].

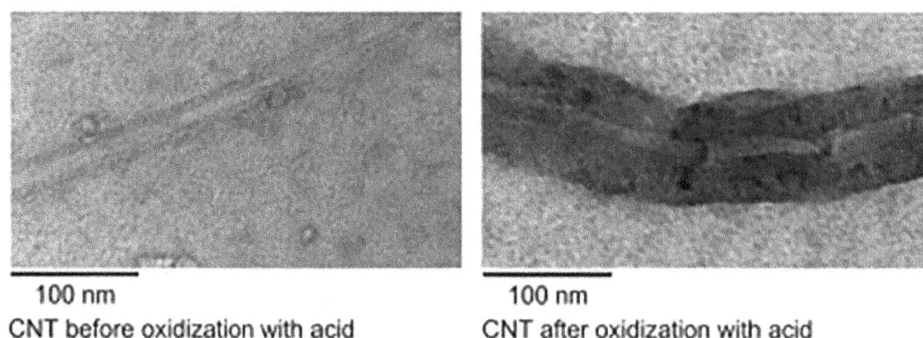

100 nm
CNT before oxidization with acid

100 nm
CNT after oxidization with acid

FIGURE 9.6 Carbon nanotubes (CNTs) before and after oxidization using a combination of nitric acid and sulfuric acid. This method resulted in chemical modifications of carbon nanotubes and formation of carboxylate groups on the surface.

9.5 CNTs' BIODISTRIBUTION

Biodistribution and clearance of the CNTs are considered among the main obstacles clinical application of CNTs is facing. The utilization of CNTs for the delivery of therapeutic agents demanded studying their biodistribution to determine their organ accumulation and toxicity following systemic administration. Yang et al. have demonstrated that pristine SWNTs intravenously injected to KM mice were distributed mainly to liver, spleen, and lung 24 h post-injection [100]. The pristine MWNT-injected mice compared to naïve mice 2 days post-injection, however, the cytokine levels returned to normal 7 days post-injection [101]. In light of the research gaps highlighted in the mentioned studies, future studies could provide more conclusive assessment of the CNTs by considering critical factors such as administered doses, frequency of administration, reliability of the methods applied to track the injected CNTs, and long-term tracking following administration.

9.6 FUNCTIONALIZED CNTs AS CANCER VACCINE DELIVERY SYSTEM

Various types of particulate carriers have been utilized in vaccine delivery [102–106]. The efficacy of particulate vaccines has been assigned to a number of suggested mechanisms. Particulate delivery systems can accommodate multiple copies of the antigen and adjuvant. Hence, the uptake of particulate vaccine delivery systems by APCs could increase the antigen and adjuvant intracellular concentrations, thus the presented antigen density.

Potent antitumor immune response induction could be achieved via combinatorial therapeutic approaches consisting of tumor antigens and immune modulators capable of overcoming tumor-induced immune suppression [11,107]. Examples of nanoscopic particulates previously employed to co-deliver tumor-derived antigen and adjuvant include liposomes (spherical vesicles consisting of lipid bilayers enclosing an aqueous core) [108], lipopolyplexes (lipid and DNA complex) [109], nanoparticles made up of emulsified PLGA [110], virus-like nanoparticles (self-assembled capsid protein lacking the viral nucleic acids) [111], albumin-based nanoparticles [112], or mesoporous silica nanoparticles (synthetic nanoparticles possessing porous structure) [113]. Examples of micro-sized carriers exploited in tumor antigen and adjuvant simultaneous delivery are polymeric systems consisting of PLGA [114] or diaminosulfide [115] polymers. Despite the differences in the composition and size of these nanoparticles or microparticles, they share the property of being spherical in shape. The efficacy of particulate delivery systems to deliver cancer vaccines comprised of antigen and adjuvant has been investigated in various studies [110,112–124]. These studies have shown that nanoparticles (e.g., liposomes, PLGA nanoparticles, or albumin nanoparticles) or microparticles (e.g., PLGA or diaminosulfide-based microparticles) co-incorporating antigen and adjuvant delayed the growth of cancer cells

inoculated in mice. This observation was attributed to the capacity of the nanoparticles or microparticles to augment the antigen-specific CD8+ T cell immune response elicited by the co-loaded antigen and adjuvant as demonstrated in these studies in vitro or in vivo [110,112–124].

Inspired by the demonstrated potentials of the conventional spherical nanosystems as vaccine delivery vectors and by the CNTs' capacity to enter the cells via different mechanisms, various studies have investigated the exploitation of CNTs as vaccine nanocarriers. As summarized in Reference [1], these studies focused on functionalized CNTs using various approaches to deliver antigens expressed by cancer cells and/or adjuvants to APCs and tested the efficacy of the CNTs-delivered vaccines through the assessment of specific immune responses elicited in vitro and in vivo.

9.6.1 FUNCTIONALIZED CNTs AS DELIVERY VECTOR FOR TUMOR-DERIVED ANTIGEN

As a cancer vaccine delivery system, Sun et al. investigated the use of carboxylated MWNTs to deliver MCF7 breast cancer cells-derived tumor lysate protein (TumorP) to APCs, specifically the DCs [125]. Flow cytometry showed that the MWNTs improved the uptake of the covalently incorporated TumorP by DCs in vitro. Furthermore, DCs pretreated with MWNT-TumorP were more efficient than DCs pretreated with free TumorP in inducing lymphocyte-mediated cytotoxicity against the MCF7 cells in vitro. However, the capability of MWNT-TumorP in retarding the MCF7 breast cancer cells' growth in vivo was not studied.

Meng et al. assessed the potentials of carboxylate MWNTs to augment the antitumor immune response elicited against covalently immobilized H22 liver cancer cell-derived tumor lysate protein (H22P) [126]. The H22 cells were subcutaneously inoculated into BALB/c mice, and the mice were subcutaneously injected with MWNT-H22P or free H22P starting 2 days post-H22 cells inoculation. The injected treatments were further potentiated by the additional administration of inactivated H22 tumor cells as a tumor cell vaccine (TCV). The maximum antitumor response was observed in mice injected with MWNT-H22P. Lymphocytes isolated from MWNT-H22P-injected mice showed higher cytotoxicity against the H22 cells in vitro than lymphocytes isolated from free H22P-injected mice. Additionally, some of the mice free of H22 tumor, as a result of MWNT-H22P treatment, successfully inhibited H22 cell growth following re-administration. This was due to the induction of antigen-specific memory T cells, since challenging "cured" mice with the unrelated breast cancer cell line EMT led to successful tumor growth. The authors [1] suggested that the augmented antigen-specific immune response elicited by MWNT-H22P was due to increased uptake of MWNT-conjugated H22P by the APCs; however, the MWNTs' ability to enhance antigen uptake by the APCs in vivo was not tested. In addition, to evaluate the therapeutic efficiency of MWNT-H22P, it would have been informative to treat H22-tumor-bearing mice with the vaccine rather than to challenge mice with tumor cells post-vaccination.

In order to potentiate the immune response elicited by the poorly immunogenic Wilms' tumor protein (WT1), Villa et al. covalently conjugated WT1-derived peptide with amine-functionalized SWNTs [127]. The SWNTs were internalized by the DCs *in vitro*, as determined using live

confocal imaging, with no effects exerted on cell viability. The free WT1 peptide or SWNT-WT1 peptide conjugate was mixed with an oil-based adjuvant and then subcutaneously administered to BALB/c mice. The highest levels of anti-WT1 peptide IgG were detected in the sera collected from mice vaccinated with SWNT-WT1 peptide. However, tumor therapy experiments using WT-1 expressing cells were not carried out.

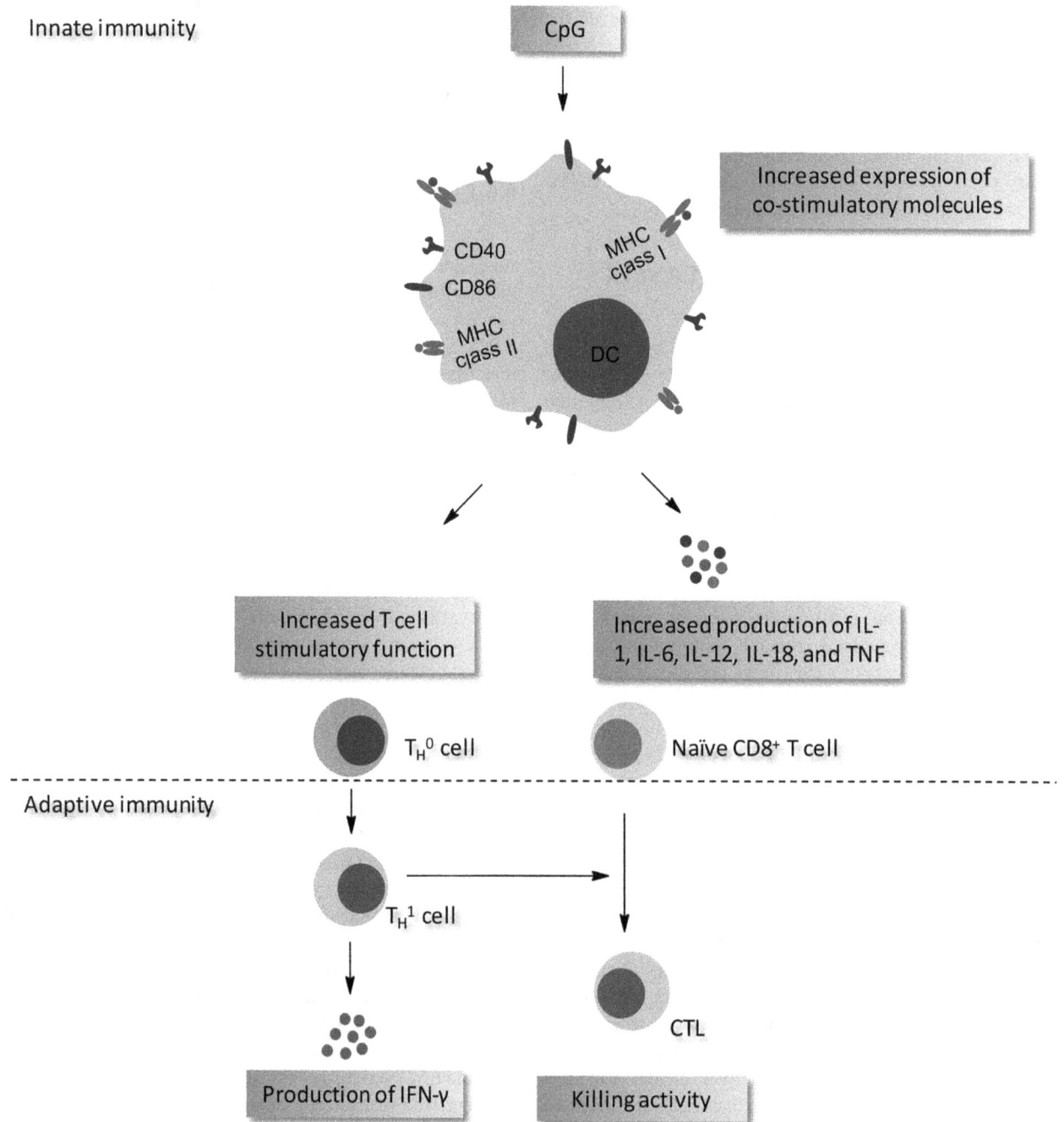

FIGURE 9.7 Immunostimulatory activities of CpG. Stimulation of the DCs' TLR9 by CpG induces DC maturation by upregulating the MHC, CD40 and CD86 expression, and provokes the immunostimulatory cytokine production that ultimately determines the DC ability to induce CD4+ and CD8+ T cell priming. (Adapted by permission from Nature (Nature Reviews Immunology) Ref. [134]. Copyright 2004.)

9.6.2 Functionalized CNTs As Delivery Vector for Adjuvants

Appropriate activation of APCs is crucial for unlocking their full T cell stimulatory capacity [128]. Innate activation of APCs is mediated by pattern recognition receptors (PRRs) such as toll-like receptors (TLRs), C-type lectin receptors (CLRs), and NOD-like receptors (NLRs) [129,130]. These receptors recognize ligands associated with invading pathogens known as pathogen-associated molecular patterns (PAMPs). Naturally occurring PAMPs or their synthetic analogues have been widely explored in vaccine formulations as adjuvants with the aim to promote immunity induction [130,131]. In particular, synthetic TLR9 agonists in form of oligodeoxynucleotides (ODN) containing unmethylated deoxycytidine-deoxyguanosine dinucleotide (CpG) motifs have been included as adjuvant in many clinically investigated cancer vaccine formulations (Figure 9.7) [132,133].

9.6.3 Functionalized CNTs As Delivery Vector for Both Tumor-Derived Antigen and Adjuvants

In 2014, Faria et al. have reported the delivery of antigen and adjuvant to APCs using CNTs [135]. In this study, the model antigen OVA and the TLR9 agonist CpG were both noncovalently linked to carboxylate MWNTs. Mice

immunized with MWNT-conjugated OVA and CpG showed higher sera levels of anti-OVA IgG and IFNγ production by *ex vivo* stimulated splenocytes than mice immunized with free OVA and CpG. The authors also tested the ability of the carboxylated MWNTs to co-deliver NY-ESO-1 (tumor antigen expressed in various human cancers) in combination with CpG to the APCs. The immune response induced *in vivo* by NY-ESO-1 and CpG was intensified following their noncovalent linkage to MWNTs. In addition, testing the ability to induce protective immunity, mice pre-injected with NY-ESO-1 and CpG-loaded MWNTs demonstrated a markedly retarded growth of NY-ESO-1 expressing B16F10 melanoma cells in subcutaneous tumor model. However, to assess the therapeutic efficacy of the designed MWNT-based vaccine, tumor-inoculated mice were vaccinated three days post-tumor cell inoculation, when tumor growth was still undetectable. Therefore, it is unclear whether therapeutic vaccination with carboxylate MWNTs co-delivering antigen in combination with CpG ODN would lead to effective remission of a well-established tumor.

It has been compared the efficacy of MWNTs functionalized using 1,3-dipolar cycloaddition, oxidation, or amide coupling reactions in delivering noncovalently immobilized OVA to APCs [136]. The MWNTs functionalized via amide coupling were more efficient in enhancing the OVA-specific immune response both *in vitro* and *in vivo*. In a follow-up study, the functionalized MWNT possessing

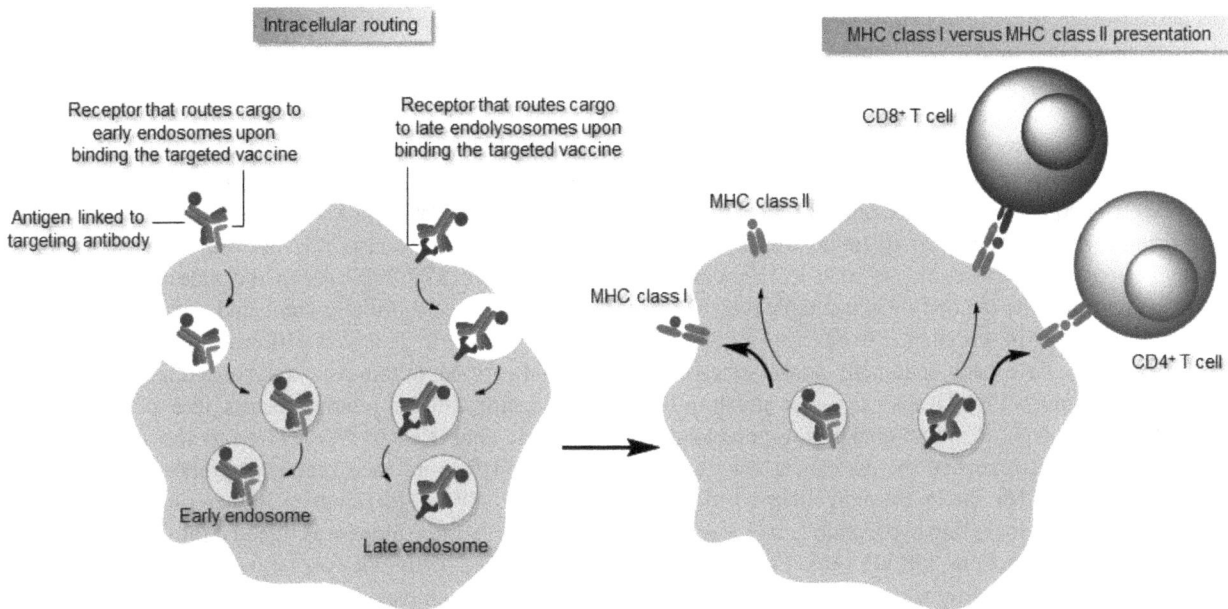

FIGURE 9.8 Impact of intracellular routing of Ab-conjugated antigen on antigen presentation. Delivering antigens through a linked targeting Ab to a specific receptor expressed by APCs is followed by cellular internalization of the formed cargo. Relying on the targeted receptor, the internalized cargo could be routed to a specific intracellular compartment. For instance, it has been found that mannose and CD40 receptors are intracellularly routed to the early endosomes, whereas CD205 receptor is routed to the late endosomes. In the late lysosome-containing endosomes, internalized antigen is subjected to rapid degradation by the lysosomal enzymes and presentation of the processed antigenic fragments via MHC class II molecules. In the early endosomes, the slow rate by which antigen is degraded could facilitate antigen escape from the endosomal to cytosolic compartments that allows proteasomal antigen degradation and, subsequently, presentation via the MHC class I molecules. The thicker arrow denotes that this route of presentation of processed antigen is more predominant than the other pathway. (Adapted by permission from Nature (Nature Reviews Immunology) Ref. [142] Copyright 2014.)

surface chemistry that was found optimal for OVA delivery was then utilized for the co-delivery of OVA along with the adjuvants CpG and anti-CD40 Ab (αCD40) to the APCs in form of a (αCD40) MWNT (OVA-CpG) conjugate [137]. In addition to the immunostimulatory properties that can be acquired by the inclusion of αCD40 [107,138,139], we hypothesized that αCD40 contained in the aforementioned conjugate will target it to the CD40 receptor on APCs, including cross-priming DC subsets, and thereby further enhance antigen cross-presentation to CD8$^+$ T cells. Previous studies have demonstrated the ability of αCD40-antigen conjugates to mediate uptake via CD40 receptor and enable translocation of the conjugate to the early endosomes [140–142]. It has been suggested that antigen translocation to early endosomes could support antigen escape into the cytosol and thereby promote antigen cross-presentation (Figure 9.8).

9.7 CNTs IN DRUG DELIVERY

Chemotherapeutic agents have some limitations due to their toxic side effects. There is a niche in the pharmaceutical market for drug delivery that does not elicit such toxicity, while still having high therapeutic efficacy. Thus, there is an unmet need to develop cell-targeting drug formulations with a wide therapeutic index. CNTs have shown great promise as nanoscaled vehicles for targeted drug delivery [48,143]. One of the main advantages of the CNT is its ability to deliver drugs directly to cancer cells [45,144]. In the past, there have been numerous experimental studies performed *in vitro* and *in vivo* using Ab-functionalized CNTs loaded with chemotherapeutic agents. Another application of CNTs for drug delivery is intravenous injection. One of the issues with injecting drugs into the body is the risk of blood vessels becoming blocked because of the large size of the drugs, which would lead to tissue toxicity. It has been suggested that CNTs could be used as nanocarriers for delivering drugs into the body via injectable routes [45]. It is beyond the scope of this chapter to describe all of them in detail, but they have been succinctly summarized in a series of recent reports [39]. Drugs can either attach to the outer surface of the CNT via functional groups or be loaded inside the CNT. Attachment of the anticancer drug to the outer surface of the CNT can be through either covalent or noncovalent bonding, including hydrophobic, π–π stacking, and electrostatic interactions [58,145,146]. Filling of the CNT with the anticancer drug is another method of incorporating drugs to CNTs, which will also be discussed in this chapter.

9.7.1 Covalent Drug Attachment to CNTs

Different methods of drug loading and attachment to the CNT suggest the need for use of a linker, with which both the drug and CNT react to form covalent bonds [147,148]. Researchers at Stanford University have delivered pacli-taxel (PTX) to cancer cells by covalent attachment of PTX

to the outer surface of the SWCNT. In this experiment, PTX was initially reacted with succinic anhydride, which resulted in the addition of carboxylic acid groups on the surface of PTX. Subsequently, SWCNTs were sonicated in a 0.2 mmol/L solution of DSPE-PEG 5000–4-arm-(PEG-amine) for 30 min using a cuphorn sonicator, followed by centrifugation at 24,000 g for 6 h. This resulted in the formation of SWCNTs noncovalently attached to PEG-NH$_2$. The product was then reacted with the carboxylic acid-coated PTX, in the presence of coupling agents, i.e., 1-ethyl-3-(3-dimethylaminopropyl) carbodiimide hydrochloride (EDC) 5 mmol/L and N-hydroxysulfosuccinimide (NHS) 5 mmol/L. Unconjugated PTX was subsequently removed by filtration. Ultraviolet–visible near-infrared spectra of SWCNTs before and after conjugation with PTX were then obtained. The absorbance peak of PTX was used to demonstrate the loading of PTX onto the SWCNTs, and the result was confirmed by radiolabel-based assay. *In vitro* delivery of PTX attached to SWCNTs showed higher efficacy in suppressing tumor growth than delivery of PTX alone. This suggests that higher concentrations of PTX were delivered to breast cancer cells using SWCNT–PTX conjugates in comparison with delivery of PTX alone [58].

Another group of researchers have attempted to deliver an antitumor agent, 10-hydroxycamptothecin (HCPT), by covalent attachment to the outer surface of the MWCNT. In the same way as above, the HCPT was reacted with succinic anhydride in order to obtain carboxylic groups on its surface. Amino groups were then introduced to the MWCNTs. CNTs coated with amino groups and HCPT functionalized by carboxylic groups were then reacted together in the presence of NHS and EDC as coupling agents. The excess HCPT was then removed using a filtration technique. Ultraviolet–visible near-infrared spectrometry was then used to confirm linkage of the MWCNTs to HCPT [145].

Platinum (IV) has also been delivered to cancer cells by conjugation to SWCNTs. As in the aforementioned studies, SWCNTs were initially sonicated with platinum (IV)-PEG-NH2 for 1 h. This was followed by centrifugation at 2.4×10^4 g for 6 h to remove catalysts and large aggregates, and ultrafiltration to remove excess free platinum (IV)-PEG-NH$_2$. The treated SWCNTs and the functionalized platinum (IV) were then reacted together. Platinum (IV) attached to SWCNTs achieved higher rates of cell death than when platinum alone was injected into the cancer cells. The enhanced cytotoxicity obtained using the platinum (IV)-SWCNT complex suggests that SWCNTs can mediate the delivery of platinum (IV) and hence improve cellular uptake of the drug [149].

9.7.2 Noncovalent Drug Attachment to CNTs

In addition to covalent attachment, anticancer drugs can also attach to the surface of the CNT by noncovalent bonding. This involves physical conjugation of the drug to CNT via π–π stacking, hydrophobic interaction, or electrostatic adsorption. Although covalent attachment is a very feasible procedure, it has been suggested that this may cause chemical changes in anticancer drugs, implying that their efficacy can potentially be altered [97]. However, one of the disadvantages of noncovalent bonding is the lack of efficient attachment, potentially resulting in release of the drug before it reaches its site of action [53,150]. An example of noncovalent attachment of an anticancer drug in this context is the attachment of doxorubicin to MWCNTs. In one experiment, MWCNTs were dispersed in 1% Pluronic® F127 solution until a final MWCNT concentration of 1 mg/mL was formed. The solution was then bath-sonicated for 30 min. Increasing concentrations of Pluronic–MWCNT (10, 20, and 40 μg/mL) were then reacted with doxorubicin 20 μg/mL. The interaction between the MWCNTs and doxorubicin was studied using luminescence spectrometry. The results showed that the fluorescence intensity of doxorubicin decreased with increasing concentrations of MWCNT. This suggests that as the concentration of the MWCNT increases, more platforms become available for noncovalent π–π interaction of doxorubicin with the surface of the MWCNT [151]. In another experiment, PEGylated CNTs were reacted with doxorubicin, resulting in doxorubicin becoming loaded onto the PEG that was covering the surfaces of the CNTs. It was suggested that, due to the aromatic nature of doxorubicin, noncovalent binding of this molecule onto the surface of the CNT was most likely because of π–π stacking and hydrophobic interactions.

SWCNTs attached noncovalently to doxorubicin were then used for *in vitro* and *in vivo* experiments. The SWCNT–doxorubicin complex showed greater toxicity than doxorubicin alone to cancer cells *in vitro*, suggesting doxorubicin release from the SWCNTs inside cell endosomes and lysosomes. In one *in vivo* study, doxorubicin alone and SWCNT–doxorubicin were injected into SCID mice bearing Raji lymphoma xenografts. The mice were sacrificed 6 h after injection, and the major organs were investigated for doxorubicin content. A larger amount of doxorubicin was found in the organs when the drug was conjugated to CNTs. This study also showed that doxorubicin was successfully delivered by SWCNTs to target organs in mice [152].

9.8 DELIVERY OF CHEMOTHERAPEUTICS

9.8.1 CNT–Doxorubicin Complexes

One of the advantages of using CNTs in cancer therapy is the capacity of their backbone to form supramolecular complexes with polycyclic aromatic molecules through π–π stacking. The most investigated anticancer drug in this context is the anthracycline doxorubicin (Dox). The earliest investigations in this regard were carried out initially with PEG-functionalized SWCNTs or copolymer-coated MWCNTs forming a supramolecular complex with doxorubicin [34,153,154]. Ali-Boucetta et al. [153] found increased cell death with the MWCNT–Dox complex compared to Dox alone, when tested *in vitro* on human breast cancer cells (MCF7). Liu et al. [154] used either SWCNT noncovalently

functionalized with a phospholipid–PEG surfactant or oxidized SWCNT covalently PEGylated through amidation of the carboxylic moieties. It was reported that the interaction between the SWCNT and doxorubicin is pH-dependent, which meant that the loading was performed at pH 9, when doxorubicin is deprotonated and hence has low water solubility, while a decrease in the pH led to the release of the drug from the SWCNT carrier due to its increased hydrophilicity. The cytotoxicity of the phospholipid–PEG wrapped SWCNT–doxorubicin construct was tested on human glioblastoma cancer cells. This derivative induced cell death, similarly to free doxorubicin at a concentration of 10 mM, although the observed IC_{50} value was higher (~8 mM for the nanotube conjugate compared to ~2 mM for the free doxorubicin). Furthermore, a targeted doxorubicin delivery was tested using a cyclic arginine–glycine–aspartic acid (RGD) peptide, which acts as a recognition motif for integrin $\alpha V b_3$ receptors, overexpressed in a wide range of solid tumors. In the noncovalent SWCNT derivative, the targeting agent was bound on the PEG chain and doxorubicin was then loaded. This conjugate, tested on integrin $\alpha V b_3$-positive cells, showed enhanced drug delivery compared to the derivative without RGD and a smaller IC_{50} value (~3 mM), compared to the constructs without RGD ligand. The behavior of this phospholipid–PEG wrapped SWCNT–doxorubicin was further studied *in vivo* into SCID mice bearing Raji lymphoma xenografts [155]. The authors observed higher tumor uptake, probably due to the prolonged circulation half-life of the construct, and a greater inhibition of tumor growth compared to the free drug. However, the therapeutic efficacy of the SWCNT–Dox construct was not better than DOXIL® (a liposomal formulation containing doxorubicin). On the other hand, the SWCNT–Dox construct caused neither significant toxicity nor mortality, allowing the use of higher doses which is not the case with DOXIL®. Treatments with 10 mg/kg of SWCNT–Dox (dose normalized on doxorubicin) instead of 5 mg/kg led to improved efficacy, without causing any severe toxicity. In comparison, 5 mg/kg of free doxorubicin or DOXIL® resulted in a definite decrease in the weight of animals and increased mortality rates of 20% and 40%, respectively. Possible reasons are that the larger size of the SWCNT–Dox constructs, compared to free doxorubicin, probably slowed down the excretion rates and the PEG coating of SWCNTs could have hidden doxorubicin from macrophages. Both these effects could determine prolonged blood circulation, thus enhancing tumor accumulation because of the EPR effect (Figure 9.1). Moreover, the slightly acidic microenvironment of tumors is expected to facilitate doxorubicin detachment from the SWCNT as previously speculated [154]. The same authors, however, observed a slow *in vivo* dissociation of doxorubicin from the SWCNT after administration, which suggests that noncovalent constructs cannot guarantee proper *in vivo* stability. Another *in vivo* targeting study was performed with PEGylated SWCNT functionalized with RGD peptide. After tail vein injection into U87MG tumor-bearing mice, the nanotubes accumulated in tumors

(13% ID g^{-1} in 24 h), with no obvious toxicity or negative health effects for the animals [156].

Zhang et al. prepared a different kind of SWCNT-based vector for doxorubicin [157]. CNTs were firstly oxidized and then derivatives by wrapping them with an anionic and a cationic polysaccharide, namely sodium alginate and chitosan, respectively. Doxorubicin was then loaded onto the modified SWCNT via electrostatic interactions and π–π stacking. The release of doxorubicin under acidic conditions (pH 5.5) was assessed in order to mimic the typical environment of lysosomes or cancer tissues. A release was found of almost 40% in 72 h, while the construct was stable at pH 7.4. Finally, an identical conjugate bearing folic acid (linked to chitosan) was prepared to target tumor cells overexpressing the folate receptor. *In vitro* cytotoxicity tests and cellular uptake studies were performed on human cervical carcinoma (HeLa) cells. The construct caused a significant reduction in cell viability compared to the drug itself, which proves its efficacy as a targeted delivery system.

A triply functionalized SWCNT derivative was prepared, bearing doxorubicin, fluorescein, and a targeting Ab that recognizes the carcinoembryonic antigen (CEA), a tumor marker for a variety of adenocarcinomas [158]. Doxorubicin was noncovalently loaded onto the oxidized SWCNT by π–π stacking. A fluorescein-labeled BSA was then covalently attached through its amines to the carboxylic groups present on the oxidized SWCNT, via an amidation reaction. Finally, the Ab was tethered through its amines to the BSA carboxylic groups again with an amidation step. In this way, the authors designed a construct that targets CEA-overexpressing cancer cells and is then internalized by endocytosis releasing doxorubicin at lysosomal acidic pH. The fluorescein unit was introduced to localize the SWCNT construct by the fluorescent signal after doxorubicin release. The internalization by WiDr human colon cancer cells was studied by confocal microscopy. After a 4-h treatment, the fluorescently labeled SWCNTs were found in the cytoplasm, while doxorubicin was localized in the nucleus, where the drug exerts its activity. As a control, the fluorescein-labeled BSA did not show internalization to the same high extent, indicating the good carrier ability of CNTs. Nevertheless, no information on the cytotoxicity of the complex was reported, nor any stability study to evaluate the release of doxorubicin from the CNT.

In a different approach, doxorubicin was linked to pyrene and this system was noncovalently attached to the SWCNT via π–π bonding driven by the polyaromatic unit of pyrene [159]. The linker between doxorubicin and pyrene was a short chain with a carbamate group, designed to be enzymatically cleaved inside lysosomes. *In vitro* studies on a mouse melanoma cell line were performed to assess the internalization of the construct and its cellular toxicity. The construct was found to accumulate in the lysosomes and caused a time- and dose-dependent cytotoxicity. Furthermore, the therapeutic efficacy was evaluated *in vivo* on B16F10 melanoma-bearing mice. Free doxorubicin and SWCNT–doxorubicin induced similar reduction in tumor

volume, with a significant decrease in the systemic toxicity for the CNT–Dox construct. In this case also the release of the drug from the CNT was studied, comparing the effect of incubation with cell lysate to the use of a normal buffer. Though the former system was significantly more efficient, proving that intracellular enzymes play a fundamental role, a release was also observed in the latter case, demonstrating that a noncovalent construct is not totally stable in a biological environment.

With the double aim of obtaining a targeted drug delivery system while overcoming the MDR effect, SWCNTs were functionalized via amidation with an Ab directed toward P-gp, one of the main players in MDR [160]. Subsequently, the Ab–SWCNT construct was noncovalently loaded with doxorubicin, via p–p stacking. This construct was tested *in vitro* on human leukemia cells, overexpressing P-gp on their surface and therefore being resistant to doxorubicin. Cells were exposed to NIR radiation to trigger doxorubicin release. As a consequence of NIR absorption by SWCNT, the amount of doxorubicin released in 24 h was tripled (nevertheless, a partial release was observed without NIR radiation as well). The Ab–SWCNT construct appeared bound to the cell membrane, while doxorubicin was localized inside cells in much higher quantities with respect to treatments with the free drug. Doxorubicin alone or together with the anti-P-gp antibodies (at a concentration of 5 µg/mL) could partially inhibit cell growth. Increasing the incubation time after treatment from 24 h to 48 h and 72 h, cells gradually recovered and began to proliferate. The SWCNT construct, on the other hand, used with an equivalent concentration of Dox, inhibited cell growth more efficiently than the free drug and in a time-dependent manner, probably due to a slow drug release from the vector surface. Since the first publications by Ali-Boucetta et al. [153] and Liu et al. [154], a lot of proof-of-principle studies on the use of CNT–Dox constructs for cancer therapy have been performed, while this research is still ongoing [161–165].

9.8.2 CNT–Methotrexate Constructs

Another clinically used anticancer drug that was investigated with CNT for cancer therapy is MTX. MTX suffers alike others from low bioavailability and toxic side effects. Preliminary studies of CNT-based drug delivery with this drug have been performed in our laboratories [166]. MWCNTs were covalently functionalized simultaneously with MTX and fluorescein [34]. Although a rapid internalization of the constructs in human Jurkat T lymphocytes was observed, the efficacy of the CNT–MTX construct was lower than the free drug. In a more recent study, the same drug (MTX) was bound to the MWCNT through cleavable linkers [167]. The use of a peptide linker recognized by intracellular proteases led to a significant decrease in MCF-7 breast cancer cell viability compared to free MTX. It is therefore possible to conclude that the lower efficacy in the first approach was probably due to the lack of drug release once the construct was internalized.

9.8.3 CNT–Taxane Constructs

Taxanes represent another class of antineoplastic drugs that have already been conjugated to CNT as a new platform for cancer therapy. PTX, a representative molecule of this class, was covalently bound through an ester bond to the PEG of the noncovalently PEGylated SWCNT and intravenously (i.v.) injected into xenograft tumor-bearing mice (a PTX-resistant 4T1 murine breast cancer mice model) to test the *in vivo* efficacy of the CNT–PTX construct [34,168]. Results were promising, showing a tumor growth inhibition value of almost 60% for the SWCNT–PTX derivative, which is two or three times higher than that reported for Taxol® and PEG-PTX (28% and 21%, respectively). Higher apoptosis levels and lower cellular proliferation were observed with the SWCNT–PTX construct compared to the drug alone. It is important to underline the lack of toxicity in mice for these PEGylated SWCNTs themselves, which has been demonstrated by the same authors in another study [24]. Evaluation of the pharmacokinetics showed that SWCNT–PTX has a longer blood circulation half-life coherently with the enhanced hydrophilicity of the conjugate with respect to the drug itself. However, a much higher PTX presence in reticuloendothelial system (RES) organs (liver/spleen) and intestine was also observed 2 h after injection. This is a predictable behavior for nanomaterial in general and could raise concerns about the toxicity toward these organs. Nevertheless, the authors reported differences between the biodistribution of SWCNT and PTX, indicating a rapid release of the drug from the conjugate probably due to ester cleavage by carboxylesterases. As a consequence, the drug seemed to be rapidly excreted, lowering its toxicity. At the same time, PTX levels in tumors were ten times higher for the SWCNT–PTX derivative than for the free Taxol®, 2 h post-injection, and the tumor-to-normal organ/tissue PTX uptake ratio was bigger, thus indicating a better selectivity of the CNT-delivered drug.

In a recently published paper, another kind of CNT–PTX construct was prepared [169]. MWCNTs were first oxidized and covalently functionalized with hyperbranched poly(citric acid) (PCA). Then, PTX was bound to PCA carboxyl groups with a cleavable ester bond, able to release the drug at acidic pH and through enzymatic hydrolysis. Finally, the *in vitro* activity of the construct toward SKOV3 ovary and A549 lung cancer cell lines was assessed. Earlier cytotoxic effects, even though comparable in intensity, were reported for the construct with respect to PTX alone, the fact being ascribed by the authors to an improved cell penetration for the CNT-based construct.

Another study with the same class of therapeutic compounds was performed. This was a case of a covalent SWCNT derivative bearing a toxoid molecule, derivatives with biotin as targeting unit toward cancer cells [170]. This construct was intended to be a prodrug, driven by the biotin to cancer cells, which overexpress the specific receptor on their surface and thus internalized by receptor-mediated endocytosis. Once inside the cell, the prodrug liberates its cargo upon reduction of the disulfide bond by endogenous thiols such as glutathione (GSH), whose concentrations are typically more than one order of magnitude higher in tumor tissues than in blood plasma. The system should act specifically on cancer cells leading the taxoid to carry out its mitosis inhibition action only in the desired sites. By means of confocal fluorescence microscopy, thanks to the presence of a fluorescent tag covalently bound to the taxoid molecule, the authors demonstrated the actual internalization of the whole conjugate in leukemia L1210FR cells. Moreover, in the case of a control SWCNT derivative without biotin, they observed a temperature-dependent but an energy-independent internalization. This is coherent with a non-endocytotic mechanism and is in accordance with the hypothesis of a needle-like diffusion of CNTs through cell membranes [19]. The biotin conjugate, as foreseen, was instead internalized by receptor-mediated endocytosis, the uptake being far higher than in cells not expressing the biotin receptor. The release of the drug by GSH and its binding to the microtubule network, where it exerts its cytotoxic action, were efficient, with an IC_{50} value smaller than the one for the drug alone, probably due to an increase in intracellular delivery.

9.8.4 CNT–Platinum Constructs

Platinum (Pt) analogues have also been investigated for drug delivery using CNTs for cancer treatment. Feazell et al. reported that the preparation of a Pt (IV)-based SWCNT prodrug led to intracellular concentrations six times higher than those reached when treating the cells with the free drug [34,171]. More recently, the same authors built another Pt-based targeted prodrug system using SWCNT as a longboat for the delivery of Pt [172]. The derivative was prepared by binding folic acid, as targeting agent, to a Pt(IV) compound, and tethering this conjugate through an amide coupling with terminal amines of phospholipid–PEG chains wrapped around the CNT. The Pt(IV) can be reduced inside the endosome, then losing the two axial ligands and leading to the active Pt(II) compound. The authors demonstrated that the internalization of this construct takes place by folate receptor-mediated endocytosis. The system was active in killing cancer cells (human choriocarcinoma and human nasopharyngeal carcinoma) with IC_{50} values more than eight times lower than cisplatin alone. The authors thus proved the actual ability of the system to act as a prodrug, generating the cytotoxic derivative (cisplatin) once internalized, and thus killing in a selective way folate receptor overexpressing cells.

Bhirde et al. described the targeted killing of cancer cells using a cisplatin-delivery system based on drug–SWCNT covalent conjugates [173]. The interaction of an epidermal growth factor (EGF) ligand with its receptor (EGFR), which is overexpressed in cancer cells, was exploited to target CNTs both *in vitro* and *in vivo*. The efficient *in vitro* internalization in head and neck squamous carcinoma cells of the SWCNT–EGF conjugate was proven and was found to be mediated by the EGF–EGFR interaction. Furthermore, quantum dot (QD)-functionalized SWCNTs were administrated to tumor-bearing athymic mice to study the short-term biodistribution profile of this construct. The EGF–CNT conjugate showed a much higher accumulation within the tumor compared to the control conjugate without EGF. Small amounts of CNT were found within spleen, lungs, liver, kidneys, and heart, regardless of the presence of EGF. Moreover, the animals treated with SWCNT–cisplatin–EGF showed a decrease in tumor growth compared with the untargeted SWCNT–cisplatin conjugate. This demonstrated that the SWCNT can effectively and selectively deliver cisplatin toward EGFR overexpressing tumors.

Another interesting approach for the functionalization of CNTs, also used in oncology, is the filling of the internal empty cavity of the nanotubes. This method was first investigated by the Green Group in 1994 and involves the opening of MWCNT caps by nitric acid treatment and filling of the inner cavity with different materials through a wet chemistry approach [174]. By applying the same method, Hampel et al. filled the nanotubes with carboplatin, a widely used chemotherapeutic agent for cancer treatment [175]. This derivative was then tested on human bladder cancer cells and a reduced cell viability compared to the drug alone was observed. More recently, cisplatin was also encapsulated into a SWCNT [176]. The release of the drug in physiological solution was studied, and it was found to start after 24 h and to continue up to 72 h. However, the inhibition of cell growth with this construct on two prostate cell lines (DU145 and PC3) was comparable to the free drug.

9.8.5 CNT–Camptothecin Constructs

Another antineoplastic drug, 10-hydroxycamptothecine (HCPT), was covalently attached to the MWCNT to study the influence of CNT on drug efficacy [34,177]. MWCNTs were first oxidized, and the generated carboxylic groups underwent an amidation step to introduce a spacer bearing an amino group to which a tethered derivative of HCPT was bound through another amidic bond. The tether presented an ester linkage, hydrolytically unstable, and was introduced to subsequently trigger the release of the drug. The authors observed a reduced drug release (<15% after 5 days) under both acidic and basic conditions, but a much improved release (80% after 5 days) when incubating the construct with fetal bovine serum, which contains esterase that could catalyze the hydrolysis. Furthermore, a fluorescein moiety was bound to the unreacted amine after HCPT conjugation, for *in vitro* imaging on human gastric carcinoma cells. Fluorescence confocal microscopy showed that the constructs localize intracellularly with a uniform distribution in the cytoplasm. Cell viability (WST-1) assay revealed a significantly improved cytotoxicity with respect to equal concentrations of HCPT, whereas CNT alone did not cause any decrease in cell viability. Finally, a different construct bearing DTPA was prepared, in order to chelate a radioactive nuclide (Tc) for *in vivo* biodistribution studies

in tumor-bearing mice. High uptake was found in the liver, spleen, lungs, kidneys, stomach, femur, and tumor. In the latter, the maximum uptake level (3.6% ID g^{-1}) was reached within 4 h post-injection. The observed blood circulation half-life was 3.6 h, versus 30 min reported for HCPT. Since the *in vitro* drug release tests showed that 4 h after incubation with serum only 12% of the HCPT was released, the authors considered that the majority of the conjugate could reach the different organs (and the tumor) without releasing a large amount of drug into the bloodstream. The *in vivo* antitumor performance of the HCPT-bound MWCNT was also studied, finding tumor growth inhibition much more efficient than HCPT alone, without causing any severe toxicity to the animals.

9.8.6 CNT–Gemcitabine Constructs

A MWCNT–gemcitabine construct was delivered to lymphatic vessels, exploiting the EPR effect together with the use of an external magnetic field [34,178]. MWCNTs were first functionalized with poly(acrylic) acid and then decorated with magnetite nanoparticles (FeO.Fe$_2$O$_3$) by a co-precipitation step with Fe^{2+} and Fe^{3+}. Three hours after subcutaneous injection in rats, the construct was able to reach popliteal lymph nodes without accumulation in the major organs such as the liver, spleen, kidneys, heart, and lungs, simply by the EPR effect. The same CNTs were loaded with the antineoplastic drug gemcitabine by physical adsorption. The system was guided *in vivo* by applying a permanent magnet on the projection surface of one popliteal lymph node. Very high accumulation of gemcitabine was detected in the lymph nodes after 24 h. At the same time, blood concentration was lower, when compared to gemcitabine alone, to the treatment without the magnetic field, and also to a control represented by nanosized activated carbon decorated with magnetic nanoparticles.

9.9 DELIVERY OF IMMUNOTHERAPEUTIC

CNT-based antitumor immunotherapy has also been explored. This approach employs TCV made of inactivated cancer cells or dendritic cells presenting tumor antigens to trigger the immune response of the patient against the tumor itself [179]. With the aim of improving the efficacy of TCV, tumor lysate proteins were covalently coupled to oxidized MWCNTs via an amide bond [34]. The conjugate was injected subcutaneously into H22 hepatoma-bearing mice treated with TCV. Controls were performed with TCV+CNT only and TCV+tumor lysate proteins only. The cure rate was significantly increased with respect to animals treated only with TCV or with TCV+tumor lysate proteins, even if a partial effect was exerted by CNT alone. To assess whether the immunity was tumor-specific, the animals that survived after treatment with tumor lysate protein-bearing MWCNTs were challenged again with a subcutaneous injection of tumor cells. In the case of H22 cells, the animals rejected the tumor, while they did not reject another mouse breast cancer, proving how the therapeutic system made them develop specific immune responses.

In the same therapeutic context, Villa et al. studied the ability of SWCNTs to act as antigen-presenting carriers, in order to improve the response to weakly immunogenic peptides [180]. The Wilms tumor protein (WT1), which attracted attention as a vaccine target for many human leukemias and cancers (currently in human clinical trials), was covalently conjugated with SWCNT. It was found that SWCNT–WT1 was rapidly taken up in vitro by antigen-presenting cells, in a dose-dependent manner. Interestingly, in vivo immunization of BALB/c mice using SWCNT–WT1 and an adjuvant caused a specific humoral immune response, which was not seen against the peptide alone neither against the peptide mixed with the adjuvant, proving the potential of the SWCNT to deliver poorly immunogenic peptides to the immune system, thus improving vaccine therapy.

9.10   DELIVERY OF NUCLEIC ACIDS

The way the CNTs interact with nucleic acids has been extensively studied for their potential applications. Both antisense oligonucleotides and small interfering RNA (siRNA) are very promising fragments for gene silencing, applicable for the treatment of many diseases. They can in fact inhibit protein expression, potentially blocking many cellular pathways. Cancer therapy is one of the possible applications, when the targets are oncogenes or genes involved, for instance, in angiogenesis or chemotherapy resistance. One of the first studies in this field was performed a few years ago [181]. Cationic SWCNTs were used to complex siRNA, able to silence the expression of telomerase reverse transcriptase and thus inhibit cell growth. This activity was proved in vitro, on different cell lines, both murine and human, and in vivo, after intra-tumor injection in xenografted mice.

The in vivo antitumor activity of a CNT-based siRNA delivery system was also assessed by our group, using a different kind of construct [182]. MWCNTs, covalently functionalized via 1,3-dipolar cycloaddition and bearing terminal amino groups, were used as cargos for a pro-apoptotic siRNA sequence (the proprietary siTOX). The system was injected within the tumor mass on human lung carcinoma (Calu-6) xenografted mice and compared with MWCNT with a noncoding sequence (siNEG), functionalized MWCNT alone, and both siTOX and siNEG delivered with cationic liposomes. MWCNT–siTOX conjugates significantly inhibited tumor growth and prolonged animal survival compared with the controls, while cationic liposome-based systems did not affect tumor growth or preserve the animals alive.

In the context of targeted delivery, a folate-targeted DNA transporter based on CNT was prepared, as a system in principle exploitable to deliver nucleic acids to cancer cells [183]. In this case, the covalently functionalized SWCNT presented positive charges to form electrostatic interactions with nucleic acids. The authors then bound fluorescently labeled double-stranded DNA (dsDNA) to this derivative, proving by UV a strong enhancement in the loading of dsDNA for the positively charged SWCNT compared with the non-charged SWCNT. The derivative was further functionalized by wrapping a folic acid-modified phospholipid around it. The complex was tested in mouse ovarian epithelial cells, showing an increased uptake for the derivative with the folic acid, compared to the one without the targeting unit. In addition, the fluorescently labeled dsDNA alone was internalized only at a very poor level, thus demonstrating the carrier role of CNT. In a final experiment, HeLa cells were induced to overexpress folate receptors, culturing them with a folic acid-free medium. These cells showed a much higher internalization of the derivative than normal HeLa cells, confirming the efficacy of the delivery system.

In another study, oxidized MWCNTs were complexed to polyethylenimine and then coated with an oligonucleotide antisense sequence, by means of electrostatic interactions [184]. The oligonucleotide was coupled to fluorescent cadmium telluride QDs to follow the cellular trafficking of the complex. An efficient uptake was demonstrated while the complex exerted the expected apoptotic activity.

Dendrimer–CNT constructs have also been exploited for gene delivery. The anti-survivin oligonucleotide was complexed to the polyamidoamine (PAMAM) dendrimer covalently attached to the CNT and used to transfect MCF-7 cells [185]. The conjugate was distributed mainly in the cytoplasm, endosomes, and lysosomes of the cells and was able to release the antisense oligonucleotide, inducing apoptosis. The PAMAM dendron was also directly grown on the MWCNT surface and used as an anchoring point for siRNA, after introducing a trimethylammonium unit on each branch termination. Different dendron generations were prepared and an improved efficacy in delivering a fluorescent oligonucleotide was observed, as the degree of dendritic branching increased. Furthermore, the gene silencing capability of the system was confirmed [186,187].

An interesting approach was developed combining the use of CNT as a nucleic acid delivery system with photodynamic therapy [188]. This therapy represents an option to cancer treatment, and it is based on the delivery of a photosensitizer, which, upon activation by an appropriate light source, transfers light energy to tissue oxygen. Mainly, singlet oxygen is generated, which can react rapidly with cellular components, triggering cellular damage. In this study, an aptamer, a synthetic DNA/RNA probe able to recognize and bind a specific target, was covalently bound to chlorine e6 (Ce6), a well-known photosensitizer. The aptamer was subsequently wrapped around the SWCNT, the conjugate being able to quench 98% of the singlet oxygen generation (SOG) normally occurring upon excitation of Ce6. When involved in the binding to its target human a-thrombin, the aptamer was released from the CNT, and SOG was no longer quenched. Phototoxicity on human lymphoma cells treated with the construct was also studied, showing a reduction in cell viability comparable with treatment with Ce6 alone, when thrombin was added. This indicated the feasibility of a targeted SWCNT-based system for photodynamic therapy.

All the examples reported above demonstrate that both SWCNTs and MWCNTs are good vectors for nucleic acid delivery and that the transported sequences retain their activity. These results are even more attractive considering that CNTs also exert an important protective action against enzymatic digestion [189]. Indeed, oligonucleotides wrapped on SWCNTs are preserved from enzymatic cleavage and interference from nucleic acid-binding proteins, increasing their stability in cells. Moreover, it has been reported that oxidized SWCNTs induce a stabilization of the human telomeric i-motif of DNA [190]. Even though the mechanism still needs to be studied, it could be exploited in anti-neoplastic systems, since stabilization of the i-motif inhibits telomerase, an essential enzyme for the proliferation of cancer cells.

9.11 LOADING CNTs WITH ANTICANCER DRUGS

Filling CNTs with an appropriate anticancer drug is another method of delivering anticancer therapy. According to Arsawang et al., a CNT with a diameter of 80 nm can hold up to 5 million drug molecules [51]. Several strategies have been used to incorporate drugs into CNTs. One of these methods is steered molecular dynamic simulation. The

general principle of steered molecular dynamics involves applying an external force to particles in a specific direction by use of harmonic (spring-like) restraint in order to create greater change of the particle coordinates. In an experiment carried out by researchers in Thailand, gemcitabine, an anticancer drug, was loaded onto SWCNTs using a steered molecular dynamic technique. Following application of force to the gemcitabine, it was shown that the cytosine ring of gemcitabine formed π–π stacking on the internal surface of the CNT with 25 Angstrom far from one end of the SWCNT [51].

The wet chemical technique is also commonly used. An example of this method comes from a study in which a 1 mg/1 mL suspension of open-ended CNTs was placed in a 10 mg/1 mL carboplatin solution, with sonication of the mixture for 10 min, followed by stirring for 24 h. Optical investigations of the sample obtained were performed using transmission electron microscopy (Figure 9.9), energy-dispersive X-ray analysis, electron energy loss spectroscopy, and X-ray photoelectron spectroscopy, all of which established the presence of carboplatin inside the CNTs. The quantity of carboplatin was also determined by inductively coupled plasma optical emission spectrometry.

After a considerable number of investigations at temperatures of 30°C–90°C, researchers in Germany found that the amount of drug loaded onto CNTs increases at higher temperatures and that when the temperature exceeded

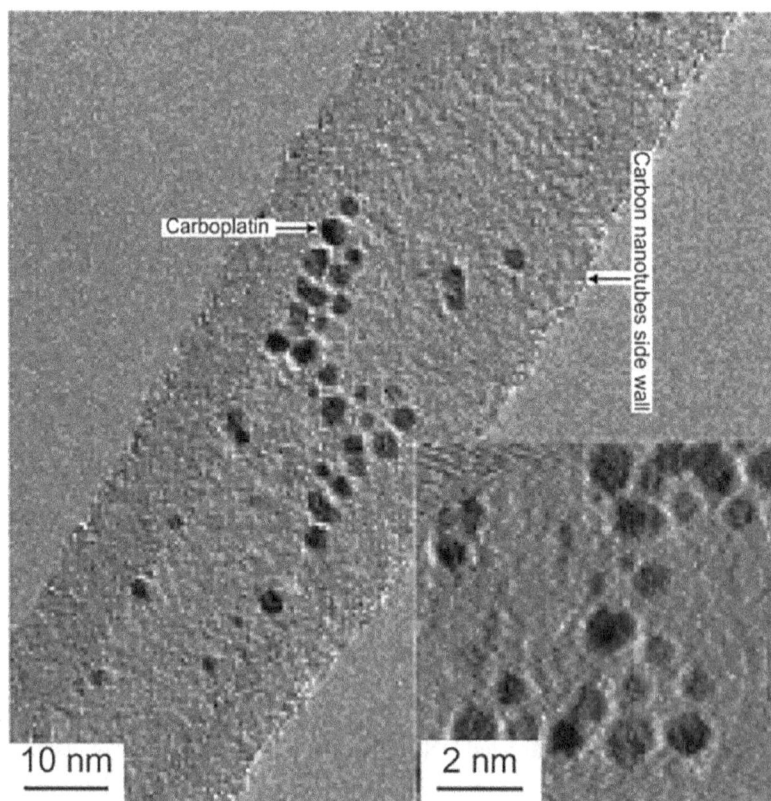

FIGURE 9.9 Loading anticancer drugs onto carbon nanotubes. A wet chemical approach is applied in which the capillary is the driving force for incorporating the anticancer drugs into the open-ended carbon nanotubes. (Adapted from Ref. [143]. Copyright 2008, Future Medicine Ltd. Reproduced with permission.)

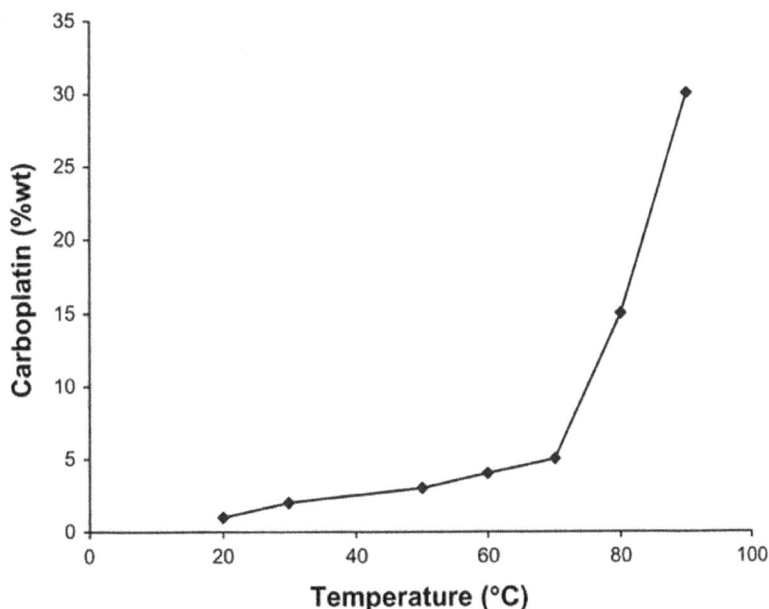

FIGURE 9.10 Relationship between temperature and anticancer drug loading. A larger amount of drug can be loaded onto carbon nanotubes as temperature increases, especially in the temperature range of 70°C–90°C. (Adapted from Ref. [143]. Copyright 2008, Future Medicine Ltd. Reproduced with permission.)

70°C, the concentration of anticancer drug inside the CNT increased dramatically (Figure 9.10).

A disadvantage of loading CNTs using the wet chemical technique is that some of the drugs bind to the exterior of the CNT. To avoid this, it has been suggested to coat the CNTs prior to loading and subsequently wash them with water and ethanol [143].

To determine the release profile of carboplatin-loaded CNTs, the conjugates were added to Dulbecco's modified Eagle's medium at varying pH for 14 days. Atomic absorption spectrometry was then used to measure carboplatin release into the culture medium. At day 0, only 3%–5% of the carboplatin was released, while approximately 55% and 68% (at pH 5 and pH 8, respectively) of the carboplatin was released from the CNTs after 14 days. This indicates a gradual and sustained release of carboplatin after loading into CNTs and possibly enhanced carboplatin release from carboplatin-loaded CNTs at higher pH values [191].

9.12   CELLULAR TARGETING AND UPTAKE OF CNTs

The question arises as to how anticancer drug-loaded CNTs can recognize their site of action and the routes by which CNTs can be delivered to target cells. A number of methods have been used by various research groups to investigate how the anticancer drug-loaded CNT might recognize the cancer cell. One of the major techniques used involves coating the surface of the CNT with a particular Ab having affinity for the target cancer cell.

According to the National Institute of Standards and Technology, all antibodies that have been used for cell targeting have been monoclonal IgG antibodies. However, experiments have recently been carried out using IgY as a substitute for IgG. IgY has shown some biochemical, immunological, and production-related advantages in comparison with IgG [192,193]. Other observations show that the attachment of antibodies to the CNT surface does not lead to alteration of Ab specificity for the target cell. It has been shown that the Ab can successfully deliver anticancer drug-loaded CNTs to the site of action. For example, Ashcroft et al. found that more than 40 CNT-anticancer drug complexes could be targeted as a result of coating the CNT with ZME-108, a specific type of skin cancer Ab [194]. In another experiment, a SWCNT functionalized by PEG and Rituxan (the monoclonal Ab against CD20, found primarily on B cells) selectively targeted the CD20 cell surface receptor on B cells with little binding to T cells [45].

In addition to coating CNT successfully with functional groups, such as antibodies, to achieve cell specificity, another important issue is being able to track the course of CNTs in the living organism. For this purpose, quantum dots, which have the ability to generate fluorescence when exposed to certain wavelengths of light [195], have been functionalized to the walls of CNTs.

There is still debate about the exact mechanism by which CNTs enter cells. However, two main routes have been described in the literature. These are passive diffusion of CNTs through the lipid bilayers of the cell membrane and attachment of CNTs to the external cell membrane, resulting in its absorption by the cell using an energy-dependent process, such as endocytosis. The exact mechanism of CNT uptake is determined by various factors, such as size, shape, degree of dispersion, and the formation of supramolecular CNT complexes.

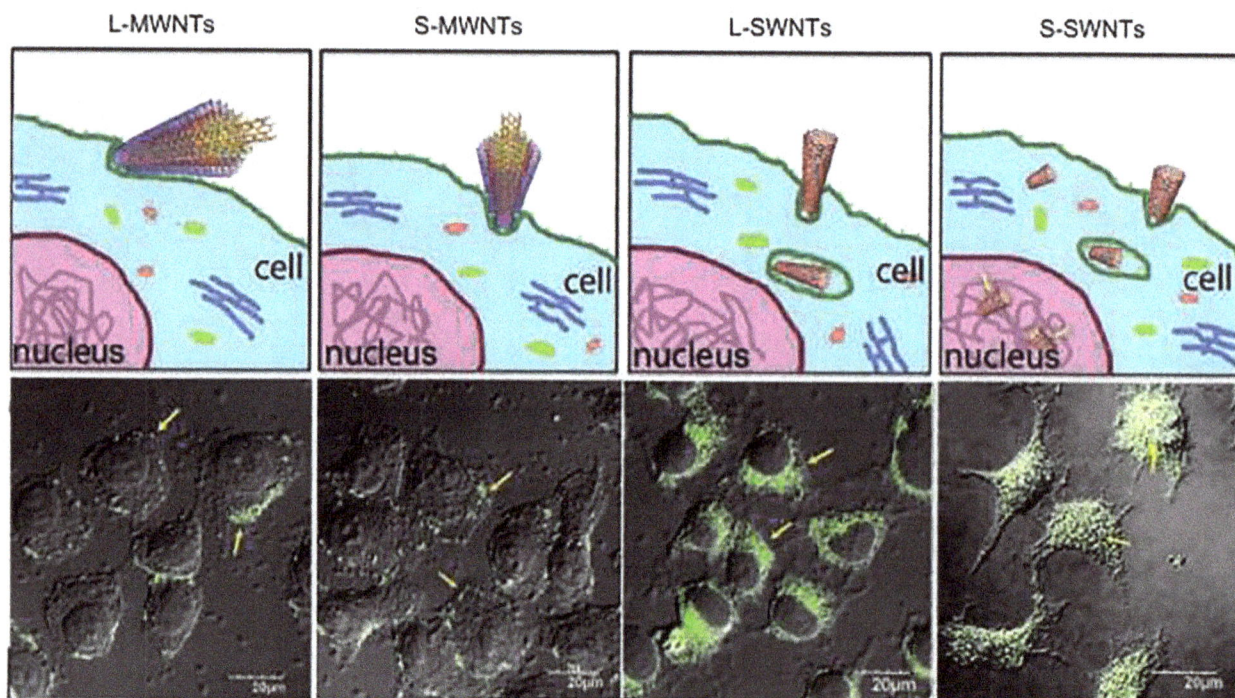

FIGURE 9.11 Confocal microscopy shows that the single-walled carbon nanotubes have the ability to be internalized into the cells whereas the multiwalled carbon nanotubes are excluded from the interior. Also, in terms of the influence of the size, it has been shown that the long single-walled carbon nanotubes are localized only in the cytoplasm but the short single-walled carbon nanotubes are transported into the nucleus. (Adapted from Ref. [197]. Copyright 2010, Wiley-VCH Verlag GmbH & Co KGaA. Reproduced with permission.)

One group of researchers has reported that small CNTs with a length of up to 400 nm are internalized by a diffusion mechanism and that CNTs larger than 400 nm in length are internalized by endocytosis [196]. It has also been suggested that CNTs attached to large proteins, such as streptavidin, staphylococcal protein A, or bovine serum albumin, are taken up via endocytosis, whereas CNTs attached to small molecules, such as ammonium, MTX, or amphotericin B, enter cells by a diffusion process [46].

MWCNTs and SWCNTs differ in their mechanism of cell penetration. Confocal microscopy imaging has shown that SWCNTs have the ability to be internalized into cells, whereas MWCNTs are excluded from the interior of the cell. Size of the CNTs also influences their cellular uptake and fate, because long SWCNTs are shown to be localized in the cytoplasm, while short SWCNTs are transported into the nucleus (Figure 9.11) [197].

9.13 DRUG RELEASE FROM CNTs

An important aspect of CNT drug delivery systems is the mechanism by which drug is released to target the cancer cell upon entry of the CNT–drug conjugate into the cell. Different modes of drug release from CNTs in the targeted cell have been described in the literature. Substantial data describing the rate and amount of drug release from CNTs are lacking. Different reports have shown that once the drug is loaded into the CNT, it will be excreted from the tube

into the cellular environment [46], but there is no accurate quantification of the amount of drug released [54]. One of the novel ideas is to load CNTs with drugs and seal the two ends of the CNT with molecules that can be cleaved off intracellularly. Alternatively, the drug can be attached to the CNT through a linker, such as disulfide, which is susceptible to cleavage under the influence of various factors, such as pH changes, heat, and reducing agents [198,199]. It has been observed that, as the environmental pH becomes acidotic, more doxorubicin is released from the CNT–doxorubicin conjugate. At a pH of 5.5, the approximate release of doxorubicin from the CNT is approximately 40% in 1 day. Because the microenvironment of the extracellular tumor tissue and intracellular lysosomes and endosomes is acidotic, the release of doxorubicin in these environments occurs with a higher magnitude [152].

In a similar experiment, small interfering RNA (siRNA) was attached to the CNT surface with the aid of disulfide bonding and delivered to the targeted cell. The results of this experiment showed that, on endocytotic entry of the CNT–siRNA, the disulfide bond was cleaved off by the thiol-reducing enzyme and siRNA was released. This process was aided by the acidic pH in the lysosomes [199].

Apart from an acidic environment, the element of heat can also be useful for the release of drugs. CNT was initially reacted with acid to form carboxyl groups at the open ends of the CNT tube, and (2-aminopethylthiol)-2-thiopyridine was then reacted with CNT–COOH to form

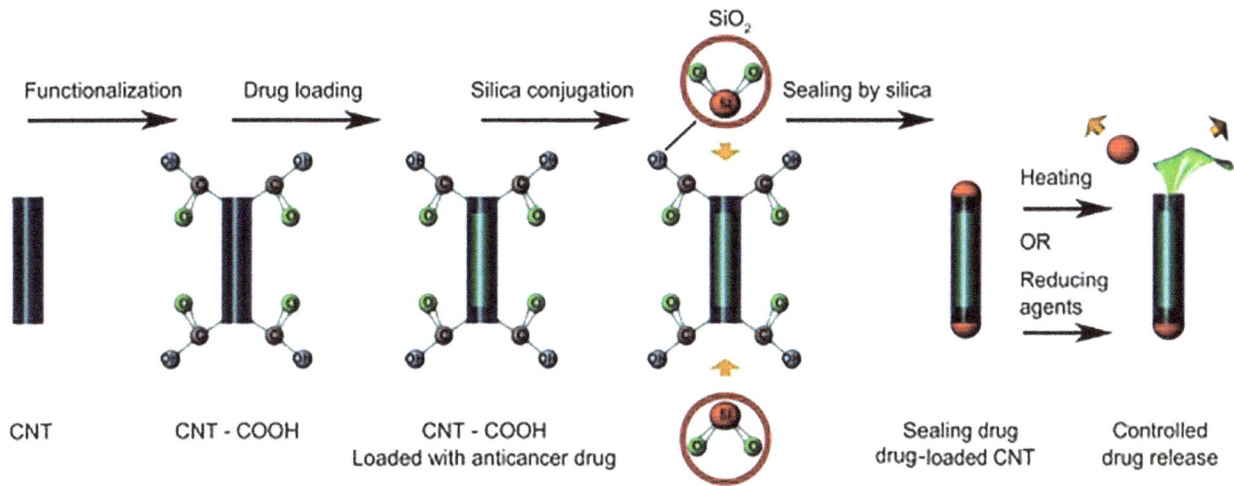

FIGURE 9.12 The picture illustrates that the silica can be used to seal the two ends of the drug-loaded carbon nanotubes (CNTs). This is used to allow the drugs to be released in a controlled manner.

thiopyridine-functionalized CNT ends. Following filling of the tube with fluorescein, the tube was then sealed by the addition of silica nanospheres. The silica was conjugated to the ends of the CNT by means of thiol groups. CNTs were shown to reopen after exposure to heat as a result of cleavage of the disulfide bonds. Once opened, the contents were released. In other words, controlled cap ejection governs the release of contents within the CNTs (Figure 9.12) [143,200].

9.14 CNTs IN THERMAL ABLATION OF CANCER CELLS

There is much interest into the use of CNTs in conjunction with radiofrequency and laser therapy in cancer treatment. Thermal ablation represents a potential form of cancer therapy that is noninvasive and harmless to normal cells, with high efficacy.

This section looks into the ways in which cancer cells can be ablated using high temperature. Generally, the thermal ablation method involves heating cells at temperatures above 55°C, which results in coagulate necrosis and protein denaturation of the cell, thus disabling functioning of the targeted cells [54,201].

Over the last years, research has been conducted into the development of nanostructures that produce heat on activation by near-infrared optical excitation. These particular nanostructures would be able to target the malignant tumor site specifically and selectively ablate tumor cells, leaving nearby healthy tissue relatively unharmed, providing a far less invasive alternative to surgery.

Exposure to modalities, such as near infrared, leads to cell death by irreversible protein denaturation or plasma membrane damage as a result of temperatures reaching over 40°C. This form of therapy has been shown to be efficacious for the treatment of numerous malignancies, including those of the lung, liver, and prostate. Zavaleta et al. observed that a modest temperature increase of 3°C–5°C was sufficient to cause protein denaturation in cells, leading to the death

of malignant cells [202]. The transmission of laser beams could be divided into two different types, i.e., short laser nanosecond exposure and long laser exposure. Nanosecond exposure is usually used for the ablation of metastatic or individual tumor cells. Although temperatures using this method can reach a maximum of 300°C, its nanosecond exposure ensures minimal damage to surrounding tissues [202,203]. The second method requires a few minutes of laser exposure and is generally used for ablation of primary cancer cells that are relatively large in size. The latter usually disables cell function by thermal protein denaturation and, unlike short laser exposure, may affect healthy cells as well as cancer cells. The temperature range for this type of laser is typically 45°C–65°C. To overcome the risk of death of healthy cells, researchers at Arkansas University produced a laser beam that generates a higher temperature in the range of 80°C–95°C. This is high enough to kill cancer cells but has a minimal effect on surrounding healthy tissue due to the shorter exposure time required [54,204]. Targeted killing of cancer cells using heat-generating lasers is performed in clinical practice at present, but current techniques have problems, such as the laser being a single point source of thermal energy that results in uneven tumor heating, or production of tumor seeding along the needle track that can result in tumor recurrence [54,205]. Various experiments have shown that CNT-mediated thermal ablation can overcome such limitations and generate effective heating and thermal ablation of tumor cells. Also, laser-stimulated CNT produces temperature gradients that extend more deeply into the tissue than laser treatment alone [206]. Exposing CNTs to radiofrequency can also increase the temperature of these materials. Gannon et al. showed in both *in vitro* and *in vivo* experiments that once CNTs are exposed to radiofrequency, they can thermally destroy cancer cells [207].

One way of finding out more about the effects of temperature changes in organs and of understanding whether the tissues are affected by heat production is to conduct a

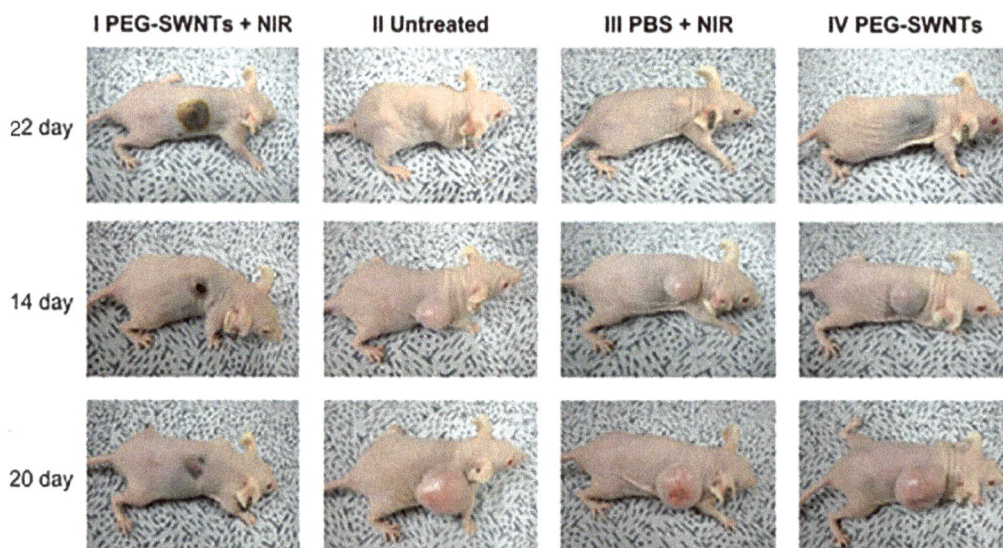

FIGURE 9.13 Regression of tumor via thermal ablation. (I) Thermal ablation and subsequent regression of tumor were seen when near infrared was administered with single-walled carbon nanotubes. There was an increase in size of tumor for untreated (II), near infrared alone (III), and carbon nanotubes alone (IV). (Reprinted with permission from Ref. [208]. Copyright 2009, American Chemical Society.) **Abbreviations**: PEG, polyethylene glycol; SWNTs, single-walled cartoon nanotubes; PBS, phosphate-buffered saline.

heat-shock protein analysis. Heat-shock protein works as an endogenous marker of thermal stress and is induced by elevated temperature (typically in excess of 43°C). Researchers have shown that when cancer cells are exposed to laser alone, heat-shock protein expression is induced proximal to the incident laser and gradually diminishes more distal to it. In contrast, when the laser is exposed to CNTs, the heat generated from these materials is high enough to increase the surface temperature of the cells and cause coagulated necrosis. As a result, heat-shock protein induction is seen in deeper tissue, indicating that CNTs can be used to extend the depth of thermal therapy [206].

The temperature of CNTs can increase to over 60°C within 2 min when they are exposed to near-infrared wavelengths of 700–1100 nm [54]. At the same time, it has been found that, because of the lack of specific chromophores, normal cells and biological systems are highly transparent to this range of wavelengths. This has led to recent interest in the effect of near-infrared light on CNTs used for thermal treatment of cancer. Carrying out the experiments *in vitro* is crucial, but there are critical issues in conducting the same experiments *in vivo*. For example, it is imperative to delineate the difference between using CNTs for thermal ablation of cancer cells *in vitro* as opposed to *in vivo*.

In one experiment, a group of mice were injected with human epidermoid cancer cells. Once the size of the tumor reached 70 mm^3, functionalized CNTs were injected into the tumors, which were then exposed to near infrared. The results showed that the cancerous cells treated with CNTs and near-infrared light disappeared within 20 days (Figure 9.13) [208]. It was also shown that a local rise in temperature increased the permeability of the tumor vasculature, which may be advantageous for selective delivery of drugs to the tumor site from the systemic circulation [206,209].

In addition to CNT, magnetic nanoparticles can also be used for thermal treatment of cancer. Magnetic nanoparticles can be localized in deep tissue, an external magnetic field can then fix them at a specific position, and alteration of the AC field can be used to change the temperature of the magnetic nanoparticles. However, toxicity and oxidation of the magnetic nanoparticles in the biological setting must be avoided.

Insertion of magnetic nanoparticles inside the CNTs could be a way to overcome this issue. The CNT could act as a shell, protecting the biological environment against oxidation and toxicity of the magnetic nanoparticles. The other benefit of using CNTs is the fact that the magnetic properties of these materials are not altered by their insertion into CNTs, and so they can still be used for thermal ablation of cancer [210].

9.15 ALTERNATIVE ANTICANCER STRATEGIES: THERMAL ABLATION AND RADIOTHERAPY

Cancer treatments may deal not only with the administration of drugs but can cover other possibilities. Among these, a very interesting strategy, named thermal ablation, arises from the intrinsic optical properties of CNT that allows for the development of hyperthermia. The optical absorbance of CNT is in fact very high in the NIR region, 700–1100 nm, where biological systems are transparent.

It is worthy of note that gold nanoshells and gold nanoparticles, to the best of our knowledge, represent the only other materials which have provided good results in photothermal cancer treatment with NIR radiations [211–213]. The laser intensity and radiation time used, however, are often higher than those needed to kill the cells with CNT. This observation makes CNT an even more promising material in the field, opening the way for further exploration, to reach a maximum laser energy level corresponding to a peak fluence of 35–45 mJ/cm^2, established as the safety standard for medical lasers [214].

Among the studies carried out so far, it is important to distinguish the non-targeted approaches, both *in vitro* [215,216] and *in vivo*, when CNTs were directly injected into the tumor [217,218] from those where CNTs were specifically targeted to tumor cells. The first paper reporting this use of CNT was published by the Dai group [219]. SWCNTs were noncovalently functionalized with phospholipid–PEG chains bearing a fluorescent tag or a folic acid molecule. The complex was then administered to HeLa cells overexpressing the folate receptor (FR+ cells) and to normal HeLa cells as a control. The FR+ cells showed a high internalization of the folic acid–SWCNT derivative, imaged by fluorescence microscopy, while the normal cells showed poor uptake. Cells were then irradiated by an 808 nm laser (1.4 W/cm^2) for 2 min [34]. This treatment resulted in extensive FR$^+$ cell death, while normal proliferation behavior was found for the cells, which did not internalize CNTs.

A multicomponent targeting system was also created by binding to the SWCNT two different monoclonal antibodies specific for breast cancer cell antigens IGF1R and HER2 [220]. The double targeting ensures high efficacy and selectivity. The derivatives were prepared by functionalizing CNT with 1-pyrenebutanoyl succinimide, which is able to interact strongly with the aromatic surface of the nanotubes by π–π stacking, as already mentioned, and bears an anchoring point to link the antibodies. The cells incubated with this conjugate were excited by 808 nm photons at 800 mW/cm^2 for 3 min [34]. After this treatment, all cells incubated with the IGF1R and HER2 Ab–SWCNT hybrids were destroyed. At the same time, 80% of the cells incubated with non-specific Ab–SWCNT hybrids survived.

Noncovalent SWCNT–Ab derivatives were also prepared exploiting the strong binding between NeutrAvidin attached to the Ab and biotin present on the polymer-coated SWCNT [221]. The constructs were targeted to human cells presenting the specific antigen for the Ab and subsequently treated with a NIR laser (808 nm, 5 W/cm^2) for 7 min [34]. This resulted in a significant decrease in cell viability. Since the disadvantage of noncovalent constructs is, as mentioned, the possible dissociation in biological fluids, the same authors prepared a covalent SWCNT–Ab construct. They formed amide bonds between the carboxylic groups of oxidized SWCNT and the amines of two different monoclonal Abs (anti-CD22 or anti-CD25) [222]. To assess the specific binding to human Burkitt's lymphoma cells (CD22$^+$CD25$^-$) and phytohemagglutinin-activated normal human peripheral blood mononuclear cells (CD22$^-$CD25$^+$), after incubation with the constructs, the cells were treated with fluorescein-conjugated goat anti-mouse immunoglobulin (FITC-GAMIg) and analyzed through flow cytometry. The results clearly showed specific recognition of the correspondent cell receptor by the two Ab–SWCNT conjugates. Finally, thermal ablation of the specifically targeted cells was achieved after exposure to NIR radiation (808 nm laser, 9.5 W/cm^2) for 4 min [34].

Among cancer thermal ablation studies involving CNTs, another interesting option was proposed [223]. Targeting cancer could be translated more specifically into targeting cancer stem cells. These cells are responsible for the formation of metastases, resistance to therapies, and restoration of tumors. They therefore represent a very important target to study, and more efforts should be made in this direction. The chosen target was the CD133$^+$ glioblastoma cell line presenting high tumorigenicity and cancer stem-like properties. SWCNTs were wrapped with chitosan, which was covalently coupled to a CD133 monoclonal Ab. These CNTs were tested *in vitro* on both CD133$^+$ and CD133$^-$ glioblastoma cells. Internalization was observed only by the CD133+ cells, which were specifically killed after exposure to NIR laser radiation (808 nm, 2 W/cm^2) for 5 min [34]. Furthermore, the treatment with CNT followed by NIR radiation inhibited spheroid body formation, which represents an index of cell self-renewal. To partially translate the study *in vivo*, CNT-treated or untreated cells were used to induce tumor formation in nude mice. Two days after a subcutaneous injection, the mice were subjected to NIR laser radiation, resulting in significant inhibition of tumor growth when CNTs were used.

Another promising anticancer strategy is radiotherapy. As mentioned above, the main purpose of attaching radioisotopes to the CNT is for imaging studies, to determine their biodistribution following radioisotope traces. A therapeutic application, however, can also be envisaged. The preparation of a SWCNT derivative bearing an ^{111}In chelate was reported and its biodistribution was analyzed, finding accumulation mainly in the kidney, spleen, and liver [224]. The same derivative was then further functionalized with a tumor-specific monoclonal Ab, and it was delivered *in vivo* to a murine model of disseminated human lymphoma, showing selective tumor targeting. Therefore, the replacement of indium with a proper radionuclide would render these constructs ideal for their application in radiotherapy. Indeed, the preparation of covalent CNT–Ab constructs intended to target tumor neovasculature for radiotherapy was subsequently reported by the same authors [225]. Angiogenic endothelial cells express on their surface a monomeric cadherin that, after forming dimers on nearby cells, constitutes the tight junctions of normal vascular endothelium. In tumors, these cells are poorly connected (this being one of the reasons for the EPR effect). Thus, the cadherin is in monomeric form, which is the only one recognized by the Ab E4G10. Doubly functionalized SWCNTs were prepared, by binding to the CNT both the specific Ab and the alpha particle-emitting ^{225}Ac, able to kill the targeted cell and the tissue in its proximity. The conjugate was tested *in vivo*, *via* intravenous injection in xenografted tumor mice, demonstrating its specific ability to reduce tumor growth and improve mice survival compared with controls bearing a different Ab. The success of this approach seems to be very promising as in principle targeting of tumor vasculature renders these kinds of constructs suitable for any species of solid tumor.

9.16   TUMOR-TARGETED CNT

As seen from the studies already mentioned above, various ligands have been attached to CNTs to improve their tumor specificity and achieve active targeting onto specific cell receptors. Some other works focused mainly on the targeting issue, as a proof of principle, without proposing any specific therapeutic approach.

Specific recognition of membrane receptors has been achieved with Ab-functionalized SWCNTs [226]. Nanotubes were first functionalized with a phospholipid–PEG to increase solubility and to prevent non-specific binding in the biological environment. Then, terminal amines of the PEG units were covalently functionalized with two different antibodies (rituximab and trastuzumab). After incubation, binding to the corresponding membrane receptors (CD20 on B-cells, and HER2/neu on breast cancer cells, respectively) was proved, exploiting the intrinsic near-infrared fluorescence of CNT. This study demonstrated the feasibility of using antibodies as targeting agents in applications such as imaging or drug delivery. Raman spectroscopy was also used as an imaging technique for CNT [227]. In this case, a phospholipid–PEG–CNT construct bound to different antibodies or to an RGD peptide was prepared using SWCNTs with a different isotope composition, which display well-shifted Raman G-band peaks. As a consequence, it was possible to distinguish the different CNT constructs in mixed cellular populations, proving that they were able to selectively recognize their specific target. Raman imaging was used also for both *in vitro* and direct *in vivo* studies exploiting PEGylated SWCNT functionalized with RGD peptide [156,228]. *In vitro* data showed that $\alpha_v\beta_3$ integrin-positive tumor cells (U87MG) internalized the construct much better than the SWCNT without RGD and then $\alpha_v\beta_3$ integrin-negative cells (HT29) do. *In vivo* data showed selective prolonged accumulation of the RGD-targeted SWCNT in the tumor, while for the non-targeted SWCNT, an initial tumor accumulation was observed, followed by a rapid decrease. Using a different approach, SWCNTs with phospholipid–PEG–COOH were bound to protein A by amidation, and then, an anti-integrin Ab, previously marked with fluorescein, was linked to the system exploiting the high affinity interaction of the Fc (fragment crystallizable) region of the Ab with protein A [229]. The chosen Ab recognizes a specific integrin overexpressed on various cancer cells, rendering the construct suitable for cancer targeting. After demonstrating that the construct was not cytotoxic, its internalizations and targeting were studied using fluorescence confocal microscopy in both integrin-positive (U87MG human glioblastoma cancer cells) and integrin-negative (MCF-7 human breast cancer cells) cell lines. Only U87MG cells internalized the SWCNT construct, while no intracellular fluorescence was detected for MCF-7 cells nor for U87MG cells after a pretreatment with the Ab alone. An integrin-mediated endocytosis uptake mechanism for CNTs was therefore hypothesized.

Bottini et al. studied the internalizations of SWCNT–QD–streptavidin complexes by CD3-positive leukemia cells based on monitoring the intracellular QD fluorescence [230]. In this case, the uptake mechanism was rather complex, being mediated by a multicomponent recognition. Initially, a biotinylated anti-CD3 Ab was allowed to bind to the CD3 receptor on the cell membrane. Then, the streptavidin-loaded SWCNT connected to the biotinylated Ab, showing high internalization. In contrast, poor uptake was observed when: (i) the Ab was absent; (ii) a non-biotinylated Ab was used; (iii) the experiments were carried out at 4°C; and (iv) CD3-negative cell lines were used. All these data suggest a receptor-mediated endocytosis for this construct.

9.17   CNTs IN GENE THERAPY

As mentioned in the previous section, drug delivery is one of the main applications of CNTs for the treatment of cancer. It has also been discovered that gene delivery, leading to gene therapy and eventually the treatment of cancer, could also be achieved using CNTS [231].

As a very general definition, gene therapy involves transport of the correct gene by viral or nonviral vectors to the affected area. However, the problem with viral vectors is side effects on the cells, such as inflammation and undesired immune responses. Nonviral vectors, such as liposomes and microparticles, seem to be a safer option, but can also have problems related to a poor pharmacokinetic profile of the administered oligonucleotide and conjugated plasmid DNA [231]. In other words, due to the lack of ability of nonviral vectors to reach and cross the nuclear membrane, the efficiency of gene expression by these vectors is lower compared with viral vectors [41,231,232].

CNTs seem to represent a very good nonviral vector for gene therapy, because they can cross the cell membrane by an endocytosis process, and also, because of the functionalization of CNTs, the DNA can be transferred without any degradation [233]. One of the relevant experiments has investigated delivery of siRNA for the treatment of tumor cells using functionalized MWCNTs and liposomes. The findings showed that the siRNA delivered via MWCNTs achieved significant inhibition of tumor growth [234].

9.18   TOXICITY OF CNT

From much research carried out over recent decades, mankind has seen vital and beneficial changes in science, and one of the most important of these has been nanotechnology. With its promising applications, nanotechnology has demonstrated to scientists that it has the potential to revolutionize many scientific disciplines. CNT is one of the interesting areas of nanotechnology, due to its many physical and chemical properties mentioned in the previous sections [235].

There are many benefits of CNTs, but alongside the positives come a few drawbacks. One of the main concerns for researchers is the fact that nanoparticles, especially CNTs, could be hazardous to human and environmental health [236]. Therefore, this technology must be monitored in order to assess the potential risk it may hold, and nanotoxicology studies of CNT should be undertaken to investigate the safety of these nanoparticles.

According to different investigations, various factors, such as size of the nanoparticles, and their surface chemistry, dosage, morphology, and chemical components, impact the magnitude of their toxicity. Clearly, the toxicity of CNTs has to be kept at a certain level in order for this technology to be safe. Researchers are always interested in finding new ways in which they can adjust toxicity levels to protect human health.

Various factors impact the toxicity of nanoparticles. It has been shown that, as the particle size decreases, the surface area of the particles increases. This means that there will be more area available for chemical interactions to take place, which would enhance the toxicity of the particles [236,237].

Various investigations have been carried out on surface chemistry and chemical components of CNTs. These investigations have shown that, despite the biological advantages of these materials, there are also limitations to their biomedical usage because their surfaces are severely contaminated with metal catalysts and amorphous carbon. One of the studies showed that when murine epidermal cells were exposed to unpurified SWCNTS containing 30% iron, significant dose-dependent activation of transcription factor AP-1 occurred. However, when SWCNTs containing 0.23% iron were added to the same epidermal cells, no significant changes in AP-1 activation were detected. In other words, when there is a large amount of iron present on the surface of SWCNTs, changes in AP-1 are more easily detectable than when there is hardly any iron present [238].

The functionalization process refers to the attachment of appropriate molecules to the CNT surface in order to make these materials less toxic and more biocompatible [239]. Different studies have shown that a high degree of functionalization dramatically reduces the toxicity of CNTs. This is a desirable feature and needs further research to avoid the problem of toxicity [240]. The amount of nanoparticles entering the body also has a major impact on toxicity. Results have shown that, regardless of the size of the particles, a high dose of nanoparticles would be toxic to the body. A number of studies have been done by different research groups on toxicology of CNTs *in vitro*. The results have suggested that, upon the addition of CNTs to cells, genes involved in cellular transport, metabolism, cell cycle regulation, stress response, inflammation, and the immune response may be activated. It has also been suggested that the addition of CNT could activate genes enabling the cell death program to commence. According to various researchers, upon the addition of CNTs to cells, CNTs could enter the cells and be toxic to their functions

[241]. This would have negative implications for the genetic makeup of the cell. Therefore, further research needs to be done in order to reach definitive conclusions.

In another experiment, five concentrations ranging from 0.25 to 100 µg/mL of SWCNTs, MWCNTs, and carbon black were added to RAW 264.7 cells obtained from mice. Results of transmission electron microscopy showed that CNT incubation can eventually induce cell necrosis and apoptosis. Also, 24 h after the addition of CNTs to the RAW 264.7 cells, transmission electron microscopy indicated more phagocytic activity in comparison with normal cells, as shown by changes in nucleus morphology [241]. However, as mentioned earlier, the functionalization technique used will dramatically attenuate the toxicity of CNTs [239].

Morphology of the particles also plays a major role in their toxicity [242]. As an example, the CNTs are known to have a high length to diameter (aspect) ratio, which means that they have the characteristics of both nanoparticles and fibers. Given that CNTs have fibrous characteristics, an extremely high aspect ratio, and low solubility, their behavior can be likened to that of asbestos [236,242]. Fibers are defined as elongated structures with an aspect ratio ≥ 1:3, a length > 5 µm, and diameter ≤ 3 µm. The aspect ratios of CNTs have been found to be up to 100 [243]. The apparent similarities between CNTs and asbestos have led to several groups spearheading investigations into the effects of CNT exposure on the respiratory system. Due to the size of the CNTs, these particles can easily become airborne and inhaled [241]. It has been suggested that widespread distribution of CNTs in the respiratory system could lead to symptoms similar to those that develop after exposure to asbestos [243]. Inhalation of asbestos fibers is known to induce chronic inflammation, scarring of the lungs (asbestosis), and malignant mesothelioma [235]. It has been reported that CNTs delivered to the abdominal cavity of mice can induce a response similar to that associated with exposure to asbestos fibers [244].

In an experiment carried out in the USA, mice were intratracheally instilled with a single dose of CNTs 0, 0.1, or 0.5 mg, using carbon black as a negative control and quartz as a positive control, and euthanized 7 or 90 days later for histopathological study of the lungs. The results showed that CNTs were much more toxic to the lungs at all concentrations in comparison with carbon black and quartz. The CNTs also induced epithelioid granulomas in a dose-dependent manner and, in some cases, caused interstitial inflammation. Peribronchial inflammation and, in some cases, necrosis extending into the alveolar septa were also observed.

In a similar experiment carried out in guinea pigs by a group of researchers at Peking University, various concentrations of SWCNTs, MWCNTs, and C60 were added to alveolar macrophages. Cytotoxicity testing showed that, as the CNT dose increased, more cells became affected by toxicity, demonstrating that necrosis occurs more frequently with increasing CNT dosage. SWCNTs also produced greater toxicity in comparison with MWCNTs at the

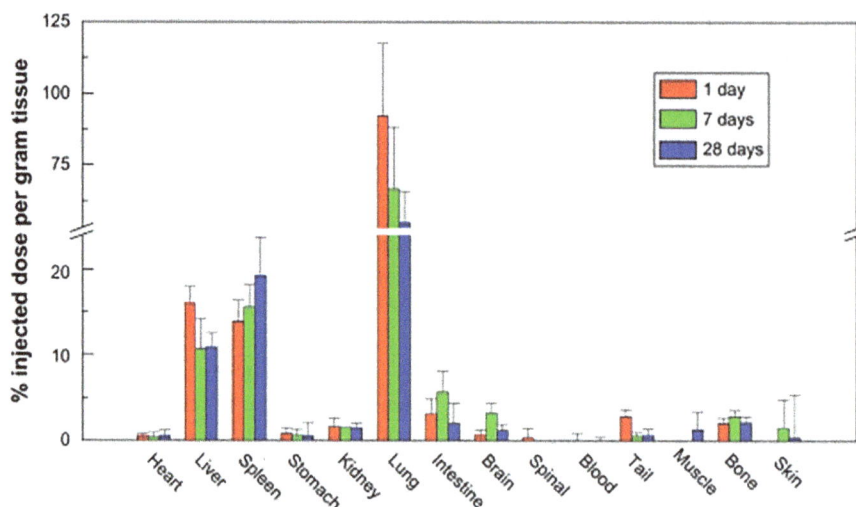

FIGURE 9.14 The biodistribution of carbon nanotubes in different organs. A high biodistribution of carbon nanotubes is seen in the liver, spleen, and lung. (Reprinted with permission from [100]. Copyright 2007, American Chemical Society.)

same doses. Unlike MWCNTs and SWCNTs, C60 did not show any toxicity [245].

Once nanoparticles are inhaled, they deposit on the surface of the lungs and interact with lung surfactants. Upon deposition, they either penetrate the lung tissues or get phagocytosed [242]. CNTs have been associated with defective phagocytosis, leading to chronic inflammation [246], most likely because of their high aspect ratio, which is a property they have in common with asbestos [247].

In another experiment, 50 μg of non-functionalized MWCNTs of different lengths was dispersed in saline with bovine serum albumin and injected into normal mice intraperitoneally. MWCNTs with lengths 0.20 μm accumulated in significant amounts in the diaphragmatic mesothelium, unlike entangled nanotube aggregates or negative control-containing compounds with low aspect ratios and not needle-shaped. This result would indicate that because the long-length CNTs could not be engulfed by macrophages, they would have a higher risk of toxicity [244]. A major question that remains to be answered is the fate of CNTs in biological systems (Figure 9.14). There is evidence to suggest that the clearance rate of CNTs in the body is rather low, which could lead to the formation of granulomas [100].

9.19 FUTURE PERSPECTIVE OF CNTs AS VACCINE DELIVERY SYSTEMS

As with all cancer vaccines, their success, or failure, is dependent on finding the right combination of antigen, adjuvant, and delivery vehicle. The future of CNTs as a delivery platform/adjuvant is dependent on their relative potency compared to other modalities, while the future of the field itself is inextricably linked to the identification of novel antigens or vaccine regimes. In the immediate future, CNTs need to be comprehensively assessed against other vaccine formulations to establish where they belong on the "spectrum of adjuvanticity." These studies are seldom performed

(or at least seldom published) on novel adjuvant candidates due to the fear of coming up short against current formulations and thus losing funding/interest. However, it has made assessing whether an adjuvant is clinically viable over an alternate, near impossible.

Whether the outcome of these studies is positive or negative, it should be noted CNTs have two distinct advantages over traditional adjuvants; the first is their mode of entry into cells. As previously reviewed, CNTs have direct access to the cytosol through the proposed nanoneedle mechanism. The implications of this in the context of vaccine adjuvants should not be understated. The ability to initiate a strong cytotoxic MHC class I restricted immune response to a soluble antigen has been seen as the Holy Grail for vaccine adjuvants. This is especially the case for cancer vaccines but also for vaccines against certain infectious agents [248,249]. In addition, efficient delivery of payload to the cytosol may make other types of vaccines, specifically nucleic acid-based vaccine including DNA and recently mRNA vaccines, more viable. The nanoneedle mechanism is poorly understood with many groups reporting differing outcomes following administration of CNTs depending on a multitude of factors such as surface chemistry, size, and aspect ratios as previously discussed. The first step in the rational design of a CNT-based delivery vehicle should be the systematic evaluation of physical traits and surface modifications in order to improve cytosolic delivery. Our group has looked into some of the modifications of CNTs and has shown that relatively minor changes in structure can cause vast differences in immunogenicity though we have not been able to attribute this to improved cytosolic delivery [136]. Future work should continue and expand upon this.

The second key advantage of CNTs over traditional carriers is their large surface area. According to the current rationale for the use of CNTs, this enables the delivery of large amounts of antigen/adjuvant to APCs. Expanding on this theory, it has recently been shown that particulates can bind to antigen within the tumor environments following intratumoral inoculation [250]. For instance, Min et al. recently demonstrated that an injection of nanoparticle intratumorally, prior to radio ablation of the tumor, served to enhance the so-called abscopal effect: the phenomenon whereby following the ablation of a tumor a systemic immune response is triggered against the released antigen/immune stimulants resulting in remission of distal tumors. One hypothesis is that the particles are retained within the tumor "mopping up" antigen and immune active molecules. When the tumor is subsequently ablated, the particles are released and are taken up by APCs in the tumor-draining lymph nodes [250]. The high surface area of the CNTs and the ability to form strong noncovalent associations with proteins specifically lend them to this purpose. Indeed, it has been shown that GO formulated with CpG can be used for photothermal ablation; though the assessment of the abscopal effect was not measured, there is clearly an immune component [251]. There have been some studies assessing the "protein corona" following administration of CNT intravenously; it would be interesting to perform these studies following intra-tumoral administration to determine how much tumor antigen can be absorbed directly from the tumor tissue in comparison with other carriers [252,253]. Supporting this general hypothesis, it has been shown that CNTs, when formulated *in vitro* with tumor cell lysate, can serve to protect from tumor challenge [126].

Another intra-tumoral approach is the concept of *in situ* vaccination. Here, an agent is injected into the tumor leading to activation of the immune system to antigens present on the tumor/in the microenvironment. This relatively simple concept has led to miraculous results preclinically; notably, the use of CpG and anti-OX40 in combination is particularly potent [254]. It would be interesting to compare anti-OX40 to anti-CD40 Ab plus CpG in combination with CNT in a preclinical model to identify which approach is more efficient in eliciting antitumor immunity. It also would be interesting to compare the efficacy of synthetic CNT vaccines to biological vaccines such as plant virus-based vaccines. Filamentous and spherical plant viruses have been explored as *in situ* vaccines [255,256]. In contrast to plant viruses, which are complex biological entities, CNTs may provide a better-controllable synthetic platform to explore the relationship between morphology and immunogenicity. In addition, CNT vaccines allow different combinations of TLR agonists to be used and thereby enable the dissection of the requirements for optimal formulation.

In more general terms, it is likely that all future cancer vaccine candidates will be trialed in combination with a checkpoint inhibitor at some stage during their clinical assessment. To date, two checkpoint inhibitors have been clinically approved and these are targeted against inhibitory molecules PD-1 and CTLA4 and their purported mechanism has been reviewed elsewhere [10]. However, new classes of stimulatory checkpoint molecules including agonistic anti-OX40 and anti-4-1-BBL antibodies are showing efficacy in preclinical trials [139]. This has led to

the concept of an "immune switch"; this is a biomaterial containing both an immunostimulatory Ab and an anti-inhibitory Ab [257]. In this study, the authors [1] show that the immune switch is more potent than either of the two antibodies when administered in their soluble form. Again, due to their high surface area and ease at forming noncovalent attachments to proteins, CNTs could be the preferred vehicle for this purpose. Other than checkpoint blockade, it could be argued that the generation of personalized vaccines becomes more feasible as DNA sequencing becomes faster and cheaper. The antigenic payload of personalized vaccines will likely be peptides or nucleic acid due to ease of synthesis and quality control. However, both of these modalities are typically poorly immunogenic and require a delivery platform and adjuvant. In a proof-of-concept study, the group of Kuai et al. sequenced murine tumors to detect mutations and these neopeptides were synthesized and loaded onto lipid nanodisks [258]. The resulting particles were shown to protect against tumor challenge. In this approach, it could be envisioned that the adjuvant/delivery platform will be prepared in a ready-to-use "off-the-shelf" format and simply mixed with individual tumor neoantigens as determined by high throughput sequencing. CNTs represent a candidate platform for this approach as they can be synthesized in bulk and stored for long durations with little degradation; furthermore, they can be made positively charged or amine reactive for binding of nucleic acid or peptide, respectively, as previously discussed.

9.20 CONCLUSION AND FUTURE DIRECTIONS

CNTs have cylindrical shape and belong to the fullerene family of carbon allotropes [259,260], consisting of a hexagonal arrangement of sp2-hybridized carbon atoms. The wall of CNTs is formed from single or multiple layers of graphene sheets. When a single sheet is rolled up, it forms SWCNTs, and MWCNTs are obtained by rolling up more than one sheet [261]. CNTs display abilities for drug loading on the surface or in the inner core through covalent and noncovalent interactions. These nanoparticles are able to immobilize therapeutic agents such as drugs, proteins, DNA, and antibodies on the outer wall, or encapsulate them inside the nanotubes, decreasing the cytotoxicity for healthy tissues. Due to their nanoneedle-like structure, carbon nanoparticles are efficiently taken up and translocated into the cytoplasm of target cells without causing cell death. Their applications are limited due to the fact that CNTs are hydrophobic in nature and insoluble in water and are accumulated in internal organs, having a low degradation rate [262]. To eliminate the undesirable effects and to facilitate their use in medical applications, various methods of functionalization of CNTs, such as adsorption and electrostatic and covalent interaction, are used. To increase the systemic retention, circulation time, and solubility of CNTs, a hydrophilic biocompatible polymer with neutral charge such as PEG or polyethylene oxide is used [263,264].

The utilization of CNTs in cancer therapy has expanded dramatically in recent years. Encouraging proof-of-principle studies have been conducted so far, showing great promise for CNT-based therapeutic systems in various cancer treatment modalities. The main advantage is related to the capability of CNTs to deliver cargos intracellularly, and most efforts have concentrated on the development of specific tumor cell targeting following different therapeutic approaches. It has to be emphasized that the development of CNTs is not an end in itself, but part of a broader concerted effort from the wider research community to utilize the different capabilities that various types of nanoscale systems have revealed and can offer to cancer therapy [265]. In that respect, CNTs have been shown to provide with: (i) capability to deliver biologically active molecules cytoplasmatically, bypassing a lot of biological barriers and acting as a cellular needle; (ii) large surface area and internal cavity that can be decorated with targeting ligands and filled with therapeutic or diagnostic agents; and (iii) unprecedented electrical and thermal conductivity properties. However, it is not always possible to precisely compare the many therapeutic approaches, nor the different nanomaterials due to the great diversity among the constructs used. Further work is certainly necessary, both from the chemical point of view, in the preparation of well-characterized constructs with the desired properties, and in terms of biological activity, for a full comprehension of the potential CNT can offer to clinically relevant cancer therapy [67].

The better understanding of tumor immunology has allowed the development of cancer vaccines. However, tumor-induced immunosuppression has constituted a major hurdle to the capacity of these formulations to enhance the immune response. Attempts applied to augment antitumor immune response potency have included the delivery of the aforementioned vaccine formulations via nanocarriers. CNTs demonstrated characteristic cellular uptake properties that encouraged the exploitation of their nanoneedle properties. Preclinical studies highlight that CNTs represent a competent cancer vaccine delivery system. Nevertheless, future studies are required to investigate the uniqueness that these CNTs possess as vaccine carrier over other vectors such as liposomes. In addition, despite the encouraging results reported in preclinical studies, clinical studies are hindered by the conflicting reports on CNTs' biocompatibility and biodegradability.

The novel properties of CNTs allow them to be multifunctional therapeutic agents in cancer treatment. However, one major hurdle that needs to be addressed is the issue of toxicity. It is highly probable that functionalizing CNTs would allow them to be biocompatible for clinical applications. Despite this, the advances made in both *in vivo* and *in vitro* animal models, however small, are very real and are of great significance in our understanding of the biological effects of nanoparticles. Therefore, more rigorous *in vitro* and *in vivo* testing is not only worth pursuing, but necessary.

Finally, fortification of the vaccine formulations via the inclusion of multiple adjuvants, APCs targeting ligands and

combining this approach with a checkpoint inhibitor, could dramatically reduce the required CNTs' doses and encourage their clinical assessment. We hope that future research will confirm the promise toward the achievement of this new technology platform, able to help fight cancer in a more selective and effective way.

REFERENCES

1. H.A.F.M. Hassan, S.S. Diebold, L.A. Smyth, A.A. Walters, G. Lombardi, K.T. Al-Jamal. Application of carbon nanotubes in cancer vaccines: Achievements, challenges and chances, *J. Control. Release* 297 (2019) 79–90.
2. C.R. Parish, Cancer immunotherapy: the past, the present and the future, *Immunol. Cell Biol.* 81 (2003) 106–113.
3. P.G. Coulie, B.J. Van den Eynde, P. van der Bruggen, T. Boon, Tumour antigens recognized by T lymphocytes: at the core of cancer immunotherapy, *Nat. Rev. Cancer* 14 (2014) 135–146.
4. M.R. Stratton, P.J. Campbell, P.A. Futreal, The cancer genome, *Nature* 458 (2009) 719–724.
5. J. Schlom, P.M. Arlen, J.L. Gulley, Cancer vaccines: moving beyond current paradigms, Clinical cancer research: an official journal of the American Association for, *Cancer Res.* 13 (2007) 3776–3782.
6. F. Pages, A. Berger, M. Camus, F. Sanchez-Cabo, A. Costes, R. Molidor, B. Mlecnik, A. Kirilovsky, M. Nilsson, D. Damotte, T. Meatchi, P. Bruneval, P.H. Cugnenc, Z. Trajanoski, W.H. Fridman, J. Galon, Effector memory T cells, early metastasis, and survival in colorectal cancer, *N. Engl. J. Med.* 353 (2005) 2654–2666.
7. K. Palucka, J. Banchereau, Cancer immunotherapy via dendritic cells, *Nat. Rev. Cancer* 12 (2012) 265–277.
8. O.J. Finn, Cancer vaccines: between the idea and the reality, *Nat. Rev. Immunol.* 3 (2003) 630–641.
9. W. Zou, Immunosuppressive networks in the tumour environment and their therapeutic relevance, *Nat. Rev. Cancer* 5 (2005) 263–274.
10. A. Ribas, J.D. Wolchok, Cancer immunotherapy using checkpoint blockade, *Science* 359 (2018) 1350–1355.
11. I. Mellman, G. Coukos, G. Dranoff, Cancer immunotherapy comes of age, *Nature* 480 (2011) 480–489
12. D.S.-W. Tan, M. Gerlinger, B.-T. The, C. Swanton, Anticancer drug resistance: Understanding the mechanisms through the use of integrative genomics and functional RNA interference *Eur. J. Cancer* 46(12) (2010) 2166–2177. doi:10.1016/j.ejca.2010.03.019.
13. S.V. Ambudkar, S. Dey, C.A. Hrycyna, M. Ramachandra, I. Pastan, M.M. Gottesman, Biochemical, cellular, and pharmacological aspects of the multidrug transporter, *Annu. Rev. Pharmacol. Toxicol.* 39 (1999) 361–398. doi:10.1146/annurev.pharmtox.39.1.361.
14. Y. Matsumura, H. Maeda, A new concept for macromolecular therapeutics in cancer chemotherapy: mechanism of tumoritropic accumulation of proteins and the antitumor agent smancs, *Cancer Res.* 46(12) Part 1 (1986) 6387–6392. http://cancerres.aacrjournals.org/content/46/12_Part_1/6387
15. A.K. Iyer, G. Khaled, J. Fang, H. Maeda, Exploiting the enhanced permeability and retention effect for tumor targeting, *Drug Disc. Today* 11 (17–18) (2006) 812–818. doi:10.1016/j.drudis.2006.07.005.

16. K.T. Oh, H.J. Baik, A.H. Lee, Y.T. Oh, Y.S. Youn, E.S. Lee, The reversal of drug-resistance in tumors using a drug-carrying nanoparticular system, *Int. J. Mol. Sci.* 10(9) (2009) 3776–3792. doi:10.3390/ijms10093776.

17. L.S. Jabr-Milane, L.E. van Vlerken, S. Yadav, M.M. Amiji, Multi-functional nanocarriers to overcome tumor drug resistance, *Cancer Treat. Rev.* 34 (7) (2008) 592–602. doi:10.1016/j.ctrv.2008.04.003.

18. N.W.S. Kam, Z. Liu, H. Dai, Carbon nanotubes as intracellular transporters for proteins and DNA: an investigation of the uptake mechanism and pathway, *Angew. Chem. Int. Ed.* 45(4) (2006) 577–581. doi:10.1002/anie.200503389.

19. K. Kostarelos, L. Lacerda, G. Pastorin, W. Wu, S. Wieckowski, J. Luangsivilay, S. Godefroy, D. Pantarotto, J.-Paul Briand, S. Muller, M. Prato, A. Bianco, Cellular uptake of functionalized carbon nanotubes is independent of functional group and cell type, *Nat. Nanotechnol.* 2(2) (2007) 108–113. doi:10.1038/nnano.2006.209.

20. R. Singh, D. Pantarotto, L. Lacerda, G. Pastorin, C. Klumpp, M. Prato, A. Bianco, K. Kostarelos, Tissue biodistribution and blood clearance rates of intravenously administered carbon nanotube radiotracers, *Proc. Natl. Acad. Sci. U. S. A.* 103(9) (2006) 3357–3362. doi:10.1073/pnas.0509009103.

21. L. Lacerda, H. Ali-Boucetta, M.A. Herrero, G. Pastorin, A. Bianco, M. Prato, K. Kostarelos, Tissue histology and physiology following intravenous administration of different types of functionalized multiwalled carbon nanotubes, *Nanomedicine* 3(2) (2008) 149–161. doi:10.2217/17435889.3.2.149.

22. L. Lacerda, M.A. Herrero, K. Venner, A. Bianco, M. Prato, K. Kostarelos, Carbon nanotube shape and individualization critical for renal excretion, *Small* 4(8) (2008) 1130–1132.

23. M.R. McDevitt, D. Chattopadhyay, J.S. Jaggi, R.D. Finn, P.B. Zanzonico, C. Villa, D. Rey, J. Mendenhall, C.A. Batt, J.T. Njardarson, D.A. Scheinberg, PET imaging of soluble yttrium-86-labeled carbon nanotubes in mice, *PLoS One* 2(9) (2007) e907. doi:10.1371/journal.pone.0000907.

24. Z. Liu, C. Davis, W. Cai, L. He, X. Chen, H. Dai, Circulation and long-term fate of functionalized, biocompatible single-walled carbon nanotubes in mice probed by Raman spectroscopy, *Proc. Natl. Acad. Sci. U. S. A.* 105(5) (2008) 1410–1415. doi:10.1073/pnas.0707654105.

25. K. Kostarelos, A. Bianco, M. Prato, Promises, facts and challenges for carbon nanotubes in imaging and therapeutics, *Nat. Nanotechnol.* 4 (2009) 627–633. doi:10.1038/nnano.2009.241.

26. A. Ruggiero, C.H. Villa, E. Bander, D.A. Rey, M. Bergkvist, C.A. Batt, K. Manova Todorova, W.M. Deen, D.A. Scheinberg, M.R. McDevitt, Paradoxical glomerular filtration of carbon nanotubes, *Proc. Natl. Acad. Sci. U. S. A.* 107(27) (2010) 12369–12374. doi:10.1073/pnas.0913667107.

27. C.A. Poland, R. Duffin, I. Kinloch, A. Maynard, W.A.H. Wallace, A. Seaton, V. Stone, S. Brown, W. Macnee, K. Donaldson, Carbon nanotubes introduced into the abdominal cavity of mice show asbestos-like pathogenicity in a pilot study, *Nat. Nanotechnol.* 3(7) (2008) 423–428. doi:10.1038/nnano.2008.111.

28. H. Nagai, Y. Okazaki, S.H. Chew, N. Misawa, Y. Yamashita, S. Akatsuka, T. Ishihara, K. Yamashita, Y. Yoshikawa, H. Yasui, L. Jiang, H. Ohara, T. Takahashi, G. Ichihara, K. Kostarelos, Y. Miyata, H. Shinohara, S. Toyokuni, Diameter and rigidity of multiwalled carbon nanotubes are critical factors in mesothelial injury and carcinogenesis, *Proc. Natl. Acad. Sci. U. S. A.* 108(49) (2011) E1330–E1338. doi:10.1073/pnas.1110013108.

29. C.M. Sayes, F. Liang, J.L. Hudson, J. Mendez, W. Guo, J.M. Beach, V.C. Moore, C.D. Doyle, J.L. West, W.E. Billups, K.D. Ausman, V.L. Colvin, Functionalization density dependence of single-walled carbon nanotubes cytotoxicity in vitro, *Toxicol. Lett.* 161(2) (2006) 135–142. doi:10.1016/j.toxlet.2005.08.011.

30. H. Ali-Boucetta, K.T. Al-Jamal, K.H. Mu¨ller, S. Li, A.E. Porter, A. Eddaoudi, M. Prato, A. Bianco, K. Kostarelos, Cellular Uptake and Cytotoxic Impact of Chemically Functionalized and Polymer-Coated Carbon Nanotubes, *Small* 7(22) (2011) 3230–3238. doi:10.1002/smll.201101004.

31. L.W. Zhang, L. Zeng, A.R. Barron, N.A. Monteiro-Riviere, Biological interactions of functionalized single-wall carbon nanotubes in human epidermal keratinocytes, *Int. J. Toxicol.* 26(2) (2008) 103–113. doi:10.1080/10915810701225133.

32. A. Bianco, K. Kostarelos, M. Prato, Making carbon nanotubes biocompatible and biodegradable, *Chem. Commun.* 47 (2011) 10182–10188. doi:10.1039/C1CC13011K

33. A. Nunes, C. Bussy, L. Gherardini, M. Meneghetti, M.A. Herrero, A. Bianco, M. Prato, T. Pizzorusso, K.T. Al-Jamal, K. Kostarelos, In vivo degradation of functionalized carbon nanotubes after stereotactic administration in the brain cortex, *Nanomedicine* 7(10) (2012) 1485–1494. doi: 10.2217/NNM.12.33.

34. C. Fabbro, H. Ali-Boucetta, T. Da Ros, K. Kostarelos, A. Bianco, M. Prato. Targeting carbon nanotubes against cancer, *Chem. Commun.* 48 (2012) 3911–3926. This journal is © The Royal Society of Chemistry 2012 www.rsc.org/chemcomm.

35. H. Ghanbari, A. de Mel, A.M. Seifalian, Cardiovascular application of polyhedral oligomeric silsesquioxane nanomaterials: A glimpse into prospective horizons, *Int. J. Nanomed.* 6 (2011) 775–786.

36. T. Jamieson, R. Bakhshi, D. Petrova, R. Pocock, M. Imani, A.M. Seifalian, Biological applications of quantum dots, *Biomaterials* 28 (2007) 4717–4732.

37. A. Tan, H. De La Pena, A.M. Seifalian, The application of exosomes as a nanoscale cancer vaccine, *Int. J. Nanomed.* 5 (2010) 889–900.

38. T.M. Chang, S. Prakash, Procedures for microencapsulation of enzymes, cells and genetically engineered microorganisms, *Mol. Biotechnol.* 17 (2001) 249–260.

39. S.Y. Madani, N. Naderi, O. Dissanayake, A. Tan, A.M. Seifalian. A new era of cancer treatment: carbon nanotubes as drug delivery tools, *Int. J. Nanomed.* 6 (2011) 2963–2979.

40. N.G. Sahoo, H. Bao, Y. Pan, et al., Functionalized carbon nanomaterials as nanocarriers for loading and delivery of a poorly water-soluble anticancer drug: A comparative study, *Chem. Commun (Camb).* 47 (2011) 5235–5237.

41. C. Klumpp, K. Kostarelos, M. Prato, A. Bianco, Functionalized carbon nanotubes as emerging nanovectors for the delivery of therapeutics, *Biochim. Biophys. Acta.* 1758 (2006) 404–412.

42. E. Bekyarova, Y. Ni, E.B. Malarkey, et al., Applications of carbon nanotubes in biotechnology and biomedicine, *J. Biomed Nanotechnol.* 1 (2005) 3–17.

43. P. Utreja, S. Jain, A.K. Tiwary. Novel drug delivery systems for sustained and targeted delivery of anti-cancer drugs: Current status and future prospects, *Curr. Drug Deliv.* 7 (2010) 152–161.

44. C. Lamprecht, I. Liashkovich, V. Neves, et al., AFM imaging of functionalized carbon nanotubes on biological membranes, *Nanotechnology* 20 (2009) 434001.

45. S. Beg, M. Rizwan, A.M. Sheikh, M.S. Hasnain, K. Anwer, K. Kohli, Advancement in carbon nanotubes: Basics, biomedical applications and toxicity, *J. Pharm. Pharmacol.* 63 (2011) 141–163.

46. V. Raffa, G. Ciofani, O. Vittorio, C. Riggio, A. Cuschieri, Physicochemical properties affecting cellular uptake of carbon nanotubes, *Nanomedicine (Lond).* 5 (2010) 89–97.

47. A.E. Porter, M. Gass, K. Muller, J.N. Skepper, P.A. Midgley, M. Welland, Direct imaging of single-walled carbon nanotubes in cells, *Nat. Nanotechnol.* 2 (2007) 713–717.

48. A. Bianco, K. Kostarelos, M. Prato, Applications of carbon nanotubes in drug delivery, *Curr. Opin. Chem. Biol.* 9 (2005) 674–679.

49. D. Pantarotto, J.P. Briand, M. Prato, A. Bianco, Translocation of bioactive peptides across cell membranes by carbon nanotubes, *Chem. Commun (Camb)* 1 (2004) 16–17.

50. J.F. Campbell, I. Tessmer, H.H. Thorp, D.A. Erie, Atomic force microscopy studies of DNA-wrapped carbon nanotube structure and binding to quantum dots, *J. Am. Chem. Soc.* 130 (2008) 10648–10655.

51. N.W. Kam, H. Dai, Carbon nanotubes as intracellular protein transporters: Generality and biological functionality, *J. Am. Chem. Soc.* 127 (2005) 6021–6026.

52. U. Arsawang, O. Saengsawang, T. Rungrotmongkol, et al., How do carbon nanotubes serve as carriers for gemcitabine transport in a drug delivery system? *J. Mol. Graph. Model* 2011 (29) 591–596.

53. N.W. Shi Kam, T.C. Jessop, P.A. Wender, H. Dai, Nanotube molecular transporters: Internalization of carbon nanotube-protein conjugates into mammalian cells, *J. Am. Chem. Soc.* 126 (2004) 6850–6851.

54. N.W. Kam, M. O'Connell, J.A. Wisdom, H. Dai, Carbon nanotubes as multifunctional biological transporters and near-infrared agents for selective cancer cell destruction, *Proc. Natl. Acad. Sci. U. S. A.* 102 (2005) 11600–11605.

55. D. Danailov, P. Keblinski, S. Nayak, P.M. Ajayan, Bending properties of carbon nanotubes encapsulating solid nanowires, *J. Nanosci. Nanotechnol.* 2 (2002) 503–507.

56. T.W. Ebbesen, P.M. Ajayan, Large-scale synthesis of carbon nanotubes, *Nature* 358 (1992) 220–222.

57. R.P. Feazell, N. Nakayama-Ratchford, H. Dai, S.J. Lippard, Soluble singlewalled carbon nanotubes as longboat delivery systems for platinum (IV) anticancer drug design, *J. Am. Chem. Soc.* 129 (2007) 8438–8439.

58. Z. Liu, K. Chen, C. Davis, et al., Drug delivery with carbon nanotubes for in vivo cancer treatment, *Cancer Res.* 68 (2008) 6652–6660.

59. Z. Liu, C. Davis, W. Cai, L. He, X. Chen, H. Dai, Circulation and long-term fate of functionalized, biocompatible single-walled carbon nanotubes in mice probed by Raman spectroscopy, *Proc. Natl. Acad. Sci. U. S. A.* 105 (2008) 1410–1415.

60. A. Hartschuh, H.N. Pedrosa, L. Novotny, T.D., Simultaneous fluorescence and Raman scattering from single carbon nanotubes, *Science* 301 (2003) 1354–1356.

61. L.R. Hirsch, R.J. Stafford, J.A. Bankson, et al., Nanoshell-mediated nearinfrared thermal therapy of tumors under magnetic resonance guidance, *Proc. Natl. Acad. Sci. U. S. A.* 100 (2003) 13549–13554.

62. A. Hirsch, The era of carbon allotropes, *Nat. Mater.* 9 (2010) 868–871.

63. H.W. Kroto, J.R. Heath, S.C. O'Brien, R.F. Curl, R.E. Smalley, C60: Buckminsterfullerene, *Nature* 318 (1985) 162–163.

64. K.S. Novoselov, A.K. Geim, S.V. Morozov, D. Jiang, Y. Zhang, S.V. Dubonos, I.V. Grigorieva, A.A. Firsov, Electric field effect in atomically thin carbon films, *Science* 306 (2004) 666–669.

65. S. Iijima, Helical microtubules of graphitic carbon, *Nature* 354 (1991) 56–58.

66. E.T. Thostenson, Z. Ren, T.-W. Chou, Advances in the science and technology of carbon nanotubes and their composites: a review, *Compos. Sci. Technol.* 61 (2001) 1899–1912.

67. L. Xu, Y. Liu, Z. Chen, W. Li, Y. Liu, L. Wang, L. Ma, Y. Shao, Y. Zhao, C. Chen, Morphologically virus-like fullerenol nanoparticles act as the dual-functional nanoadjuvant for HIV-1 vaccine, *Adv. Mater.* 25 (2013) 5928–5936.

68. B.G. Trewyn, J.A. Nieweg, Y. Zhao, V.S.Y. Lin, Biocompatible mesoporous silica nanoparticles with different morphologies for animal cell membrane penetration, *Chem. Eng. J.* 137 (2008) 23–29.

69. X. Huang, X. Teng, D. Chen, F. Tang, J. He, The effect of the shape of mesoporous silica nanoparticles on cellular uptake and cell function, *Biomaterials* 31 (2010) 438–448.

70. K.-C. Mei, A. Ghazaryan, E.Z. Teoh, H.D. Summers, Y. Li, B. Ballesteros, J. Piasecka, A. Walters, R.C. Hider, V. Mailänder, K.T. Al-Jamal, Protein-corona-by-design in 2D: a reliable platform to decode bio–nano interactions for the next generation quality-by-design nanomedicines, *Adv. Mater.* 30 (2018) 1802732.

71. N. Rubio, K.C. Mei, R. Klippstein, P.M. Costa, N. Hodgins, J.T. Wang, F. Festy, V. Abbate, R.C. Hider, K.L. Chan, K.T. Al-Jamal, Solvent-free click-mechanochemistry for the preparation of cancer cell targeting graphene oxide, *ACS Appl. Mater. Interfaces* 7 (2015) 18920–18923.

72. K.C. Mei, Y. Guo, J. Bai, P.M. Costa, H. Kafa, A. Protti, R.C. Hider, K.T. Al-Jamal, Organic solvent-free, one-step engineering of graphene-based magnetic-responsive hybrids using design of experiment-driven mechanochemistry, *ACS Appl. Mater. Interfaces* 7 (2015) 14176–14181.

73. K.C. Mei, N. Rubio, P.M. Costa, H. Kafa, V. Abbate, F. Festy, S.S. Bansal, R.C. Hider, K.T. Al-Jamal, Synthesis of double-clickable functionalised grapheme oxide for biological applications, *Chem. Commun. (Camb.)* 51 (2015) 14981–14984.

74. H. Yue, W. Wei, Z. Gu, D. Ni, N. Luo, Z. Yang, L. Zhao, J.A. Garate, R. Zhou, Z. Su, G. Ma, Exploration of graphene oxide as an intelligent platform for cancer vaccines, *Nanoscale* 7 (2015) 19949–19957.

75. A. Sinha, B.G. Cha, Y. Choi, T.L. Nguyen, P.J. Yoo, J.H. Jeong, J. Kim, Carbohydrate-functionalized rGO as an effective cancer vaccine for stimulating antigen-specific cytotoxic T cells and inhibiting tumor growth, *Chem. Mater.* 29 (2017) 6883–6892.

76. X. Zhang, W. Hu, J. Li, L. Tao, Y. Wei, A comparative study of cellular uptake and cytotoxicity of multi-walled carbon nanotubes, graphene oxide, and nanodiamond, *Toxicol. Res.* 1 (2012) 62–68.

77. K. Kostarelos, L. Lacerda, G. Pastorin, W. Wu, S. Wieckowski, J. Luangsivilay, S. Godefroy, D. Pantarotto, J.P. Briand, S. Muller, M. Prato, A. Bianco, Cellular uptake

of functionalized carbon nanotubes is independent of functional group and cell type, *Nat. Nanotechnol.* 2 (2007) 108–113.

78. Q. Mu, D.L. Broughton, B. Yan, Endosomal leakage and nuclear translocation of multiwalled carbon nanotubes: developing a model for cell uptake, *Nano Lett.* 9 (2009) 4370–4375.

79. J.A. Villadangos, P. Schnorrer, Intrinsic and cooperative antigen-presenting functions of dendritic-cell subsets in vivo, *Nat. Rev. Immunol.* 7 (2007) 543–555.

80. C.F. Lopez, S.O. Nielsen, P.B. Moore, M.L. Klein, Understanding nature's design for a nanosyringe, *Proc. Natl. Acad. Sci. U. S. A.* 101 (2004) 4431–4434.

81. J. Tschopp, K. Schroder, NLRP3 inflammasome activation: the convergence of multiple signalling pathways on ROS production? *Nat. Rev. Immunol.* 10 (2010) 210–215.

82. Y. He, H. Hara, G. Nunez, Mechanism and regulation of NLRP3 inflammasome activation, *Trends Biochem. Sci.* 41 (2016) 1012–1021.

83. D. Cui, F. Tian, C.S. Ozkan, M. Wang, H. Gao, Effect of single wall carbon nanotubes on human HEK293 cells, *Toxicol. Lett.* 155 (2005) 73–85.

84. B.M. Rotoli, O. Bussolati, M.G. Bianchi, A. Barilli, C. Balasubramanian, S. Bellucci, E. Bergamaschi, Non-functionalized multi-walled carbon nanotubes alter the paracellular permeability of human airway epithelial cells, *Toxicol. Lett.* 178 (2008) 95–102.

85. P.-X. Hou, C. Liu, H.-M. Cheng, Purification of carbon nanotubes, *Carbon* 46 (2008) 2003–2025.

86. R. Li, X. Wang, Z. Ji, B. Sun, H. Zhang, C.H. Chang, S. Lin, H. Meng, Y.P. Liao, M. Wang, Z. Li, A.A. Hwang, T.B. Song, R. Xu, Y. Yang, J.I. Zink, A.E. Nel, T. Xia, Surface charge and cellular processing of covalently functionalized multiwall carbon nanotubes determine pulmonary toxicity, *ACS Nano* 7 (2013) 2352–2368.

87. A.E. Porter, M. Gass, J.S. Bendall, K. Muller, A. Goode, J.N. Skepper, P.A. Midgley, M. Welland, Uptake of non-cytotoxic acid-treated single-walled carbon nanotubes into the cytoplasm of human macrophage cells, *ACS Nano* 3 (2009) 1485–1492.

88. V.E. Kagan, Y.Y. Tyurina, V.A. Tyurin, N.V. Konduru, A.I. Potapovich, A.N. Osipov, E.R. Kisin, D. Schwegler-Berry, R. Mercer, V. Castranova, A.A. Shvedova, Direct and indirect effects of single walled carbon nanotubes on RAW 264.7 macrophages: role of iron, *Toxicol. Lett.* 165 (2006) 88–100.

89. K. Pulskamp, S. Diabaté, H.F. Krug, Carbon nanotubes show no sign of acute toxicity but induce intracellular reactive oxygen species in dependence on contaminants, *Toxicol. Lett.* 168 (2007) 58–74.

90. J. Palomäki, E. Välimäki, J. Sund, M. Vippola, P.A. Clausen, K.A. Jensen, K. Savolainen, S. Matikainen, H. Alenius, Long, needle-like carbon nanotubes and asbestos activate the NLRP3 inflammasome through a similar mechanism, *ACS Nano* 5 (2011) 6861–6870.

91. J. Wang, R.H. Sun, N. Zhang, H. Nie, J.H. Liu, J.N. Wang, H. Wang, Y. Liu, Multiwalled carbon nanotubes do not impair immune functions of dendritic cells, *Carbon* 47 (2009) 1752–1760.

92. H. Dumortier, S. Lacotte, G. Pastorin, R. Marega, W. Wu, D. Bonifazi, J.P. Briand, M. Prato, S. Muller, A. Bianco, Functionalized carbon nanotubes are non-cytotoxic and preserve the functionality of primary immune cells, *Nano Lett.* 6 (2006) 1522–1528.

93. M. Pescatori, D. Bedognetti, E. Venturelli, C. Ménard-Moyon, C. Bernardini, E. Muresu, A. Piana, G. Maida, R. Manetti, F. Sgarrella, A. Bianco, L.G. Delogu, Functionalized carbon nanotubes as immunomodulator systems, *Biomaterials* 34 (2013) 4395–4403.

94. K. Medepalli, B. Alphenaar, A. Raj, P. Sethu, Evaluation of the direct and indirect response of blood leukocytes to carbon nanotubes (CNTs), *Nanomedicine* 7 (2011) 983–991.

95. M. Prato, K. Kostarelos, A. Bianco, Functionalized carbon nanotubes in drug design and discovery. *Acc. Chem. Res.* 41 (2008) 60–68.

96. I.D. Rosca, F. Watari, M. Uo, T. Akaska, Oxidation of multiwalled carbon nanotubes by nitric acid. *Carbon* 2005;43:3124–3131.

97. Z. Liu, X. Sun, N. Nakayama-Ratchford, H. Dai, Supramolecular chemistry on water-soluble carbon nanotubes for drug loading and delivery, *ACS Nano.* 2007;1:50–56.

98. S. Niyogi, M.A. Hamon, H. Hu, et al., Chemistry of single-walled carbon nanotubes, *Acc. Chem. Res.* 35 (2002) 1105–1113.

99. Z. Liu, S.M. Tabakman, Z. Chen, H. Dai, Preparation of carbon nanotube bioconjugates for biomedical applications, *Nat Protoc.* 4 (2009) 1372–1382.

100. S.-t. Yang, W. Guo, Y. Lin, X.-y. Deng, H.-f. Wang, H.-f. Sun, Y.-f. Liu, X. Wang, W. Wang, M. Chen, Y.-p. Huang, Y.-P. Sun, Biodistribution of pristine singlewalled carbon nanotubes in vivo, *J. Phys. Chem. C* 111 (2007) 17761–17764.

101. J. Meng, M. Yang, F. Jia, Z. Xu, H. Kong, H. Xu, Immune responses of BALB/c mice to subcutaneously injected multi-walled carbon nanotubes, *Nanotoxicology* 5 (2011) 583–591.

102. M.L. De Temmerman, J. Rejman, J. Demeester, D.J. Irvine, B. Gander, S.C. De Smedt, Particulate vaccines: on the quest for optimal delivery and immune response, *Drug Discov. Today* 16 (2011) 569–582.

103. M.F. Bachmann, G.T. Jennings, Vaccine delivery: a matter of size, geometry, kinetics and molecular patterns, *Nat. Rev. Immunol.* 10 (2010) 787–796.

104. D.M. Smith, J.K. Simon, J.R. Baker Jr., Applications of nanotechnology for immunology, *Nat. Rev. Immunol.* 13 (2013) 592–605.

105. D.J. Irvine, M.A. Swartz, G.L. Szeto, Engineering synthetic vaccines using cues from natural immunity, *Nat. Mater.* 12 (2013) 978–990.

106. Y. Krishnamachari, S.M. Geary, C.D. Lemke, A.K. Salem, Nanoparticle delivery systems in cancer vaccines, *Pharm. Res.* 28 (2010) 215–236.

107. M.J. Smyth, S.F. Ngiow, A. Ribas, M.W. Teng, Combination cancer immunotherapies tailored to the tumour microenvironment, *Nat. Rev. Clin. Oncol.* 13 (2016) 143–158.

108. V.P. Torchilin, Recent advances with liposomes as pharmaceutical carriers, *Nat. Rev. Drug Discov.* 4 (2005) 145–160.

109. M.M. Whitmore, S. Li, L. Falo Jr., L. Huang, Systemic administration of LPD prepared with CpG oligonucleotides inhibits the growth of established pulmonary metastases by stimulating innate and acquired antitumor immune responses, *Cancer Immunol. Immunother.* 50 (2001) 503–514.

110. S. Hamdy, O. Molavi, Z. Ma, A. Haddadi, A. Alshamsan, Z. Gobti, S. Elhasi, J. Samuel, A. Lavasanifar, Co-delivery of cancer-associated antigen and Toll-like receptor 4 ligand in PLGA nanoparticles induces potent CD8+ T cell-mediated anti-tumor immunity, *Vaccine* 26 (2008) 5046–5057.

111. A. Zeltins, Construction and characterization of virus-like particles: a review, *Mol. Biotechnol.* 53 (2013) 92–107.

112. G. Zhu, G.M. Lynn, O. Jacobson, K. Chen, Y. Liu, H. Zhang, Y. Ma, F. Zhang, R. Tian, Q. Ni, S. Cheng, Z. Wang, N. Lu, B.C. Yung, L. Lang, X. Fu, A. Jin, I.D. Weiss, H. Vishwasrao, G. Niu, H. Shroff, D.M. Klinman, R.A. Seder, X. Chen, Albumin/vaccine nanocomplexes that assemble in vivo for combination cancer immunotherapy, *Nat. Commun.* 8 (2017) 1954.

113. B.G. Cha, J.H. Jeong, J. Kim, Extra-large pore mesoporous silica nanoparticles enabling co-delivery of high amounts of protein antigen and toll-like receptor 9 agonist for enhanced cancer vaccine efficacy, *ACS Central Sci.* 4 (2018) 484–492.

114. M. Mueller, E. Schlosser, B. Gander, M. Groettrup, Tumor eradication by immunotherapy with biodegradable PLGA microspheres–an alternative to incomplete Freund's adjuvant, *Int. J. Cancer* 129 (2011) 407–416.

115. S.M. Geary, Q. Hu, V.B. Joshi, N.B. Bowden, A.K. Salem, Diaminosulfide based polymer microparticles as cancer vaccine delivery systems, *J. Control. Release* 220 (2015) 682–690.

116. D. Wakita, K. Chamoto, Y. Zhang, Y. Narita, D. Noguchi, H. Ohnishi, T. Iguchi, T. Sakai, H. Ikeda, T. Nishimura, An indispensable role of type-1 IFNs for inducing CTL-mediated complete eradication of established tumor tissue by CpG-liposome co-encapsulated with model tumor antigen, *Int. Immunol.* 18 (2006) 425–434.

117. B. Ludewig, F. Barchiesi, M. Pericin, R.M. Zinkernagel, H. Hengartner, R.A. Schwendener, In vivo antigen loading and activation of dendritic cells via a liposomal peptide vaccine mediates protective antiviral and anti-tumour immunity, *Vaccine* 19 (2000) 23–32.

118. W. Chen, W. Yan, L. Huang, A simple but effective cancer vaccine consisting of an antigen and a cationic lipid, *Cancer Immunol. Immunother.* 57 (2007) 517–530.

119. S. Shariat, A. Badiee, S.A. Jalali, M. Mansourian, M. Yazdani, S.A. Mortazavi, M.R. Jaafari, P5 HER2/neu-derived peptide conjugated to liposomes containing MPL adjuvant as an effective prophylactic vaccine formulation for breast cancer, *Cancer Lett.*, 355 (2014) 54–60.

120. Z. Zhang, S. Tongchusak, Y. Mizukami, Y.J. Kang, T. Ioji, M. Touma, B. Reinhold, D.B. Keskin, E.L. Reinherz, T. Sasada, Induction of anti-tumor cytotoxic T cell responses through PLGA-nanoparticle mediated antigen delivery, *Biomaterials* 32 (2011) 3666–3678.

121. K.K. Ahmed, S.M. Geary, A.K. Salem, Development and evaluation of biodegradable particles coloaded with antigen and the toll-like receptor agonist, pentaerythritol lipid a, as a cancer vaccine, *J. Pharm. Sci.* 105 (2016) 1173–1179.

122. R.A. Rosalia, L.J. Cruz, S. van Duikeren, A.T. Tromp, A.L. Silva, W. Jiskoot, T. de Gruijl, C. Lowik, J. Oostendorp, S.H. van der Burg, F. Ossendorp, CD40-targeted dendritic cell delivery of PLGA-nanoparticle vaccines induce potent anti-tumor responses, *Biomaterials* 40 (2015) 88–97.

123. N.M. Molino, M. Neek, J.A. Tucker, E.L. Nelson, S.W. Wang, Viral-mimicking protein nanoparticle vaccine for eliciting anti-tumor responses, *Biomaterials* 86 (2016) 83–91.

124. M. Mueller, W. Reichardt, J. Koerner, M. Groettrup, Coencapsulation of tumor lysate and CpG-ODN in PLGA-microspheres enables successful immunotherapy of prostate carcinoma in TRAMP mice, *J. Control. Release* 162 (2012) 159–166.

125. Z. Sun, W. Wang, J. Meng, S. Chen, H. Xu, X.D. Yang, Multi-walled carbon nanotubes conjugated to tumor protein enhance the uptake of tumor antigens by human dendritic cells in vitro, *Cell Res.* 20 (2010) 1170–1173.

126. J. Meng, J. Duan, H. Kong, L. Li, C. Wang, S. Xie, S. Chen, N. Gu, H. Xu, X.D. Yang, Carbon nanotubes conjugated to tumor lysate protein enhance the efficacy of an antitumor immunotherapy, *Small* 4 (2008) 1364–1370.

127. C.H. Villa, T. Dao, I. Ahearn, N. Fehrenbacher, E. Casey, D.A. Rey, T. Korontsvit, V. Zakhaleva, C.A. Batt, M.R. Philips, D.A. Scheinberg, Single-walled carbon nanotubes deliver peptide antigen into dendritic cells and enhance igg responses to tumor-associated antigens, *ACS Nano* 5 (2011) 5300–5311.

128. S.S. Diebold, Determination of T-cell fate by dendritic cells, *Immunol. Cell Biol.* 86 (2008) 389–397.

129. C.A. Janeway Jr., R. Medzhitov, Innate immune recognition, *Annu. Rev. Immunol.* 20 (2002) 197–216.

130. N.W. Palm, R. Medzhitov, Pattern recognition receptors and control of adaptive immunity, *Immunol. Rev.* 227 (2009) 221–233.

131. S. Gordon, Pattern recognition receptors: doubling up for the innate immune response, *Cell* 111 (2002) 927–930.

132. A.M. Krieg, Toll-like receptor 9 (TLR9) agonists in the treatment of cancer, *Oncogene* 27 (2008) 161–167.

133. F. Steinhagen, T. Kinjo, C. Bode, D.M. Klinman, TLR-based immune adjuvants, *Vaccine* 29 (2011) 3341–3355.

134. D.M. Klinman, Immunotherapeutic uses of CpG oligodeoxynucleotides, *Nat. Rev. Immunol.* 4 (2004) 249–258.

135. P.C.B. de Faria, L.I. dos Santos, J.P. Coelho, H.B. Ribeiro, M.A. Pimenta, L.O. Ladeira, D.A. Gomes, C.A. Furtado, R.T. Gazzinelli, Oxidized multiwalled carbon nanotubes as antigen delivery system to promote superior CD8(+) T cell response and protection against cancer, *Nano Lett.* 14 (2014) 5458–5470.

136. H.A.F.M. Hassan, L. Smyth, N. Rubio, K. Ratnasothy, J.T.W. Wang, S.S. Bansal, H.D. Summers, S.S. Diebold, G. Lombardi, K.T. Al-Jamal, Carbon nanotubes' surface chemistry determines their potency as vaccine nanocarriers in vitro and in vivo, *J. Control. Release* 225 (2016) 205–216.

137. H.A.F.M. Hassan, L. Smyth, J.T.W. Wang, P.M. Costa, K. Ratnasothy, S.S. Diebold G. Lombardi, K.T. Al-Jamal, Dual stimulation of antigen presenting cells using carbon nanotube-based vaccine delivery system for cancer immunotherapy, *Biomaterials* 104 (2016) 310–322.

138. C. van Kooten, J. Banchereau, CD40-CD40 ligand, *J. Leukoc. Biol.* 67 (2000) 2–17.

139. I. Melero, S. Hervas-Stubbs, M. Glennie, D.M. Pardoll, L. Chen, Immunostimulatory monoclonal antibodies for cancer therapy, *Nat. Rev. Cancer* 7 (2007) 95–106.

140. B. Chatterjee, A. Smed-Sorensen, L. Cohn, C. Chalouni, R. Vandlen, B.C. Lee, J. Widger, T. Keler, L. Delamarre, I. Mellman, Internalization and endosomal degradation of receptor-bound antigens regulate the efficiency of cross presentation by human dendritic cells, *Blood* 120 (2012) 2011–2020.

141. L. Cohn, B. Chatterjee, F. Esselborn, A. Smed-Sorensen, N. Nakamura, C. Chalouni, B.C. Lee, R. Vandlen, T. Keler, P. Lauer, D. Brockstedt, I. Mellman, L. Delamarre, Antigen delivery to early endosomes eliminates the superiority of human blood BDCA3+ dendritic cells at cross presentation, *J. Exp. Med.* 210 (2013) 1049–1063.

142. W. Kastenmuller, K. Kastenmuller, C. Kurts, R.A. Seder, Dendritic cell-targeted vaccines–hope or hype? *Nat. Rev. Immunol.* 14 (2014) 705–711.

143. S. Hampel, D. Kunze, D. Haase, et al., Carbon nanotubes filled with a chemotherapeutic agent: A nanocarrier mediates inhibition of tumor cell growth, *Nanomedicine (Lond).* 3 (2008) 175–182.

144. H. Jin, D.A. Heller, M.S. Strano, Single-particle tracking of endocytosis and exocytosis of single-walled carbon nanotubes in NIH-3T3 cells, *Nano Lett.* 8 (2008) 1577–1585.

145. W. Wu, R. Li, X. Bian, et al., Covalently combining carbon nanotubes with anticancer agent: Preparation and antitumor activity, *ACS Nano.* 2009; 3:2740–2750.

146. Y. Li, B.G. Cousins, R.V. Ulijn, I.A. Kinloch, A study of the dynamic interaction of surfactants with graphite and carbon nanotubes using Fmoc-amino acids as a model system, *Langmuir* 25 (2009) 11760–11767.

147. H. Xu, J. Meng, H. Kong, What are carbon nanotube roles in anti-tumor therapies? *Sci. China* 53 (2010) 2250–2256.

148. H.M. Deutsch, J.A. Glinski, M. Hernandez, et al., Synthesis of congeners and prodrugs. 3. Water-soluble prodrugs of taxol with potent antitumor activity, *J. Med. Chem.* 32 (1989) 788–792.

149. S. Dhar, Z. Liu, J. Thomale, H. Dai, S.J. Lippard, Targeted single-wall carbon nanotube-mediated Pt(IV) prodrug delivery using folate as a homing device, *J. Am. Chem. Soc.* 130 (2008) 11467–11476.

150. M.M. Gottesman, T. Fojo, S.E. Bates, Multidrug resistance in cancer: Role of ATP-dependent transporters, *Nat. Rev. Cancer.* 2 (2002) 48–58.

151. H. li-Boucetta, K.T. Al-Jamal, D. McCarthy, M. Prato, A. Bianco, K. Kostarelos, Multiwalled carbon nanotube-doxorubicin supramolecular complexes for cancer therapeutics, *Chem. Commun (Camb).* 4 (2008) 459–461.

152. Liu Z, Fan AC, Rakhra K, et al., Supramolecular stacking of doxorubicin on carbon nanotubes for in vivo cancer therapy, *Angew. Chem. Int. Ed. Eng.* 48 (2009) 7668–7672.

153. H. Ali-Boucetta, K.T. Al-Jamal, D. McCarthy, M. Prato, A. Bianco, K. Kostarelos, Multiwalled carbon nanotube–doxorubicin supramolecular complexes for cancer therapeutics, *Chem. Commun.* 4 (2008) 459–461. doi:10.1039/B712350G.

154. Z. Liu, X. Sun, N. Nakayama-Ratchford, H. Dai, Supramolecular chemistry on water-soluble carbon nanotubes for drug loading and delivery, *ACS Nano* 1(1) (2007) 50–56. doi:10.1021/nn700040t.

155. Z. Liu, A.C. Fan, K. Rakhra, S. Sherlock, A. Goodwin, X. Chen, Q. Yang, D.W. Felsher, H. Dai, Supramolecular stacking of doxorubicin on carbon nanotubes for in vivo cancer therapy, *Angew. Chem., Int. Ed.* 48(41) (2009) 7668–7672. doi:10.1002/anie.200902612.

156. Z. Liu, W. Cai, L. He, N. Nakayama, K. Chen, X. Sun, X. Chen, H. Dai, In vivo biodistribution and highly efficient tumour targeting of carbon nanotubes in mice, *Nat. Nanotechnol.* 2 (2007) 47–52. doi:10.1038/nnano.2006.170.

157. X. Zhang, L. Meng, Q. Lu, Z. Fei, P.J. Dyson, Targeted delivery and controlled release of doxorubicin to cancer cells using modified single wall carbon nanotubes, *Biomaterials* 30(30) (2009) 6041–6047. doi:10.1016/j.biomaterials.2009.07.025.

158. E. Heister, V. Neves, C. Tîlmaciu, K. Lipert, V.S. Beltran, H.M. Coley, S.R.P. Silva, J. McFadden, Triple functionalisation of single-walled carbon nanotubes with doxorubicin, a monoclonal antibody, and a fluorescent marker for targeted cancer therapy, *Carbon* 47(9) (2009) 2152–2160. doi:10.1016/j.carbon.2009.03.057.

159. P. Chaudhuri, S. Soni, S. Sengupta, Single-walled carbon nanotube-conjugated chemotherapy exhibits increased therapeutic index in melanoma, *Nanotechnology* 21(2) (2010) 025102 (11pp). doi:10.1088/0957-4484/21/2/025102.

160. R. Li, R. Wu, L. Zhao, M. Wu, L. Yang, H. Zou, P-Glycoprotein antibody functionalized carbon nanotube overcomes the multidrug resistance of human leukemia cells, *ACS Nano* 4(3) (2010) 1399–1408. doi:10.1021/nn9011225.

161. A. Di Crescenzo, D. Velluto, J.a. Hubbell, A. Fontana, Biocompatible dispersions of carbon nanotubes: a potential tool for intracellular transport of anticancer drugs, *Nanoscale* 3 (2011) 925–928. doi:10.1039/C0NR00444H.

162. Z. Ji, G. Lin, Q. Lu, L. Meng, X. Shen, L. Dong, C. Fu, X. Zhang, Targeted therapy of SMMC-7721 liver cancer in vitro and in vivo with carbon nanotubes based drug delivery system, *J. Colloid Interface Sci.* 365(1) (2012) 143–149. doi:10.1016/j.jcis.2011.09.013.

163. Y.-J. Lu, K.-C. Wei, C.-C. Ma, S.-Y. Yang, J.-P. Chen, Dual targeted delivery of doxorubicin to cancer cells using folate-conjugated magnetic multi-walled carbon nanotubes, *Colloids Surf., B* 89 (2011) 1–9. doi:10.1016/j.colsurfb.2011.08.001.

164. Y.-J. Gu, J. Cheng, J. Jin, S.H. Cheng, W.-T. Wong, Development and evaluation of pH-responsive single-walled carbon nanotube-doxorubicin complexes in cancer cells, *Int. J. Nanomed.* 6 (2011) 2889–2898. doi:10.2147/IJN.S25162.

165. H. Huang, Q. Yuan, J.S. Shah, R.D.K. Misra, A new family of folate-decorated and carbon nanotube-mediated drug delivery system: synthesis and drug delivery response, *Adv. Drug Deliv. Rev.* 63(14–15) (2011) 1332–1339. doi:10.1016/j.addr.2011.04.001.

166. G. Pastorin, W. Wu, S. Wieckowski, J.-P. Briand, K. Kostarelos, M. Prato, A. Bianco, Double functionalization of carbon nanotubes for multimodal drug delivery, *Chem. Commun.* (11) (2006) 1182–1184. doi:10.1039/b516309a.

167. C. Samorì, H. Ali-Boucetta, R. Sainz, C. Guo, M.F. Toma, C. Fabbro, T. Da Ros, M. Prato, K. Kostarelos, A. Bianco, Enhanced anticancer activity of multi-walled carbon nanotube–methotrexate conjugates using cleavable linkers, *Chem. Commun.* 46 (2010) 1494–1496. doi:10.1039/B923560D.

168. Z. Liu, K. Chen, C. Davis, S. Sherlock, Q. Cao, X. Chen, H. Dai, Drug delivery with carbon nanotubes for in vivo cancer treatment *Cancer Res.* 68(16) (2008) 6652–6660. doi:10.1158/0008-5472.CAN-08-1468.

169. Z. Sobhani, R. Dinarvand, F. Atyabi, M. Ghahremani, M. Adeli, Increased paclitaxel cytotoxicity against cancer cell lines using a novel functionalized carbon nanotube, *Int. J. Nanomed.* 6 (2011) 705–719. doi:10.2147/IJN.S17336.

170. J. Chen, S. Chen, X. Zhao, L.V. Kuznetsova, S.S. Wong, I. Ojima, Functionalized single-walled carbon nanotubes as rationally designed vehicles for tumor-targeted drug delivery, *J. Am. Chem. Soc.* 130(49) (2008) 16778–16785. doi:10.1021/ja805570f.

171. R.P. Feazell, N. Nakayama-Ratchford, H. Soluble single-walled carbon nanotubes as longboat delivery systems for platinum(IV) anticancer drug design, *Am. Chem. Soc.* 129(27) (2007) 8438–8439. doi:10.1021/ja073231f.

172. S. Dhar, Z. Liu, J. Thomale, H. Dai, S.J. Lippard, Targeted single-wall carbon nanotube-mediated Pt(IV) prodrug delivery using folate as a homing device, *J. Am. Chem. Soc.* 130(34) (2008) 11467–11476. doi:10.1021/ja803036e.

173. A.A. Bhirde, V. Patel, J. Gavard, G. Zhang, A.A. Sousa, A. Masedunskas, R.D. Leapman, R. Weigert, J.S. Gutkind, J.F. Rusling, Targeted killing of cancer cells in vivo and in vitro with EGF-directed carbon nanotube-based drug delivery, *ACS Nano* 3(2) (2009) 307–316. doi:10.1021/nn800551s.

174. S.C. Tsang, Y.K. Chen, P.J.F. Harris, M.L.H. Green, A simple chemical method of opening and filling carbon nanotubes, *Nature* 372 (1994) 159–162. doi:10.1038/372159a0.

175. S. Hampel, D. Kunze, D. Haase, K. Krämer, M. Rauschenbach, M. Ritschel, A. Leonhardt, J. Thomas, S. Oswald, V. Hoffmann, B. Büchner, Carbon nanotubes filled

with a chemotherapeutic agent: a nanocarrier mediates inhibition of tumor cell growth, *Nanomedicine* 3(2) (2008) 175–182. doi:10.2217/17435889.3.2.175.

176. C. Tripisciano, K. Kraemer, A. Taylor, E. Borowiak-Palen, Single-wall carbon nanotubes based anticancer drug delivery system, *Chem. Phys. Lett.* 478(4–6) (2009) 200–205. doi:10.1016/j.cplett.2009.07.071.

177. W. Wu, R. Li, X. Bian, Z. Zhu, D. Ding, X. Li, Z. Jia, X. Jiang, Y. Hu, Covalently combining carbon nanotubes with anticancer agent: preparation and antitumor activity, *ACS Nano* 3(9) (2009) 2740–2750. doi:10.1021/nn9005686.

178. D. Yang, F. Yang, J. Hu, J. Long, C. Wang, D. Fu, Q. Ni, Hydrophilic multi-walled carbon nanotubes decorated with magnetite nanoparticles as lymphatic targeted drug delivery vehicles, *Chem. Commun.* 29 (2009) 4447–4449. doi:10.1039/B908012K.

179. J. Meng, J. Meng, J. Duan, H. Kong, L. Li, C. Wang, S. Xie, S. Chen, N. Gu, H. Xu, X. da Yang, Carbon nanotubes conjugated to tumor lysate protein enhance the efficacy of an antitumor immunotherapy, *Small* 4(9) (2008) 1364–1370. doi:10.1002/smll.200701059.

180. C.H. Villa, T. Dao, I. Ahearn, N. Fehrenbacher, E. Casey, D.A. Rey, T. Korontsvit, V. Zakhaleva, C.a. Batt, M.R. Philips, D.a. Scheinberg, Single-walled carbon nanotubes deliver peptide antigen into dendritic cells and enhance IgG Responses to tumor-associated antigens, *ACS Nano* 5(7) (2011) 5300–5311. doi:10.1021/nn200182x.

181. Z. Zhang, Y. Zhang, B. Zeng, S. Wang, T. Zhu, R.B.S. Roden, Y. Chen, R. Yang, Delivery of telomerase reverse transcriptase small interfering RNA in complex with positively charged single-walled carbon nanotubes suppresses tumor growth, *Clin. Cancer Res.* 12(16) (2006) 4933–4939. doi:10.1158/1078-0432.CCR-05-2831.

182. J.E. Podesta, K.T. Al-Jamal, M.A. Herrero, B. Tian, H. Ali-Boucetta, V. Hegde, A. Bianco, M. Prato, K. Kostarelos, Antitumor activity and prolonged survival by carbon-nanotube-mediated therapeutic siRNA silencing in a human lung xenograft model, *Small* 5(10) (2009) 1176–1185. doi:10.1002/smll.200801572.

183. X. Yang, Z. Zhang, Z. Liu, Y. Ma, R. Yang, Y. Chen, Multi-functionalized single-walled carbon nanotubes as tumor cell targeting biological transporters, *J. Nanopart. Res.* 10 (2008) 815–822. doi:10.1007/s11051-007-9316-5.

184. N. Jia, Q. Lian, H. Shen, C. Wang, X. Li, Z. Yang, Intracellular delivery of quantum dots tagged antisense oligodeoxynucleotides by functionalized multiwalled carbon nanotubes, *Nano Lett.* 7(10) (2007) 2976–2980. doi:10.1021/nl071114c.

185. B. Pan, F. Liu, Q. Li, T. Huang, X. You, J. Shao, C. Bao, D. Cui, P. Xu, H. Chen, F. Gao, R. He, M. Shu, Y. Ma, Design of dendrimer modified carbon nanotubes for gene delivery, *Chin. J. Cancer Res.* 19 (2007) 1–6. doi:10.1007/s11670-007-0001-0.

186. M.A. Herrero, F.M. Toma, K.T. Al-Jamal, K. Kostarelos, A. Bianco, T. Da Ros, F. Bano, L. Casalis, G. Scoles, M. Prato, Synthesis and characterization of a carbon nanotube–dendron series for efficient siRNA delivery, *J. Am. Chem. Soc.* 131(28) (2009) 9843–9848. doi:10.1021/ja903316z.

187. K.T. Al-Jamal, F.M. Toma, A. Yilmazer, H. Ali-Boucetta, A. Nunes, M.-A. Herrero, B. Tian, A. Eddaoui, W.T. Al-Jamal, A. Bianco, M. Prato, K. Kostarelos, Enhanced cellular internalization and gene silencing with a series of cationic dendron-multiwalled carbon nanotube:siRNA complexes, *FASEB J.* 24(11) (2010) 4354–4365. doi:10.1096/fj.09-141036.

188. Z. Zhu, Z. Tang, J.A. Phillips, R. Yang, H. Wang, W. Tan, Regulation of singlet oxygen generation using single-walled carbon nanotubes, *J. Am. Chem. Soc.* 130(33) (2008) 10856–10857. doi:10.1021/ja802913f.

189. Y. Wu, J.A. Phillips, H. Liu, R. Yang, W. Tan, Carbon nanotubes protect DNA strands during cellular delivery, *ACS Nano* 2(10) (2008) 2023–2028. doi:10.1021/nn800325a.

190. X. Li, Y. Peng, J. Ren, X. Qu, Carboxyl-modified single-walled carbon nanotubes selectively induce human telomeric i-motif formation, *Proc. Natl. Acad. Sci. U. S. A.* 103(52) (2006) 19658–19663. doi:10.1073/pnas.0607245103.

191. M. Arlt, D. Haase, S. Hampel, et al., Delivery of carboplatin by carbon based nanocontainers mediates increased cancer cell death, *Nanotechnology* 21 (2010) 335101.

192. Y. Xiao, X.G. Gao, O. Taratula, et al., Anti-HER2 IgY antibody-functionalized single-walled carbon nanotubes for detection and selective destruction of breast cancer cells, *BMC Cancer* 95 (2009) 351.

193. V.K. Prajapati, K. Awasthi, S. Gautam, et al., Targeted killing of *Leishmania donovani* in vivo and in vitro with amphotericin B attached to functionalized carbon nanotubes, *J. Antimicrob. Chemother.* 66 (2011) 874–879.

194. J.M. Ashcroft, D.A. Tsyboulski, K.B. Hartman, et al., Fullerene (C60) immunoconjugates: Interaction of water-soluble C60 derivatives with the murine anti-gp240 melanoma antibody, *Chem. Commun. (Camb).* 28 (2006) 3004–3006.

195. D.L. Shi, H.S. Cho, C. Huth, et al., Conjugation of quantum dots and Fe$_3$O$_4$ on carbon nanotubes for medical diagnosis and treatment, *Appl. Phys. Lett.* 95 (2009) 223702.

196. A. Antonelli, S. Serafini, M. Menotta, et al., Improved cellular uptake of functionalized single-walled carbon nanotubes, *Nanotechnology* 21 (2010) 425101.

197. B. Kang, S. Chang, Y. Dai, D. Yu, D. Chen, Cell response to carbon nanotubes: Size-dependent intracellular uptake mechanism and subcellular fate, *Small* 6 (2010) 2362–2366.

198. C. Samori, H. li-Boucetta, R. Sainz, et al., Enhanced anticancer activity of multi-walled carbon nanotube-methotrexate conjugates using cleavable linkers, *Chem. Commun (Camb).* 46 (2010) 1494–1496.

199. N.W. Kam, Z. Liu, H. Dai, Functionalization of carbon nanotubes via cleavable disulfide bonds for efficient intracellular delivery of siRNA and potent gene silencing, *J. Am. Chem. Soc.* 127 (2005) 12492–12493.

200. X. Chen, H. Chen, C. Tripisciano, et al., Carbon-nanotube-based stimuli-responsive controlled-release system, *Chemistry* 17 (2011) 4454–4459.

201. D.P. O'Neal, L.R. Hirsch, N.J. Halas, J.D. Payne, J.L. West, Photo-thermal tumor ablation in mice using near infrared-absorbing nanoparticles, *Cancer Lett.* 209 (2004) 171–176.

202. C. Zavaleta, A. de la Zerda, Z. Liu, et al., Noninvasive Raman spectroscopy in living mice for evaluation of tumor targeting with carbon nanotubes, *Nano Lett.* 8 (2008) 2800–2805.

203. V.P. Zharov, E.N. Galitovskaya, C. Johnson, T. Kelly, Synergistic enhancement of selective nanophotothermolysis with gold nanoclusters: Potential for cancer therapy, *Lasers Surg. Med.* 37 (2005) 219–226.

204. A.S. Biris, D. Boldor, J. Palmer, et al., Nanophotothermolysis of multiple scattered cancer cells with carbon nanotubes guided by time-resolved infrared thermal imaging, *J. Biomed. Opt.* 14 (2009) 021007.

205. J. Imamura, R. Tateishi, S. Shiina, et al., Neoplastic seeding after radiofrequency ablation for hepatocellular carcinoma, *Am. J. Gastroenterol.* 103 (2008) 3057–3062.

206. A. Burke, X. Ding, R. Singh, et al., Long-term survival following a single treatment of kidney tumors with multi-walled carbon nanotubes and near-infrared radiation, *Proc. Natl. Acad. Sci. USA.* 106 (2009) 12897–12902.

207. C.J. Gannon, P. Cherukuri, B.I. Yakobson, et al., Carbon nanotube-enhanced thermal destruction of cancer cells in a noninvasive radiofrequency field, *Cancer* 110 (2007) 2654–2665.

208. H.K. Moon, S.H. Lee, H.C. Choi, In vivo near-infrared mediated tumor destruction by photothermal effect of carbon nanotubes, *ACS Nano* 3 (2009) 3707–3713.

209. Z. Liu, W. Cai, L. He, et al., In vivo biodistribution and highly efficient tumour targeting of carbon nanotubes in mice, *Nat. Nanotechnol.* 2 (2007) 47–52.

210. R. Klingeler, S. Hampel, B. Buchner, Carbon nanotube based biomedical agents for heating, temperature sensoring and drug delivery, *Int. J. Hyperthermia.* 24 (2008) 496–505.

211. L.R. Hirsch, R.J. Stafford, J.A. Bankson, S.R. Sershen, B. Rivera, R.E. Price, J.D. Hazle, N.J. Halas, J.L. West, Nanoshell-mediated near-infrared thermal therapy of tumors under magnetic resonance guidance, *Proc. Natl. Acad. Sci. U. S. A.*, 2003, 100(23), 13549–13554. doi:10.1073/pnas.2232479100.

212. X. Huang, I.H. El-sayed, W. Qian, M.A. El-Sayed, Cancer cell imaging and photothermal therapy in the near-infrared region by using gold nanorods, *J. Am. Chem. Soc.* 128(6) (2006) 2115–2120. doi:10.1021/ja057254a.

213. D.P. O'Neal, L.R. Hirsch, N.J. Halas, J.D. Payne, J.L. West, Photo-thermal tumor ablation in mice using near infrared-absorbing nanoparticles, *Cancer Lett.* 209(2) (2004) 171–176. doi:10.1016/j.canlet.2004.02.004.

214. R.J. Thomas and B.A. Rockwell, A procedure for laser hazard classification under the Z136.1-2000 American National Standard for Safe Use of Lasers. ANSI Z136.1, 2000, *J. Laser Appl.* 14 (2002) 57. doi:10.2351/1.1436484.

215. S.V. Torti, F. Byrne, O. Whelan, N. Levi, B. Ucer, M. Schmid, F.M. Torti, S. Akman, J. Liu, P.M. Ajayan, O. Nalamasu, D.L. Carroll, Thermal ablation therapeutics based on CN(x) multi-walled nanotubes, *Int. J. Nanomed.* 2(4) (2007) 707–714. PMCID: PMC2676813.

216. L. Gomez-De Arco, M. tse Chen, W. Wang, T. Vernier, P. Pagnini, T. Chen, M. Gundersen, C. Zhou, Optical properties of carbon nanotubes: near-infrared induced hyperthermia as therapy for brain tumors, *Mater. Res. Soc. Symp. Proc.* 1065 (2008) QQ04–QQ07. Article number: 407. doi:10.1557/PROC-1065-QQ04-07.

217. H.K. Moon, S.H. Lee, H.C. Choi, In vivo near-infrared mediated tumor destruction by photothermal effect of carbon nanotubes, *ACS Nano* 3(11) (2009) 3707–3713. doi:10.1021/nn900904h.

218. S. Ghosh, S. Dutta, E. Gomes, D. Carroll, R. D'Agostino, J. Olson, M. Guthold, W.H. Gmeiner, Increased heating efficiency and selective thermal ablation of malignant tissue with DNA-encased multiwalled carbon nanotubes, *ACS Nano* 3(9) (2009) 2667–2673. https://doi.org/10.1021/nn900368b.

219. N. Wong, S. Kam, M.O. Connell, J.A. Wisdom, H. Dai, Carbon nanotubes as multifunctional biological transporters and near-infrared agents for selective cancer cell destruction, *Proc. Natl. Acad. Sci. U. S. A.* 102(33) (2005) 11600–11605. doi:10.1073/pnas.0502680102.

220. N. Shao, S. Lu, E. Wickstrom, B. Panchapakesan, Integrated molecular targeting of IGF1R and HER2 surface receptors and destruction of breast cancer cells using single wall carbon nanotubes, *Nanotechnology* 18(31) (2007) 315101 (9pp). doi:10.1088/0957-4484/18/31/315101.

221. P. Chakravarty, R. Marches, N.S. Zimmerman, A.D.E. Swafford, P. Bajaj, I.H. Musselman, P. Pantano, R.K. Draper, E.S. Vitetta, Thermal ablation of tumor cells with antibody-functionalized single-walled carbon nanotubes, *Proc. Natl. Acad. Sci. U. S. A.* 105(25) (2008) 8697–8702. doi:10.1073/pnas.0803557105.

222. R. Marches, P. Chakravarty, I.H. Musselman, P. Bajaj, R.N. Azad, P. Pantano, R.K. Draper, E.S. Vitetta, Specific thermal ablation of tumor cells using single-walled carbon nanotubes targeted by covalently-coupled monoclonal antibodies, *Int. J. Cancer* 125(12) (2009) 2970–2977. doi:10.1002/ijc.24659.

223. C.-H. Wang, S.-H. Chiou, C.-P. Chou, Y.-C. Chen, Y.-J. Huang, C.-A. Peng, Photothermolysis of glioblastoma stem-like cells targeted by carbon nanotubes conjugated with CD133 monoclonal antibody, *Nanomed.: Nanotechnol., Biol., Med.* 7(1) (2011) 69–79. doi:10.1016/j.nano.2010.06.010.

224. M.R. Mcdevitt, D. Chattopadhyay, B.J. Kappel, J.S. Jaggi, S.R. Schiffman, C. Antczak, J.T. Njardarson, R. Brentjens, D.A. Scheinberg, Tumor targeting with antibody-functionalized, radiolabeled carbon nanotubes, *J. Nucl. Med.* 48(7) (2007) 1180–1189. doi:10.2967/jnumed.106.039131.

225. A. Ruggiero, C.H. Villa, J.P. Holland, S.R. Sprinkle, C. May, J.S. Lewis, D.A. Scheinberg, M.R. McDevitt, Imaging and treating tumor vasculature with targeted radiolabeled carbon nanotubes, *Int. J. Nanomed.* 5 (2010) 783–802. doi:10.2147/IJN.S13300.

226. K. Welsher, Z. Liu, D. Daranciang, H. Dai, Selective probing and imaging of cells with single walled carbon nanotubes as near-infrared fluorescent molecules, *Nano Lett.* 8(2) (2008) 586–590. doi:10.1021/nl072949q.

227. Z. Liu, X. Li, S.M. Tabakman, K. Jiang, S. Fan, H. Dai, Multiplexed multicolor Raman imaging of live cells with isotopically modified single walled carbon nanotubes, *J. Am. Chem. Soc.* 130(41) (2008) 13540–13541. doi:10.1021/ja806242t.

228. C. Zavaleta, A. de La Zerda, Z. Liu, S. Keren, Z. Cheng, M. Schipper, X. Chen, H. Dai, S.S. Gambhir, Noninvasive Raman Spectroscopy in Living Mice for Evaluation of Tumor Targeting with Carbon Nanotubes, *Nano Lett.* 8(9) (2008) 2800–2805. doi:10.1021/nl801362a.

229. Z. Ou, B. Wu, D. Xing, F. Zhou, H. Wang, Y. Tang, Functional single-walled carbon nanotubes based on an integrin αvβ3 monoclonal antibody for highly efficient cancer cell targeting, *Nanotechnology* 20(10) (2009) 105102 (7pp). doi:10.1088/0957-4484/20/10/105102.

230. M. Bottini, F. Cerignoli, M.I. Dawson, A. Magrini, N. Rosato, T. Mustelin, Full-Length single-walled carbon nanotubes decorated with streptavidin-conjugated quantum dots as multivalent intracellular fluorescent nanoprobes, *Biomacromolecules* 7(8) (2006) 2259–2263. doi:10.1021/bm0602031.

231. K. Osada, R.J. Christie, K. Kataoka, Polymeric micelles from poly(ethylene glycol)-poly(amino acid) block copolymer for drug and gene delivery, *J. R. Soc. Interface.* 6(Suppl 3) (2009) S325–S329.

232. A. de Mel, F. Murad, A.M. Seifalian, Nitric oxide: A guardian for vascular grafts? *Chem. Rev.* 111 (2011) 5742–5767.

233. D. Cai, J.M. Mataraza, Z.H. Qin, et al., Highly efficient molecular delivery into mammalian cells using carbon nanotube spearing, *Nat. Methods.* 2 (2005) 449–454.

234. J.E. Podesta, K.T. Al-Jamal, M.A. Herrero, et al., Antitumor activity and prolonged survival by carbon-nanotube-mediated therapeutic siRNA silencing in a human lung xenograft model, *Small* 5 (2009) 1176–1185.

235. J.S. Kim, K.S. Song, J.H. Lee, I.J. Yu, Evaluation of biocompatible dispersants for carbon nanotube toxicity tests, *Arch. Toxicol.* 85 (2011) 1499–1508. [Epub ahead of print.]

236. D. Berhanu, A. Dybowska, S.K. Misra, et al., Characterisation of carbon nanotubes in the context of toxicity studies, *Environ Health.* 8(Suppl 1) (2009) S3.

237. J. Ai, E. Biazar, M. Jafarpour, et al., Nanotoxicology and nanoparticle safety in biomedical designs, *Int. J. Nanomedicine.* 6 (2011) 1117–1127.

238. E.J. Park, J. Roh, S.N. Kim, et al., A single intratracheal instillation of singlewalled carbon nanotubes induced early lung fibrosis and subchronic tissue damage in mice, *Arch. Toxicol.* 85 (2011) 1121–1131.

239. B. Fei, H.F. Lu, Z.G. Hu, J.H. Xin, Solubilization, purification and functionalization of carbon nanotubes using polyoxometalate, *Nanotechnology* 17 (2006) 1589–1593.

240. T. Coccini, E. Roda, D.A. Sarigiannis, et al., Effects of water-soluble functionalized multi-walled carbon nanotubes examined by different cytotoxicity methods in human astrocyte D384 and lung A549 cells, *Toxicology* 269 (2010) 41–53.

241. M.L. Di Giorgio, S.D. Bucchianico, A.M. Ragnelli, P. Aimola, S. Santucci, A. Poma, Effects of single and multi walled carbon nanotubes on macrophages: Cyto and genotoxicity and electron microscopy, *Mutat. Res.* 722 (2011) 20–31.

242. R. Wang, C. Mikoryak, S. Li, et al., Cytotoxicity screening of single-walled carbon nanotubes: Detection and removal of cytotoxic contaminants from carboxylated carbon nanotubes, *Mol. Pharm.* 8 (2011) 1351–1361.

243. C.A. Poland, R. Duffin, I. Kinloch, et al., Carbon nanotubes introduced into the abdominal cavity of mice show asbestos-like pathogenicity in a pilot study, *Nat. Nanotechnol.* 3 (2008) 423–428.

244. K. Kostarelos, The long and short of carbon nanotube toxicity, *Nat. Biotechnol.* 26 (2008) 774–776.

245. C.W. Lam, J.T. James, R. McCluskey, R.L. Hunter, Pulmonary toxicity of single-wall carbon nanotubes in mice 7 and 90 days after intratracheal instillation, *Toxicol. Sci.* 77 (2004) 126–134.

246. D.M. Brown, I.A. Kinloch, U. Bangert, et al., An in vitro study of the potential of carbon nanotubes and nanofibres to induce inflammatory mediators and frustrated phagocytosis, *Carbon* 45 (2007) 1743–1756.

247. K. Donaldson, R. Aitken, L. Tran, et al., Carbon nanotubes: A review of their properties in relation to pulmonary toxicology and workplace safety, *Toxicol. Sci.* 92 (2006) 5–22.

248. J. Wen, A. Elong Ngono, J.A. Regla-Nava, K. Kim, M.J. Gorman, M.S. Diamond, S. Shresta, Dengue virus-reactive CD8(+) T cells mediate cross-protection against subsequent Zika virus challenge, *Nat. Commun.* 8 (2017) 1459.

249. N. Van Braeckel-Budimir, J.T. Harty, CD8 T-cell-mediated protection against liverstage malaria: lessons from a mouse model, *Front. Microbiol.* 5 (2014) 272.

250. Y. Min, K.C. Roche, S. Tian, M.J. Eblan, K.P. McKinnon, J.M. Caster, S. Chai, L.E. Herring, L. Zhang, T. Zhang, J.M. DeSimone, J.E. Tepper, B.G. Vincent, J.S. Serody, A.Z. Wang, Antigen-capturing nanoparticles improve the abscopal effect and cancer immunotherapy, *Nat. Nanotechnol.* 12 (2017) 877–882.

251. Y. Tao, E. Ju, J. Ren, X. Qu, Immunostimulatory oligonucleotides-loaded cationic grapheme oxide with photothermally enhanced immunogenicity for photothermal/immune cancer therapy, *Biomaterials* 35 (2014) 9963–9971.

252. X. Cai, R. Ramalingam, H.S. Wong, J. Cheng, P. Ajuh, S.H. Cheng, Y.W. Lam, Characterization of carbon nanotube protein corona by using quantitative proteomics, *Nanomedicine* 9 (2013) 583–593.

253. S.H. De Paoli, L.L. Diduch, T.Z. Tegegn, M. Orecna, M.B. Strader, E. Karnaukhova, J.E. Bonevich, K. Holada, J. Simak, The effect of protein corona composition on the interaction of carbon nanotubes with human blood platelets, *Biomaterials* 35 (2014) 6182–6194.

254. I. Sagiv-Barfi, D.K. Czerwinski, S. Levy, I.S. Alam, A.T. Mayer, S.S. Gambhir, R. Levy, Eradication of spontaneous malignancy by local immunotherapy, *Sci. Transl. Med.* 10 (2018).

255. P.H. Lizotte, A.M. Wen, M.R. Sheen, J. Fields, P. Rojanasopondist, N.F. Steinmetz, S. Fiering, In situ vaccination with cowpea mosaic virus nanoparticles suppresses metastatic cancer, *Nat. Nanotechnol.* 11 (2016) 295–303.

256. A.A. Murray, C. Wang, S. Fiering, N.F. Steinmetz, In situ vaccination with cowpea vs tobacco mosaic virus against melanoma, *Mol. Pharm.* 15 (2018) 3700–3716.

257. A.K. Kosmides, J.W. Sidhom, A. Fraser, C.A. Bessell, J.P. Schneck, Dual targeting nanoparticle stimulates the immune system to inhibit tumor growth, *ACS Nano* 11 (2017) 5417–5429.

258. R. Kuai, L.J. Ochyl, K.S. Bahjat, A. Schwendeman, J.J. Moon, Designer vaccine nanodiscs for personalized cancer immunotherapy, *Nat. Mater.* 16 (2017) 489–496.

259. A. Jurj, C. Braicu, L.-A. Pop, C. Tomuleasa, C.D. Gherman, I. Berindan-Neagoe, The new era of nanotechnology, an alternative to change cancer treatment, *Drug Design, Dev. Ther.* 11 (2017) 2871–2890.

260. W. Zhang, Z. Zhang, Y. Zhang, The application of carbon nanotubes in target drug delivery systems for cancer therapies, *Nanoscale Res. Lett.* 6 (2011) 555.

261. S.K.S. Kushwaha, S. Ghoshal, A.K. Rai, S. Singh, Carbon nanotubes as a novel drug delivery system for anticancer therapy: a review, *Braz. J. Pharm. Sci.* 49(4) (2013) 629–643.

262. C. Gherman, M.C. Tudor, B. Constantin, et al., Pharmacokinetics evaluation of carbon nanotubes using FTIR analysis and histological analysis, *J. Nanosci. Nanotechnol.* 15(4) (2015) 2865–2869.

263. B.V. Farahani, G.R. Behbahani, N. Javadi, Functionalized multi walled carbon nanotubes as a carrier for doxorubicin: drug adsorption study and statistical optimization of drug loading by factorial design methodology, *J. Braz. Chem. Soc.* 27(4) (2016) 694–705.

264. C.D.M. Fletcher, J.A. Bridge, P. Hogendoorn, F. Mertens, *WHO Classification of Tumours of Soft Tissue and Bone.* 4th ed. Lyon: IARC Press; 2013.

265. D. Peer, J.M. Karp, S. Hong, O.C. Farokhzad, R. Margalit, R. Langer, *Nat. Nanotechnol.* 2 (2007) 751–760.

10 Development of Oligonucleotide Delivery, (siRNAs), and (miRNA) Systems for Anticancer Therapeutic Strategy Immunotherapy

Successful nanomedicines should be based on sound drug delivery systems (DDS) that permit intracellular trafficking as well as the biodistribution of cargos to be controlled. It has been developing new types of DDS that are multifunctional envelope-type nanodevices referred to as MENDs. The YSK-MEND is capable of inducing efficient silencing activity in hepatocytes and can be used to cure mice that are infected with hepatitis C or B. The findings indicate that, as predicted, these compounds, when encapsulated in the YSK-MEND, can be delivered to the site of action and induce immune activation through different mechanisms.

Hematological malignancies are a group of diseases characterized by clonal proliferation of blood-forming cells. Malignant blood cells are classified as myeloid or lymphoid cells depending on their stem cell origin. Lymphoid malignancies are characterized by lymphocyte accumulation in the bloodstream, bone marrow, or in lymphatic nodes and organs. Several of these diseases are associated with chromosomal translocations, which cause gene fusion and amplification of expression, while others are characterized with an aberrant expression of oncogenes. Overall, these genes play a major role in the development and maintenance of malignant clones. Finally, a MITO-Porter, a membrane fusion-based delivery system to mitochondria, is introduced as an organelle targeting DDS, and a new strategy for cancer therapy is proposed by delivering gentamicin to the mitochondria of cancer cells. These new technologies are expected to extend the therapeutic area of nanomedicine by increasing the power of DDS, especially from the viewpoint of controlled intracellular trafficking.

10.1 DRUG DELIVERY SYSTEMS

The concept of DDS was born in the 20th century and Doxil is now recognized as one of the most successful achievements in the history of DDS for delivering anticancer agents to the tumor tissue with its distribution to normal tissue, such as the heart, kidney, etc., being decreased. This targeting strategy relies on the enhanced permeability and retention effect and is classified as passive targeting. In the case of doxorubicin (DOX), there is no need to control the cellular uptake and intracellular trafficking of DOX since DOX efficiently enters the cancer cells and reaches

the nucleus where its pharmacological action is exerted. To expand the therapeutic scope of DDS from low-molecular compounds such as DOX to peptides, proteins, and nucleic acids, more sophisticated types of DDS are required to enhance their cellular uptake and intracellular trafficking. Nucleic acids are expected to be the next-generation medicine since their action is very selective due to the very specific recognition of sequences of nucleic acid base pairs as well as the direct action against the causes of diseases at the DNA/RNA level.

We have been developing a multifunctional envelope-type nanodevice (MEND) for use as an intelligent DDS that will permit not only the biodistribution but also the intracellular trafficking of cargos (nucleic acids, proteins, peptides, etc.) to be controlled [1]. An octaarginine peptide known as a cell-penetrating peptide can be incorporated into the MEND for surface modification in the form of stearylated octaarginine (R8). The R8-MEND has the ability to enhance the cellular uptake and transfection activity of pDNA/short-interfering RNA (siRNA) in most dividing cells, but its application was limited to cellular conditions since cationically charged nanoparticles are taken up by the liver and spleen once they are introduced into the blood circulation. YSK lipids are new types of pH-responsive cationic lipids in which the cationic charge is eliminated at normal pH but develops a cationic charge in the acidic conditions in endosomes after cellular internalization. Such types of environmentally responsive materials have the ability to efficiently escape from endosomes as well as being rapidly taken up by hepatocytes in *in vivo* conditions [2]. This family of YSK lipids has been used to stimulate immune action by delivering a variety of compounds such as a low-molecular compound, siRNA, or lipid antigens through different mechanisms.

We are also in the process of developing a MITO-Porter, a membrane fusion–type DDS, that targets mitochondria. Mitochondrial dysfunction is known to be associated with many kinds of diseases, including diabetes, obesity, neurodegenerative diseases, cardiac infarction, and cancer. In spite of this, developing a DDS that can reach the matrix of the mitochondria where transcription/translation of the mitochondria genome occurs remains a formidable task. A MITO-Porter for achieving this was developed based

DOI: 10.1201/9781003229674-10

on lipid compositions that were screened based on *in vitro* fusion assays using isolated mitochondria and have been shown to fuse efficiently with mitochondrial membranes [3]. The MITO-Porter was shown to be capable of delivering peptides, proteins, and nucleic acids to mitochondria via membrane fusion. A new strategy for cancer therapy is therefore now possible by using the MITO-Porter as an organelle targeting DDS.

10.2 SHORT-INTERFERENCE RNA AS A POTENTIAL TREATMENT OF LIVER DISEASES

It is estimated that >4000 diseases are the result of genetic disorders in liver tissue [4]. Moreover, it is estimated that >200 million persons are infected with hepatotropic viruses, including the hepatitis B virus (HBV) and the hepatitis C virus (HCV) [5]. siRNA can induce the sequence-dependent specific silencing of gene expression through RNA interference (RNAi) [6]. siRNA theoretically can target all endogenous mRNAs and exogenous RNAs as well, including viral RNAs. Therefore, the realization of RNAi-based therapy for liver-related diseases appears to be a realistic and achievable goal. Alnylam Pharmaceuticals, a leading RNAi therapeutics company, started a phase I clinical study for the treatment of transthyretin (TTR)-mediated amyloidosis (ATTR) in 2010 [7], and phase III clinical studies are now ongoing with investigational RNAi therapeutics, patisiran and revusiran, which target TTR. ALN-PSCsc, an investigational therapeutic targeting proprotein convertase subtilisin/kexin type 9 (PCSK9) for the treatment of hypercholesterolemia [8], is now in a phase II clinical study. Furthermore, ALN-AT3SC, ALN-CC5, ALN-AS1, ALN-AAT, and ALN-GO1 are also in phase I clinical studies for the treatment of hemophilia, complement-related diseases, hepatic porphyrias, alpha-1 antitrypsin deficiency, and primary hyperoxaluria type 1, respectively. Moreover, Arbutus Biopharma (formerly Tekmira Pharmaceuticals) focused on the treatment of HBV infections and advanced their RNAi product (ARB-1467) into phase I clinical studies in early 2015. In this way, several RNAi-based therapeutics for liver diseases have been tested in several clinical studies. However, no RNAi-based therapeutics has been approved as of this writing [9].

10.2.1 CURRENT REPORTS REGARDING DELIVERY OF siRNA TO LIVER TISSUE

Because of the physicochemical properties of the siRNA, which includes a high molecular weight, a polyanionic charge, and hydrophilicity, the siRNA itself cannot pass through the cell membrane and reach the cytosol. Moreover, in the blood circulation, siRNA can be degraded by RNases and therefore cannot be easily removed by renal filtration. Therefore, in order to overcome these severe limitations and to apply siRNA to *in vivo* situations, an adequate delivery technology that permits the siRNA to be stabilized and reach the cytosol

of target cells is needed. Among several tissues, the liver has a unique blood vessel structure, referred to as discontinuous sinusoidal capillaries, which has a number of pores with diameters of about 100 nm (fenestrae) [10]. Because of this structural characteristic, nanoparticles with diameters of 100 nm or less are able to reach parenchymal cells (hepatocytes), and thus attempts to develop siRNA delivery systems to hepatocytes have widely been advancing [11–16]. Zimmermann et al. first reported on RNAi-mediated specific gene silencing in the liver in nonhuman primates (nonrodent species) [17]. They administered an apolipoprotein B (APOB)-specific siRNA formulated in lipid-based nanoparticles, stable nucleic acid lipid particles (SNALPs), and confirmed APOB gene silencing (>90%) and pharmacological effects including the reduction of total serum cholesterol concentrations and serum low-density lipoprotein particle concentrations. The SNALP contains 1,2-dilinoleyloxy-N, N-dimethyl-3-aminopropane (DLinDMA) as an ionizable amino lipid, which is electrostatically neutral at physiological pH (e.g., in the blood circulation) and changes to a cationic form in weakly acidic conditions (e.g., endosome/lysosome) [18]. The DLinDMA is a key component to facilitate endosomal escape through membrane fusion between the SNALP and the endosomal membranes. In 2010, Semple and Akinc et al. rationally designed some amino lipids and developed DLin-KC2-DMA [19]. The DLin-KC2-DMA contains a ketal linker to emphasize the cone shape of the lipid for the disruption of endosomal membranes, and a lipid nanoparticle (LNP) containing the DLin-KC2-DMA achieved a 50% effective dose (ED_{50}) for coagulation factor 7 (F7) gene silencing at 0.02 mg/kg, which is approximately a 50-fold higher activity compared to the DLin-DMA benchmark. More recently, Jayaraman et al. identified an active amino lipid, dilinoleylmethyl-4-dimethylaminobutyrate (DLin-MC3-DMA), which is currently in clinical trials [20]. On the other hand, lipid-like materials, termed lipidoids, have been developed through a combinatorial synthesis approach. In this approach, amine-containing head groups and nonpolar hydrocarbon tails are reacted via the ring opening of epoxides or the addition of alkyl acrylates or alkyl acrylamides [21,22]. Through parallel synthesis and high throughput screening, Love and Mahon et al. identified the most potent lipidoid, C12-200, which achieved an ED_{50} of 0.01mg/kg for F7 gene silencing [22]. More recently, the same research group developed lipopeptide nanoparticles containing cKK-E12 which achieved an ED_{50} of 0.002 mg/kg for F7 gene silencing [23].

For polymer-based siRNA delivery technology, Rozema et al. reported the development of siRNA Dynamic PolyConjugates. This formulation contains PBAVE, an endosomolytic cationic polymer. In order to increase the stealth function and targeting ability to hepatocytes, a shielding agent, polyethylene glycol (PEG), and a hepatocyte-targeting agent, N-acetylgalactosamine (NAG), were conjugated through a maleamate linkage, a bond that is labile at an acidic pH [24]. The siRNAs are also attached to the PBAVE polymer through a disulfide linkage, which is labile under reducing conditions (e.g., the cytosol). The PBAVE formulation containing ApoB siRNA showed ApoB gene silencing with an ED_{50} of ~1 mg/kg [25]. More recently, Wooddell et al. reported the development of a hepatocyte-targeted NAG-conjugated endosomolytic melittin-like peptide (MLP) [26]. In this system, the NAG-MLPs were co-injected with hepatotropic cholesterol-conjugated siRNAs (chol-siRNAs). The system achieved an ED_{50} of 0.01 mg/kg for F7 gene silencing in mice and showed therapeutic efficacy in transient and transgenic mouse models of HBV infections.

10.2.2 YSK-MEND, LIPID NANOPARTICLES FOR THE DELIVERY OF siRNA TO THE LIVER

It has been recently reported [27] the development of an original siRNA delivery system, a MEND, containing a pH-sensitive cationic lipid, referred to as YSK lipid (Figure 10.1). As a first-generation device, we developed YSK05, which contains a small pH-sensitive structure (N-methylpiperidine) and two long unsaturated carbon chains and has a tendency to form an inverted hexagonal phase with anionic lipids at an acidic pH because of its cationic properties and cone-shaped structure. It is well known that membrane fusion can be achieved by a phase transition from a lamella to an inverted hexagonal phase. Therefore, a MEND that contained YSK05 would be expected to fuse with anionic lipid-containing endosomal membranes, resulting in efficient release of siRNAs into the cytosol (Figure 10.1). The YSK05 was

compared with a conventional cationic lipid, 1,2-dioleoyl-3-trimethylammonium propane (DOTAP), and a conventional pH-sensitive cationic lipid, 1,2-dioleoyl-3-dimethylammonium propane (DODAP), in *in vitro* experiments [28]. The MENDs were composed of a (pH-sensitive) cationic lipid, DOPE, cholesterol, and 1,2-dimyristoyl-sn-glycerol, methoxypolyethyleneglycol 2000 (PEG-DMG), at a molar ratio of 30/40/30/3. The DODAP-MEND and YSK05-MEND showed lower cellular uptake compared to the DOTAP-MEND because each pH-sensitive cationic MEND has an acid dissociation value (pKa) (5.8 for DODAP-MEND and 6.6 for YSK05-MEND) and is nearly neutrally charged in media. However, the YSK05-MEND showed the highest half-maximal inhibitory concentration (IC_{50}) value (30 nM), which was approximately 10-fold higher than that for the DOTAP-MEND. Hemolytic activity, which is an indicator of fusogenic activity with endosomal membranes, was well correlated with gene silencing activity. After optimization of the lipid composition of the YSK05-MEND (YSK05, 1-palmitoyl-2-oleoyl-sn-glycero-3-phosphoethanolamine, cholesterol, and PEG-DMG at a molar ratio of 50/25/25/3), the gene silencing activity and hemolytic activity, but not cellular uptake, were further increased. In this manner, the endosomal escape of siRNA is a rate-limiting step in inducing RNAi-mediated gene silencing. Moreover, the YSK05-MEND was applied *in vivo* to the liver, and an ED50 of 0.06 mg/kg for F7 gene silencing was reported, after optimization of the lipid composition (YSK05, cholesterol, and PEG-DMG at a molar ratio of

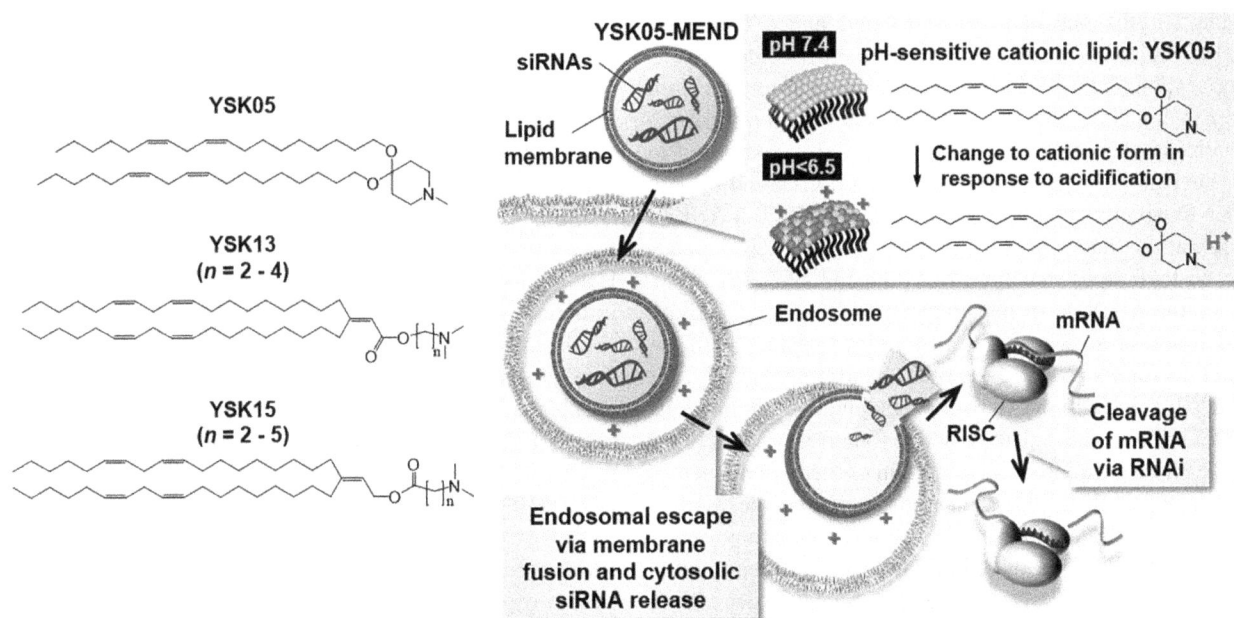

FIGURE 10.1 Structure of the YSK-lipids and a schematic illustration of the mechanism for the cytosolic delivery of siRNA by the YSK05-MEND. A pH-sensitive cationic lipid, YSK05, changes to a cationic form in response to the acidic environment of the endosomal compartment. Encapsulated siRNAs are released to the cytosol through membrane fusion between the cationized YSK05-MEND and anionic endosomal membranes. The released siRNAs form RNA-induced silencing complexes (RISC), that bind to the target mRNA, and cleave it.

70/30/3) [29]. In order to confirm the applicability of the YSK05-MEND for use in the treatment of liver diseases, we examined its therapeutic efficacy in an HCV infection. Since siRNA can directly target the genomic RNA of the HCV which is a positive-sense single-stranded RNA virus, the delivery of siRNA to the HCV-infected hepatocytes leads to the suppression of HCV production and hepatic inflammation. Two intravenous administrations of the optimized YSK05-MEND containing encapsulated siRNA against HCV genomic RNA resulted in a significant and durable reduction of the concentration of HCV genomic RNA in mice with persistent HCV infections [29]. Moreover, we confirmed that the administration of the YSK05-MEND resulted in the suppression of the intrahepatic infiltration of leukocytes and normalization of chronically inflamed liver tissue caused by HCV [29]. These facts prompted us to develop next-generation pH-sensitive cationic lipids with higher fusogenic activity with the goal of further improving gene silencing activity.

The YSK13 and YSK15 series were developed as second-generation [30]. Both YSK13 and YSK15 contain two long unsaturated carbon chains which are linked to the same sp^2 carbon atom. Based on this structure, the cone shape structure of both lipids is emphasized and would be predicted to enhance membrane disruption activity because the bond angle of the sp^2 carbon is fixed at 120°, which is larger than that of an sp^3 carbon (~109.5). In order to examine the effect of the apparent pKa value of the MEND on *in vivo* gene silencing activity and cell specificity, the YSK13 and YSK15 preparations include three and four kinds of structures that contain carbon chains with different lengths between an ester bond and a dimethylamine moiety. We first confirmed that all three YSK13 preparations show a lower phase transition temperature from a lamellar phase to an inverted hexagonal phase, which indicates a higher fusogenic activity, compared to DODAP and YSK05 under acidic conditions (pH 4.0). The MEND which is composed of different YSK13 or YSK15 preparations had a pKa value from 5.70 to 7.25, depending on their lipid structure. For the gene silencing activity of the MENDs in hepatocytes, the maximal activity was found at a pKa of 6.4, a finding consistent with the previous report [20]. On the other hand, interestingly, for gene silencing activity in liver sinusoidal endothelial cells (LSECs), the maximal activity was found at a pKa of 7.0 or higher. The intrahepatic distribution of the MEND clearly depended on their pKa values. Specifically, the MEND with a lower pKa value (<6.0) showed a hepatocyte-specific distribution. On the other hand, the intrahepatic distribution of the MENDs was shifted to LSECs depending on the extent of increase in their pKa value. Notably, only a 0.3-point difference in the pKa value resulted in a different intrahepatic distribution. Therefore, based on our findings, we conclude that fine-tuning of the pKa value is essential, not only for gene silencing activity in target cells but also for cell specificity. Moreover, we found that

an ester bond in the YSK13 lipid structure can be cleaved by the phospholipase A1 activity of endothelial lipases, which are present on the surface of the endothelial cells but not on hepatocytes, and the YSK13-MEND was inactivated only in LSECs. Based on this fact, the hepatocyte specificity of the YSK13-C3-MEND on gene silencing was increased by >67-fold against LSECs, which was much higher than that of the YSK05-MEND (8.3-fold). Taken together, both the pKa value and lipase sensitivity of the lipid component are key determinants of the quality of siRNA delivery to hepatocytes.

10.2.3 CHALLENGE TO TREATING HBV INFECTIONS USING THE YSK-MEND

Through the above findings, it has been identified the most potent formulation (YSK13-C3-MEND) with an ED50 of 0.015 mg/kg for F7 gene silencing, which is a 4-fold higher activity compared to the first-generation YSK05-MEND [30]. This fact prompted us to apply the YSK13-C3-MEND to the treatment of chronic HBV infections. It is estimated that approximately 350 million persons are infected with HBV, which causes hepatitis B–related deaths of 0.6 million persons every year worldwide [31]. Despite this severe situation, only two classes of treatment, namely, interferon (IFN)-α and viral reverse transcriptase (RT) inhibitors are available. The IFN-α treatment frequently causes severe side effects including flu-like symptoms. The viral RT inhibitor treatment efficiently controls the HBV infection but does not inhibit HBV mRNAs derived from a covalently closed circular DNA [32]. It is known that HBV antigens, which are translated from the mRNAs, are involved in the suppression of the immune response [33–35]. Because a viral RT inhibitor suppresses only HBV DNA and not other HBV antigens, the drug cannot eliminate HBV in patients. Therefore, the development of new approaches for the treatment of HBV infections would be highly desirable. Because siRNA can target viral RNA, RNAi therapy for HBV infections represents an appropriate strategy for inducing reactivation of the acquired immune response, resulting in efficient elimination of HBV by the suppression of HBV antigens [36,37]. The YSK13-C3-MEND encapsulating a mixture of three kinds of siRNAs targeting HBV mRNA was intravenously administered to mice with persistent HBV infections. Reduction of HBV DNA, HBV surface protein (HBsAg), and HBV e antigen (HBeAg) was observed for a period of 2 weeks after a single injection [38]. On the other hand, daily administration of entecavir, which is one of the most frequently used viral RT inhibitors used for patients, sharply inhibited HBV DNA but failed to reduce serum levels of HBsAg and HBeAg. These results suggest that the RNAi-mediated HBV treatment can control HBV more efficiently than entecavir. In the light of the application of the YSK-MEND for the treatment of hepatitis, the issue of whether the formulation can actually be tolerated needs to be confirmed. Regarding the YSK05-MEND, we evaluated its hepatotoxicity after four repeat doses at a dose of 1 mg/kg in mice with humanized livers. No signs of toxicity, including decreased human albumin levels or elevated levels of alanine aminotransferase, were found [29]. A similar result was obtained after a single injection of the YSK13-C3-MEND to the mice with a persistent HBV infection at a dose of 5 mg/kg [38]. Taken together, the YSK-MENDs appear to be well tolerated under the experimental conditions of this study. We are currently investigating the toxicity profile and the effects of using higher doses of the YSK-MENDs.

10.3 MEND SYSTEM MEETS TO CANCER IMMUNOTHERAPY

Cancer immunotherapy has been received with skepticism for a long time because of the insufficient therapeutic effects reported in clinical trials. However, in the past decade, this has drastically changed because of the appearance of immune checkpoint inhibitors [39] and adoptive T-cell therapy [40]. It can now be said that cancer immunotherapy is now established as the 4th most effective cancer therapy following surgical therapy, chemotherapy, and radiation therapy. However, the immunomodulatory drugs (e.g., cytokines, antibodies, adjuvants, antigens, siRNA, DNA, etc.) including approved drugs are accompanied by serious toxic side effects. In virtually all cases, the toxicities arise from on-target, the off-tumor broad stimulation of immune cells (or nonimmune cells) in the bloodstream or distal organs because these drugs are generally administered systemically. To avoid such undesirable aspects, immunomodulatory drugs need to be developed such that they affect only the right cells in the right tissue microenvironments, resulting in a decrease of the dose and minimization of systemic exposure and the dissemination of the drug. Potent delivery systems and engineered materials are currently under development and these have been reviewed elsewhere [41,42]. Likewise, our MEND system has been applied to cancer immunotherapy [2,43]. In this chapter, the recent efforts regarding cancer immunotherapy using the MEND system are reviewed.

10.3.1 STING LIGAND, CYCLIC DI-GMP, LOADED NANOPARTICLES FOR CANCER IMMUNOTHERAPY

The infiltration of preexisting T cells into tumor microenvironments affects the prognostic benefits of cancer patients [44–46]. That is, spontaneous immune responses against cancer greatly contribute to the control of tumor growth. A recent report has shown that the stimulator of interferon gene (STING) pathway, but not other innate sensors such as toll-like receptors (TLRs), dominated spontaneous immune responses against cancer [47]. Therefore, an adjuvant for activating the STING pathway represents a potential weapon for cancer immunotherapy.

The STING pathway functions as an innate sensor of double-stranded DNA in the cytosol [48]. STING recognizes 2′3′-cGAMP, a cyclic dinucleotide, which is produced by the action of cyclic-GMP-AMP (cGAMP) synthase (cGAS) and results in the production of type I interferons (IFNs) via the signal activation of the tank binding kinase 1 (TBK1)-interferon regulator factor 3 (IRF3) pathway.

Cyclic di-GMP (c-di-GMP) is a cyclic dinucleotide and functions as a STING ligand [49]. The c-di-GMP binds to ATP-dependent RNA helicase (DDX41) in the cytosol and forms a complex with STING, leading to the activation of the TBK1-IRF3 pathway [50]. Therefore, c-di-GMP represents one of the potent candidates for the adjuvant stimulating STING pathway. However, cyclic dinucleotides such as c-di-GMP are negatively charged due to the presence of phosphate groups and, as a result, their transport across the cell membrane is hampered. Thus, to maximize the function of c-di-GMP, efficient delivery systems are needed. We recently succeeded in developing c-di-GMP-loaded nanoparticles and their use in inducing antitumor immunity [51]. This is the first report to show that c-di-GMP represents a potent adjuvant for use in cancer therapy. The c-di-GMP-loaded nanoparticles contain our original lipid, YSK05, which has pH-dependent characteristics and a high fusogenic activity (Figure 10.2a). The c-di-GMP-loaded YSK05 nanoparticles (c-di-GMP/YSK05-NP) efficiently delivered c-di-GMP to the cytosol of antigen-presenting cells (APCs), resulting in high levels of IFN-β production compared with Lipofectamine 2000 (LF2000). IFN-β production was dependent on the TBK1-IRF3 pathway. In addition, in vivo experiments revealed that c-di-GMP/YSK05-NP efficiently induced antigen-specific antitumor immune responses. The administration of a mixture of c-di-GMP/YSK05-NP and ovalbumin (OVA), a model antigen, to mice facilitated OVA-specific cytotoxic T cell (CTL) responses and the inhibition of tumor growth in an E.G7-OVA-bearing mouse model (Figure 10.2b).

CTL is the main effector cell in cancer immune responses and participates in antigen-specific killing by recognizing the antigen peptide present on major histocompatibility complex class I (MHC-I) in cancer cells. On the other hand, some cancer cells escape from the immunosurveillance by CTL by the loss/downregulation of MHC-I expression [52]. Malignant melanoma, a very aggressive tumor and rapidly progresses to a metastatic stage, is the best-known example of this. Natural killer (NK) cells can be major effector cells against tumors with the loss/downregulation of MHC-I such as malignant melanomas. In a recent study, we investigated the induction of antitumor immune responses via NK cells against malignant melanomas by c-di-GMP/YSK05-NP [53]. The intravenous administration of c-di-GMP/YSK05-NP to mice caused efficient induction of IFN-β (Figure 10.2b) and activation of NK cells. Moreover, we prepared a lung metastatic mouse model by intravenously injecting B16-F10 melanoma cells and intravenously administered c-di-GMP/YSK05-NP to the mice on days 2, 4, and 8. As a result, a significant decrease

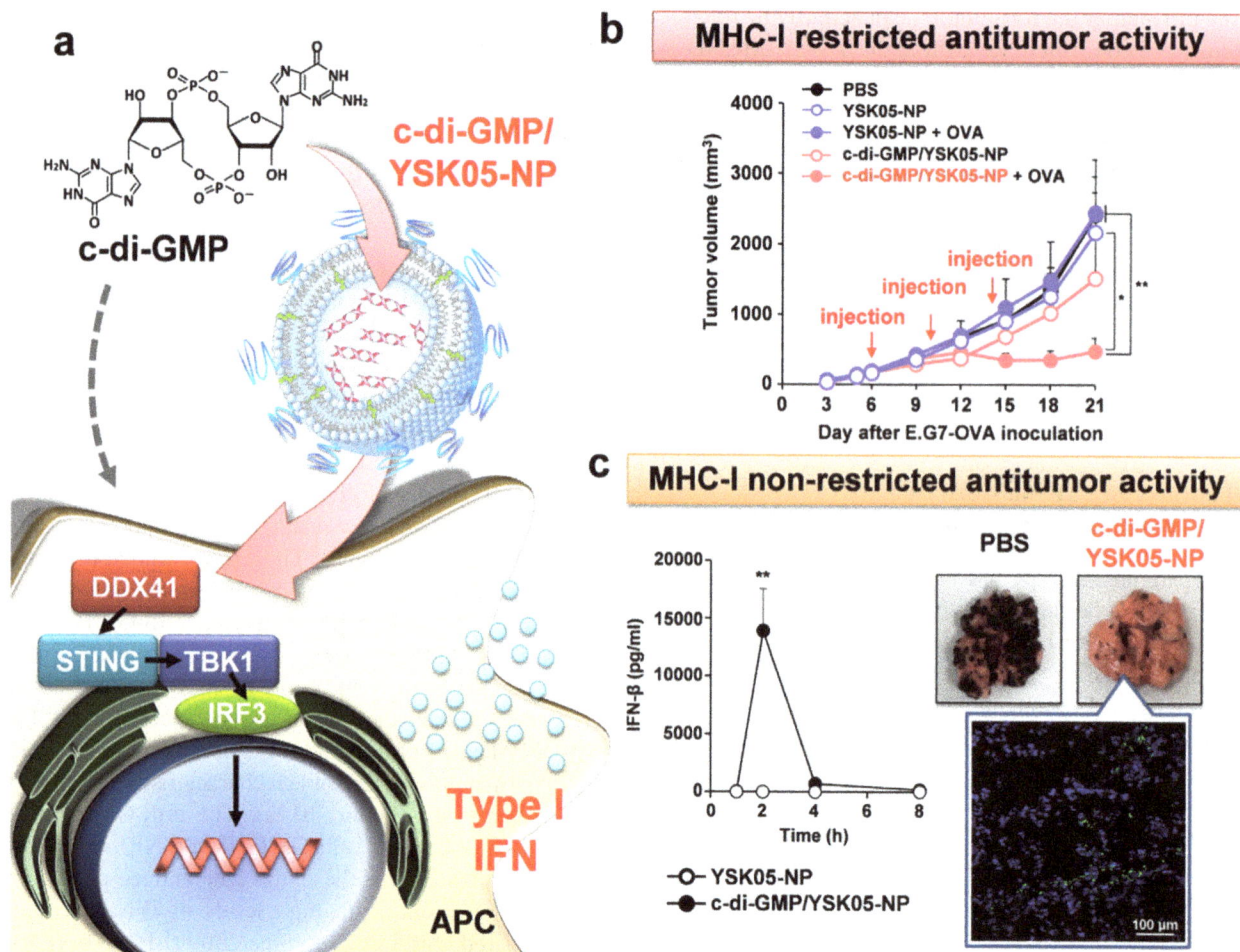

FIGURE 10.2 Cancer immunotherapy using c-di-GMP/YSK05-NP. (a) Conceptual image of c-di-GMP/YSK05-NP. YSK05-NP efficiently delivers c-di-GMP to the cytosol, resulting in the activation of the STING pathway. (b) MHC-I restricted antitumor effect by c-di-GMP/YSK05-NP. The c-di-GMP/YSK05-NP and OVA were subcutaneously injected into the mice bearing E.G7-OVA tumors (mean±SEM, n=5, **P b 0.01, *P b 0.05). (c) MHC-I non-restricted antitumor effect by c-di-GMP/YSK05-NP. Left: the IFN-β production in mice intravenously treated with cdi-GMP/YSK05-NP (mean±SEM, n=3, **P b 0.01). Right: mice with B16-F10 melanomas were intravenously treated with c-di-GMP/YSK05-NP. The tumor colony of the lungs was observed on day 21. The infiltration of NK cells was observed in the lungs of mice with B16-F10 on day 9. Green fluorescence and blue fluorescence show NK cell (Cy5) and nuclei (Hoechst 33342), respectively. Bar=100 μm. (Reproduced from a part of our previous report [53]. Copyright 2016 Elsevier B. V.)

in tumor colonies was observed in the mouse group that had been treated with c-di-GMP/YSK05-NP (Figure 10.2b), and the NK cells were critical for the antitumor effect mediated by cdi-GMP/YSK05-NP. The depletion of NK cells reduced antitumor activity and the efficient infiltration of NK cells was observed in the lungs of mice with B16-F10 treated with c-di-GMP/YSK05-NP (Figure 10.2b). This study represents the first demonstration of immunotherapy via NK cell activation against MHC-I-negative tumors, mediated by c-di-GMP.

Based on the reports [27], c-di-GMP/YSK05-NP efficiently induces MHC-I-restricted and -nonrestricted antitumor immune responses (Figure 10.2). In addition, the mechanism responsible for the stimulation of immune systems by c-di-GMP/YSK05-NP may be advantageous and potent compared with other adjuvants. Therefore, c-di-GMP/YSK05-NP promises to be a powerful adjuvant system for use in cancer immunotherapy against various tumors.

10.3.2 ENHANCEMENT OF DENDRITIC CELL –BASED IMMUNOTHERAPY AGAINST CANCER BY siRNA-MEDIATED GENE SILENCING

Dendritic cell–based immunotherapy is one of the potent cancer immunotherapies. DCs are differentiated from monocytes in the blood of cancer patients and are treated with antigens or cytokines. DCs are then administered to cancer patients. PROVENGE was first approved in 2010 by the US FDA as a DC-based cancer vaccine. However, its effectiveness has been questioned because of insufficient therapeutic effects [54]. Therefore, several clinical trials using strategies different from PROVENGE, such as different DC subsets or combination with an adjuvant, cytokines, antibodies, and chemo drugs, are currently underway [55]. One of the potent strategies for enhancing DC-based immunotherapy involves gene silencing mediated by RNAi. Some reports have demonstrated that gene silencing of negative regulators, such as a suppressor of cytokine signaling 1 (SOCS1) and A20, in DCs drastically enhanced the antitumor effects of DC-based therapy [56,57]. In these studies, a lentivirus vector expressing short hairpin RNA was used for silencing the target gene because gene silencing in DCs is quite difficult when conventional reagents are used. In the case of clinical applications, however, a nonviral approach might well be more desirable. Gene silencing in DCs using nonviral vectors such as LF2000 have been reported, but siRNA doses used in these reported studies were 100 nM–4 μM for transfection [58–63]. These siRNA doses are considerably higher than the doses used for transfection to other cell lines. The cause of the low gene silencing efficiency when nonviral reagents are used remains unclear. Thus, we recently attempted to identify the cause by comparing the intracellular fates of LF2000 between mouse DC and some cell lines (Hepa1c1c7 and B16F1) [64]. Major factors that determine *in vitro* gene silencing efficiency are the extent of cellular internalization and endosomal escape. We performed comparative analyses of cellular uptake, intracellular trafficking, the amount of intracellular-intact siRNA, and gene silencing efficiency. Contrary to our expectations, cellular uptake, intracellular trafficking, and the amount of intracellular-intact siRNA in mouse DC were comparable or high compared with those of the cell lines used. Nevertheless, a gene silencing efficiency of only 50% was observed in mouse DC, even when a high siRNA dose at which >70% gene silencing was used. Consequently, we concluded that the rate-limiting step associated with the low gene silencing efficiency in mouse DC was a process following the endosomal escape, namely the intracellular pharmacodynamics of siRNA. Although further studies will be needed to clarify the mechanism responsible for this, this finding provides new insights into developing nanoparticles for delivering siRNA to DCs.

Subsequently, the plan to find success [27] in the efficient siRNA delivery to mouse DC is via the use of a novel synthetic lipid, YSK12-C4 (Figure 10.3a). YSK12-C4 was designed so as to have cationic properties for efficient *in vitro* siRNA transfection in addition to unsaturated carbon chains, based on YSK05 [28]. In the study, we constructed an siRNA-loaded MEND containing YSK12-C4 (YSK12-MEND) and investigated the potential of YSK12-MEND in DC-based therapy [65]. The YSK12-MEND resulted in an efficient gene silencing in excess of 90%, with a median ED_{50} of 1.5 nM, in mouse DC, whereas the maximum gene silencing efficiency of Lipofectamine RNAiMAX (RNAiMAX), a powerful siRNA transfection reagent, was <60% and the ED_{50} was 25 nM (Figure 10.3b). The cause of the efficient gene silencing by YSK12-MEND in mouse DC was likely due to the enhancement of endosomal escape caused by the high membrane disruption activity of YSK12-MEND. The YSK12-MEND also succeeded in silencing the SOCS1 gene in excess of 80% and SOCS1 silencing by the YSK12-MEND drastically facilitated cytokine production in mouse DC. Furthermore, to apply it to a DC-based therapy, the preventative and therapeutic antitumor effects were investigated in a mouse model bearing E.G7-OVA tumors. In the preventative experiment, E.G7-OVA cells in mice that had already been immunized with SOCS1-silenced DC were subcutaneously inoculated, resulting in complete inhibition of tumor growth in mice treated with SOCS1-silenced DC by the YSK12-MEND. In a therapeutic experiment, SOCS1-silenced DC was injected into mice bearing E.G7-OVA tumors. Significant inhibition of tumor growth was observed compared with the control group in mice treated with SOCS1-silenced DC by the YSK12-MEND, but not RNAiMAX. The findings clearly suggest that the YSK12-MEND is a highly potent nonviral vector for delivering siRNA to DCs and is also a powerful tool for controlling DC functions in DC-based therapy. Furthermore, in the future, we plan to apply YSK12-MEND to delivering siRNA to human immune cells.

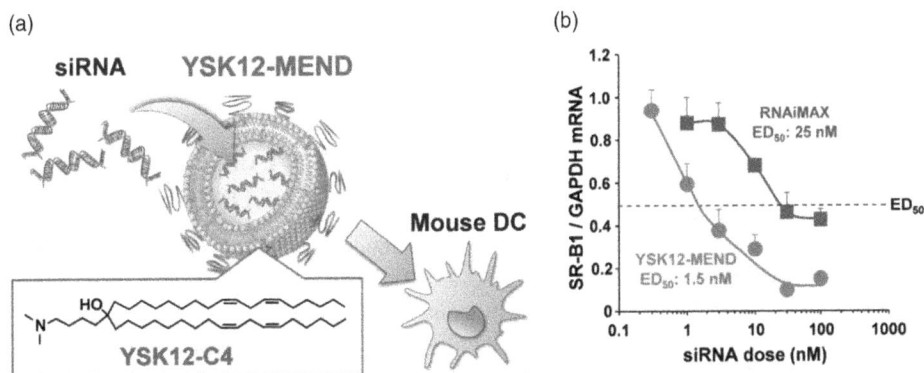

FIGURE 10.3 Delivering siRNA to mouse DCs by the YSK12-MEND. (a) Conceptual image of our strategy. YSK12-MEND contains the YSK12-C4 lipid and efficiently delivers siRNA to mouse DCs. (b) Dose-response curve for gene silencing efficiency by the YSK12-MEND in mouse DCs. The target gene was the scavenger receptor class B type 1 (SR-B1). The vertical axis shows the relative SR-B1/GAPDH mRNA level, in which the mean of the no-treatment mouse DCs was assumed to be 1.0. Data are the mean±SEM (n=3−5). (Reproduced from part of the previous report [65]. Copyright 2016 Elsevier B.V.)

10.3.3 LIPID ANTIGEN DELIVERY: NEW STRATEGY FOR IMMUNOTHERAPY

As mentioned above [27], the MHC-I molecule binds the peptide derived from a protein antigen and presents it to T cells. However, we now know that a new paradigm exists for antigen presentation, which is the recognition of nonpeptide antigens, lipid-based antigens that are present on CD1 molecules by T cells or NKT cells [66]. A recent study also revealed that MHC-I molecules presented lipopeptide antigens in addition to peptide antigens [67]. The expression of CD1 was different between human and muroid rodents. The human CD1 family is composed of CD1a, CD1b, CD1c, CD1d, and CD1e, whereas only CD1d is expressed by muroid rodents [68]. These CD1 molecules, which are prominently expressed in APCs, bind lipids such as fatty acids, glycolipids, and lipopeptides. The lipid antigens would be expected to function as a new vaccine against bacterial infections because lipid antigens are mainly found in bacteria, particularly mycobacteria, and induce lipid antigen–specific T cell responses. However, it has been difficult to develop and utilize them as vaccines or tools because of their poor solubility in water. We hypothesized that the lipid antigens would be excellent with LNPs and that a lipid antigen could be incorporated into octaarginine (R8)-modified nanoparticles (R8-NP). R8-NP has a high affinity for cells, efficiently delivers antigens to APCs, and is a potent vaccine carrier [69–71]. It has been recently reported that R8-NP was a potent carrier for lipid antigens [72–78].

Alpha-galactosylceramide (α-GC) is a ligand of CD1d and its presentation via CD1d strongly activates NKT cells [79]. The activation of NKT cells by α-GC would be expected to be a powerful cancer immunotherapy because activated NKT cells produce large amounts of IFN-γ. However, the intravenous administration of α-GC failed to induce any measurable clinical benefits [80]. The cause for this appears to be that insufficient α-GC was delivered because of its poor solubility in water. To overcome this problem, we incorporated α-GC into R8-NP and investigated its functions. The intravenously administered α-GC-loaded R8-NP (α-GC/R8-NP) drastically facilitated the production of IFN in vivo compared with free α-GC [73]. This enhancement was due to an increase in the accumulation of α-GC/R8-NP to the spleen by modifying R8 and controlling particle size. The α-GC/R8-NP treatment also increased the presentation of α-GC on CD1d in APCs and the proliferation of NKT cells in vivo, resulting in significant inhibition of tumor growth in a B16-F10 lung metastasis mouse model, compared to free α-GC.

Furthermore, it has been examined [27] the effect of a combination of interleukin (IL)-12 and α-GC/R8-NP [72]. In addition to the activation signal via the α-GC presentation of CD1d, a cytokine signal also was found to induce NKT cell activation [81]. IL-12 is the best-described cytokine mediator of NKT cell activation [82]. The IL-12 combination enhanced IFN-γ production from splenocytes stimulated with α-GC/R8-NP in vitro in a dose-dependent manner. In contrast, and interestingly, the in vivo production of IFN-γ by ta α-GC/R8-NP treatment was enhanced at a low dose of IL-12. That is, in vivo IFN-γ production appears to be inversely correlated with the dose of IL-12 during the dual-signal stimulation of NKT cells by both α-GC/R8-NP and IL-12.

It has been also analyzed the relationship between the efficiency of α-GC presentation and the character of α-GC/R8-NP in vitro using JAWSII, a murine DC line [83]. The 3 types of α-GC/R8-NP were prepared with DOPE/cholesterol/R8, egg phosphatidylcholine (EPC)/cholesterol/R8, or distearoylphosphatidylcholine (DSPC)/cholesterol/R8. As expected, the DOPE-based α-GC/R8-NP, showing a high endosomal escape activity, decreased the α-GC presentation compared with the EPC-based α-GC/R8-NP because CD1d is mainly expressed in endosomes and lysosomes. On the other hand, contrary to our expectations, the stability of nanoparticles had no effect on α-GC presentation. The EPC-based α-GC/R8-NP was degraded in endosomes and lysosomes, whereas the DSPC-based α-GC/R8-NP remained intact in endosomes and lysosomes. Nevertheless, their α-GC presentations were comparable. These α-GC presentations that were independent of the degradation of α-GC/R8-NP were dominated by saposins, sphingolipid activator proteins. These findings suggest that delivering α-GC to endosomes and lysosomes is important for achieving efficient α-GC presentation, regardless of whether nanoparticle degradation occurs.

In addition to the use of α-GC in cancer immunotherapy, R8-NP was applied to analysis of immune defense against tuberculosis infections by incorporating mycobacterial lipid antigens, such as glucose monomycolate and glycerol monomycolate in guinea pigs and rhesus macaques [74–78]. These findings would contribute to the development of new tuberculosis vaccines. Taken together, R8-NP represents a powerful delivery system for achieving efficient immunotherapy using lipid antigens against cancer and infectious diseases.

10.4 MITOCHONDRIA, A CANDIDATE FOR A TARGET ORGANELLE IN CANCER THERAPY

Mitochondria have been implicated in cancer cell proliferation, invasion, metastasis, and even drug resistance mechanisms [84–86], making them a potential target organelle for cancer therapy. It has summarized the current status of mitochondrial DDS directed to cancer therapy (Table 10.1). In addition, our recent efforts regarding the validation of cancer therapeutic strategy using our original mitochondrial DDS, MITO-Porter, are described.

TABLE 10.1

Current Reports of Mitochondrial DDS to Validate a Cancer Therapeutic Strategy by the Mitochondrial Delivery of DOX

Category	Device and DOX Loading Manner	Delivery Mechanism to Mitochondria	Target to Exert Therapeutic Effect	
			Cell Line	Model Animal
Chemical conjugation	MPP [mitochondrial-penetrating peptide conjugated DOX]	Permeating the hydrophobic mitochondria using alternating cationic and hydrophobic residues	A2780ADR [DOX-resistant human ovarian cancer cell line]	–
	TPP [triphenylphosphine conjugated with DOX]	Driven by the large negative potential, across the mitochondrial membrane	MDA-MB-435/DOX [DOX-resistant human breast cancer cell line]	–
Complexed particles	TPP-linked PEI to form PEI-TPP-DOX, where DOX is encapsulated	Mitochondrial delivery via TPP-mediated import machinery	DU145 [human prostate carcinoma cell line]	–
	TPP-modified mesoporous silica nanoparticles (TPP-MSNP) to encapsulate DOX		HeLa [human cervical cancer cell line]	–
	Folate-terminated polyrotaxanes along with DQA to form functional DOX nanoparticles, where DOX is encapsulated	Mitochondrial delivery via DQA-mediated import machinery, driven by transmembrane electric potential	MCF-7/Adr [DOX-resistant human breast carcinoma cell line]	MCF-7/Adr-bearing mouse
	DSPE-hyd-PEG-AA to form DOX/DQA-DOX@DSPE-hyd-PEG-AA where both DOX and DQA-DOX are encapsulated	After the micelle is disassembled, DQA-DOX is delivered to the mitochondria via DQA-mediated import machinery	MDA-MB-231/Adr [DOX-resistant human breast carcinoma cell line]	MDA-MB-231/Adr-bearing mouse

10.4.1 Current State of Our Knowledge Regarding Mitochondrial DDS Focusing on Cancer Therapy

Most anticancer drugs that are in clinical use are intended to function in the nucleus and are intended to kill cancer cells. Mitochondria, the energy plant of a cell, can also be considered to be a target organelle for cancer therapy. If toxins could be delivered to mitochondria, the cell energy plant would be destroyed, resulting in the arrest of the energy supply and the death of the cancer cells. To achieve such an innovative therapeutic strategy, the development of a mitochondrial DDS targeted at cancer cells is needed. To date, there have been many reports of cancer therapeutic strategies by mitochondrial targeting, and these studies are summarized in excellent, previous reviews [87,88]. In this section, we focus on the mitochondrial delivery of DOX, which is an anthracycline antitumor drug and the cargo of Doxil, world's first liposomal formulation [89].

Several groups reported that the mitochondrial delivery of DOX was achieved via the direct chemical conjugation of the cargo with mitochondrial targeting ligands. S.O. Kelley and colleagues synthesized a mitochondrial targeted version of DOX (mtDOX), which is made up of DOX conjugated with mitochondrial-penetrating peptides (MPP) [90]. MPP is a short cationic sequence designed by the S.O. Kelley group and achieves mitochondrial delivery using its alternating cationic and hydrophobic residues [91,92]. The authors investigated the cell toxicity of mtDOX using a DOX-resistant human ovarian cancer cell line (A2780ADR) and confirmed that mtDOX showed a higher toxicity than naked DOX [90]. M. Han et al. reported on the mitochondrial delivery of DOX via a lipophilic triphenylphosphine (TPP) modification [93]. TPP, originally designed by M.P. Murphy, is a mitochondriotropic ligand that is taken up by the mitochondrial membrane potential because of its high lipophilicity and stable cationic charge [94]. Han et al. synthesized a TPP-modified DOX and investigated its mitochondrial targeting and cytotoxicity using a DOX-resistant human breast cancer cell line (MDA-MB-435/DOX). The findings indicated that the TPP-modified DOX was delivered to the mitochondria of MDA-MB-435/DOX more effectively than naked DOX, and the TPP-DOX showed more cytotoxicity compared with the naked DOX at lower applied concentrations of DOX. These reports indicate that the mitochondrial delivery of DOX represents a potentially useful cancer therapeutic strategy for targeting DOX-resistant cells.

Polymeric nanoparticles offer certain advantages over other materials because they are easily chemically modified and conjugated to targeting ligands. T.A. Theodossiou et al. developed TPP linked to a poly(ethylene imine)-hyperbranched polymer (PEI) to produce a PEITPP-DOX, which is DOX loaded in a nanoparticle via the hydrophobic assembly of TPP-linked PEI [95]. Using a human prostate carcinoma cell line (DUI45), intracellular observations showed that PEI-TPP-DOX efficiently accumulated in mitochondria. Moreover, the authors found that PEI-TPP-DOX triggered a rapid and severe cytotoxicity in DUI45 cells. Q. Qiuyu reported on the preparation of mesoporous silica nanoparticles (MSNPs) modified with TPP (TPP-MSNPs) [96]. They showed that DOX-loaded TPP-MSNPs could be delivered to the mitochondria of a human cervical cancer cell line (HeLa) and showed higher cellular toxicity than DOX-loaded MSNPs without TPP.

As described above [27], the utility of cancer therapeutic strategies involving the mitochondrial delivery of DOX has been demonstrated in living cells in an *in vitro* experiment. To accelerate the development of innovative cancer medicines, the utility of this concept needs to be validated using model animals in *in vivo* experiments. H. Wang et al. developed functional DOX nanoparticles using folate-terminated polyrotaxanes along with dequalinium (DQA) [97]. DQA is an amphipathic, cationic compound and selectively accumulates in mitochondria via electrostatic interactions [98]. The authors showed that the functional DOX nanoparticles exhibited a stronger anticancer efficacy *in vitro* and in a DOX-resistant human breast carcinoma cell line (MCF-7/Adr) xenograft tumor model mice compared with naked DOX and DOX nanoparticles without DQA. Y.F. Song et al. attempted to deliver DOX to nuclei and mitochondria using a pH-sensitive micelle (DOX/DQA-DOX@DSPE-hyd-PEG-AA) to overcome drug-resistant cells and enhance the antitumor activity of DOX [99]. The authors synthesized an amphiphilic pH-sensitive material DSPE-hyd-PEG-AA, a lipid PEG conjugate with anisamide, a tumor cell targeting ligand, and formed DSPE-hyd-PEG-AA micelle loaded with DOX and DQA-DOX (DOX/DQA-DOX@DSPE-hyd-PEG-AA). The DOX/DQA-DOX@DSPE-hyd-PEGAA showed a higher cytotoxicity in a DOX-resistant human breast cancer (MDA-MB-231/ADR) and inhibited the growth of DOX-resistant tumors in tumor-bearing mice compared with naked DOX.

Promising reports as described above [27] should promote the development of mitochondrial targeting nanomedicines for cancer therapy and related research. Doxil is a conventional useful liposomal formulation for cancer therapy and accumulates at increased levels in cancer cells, permitting its therapeutic effect to be enhanced by regulating its biodistribution in the human body [89]. Thus, a comparison of cancer therapeutic effects between mitochondrial targeting complex nanoparticles and Doxil should accelerate the development of new conceptual nanomedicines via mitochondrial toxicity.

As described above [27], there are several reports of mitochondrial targeting complexed particles for cancer therapy, but few reports of useful mitochondrial targeting liposomal carriers for cancer therapy and no reports of DOX-resistant tumor-bearing model animals in *in vivo* experiments. As liposomal carriers for mitochondrial delivery, it has been reported that DQAsomes and a TPP-modified liposome (TPP-LP), developed by Weissig and coworkers [100,101], and the MITO-Porter, developed in the laboratory [2,102] are both viable vesicles. In the following section, we discuss the efforts regarding mitochondrial drug delivery using a MITO-Porter and validation of a cancer therapeutic strategy.

10.4.2 MITO-PORTER: A LIPOSOME FOR MITOCHONDRIAL DELIVERY

It has been recently reported [27] on the development of a MITO-Porter, a liposome-based nanocarrier, that delivers its cargo to mitochondria via a membrane-fusion mechanism (Figure 10.4a) [2,102,103]. The MITO-Porter, which is modified with a cell-penetrating peptide, octaarginine (R8), is first internalized into the cytosol via macropinocytosis. The MITO-Porter then binds to mitochondria via electrostatic interactions between the cationic R8 and negatively charged mitochondria. Finally, the cargoes are delivered to the mitochondria via membrane fusion. Mitochondria actively repeat fusion and fission to share biomacromolecules in living cells. Therefore, we hypothesized that a strategy involving membrane fusion via a MITO-Porter system would permit the delivery of a cargo to the mitochondria, independent of particle size and physical properties.

To determine the optimal mitochondrial fusogenic lipid compositions, it has been screened for fusogenic activities directed at mitochondria by monitoring the cancellation of FRET [102]. As a result, we succeeded in identifying liposomes with a high mitochondrial fusogenic activity and denoted the nanocapsule as a MITO-Porter. The successful MITO-Porter had the following lipid composition: DOPE/sphingomyelin (SM)/stearylated R8 (STR-R8) [9:2:1, molar ratio] or DOPE/phosphatidic acid (PA)/STR-R8 [9:2:1,

molar ratio] [102]. Moreover, lipid compositions containing SM had a lower cytotoxicity than that of PA, indicating that the lipid composition, DOPE/SM/R8 (9:2:1), was optimal for mitochondrial delivery (Figure 10.4b) [106].

To evaluate the mitochondrial delivery of the MTIO-Porter to living cells, we observed intracellular trafficking using confocal laser scanning microscopy. It has been confirmed that the green fluorescent protein, used as a model macromolecule, that was encapsulated in the MITO-Porter was co-localized with the mitochondria [102]. It has been also performed electron microscopy analyses and observed that the MITO-Porter successfully delivered colloidal gold particles as model macromolecules into the mitochondria (Figure 10.4c) [102]. These results verify that the MITO-Porter is capable of delivering macromolecules into the mitochondria of living cells.

More recently, it has been evaluated [27] the utility of mitochondrial targeting functional peptides as a ligand for delivering carriers using isolated mitochondria, homogenates, and living cells [105]. The MITO-Porter modified with the S2 peptide (Dmt-D-Arg-FK-Dmt-D-Arg-FK-NH$_2$) showed a high mitochondrial targeting activity in both homogenates and living cells. In addition, the S2 peptide possessed a low cellular toxicity compared to R8 while the mitochondrial targeting activity in homogenates and living cells was similar to that of R8. The findings reported herein indicate that the S2 peptide can be considered an ideal modifier for a mitochondrial targeting nanocapsule. Mitochondrial delivery of therapeutics is considered an important issue in the development of mitochondrial medicine. To achieve these goals, our research then focused on

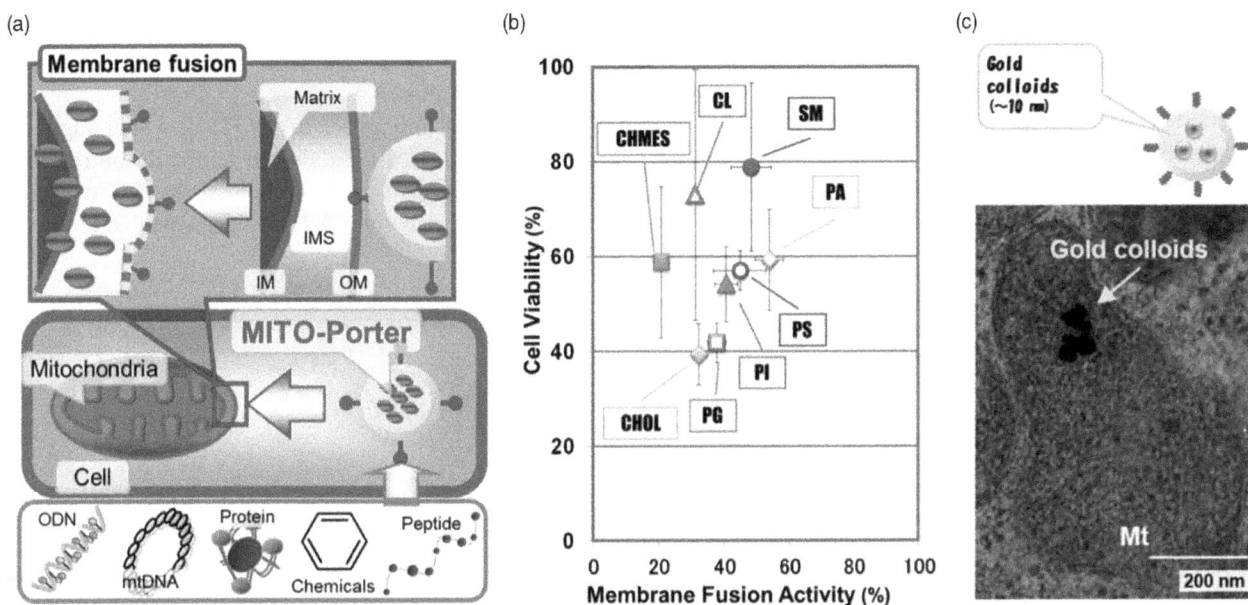

FIGURE 10.4 Summary of our research on mitochondrial delivery by the MITO-Porter system. (a) Schematic image of mitochondrial delivery by the MITO-Porter via membrane fusion [102,104]. (b) Relationship between mitochondrial membrane fusion and cell viability [105]. CL, cardiolipin; PI, phosphatidyl inositol; PG, phosphatidyl glycerol; PS, phosphatidyl serine; PA, phosphatidic acid; CHEMS, cholesteryl hemisuccinate (5-cholesten-3-ol 3-hemisuccinate); SM, sphingomyelin; Chol, cholesterol. (c) Electron microscopy analysis for the mitochondrial delivery of gold colloid particles in living cells [102,104]. Mt. indicates mitochondria. (These figures are also reproduced, in part, with permission from Elsevier and nature publishing group.)

the development of a mitochondrial medicine based on an established MITO-Porter system. It has been first attempted to validate the therapeutic strategy using model disease cells in *in vitro* experiments that involved the mitochondrial delivery of superoxide dismutase [107], an antioxidant enzyme and bongkrekic acid [108], an antiapoptosis chemical. The result indicated that the MITO-Porter represents a potentially useful carrier for use as a mitochondrial medicine, based on the results of *in vitro* experiments [107,108]. To accelerate the development of mitochondrial medicine, it has been evaluated the antioxidant effect conferred by the mitochondrial delivery of coenzyme Q_{10} (CoQ_{10}) using an ischemic/reperfusion injury model mouse in *in vivo* experiments [109]. As a result, we confirmed that the systemic injection of the CoQ_{10}-MITO-Porter resulted in a significant therapeutic effect compared with the naked CoQ_{10} and other carriers [109]. The results indicate that the MITO-Porter represents a potentially useful carrier for use as a mitochondrial medicine.

10.4.3 CHALLENGE TO CANCER THERAPY BY THE MITOCHONDRIAL DELIVERY OF THERAPEUTICS USING A MITO-PORTER

In this chapter, we introduce [27] the efforts regarding validating the utility of a cancer therapeutic strategy by mitochondrial delivery of toxic compounds [110]. As a mitochondrial toxic cargo, it has been chosen gentamicin (GM), an aminoglycoside drug (AG), which is a small molecule that functions as an antibiotic and has ototoxic and nephrotoxic characteristics via mitochondrial toxicity. Thus, we hypothesized that the cellular uptake of GM would kill cancer cells via mitochondrial toxicity, which would lead to an effective strategy for treating cancer using a different approach from that for conventional anticancer agents. To date, our knowledge of the antitumor effect of AG remains limited, probably because the internalization of AG into cancer cells would be difficult. Thus, it has been

attempted [27] the mitochondrial delivery of GM using the MITO-Porter in HeLa cells. To date, we have shown that the MITO-Porter was efficiently taken up by HeLa cells, and that biofunctional cargoes could be delivered to the mitochondria [106–108].

In order to investigate the intracellular dynamics and cellular toxicity of GM using cancer HeLa cells, we constructed a GM-MITO-Porter, in which GM was conjugated with 7-nitrobenz-2-oxa-1,3-diazole (NBD) (a fluorescent dye) and was then encapsulated into the MITO-Porter to achieve a high cellular uptake and mitochondrial fusion activities. In this experiment [27], it has been also prepared a GM-R8-EPC-LP containing the lipid composition: EPC/SM/STR-R8 [9:2:1, molar ratio] with high cellular uptake and low mitochondrial fusion activities. Flow cytometry analyses permitted us to confirm that the GM–MITO-Porter and GM-R8-EPC-LP were efficiently taken up by HeLa cells, while naked GM was not. Moreover, fluorescent microscopy observations showed that the GM–MITO-Porter had accumulated in mitochondria more efficiently than GM-R8-EPC-LP [110].

It has been then evaluated [27] cellular toxicity by means of a cell viability assay of HeLa cells after the mitochondrial delivery of NBD-GM by the MITO-Porter. The results showed that cell viability was decreased with increasing applied dose of GM-MITO-Porter (circles), while cell viability was not decreased in the case of GM-R8-EPC-LP (squares) or NBD-GM (diamonds) (Figure 10.5a). It has been also validated the relationship between cellular toxicity and the mitochondrial accumulation of NBD-GM and found that the toxicity steadily increased in proportion to the amount of NBD-GM in mitochondria (Figure 10.5b).

There have been many reports regarding multidrug-resistant cancer cells and the complex mechanisms associated with this effect [111], e.g., P-glycoproteins as efflux pumps of anticancer drugs [112], which suggests that there are some limitations to clinically untreatable cancers by using conventional chemotherapy. The use of a MITO-Porter system for delivering agents that are toxic

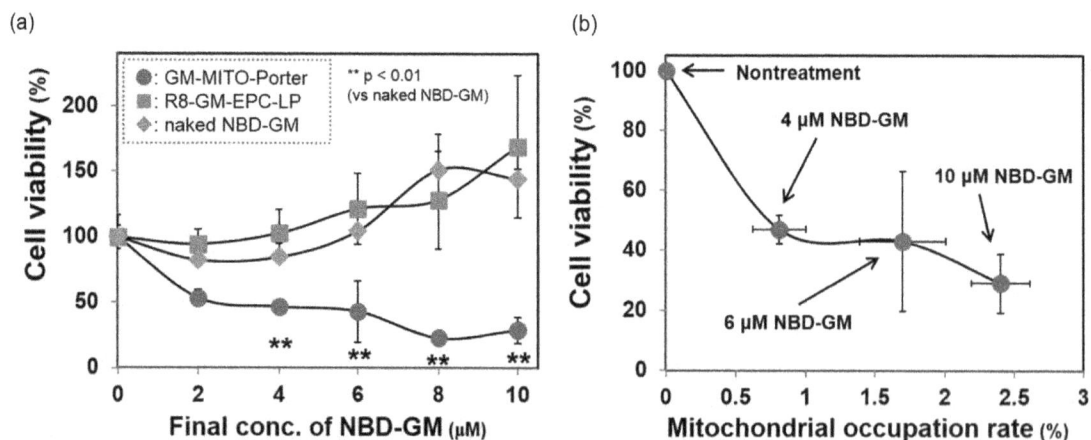

FIGURE 10.5 Evaluation of the cellular toxicity of the GM-MITO-Porter in HeLa cells [110]. (a) Comparison of cellular toxicity among the GM-MITO-Porter, R8-GM-EPC-LP and naked NBD-GMat various applied doses. **P b 0.01 (vs. naked NBD-GM). (b) Relationship between mitochondrial occupation rate and cell viability. (These figures are reproduced, in part, with permission from Wiley.)

to mitochondria, such as GMs, may be an alternative anti-cancer therapeutic strategy. To use the GM-MITO-Porter as a clinical application for cancer therapy, selective targeting to cancer cells in the body is required. Thus, we plan to equip the GM-MITO-Porter with *in vivo* cancer targeting ability.

10.5 IMMUNOMODULATION OF HEMATOLOGICAL MALIGNANCIES

Hematological malignances are a group of diseases characterized by clonal proliferation of blood-forming cells that collectively represent 9% of all cancers and affect people of all ages. Malignant blood diseases are classified as myeloid or lymphoid depending on their stem cells of origin and as acute or chronic based on the clinical course. The myeloid lineage normally produces granulocytes, erythrocytes, thrombocytes, macrophages, and mast cells. The myeloid neoplasms are a group of diseases that primarily develop and expand in the bone marrow and can home to peripheral hematopoietic tissues. Myeloid neoplasms include myeloproliferative neoplasm (chronic myelogenous leukemia [CML], chronic neutrophilic leukemia, polycythemia vera, primary myelofibrosis, and essential thrombocythemia), myelodysplastic syndromes, and acute myelogenous leukemia (AML). The lymphoid lineage produces B lymphocytes, T lymphocytes, natural killer, and plasma cells. Lymphoid neoplasms are characterized by lymphocyte accumulation in the bloodstream, the bone marrow, or in lymphatic nodes and organs. Lymphoid neoplasms include acute leukemia of uncertain lineage, mature B-cell neoplasms, acute B and T leukemias (ALL), B and T lymphoblastic leukemia/lymphoma, chronic lymphocytic leukemia (CLL), lymphoma, and multiple myeloma (MM). In adults, AML and CLL are the most common types of leukemia. Leukemia is the most commonly diagnosed cancer in children aged 0–14 years, accounting for up to 35% of all cancers, 77% of which are ALL [113]. Although hematological malignancies represent >60 distinct disease types, each having particular clinical features, treatment pathways, and outcomes, these diseases are related in the sense that they may all result from acquired mutations to the DNA of a single lymph- or blood-forming stem cell. Several of these diseases are associated with chromosomal translocations, which cause gene fusion and amplification of expression, while others are characterized by an aberrant expression of oncogenes. Overall, these genes play a major role in the development and maintenance of malignant clones.

The current treatment of most hematologic malignancies is still based on various combinations of chemotherapeutic agents. However, the treatment landscape for hematologic malignancies is evolving rapidly, as recent insights into the genetic signatures of the disease continue to appraise the development of targeted therapies in the form of specific small molecules and antibodies against various epitopes expressed on malignant cells. These potent therapies are more effective and potentially safer than standard chemotherapy because they target specific proteins and mutated gene products while leaving other cells unharmed.

Silencing genes using inhibitory oligonucleotides is an attractive therapeutic strategy for the treatment of hematological malignancies. This approach includes small interfering RNAs (siRNAs), microRNA (miRNA), anti-miRNA oligonucleotides (AMOs), and antisense oligonucleotides (ASOs). siRNAs are produced by cleaving long double-stranded RNA (Dicer substrate) by the endonuclease Dicer into the molecules of 21–23 nucleotides in length. siRNAs are double-stranded RNAs with an antisense active strand that is exactly complementary to a sequence anywhere in the target mRNA and a sense strand [114]. Inside the cell cytoplasm, siRNA associates with an Argonaute (AGO) protein within the precursor RNAi-induced silencing complex (pre-RISC) which cleaves the sense siRNA strand. The mature RISC contains the antisense strand which directs the complex to the target mRNA for post-transcriptional gene silencing [115]. miRNA is recruited to the RISC and regulates gene expression of protein-coding genes through diverse mechanisms. The interaction of miRNAs with the 3′ untranslated region of protein-coding genes is considered the main mechanism, which usually leads to a decrease in protein output either by mRNA degradation or by translational repression [116]. AMOs act by blocking the interactions between miRNA and their target mRNAs through competitive binding, therefore neutralizing specific miRNAs. ASOs are single strand, chemically modified oligonucleotides that bind to complementary sequences in target mRNAs and reduce gene expression both by RNase H-mediated cleavage of the target RNA and by inhibition of translation by steric blockade of ribosomes [117].

Since the discovery of RNAi in mammalian cells, RNAi has become an important tool in understanding gene expression and function in many types of cells. The main advantage of using this strategy is that it can silence in principle any gene with high specificity and selectivity, including "undruggable" target genes, which are uniquely expressed in different types of hematological malignancies, translocated genes, overexpressed genes, as well as mutated genes. Therefore, RNAi molecules may represent the future medicine of targeted therapeutics for hematological malignancies.

Despite this promise, utilizing RNAi for therapeutics is not a trivial task. For example, due to their large molecular weight, the net negative charge, and their hydrophilicity, the efficiency with which naked RNA molecules cross the plasma membrane and enter the cell cytoplasm is very low. Furthermore, RNA molecules are easily excreted from the kidneys and extremely susceptible to nuclease degradation in plasma [118,119]. In addition, RNA molecules bind to innate immune cell receptors responsible for nucleic acid recognition: the transmembrane toll-like receptors and the cytoplasmic sensors retinoic acid–inducible gene I (RIG-I)-like helicase family receptors [120]. Activation of innate immune cells may lead to immuno-toxicity by the secretion of IFN and pro-inflammatory cytokines [121,122]. To avoid innate immune recognition and increase therapeutic RNAi molecule stability, engineered molecules that include nucleotide chemical modifications have been developed, such as short interfering ribonucleic neutrals (siRNNs), whose phosphate backbone contains neutral phosphotriester groups [123] and conversion of one nucleotide to phosphorodithioate (PS2) and 2′-OMethyl (2′-OMe) MePS2 [124]. Encapsulation of modified RNAi molecules in nanocarriers (NCs) provides additional benefits, as NCs can condense their charge and could be surface-decorated with targeting ligands to endow these carriers the ability to deliver the payloads to specific cell types. To this end, the use of nanotechnology strategies might be highly beneficial [125].

Nanotechnology offers a variety of conjugate and particle packaging methods that utilize the special characteristics of nucleic acids and could mediate the delivery of oligonucleotides directly into blood cancer cells. While most of these developments were able to silence genes in various blood cancer cell lines *in vitro*, only a few of them demonstrated *in vivo* gene silencing, in dispersed mouse model of leukemia/lymphoma, or *ex-vivo*, in patients' primary cells and in clinical trials. In this chapter, we will survey the latest progress in the field of oligonucleotide-based nanomedicine in the heterogeneous group of hematological malignancies. We will describe the most advanced nonviral NCs for oligonucleotide delivery to malignant blood cells and special emphasis will be made on the ex-vivo, *in vivo*, and clinical trials, which are currently under development.

10.6 THE REQUIREMENTS FROM OLIGONUCLEOTIDE DELIVERY SYSTEMS FOR SITE-SPECIFIC TARGETING TO MALIGNANT LEUKOCYTES

The major obstacle preventing clinical translation of this powerful technology from revolutionizing treatments of hematological malignancies is the difficulty to introduce oligonucleotides into malignant blood cells. The field of systemic drug delivery into tumor cells has emerged extensively during recent years. However, the science of delivery into the dispersed population of blood cells remains a challenge. Seemingly, systemic drug delivery to leukocytes should be less challenging in comparison to solid tumors, as there are fewer barriers to cross. Upon targeting solid tumors, the intact drug should cross into the blood vessels surrounding the tumor, then pass through the extracellular matrix, bind and internalize into the tumor cell, and enter into the cell cytoplasm. However, due to the fact that blood cells, especially leukocytes, are notoriously hard to transfect and are spread not only in peripheral blood but also in the bone marrow, lymph nodes, and lymphatic organs, there is an unmet need for developing designated delivery strategies to leukocytes [126].

10.7 SYSTEMIC DELIVERY OF INHIBITORY OLIGONUCLEOTIDES TO MALIGNANT LEUKOCYTES

10.7.1 ASOs AND siRNA-CpG

ASOs are single-strand, chemically modified oligonucleotides that bind to complementary sequences in target mRNAs and reduce gene expression both by RNase H-mediated cleavage of the target mRNA and by inhibition of translation by steric blockade of ribosomes [117]. Several attempts have been made to treat hematological malignancies with unformulated ASOs constituting unmethylated CpG motifs as an integral part of their design or with siRNA molecules chemically conjugated to CpG sequences (CpG-siRNA) (Figure 10.6). CpG oligonucleotides are efficiently internalized by antigen-presenting cells. Upon internalization, these motifs are recognized by the endosomal TLR9, which is expressed on B cells and plasmacytoid dendritic cells and regulates different immune responses [127]. TLR9 is also present in primary malignant blood cells, such as MM, CLL, and AML [62,128,129]. Conjugation of CpG oligonucleotide to siRNA therefore creates a molecule capable of both delivering siRNA and activating therapeutic antitumor immune responses [130]. This immune stimulation may be beneficial in immunosuppressive illnesses such as blood cancers. Zhang et al. [62] synthesized CpG-siRNA STAT3 to target both malignant MM and AML cells and innate immune cells. Using systemic delivery of CpG-siRNA STAT3, they demonstrated a reduced level of STAT3 mRNA and antileukemic effects both *in vitro* and *in vivo* using subcutaneous mouse MM and AML xenograft models, without significant toxic side effects. A recent study utilized CpG-siRNA STAT3 for the systemic treatment of AML and demonstrated a regression of disseminated orthotopic AML in mouse models, which require host's effector CD8+T lymphocytes but not TLR9-positive antigen-presenting cells. Interestingly, the investigators reported that CpG-Stat3 siRNA has a direct immunogenic effect on AML cells *in vivo* by upregulating major histocompatibility complex class-II, co-stimulatory and pro-inflammatory mediators, while also downregulating co-inhibitory PD-L1 molecule. Multiple administrations of unformulated CpG-Stat3 siRNA conjugates generated tumor remission of disseminated AML in 60% of mice. Nevertheless, the systemic administration of naked CpG–siRNA might lead to unwanted immune responses, which can result in severe adverse reactions and treatment failure [131].

ASOs that hybridize with and downregulate targeted mRNAs have shown promise in the range of hematological diseases. F. M. Uckun et al. [132] used an immunoconjugate of anti-CD19 antibody and ASO targeting one of the most common chromosomal translocations in acute lymphoblastic leukemia [t(1;19)(q23;p13)], which results in the expression of the oncogenic protein E2A–PBX1. Treatment of E2A–PBX1+ leukemia cells with aCD19–ASO resulted

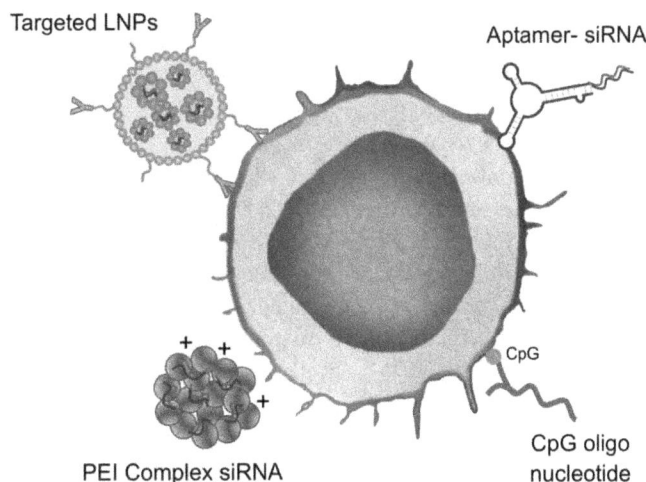

FIGURE 10.6 The most advanced strategies to deliver RNAi to malignant blood cells. Antisense oligonucleotides comprised of CpG motifs as an integral part of their design. Aptamer and siRNA are selective to malignant blood cell antigens and link to siRNA molecules. Polyethylenimine nanoparticles that contain siRNA molecules (PEI complex siRNA). LNPs encapsulated with siRNA molecules and coated with specific targeted ligands for malignant blood cell antigens (targeted LNPs).

in downregulation of E2A–PBX1 transcripts and promoted apoptosis *in vitro* and *in vivo*. Furthermore, continuous infusion of aCD19–ASO for 14 days using a micro-osmotic pump resulted in the double median survival rate of SCID mice challenged with radio- and chemotherapy-resistant highly aggressive human E2A–PBX1+B-lineage leukemia compared to controlled treated mice. Recently, D. Hong et al. [133] reported next generation of ASO-targeting human STAT3 (AZD9150). They have evaluated the efficacy of this new ASO in several preclinical tumor models including subcutaneous cell line–derived xenografts, a systemically disseminated xenograft model of large cell lymphoma, and lymphoma patient-derived tumor explant. Systemic administration of AZD9150 resulted in STAT3 mRNA knockdown of ~40, 50, or 37%, respectively. Human STAT3 inhibition by AZD9150 resulted in significant tumor growth inhibition in the subcutaneous tumor model and reduced tumor burden of the disseminated model with no effect on the mice's bodyweight. Next, they evaluated the safety of AZD9150 in a phase I dose-escalation study, which included 12 advanced lymphoma patients (of 25 overall patients). Although partial clinical responses have been achieved in several refractory patients to frontline therapies, severe drug-related adverse events occurred in >5% of patients.

Several other types of ASOs are currently under clinical evaluation in various hematological malignancy indications [134]. In most of these trials, ASOs were not used as a single therapy but rather added to chemotherapy, radiotherapy, or immunotherapy treatments. A modest response was observed in phase II clinical study where the response of relapsed/refractory AML patients to an addition of ASO targeting p53 (cenersen™) with idarubicin® with or without cytarabine® treatment was measured [135]. Addition of an ASO-targeting Bcl-2 (oblimersen™) to fludarabine® and cyclophosphamide® treatment was associated with a significant increase in complete response vs. nodular partial

response in a phase III study of relapsed/refractory CLL patients [136]. Nevertheless, the addition of oblimersen™ to dexamethasone® in a phase III clinical trial for relapsed/refractory MM patients did not improve time to tumor progression [137]. These results emphasize both the great potential and the challenges of using nonformulated ASOs in the clinic. Nonformulated siRNAs or ASOs are well tolerated in murine models in high doses; however, in clinical evaluations significantly lower doses result in various adverse events. In this chapter, it can be resolved by formulating ASOs and CpG–siRNAs in NCs. Additional advantages of the formulation are prolonged nucleotide stability, altered biodistribution, decreased potential immune activation, and increased specific targeting to the desired cells. All of the above could augment the therapeutic efficacy of blood cancer patients.

10.7.2 Aptamers

Aptamers are small structured RNAs or DNAs selected for high-affinity binding of target proteins [138]. Aptamers specific to leukocyte antigens can be linked to inhibitory oligonucleotides to produce multifunctional compounds for targeting immune cells and modulation of gene expression (Figure 10.6). Several recent preclinical studies have demonstrated a promising ability of aptamer-conjugated siRNA chimeras (AsiCs) to promote *in vivo* gene silencing of T-lymphocytes. Wheeler et al. [139] showed that pretreatment of humanized mice with CD4-siRNA-CCR5 AsiCs targeted the HIV coreceptor CCR5 in CD4+ T lymphocytes and prevented genital transmission of HIV. Recently, J. Zhou et al. generated a novel CCR5-siRNA-CCR5 AsiCs capable of specifically targeting HIV-susceptible cells (CD4+ T lymphocytes and monocytes) via CCR5 receptor and inhibiting HIV infectivity via block of the CCR5 expression [140].

AsiCs that induce efficient cell-specific knockdown can be used as an immunomodulating therapeutic for hematological malignancies. A. Herrmann et al. [141] recently reported the use of this strategy where CTLA4-siRNA-STAT3 AsiCs used to target human T large cell lymphoma in a mouse xenograft model. Intravenous administration of CTLA4-siRNASTAT3 AsiCs demonstrated tumor growth inhibition as well as reduced STAT3 activity. Overall, while there are clearly important challenges remaining, aptamer-siRNA chimera technology has the potential to become an attractive tool for therapeutic application in hematological malignancies.

10.8 SUPRAMOLECULAR NCs FOR SYSTEMIC DELIVERY OF INHIBITORY OLIGONUCLEOTIDES INTO BLOOD CANCERS

NCs offer effective delivery platforms for the negatively charged oligonucleotides, providing protection against both rapid renal excretion and nuclease cleavage, reduced unwanted immune response (either suppression or activation), having the ability to deliver oligonucleotides in combination with either soluble or insoluble drugs, controlled drug release mechanisms, and improved intracellular penetration [142]. NCs come in different "flavors" and can be controlled by adjusting their size, surface chemistry, and shape. For instance, formulations of NCs that range between 100 and 200 nm have been determined to be optimal for long circulation in the bloodstream since at this specific size range they can avoid uptake by the reticuloendothelial system, also known as the mononuclear phagocytic system. In addition, the hydrophilic surface achieved by coating NCs with either polyethylene glycol (PEG) or hyaluronan protects them from protein opsonization—a process which tags the NC for removal from circulation by specialized macrophages [143]. NCs also provide mechanisms for the release of the therapeutic cargo, such as activated release that breaks the bonds between the drug and NC or leads to particle degradation or efflux of the drug from the NC. All the above have been shown to improve the therapeutic efficacy in comparison to nonformulated oligonucleotides under several parameters such as improved gene silencing and increased therapeutic outcome with minimal adverse effects. Although a variety of NCs are being developed (liposomes, lipid-based particles, polyplex, lipoplex, dendrimers, polymeric nanoconjugates, and more) for delivering therapeutic nucleotides to tumors, only several of them have been shown to effectively silence malignant blood cells, and only a few are in the advanced stage of clinical trials [134,144].

10.8.1 POLYMER-BASED DELIVERY SYSTEMS

Several polymer-based particles were recently suggested to deliver therapeutic oligonucleotides to malignant blood cells. The most advanced system which is now under clinical studies (phase I/II) for the treatment of relapsed or refractory MM and B cell lymphoma named SNS01-T [145]. SNS01-T are polyethylenimine (PEI) nanoparticles that contain both siRNA and a decoy DNA plasmid (Figure 10.6). The siRNA sequence targets the eukaryotic translation initiation factor 5A (eIF5A) while the plasmid DNA expresses a non-hypusinable mutant of eIF5A (K50R), which induces apoptosis under a B-cell-specific promoter. Although these positively charged nanoparticles are untargeted, the enhanced tumor cell uptake and relatively low toxicity suggest that SNS01-T preferentially targets malignant cells. Using local and systemic administration methods of the siRNA-DNA chimeric NPs, S. Francis et al. showed a significant growth inhibition of MM tumors and increased survival rate in the human myeloma xenograft mouse model [146].

siRNA potency and half-life of the targeted protein are other critical components that play a crucial role in the success rate of RNAi-based therapy. New siRNA optimization strategies are needed in order to design more potent siRNA sequences for proteins with long half-lives. K. Gavrilov et al. [147] leveraged the siRNA potency of BCR-ABL-TMPRSS2 fusion genes by incorporating terminus modifications and targeted the junction site of the BCR-ABL/TMPRSS2 fusion oncoproteins. They developed a "slow release" and nontoxic delivery system based on poly lactic-co-glycolic acid (PLGA) polymer NPs, which demonstrate a robust killing effect of human CML leukemic cell line. However, further in vivo analysis and primary cell-based assays are needed in order to test the effectiveness of this modified junction site-targeted siRNAs against fusion genes.

Overexpression of oncogenic miRNAs that are particular to hematological malignancies and correlate with poor prognosis is considered a favorable target for NP delivery systems of AMOs. MiRNA-155 is one of these candidates. Babar et al. used PLGA NPs with a cell-penetrating peptide in order to deliver anti-miR-155 molecules in a safe manner to the tumor cells and showed an antitumor effect in a mIR-155 cre-lox P inducible lymphoma mouse model [148]. Yet, in these experiments, the particles were injected locally, and continued research will be needed in order to evaluate their effectiveness systemically.

Another nonconventional attempt to deliver siRNA to uneasily transfect human primary T lymphocytes is the use of multiarm (star) polycationic NPs made of poly 2-dimethylamino ethyl methacrylate (PDMAEMA). The researchers showed >40% gene silencing in these cells [149]. However, only in vivo studies will confirm if these star-shaped NPs can successfully overcome the challenge of transfecting T lymphocytes.

10.8.2 LIPID-BASED DELIVERY SYSTEMS

Lipid-based NCs are the first nano delivery systems to make the transition from concept to the clinical application [150]. This can be attributed to their attractive biological properties, which include general biocompatibility, biodegradability, isolation of drugs from the surrounding environment, and the ability to entrap both hydrophilic and hydrophobic drugs [142,150]. Multiple properties of lipid-based NCs can be altered via surface chemistry including their size, charge, and surface functionality [142].

10.8.2.1 Liposomes

Liposomal formulations are the veteran drug NCs, with >13 approved clinical products. They are spherical, self-closed structures formed by one or several concentric lipid bilayers with an aqueous phase inside and between different shells of multilayered particles. Liposomes possess many attractive characteristics as they can entrap water-soluble (hydrophilic) pharmaceutical agents in their internal water compartment and water-insoluble (hydrophobic) pharmaceuticals into the membrane [151]. Therefore, liposomes provide a unique opportunity to deliver pharmaceuticals into cells. Furthermore, the size, charge, and surface properties of liposomes can be easily changed simply by adding new ingredients into the lipid mixture before liposome preparation and/or by variation of the preparation method.

A novel amphoteric liposomal delivery system for nucleic acid named SMARTICLES, developed by Marina Biotech is currently under clinical trial, phase I, dose-escalation study for the delivery of miR34 (MRX34) in advanced cancer patients with primary liver and hematological malignancies; MM, and lymphoma. SMARTICLES are composed of unique combinations of lipids having anionic and cationic groups that work together to enable cell uptake, provide serum stability, and provide pH-triggered endosomal escape.

An antibody-targeted liposomal delivery system was recently reported to specifically deliver antisense ASO-targeting BCL-2 mRNA (G3139) into CD20-positive CLL B cells. The researchers post inserted micelles bound to anti-CD20 (rituximab) into liposomes encapsulating G3139. Using this formulation, they demonstrated that the adverse systemic immunostimulatory responses of the ASO were abrogated. Furthermore, BCL-2 protein levels were significantly reduced, which enhanced fludarabine-induced apoptosis in CLL B cells and achieved a significant therapeutic effect *in vivo* in an orthotopic B-cell lymphoma xenograft mouse model [152].

10.8.2.2 Stabilized Nucleic Acid Lipid Particles

A family of LNPs known as SNALPs are one of the most advanced strategies for siRNA delivery due to their high siRNA encapsulation efficiency and low immunogenic properties and potent gene knockdown in humans [7,153]. LNPs are ionizable particles that contain mixtures of polyethylene glycol-conjugated (PEGylated) lipids, cholesterol, and nucleic acids [154]. Ionizable LNPs are neutral in the circulation, where they associate with apolipoproteins (in particular, apolipoprotein E3), which mediates their endocytosis, primarily by hepatocytes and monocytes [155,156]. The lipids become protonated at low pH in endosomes, which triggers endosomal membrane destabilization and subsequent cytosolic release of some of their nucleic acid cargo. A first-generation LNP, DLinDMA, which potently knocked down liver gene expression in rodents and nonhuman primates [17], showed limited liver gene knockdown in initial clinical studies and caused some toxicity (complement and innate immune activation). Second-generation LNPs show substantially improved siRNA delivery and knockdown in the liver. Constructed with the anionic lipid DLin-MC3-DMA, they mediate potent gene knockdown in humans at reduced doses compared with first-generation LNPs [7]. When systematically administered, most SNALPs were trapped by hepatocytes. It is therefore logical to utilize them to treat liver diseases [154], but it is more ambitious to apply this technology for disseminated diseases, such as leukemia and lymphoma. Such an effort was recently initiated in a dose-escalation phase I study by Dicerna Pharmaceuticals, using a dicer substrate RNAi-based therapy encapsulated in SNALPs that is designed to silence the Myc oncogene in liver tumors and selected solid tumors, but also in MM and non-Hodgkin's lymphoma patients.

A more promising approach is to construct LNPs that will target specifically malignant blood cells (Figure 10.6). In a recent study, we describe a novel strategy to specifically deliver siRNAs to murine CD4(+) T cells using targeted lipid nanoparticles (tLNPs). The tLNPs were surface-functionalized with anti-CD4 monoclonal antibodies to permit the delivery of siRNAs specifically to CD4(+) T lymphocytes. Systemic intravenous administration of these particles led to efficient binding and uptake into CD4(+) T lymphocytes, which was followed by CD45 silencing [157]. A similar strategy was recently described by S. Weinstein et al. [158] to specifically deliver siRNAs against cyclin D1 to mantle cell lymphoma cells (MCL) in human MCL-xenografted mice. LNPs coated with anti-CD38 monoclonal antibodies and loaded with siRNAs against cyclin D1 induced gene silencing in MCL cells and prolonged survival of tumor-bearing mice with no observed adverse effects. These results present a novel RNAi delivery system that opens new therapeutic opportunities for treating MCL and other B-cell malignancies.

As of January 2020, ten oligonucleotide drugs have received regulatory approval from the FDA (Figure 10.7). However, a major obstacle preventing widespread usage of oligonucleotide therapeutics is the difficulty of achieving efficient delivery to target organs and tissues other than the liver. In addition, off-target interactions [159–163], sequence and chemistry-dependent toxicity, and saturation of endogenous RNA-processing pathways [164] must also be carefully considered. The most commonly used strategies employed to improve nucleic acid drug delivery include chemical modification to improve "drug-likeness," covalent conjugation to cell-targeting or cell-penetrating moieties, and nanoparticle formulation. More recently developed approaches such as endogenous vesicle (that is, exosome) loading, spherical nucleic acids, nanotechnology applications (for example, DNA cages), and "smart" materials are also being pursued.

a Fomivirsen

5′ G-C-G-T-T-T-G-C-T-C-T-T-C-T-T-C-T-T-G-C-G 3′
1   10   20

b Mipomersen

5′ G-C-C-U-C-A-G-T-C-T-G-C-T-T-C-G-C-A-C-C 3′
1   10   20

c Inotersen

5′ U-C-U-U-G-G-T-T-A-C-A-T-G-A-A-A-U-C-C-C 3′
1   10   20

d Eteplirsen

5′ C-T-C-C-A-A-C-A-T-C-A-A-G-G-A-A-G-A-T-G-G-C-A-T-T-T-C-T-A-G 3′
1   10   20   30

e Golodirsen

5′ G-T-T-G-C-C-T-C-C-G-G-T-T-C-T-G-A-A-G-G-T-G-T-T-C 3′
1   10   20

f Nusinersen

5′ U-C-A-C-U-U-U-C-A-U-A-A-U-G-C-U-G-G 3′
1   10

g Patisiran

Passenger strand
1   10   20
5′ G-U-A-A-C-C-A-A-G-A-G-U-A-U-U-C-C-A-U-T-T 3′
3′ T-T-C-A-U-U-G-G-U-U-C-U-C-A-U-A-A-G-G-U-A 5′
20   10   1
Guide strand

h Givosiran

Passenger strand
1   10   20
5′ C-A-G-A-A-A-G-A-G-U-G-U-C-U-C-A-U-C-U-U-A 3′ —GalNAc
3′ U-G-G-U-C-U-U-U-C-U-C-A-C-A-G-A-G-U-A-G-A-A-U 5′
        20   10   1
Guide strand

i Pegaptanib

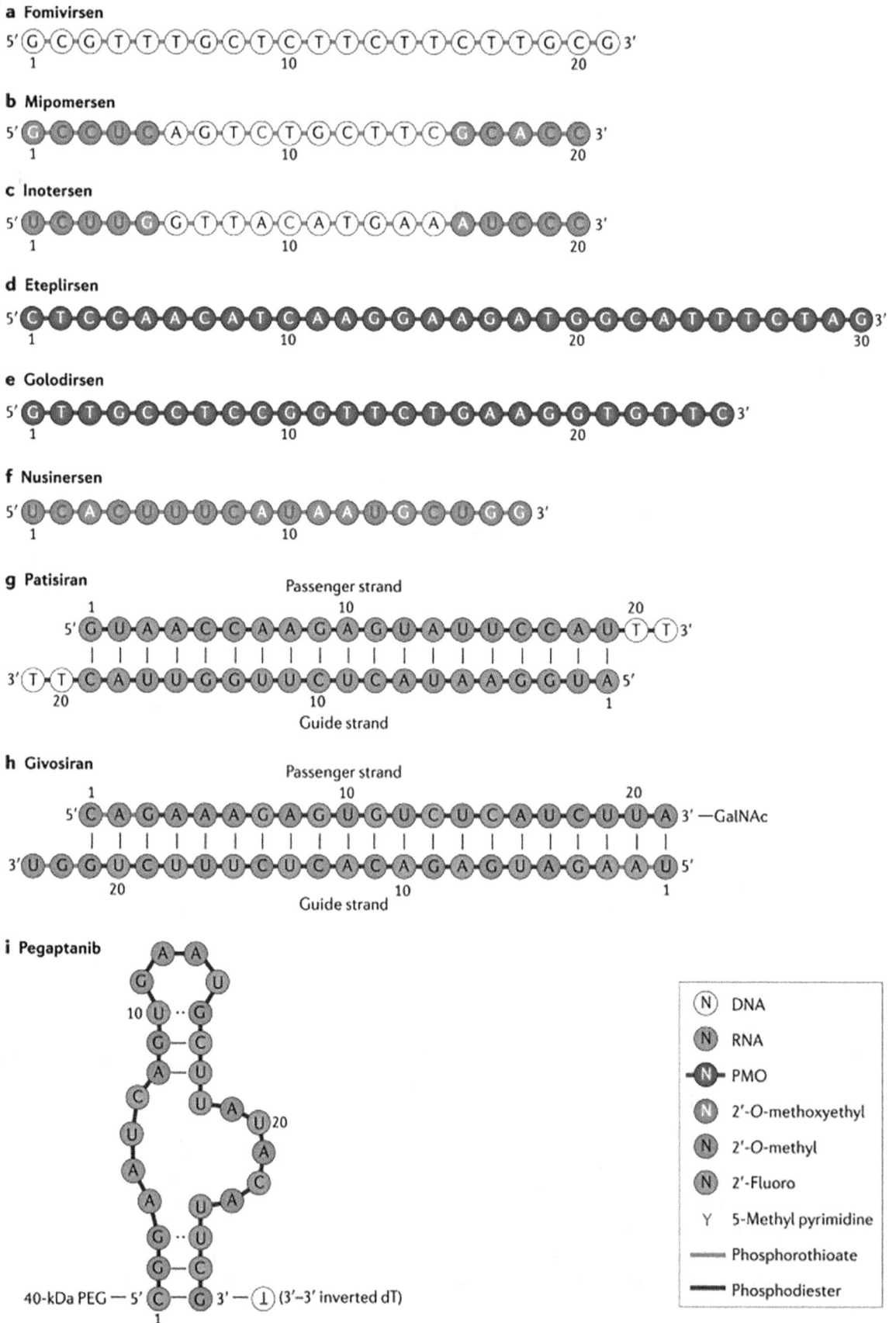

40-kDa PEG — 5′ C—G 3′ — (I) (3′–3′ inverted dT)

Legend:
N DNA
N RNA
N PMO
N 2′-O-methoxyethyl
N 2′-O-methyl
N 2′-Fluoro
Y 5-Methyl pyrimidine
— Phosphorothioate
— Phosphodiester

FIGURE 10.7   Chemistry of FDA-approved oligonucleotide drugs.

Chemical composition of the FDA-approved oligonucleotide drugs fomivirsen (part a), mipomersen (part b), inotersen (part c), eteplirsen (part d), golodirsen (part e), nusinersen (part f), patisiran (part g), givosiran (part h), and pegaptanib (part i). Drugs are ordered by mechanism of action. Drug names, trade names, principal developing company, modality, and RNA target are described in [165] for each compound. The drug defibrotide consists of a mixture of single-stranded and double-stranded ribonucleotides of variable length and sequence composition harvested from the pig intestine. It therefore cannot be easily represented in the same manner as the other oligonucleotide drugs and so is not shown here. GalNAc, N-acetylgalactosamine; PEG, polyethylene glycol; PMO, phosphorodiamidate morpholino oligonucleotide. Part i structure adapted from Ref. [166], Springer Nature Limited.

10.9   FUTURE OUTLOOK

Only limited success has been currently achieved upon careful examination of ASOs in clinical trials for the treatment of hematological malignancies. This may be attributed to the fact that unlike siRNA in which RISC provides a catalytic mechanism and each siRNA molecule can be used multiple times to target mRNA degradation following cell penetration, ASOs utilize a stoichiometric mechanism, with each ASO blocking one mRNA molecule. Therefore, ASOs are only effective at much higher than siRNA doses (200–900 vs. 10–200 nM) [167]. In addition, most clinical trials are currently utilizing unpackaged ASOs, for which both cell penetration and circulation time may be very limited.

Moreover, it is important to note that even if the target gene is silenced at the mRNA level, it does not necessarily mean a decrease in the protein level that is required for a robust phenotypic change such as blocking the cell cycle (when blocking such proteins) or apoptotic genes that will result in cell death. The targeted protein half-life plays a crucial role in this respect together with a toxicity window, which might be caused by the delivery system itself and can be confused with the specific killing effect of the target cell. The ability to load the siRNA effectively and release the drug (e.g., siRNA) in the specific target cell (e.g., tumor "neighborhood" cells) in a sustained release manner will influence the therapeutic window dramatically. This requires smart targeted NPs, which will have the capacity to release its cargo in the right target cell on an appropriate release schedule.

We have recently [168–171] shown that the combination of binding-specific targeting moieties (thus creating targeted LNPs, tLNPs) and grafting hydrophilic polymers on the surface of tLNPs (therefore preventing opsonization) are necessary in order to overcome the recognition of LNPs by liver cells and the mononuclear phagocytic system [157,158,172,173]. Therefore, passive targeting systems may not be the best choice to deliver NCs to blood cancer cells. It is also important to consider the expression levels of the receptor of interest on the targeted cells. The robust expression on both diseased and healthy cells reduces the targeting efficiency of NCs, as therapeutic uptake occurs in healthy cells as well. Though the side effects should be significantly less profound than those of chemotherapy, it is still vital to consider maximizing targeted therapy.

Recently, S. Wilhelm et al. published a perspective examining the success of nanoparticle delivery to tumors [174]. In this chapter, it was stipulated that <1% of nanoparticles actually reach their desired site. This stresses the importance of an efficient active targeting system that will have extremely high specificity for the ligand of interest. Moreover, because many hematological malignancies are cells in constant circulation, molecular targeting becomes increasingly important as opposed to organ localization methods. Thus, we suggest that novel strategies built on selective targeting to hematological malignancies will be developed taking into account the expression level of the specific receptor, its ability to internalize cargo based on ligand binding, and the kinetics of internalization. These strategies necessitate the interaction of hematologists with fundamental cell biologists, immunologists, and material scientists to focus on a better understanding of current pathology and potential opportunities to develop novel therapies based on receptor expression and biology.

Though these novel strategies increase the complexity of delivery systems and will need approval for therapeutic use in humans, they may pave the way for improved RNA therapy in hematological malignancies and other leukocyte-related diseases.

REFERENCES

1. Y. Sato, T. Nakamura, Y. Yamada, H. Akita, H. Harashima, Multifunctional enveloped nanodevices (MENDs), *Adv. Genet.* 88 (2014) 139–204.
2. K. Kajimoto, Y. Sato, T. Nakamura, Y. Yamada, H. Harashima, Multifunctional envelope-type nano device for controlled intracellular trafficking and selective targeting in vivo, *J. Control. Release* 190 (2014) 593–606.
3. Y. Yamada, H. Akita, H. Harashima, Multifunctional envelope-type nano device (MEND) for organelle targeting via a stepwise membrane fusion process, *Methods Enzymol.* 509 (2012) 301–326.
4. J. McClellan, M.C. King, Genetic heterogeneity in human disease, *Cell* 141 (2010) 210–217.
5. S.K. Basnayake, P.J. Easterbrook, Wide variation in estimates of global prevalence and burden of chronic hepatitis B and C infection cited in published literature, *J. Viral Hepat.* (2016). doi: 10.1111/jvh.12519
6. S.M. Elbashir, J. Harborth, W. Lendeckel, A. Yalcin, K.Weber, T. Tuschl, Duplexes of 21-nucleotide RNAs mediate RNA interference in cultured mammalian cells, *Nature* 411 (2001) 494–498.
7. T. Coelho, D. Adams, A. Silva, P. Lozeron, P.N. Hawkins, T. Mant, J. Perez, J. Chiesa, S. Warrington, E. Tranter, M. Munisamy, R. Falzone, J. Harrop, J. Cehelsky, B.R. Bettencourt, M. Geissler, J.S. Butler, A. Sehgal, R.E. Meyers, Q. Chen, T. Borland, R.M. Hutabarat, V.A. Clausen, R. Alvarez, K. Fitzgerald, C. Gamba-Vitalo, S.V.

Nochur, A.K. Vaishnaw, D.W. Sah, J.A. Gollob, O.B. Suhr, Safety and efficacy of RNAi therapy for transthyretin amyloidosis, *N. Engl. J. Med.* 369 (2013) 819–829.

8. K. Fitzgerald, M. Frank-Kamenetsky, S. Shulga-Morskaya, A. Liebow, B.R. Bettencourt, J.E. Sutherland, R.M. Hutabarat, V.A. Clausen, V. Karsten, J. Cehelsky, S.V. Nochur, V. Kotelianski, J. Horton, T. Mant, J. Chiesa, J. Ritter, M. Munisamy, A.K. Vaishnaw, J.A. Gollob, A. Simon, Effect of an RNA interference drug on the synthesis of proprotein convertase subtilisin/kexin type 9 (PCSK9) and the concentration of serum LDL cholesterol in healthy volunteers: a randomised, single-blind, placebo-controlled, phase 1 trial, *Lancet* 383 (2014) 60–68.

9. Y. Singh, S. Tomar, S. Khan, J.G. Meher, V.K. Pawar, K. Raval, K. Sharma, P.K. Singh, M. Chaurasia, B. Surendar Reddy, M.K. Chourasia, Bridging small interfering RNA with giant therapeutic outcomes using nanometric liposomes, *J. Control. Release* 220 (2015) 368–387.

10. J. Snoeys, J. Lievens, E. Wisse, F. Jacobs, H. Duimel, D. Collen, P. Frederik, B. De Geest, Species differences in transgene DNA uptake in hepatocytes after adenoviral transfer correlate with the size of endothelial fenestrae, *Gene Ther.* 14 (2007) 604–612.

11. C.L. Walsh, J. Nguyen, M.R. Tiffany, F.C. Szoka, Synthesis, characterization, and evaluation of ionizable lysine-based lipids for siRNA delivery, *Bioconjug. Chem.* 24 (2013) 36–43.

12. B. Yu, S.H. Hsu, C. Zhou, X. Wang, M.C. Terp, Y. Wu, L. Teng, Y. Mao, F. Wang, W. Xue, S.T. Jacob, K. Ghoshal, R.J. Lee, L.J. Lee, Lipid nanoparticles for hepatic delivery of small interfering RNA, *Biomaterials* 33 (2012) 5924–5934.

13. R.C. Adami, S. Seth, P. Harvie, R. Johns, R. Fam, K. Fosnaugh, T. Zhu, K. Farber, M. McCutcheon, T.T. Goodman, Y. Liu, Y. Chen, E. Kwang, M.V. Templin, G. Severson, T. Brown, N. Vaish, F. Chen, P. Charmley, B. Polisky, M.E. Houston, An amino acid-based amphoteric liposomal delivery system for systemic administration of siRNA, *Mol. Ther.* 19 (2011) 1141–1151.

14. A. Akinc, M. Goldberg, J. Qin, J.R. Dorkin, C. Gamba-Vitalo, M. Maier, K.N. Jayaprakash, M. Jayaraman, K.G. Rajeev, M. Manoharan, V. Kotelianski, I. Röhl, E.S. Leshchiner, R. Langer, D.G. Anderson, Development of lipidoid-siRNA formulations for systemic delivery to the liver, *Mol. Ther.* 17 (2009) 872–879.

15. J. Soutschek, A. Akinc, B. Bramlage, K. Charisse, R. Constien, M. Donoghue, S. Elbashir, A. Geick, P. Hadwiger, J. Harborth, M. John, V. Kesavan, G. Lavine, R.K. Pandey, T. Racie, K.G. Rajeev, I. Röhl, I. Toudjarska, G. Wang, S. Wuschko, D. Bumcrot, V. Kotelianski, S. Limmer, M. Manoharan, H.P. Vornlocher, Therapeutic silencing of an endogenous gene by systemic administration of modified siRNAs, *Nature* 432 (2004) 173–178.

16. C. Wolfrum, S. Shi, K.N. Jayaprakash, M. Jayaraman, G. Wang, R.K. Pandey, K.G. Rajeev, T. Nakayama, K. Charrise, E.M. Ndungo, T. Zimmermann, V. Kotelianski, M. Manoharan, M. Stoffel, Mechanisms and optimization of in vivo delivery of lipophilic siRNAs, *Nat. Biotechnol.* 25 (2007) 1149–1157.

17. T.S. Zimmermann, A.C. Lee, A. Akinc, B. Bramlage, D. Bumcrot, M.N. Fedoruk, J. Harborth, J.A. Heyes, L.B. Jeffs, M. John, A.D. Judge, K. Lam, K. McClintock, L.V. Nechev, L.R. Palmer, T. Racie, I. Röhl, S. Seiffert, S. Shanmugam, V. Sood, J. Soutschek, I. Toudjarska, A.J. Wheat, E. Yaworski, W. Zedalis, V. Kotelianski, M. Manoharan, H.P. Vornlocher, I. MacLachlan, RNAi-mediated gene silencing in non-human primates, *Nature* 441 (2006) 111–114.

18. J. Heyes, L. Palmer, K. Bremner, I. MacLachlan, Cationic lipid saturation influences intracellular delivery of encapsulated nucleic acids, *J. Control. Release* 107 (2005) 276–287.

19. S.C. Semple, A. Akinc, J. Chen, A.P. Sandhu, B.L.Mui, C.K. Cho, D.W. Sah, D. Stebbing, E.J. Crosley, E. Yaworski, I.M. Hafez, J.R. Dorkin, J. Qin, K. Lam, K.G. Rajeev, K.F. Wong, L.B. Jeffs, L. Nechev, M.L. Eisenhardt, M. Jayaraman, M. Kazem, M.A. Maier, M. Srinivasulu, M.J. Weinstein, Q. Chen, R. Alvarez, S.A. Barros, S. De, S.K. Klimuk, T. Borland, V. Kosovrasti, W.L. Cantley, Y.K. Tam, M. Manoharan, M.A. Ciufolini, M.A. Tracy, A. de Fougerolles, I. MacLachlan, P.R. Cullis, T.D. Madden, M.J. Hope, Rational design of cationic lipids for siRNA delivery, *Nat. Biotechnol.* 28 (2010) 172–176.

20. M. Jayaraman, S.M. Ansell, B.L. Mui, Y.K. Tam, J. Chen, X. Du, D. Butler, L. Eltepu, S. Matsuda, J.K. Narayanannair, K.G. Rajeev, I.M. Hafez, A. Akinc, M.A. Maier, M.A. Tracy, P.R. Cullis, T.D. Madden, M. Manoharan, M.J. Hope, Maximizing the potency of siRNA lipid nanoparticles for hepatic gene silencing in vivo, *Angew. Chem. Int. Ed. Eng.* 51 (2012) 8529–8533.

21. A. Akinc, A. Zumbuehl, M. Goldberg, E.S. Leshchiner, V. Busini, N. Hossain, S.A. Bacallado, D.N. Nguyen, J. Fuller, R. Alvarez, A. Borodovsky, T. Borland, R. Constien, A. de Fougerolles, J.R. Dorkin, K.N. Jayaprakash, M. Jayaraman, M. John, V. Kotelianski, M. Manoharan, L. Nechev, J. Qin, T. Racie, D. Raitcheva, K.G. Rajeev, D.W. Sah, J. Soutschek, I. Toudjarska, H.P. Vornlocher, T.S. Zimmermann, R. Langer, D.G. Anderson, A combinatorial library of lipid-like materials for delivery of RNAi therapeutics, *Nat. Biotechnol.* 26 (2008) 561–569.

22. K.T. Love, K.P. Mahon, C.G. Levins, K.A. Whitehead, W. Querbes, J.R. Dorkin, J. Qin, W. Cantley, L.L. Qin, T. Racie, M. Frank-Kamenetsky, K.N. Yip, R. Alvarez, D.W. Sah, A. de Fougerolles, K. Fitzgerald, V. Kotelianski, A. Akinc, R. Langer, D.G. Anderson, Lipid-like materials for low-dose, in vivo gene silencing, *Proc. Natl. Acad. Sci. U. S. A.* 107 (2010) 1864–1869.

23. Y. Dong, K.T. Love, J.R. Dorkin, S. Sirirungruang, Y. Zhang, D. Chen, R.L. Bogorad, H. Yin, Y. Chen, A.J. Vegas, C.A. Alabi, G. Sahay, K.T. Olejnik, W. Wang, A. Schroeder, A.K. Lytton-Jean, D.J. Siegwart, A. Akinc, C. Barnes, S.A. Barros, M. Carioto, K. Fitzgerald, J. Hettinger, V. Kumar, T.I. Novobrantseva, J. Qin, W. Querbes, V. Kotelianski, R. Langer, D.G. Anderson, Lipopeptide nanoparticles for potent and selective siRNA delivery in rodents and nonhuman primates, *Proc. Natl. Acad. Sci. U. S. A.* 111 (2014) 3955–3960.

24. D.B. Rozema, K. Ekena, D.L. Lewis, A.G. Loomis, J.A. Wolff, Endosomolysis by masking of a membrane-active agent (EMMA) for cytoplasmic release of macromolecules, *Bioconjug. Chem.* 14 (2003) 51–57.

25. D.B. Rozema, D.L. Lewis, D.H.Wakefield, S.C.Wong, J.J. Klein, P.L. Roesch, S.L. Bertin, T.W. Reppen, Q. Chu, A.V. Blokhin, J.E. Hagstrom, J.A. Wolff, Dynamic polyconjugates for targeted in vivo delivery of siRNA to hepatocytes, *Proc. Natl. Acad. Sci. U. S. A.* 104 (2007) 12982–12987.

26. C.I. Wooddell, D.B. Rozema, M. Hossbach, M. John, H.L. Hamilton, Q. Chu, J.O. Hegge, J.J. Klein, D.H. Wakefield, C.E. Oropeza, J. Deckert, I. Roehl, K. Jahn-Hofmann, P. Hadwiger, H.P. Vornlocher, A. McLachlan, D.L. Lewis, Hepatocyte-targeted RNAi therapeutics for the treatment of chronic hepatitis B virus infection, *Mol. Ther.* 21 (2013) 973–985.

27. Y. Sato, T. Nakamura, Y. Yamada, H. Harashima, Development of a multifunctional envelope-type nano device and its application to nanomedicine, *J. Control. Release* 244 (2016) 194–204.

28. Y. Sato, H. Hatakeyama, Y. Sakurai, M. Hyodo, H. Akita, H. Harashima, A pH-sensitive cationic lipid facilitates the delivery of liposomal siRNA and gene silencing activity in vitro and in vivo, *J. Control. Release* 163 (2012) 267–276.

29. T. Watanabe, H. Hatakeyama, C. Matsuda-Yasui, Y. Sato, M. Sudoh, A. Takagi, Y. Hirata, T. Ohtsuki, M. Arai, K. Inoue, H. Harashima, M. Kohara, In vivo therapeutic potential of Dicer-hunting siRNAs targeting infectious hepatitis C virus, *Sci. Rep.* 4 (2014) 4750.

30. Y. Sato, H. Hatakeyama, M. Hyodo, H. Harashima, Relationship between the physicochemical properties of lipid nanoparticles and the quality of siRNA delivery to liver cells, *Mol. Ther.* 24 (2016) 788–795.

31. M.S. Weinberg, P. Arbuthnot, Progress in the use of RNA interference as a therapy for chronic hepatitis B virus infection, *Genitourin. Med.* 2 (2010) 28.

32. J. Fung, C.L. Lai, J. Young, D.K.Wong, J. Yuen, W.K. Seto, M.F. Yuen, Quantitative hepatitis B surface antigen levels in patients with chronic hepatitis B after 2 years of entecavir treatment, *Am. J. Gastroenterol.* 106 (2011) 1766–1773.

33. C. Jochum, R. Voth, S. Rossol, K.H.M.Z. Buschenfelde, G. Hess, H. Will, H.C. Schroder, R. Steffen, W.E. Muller, Immunosuppressive function of hepatitis B antigens in vitro: role of endoribonuclease V as one potential trans inactivator for cytokines in macrophages and human hepatoma cells, *J. Virol.* 64 (1990) 1956–1963.

34. K. Nagaraju, S.R. Naik, S. Naik, Functional implications of hepatitis B surface antigen (HBsAg) in the T cells of chronic HBV carriers, *J. Viral Hepat.* 4 (1997) 221–230.

35. M.T. Chen, J.N. Billaud, M. Sallberg, L.G. Guidotti, F.V. Chisari, J. Jones, J. Hughes, D.R. Milich, A function of the hepatitis B virus precore protein is to regulate the immune response to the core antigen, *Proc. Natl. Acad. Sci. U. S. A.* 101 (2004) 14913–14918.

36. D. Ivacik, A. Ely, P. Arbuthnot, Countering hepatitis B virus infection using RNAi: how far are we from the clinic? *Rev. Med. Virol.* 21 (2011) 383–396.

37. Y. Chen, G. Cheng, R.I. Mahato, RNAi for treating hepatitis B viral infection, *Pharm. Res.* 25 (2008) 72–86.

38. N. Yamamoto, Y. Sato, T. Munakata, M. Kakuni, C. Tateno, T. Sanada, Y. Hirata, S. Murakami, Y. Tanaka, K. Chayama, H. Hatakeyama, M. Hyodo, H. Harashima, M. Kohara, Novel pH-sensitive multifunctional envelope-type nanodevice for siRNAbased treatments for chronic HBV infection, *J. Hepatol.* 64 (2016) 547–555.

39. D.M. Pardoll, The blockade of immune checkpoints in cancer immunotherapy, *Nat. Rev. Cancer* 12 (2012) 252–264.

40. C.S. Hinrichs, S.A. Rosenberg, Exploiting the curative potential of adoptive T-cell therapy for cancer, *Immunol. Rev.* 257 (2014) 56–71.

41. D.J. Irvine, M.C. Hanson, K. Rakhra, T. Tokatlian, Synthetic nanoparticles for vaccines and immunotherapy, *Chem. Rev.* 115 (2015) 11109–11146.

42. A.S. Cheung, D.J. Mooney, Engineered materials for cancer immunotherapy, *Nano Today* 10 (2015) 511–531.

43. T. Nakamura, H. Akita, Y. Yamada, H. Hatakeyama, H. Harashima, A multifunctional envelope-type nanodevice for use in nanomedicine: concept and applications, *Acc. Chem. Res.* 45 (2012) 1113–1121.

44. T.F. Gajewski, J. Louahed, V.G. Brichard, Gene signature in melanoma associated with clinical activity: a potential clue to unlock cancer immunotherapy, *Cancer J.* 16 (2010) 399–403.

45. O. Hamid, H. Schmidt, A. Nissan, L. Ridolfi, S. Aamdal, J. Hansson, M. Guida, D.M. Hyams, H. Gomez, L. Bastholt, S.D. Chasalow, D. Berman, A prospective phase II trial exploring the association between tumor microenvironment biomarkers and clinical activity of ipilimumab in advanced melanoma, *J. Transl. Med.* 9 (2011) 204.

46. H. Harlin, Y. Meng, A.C. Peterson, Y. Zha, M. Tretiakova, C. Slingluff, M. McKee, T.F. Gajewski, Chemokine expression in melanoma metastases associated with CD8+T-cell recruitment, *Cancer Res.* 69 (2009) 3077–3085.

47. S.R. Woo, M.B. Fuertes, L. Corrales, S. Spranger, M.J. Furdyna, M.Y. Leung, R. Duggan, Y. Wang, G.N. Barber, K.A. Fitzgerald, M.L. Alegre, T.F. Gajewski, STING-dependent cytosolic DNA sensing mediates innate immune recognition of immunogenic tumors, *Immunity* 41 (2014) 830–842.

48. G.N. Barber, STING: infection, inflammation and cancer, *Nat. Rev. Immunol.* 15 (2015) 760–770.

49. D.L. Burdette, K.M. Monroe, K. Sotelo-Troha, J.S. Iwig, B. Eckert, M. Hyodo, Y. Hayakawa, R.E. Vance, STING is a direct innate immune sensor of cyclic di-GMP, *Nature* 478 (2011) 515–518.

50. K. Parvatiyar, Z. Zhang, R.M. Teles, S. Ouyang, Y. Jiang, S.S. Iyer, S.A. Zaver, M. Schenk, S. Zeng, W. Zhong, Z.J. Liu, R.L. Modlin, Y.J. Liu, G. Cheng, The helicase DDX41 recognizes the bacterial secondary messengers cyclic di-GMP and cyclic di-AMP to activate a type I interferon immune response, *Nat. Immunol.* 13 (2012) 1155–1161.

51. H. Miyabe, M. Hyodo, T. Nakamura, Y. Sato, Y. Hayakawa, H. Harashima, A new adjuvant delivery system 'cyclic di-GMP/YSK05 liposome' for cancer immunotherapy, *J. Control. Release* 184 (2014) 20–27.

52. M. Ahmad, R.C. Rees, S.A. Ali, Escape from immunotherapy: possible mechanisms that influence tumor regression/progression, *Cancer Immunol. Immunother.* 53 (2004) 844–854.

53. T. Nakamura, H.Miyabe, M. Hyodo, Y. Sato, Y. Hayakawa, H. Harashima, Liposomes loaded with a STING pathway ligand, cyclic di-GMP, enhance cancer immunotherapy against metastatic melanoma, *J. Control. Release* 216 (2015) 149–157.

54. M.L. Huber, L. Haynes, C. Parker, P. Iversen, Interdisciplinary critique of sipuleucel-T as immunotherapy in castration-resistant prostate cancer, *J. Natl. Cancer Inst.* 104 (2012) 273–279.

55. S. Anguille, E.L. Smits, E. Lion, V.F. van Tendeloo, Z.N. Berneman, Clinical use of dendritic cells for cancer therapy, *Lancet Oncol.* 15 (2014) e257–e267.

56. L. Shen, K. Evel-Kabler, R. Strube, S.Y. Chen, Silencing of SOCS1 enhances antigen presentation by dendritic cells and antigen-specific anti-tumor immunity, *Nat. Biotechnol.* 22 (2004) 1546–1553.

57. X.T. Song, K. Evel-Kabler, L. Shen, L. Rollins, X.F. Huang, S.Y. Chen, A20 is an antigen presentation attenuator, and its inhibition overcomes regulatory T cell-mediated suppression, *Nat. Med.* 14 (2008) 258–265.

58. X. Gu, J. Xiang, Y. Yao, Z. Chen, Effects of RNA interference on CD80 and CD86 expression in bone marrow-derived murine dendritic cells, *Scand. J. Immunol.* 64 (2006) 588–594.

59. M.H. Karimi, P. Ebadi, A.A. Pourfathollah, Z.S. Soheili, S. Samiee, Z. Ataee, S.Z. Tabei, S.M. Moazzeni, Immune modulation through RNA interference-mediated silencing of CD40 in dendritic cells, *Cell. Immunol.* 259 (2009) 74–81.

60. M.B. Heo, Y.T. Lim, Programmed nanoparticles for combined immunomodulation, antigen presentation and tracking of immunotherapeutic cells, *Biomaterials* 35 (2014) 590–600.

61. W. Jiang, Blockade of B7-H1 enhances dendritic cell-mediated T cell response and antiviral immunity in HBV transgenic mice, *Vaccine* 30 (2012) 758–766.

62. Q. Zhang, D.M. Hossain, S. Nechaev, A. Kozlowska, W. Zhang, Y. Liu, C.M. Kowolik, P. Swiderski, J.J. Rossi, S. Forman, S. Pal, R. Bhatia, A. Raubitschek, H. Yu, M. Kortylewski, TLR9-mediated siRNA delivery for targeting of normal and malignant human hematopoietic cells in vivo, *Blood* 121 (2013) 1304–1315.

63. W. Hobo, T.I. Novobrantseva, H. Fredrix, J. Wong, S. Milstein, H. Epstein-Barash, J. Liu, N. Schaap, R. van der Voort, H. Dolstra, Improving dendritic cell vaccine immunogenicity by silencing PD-1 ligands using siRNA-lipid nanoparticles combined with antigen mRNA electroporation, *Cancer Immunol. Immunother.* 62 (2013) 285–297.

64. T. Nakamura, Y. Fujiwara, S. Warashina, H. Harashima, The intracellular pharmacodynamics of siRNA is responsible for the low gene silencing activity of siRNA-loaded nanoparticles in dendritic cells, *Int. J. Pharm.* 494 (2015) 271–277.

65. S. Warashina, T. Nakamura, Y. Sato, Y. Fujiwara, M. Hyodo, H. Hatakeyama, H. Harashima, A lipid nanoparticle for the efficient delivery of siRNA to dendritic cells, *J. Control. Release* 225 (2016) 183–191.

66. M. Sugita, M. Cernadas, M.B. Brenner, New insights into pathways for CD1-mediated antigen presentation, *Curr. Opin. Immunol.* 16 (2004) 90–95.

67. D. Morita, Y. Yamamoto, T. Mizutani, T. Ishikawa, J. Suzuki, T. Igarashi, N. Mori, T. Shiina, H. Inoko, H. Fujita, K. Iwai, Y. Tanaka, B.Mikami, M. Sugita, Crystal structure of the N-myristoylated lipopeptide-bound MHC class I complex, *Nat. Commun.* 7 (2016) 10356.

68. D.C. Barral, M.B. Brenner, CD1 antigen presentation: how it works, *Nat. Rev. Immunol.* 7 (2007) 929–941.

69. T. Nakamura, R. Moriguchi, K. Kogure, H. Harashima, Incorporation of polyinosinepolycytidylic acid enhances cytotoxic T cell activity and antitumor effects by octaarginine-modified liposomes encapsulating antigen, but not by octaarginine-modified antigen complex, *Int. J. Pharm.* 441 (2013) 476–481.

70. T. Nakamura, R. Moriguchi, K. Kogure, N. Shastri, H. Harashima, Efficient MHC class I presentation by controlled intracellular trafficking of antigens in octaarginine-modified liposomes, *Mol. Ther.* 16 (2008) 1507–1514.

71. T. Nakamura, K. Ono, Y. Suzuki, R. Moriguchi, K. Kogure, H. Harashima, Octaarginine-modified liposomes enhance cross-presentation by promoting the C-terminal trimming of antigen peptide, *Mol. Pharm.* 11 (2014) 2787–2795.

72. H. Abdelmegeed, T. Nakamura, H. Harashima, In vivo inverse correlation in the activation of natural killer T cells through dual-signal stimulation via a combination of alpha-galactosylceramide-loaded liposomes and interleukin-12, *J. Pharm. Sci.* 105 (2016) 250–256.

73. T. Nakamura, D. Yamazaki, J. Yamauchi, H. Harashima, The nanoparticulation by octaarginine-modified liposome improves alpha-galactosylceramide-mediated antitumor therapy via systemic administration, *J. Control. Release* 171 (2013) 216–224.

74. Y. Hattori, I. Matsunaga, T. Komori, T. Urakawa, T. Nakamura, N. Fujiwara, K. Hiromatsu, H. Harashima, M. Sugita, Glycerol monomycolate, a latent tuberculosis-associated mycobacterial lipid, induces eosinophilic hypersensitivity responses in Guinea pigs, *Biochem. Biophys. Res. Commun.* 409 (2011) 304–307.

75. T. Komori, T. Nakamura, I.Matsunaga, D. Morita, Y. Hattori, H. Kuwata, N. Fujiwara, K. Hiromatsu, H. Harashima, M. Sugita, A microbial glycolipid functions as a new class of target antigen for delayed-type hypersensitivity, *J. Biol. Chem.* 286 (2011) 16800–16806.

76. D. Morita, Y. Hattori, T. Nakamura, T. Igarashi, H. Harashima, M. Sugita, Major T cell response to a mycolyl glycolipid is mediated by CD1c molecules in rhesus macaques, *Infect. Immun.* 81 (2013) 311–316.

77. D.Morita, A.Miyamoto, Y.Hattori, T.Komori, T.Nakamura, T. Igarashi, H. Harashima, M. Sugita, Th1-skewed tissue responses to a mycolyl glycolipid in mycobacteria-infected rhesus macaques, *Biochem. Biophys. Res. Commun.* 441 (2013) 108–113.

78. Y. Hattori, D. Morita, N. Fujiwara, D. Mori, T. Nakamura, H. Harashima, S. Yamasaki, M. Sugita, Glycerol monomycolate is a novel ligand for the human, but not mouse macrophage inducible C-type lectin, Mincle, *J. Biol. Chem.* 289 (2014) 15405–15412.

79. M.M. Venkataswamy, S.A. Porcelli, Lipid and glycolipid antigens of CD1d-restricted natural killer T cells, *Semin. Immunol.* 22 (2010) 68–78.

80. J.W. Molling, M.Moreno, H.J. van der Vliet, A.J. van den Eertwegh, R.J. Scheper, B.M. von Blomberg, H.J. Bontkes, Invariant natural killer T cells and immunotherapy of cancer, *Clin. Immunol.* 129 (2008) 182–194.

81. P.J. Brennan, M. Brigl, M.B. Brenner, Invariant natural killer T cells: an innate activation scheme linked to diverse effector functions, *Nat. Rev. Immunol.* 13 (2013) 101–117.

82. H. Kitamura, K. Iwakabe, T. Yahata, S. Nishimura, A. Ohta, Y. Ohmi, M. Sato, K. Takeda, K. Okumura, L. Van Kaer, T. Kawano, M. Taniguchi, T. Nishimura, The natural killer T (NKT) cell ligand alpha-galactosylceramide demonstrates its immunopotentiating effect by inducing interleukin (IL)-12 production by dendritic cells and IL-12 receptor expression on NKT cells, *J. Exp. Med.* 189 (1999) 1121–1128.

83. T. Nakamura, M. Kuroi, H. Harashima, Influence of endosomal escape and degradation of alpha-galactosylceramide loaded liposomes on CD1d antigen presentation, *Mol. Pharm.* 12 (2015) 2791–2799.

84. D.C. Wallace, Mitochondria and cancer, *Nat. Rev. Cancer* 12 (2012) 685–698.

85. K. Ishikawa, K. Takenaga, M. Akimoto, N. Koshikawa, A. Yamaguchi, H. Imanishi, K. Nakada, Y. Honma, J. Hayashi, ROS-generating mitochondrial DNA mutations can regulate tumor cell metastasis, *Science* 320 (2008) 661–664.

86. A. Ashkenazi, Targeting the extrinsic apoptotic pathway in cancer: lessons learned and future directions, *J. Clin. Invest.* 125 (2015) 487–489.

87. S. Fulda, L. Galluzzi, G. Kroemer, Targeting mitochondria for cancer therapy, *Nat. Rev. Drug Discov.* 9 (2010) 447–464.

88. J.S. Modica-Napolitano, V. Weissig, Treatment strategies that enhance the efficacy and selectivity of mitochondria-targeted anticancer agents, *Int. J. Mol. Sci.* 16 (2015) 17394–17421.

89. N. Oku, K. Doi, Y. Namba, S. Okada, Therapeutic effect of adriamycin encapsulated in long-circulating liposomes on Meth-A-sarcoma-bearing mice, *Int. J. Cancer* 58 (1994) 415–419.

90. G.R. Chamberlain, D.V. Tulumello, S.O. Kelley, Targeted delivery of doxorubicin to mitochondria, *ACS Chem. Biol.* 8 (2013) 1389–1395.

91. K.L. Horton, K.M. Stewart, S.B. Fonseca, Q. Guo, S.O. Kelley, Mitochondria-penetrating peptides, *Chem. Biol.* 15 (2008) 375–382.

92. K.L. Horton, M.P. Pereira, K.M. Stewart, S.B. Fonseca, S.O. Kelley, Tuning the activity of mitochondria-penetrating peptides for delivery or disruption, *Chembiochem* 13 (2012) 476–485.

93. M. Han, M.R. Vakili, H. Soleymani Abyaneh, O. Molavi, R. Lai, A. Lavasanifar, Mitochondrial delivery of doxorubicin via triphenylphosphine modification for overcoming drug resistance in MDA-MB-435/DOX cells, *Mol. Pharm.* 11 (2014) 2640–2649.

94. M.P. Murphy, R.A. Smith, Targeting antioxidants to mitochondria by conjugation to lipophilic cations, *Annu. Rev. Pharmacol. Toxicol.* 47 (2007) 629–656.

95. T.A. Theodossiou, Z. Sideratou, M.E. Katsarou, D. Tsiourvas, Mitochondrial delivery of doxorubicin by triphenylphosphonium-functionalized hyperbranched nanocarriers results in rapid and severe cytotoxicity, *Pharm. Res.* 30 (2013) 2832–2842.

96. Q. Qu, X. Ma, Y. Zhao, Targeted delivery of doxorubicin to mitochondria using mesoporous silica nanoparticle nanocarriers, *Nanoscale* 7 (2015) 16677–16686.

97. H. Wang, H. Yin, F. Yan, M. Sun, L. Du, W. Peng, Q. Li, Y. Feng, Y. Zhou, Folate-mediated mitochondrial targeting with doxorubicin-polyrotaxane nanoparticles overcomes multidrug resistance, *Oncotarget* 6 (2015) 2827–2842.

98. G.G. D'Souza, R. Rammohan, S.M. Cheng, V.P. Torchilin, V. Weissig, DQAsome-mediated delivery of plasmid DNA toward mitochondria in living cells, *J. Control. Release* 92 (2003) 189–197.

99. Y.F. Song, D.Z. Liu, Y. Cheng, M. Liu, W.L. Ye, B.L. Zhang, X.Y. Liu, S.Y. Zhou, Dual subcellular compartment delivery of doxorubicin to overcome drug resistant and enhance antitumor activity, *Sci. Rep.* 5 (2015) 16125.

100. V. Weissig, G.G. D'Souza, V.P. Torchilin, DQAsome/DNA complexes release DNA upon contact with isolated mouse liver mitochondria, *J. Control. Release* 75 (2001) 401–408.

101. V. Weissig, From serendipity to mitochondria-targeted nanocarriers, *Pharm. Res.* 28 (2011) 2657–2668.

102. Y. Yamada, H. Akita, H. Kamiya, K. Kogure, T. Yamamoto, Y. Shinohara, K. Yamashita, H. Kobayashi, H. Kikuchi, H. Harashima, MITO-Porter: a liposome-based carrier system for delivery of macromolecules into mitochondria via membrane fusion, *Biochim. Biophys. Acta* 1778 (2008) 423–432.

103. Y. Yamada, H. Harashima, Mitochondrial drug delivery systems for macromolecule and their therapeutic application to mitochondrial diseases, *Adv. Drug Deliv. Rev.* 60 (2008) 1439–1462.

104. Y. Yamada, Mitochondrial DDS opens innovative pharmaceutics, *Yakugaku Zasshi* 136 (2016) 55–62.

105. E. Kawamura, Y. Yamada, H. Harashima, Mitochondrial targeting functional peptides as potential devices for the mitochondrial delivery of a DF-MITO-Porter, *Mitochondrion* 13 (2013) 610–614.

106. Y. Yamada, R. Furukawa, Y. Yasuzaki, H. Harashima, Dual function MITO-Porter, a nano carrier integrating both efficient cytoplasmic delivery and mitochondrial macromolecule delivery, *Mol. Ther.* 19 (2011) 1449–1456.

107. R. Furukawa, Y. Yamada, M. Takenaga, R. Igarashi, H. Harashima, Octaarginine-modified liposomes enhance the anti-oxidant effect of lecithinized superoxide dismutase by increasing its cellular uptake, *Biochem. Biophys. Res. Commun.* 404 (2011) 796–801.

108. Y. Yamada, K. Nakamura, R. Furukawa, E. Kawamura, T. Moriwaki, K. Matsumoto, K. Okuda, M. Shindo, H. Harashima, Mitochondrial delivery of bongkrekic acid using a MITO-porter prevents the induction of apoptosis in human hela cells, *J. Pharm.* 102 (2013) 1008–1015.

109. Y. Yamada, K. Nakamura, J. Abe, M. Hyodo, S. Haga, M. Ozaki, H. Harashima, Mitochondrial delivery of Coenzyme Q10 via systemic administration using a MITO-Porter prevents ischemia/reperfusion injury in the mouse liver, *J. Control. Release* 213 (2015) 86–95.

110. J. Abe, Y. Yamada, H. Harashima, Validation of a strategy for cancer therapy: delivering aminoglycoside drugs to mitochondria in HeLa cells, *J. Pharm. Sci.* 105 (2016) 734–740.

111. B.C. Baguley, Multiple drug resistance mechanisms in cancer, *Mol. Biotechnol.* 46 (2010) 308–316.

112. H.M. Abdallah, A.M. Al-Abd, R.S. El-Dine, A.M. El-Halawany, P-glycoprotein inhibitors of natural origin as potential tumor chemo-sensitizers: a review, *J. Adv. Res.* 6 (2015) 45–62.

113. D.A. Arber, A. Orazi, R. Hasserjian, J. Thiele, M.J. Borowitz, M.M. Le Beau, C.D. Bloomfield, M. Cazzola, J.W. Vardiman, The 2016 revision to the World Health Organization classification of myeloid neoplasms and acute leukemia, *Blood* 127 (2016) 2391–2405.

114. S. Weinstein, D. Peer, RNAi nanomedicines: challenges and opportunities within the immune system, *Nanotechnology* 21 (2010) 232001.

115. B.L. Davidson, P.B. McCray Jr., Current prospects for RNA interference-based therapies, *Nat. Rev. Genet.* 12 (2011) 329–340.

116. H. Ling, M. Fabbri, G.A. Calin, MicroRNAs and other noncoding RNAs as targets for anticancer drug development, *Nat. Rev. Drug Discov.* 12 (2013) 847–865.

117. A. Wittrup, J. Lieberman, Knocking down disease: a progress report on siRNA therapeutics, *Nat. Rev. Genet.* 16 (2015) 543–552.

118. Y. Dorsett, T. Tuschl, siRNAs: applications in functional genomics and potential as therapeutics, *Nat. Rev. Drug Discov.* 3 (2004) 318–329.

119. R. Juliano, M.R. Alam, V. Dixit, H. Kang, Mechanisms and strategies for effective delivery of antisense and siRNA oligonucleotides, *Nucleic Acids Res.* 36 (2008) 4158–4171.

120. M. Schlee, G. Hartmann, The chase for the RIG-I ligand – recent advances, *Mol. Ther.* 18 (2010) 1254–1262.

121. V. Hornung, M. Guenthner-Biller, C. Bourquin, A. Ablasser, M. Schlee, S. Uematsu, A. Noronha, M. Manoharan, S. Akira, A. de Fougerolles, S. Endres, G. Hartmann, Sequence-specific potent induction of IFN-alpha by short interfering RNA in plasmacytoid dendritic cells through TLR7, *Nat. Med.* 11 (2005) 263–270.

122. A.D. Judge, V. Sood, J.R. Shaw, D. Fang, K. McClintock, I. MacLachlan, Sequence-dependent stimulation of the mammalian innate immune response by synthetic siRNA, *Nat. Biotechnol.* 23 (2005) 457–462.

123. B.R. Meade, K. Gogoi, A.S. Hamil, C. Palm-Apergi, A. van den Berg, J.C. Hagopian, A.D. Springer, A. Eguchi, A.D. Kacsinta, C.F. Dowdy, A. Presente, P. Lonn, M. Kaulich, N. Yoshioka, E. Gros, X.S. Cui, S.F. Dowdy, Efficient delivery of RNAi prodrugs containing reversible charge-neutralizing phosphotriester backbone modifications, *Nat. Biotechnol.* 32 (2014) 1256–1261.

124. S.Y. Wu, X. Yang, K.M. Gharpure, H. Hatakeyama, M. Egli, M.H. McGuire, A.S. Nagaraja, T.M. Miyake, R. Rupaimoole, C.V. Pecot, M. Taylor, S. Pradeep, M. Sierant, C. Rodriguez-Aguayo, H.J. Choi, R.A. Previs, G.N. Armaiz-Pena, L. Huang, C. Martinez, T. Hassell, C. Ivan, V. Sehgal, R. Singhania, H.D. Han, C. Su, J.H. Kim, H.J. Dalton, C. Kovvali, K. Keyomarsi, N.A. McMillan, W.W. Overwijk, J. Liu, J.S. Lee, K.A. Baggerly, G. Lopez-Berestein, P.T. Ram, B. Nawrot, A.K. Sood, 2'-OMephosphorodithioate-modified siRNAs show increased loading into the RISC complex and enhanced anti-tumour activity, *Nat. Commun.* 5 (2014) 3459.

125. D. Peer, E.J. Park, Y. Morishita, C.V. Carman, M. Shimaoka, Systemic leukocyte-directed siRNA delivery revealing cyclin D1 as an anti-inflammatory target, *Science* 319 (2008) 627–630.

126. D. Peer, M. Shimaoka, Systemic siRNA delivery to leukocyte-implicated diseases, *Cell Cycle* 8 (2009) 853–859.

127. A.M. Krieg, The role of CpG motifs in innate immunity, *Curr. Opin. Immunol.* 12 (2000) 35–43.

128. J. Abdi, T.Mutis, J. Garssen, F. Redegeld, Characterization of the Toll-like receptor expression profile in human multiple myeloma cells, *PLoS One* 8 (2013), e60671.

129. P.K. Mongini, R. Gupta, E. Boyle, J. Nieto, H. Lee, J. Stein, J. Bandovic, T. Stankovic, J. Barrientos, J.E. Kolitz, S.L. Allen, K. Rai, C.C. Chu, N. Chiorazzi, TLR-9 and IL-15 synergy promotes the in vitro clonal expansion of chronic lymphocytic leukemia B cells, *J. Immunol.* 195 (2015) 901–923.

130. M. Kortylewski, P. Swiderski, A. Herrmann, L. Wang, C. Kowolik, M. Kujawski, H. Lee, A. Scuto, Y. Liu, C. Yang, J. Deng, H.S. Soifer, A. Raubitschek, S. Forman, J.J. Rossi, D.M. Pardoll, R. Jove, H. Yu, In vivo delivery of siRNA to immune cells by conjugation to a TLR9 agonist enhances antitumor immune responses, *Nat. Biotechnol.* 27 (2009) 925–932.

131. D.M. Hossain, C. Dos Santos, Q. Zhang, A. Kozlowska, H. Liu, C. Gao, D. Moreira, P. Swiderski, A. Jozwiak, J. Kline, S. Forman, R. Bhatia, Y.H. Kuo, M. Kortylewski, Leukemia cell-targeted STAT3 silencing and TLR9 triggering generate systemic antitumor immunity, *Blood* 123 (2014) 15–25.

132. F.M. Uckun, S. Qazi, I. Dibirdik, D.E. Myers, Rational design of an immunoconjugate for selective knock-down of leukemia-specific E2A-PBX1 fusion gene expression in human Pre-B leukemia, *Integr. Biol.* 5 (2013) 122–132.

133. D. Hong, R. Kurzrock, Y. Kim, R.Woessner, A. Younes, J. Nemunaitis, N. Fowler, T. Zhou, J. Schmidt, M. Jo, S.J. Lee, M. Yamashita, S.G. Hughes, L. Fayad, S. Piha-Paul, M.V. Nadella, M. Mohseni, D. Lawson, C. Reimer, D.C. Blakey, X. Xiao, J. Hsu, A. Revenko, B.P. Monia, A.R. MacLeod, AZD9150, a next-generation antisense oligonucleotide inhibitor of STAT3 with early evidence of clinical activity in lymphoma and lung cancer, *Sci. Transl. Med.* 7 (2015) 314ra185.

134. I. Hazan-Halevy, D. Landesman-Milo, D. Rosenblum, S. Mizrahy, B.D. Ng, D. Peer, Immunomodulation of hematological malignancies using oligonucleotides based-nanomedicines, *J. Control. Release* 244 (2016) 149–156.

135. J. Cortes, H. Kantarjian, E.D. Ball, J. Dipersio, J.E. Kolitz, H.F. Fernandez, M. Goodman, G. Borthakur, M.R. Baer, M. Wetzler, Phase 2 randomized study of p53 antisense oligonucleotide (cenersen) plus idarubicin with or without cytarabine in refractory and relapsed acute myeloid leukemia, *Cancer* 118 (2012) 418–427.

136. S. O'Brien, J.O. Moore, T.E. Boyd, L.M. Larratt, A. Skotnicki, B. Koziner, A.A. Chanan-Khan, J.F. Seymour, R.G. Bociek, S. Pavletic, K.R. Rai, Randomized phase III trial of fludarabine plus cyclophosphamide with or without oblimersen sodium (Bcl-2 antisense) in patients with relapsed or refractory chronic lymphocytic leukemia, *J. Clin. Oncol.* 25 (2007) 1114–1120.

137. A.A. Chanan-Khan, R. Niesvizky, R.J. Hohl, T.M. Zimmerman, N.P. Christiansen, G.J. Schiller, N. Callander, J. Lister, M. Oken, S. Jagannath, Phase III randomised study of dexamethasone with or without oblimersen sodium for patients with advanced multiple myeloma, *Leuk. Lymphoma* 50 (2009) 559–565.

138. J. Lieberman, Manipulating the in vivo immune response by targeted gene knockdown, *Curr. Opin. Immunol.* 35 (2015) 63–72.

139. L.A. Wheeler, V. Vrbanac, R. Trifonova, M.A. Brehm, A. Gilboa-Geffen, S. Tanno, D.L. Greiner, A.D. Luster, A.M. Tager, J. Lieberman, Durable knockdown and protection from HIV transmission in humanized mice treated with gel-formulated CD4 aptamer-siRNA chimeras, *Mol. Ther.* 21 (2013) 1378–1389.

140. J. Zhou, S. Satheesan, H. Li, M.S. Weinberg, K.V. Morris, J.C. Burnett, J.J. Rossi, Cell-specific RNA aptamer against human CCR5 specifically targets HIV-1 susceptible cells and inhibits HIV-1 infectivity, *Chem. Biol.* 22 (2015) 379–390.

141. A. Herrmann, S.J. Priceman, P. Swiderski, M. Kujawski, H. Xin, G.A. Cherryholmes, W. Zhang, C. Zhang, C. Lahtz, C. Kowolik, S.J. Forman, M. Kortylewski, H. Yu, CTLA4 aptamer delivers STAT3 siRNA to tumor-associated and malignant T cells, *J. Clin. Invest.* 124 (2014) 2977–2987.

142. D. Peer, J.M. Karp, S. Hong, O.C. Farokhzad, R. Margalit, R. Langer, Nanocarriers as an emerging platform for cancer therapy, *Nat. Nanotechnol.* 2 (2007) 751–760.

143. D. Peer, A daunting task: manipulating leukocyte function with RNAi, *Immunol. Rev.* 253 (2013) 185–197.

144. D. Landesman-Milo, D. Peer, Transforming nanomedicines from lab scale production to novel clinical modality, *Bioconjug. Chem.* 27 (2016) 855–862.

145. S.T. Chou, A.J. Mixson, siRNA nanoparticles: the future of RNAi therapeutics for oncology?, *Nanomedicine* 9 (2014) 2251–2254.

146. S.M. Francis, C.A. Taylor, T. Tang, Z. Liu, Q. Zheng, R. Dondero, J.E. Thompson, SNS01-T modulation of eIF5A inhibits B-cell cancer progression and synergizes with bortezomib and lenalidomide, *Mol. Ther.* 22 (2014) 1643–1652.

147. K. Gavrilov, Y.E. Seo, G.T. Tietjen, J. Cui, C.J. Cheng, W.M. Saltzman, Enhancing potency of siRNA targeting fusion genes by optimization outside of target sequence, *Proc. Natl. Acad. Sci. U. S. A.* 112 (2015) E6597–E6605.

148. I.A. Babar, C.J. Cheng, C.J. Booth, X. Liang, J.B. Weidhaas, W.M. Saltzman, F.J. Slack, Nanoparticle-based therapy in an in vivo microRNA-155 (miR-155)-dependent mouse model of lymphoma, *Proc. Natl. Acad. Sci. U. S. A.* 109 (2012) E1695–E1704.

149. A. Schallon, C.V. Synatschke, V. Jerome, A.H. Muller, R. Freitag, Nanoparticulate nonviral agent for the effective delivery of pDNA and siRNA to differentiated cells and primary human T lymphocytes, *Biomacromolecules* 13 (2012) 3463–3474.

150. A.Z. Badros, O. Goloubeva, A.P. Rapoport, B. Ratterree, N. Gahres, B. Meisenberg, N. Takebe, M. Heyman, J. Zwiebel, H. Streicher, C.D. Gocke, D. Tomic, J.A. Flaws, B. Zhang, R.G. Fenton, Phase II study of G3139, a Bcl-2 antisense oligonucleotide, in combination with dexamethasone and thalidomide in relapsed multiple myeloma patients, *J. Clin. Oncol.* 23 (2005) 4089–4099.

151. J. Durig, U. Duhrsen, L. Klein-Hitpass, J. Worm, J.B. Hansen, H. Orum, M. Wissenbach, The novel antisense Bcl-2 inhibitor SPC2996 causes rapid leukemic cell clearance and immune activation in chronic lymphocytic leukemia, *Leukemia* 25 (2011) 638–647.

152. B. Yu, Y. Mao, L.Y. Bai, S.E. Herman, X.Wang, A. Ramanunni, Y. Jin, X. Mo, C. Cheney, K.K. Chan, D. Jarjoura, G. Marcucci, R.J. Lee, J.C. Byrd, L.J. Lee, N. Muthusamy, Targeted nanoparticle delivery overcomes off-target immunostimulatory effects of oligonucleotides and improves therapeutic efficacy in chronic lymphocytic leukemia, *Blood* 121 (2013) 136–147.

153. J. Tabernero, G.I. Shapiro, P.M. LoRusso, A. Cervantes, G.K. Schwartz, G.J. Weiss, L. Paz-Ares, D.C. Cho, J.R. Infante, M. Alsina, M.M. Gounder, R. Falzone, J. Harrop, A.C. White, I. Toudjarska, D. Bumcrot, R.E. Meyers, G. Hinkle, N. Svrzikapa, R.M. Hutabarat, V.A. Clausen, J. Cehelsky, S.V. Nochur, C. Gamba-Vitalo, A.K. Vaishnaw, D.W. Sah, J.A. Gollob, H.A. Burris III, First-in-humans trial of an RNA interference therapeutic targeting VEGF and KSP in cancer patients with liver involvement, *Cancer Discov.* 3 (2013) 406–417.

154. D.V. Morrissey, J.A. Lockridge, L. Shaw, K. Blanchard, K. Jensen, W. Breen, K. Hartsough, L. Machemer, S. Radka, V. Jadhav, N. Vaish, S. Zinnen, C. Vargeese, K. Bowman, C.S. Shaffer, L.B. Jeffs, A. Judge, I. MacLachlan, B. Polisky, Potent and persistent in vivo anti-HBV activity of chemically modified siRNAs, *Nat. Biotechnol.* 23 (2005) 1002–1007.

155. A. Akinc, W. Querbes, S. De, J. Qin, M. Frank-Kamenetsky, K.N. Jayaprakash, M. Jayaraman, K.G. Rajeev, W.L. Cantley, J.R. Dorkin, J.S. Butler, L. Qin, T. Racie, A. Sprague, E. Fava, A. Zeigerer, M.J. Hope, M. Zerial, D.W. Sah, K. Fitzgerald, M.A. Tracy, M. Manoharan, V. Koteliansky, A. Fougerolles, M.A. Maier, Targeted delivery of RNAi therapeutics with endogenous and exogenous ligand-based mechanisms, *Mol. Ther.* 18 (2010) 1357–1364.

156. T.I. Novobrantseva, A. Borodovsky, J. Wong, B. Klebanov, M. Zafari, K. Yucius, W. Querbes, P. Ge, V.M. Ruda, S. Milstein, L. Speciner, R. Duncan, S. Barros, G. Basha, P. Cullis, A. Akinc, J.S. Donahoe, K. Narayanannair Jayaprakash, M. Jayaraman, R.L. Bogorad, K. Love, K. Whitehead, C. Levins, M. Manoharan, F.K. Swirski, R. Weissleder, R. Langer, D.G. Anderson, A. de Fougerolles, M. Nahrendorf, V. Koteliansky, Systemic RNAi-mediated gene silencing in nonhuman primate and rodent myeloid cells, *Mol. Ther. Nucleic Acids* 1 (2012) e4.

157. S. Ramishetti, R. Kedmi, M. Goldsmith, F. Leonard, A.G. Sprague, B. Godin, M. Gozin, P.R. Cullis, D.M. Dykxhoorn, D. Peer, Systemic gene silencing in primary T lymphocytes using targeted lipid nanoparticles, *ACS Nano* 9 (2015) 6706–6716.

158. S. Weinstein, I.A. Toker, R. Emmanuel, S. Ramishetti, I. Hazan-Halevy, D. Rosenblum, M. Goldsmith, A. Abraham, O. Benjamini, O. Bairey, P. Raanani, A. Nagler, J. Lieberman, D. Peer, Harnessing RNAi-based nanomedicines for therapeutic gene silencing in B-cell malignancies, *Proc. Natl. Acad. Sci. U. S. A.* 113 (2016) E16–E22.

159. A.L. Jackson, et al., Expression profiling reveals off-target gene regulation by RNAi, *Nat. Biotechnol.* 21, 635–637 (2003).

160. A.L. Jackson, et al., Widespread siRNA 'off-target' transcript silencing mediated by seed region sequence complementarity, *RNA* 12 (2006) 1179–1187.

161. P.C. Scacheri, et al., Short interfering RNAs can induce unexpected and divergent changes in the levels of untargeted proteins in mammalian cells, *Proc. Natl. Acad. Sci. U. S. A.* 101 (2004) 1892–1897.

162. S.P. Persengiev, X. Zhu, M.R. Green, Nonspecific, concentration-dependent stimulation and repression of mammalian gene expression by small interfering RNAs (siRNAs). *RNA* 10 (2004) 12–18.

163. J.G. Doench, C.P. Petersen, P.A. Sharp, siRNAs can function as miRNAs. *Genes Dev.* 17 (2003) 438–442.

164. D. Grimm, et al., Fatality in mice due to oversaturation of cellular microRNA/short hairpin RNA pathways. *Nature* 441 (2006) 537–541.

165. T.C. Roberts, R. Langer & Matthew J. A. Wood. Advances in oligonucleotide drug delivery. *Nat. Rev. Drug Discov.* 19 (2020) 673–694.

166. E.W.M. Ng, et al., Pegaptanib, a targeted anti-VEGF aptamer for ocular vascular disease. *Nat. Rev. Drug Discov.* 5 (2006) 123–132.

167. A.L. Ramon, C. Malvy, Anticancer oligonulceotides. In *Macromolecular Anticancer Therapeutics* (eds. L.H. Reddy, P. Couvreur) 539–568 (Springer, New York, 2010).

168. Loutfy H. Madkour, *Reactive Oxygen Species (ROS), Nanoparticles, and Endoplasmic Reticulum (ER) Stress-Induced Cell Death Mechanisms* (2020). Paperback ISBN: 9780128224816 Imprint: Academic Press. Published Date: 1st August 2020. https://www.elsevier.com/books/reactive-oxygen-species-ros-nanoparticles-and-endoplasmic-reticulum-er-stress-induced-cell-death-mechanisms/madkour/978-0-12-822481-6

169. Loutfy H. Madkour, *Nanoparticles Induce Oxidative and Endoplasmic Reticulum Antioxidant Therapeutic Defenses* (2020). Copyright 2020 Publisher Springer International Publishing Copyright Holder Springer Nature Switzerland AG eBook ISBN 978-3-030-37297-2. doi:10.1007/978-3-030-37297-2. Hardcover ISBN 978-3-030-37296-5. Series ISSN 2194-0452. Edition Number 1. https://www.springer.com/gp/book/9783030372965?utm_campaign=3_pier05_buy_print&utm_content=en_08082017&utm_medium=referral&utm_source=google_books#other version=

170. Loutfy H. Madkour, *Nucleic Acids as Gene Anticancer Drug Delivery Therapy*. 1st Edition. Publishing House: Elsevier (2020). Paperback ISBN: 9780128197776. Imprint: Academic Press Published Date: 2nd January 2020 Imprint: Academic Press Copyright: Paperback ISBN: 9780128197776. © Academic Press 2020 Published: 2nd January 2020. Imprint: Academic Press Paperback ISBN: 9780128197776. https://www.elsevier.com/books/nucleic-acids-as-gene-anticancer-drug-delivery therapy/madkour/978-0-12-819777-6

171. Loutfy H. Madkour, *Nanoelectronic Materials: Fundamentals and Applications (Advanced Structured Materials)* 1st Edition. 2019 Edition. https://link.springer.com/book/10.1007%2F978-3-030-21621-4. Series Title: Advanced Structured Materials Series Volume 116. Copyright 2019 Publisher. Springer International Publishing Copyright Holder Springer Nature Switzerland AG. eBook ISBN 978-3-030-21621-4. doi:10.1007/978-3-030-21621-4. Hardcover ISBN 978-3-030-21620-7. Series ISSN 1869-8433. Edition Number 1. Number of Pages XLIII, 783 Number of Illustrations 122 b/w illustrations, 494 illustrations in colour Topics. ISBN-10: 3030216209. ISBN-13: 978-3030216207 #117 in Nanotechnology (Books) #725 in Materials Science (Books) #187336 in Textbooks. https://books.google.com.eg/books/about/Nanoelectronic_Materials.html?id=YQXCxAEACAAJ&source=kp_book_description&redir_esc=y

172. Z.R. Cohen, S. Ramishetti, N. Peshes-Yaloz, M. Goldsmith, A. Wohl, Z. Zibly, D. Peer, Localized RNAi therapeutics of chemoresistant grade IV glioma using hyaluronangrafted lipid-based nanoparticles, *ACS Nano.* 9 (2015) 1581–1591.

173. S. Ramishetti, D. Landesman-Milo, D. Peer, Advances in RNAi therapeutic delivery to leukocytes using lipid nanoparticles. *J. Drug Target.* (2016) 1–7.

174. S. Wilhelm, A.J. Tavares, Q. Dai, S. Ohta, J. Audet, H.F. Dvorak, W.C.W. Chan, Analysis of nanoparticles delivery to tumors, *Nat. Rev. Mater.* 1 (2016) 1–12.

11 Pharmacogenomics Synergistic Strategies Using a Chimerical Peptide for Enhanced Chemotherapy Based on ROS and DNA Nanosystem

Here, an amphiphilic chimeric peptide (Fmoc)$_2$KH$_7$-TAT with pH responsibility for gene and drug delivery was designed and fabricated. As a drug carrier, the micelles self-assembled from the peptide exhibited a much faster doxorubicin (DOX) release rate at pH 5.0 than that at pH 7.4. As a nonviral gene vector, (Fmoc)$_2$KH$_7$-TAT peptide could satisfactorily mediate transfection of pGL-3 reporter plasmid with or without the existence of serum in both 293T and HeLa cell lines. Besides, the endosome escape capability of peptide/DNA complexes was investigated by confocal laser scanning microscopy (CLSM). To evaluate the codelivery efficiency and the synergistic antitumor effect of gene and drug, p53 plasmid and DOX were simultaneously loaded in the peptide micelles to form micelleplexes during the self-assembly of the peptide. Cellular uptake and intracellular delivery of gene and drug were studied by CLSM and flow cytometry respectively and p53 protein expression was determined via Western blot analysis. The *in vitro* cytotoxicity and *in vivo* tumor inhibition effect were also studied. The results [1] suggest that the codelivery of the gene and drug from peptide micelles resulted in effective cell growth inhibition *in vitro* and significant tumor growth restraining *in vivo*. The chimeric peptide-based gene and drug codelivery system will find great potential for tumor therapy.

The mesoporous silica nanoparticles (MSNs)-based nanocarriers were gated by β-cyclodextrin (β-CD) through the ROS-cleavable thioketal (TK) linker to encapsulate the anticancer drug doxorubicin hydrochloride (DOX HCL) and ROS-producing agent α-tocopheryl succinate (α-TOS), whose surface was further anchored with adamantane-conjugated polyethylene glycol chain (AD-PEG) via host–guest interaction. Both *in vitro* and *in vivo* experiments demonstrated that T/D@RSMSNs exhibited more significant antitumor activity in human breast cancer than the traditional single DOX-loaded ROS-responsive nanocarrier.

11.1 CHEMOTHERAPY AS SYNERGISTIC GENE

Chemotherapy as a dominant approach for the treatment of tumors has been widely used in clinical trials [2,3]. However, the curative effect of chemotherapy is severely dampened due to severe systemic toxicity, low bioavailability of antitumor drugs, as well as the emergence of drug resistance

of tumor cells after repeated administration of antitumor drugs [4]. Gene therapy, which focuses on the modulation and repair of particular gene defects, provides a new avenue for tumor therapy at the gene level. Unfortunately, the biosecurity concerns of viral vectors and the low transfection efficiency of nonviral vectors greatly limit its application. Recently, synergistic therapy based on the coadministration of the gene and drug has emerged rapidly as a promising modality for tumor treatment. Decreased drug dosage, negligible side effects, and high inhibition efficacy are hopeful to achieve, mostly because of the synergistic effect [5] or reversal of drug resistance to some extent via specific gene [6] by the codelivery systems.

The key point of synergistic therapy was to transport the gene and drug to the same cells and tissues. Considerable efforts have been devoted to developing delivery systems and various carriers based on dendrimers [7], liposomes [8], polymers [9,10], and nanoscaled inorganic particles [11] were proposed. But the barriers such as unsatisfactory cellular uptake, endosome escape, and vector-induced toxicity [12] are still fatal problems for these delivery systems. Especially in the gene delivery process, the major DNA-loaded complex internalized into cells through endocytosis is believed to traffic from endosome to lysosome. The milieu in the lysosome is hostile to DNA due to the existence of various enzyme systems, which may lead to the degradation of DNA/vector and failure in gene transfection [13]. Strategies based on the proton sponge hypothesis are widely used to overcome the endosome escape barrier [14]. Generally, carriers with satisfied buffering ability are always accompanied by severe cytotoxicities, such as polyethylenimine (PEI) and chloroquine.

Amphiphilic peptide-based micelles with a typical core–shell structure are an important class of promising codelivery systems for the gene and drug [15,16]. The peptide-based hydrophobic core can be used to encapsulate hydrophobic drugs, while the cationic peptide shells can be utilized to condense DNA. Additionally, benefiting from the blossom of modern molecular biology, peptides with tremendously appealing bioactivity have been exploited. For instance, TAT peptide (YGRKKRRQRRR), which derives from the transactivating transcriptional activator protein of HIV-1, has been confirmed to possess the

DOI: 10.1201/9781003229674-11

ability of autonomous and receptor-independent cell membrane translocation [17,18]. Besides, many viruses utilized pH-sensitive peptides to accelerate the endosome escape [19]; pH-sensitive peptides such as GALA or histidine-rich peptides [20,21] were fabricated as promising candidates to overcome the endosome escape barrier. Since the peptide is originated from the organism and mainly composed of natural amino acids, peptide-based biomaterials can always perform undeniable biocompatibility and biodegradability.

In this chapter, we reported an amphiphilic chimeric peptide, $(Fmoc)_2KH_7$-TAT with the chemical structure indicated in Scheme 11.1, which can self-assemble into micelleplex with DNA and drug simultaneously.

As illustrated in Scheme 11.2, at the physiological pH, the hydrophobic drug DOX was encapsulated in the hydrophobic micellar core through hydrophobic interaction and π-π stacking interaction, while the DNA was combined with the cationic shell of the TAT peptide. After cell internalization, the complexes could escape from the endosome due to the protonation of hepta-histidine domain of $(Fmoc)_2KH_7$-TAT at a low pH milieu, resulting in swelling of the complexes, accelerated drug release, and the delivery of the therapeutic gene to the nucleus subsequently. The properties of peptide micelles were characterized in terms of drug/DNA-loading ability, drug release behavior *in vitro*, gene transfection ability as well as codelivery of gene/drug, etc. Furthermore, the synergistic antitumor effect both *in vitro* and *in vivo* was evaluated in detail [1].

11.2 CHARACTERIZATION OF PEPTIDE AND COMPLEXES

The condensation of DNA is crucial for gene transfection. To demonstrate the DNA-binding ability of the micelles, an agarose gel electrophoresis assay was studied. As shown in Figure 11.1, $(Fmoc)_2KH_7$-TAT could completely retard the mobility of pGL-3 DNA at a w/w of 5. The good DNA-binding ability of $(Fmoc)_2KH_7$-TAT was probably due to the formation of micelle structure since the DNA-binding ability of TAT alone was relatively poor according to our previous work [22].

Besides, the particle size and zeta potential of $(Fmoc)_2$ KH_7-TAT/pGL-3 DNA complexes were also determined as shown in Figure 11.2. The size decreased and the zeta potential increased with increasing w/w ratio, indicating the more compact complexes formed. Furthermore, the size and zeta potential of DOX/$(Fmoc)_2KH_7$-TAT/pGL-3 DNA micelleplexes were performed to investigate the influence of the loaded drug. It was found that loading of DOX brought nearly a negligible influence in zeta potential, while the loaded DOX increased the size slightly as compared with that of the $(Fmoc)_2KH_7$-TAT/pGL-3 DNA complexes, indicating that the loaded DOX swelled the micellar hydrophobic core to some extent.

In order to get direct insight into fabricated $(Fmoc)_2KH_7$-TAT micelles and evaluate the effect of DNA and/or drug loading on a peptide micelle, four corresponding

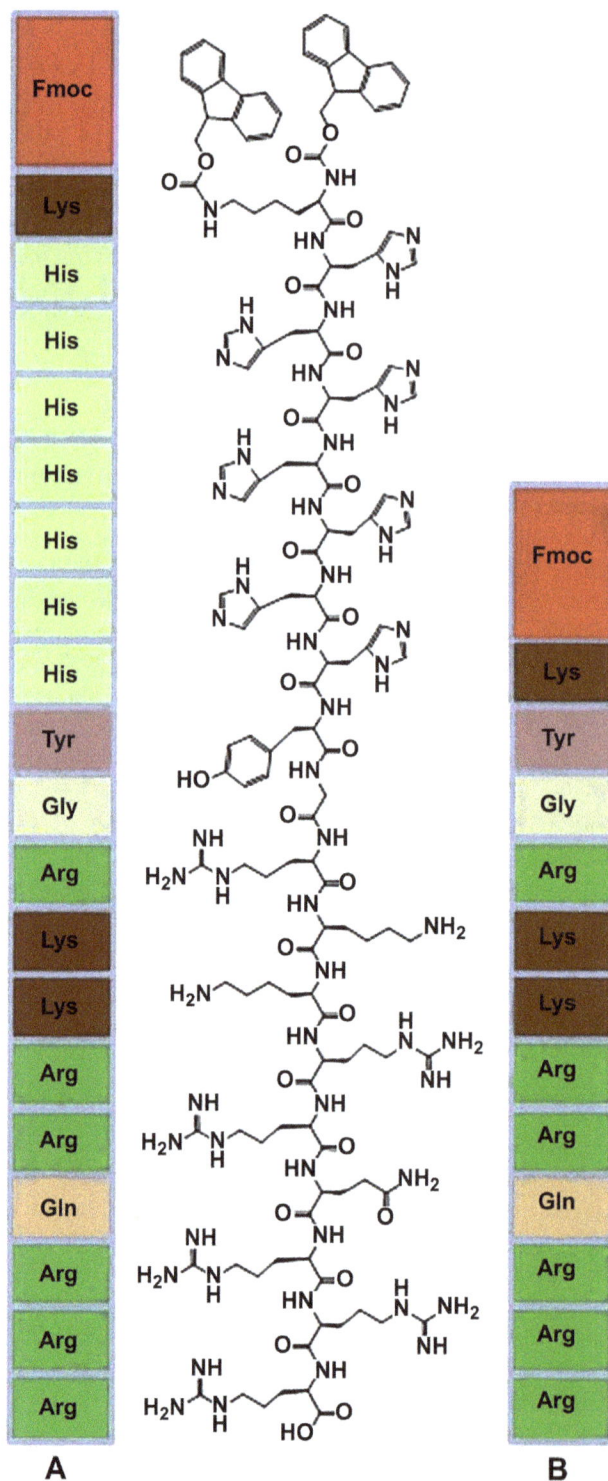

SCHEME 11.1 The chemical structure of peptide: (A) $(Fmoc)_2KH_7$-TAT; (B) $(Fmoc)_2K$-TAT.

morphologies were observed by TEM. As shown in Figure 11.3A2–D2, all the samples were well dispersed with a uniform structure. The loaded DOX increased the size of both peptide and peptide/pGL-3 DNA complexes. No matter drug was loaded or not, the condensation of DNA decreased the size of the peptide micelles. The decreased size in complexes was attributed to the

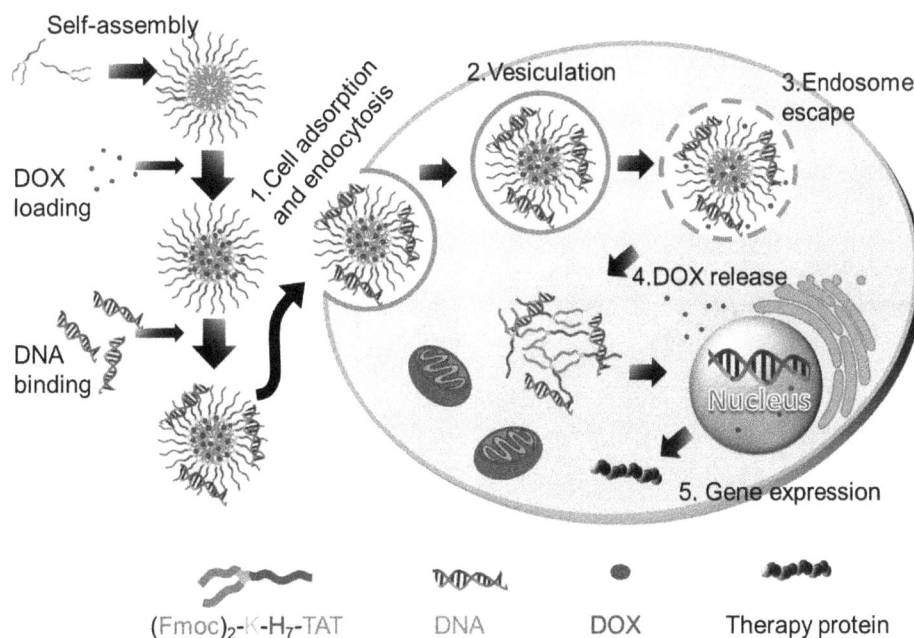

SCHEME 11.2 Codelivery and synergistic therapy of gene and drug by $(Fmoc)_2KH_7$-TAT micelleplex. (1) Endocytosis of DOX and gene-loaded $(Fmoc)_2KH_7$-TAT, (2) vesiculation of the complexes, (3) endosome escape, (4) drug release and gene delivery to nucleus and expression, (5) expression of therapy gene.

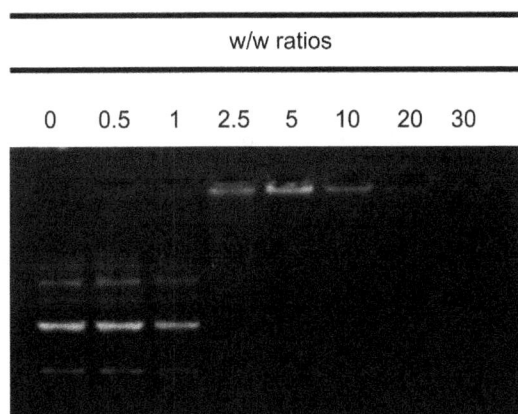

FIGURE 11.1 Agarose gel electrophoresis retardation assay of $(Fmoc)_2KH_7$-TAT/pGL-3 DNA complexes at various w/w ratios.

introduction of electrostatic interaction between cationic peptide and DNA. Furthermore, the hydrodynamic size of the four types of nanoparticles at the same peptide concentration was studied by dynamic light scattering (DLS). As shown in Figure 11.3A1–D1, the tendency in hydrodynamic size was consistent with the TEM results. Moreover, the size observed by TEM was smaller than that by DLS, and the discrepancy was ascribed to the shrinking of complexes during the preparation of TEM samples [23].

11.3 DRUG LOADING AND RELEASE BEHAVIOR *IN VITRO*

DOX was chosen [1] as the model drug to assess the drug-loading behavior, and the encapsulation efficiency and drug-loading efficiency values of peptide micelles were 21.8%

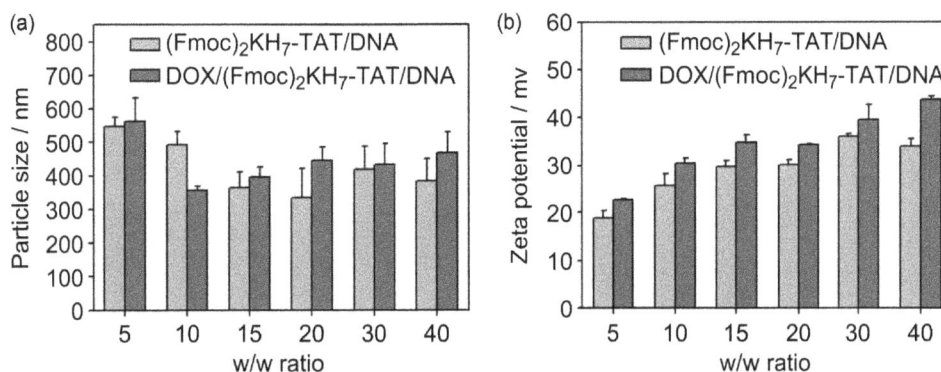

FIGURE 11.2 Size (average diameter) and zeta potential of $(Fmoc)_2KH_7$-TAT/pGL-3 DNA complexes and DOX/$(Fmoc)_2KH_7$-TAT/pGL-3 DNA micelleplexes at various w/w ratios. Data are presented as mean±S.D. (n=3).

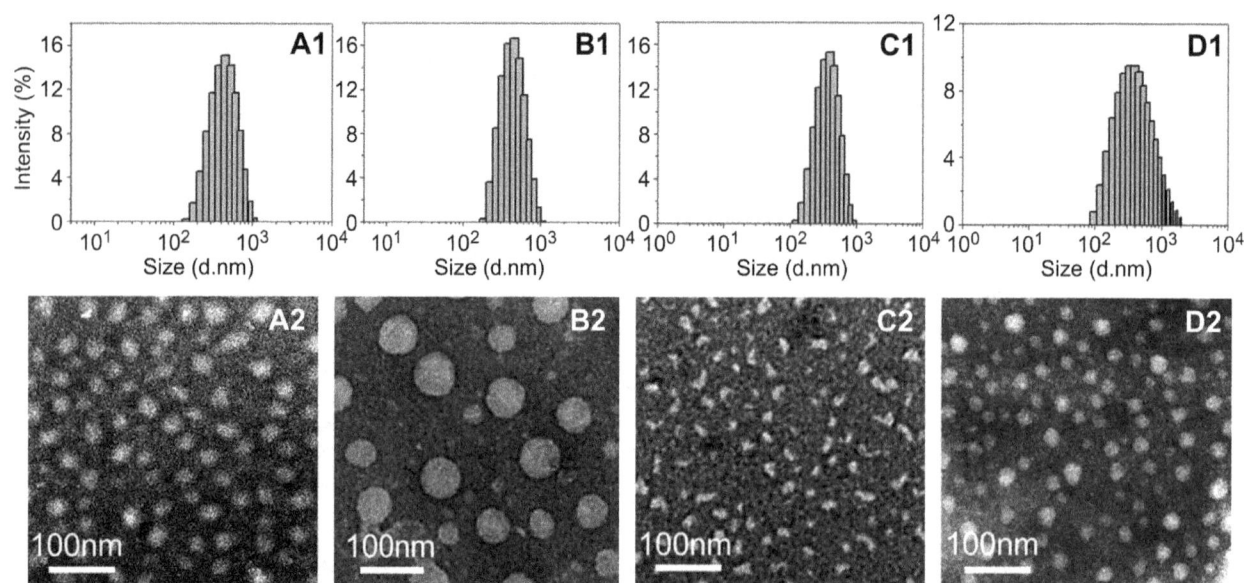

FIGURE 11.3 TEM images of (A) (Fmoc)$_2$KH$_7$-TAT; (B) drug-loaded (Fmoc)$_2$KH$_7$-TAT; (C) (Fmoc)$_2$KH$_7$-TAT/pGL-3 DNA complexes; (D) DOX/(Fmoc)$_2$KH$_7$-TAT/pGL-3 DNA micelleplexes. The w/w ratio of peptide/pGL-3 DNA complexes was 15, and the observation was under PBS buffer (pH 7.4, 5 mM).

and 11% respectively at pH 7.4. The peptide could efficiently entrap the DOX due to the π-π stacking interaction between the Fmoc group and DOX as well as the hydrophobic interaction between deprotonated histidine and DOX at a neutral pH. To demonstrate the endosome pH sensitivity of (Fmoc)$_2$KH$_7$-TAT, the drug release behaviors under different pHs were also evaluated, and pH 5.0 was chosen to imitate the endosome pH. As reflected in Figure 11.4, the cumulative release of DOX at pH 5.0 was significantly faster than that at pH 7.4. This finding was attributed to the increased hydrophilicity of the peptide at pH 5.0. Since the pKa of the imidazole group of histidine was about 6.0, the protonation of imidazole under a slightly acidic environment would vanish and destroy the hydrophobic interaction between H$_7$ and DOX, leading to the decrease in the compactness of micelles and rapid release of drugs at pH 5.0.

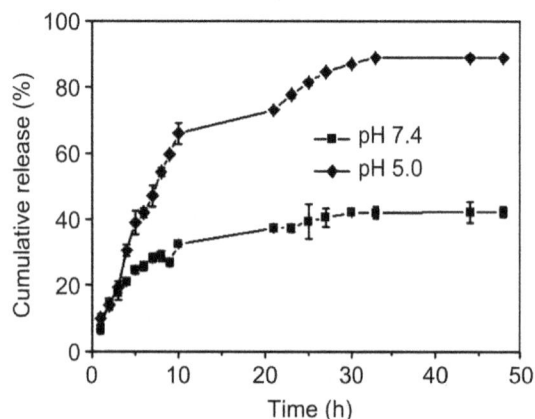

FIGURE 11.4 *In vitro* drug release behavior of DOX-loaded (Fmoc)$_2$KH$_7$-TAT micelles at different pHs (pH 7.4 and 5.0). Data are presented as mean ± S.D. (n = 3).

11.4 ENDOSOME ESCAPE CAPABILITY

Translocating through plasma membrane mediated by TAT peptide was confirmed involving the classical endocytosis uptake pathway [14]. As a result, complexes are always trafficked into endosome vesicles. Successfully conquering the endosome barrier is vital to the codelivery system. Here, CLSM observation was performed to estimate the endosome escaping ability of (Fmoc)$_2$KH$_7$-TAT/pGL-3 DNA complexes. The complexes were labeled with fluorescein isothiocyanate, while lysosome red was especially used to stain the acidic organelle lysosomes. (Fmoc)$_2$K-TAT/pGL-3 DNA was used as a negative control, and the corresponding ESI-MS of (Fmoc)$_2$K-TAT was studied [1]. As shown in Figure 11.5, only a small amount of (Fmoc)$_2$KH$_7$-TAT/pGL-3 DNA complexes was trapped in the lysosome, and the majority of complexes escaped from the endosome successfully, which was confirmed by the isolated distribution of red fluorescence and green fluorescence in Figure 11.5D2. In contrast, the existence of a large area of yellow fluorescence in Figure 11.5D1 suggested that the majority of (Fmoc)$_2$K-TAT/pGL-3 DNA complexes was localized in lysosomes.

11.5 GENE TRANSFECTION *IN VITRO*

The luciferase expression of pGL-3 DNA mediated by (Fmoc)$_2$KH$_7$-TAT was investigated in 293T and HeLa cell lines. Herein, branched 25 kDa PEI was used as a positive control. Figure 11.6A1 and B1 revealed that (Fmoc)$_2$KH$_7$-TAT performed comparable transfection efficiency to 25 kDa PEI at an optimal w/w ratio of 1.3 in both cell lines under a serum-free condition. Results demonstrated that the peptide could mediate satisfactory gene transfection.

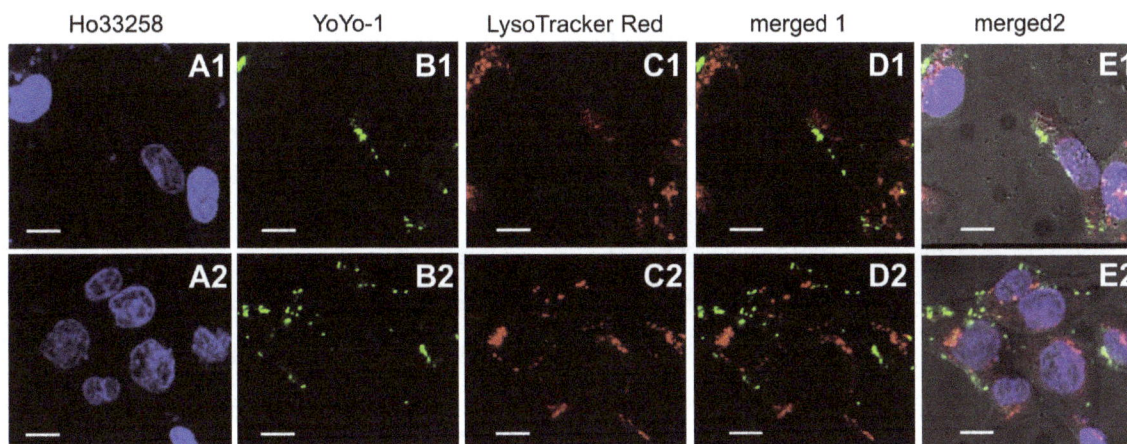

FIGURE 11.5 Endosome escape of (Fmoc)$_2$KH$_7$-TAT/pGL-3 DNA complexes (A1eE1) at a w/w ratio of 15, (Fmoc)$_2$K-TAT/pGL-3 DNA complexes (A2eE2) were used as a negative control. (A1, A2) Nucleus was stained with Hoechst 33258 (blue signal); (B1, B2) pGL3-DNA was labeled with YOYO-1 (green signal); (C1, C2) DOX (red signal); (D1) an overlay of (B1) and (C1); (D2) an overlay of (B2) and (C2). The scale bar was 10 mm and the micrographs were obtained at a magnification of 600x.

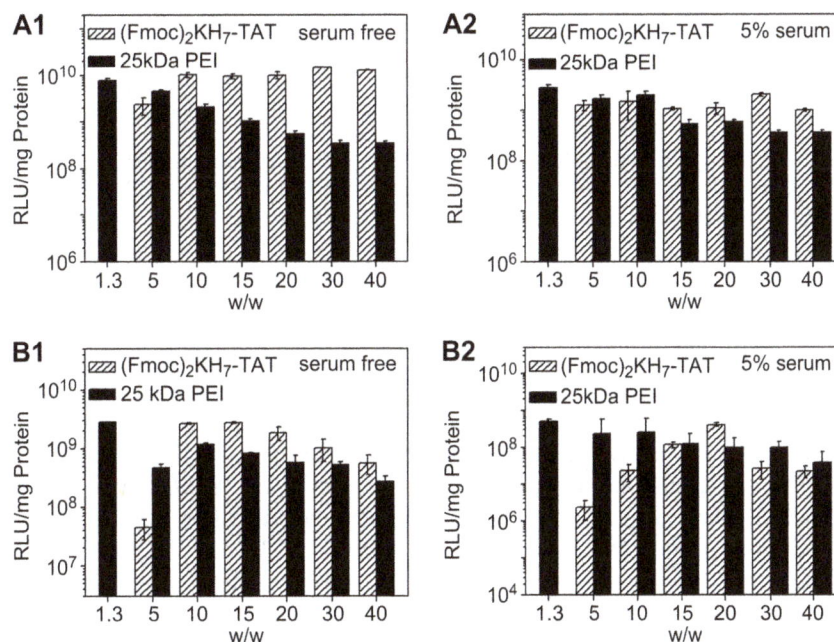

FIGURE 11.6 *In vitro* luciferase expression of (Fmoc)$_2$KH$_7$-TAT/pGL-3 DNA complexes at various w/w ratios in (A) 293T and (B) HeLa cell lines. PEI at 25 kDa was employed as a positive control. Data are presented as mean±S.D. (n=3).

The multifunctional peptide with low cytotoxicity could form micelles through self-assembly which could enhance the stability of the complexes greatly. Moreover, the excellent cellular uptake and endosome escape ability of the complexes could extremely improve their bioavailability.

The transfection ability under 5% serum-containing conditions was further assessed as shown in Figure 11.6A2 and B2. Due to the negative influence of serum on the cationic gene carrier, the transfection efficiency mediated by PEI or (Fmoc)$_2$KH$_7$-TAT decreased to some extent in both cell lines. However, the transfection efficiency of the peptide was still comparable to that of 25 kDa PEI.

11.6 *IN VITRO* CYTOTOXICITY

As a good gene carrier, the low cytotoxicity of the vector itself was essential for practical applications. Cytotoxicity of (Fmoc)$_2$KH$_7$-TAT *in vitro* was estimated against HeLa cells via a (3-(4, 5-dimethylthiazolyl-2)-2, 5-diphenyltetrazolium bromide (MTT) assay. PEI at 25 kDa was used as a negative control. As shown in Figure 11.7A, the cell viability was still above 90% when the concentration of peptide was 250 mg/L. On the contrary, the PEI showed serious cytotoxicity. Obviously, the peptide presented negligible toxicity, originating from the inherent biocompatibility of the peptide.

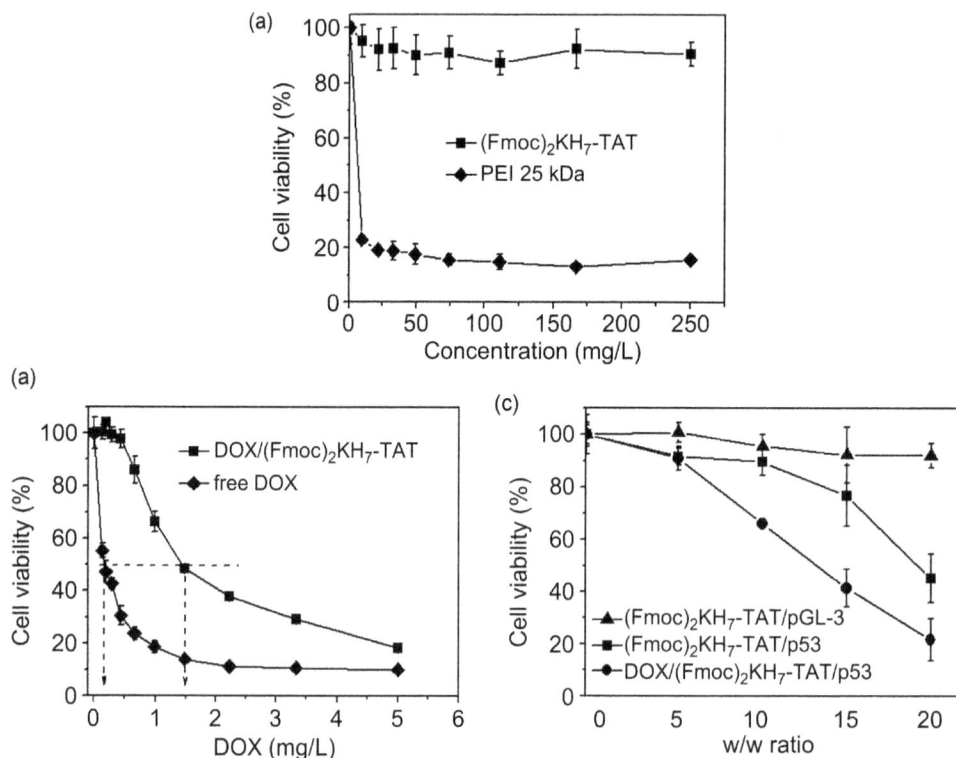

FIGURE 11.7 *In vitro* cytotoxicity against HeLa cells: (A) (Fmoc)$_2$KH$_7$-TAT and 25 kDa branched PEI; (B) free DOX and DOX-loaded (Fmoc)$_2$KH$_7$-TAT; (C) (Fmoc)$_2$KH$_7$-TAT/pGL-3 DNA complexes, (Fmoc)$_2$KH$_7$-TAT/p53 DNA complexes and DOX/(Fmoc)$_2$KH$_7$-TAT/p53 DNA micelleplexes with DOX concentration of 0.5 mg/L.

The toxicity of DOX HCl and DOX-loaded peptide system is also shown in Figure 11.7B. The IC$_{50}$ (the concentration required for 50% inhibition of cellular growth) of free DOX was 0.17 mg/L, while one of the DOX encapsulated in peptide micelles was 1.45 mg/L. Since the peptide was biocompatible, the cytotoxicity was mainly induced by the release of the loaded DOX. It was also found that at low DOX concentration, free DOX showed significantly higher cytotoxicity than a DOX-loaded peptide. With the increasing concentration of DOX, the difference in cytotoxicity between them was decreased since free DOX can be readily transported into the cytoplasm and nuclei by passive diffusion, while the DOX release from micelles was time-consuming [24].

11.7 CODELIVERY OF DRUG AND GENE *IN VITRO*

In HeLa cells, the nucleus was stained with Hoechst 33258 (blue) and pGL-3 DNA was labeled with YOYO-1 (green). The w/w ratio of (Fmoc)$_2$KH$_7$-TAT/pGL-3 DNA was 15, while the final concentration of DOX was 0.638 mg/L because the toxicity at this concentration was negligible. Cellular uptake at different times (1 h and 4 h) was performed as shown in Figure 11.8. With the increasing incubation time, the green and red fluorescence intensity increased significantly, indicating that the uptake of micelleplexes was time-dependent. Besides, the green and red

fluorescence got well overlapped after internalization for 4 h (Figure 11.8D2). In light of this finding, peptide micelles could successfully load pGL-3 DNA and DOX simultaneously. The excellent codelivery behavior may benefit from the core–shell structure of the cationic peptide micelles. Meanwhile, the image of merged 2 at 4 h revealed that the majority of DOX/peptide/pGL-3 DNA micelleplexes entered the nucleus or were around the nucleus periphery (Figure 11.8E2).

To further quantify the simultaneous delivery of gene and drug, two-color flow cytometry was performed as shown in Figure 11.9. The (Fmoc)$_2$KH$_7$-TAT micelle was used as a blank control. Here, YOYO-1-stained (Fmoc)$_2$KH$_7$-TAT/pGL-3 DNA complexes were green fluorescence positive and DOX-loaded (Fmoc)$_2$KH$_7$-TAT were red fluorescence positive. As expected, double-positive cells presented an overwhelming majority of the cells. This result demonstrated excellent ability of the peptide in the codelivery of DNA and DOX to the same cells.

11.8 SYNERGISTIC EFFECT *IN VITRO*

The key point of coadministration of gene and drug was to achieve a synergistic effect. Herein, the cell viability against HeLa cells via MTT assay was employed to evaluate the synergistic effect *in vitro*. p53 gene was chosen as a therapeutic gene to suppress the growth of the tumor. As shown in Figure 11.7C, (Fmoc)$_2$KH$_7$-TAT/pGL-3 DNA exhibited

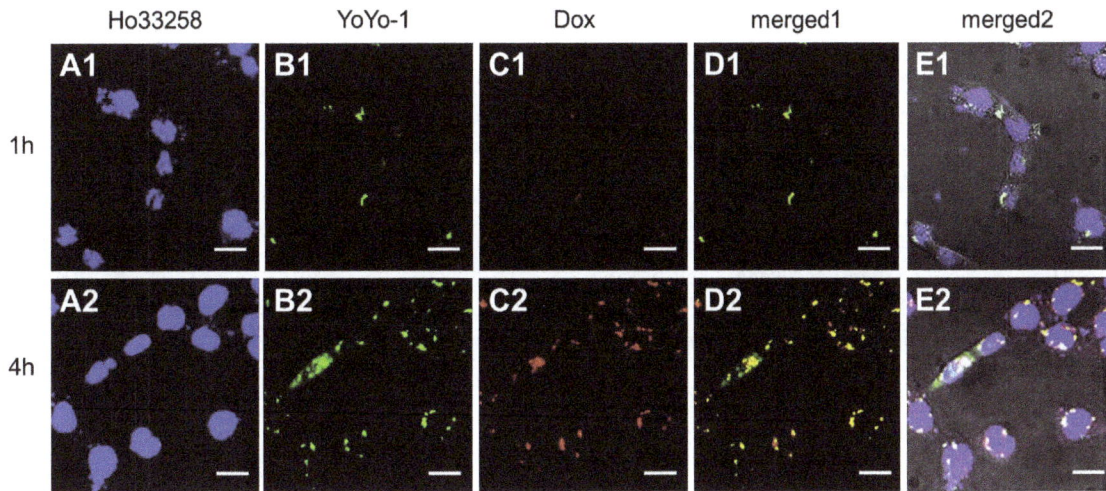

FIGURE 11.8 Codelivery of drug and gene into HeLa cells via (Fmoc)$_2$KH$_7$-TAT at different times (1 h and 4 h) by CLSM, the w/w of peptide/pGL-3 DNA complexes was 15 and the final concentration of DOX was 0.638 mg/L. (A1, A2) Nucleus was stained with Hoechst 33258 (blue signal); (B1, B2) pGL3-DNA was labeled with YOYO-1 (green signal); (C1, C2) lysosome was stained with LysoTracker Red DND-99 (red signal); (D1) an overlay of (B1) and (C1); (D2) an overlay of (B2) and (C2). The scale bar was 15 μm and the micrographs were obtained at a magnification of 600x.

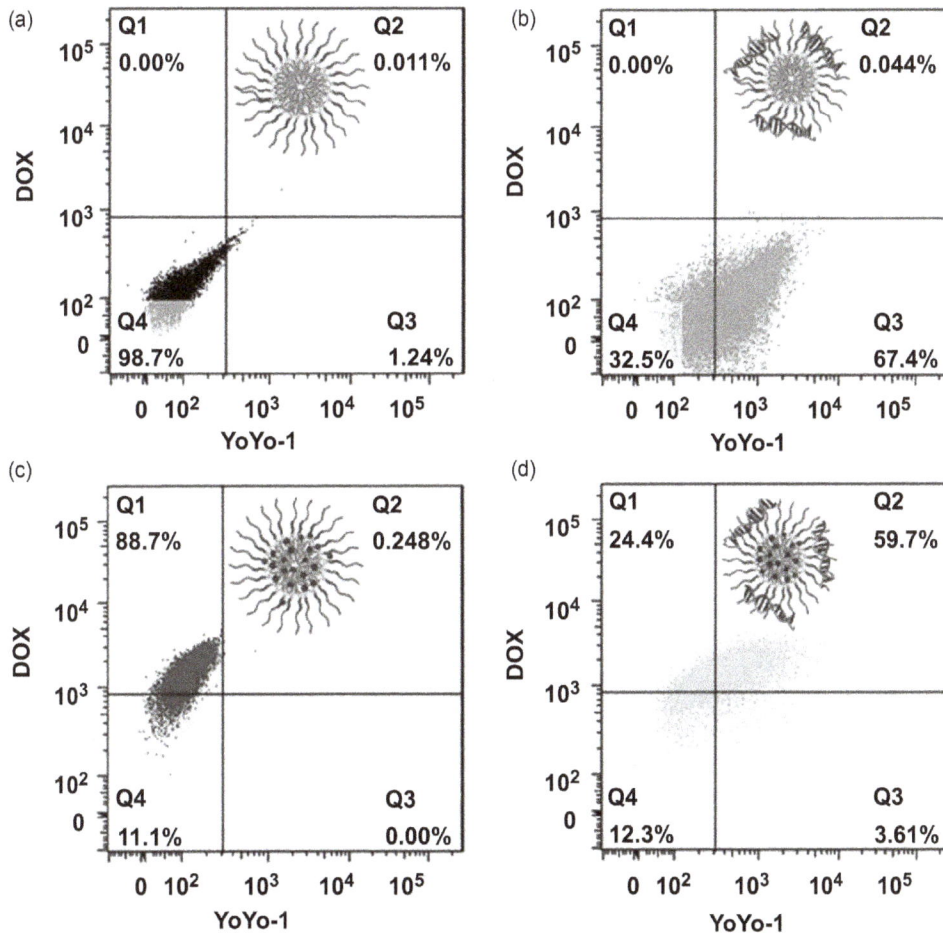

FIGURE 11.9 Codelivery of gene and drug mediated by (Fmoc)$_2$KH$_7$-TAT by two-color flow cytometry in HeLa cells. The w/w of peptide/pGL-3 DNA complexes was 15 and the final concentration of DOX was 0.638 mg/L. (A) (Fmoc)$_2$KH$_7$-TAT was used as a negative control; (B) YOYO-1-stained peptide/pGL-3 DNA complexes was green fluorescence positive; (C) DOX-loaded peptide was red fluorescence positive; (D) YOYO-1-stained DOX/peptide/pGL-3 DNA micelleplexes.

negligible toxicity in HeLa cells, while (Fmoc)$_2$KH$_7$-TAT/ p53 DNA complexes showed certain cytotoxicity. The DOX/(Fmoc)$_2$KH$_7$-TAT/p53 DNA micelleplexes presented significantly higher cytotoxicity than that of (Fmoc)$_2$KH$_7$-TAT/p53 DNA complexes. Since the concentration of loaded DOX in micelleplexes was 0.5 mg/L, the loaded DOX showed negligible cytotoxicity according to Figure 11.7B and the much-increased cytotoxicity was attributed to the synergistic effect of DOX and p53 gene. Clearly, coadministration of gene and drug exceedingly decreased the dose of DOX in peptide micelles and resulted in enhanced cell growth inhibition rate.

To further confirm the synergistic effect, the Western blot analysis was used to determine the p53 protein expression in different transfected cells. Glyceraldehyde 3-phosphate dehydrogenase (GAPDH) was used as internal control. According to Figure 11.10A, the peptide induced a very low expression level of p53 protein. Additionally, (Fmoc)$_2$KH$_7$-TAT/p53 DNA could mediate a higher expression level of p53 protein than that of 25 kDa PEI/ p53 DNA (w/w 1.3), demonstrating excellent gene transfection efficacy of (Fmoc)$_2$KH$_7$-TAT in vitro once again. Remarkably, DOX/(Fmoc)$_2$KH$_7$-TAT/p53 micelleplexes mediated considerably higher expression level of p53 protein than either (Fmoc)$_2$KH$_7$-TAT/p53 DNA complexes or DOX-loaded (Fmoc)$_2$KH$_7$-TAT. This result was consistent with that in cytotoxicity. Besides, the relative p53 protein expression was also provided in Figure 11.10B. The relative p53 protein expression was assessed as the light intensity ratio of p53 to GAPDH from Western blot results in Figure 11.10A.

11.9 ANTITUMOR EFFECT IN VIVO

The antitumor effect in vivo of PEI/p53 complexes, DOX-loaded (Fmoc)$_2$KH$_7$-TAT, (Fmoc)$_2$KH$_7$-TAT/p53 DNA complexes, and DOX/(Fmoc)$_2$KH7-TAT/p53 DNA micelleplexes was tested, and phosphate-buffered saline (PBS) was used as

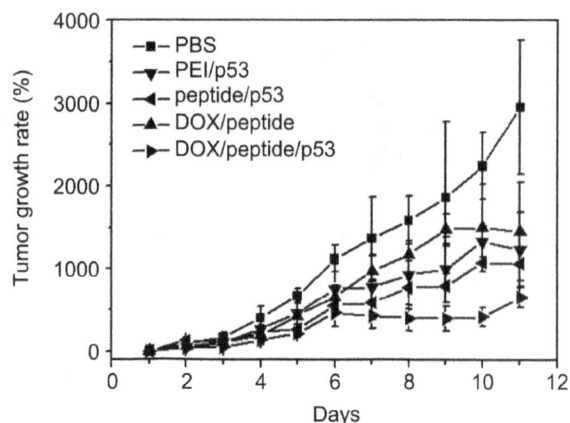

FIGURE 11.11 Antitumor effects after various treatments on H22 xenograft mice. Data are presented as mean±S.D. (n=6).

control. Figure 11.11 revealed that all testing groups showed certain antitumor effects compared to PBS control. In detail, (Fmoc)$_2$KH$_7$-TAT/p53 DNA complexes exhibited better tumor inhibition than 25 kDa PEI/p53 DNA complexes, indicating the superiority of (Fmoc)$_2$KH$_7$-TAT in gene delivery in vivo. Notably, DOX/(Fmoc)$_2$KH$_7$-TAT/p53 DNA micelleplexes performed remarkably higher efficiency in tumor inhibition than either (Fmoc)$_2$KH$_7$-TAT/p53 DNA or DOX-loaded (Fmoc)$_2$KH$_7$-TAT, attributed to the synergistic effect of codelivery of gene and drug. Similar results were also found from the tumor separated from mice on the 11th day after treatment.

The representative tumor imaging was shown in Figure 11.12. Besides, the body weight of the group that injected with DOX/(Fmoc)$_2$KH$_7$-TAT/p53 DNA micelleplexes was relatively stable, suggesting the decreased side effect of this treatment by the use of peptide as well as the satisfactory antitumor effect since the malignant growth of tumor increased the body weight to some extent.

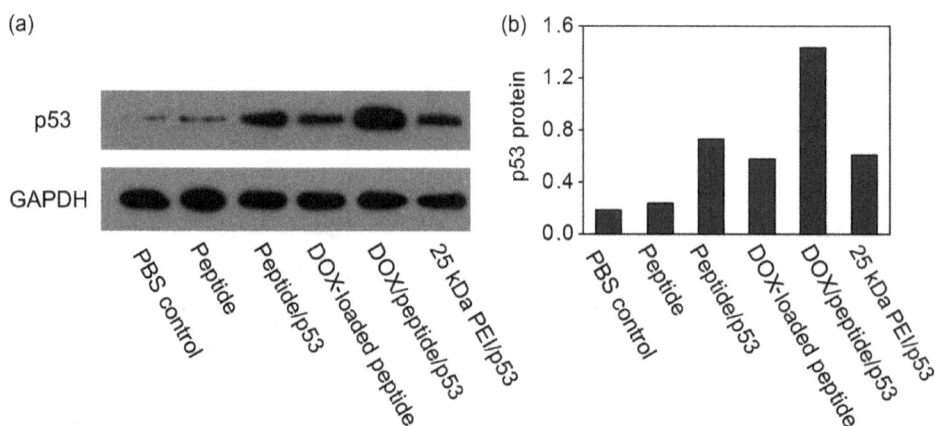

FIGURE 11.10 (A) p53 protein expression determined via Western blot analysis; (B) analysis of light intensities of p53 protein expression as the ratio of p53 to GAPDH from Western blot results, GAPDH was used as internal control.

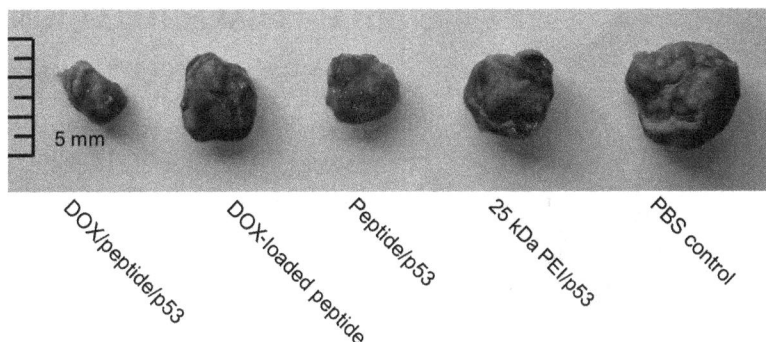

FIGURE 11.12 Imaging of the tumor on the 11th day after treatment of various formulations.

11.10 ROS-TRIGGERED SELF-ACCELERATING DRUG RELEASE NANOSYSTEM

Over the past decades, plenty of smart drug delivery systems (DDSs) have been proposed to overcome the unwanted side effects and maximize the therapeutic efficacy of tumor chemotherapy through achieving "on-demand" drug release at the tumor-targeted site under unique external or internal stimuli [25,26]. Besides the additional trigger of light and magnetic field, taking advantage of tumor-related intrinsic stimuli, including overexpressed proteases, low pH value, hyperthermia, and oversecreted glutathione, stimuli-responsive DDSs could further mediate tumor microenvironment-targeted therapy [27–32]. Recently, the relatively high level of intracellular reactive oxygen species (ROS) in the tumor environment [33–35] was also exploited as a biochemical basis for researchers to propose innovative strategies for tumor-targeted treatment [36–38]. For example, Xia et al. developed a ROS-sensitive cationic polymer poly(amino thioketal) (PATK) for targeted gene delivery. The containing TK cross-linkers could be cut away under an abundant ROS environment, leading to degradation of DNA/PATK polyplexes in PC3 cells, resulting in the release of DNA [39]. Although there are a variety of ROS cleavable bonds that have been utilized to endow the materials with ROS responsibility, very few of them exhibit sufficient sensitivity to control the drug release efficiently at a biological concentration of ROS, which is too low to trigger a reaction *in vivo* [40].

To cope with the problem mentioned above, improving the sensitivity of materials might open up appealing possibilities. A good case in point is that Sung et al. reasonably utilized H_2O_2 at a biologically relevant concentration, which could diffuse into a hollow microsphere carrier to generate CO_2 gas and disrupt the shell by reacting with a series of encapsulated molecules, resulting in the release of loaded drug [41]. However, this strategy involved complicated design and synthesis. Besides constructing the ultrasensitive ROS-responsive carriers, another prevalent approach critically relies on the generated ROS during the processes of photodynamic therapy to expand the utility of ROS-responsive reservoirs [42–45]. Nevertheless, precisely controlling the irradiation time and intensity for extra laser sources remains a hurdle. In addition, nonselectivity of ROS elevated in both normal and cancer cells under the irradiation scope could also cause lethal damage to healthy tissues.

Here, we proposed a ROS-triggered self-accelerating drug release nanosystem (defined as T/D@RSMSNs) based on a positive feedback strategy to overcome insufficient ROS generation of traditional DDSs through amplifying the intracellular ROS concentration, resulting in adequate drug release selectively in ROS abundant cancer cells *in vivo*. Firstly, as one of the most classic and primary nanocarriers, MSNs were selected as drug carriers, owing to their distinct advantages, including large pore volume for loading drugs, easy surface functionalization, and great biocompatibility [46–49]. Then, α-TOS, a vitamin E analog, which could rapidly generate ROS in cells after interacting with mitochondrial respiratory complex II and interfering with the electron transportation chain in mitochondria [50–52], and anticancer drug DOX were coencapsulated in the pores of MSNs. The gatekeeper β-CD was anchored on the surface of MSNs through the ROS-cleavable TK linker for stimuli-responsive drug release [53]. Furthermore, AD-PEG chain was introduced via host–guest interaction to enhance the stability of nanoparticles and prolong the circulation time *in vivo*. As shown in Scheme 11.3, after accumulation in tumor tissues through the enhanced permeability and retention (EPR) effect, T/D@RSMSN would be uptaken by tumor cells efficiently. At the very beginning, only limited pores were open because of the existent but insufficient intracellular ROS, resulting in simultaneous release of loaded DOX and α-TOS. Then, the released α-TOS interacted with the mitochondria in tumor cells to generate additional ROS. In other words, the intracellular ROS would be self-regenerated and amplified, which in turn facilitated the cutting of TK linkage to remove the gatekeeper β-CD and lead to more release of α-TOS as well as DOX in MSNs.

The detailed positive feedback effect with ROS-triggered self-accelerating drug release of this nanosystem was illustrated in Scheme 11.4. This novel nanosystem could not only achieve remarkable therapeutic effects but also provide a general and vital strategy to surmount the restrictions of existing ROS-responsive DDSs.

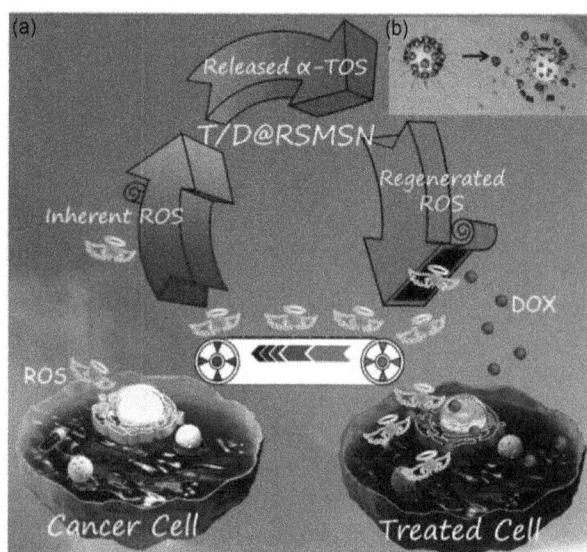

SCHEME 11.3 (A) Schematic representation of ROS-triggered self-accelerating drug release nanosystem for enhanced chemotherapy. After accumulation in tumor tissues through the EPR effect, T/D@RSMSN was uptaken by tumor cells efficiently. Initially, only limited pores were open by the stimulation of inherent ROS, resulting in the release of restricted DOX and α-TOS. Owing to the ROS-producing agent α-TOS, the intracellular ROS was self-regenerated, which could be regarded as a new trigger and in turn facilitate the procedure of cutting away the TK, leading to more α-TOS and the self-accelerating release of toxic DOX. (B) Schematic structure of T/D@RSMSN.

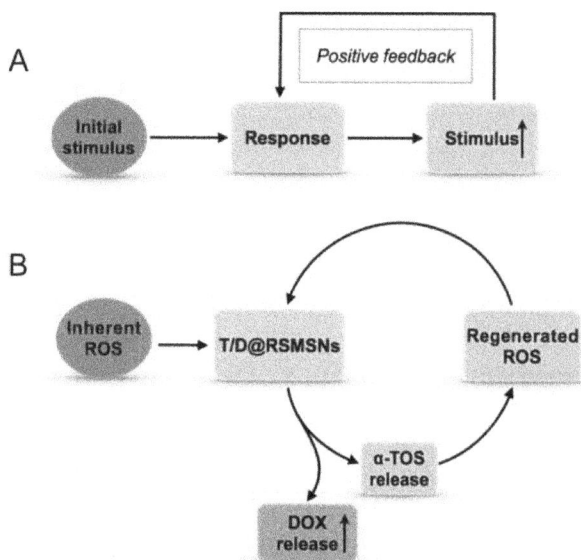

SCHEME 11.4 Schematic representation of (A) classical positive feedback loop (the response of initial stimulus could strengthen the stimulus) and (B) our ROS-triggered self-accelerating drug release nanosystem based on positive feedback strategy. After the stimulation of inherent ROS, the loaded α-TOS could be released from the pores of MSNs, which could interact with mitochondrion and produce regenerated ROS to reinforce this positive feedback loop. Along with positive circulation, the release of DOX could be accelerated.

11.11 CHARACTERIZATION OF T/D@RSMSNs

MSN was synthesized using the classic base-catalyzed cocondensation methods with several modifications according to the previous report [54]. As shown in scanning electron microcopy (Figure 11.13A) and transmission electron microscopy (TEM) (Figure 11.13B) images, well-distributed and uniform MSN with a mesoporous structure and a mean diameter of ~65 nm was prepared successfully. The hydrodynamic diameter of MSN measured by DLS [55] was 116.1 nm (PDI=0.029) and relatively larger than TEM size because of the hydrated layer surrounding the nanoparticles. The step-by-step functionalization on the surface of MSNs was monitored by zeta potential measurements (Figure 11.13C) and Fourier transforms infrared (FT-IR) spectra. As demonstrated in [55], the MSN was firstly reacted with 3-aminopropyltrimethoxysilane to obtain $MSN-NH_2$. After the surface modification of amino groups, the zeta potential of MSN-NH2 increased significantly from negative charge of MSN (−17.73 mV) to positive charge (23.36 mV). Then, the surfactant template cetrimonium chloride (CTAC) in the pores of MSN was removed completely, which was confirmed by the disappearance of the characteristic absorption peak of CeH-stretching vibrations at 2926 and 2854 cm^{-1} in FT-IR spectra. Subsequently, the ROS-cleavable TK linker [55] was introduced into the surface of $MSN-NH_2$ based on the amide condensation reaction, giving rise to the negatively charged MSN-TK nanoparticles (−14.13 mV). DOX and α-TOS were coloaded into the pores of MSNs after stirring the mixture solution of MSN-TK nanoparticles, DOX, and α-TOS vigorously. Finally, the resultant nanoparticle was modified with the gatekeeper β-CD through another amide condensation reaction and long-circulating AD-PEG5000 was further introduced via host–guest interaction to obtain T/D@MSN-TK-CD/AD-PEG5000 (defined as T/D@RSMSN). As shown in Figure 11.13D, in comparison with the distinct mesoporous structure of blank MSN, the mesostructure of T/D@RSMSN nanoparticles in TEM image was unclear and fuzzy after loading of the cargoes and surface modification. In addition, the hydrodynamic diameter of MSNs measured by DLS increased with continuous modification [55]. And the hydrodynamic diameter of T/D@RSMSN (Figure 11.13E) was 159.2 nm (PDI=0.110) with a monodisperse distribution, which was suitable for achieving the passive targeting to tumor tissue through the EPR effect. To further explore the stability of nanosystems, the hydrodynamic diameter changes of T/D@RSMSN in PBS and PBS with 10% serum after incubation for 24 h were measured. As indicated in [55], there was no significant aggregation during 24 h incubation, demonstrating good stability of T/D@RSMSN under the physiological condition. Furthermore, thermogravimetric analysis (TGA) was employed to detect the weight loss of the nanoparticles after the stepwise decoration. As illustrated in Figure 11.13F, when raising their temperature to 800°C, the weight loss of MSN-NH2, MSN-TK, and T/D@RSMSN was 11%, 20%,

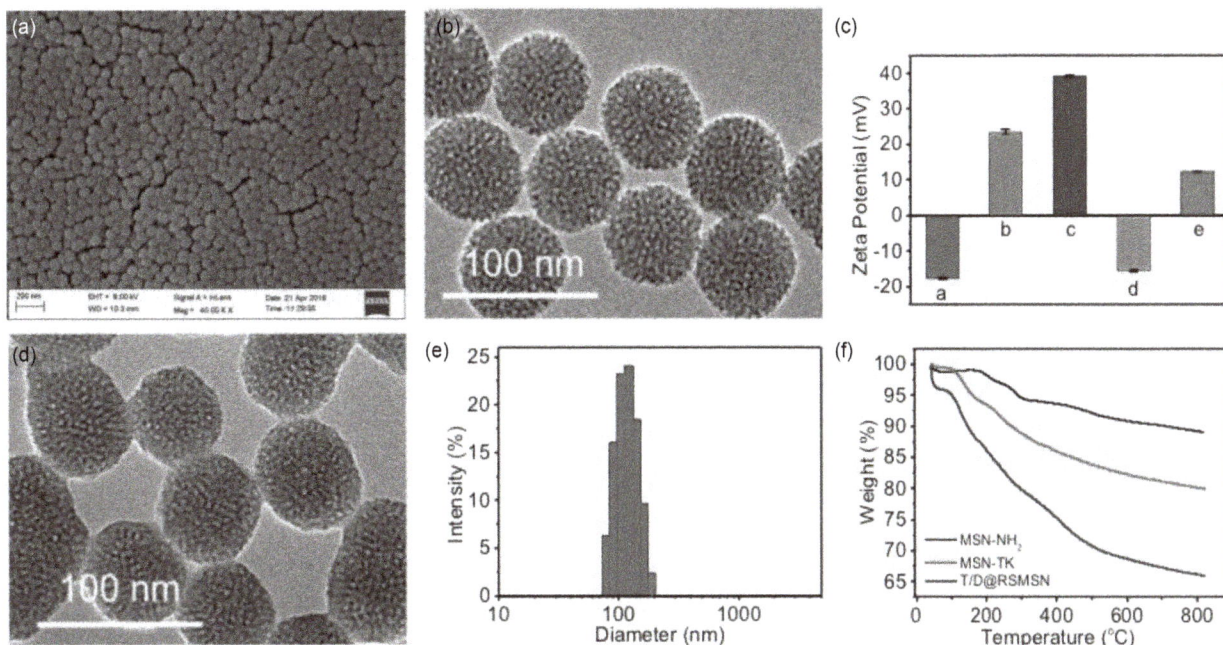

FIGURE 11.13 Characterization of T/D@RSMSN. (A) SEM image of blank MSN. (B) TEM image of blank MSN. (C) Zeta potentials of (a) CTAC@MSN, (b) CTAC@MSN-NH$_2$, (c) MSN-NH$_2$, (d) MSN-TK, (e) T/D@RSMSN. (D) TEM image of T/D@RSMSN. (E) Hydrodynamic diameter of T/D@RSMSN measured by DLS analysis. (F) TGA curves of MSN-NH$_2$, MSN-TK, and T/D@RSMSN.

and 35%, respectively, which further confirmed successful functionalization. Moreover, the mean number of CD molecules per nanoparticle was calculated to be 530 and the number of AD-PEG$_{5000}$ conjugated on T/D@RSMSN could be calculated to be 431, according to the calculation method in the previous report [56]. Besides, as measured by the RF-5301PC spectrofluorophotometer and high-performance liquid chromatography (HPLC), the loading efficiency (LE) of T/D@RSMSN was 5.1% for DOX and 2.5% for α-TOS. As to the control material D@MSNTK-CD/AD-PEG$_{5000}$ (D@RSMSN), which only encapsulated DOX, the LE was 6.7%.

11.12 EVALUATION OF ROS-RESPONSIVE DRUG RELEASE

In this study, the T/D@RSMSN was capped by b-CD/AD through the ROS-cleavable TK linkers. After stimulating ROS, the TK linkers would be broken, leading to release of the loaded drug from the pores of nanoparticles. To investigate the ROS responsibility of this nanosystem, H$_2$O$_2$ was used as a typically ROS stimulus in *in vitro* experiments [42,57], and the release profiles of the encapsulated DOX from T/D@RSMSN in PBS with different H$_2$O$_2$ concentrations were monitored by spectrofluorophotometer. As shown in Figure 11.14, without adding extra H$_2$O$_2$, T/D@RSMSN was gated by β-CD/AD effectively and less than 20% of the drug was leaked even after 72 h incubation, proving the efficiency of anchoring of nanovalves through the TK linkers. In contrast, 60% DOX was released after the incubation

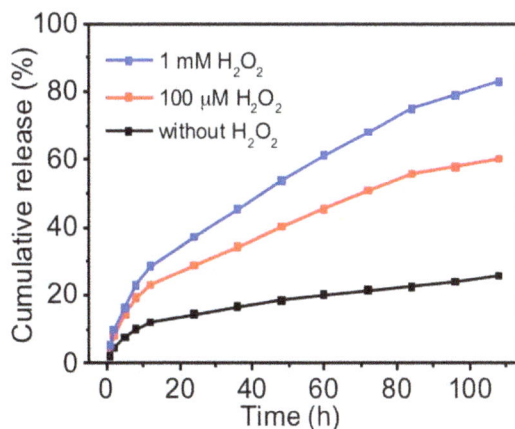

FIGURE 11.14 The drug release profiles of T/D@RSMSN incubated with different concentrations of H$_2$O$_2$.

with 100 μM H$_2$O$_2$ for 108 h. And when the nanoparticles were incubated with 1 mM H$_2$O$_2$, the release percentage of DOX reached 83% over 108 h. Apparently, the concentration of H$_2$O$_2$ had a remarkable and positive influence on the release rate and cumulative release amount of DOX, which was the basement of our self-accelerating drug release in cellular environments. Moreover, the release amount of α-TOS from T/D@RSMSN after incubating with different concentrations of H$_2$O$_2$ for 24 h was monitored by HPLC. As shown in [55], after incubating with different concentrations of H$_2$O$_2$ for 24 h, the accumulative release amount of α-TOS from T/D@RSMSN was enhanced markedly with the increased concentration of H_2O_2, confirming successful ROS-responsible release of α-TOS, which was the prerequisite for ROS generation. The results above demonstrated that the β-CD/AD could act as an effective nanovalve and open the pores after stimulating the ROS expectedly.

11.13 ANALYSIS OF THE ROS-REGENERATING ABILITY OF α-TOS *IN VITRO*

First of all, in order to better explore the feasibility of a positive feedback strategy to overcome the obstacles in ROS-responsive DDSs, the frequently used ROS abundant human breast cancer cells (MCF-7) were chosen. And the prevailing intracellular ROS-sensitive probe 2'-7'dichlorofluorescin diacetate (DCFH-DA) was utilized to confirm the ROS generation. Cell-permeable nonfluorescent DCFH-DA could be rapidly oxidized to dichlorofluorescein (DCF) with green fluorescence by the intracellular ROS [58]. As shown in Figure 11.15A_1 and B_1, the conspicuous

green fluorescence of DCF in MCF-7 cells clearly proved the inherent existence of intracellular ROS. Further, compared to the MCF-7 cells without staining (control), the fluorescence signal in MCF-7 cells incubated with DCFH-DA increased approximately 10 folds measured by the corresponding flow cytometry analysis (Figure 11.15C).

Afterward, since the ROS generation of α-TOS was the key point in this positive feedback strategy–based DDS, the intracellular ROS augmentation capability of α-TOS was also evaluated by the same ROS-sensitive probe through CLSM and flow cytometry analysis. As shown in Figure 11.15A and B, when the MCF-7 cells were incubated with α-TOS, the green fluorescent signal was noticeably stronger than that without α-TOS (blank), owing to the ROS-generating capability of α-TOS, which could restrain the bioactivity of mitochondrial respiratory complex II, resulting in electron transfer to produce ROS from oxygen. In addition, after prolonging the incubation time, the green fluorescence in MCF-7 cells incubated with a specific concentration of

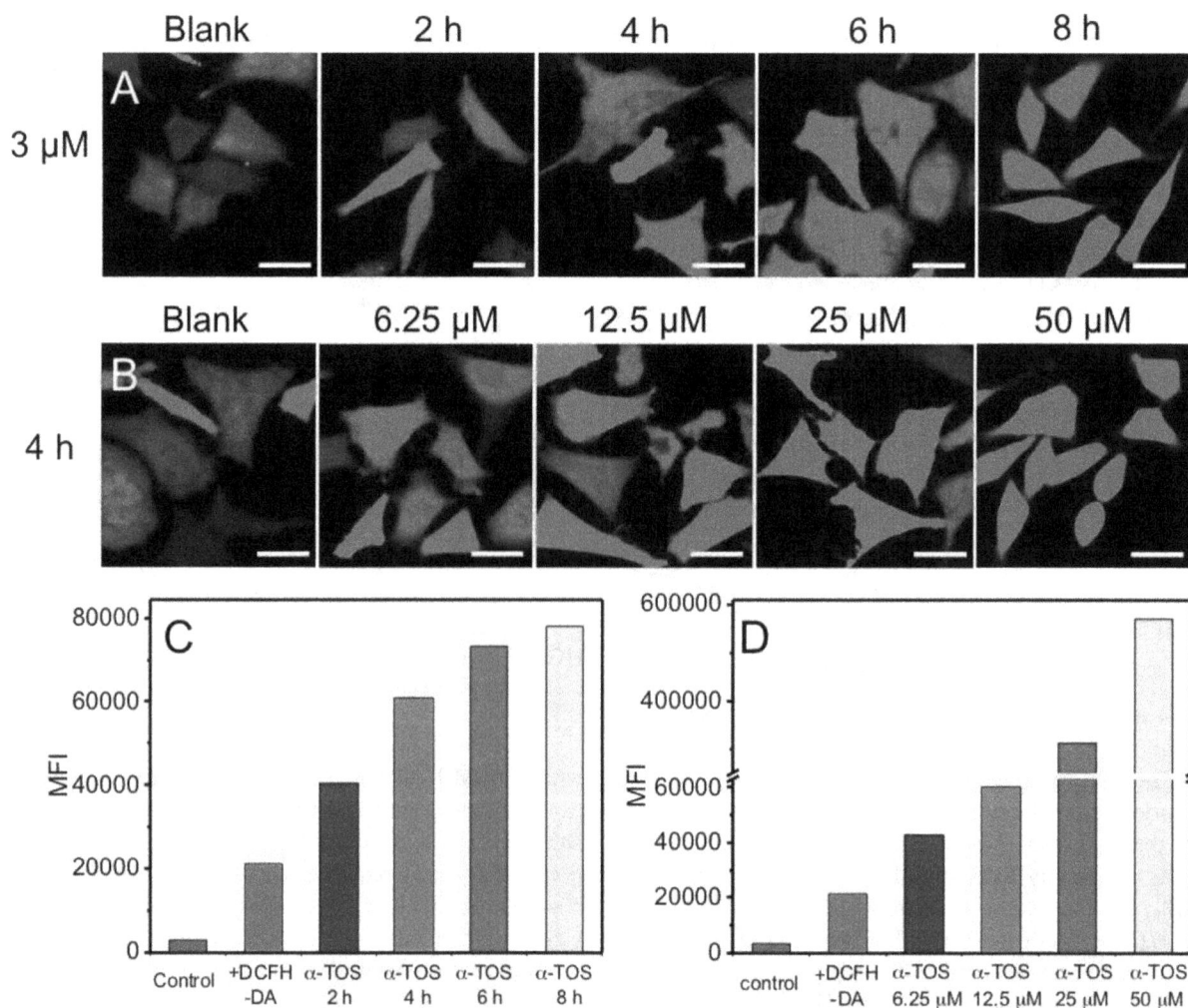

FIGURE 11.15 Evaluation of the ROS-regenerating ability of α-TOS *in vitro*. CLSM images of MCF-7 cells treated with (A_1–A_5) 3 μM α-TOS at different times and (B_1–B_5) different concentrations of α-TOS for 4 h. Green channel: DCF fluorescence illustrated intracellular ROS. Scale bar: 20 μm. Quantitative analysis of MCF-7 cells treated with (C) 3 μM α-TOS at different times and (D) different concentrations of α-TOS for 4 h by flow cytometry.

α-TOS (3 μM) became stronger (Figure 11.15A). Besides the coincubation time, the concentration of α-TOS is another factor to influence the levels of intracellular ROS. As demonstrated in Figure 11.15B, the fluorescent signal was enhanced markedly with the increased concentration of α-TOS. Thereafter, to quantitatively investigate the ROS-producing ability of α-TOS, the flow cytometry analysis was also conducted. As coincident with the CLSM results above, in the initial 2 h, the mean fluorescence intensity values in MCF-7 cells increased to 1.5-fold and up to 3.7-fold after prolonging the treated time to 8 h (Figure 11.15C). Additionally, there were 2.8-fold and 26-fold increases in the levels of ROS in MCF-7 cells treated with 12.5 and 50 μM for 4 h, respectively (Figure 11.15D). Moreover, the ROS-producing capability of α-TOS loaded in RSMSNs (T@RSMSNs) was also evaluated by CLSM. As shown in Ref. [55], with the increasing incubation time, the green fluorescence became stronger significantly, demonstrating the release of α-TOS from ROS-responsive nanocarriers. Further, no obvious change of green fluorescence indicated that possible interference of blank MSNs was excluded based on the same incubation conditions. These CLSM and flow cytometry analysis results above confirmed the intracellular ROS-producing ability of α-TOS and also revealed the possibility of loading α-TOS for positive feedback strategy–based DDS.

11.14 INTRACELLULAR ROS-TRIGGERED AMPLIFYING ROS SIGNALS AND SELF-ACCELERATING DRUG RELEASE

Encouraged by the satisfying ROS-generating capability of α-TOS, cellular coincubation experiments were further performed to estimate the intracellular ROS-triggered ROS signal amplification and self-accelerating drug release efficiency of T/D@RSMSN in vitro. To highlight the important positive feedback effect induced by the ROS-producing agent, a single DOX-loaded nanoparticle with the same modification, which was designed like a traditional ROS-responsible DDS, was employed as a control group (defined as D@RSMSN). As shown in Figure 11.16B₁–B₄, green fluorescence was found in MCF-7 treated with D@RSMSN, due to inherent ROS in MCF-7 cells. Although the green fluorescence was continuously existent, no obvious change was observed, even with increasing the incubation time from 4 to 36 h, demonstrating that without α-TOS, the intrinsic intracellular ROS was barely growing. In addition, the red fluorescence of DOX, which was released from the pores of D@RSMSN after being uptaken, was clearly detected but not enhanced significantly after prolonging the incubation time (Figure 11.16C₁–C₄). It was understandable that as a result of limited intrinsic ROS, only a part of TK linkers of D@RSMSN could be cut away, leading to partial release of DOX within the time allotted.

Compared to the unsatisfying drug release situation of the control group, the T/D@RSMSN nanoparticles

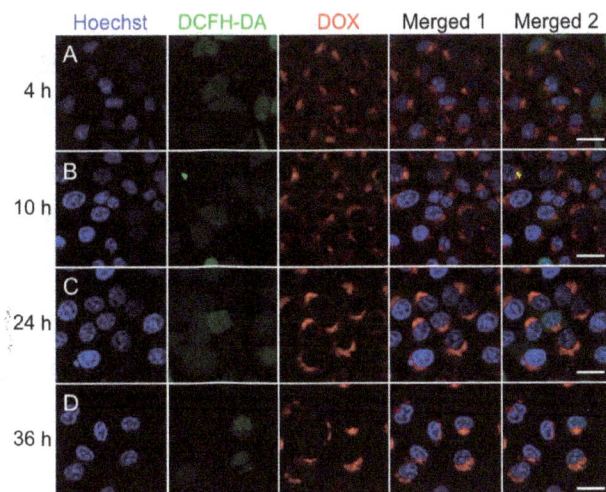

FIGURE 11.16 CLSM images of MCF-7 cells treated with control group D@RSMSN (C_DOX: 2.5 μg/mL) at different times, respectively. Blue channel: Hoechst 33342 stained nucleus. Red channel: DOX. Green channel: DCF fluorescence illustrated intracellular ROS. Scale bar: 20 μm.

have shown high efficiency of ROS-triggered ROS signal amplification and self-accelerating drug release in vitro. As illustrated in Figure 11.17B₁–B₄, the green fluorescence was stronger than that in MCF-7 cells incubated with D@RSMSN (Figure 11.17B₁–B₄) at each time point, indicating that besides the inherent intracellular ROS, the α-TOS also took effect on producing ROS. And with increasing incubation time, the green fluorescence was markedly increased, confirming that with the initial intracellular ROS triggering, the encapsulated α-TOS was released from the pores of T/D@RSMSN after the TK linkers were cleaved, resulting in ROS regeneration and replenishment. What's more, augmenting levels of intracellular ROS would in turn assist in cutting away more TK linkers and produce the positive feedback effect. As expected, during this ROS-triggered ROS amplification process, the coloaded drug DOX showed a self-accelerating release situation, which was proved by significantly increasing the red fluorescence signal with the extension of incubation time (Figure 11.17C₁–C₄). Moreover, compared to the relatively weak red fluorescence in MCF-7 cells treated with D@RSMSN mainly located in the cytoplasm after incubating for 36 h, MCF-7 cells treated with T/D@RSMSN exhibited strong red fluorescence in the cytoplasm at 4 h and 10 h, stronger red fluorescence in cytoplasm, and weak fluorescence in the nucleoplasm at 24 h, and after 36 h incubation, the red fluorescence of the released DOX spread throughout the whole MCF-7 cells (Figure 11.17E). Further, quantitative fluorescence intensity analysis by ImageJ software of red fluorescence (DOX) in MCF-7 cells showed that the released DOX amplified by α-TOS after incubation for 36 h was 1.9-fold higher than the initial-released DOX. These CLSM results demonstrated that the high efficiency of drug release in T/D@RSMSN based on ROS-triggered positive feedback effect

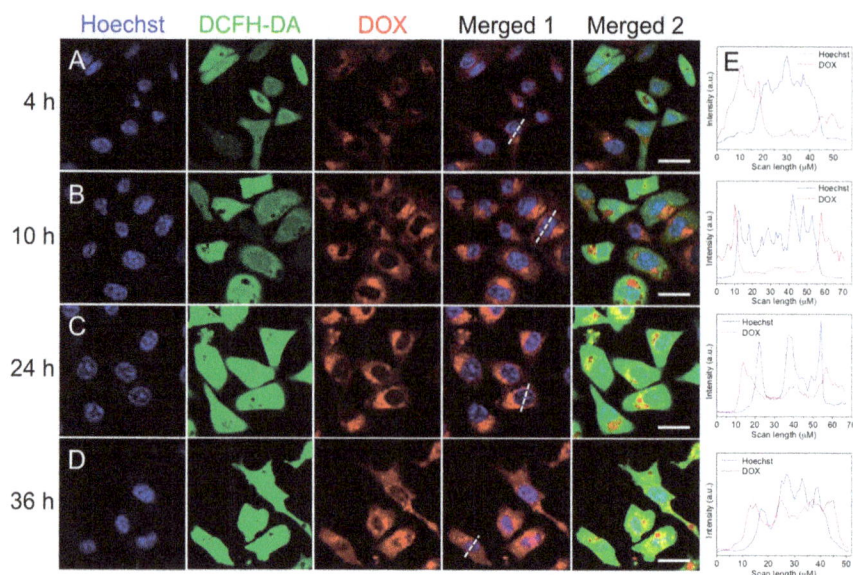

FIGURE 11.17 (AeD) CLSM images of MCF-7 cells treated with T/D@RSMSN (C_{DOX}: 2.5 μg/mL) at different times, respectively. Blue channel: Hoechst 33342 stained nucleus. Red channel: DOX. Green channel: DCF fluorescence illustrated intracellular ROS. Scale bar: 20 μm. (E) Fluorescence signals based on the white line.

could improve the discontentefficacy of omnipresent ROS-responsible DDS.

To further evaluate the ROS microenvironment selective ability of T/D@RSMSN, human embryonic kidney (293T) normal cells with relatively negligible ROS were utilized as a control group. As shown in Figure 11.18, compared to the obvious fluorescence in MCF-7 cells incubated with T/D@RSMSN or D@RSMSN, both negligible green fluorescence and red fluorescence were detected in 293T cells incubated with T/D@RSMSN or D@RSMSN, illustrating that without abundant intracellular ROS, the pores were still capped and the loaded α-TOS and DOX could avoid being prematurely released from the nanoparticles, which was coincident with the cargo release profiles above (Figure 11.3). These results further confirmed that owing to the ROS-cleavable TK linkers, the T/D@RSMSN could target the tumor cells with high levels of ROS selectively, without affecting the healthy cells.

11.15 EVALUATION OF CYTOTOXICITY *IN VITRO* OF MSN

To testify the advantages of the ROS-triggered self-accelerating drug release nanosystem, the cell viability of MCF-7 cells and 293T cells treated with T/D@RSMSN and D@RSMSN was investigated. Firstly, the cytotoxicity of blank MSNs was evaluated. The cell viability of blank MSN in two cells was higher than 90%, even up to 100 μg/mL (Figure 11.19), exhibiting low toxicity and suitability for drug delivery. Then, the cell viability of T/D@RSMSN or D@RSMSN in 293T cells had no obvious difference and was higher than 80% (Figure 11.19A$_1$ and B$_1$), due to the

nanoparticles being capped tightly without drug leakage under the really low concentration of ROS in normal cells. In comparison, the obvious cell viability was both observed in the MCF-7 cells incubated with T/D@RSMSN and D@RSMSN (Figure 11.19A$_1$). Compared to the cell viability in 293T cells, the toxicity in MCF-7 cells was noticeable because the gatekeepers of nanoparticles could be removed after being uptaken by tumor cells with relatively high levels of ROS, leading to diffusion of DOX. Also, there was a significant difference in cell toxicity between MCF-7 cells incubated with T/D@RSMSN and D@RSMSN. The cell viability of D@RSMSN in MCF-7 cells was 69%, due to the limited DOX release caused by nonsufficient ROS during the incubation time. In comparison with MCF-7 cells treated with D@RSMSN, the cell viability of T/D@RSMSN in MCF-7 cells was much lower (29%) because after the inherent ROS triggering the intracellular ROS was regenerated by the released part of α-TOS, utilized as new triggers to release much more DOX during the incubation period, which was well matched with above CLSM results (Figure 11.19A$_2$ and B$_2$). IC$_{50}$ value (half inhibitory concentration) of T/D@RSMSN was 0.84 mg/L (DOX concentration), which was much lower than D@RSMSN (>2.5 mg/L) for MCF-7 cells, indicating advantages of positive feedback strategy of T/D@RSMSN. And the IC$_{50}$ of free DOX was calculated to be 0.71 mg/L for MCF-7 cells and 0.76 mg/L for 293T cells. Furthermore, the cell viability of 293T cells or MCF-7 cells incubated with free α-TOS (Figure 11.19A$_4$ and B$_4$) was supplied for reference. Therefore, this designed nanosystem could deliver the drug targeting to the ROS abundant tumor cells and produce the cell toxicity selectively, particularly achieving enhanced chemotherapy compared to the traditional ROS-responsive nanocarriers.

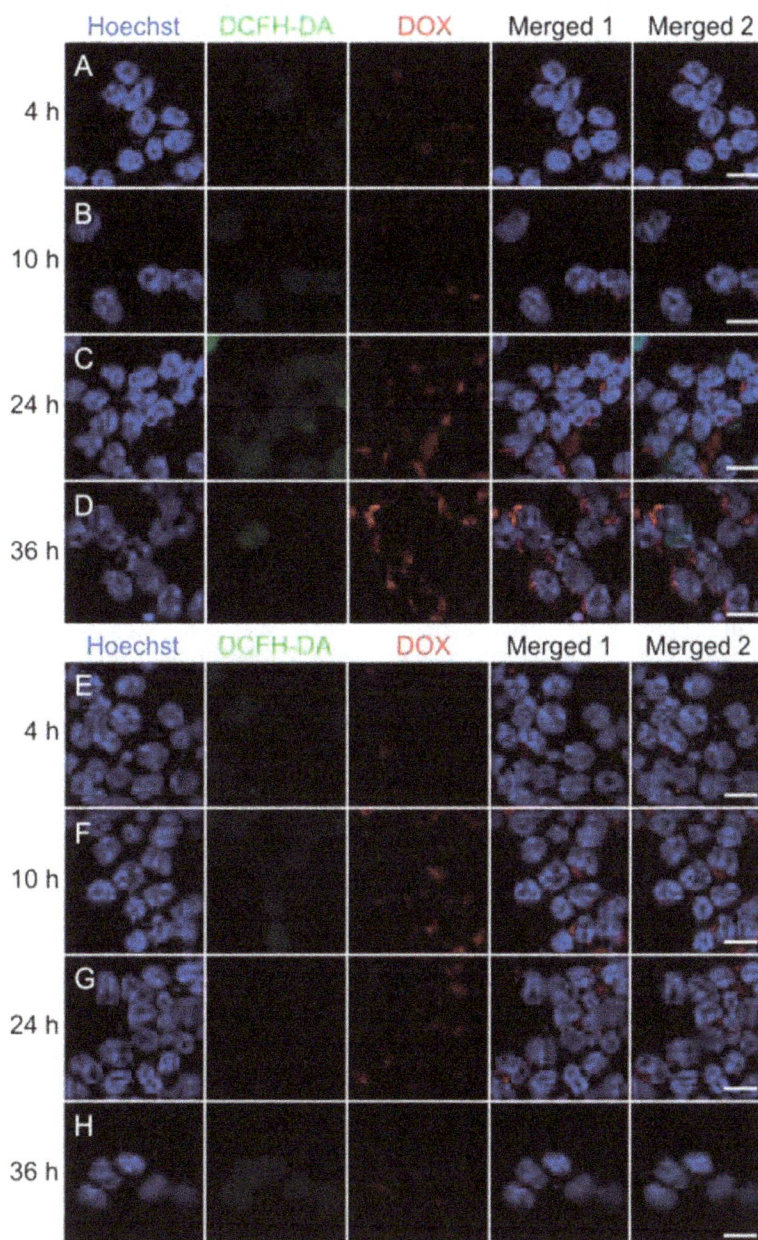

FIGURE 11.18 CLSM images of 293T normal cells treated with T/D@RSMSN (AeD) and D@RSMSN (EeH) (C_{DOX}: 2.5 µg/mL) at different times, respectively. Blue channel: Hoechst 33342 stained nucleus. Red channel: DOX. Green channel: DCF fluorescence illustrated intracellular ROS. Scale bar: 20 µm.

11.16 ANTITUMOR EXPERIMENTS *IN VIVO* VIA INTRAVENOUS INJECTION

Encouraged by the good performance in *in vitro* study, the feasibility of T/D@RSMSN in the antitumor study *in vivo* was further evaluated through intravenous injections. The MCF-7 tumor-bearing nude mice were divided into four groups randomly (n>5) and treated with PBS, free DOX, D@RSMSN, and T/D@RSMSN, respectively. No obvious body weight variation was found in the T/D@RSMSN group, confirming its good biocompatibility and nontoxicity (Figure 11.20). The continuous tumor changes of MCF-7 tumor-bearing mice in each group during the

14 days of treatment were exhibited through the digital photos (Figure 11.20A). The tumor growth in the group injected with T/D@RSMSN was noticeably inhibited, in contrast with the other three groups. As displayed in Figure 11.20C, the tumor volume in the PBS group increased rapidly and grew to 10 folds of the initial volume after 14 days of treatment. Moreover, the tumor treated with D@RSMSN could be inhibited to some extent, owing to the partial release of DOX triggered by the intracellular ROS. Compared to the free DOX, the main material T/D@RSMSN could inhibit the growth of tumors significantly, which illustrated the superiority of T/D@RSMSN in maximizing the antitumor efficiency, caused by positive

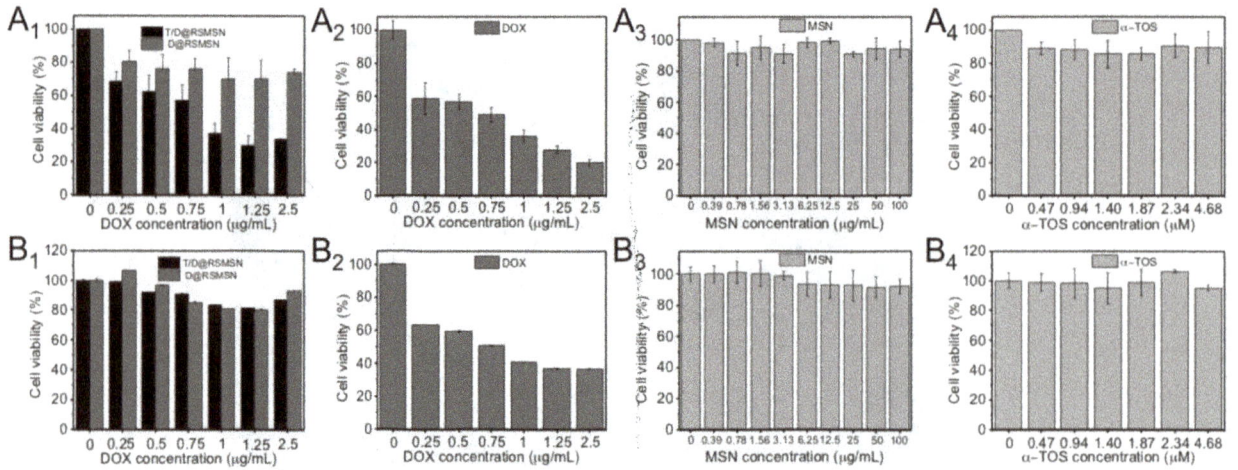

FIGURE 11.19 Cell viability of MCF-7 cells (A_1–A_4) and 293T cells (B_1–B_4) after being incubated with T/D@RSMSN and D@RSMSN (A_1, B_1), free DOX (A_2, B_2), blank MSN (A_3, B_3) and free α-TOS (A_4, B_4) for 48 h.

feedback strategy. When all the mice were sacrificed after 14 days of treatment, the tumors in each group were collected; average tumor weights (Figure 11.20D) and the representative tumor photos (Figure 11.20E) were provided to further confirm the therapeutic efficacy of T/D@RSMSN. Moreover, the therapeutic mechanism of T/D@RSMSN was studied by the terminal deoxynucleotidyl transferase dUTP nick-end labeling (TUNEL) assay (Figure 11.20F). An obvious large area of green fluorescence was displayed in the T/D@RSMSN group, in comparison with none or

a weak green fluorescent signal in other control groups, which was attributed to the cytotoxicity of the released DOX, leading to more apoptotic cells. In addition, hematoxylin and eosin (H&E) staining of tumor tissues was employed to evaluate the morphology and confirm the therapeutic efficiency of T/D@RSMSN. As exhibited in Figure 11.20G, compared to abundant and compact tumor cells in PBS group and partially destroyed tumor cells in D@RSMSN or DOX group, the tumor cells in the T/D@RSMSN group displayed a more serious damage, and many

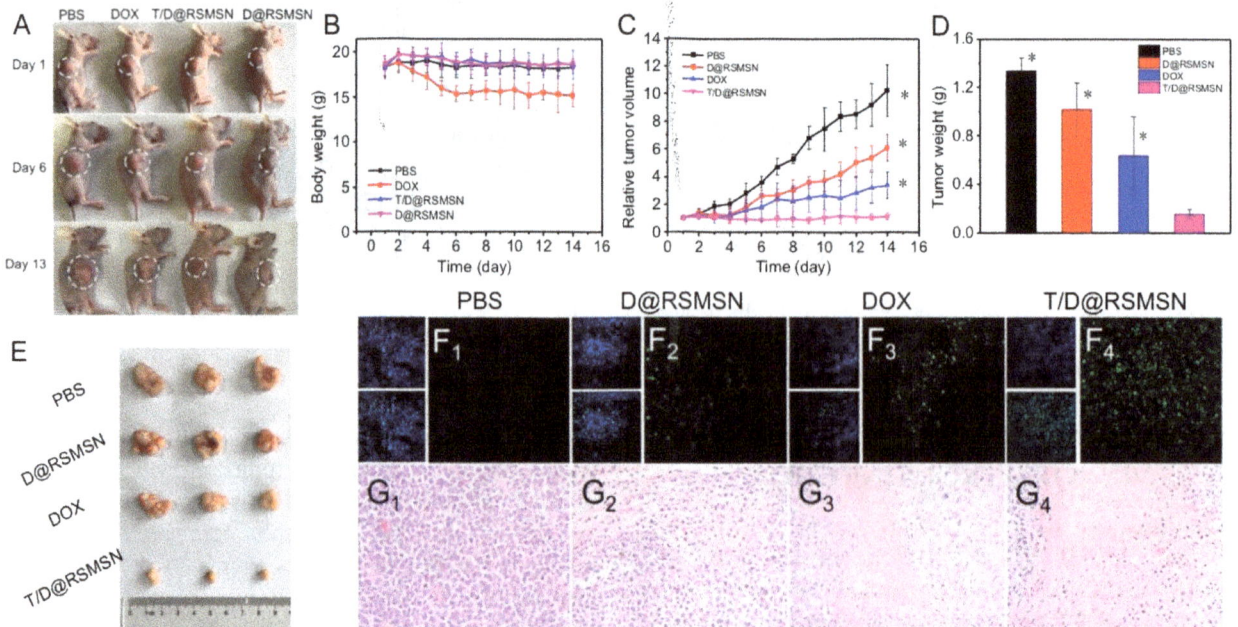

FIGURE 11.20 Antitumor experiments *in vivo* via intravenous injection. (A) Digital photos of MCF-7 tumor-bearing mice treated with PBS, free DOX, D@RSMSN, and T/D@RSMSN during the 14-day evaluation period. (B) The body weight and (C) relative tumor volume of mice after different treatments. (D) Average tumor weight on the 14th day for each group. *$p < 0.05$ was analyzed by a Student's t-test when the group compared with T/D@RSMSN, respectively. (E) Photographs of tumor tissues on the 14th day after different treatments. (F) TUNEL immunofluorescence staining and (G) H&E staining images of tumor tissues, which were sacrificed on the 14th day. H&E staining: 200x magnification.

tumor cells were dead. These H&E staining and TUNEL staining assay results were coincident with the *in vivo* data of the antitumor study above. Additionally, the low systemic toxicity of T/D@RSMSN was proved by no obvious pathological abnormalities in the heart, liver, spleen, lungs, and kidneys [55]. Furthermore, the normal myocardial five-enzyme parameters of the mice after treatment with T/D@RSMSN confirmed that T/D@RSMSN had no obvious cardiotoxicity [55]. These results above indicated that T/D@RSMSN displayed no systemic side effects and showed great potential in biomedical applications.

11.17 PLATINUM-BASED COMBINATION CHEMOTHERAPEUTIC DRUGS

Multiple randomized controlled trials during the last two decades have established combination chemotherapy (cisplatin-based) to be the standard of care as first-line treatment in recurrent or metastatic non–small-cell lung cancer (NSCLC) [59,60]. Despite these advances, response rate to first-line platinum-based therapy is approximately 30%, with median survival between 24 and 31 months [61]. Those who develop resistance to cisplatin receive pemetrexed, docetaxel, or erlotinib in the second-line setting, but response rates are only 7%–10%. Improving our ability to manage the disease by optimizing the use of existing drugs and/or developing new agents is essential in this endeavor [62]. To this end, individualizing treatments by identifying patients who will or will not respond to specific agents will potentially increase the overall effectiveness of these drugs and limit the incidence and severity of toxicities that impair the functional status of patients and their ability to tolerate further therapies.

Standard treatment for advanced NSCLC includes the use of a platinum-based chemotherapy regimen. However, response rates are highly variable. Newer agents, such as pemetrexed, have shown significant activity as second-line therapy and are currently being evaluated in the front-line setting. It has been utilized as a genomic strategy [62] to develop signatures predictive of chemotherapeutic response to both cisplatin and pemetrexed to provide a rational approach to effective individualized medicine. Using *in vitro* drug sensitivity data, coupled with microarray data, it has developed gene expression signatures predicting sensitivity to cisplatin and pemetrexed. Signatures were validated with response data from 32 independent ovarian and lung cancer cell lines as well as 59 samples from patients previously treated with cisplatin.

Since the advent of chemotherapy to treat cancer, there have been numerous advances in the development, selection, and application of these agents, sometimes with remarkable successes. In several instances, particularly in early-stage disease, combination chemotherapy in the adjuvant setting has been found to be curative. However, most patients with clinically or pathologically advanced solid tumors will eventually relapse and die as a result of their disease.

For example, in advanced NSCLC, third-generation regimens consisting of a platinum analog in combination with a second agent increases the overall response and survival when compared with older regimens [59,63,64]. However, the overall response is still only 20%–30%, [64] suggesting that a majority of the patients do not respond to a platinum analog. Subsequently, those patients who experience treatment failure with platinum-based therapy typically receive pemetrexed, docetaxel, or targeted therapies as second-line treatment, with response rates of approximately 7%–10% [65–67].

New technologies offer the potential to measure genome-wide gene activity that may serve as a powerful adjunct to the currently available clinical and biochemical markers. Such complementary approaches may better characterize the complexity of the disease and identify discrete clinical and biologically relevant phenotypes [68–70]. The ability to find structure in the data, in the form of patterns of gene expression, provides snapshots of gene activity in a cell or tissue sample that can then be used to describe a phenotype [71,72]. This transforms biology from an observational molecular science to a data-intensive quantitative genomic science [73–75]. The dimension and complexity of such data provide an opportunity to uncover patterns and trends that can distinguish subtle phenotypes in ways that traditional methods cannot.

Recently, we have described the use of gene expression profiling to develop signatures of drug sensitivity to individual chemotherapeutic drugs [76]. These signatures also reliably predicted *in vitro* and *in vivo* responses to individual cytotoxic drugs. Thus, the development of gene expression profiles that can predict the response to commonly used cytotoxic agents may provide a unique opportunity to better utilize drugs previously shown to be effective in first- or second-line therapy. Here, we describe a novel approach to rationalized drug therapy in NSCLC by developing predictors of cisplatin (a first-line agent) and pemetrexed (a second-line agent) sensitivity and demonstrating the clinical value of identifying the most appropriate drug on the basis of sensitivity profile for the treatment regimen of each individual patient, thus moving beyond empirical therapeutic choices that are now in current practice. Such an approach is likely to maximize the response to chemotherapeutic drugs and may change the current paradigm of cancer therapy, particularly in NSCLC, and possibly in other advanced cancers.

11.17.1 CELL AND RNA PREPARATION

Full details of the methods used for RNA extraction and the development of gene expression data from lung and ovarian tumors have been described previously [70,76].

Briefly, total RNA was extracted using the QIAshredder and Qiagen RNeasy Mini kit (Qiagen, Hilden, Germany), and the quality of RNA was checked by an Agilent 2100 Bioanalyzer (Agilent Technologies, Palo Alto, CA). The targets for Affymetrix DNA microarray analysis were prepared according to the manufacturer's instructions. Biotin-labeled cRNA, produced by *in vitro* transcription, was fragmented and hybridized to the Affymetrix U133A GeneChip arrays at 45°C for 16h and then washed and stained using the GeneChip Fluidics (Affymetrix). The arrays were scanned by a GeneArray Scanner (Affymetrix) and patterns of hybridization were detected as the light emitted from the fluorescent reporter groups incorporated into the target and hybridized to oligonucleotide probes. All analyses [62] were performed in a minimal information about a microarray experiment-compliant fashion, as defined in the guidelines established by microarray gene expression data.

11.17.2 CLASSIFICATION OF PLATINUM RESPONSE IN OVARIAN TUMORS

Using Affymetrix U133A GeneChips, it has measured [62] gene expression in 59 patients with advanced (International Federation of Gynecology and Obstetrics stage III/IV) serous epithelial ovarian carcinomas who received cisplatin therapy (Gene Expression Omnibus [GEO] accession number: GSE3149). All ovarian cancer specimens were obtained at initial cytoreductive surgery from patients and collected under the respective (Duke University Medical Center, Durham, NC, and H. Lee Moffitt Cancer Center, Tampa, FL) institutional review board protocols involving written informed consent.

Response to therapy was evaluated using standard criteria for patients with measurable disease, based on WHO guidelines [77]. CA-125 was used to classify responses only in the absence of a measurable lesion and based on established guidelines [78]. A complete response (CR) was defined as complete disappearance of all measurable and assessable diseases or, in the absence of measurable lesions, a normalization of the CA-125 level after salvage therapy. A partial response (PR) was considered a 50% or greater reduction in the product obtained from the measurement of each bidimensional lesion for at least 4 weeks or a drop in the CA-125 by at least 50% for at least 4 weeks. Progressive disease was defined as a 50% or greater increase in the product from any lesion documented within 8 weeks of initiation of therapy, the appearance of any new lesion within 8 weeks of initiation of therapy, or doubling of CA-125 from baseline. For the purposes of our analysis, a clinically beneficial response (i.e., "responder") included CR or PR. A patient who did not demonstrate a CR or PR was considered a "nonresponder."

11.17.3 CROSS-PLATFORM AFFYMETRIX GENECHIP COMPARISON

To map the probe sets across various generations of Affymetrix GeneChip arrays, we utilized Chip Comparer (http://tenero.duhs.duke.edu/genearray/perl/chip/chipcomparer.pl) as described previously [70,76].

11.17.4 CELL PROLIFERATION AND DRUG SENSITIVITY ASSAYS

The optimal cell number and linear range of drug concentration were determined [62] for each cell line and drug as described previously [70,76]. For drug sensitivity assay, cells were plated in non–drug-containing media in 96-well plates. After incubation for 24 h at 37°C, drugs were added to each well at a specific concentration. Cells were grown in the presence of drugs for an additional 96 h, and sensitivity to cisplatin, docetaxel, paclitaxel, and pemetrexed in the cell lines was determined by quantifying the percent reduction in growth (dimethyl sulfoxide controls) at 96 h using a standard MTT colorimetric assay (CellTiter 96 AQueous One 23 Solution Cell Proliferation Assay Kit; Promega, Madison, WI) [79,80].

11.18 DEVELOPING A GENE EXPRESSION–BASED PREDICTOR OF CISPLATIN SENSITIVITY

The experimental strategy for analysis employed in that study [62] is similar to that used for the development of oncogenic pathway and chemotherapy sensitivity signatures as described previously [70,76]. Samples representing extreme cases are used to train the expression data to develop a genomic signature that can predict drug sensitivity. A predictor of cisplatin sensitivity was developed by analyzing cell lines described by Györffy et al [81].

Using Bayesian binary regression analysis, genes highly correlated with drug sensitivity were identified and used to develop a model that could differentiate between cisplatin sensitivity and resistance. The developed model consisting of 45 genes based on cisplatin sensitivity (Figure 11.21A) was validated in a leave-one-out cross-validation. The cisplatin sensitivity predictor includes DNA repair genes such as *ERCC1* and *ERCC4*, among others, that had altered expression in the list of cisplatin sensitivity predictor genes. Interestingly, one previously described mechanism of resistance to cisplatin therapy results from the increased capacity of cancer cells to repair the DNA damage incurred, by activation of DNA repair genes [82,83].

11.18.1 DEVELOPING A GENE EXPRESSION–BASED PREDICTOR OF PEMETREXED SENSITIVITY

In NSCLC, where platinum-based therapy is the standard of care, response rates are only 30%. One approach to identifying potential drugs effective in cisplatin-resistant patients is to examine the NCI-60 dataset for agents whose IC_{50} profile showed an inverse relationship with cisplatin, focusing on those known to be effective in NSCLC. Of these drugs, an inverse correlation with cisplatin sensitivity was identified with docetaxel, abraxane, and pemetrexed. The strongest inverse correlation was found between cisplatin

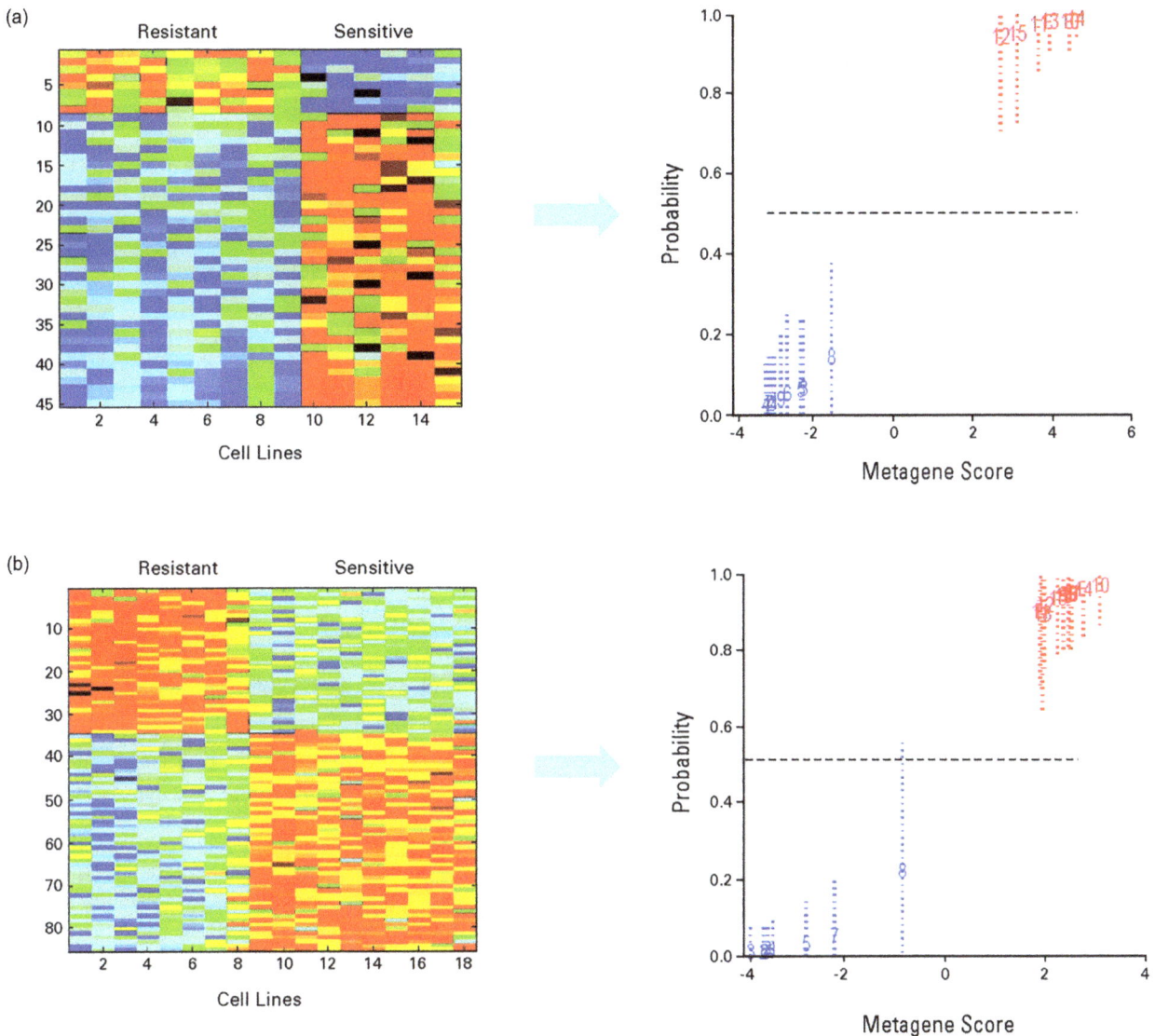

FIGURE 11.21 (A) Cisplatin and (B) pemetrexed sensitivity predictor. Left panels show the expression plot for genes discriminating the cisplatin or pemetrexed-sensitive and -resistant cell lines. Each column represents individual cell lines and each row represents individual genes in the predictors. Right panels show the accuracy in a leave-one-out cross-validation. Blue, low probability of drug sensitivity; red, high probability of drug sensitivity.

and pemetrexed sensitivity ($P < 0.001$; Pearson r value, 0.1; $\alpha = 0.05$).

Using methods previously described [76], a predictor of pemetrexed sensitivity was developed by identifying NCI-60 cell lines that were most resistant or sensitive to pemetrexed. Using Bayesian binary regression analysis, genes whose expression was most highly correlated with drug sensitivity were used to develop a predictive model that could differentiate between pemetrexed sensitivity and resistance. The developed model consisting of 85 genes based on pemetrexed sensitivity (Figure 11.21B) was validated in a leave-one-out cross-validation. Interestingly, multiple genes involved in nucleotide and cellular metabolism constituted the pemetrexed sensitivity predictor and are biologically consistent with the known mechanism of pemetrexed sensitivity, which involves interference with

cell cycle progression by reducing the pool of substrates necessary for DNA replication [84].

11.19 *IN VITRO* VALIDATION OF THE CISPLATIN AND PEMETREXED PREDICTOR

In addition to initial leave-one-out cross-validation, the true value of a predictor lies in its ability to predict sensitivity in independent *in vitro* and *in vivo* settings. In the present study [62], the predictor of cisplatin sensitivity was independently validated in a panel of 32 (lung and ovarian cancer) cell lines, using cell proliferation assays and concurrent gene expression data. As shown in Figure 11.22A, the correlation between the predicted probability of sensitivity to cisplatin (in both lung and ovarian cell lines) and

(a)

(b)

(a)

(b)

FIGURE 11.23 *In vivo* validation of cisplatin sensitivity predictor. Part (A) represents the predicted probability of cisplatin sensitivity in patients classified as responders and nonresponders. Part (B) is a single-variable scatter plot of a significance test of the predicted probabilities of sensitivity to cisplatin in the same samples (Mann–Whitney U test $P < 0.01$).

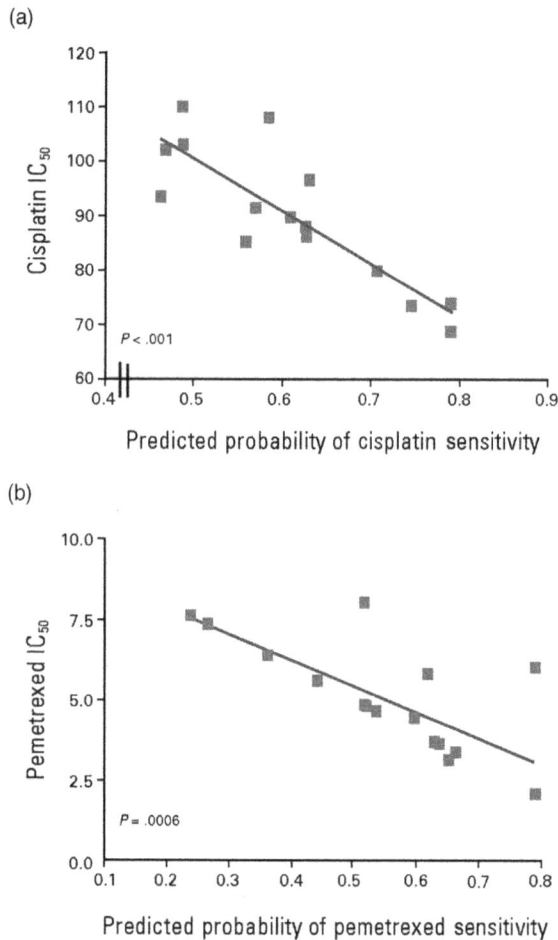

FIGURE 11.22 *In vitro* validation of the cisplatin and pemetrexed predictors. (A) Fifty percent inhibitory concentration (IC_{50}) of cisplatin plotted against predicted sensitivity to cisplatin in cell lines predicts sensitivity to the drug ($P < 0.001$ [top, ovarian] and $P = 0.03$ [bottom, lung]). (B) IC_{50} of pemetrexed plotted against the predicted probability to pemetrexed predicts sensitivity to pemetrexed in NSCLC lines ($P = 0.0006$).

the respective IC_{50} for cisplatin confirmed the capacity of the cisplatin predictor to accurately predict sensitivity to the drug in cancer cell lines.

Similar to the independent validation of the cisplatin sensitivity predictor, the pemetrexed predictor was validated using gene expression data from an independent cohort of 17 NSCLC cell lines with respective *in vitro* drug sensitivity assays. As shown in Figure 11.22B, the correlation between the predicted probability of sensitivity to pemetrexed in the 17 NSCLC cell lines and the respective IC_{50} for pemetrexed validated the ability of the pemetrexed predictor to predict sensitivity to the drug in an independent cohort of cancer cell lines.

11.19.1 *In Vivo* Validation of the Cisplatin Sensitivity Predictor

Although the ability of the cisplatin signature to predict the sensitivity in independent samples validates the

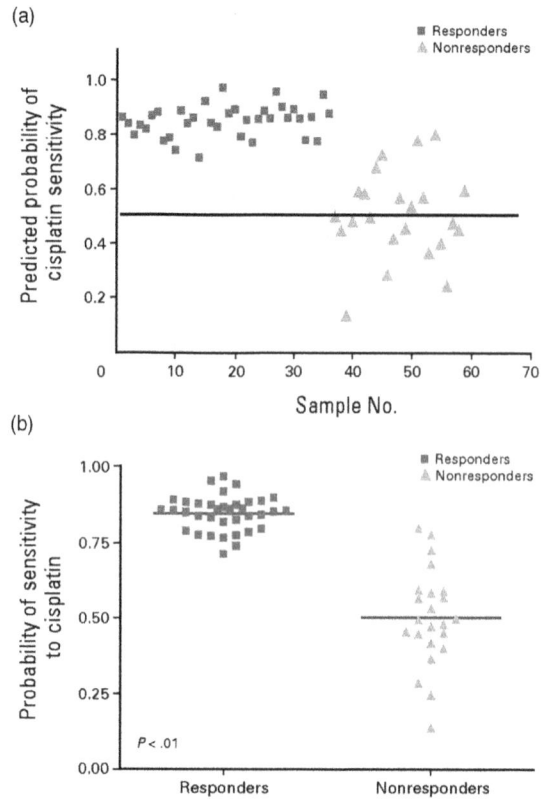

performance of the signature, it is the ability to predict response in patients that is obviously most critical. Using data from a previously published study that linked gene expression data with clinical response to cisplatin in an ovarian dataset [70] (GEO accession number: GSE3149), it has tested the ability of the *in vitro* cisplatin sensitivity predictor to accurately identify those patients who experience disease response with cisplatin. Using a predicted probability of response of 0.50 as the cutoff for predicting cisplatin sensitivity, the accuracy of the *in vitro* gene expression–based predictor of cisplatin sensitivity, based on available clinical data, was 83.1% (sensitivity, 100%; specificity, 57%; positive predictive value, 78%; negative predictive value, 100%; Figure 11.23). Furthermore, a Mann–Whitney U test revealed a significant difference in the predicted probabilities of cisplatin sensitivity between the resistant and sensitive cohorts of patients ($P < 0.01$; Figure 11.23).

11.20 PATTERNS OF PREDICTED CHEMOTHERAPY RESPONSE TO CISPLATIN AND PEMETREXED IN NSCLC

The cisplatin and pemetrexed predictors were utilized to profile the potential options of using these two drugs in a collection of 91 NSCLC described previously [85] (GEO accession number: GSE3141). These samples were first sorted according to the patterns of predicted sensitivity to cisplatin (Figure 11.24A, left panel). The pattern observed indicated that those patients resistant to cisplatin (red) were more sensitive to pemetrexed (blue). Although the data points in the scatter plot do not appear to be perfectly correlated, this analysis suggests that the relationship was statistically significant ($P=0.004$, logrank; Figure 11.24A, right panel). A similar relationship was also demonstrated in the independent cohort of NSCLC cell lines (Figure 11.24B), suggesting the possibility of alternative therapy for the treatment of advanced or metastatic NSCLC patients who would be predicted to be platinum-resistant. As a comparison, the pemetrexed signature was also applied to the ovarian cancer patient dataset. In this analysis [62], however, only two (<4%) of 59 patients were identified to have a greater than 50% of probability of being sensitive to pemetrexed.

11.21   THE SEQUENCE OF CHEMOTHERAPY MAY BE CRITICAL IN OPTIMIZING RESPONSES

Currently, first-line treatment with a platinum-based regimen is the standard of care for advanced NSCLC. Those patients developing resistance to cisplatin are treated with a taxane, pemetrexed, or erlotinib as second-line options. To explore the effect of cisplatin resistance, as well as prior treatment with potentially ineffective therapies, the IC_{50} of various lung cancer cell lines to cisplatin and pemetrexed were analyzed and revealed an inverse relationship (Figure 11.25A). Thereafter, one NSCLC cell line (H2030) that is resistant to cisplatin, paclitaxel, and docetaxel but sensitive to pemetrexed on the basis of cell proliferation assays (IC_{50}) was treated with pemetrexed, docetaxel, or paclitaxel in a systematic fashion. Interestingly, when H2030 was first treated for 4 days with a taxane (docetaxel or paclitaxel), resistance to subsequent pemetrexed exposure was

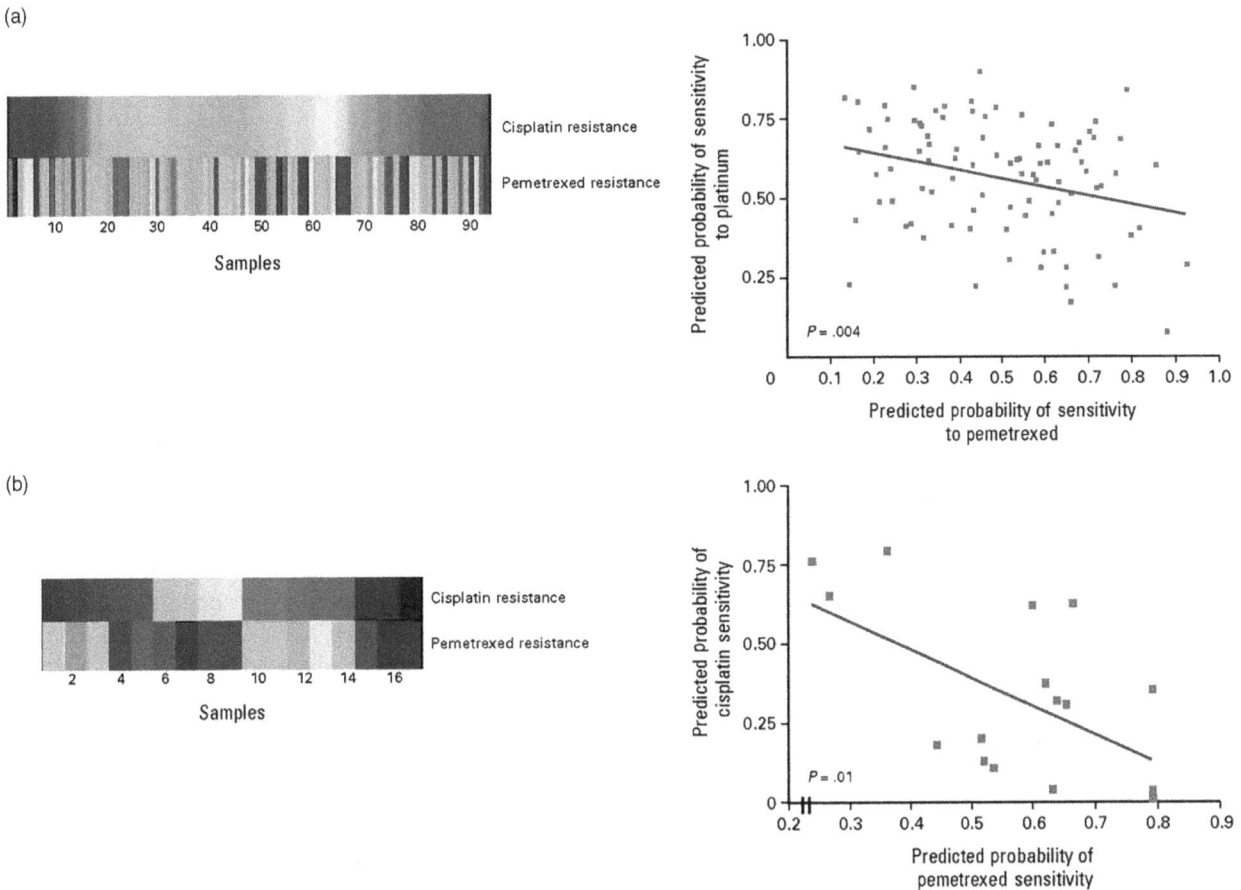

FIGURE 11.24   Correlation between cisplatin and pemetrexed sensitivity in (A) lung tumors and (B) cell lines. Top row represents the probability of cisplatin resistance and bottom row the corresponding probability of pemetrexed resistance for each sample. Right panels show the inverse relationship between predicted cisplatin and pemetrexed resistance ($P=0.004$) and cell lines ($P=0.01$).

(a)

(b)

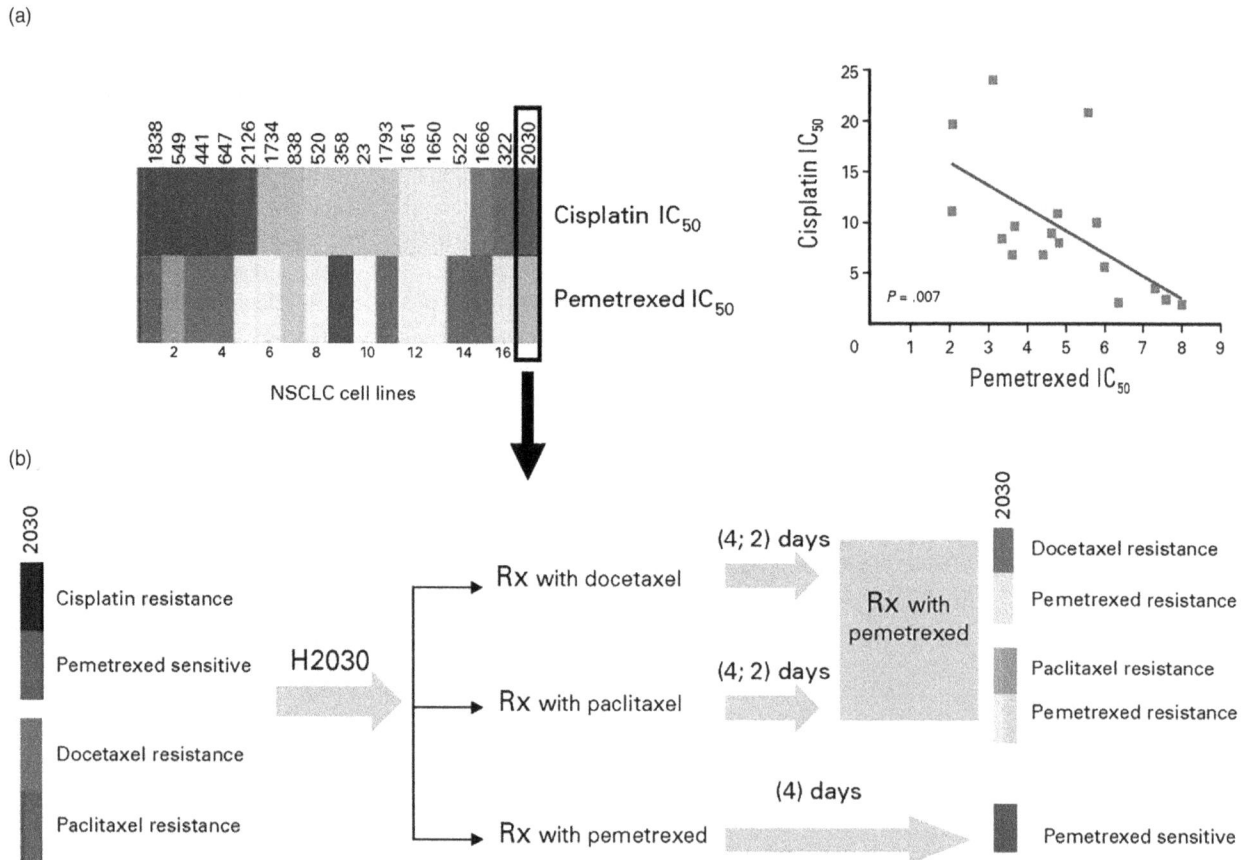

FIGURE 11.25 Sequence of chemotherapy may be critical in optimizing responses. (A) Fifty percent inhibitory concentration (IC_{50}) of lung cancer cell lines to cisplatin and pemetrexed reveal a significant inverse relationship. (B) The NSCLC cell line (H2030) is initially pemetrexed-sensitive. After exposure to a taxane for 4 days, H2030 subsequently develops resistance to pemetrexed. Rx, treatment drug.

induced (Figure 11.25B). In contrast, when H2030 was first treated with pemetrexed, H2030 was sensitive, as expected (Figure 11.25B). Although these *in vitro* observations are only hypothesis-generating at this time, this proof of principle experiment [62] suggests that the sequence of second-line chemotherapy in NSCLC may prove to be important in determining the clinical outcomes. Specifically, in tumors from cisplatin-refractory patients who are also predicted to be resistant to a taxane, treatment with a taxane (docetaxel or paclitaxel) before pemetrexed therapy may induce resistance to subsequent pemetrexed therapy. This preliminary observation, pending further validation, suggests the importance of including genomic-based, disease-specific, treatment prioritization in clinical practice.

In this study [62], the patterns of cisplatin sensitivity observed in our cohort of 91 NSCLC tumors suggest that not all patients may initially respond to first-line cisplatin-based therapy. As described herein, response rates to first-line platinum-based therapy is approximately 30%, with median survival between 24 and 31 months [61]. We have made use of *in vitro* drug sensitivity data in cancer cell lines, coupled with Affymetrix expression data, to develop gene expression signatures reflecting sensitivity to cisplatin and pemetrexed. The capacity of these signatures to predict

the response in independent sets of cell lines and patient studies begins to define a strategy that addresses the potential to identify cytotoxic agents that best match individual patients with advanced NSCLC and other advanced cancers (ovarian cancer). In addition, it can potentially be applied to patients with early-stage NSCLC to predict who may benefit from adjuvant cisplatin-based therapy. However, as promising as these approaches may seem, these strategies need to be first validated in a prospective clinical trial that would evaluate the performance of a genomic signature-based selection as an initial step in the individualized treatment strategy for patients with advanced NSCLC (Figure 11.26).

11.22 CONCLUSIONS

In conclusion, the development of signatures of drug sensitivity provides an opportunity to optimize therapy for patients with NSCLC and perhaps other patients with advanced cancer where cisplatin-based therapy is considered the standard of care.

In this chapter, an amphiphilic chimeric peptide (Fmoc)$_2$KH$_7$-TAT was designed and synthesized. (Fmoc)$_2$ KH$_7$-TAT peptide possessed a good capacity of loading DNA and DOX simultaneously. The existence of H$_7$

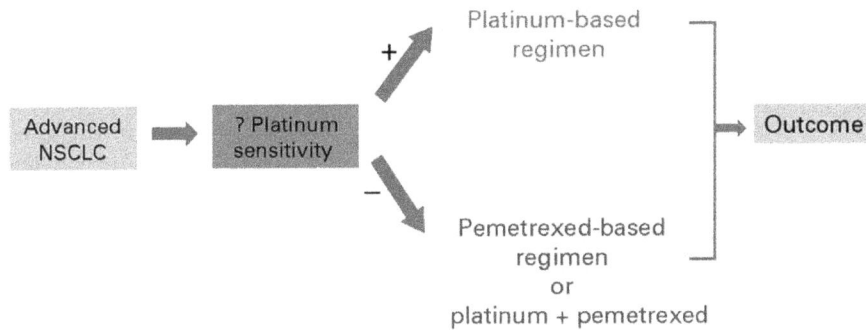

FIGURE 11.26 An example of a possible future treatment strategy for patients with advanced NSCLC. +, sensitive to cisplatin; –, resistant to cisplatin.

sequence in (Fmoc)$_2$KH$_7$-TAT peptide led to a much higher DOX release rate from (Fmoc)$_2$KH$_7$-TAT peptide at pH 5.0 than that at pH 7.4. At the same time, the H7 sequence endowed the peptide/DNA complexes with good endosome escaping ability. (Fmoc)$_2$KH$_7$-TAT peptide mediated excellent transfection efficacy both in 293T and HeLa cell lines under serum-free and serum-containing conditions. Besides, (Fmoc)$_2$KH$_7$-TAT micelle exhibited much superiority in transporting gene and drug to the same cells simultaneously and exhibited satisfactory synergistic effect both *in vitro* and *in vivo*. The results demonstrated a promising peptide-based micelle nanoplatform for efficient delivery [86–89] of gene and drug simultaneously and synergistic therapy in the realm of tumor treatment.

In summary, a novel ROS-triggered self-accelerating drug release nanosystem by amplifying the intracellular ROS concentration based on the positive feedback strategy was designed for enhanced tumor chemotherapy. It was found that owing to the ROS-cleavable TK linkers, this designed nanosystem could deliver the drug to the ROS abundant tumor cells and produce the cell toxicity selectively, without affecting the normal cells. Moreover, both *in vitro* and *in vivo* studies proved that in MCF-7 cells, T/D@RSMSNs could not only release DOX and α-TOS initiatively but also lead to the augmented concentration of intracellular ROS by α-TOS and accelerating release of DOX, displaying more remarkable antitumor activity than the traditional ROS-responsive nanocarriers. This novel ROS-triggered self-accelerating drug release nanosystem with enhanced tumor therapeutic efficiency could provide a general strategy to branch out the applications of existing ROS-responsible DDSs.

REFERENCES

1. K. Han, S. Chen, W-H. Chen, Q. Lei, Y. Liu, R-X. Zhuo, X-Z. Zhang. Synergistic gene and drug tumor therapy using a chimeric peptide, *Biomaterials* 34 (2013) 4680–4689.
2. B. Jones. Tumor genetics: evaluating oncogene cooperativities. *Nat. Rev. Genet.* 13 (2012) 598.
3. D.S. Chi, F. Musa, F. Dao, O. Zivanovic, Y. Sonoda, R.R. Barakat, et al., An analysis of patients with bulky advanced stage ovarian, tubal, and peritoneal carcinoma treated with primary debulking surgery (PDS) during an identical time period as the randomized EORTC-NCIC trial of PDS vs neoadjuvant chemotherapy (NACT), *Gynecol. Oncol.* 124 (2012) 10–14.
4. C. Bock, T. Lengauer, Managing drug resistance in tumor: lessons from HIV therapy, *Nat. Rev. Cancer* 12 (2012) 494–501.
5. T.M. Sun, J.Z. Du, Y.D. Yao, C.Q. Mao, S. Dou, J. Wang, et al., Simultaneous delivery of siRNA and paclitaxel via a "two-in-one" micelleplex promotes synergistic tumor suppression, *ACS Nano* 5 (2011) 1483–1494.
6. J.A. MacDiarmid, N.B. Amaro-Mugridge, J. Madrid-Weiss, I. Sedliarou, S. Wetzel, H. Brahmbhatt, et al., Sequential treatment of drug-resistant tumors with targeted minicells containing siRNA or a cytotoxic drug, *Nat. Biotechnol.* 27 (2009) 643–651.
7. L. Han, R.Q. Huang, J.F. Li, S.H. Liu, S.X. Huang, C. Jiang, Plasmid pORF-hTRAIL and doxorubicin co-delivery targeting to tumor using peptide-conjugated polyamidoamine dendrimer, *Biomaterials* 32 (2011) 1242–1252.
8. H.J. Wang, P.Q. Zhao, W.Y. Su, S. Wang, Z.Y. Liao, J. Chang, et al., PLGA/polymeric liposome for targeted drug and gene co-delivery, *Biomaterials* 31 (2010) 8741–8748.
9. S.H. Liu, Y.B. Guo, R.Q. Huang, J.F. Li, S.X. Huang, C. Jiang, Gene and doxorubicin co-delivery system for targeting therapy of glioma, *Biomaterials* 33 (2012) 4907–4916.
10. X. Lu, Q.Q. Wang, F.J. Xu, G.P. Tang, W.T. Yang, A cationic prodrug/therapeutic gene nanocomplex for the synergistic treatment of tumors, *Biomaterials* 32 (2011) 4849–4856.
11. H. Meng, M. Liong, T. Xia, Z.X. Li, Z.X. Ji, A.E. Nel, et al., Engineered design of mesoporous silica nanoparticles to deliver doxorubicin and P-glycoprotein siRNA to overcome drug resistance in a tumor cell line, *ACS Nano* 4 (2010) 4539–4550.
12. H.T. Lv, S.B. Zhang, B. Wang, S.H. Cui, J. Yan, Toxicity of cationic lipids and cationic polymers in gene delivery, *J. Control. Release* 114 (2006) 100–109.
13. D.W. Pack, A.S. Hoffman, S. Pun, P.S. Stayton, Design and development of polymers for gene delivery, *Nat. Rev. Drug. Discov.* 4 (2005) 581–593.
14. I. Nakase, S. Kobayashi, S. Futaki, Endosome-disruptive peptides for improving cytosolic delivery of endosome-disruptive peptide, *Biopolymers* 94 (2010) 763–770.
15. Y. Wang, S.J. Gao, W.H. Ye, H.S. Yoon, Y.Y. Yang, Co-delivery of drugs and DNA from cationic coreeshell nanoparticles self-assembled from a biodegradable copolymer, *Nat. Mater.* 5 (2006) 791–796.

16. X.B. Xiong, A. Lavasanifar, Traceable multifunctional micellar nanocarriers for tumor-targeted co-delivery of MDR-1 siRNA and doxorubicin, *ACS Nano* 5 (2011) 5202–5213.

17. F. Alexis, S.L. Lo, S. Wang, Covalent attachment of low molecular weight poly(ethyleneimine) improves Tat peptide mediated gene delivery, *Adv. Mater.* 18 (2006) 2174–2178.

18. J. Hoyer, I. Neundorf, Peptide vectors for the nonviral delivery of nucleic acids, *Acc. Chem. Res.* 45 (2012) 1048–1056.

19. P. Seth, M.C. Willingham, I. Pastan, Binding of adenovirus and its external proteins to Triton X-114, *J. Biol. Chem.* 260 (1985) 14431–14434.

20. T. Kakudo, S. Chaki, S. Futaki, I. Nakase, K. Akaji, H. Harashima, et al., Transferrinmodified liposomes equipped with a pH-sensitive fusogenic peptide: an artificial viral-like delivery system, *Biochemistry* 43 (2004) 5618–5628.

21. A. Kichler, C. Leborgne, J. Marz, O. Danos, B. Bechinger, Histidine-rich amphipathic peptide antibiotics promote efficient delivery of DNA into mammalian cells, *Proc. Natl. Acad. Sci. U. S. A.* 100 (2003) 1564–1568.

22. W.J. Yi, J. Yang, C. Li, H.Y. Wang, R.X. Zhuo, X.Z. Zhang, et al., Enhanced nuclear import and transfection efficiency of TAT peptide based gene delivery systems modified by additional nuclear localization signals, *Bioconjug. Chem.* 23 (2012) 125–134.

23. K. Han, J. Yang, S. Chen, C.J. Chen, R.X. Zhuo, X.Z. Zhang, et al., Novel gene transfer vectors based on artificial recombinant multi-functional oligopeptides, *Int. J. Pharm.* 436 (2012) 555–563.

24. D.X. Lu, X.T. Wen, J. Liang, Z.W. Gu, X.D. Zhang, Y.U. Fan, A pH-sensitive nano drug delivery system derived from pullulan/Doxorubicin conjugate, *J. Biomed. Mater. Res. B* 89B (2009) 177–183.

25. S. Mura, J. Nicolas, P. Couvreur, Stimuli-responsive nanocarriers for drug delivery, *Nat. Mater.* 12 (2013) 991–1003.

26. J. Du, L.A. Lane, S. Nie, Stimuli-responsive nanoparticles for targeting the tumor microenvironment, *J. Control. Release* 219 (2015) 205–214.

27. J.J. Hu, L.H. Liu, Z.Y. Li, R.X. Zhuo, X.Z. Zhang, MMP-responsive theranostic nanoplatform based on mesoporous silica nanoparticles for tumor imaging and targeted drug delivery, *J. Mater. Chem. B* 4 (2016) 1932–1940.

28. J. Zhang, Z.F. Yuan, Y. Wang, W.H. Chen, G.F. Luo, S.X. Cheng, et al., Multifunctional envelope-type mesoporous silica nanoparticles for tumor-triggered targeting drug delivery, *J. Am. Chem. Soc.* 135 (2013) 5068–5073.

29. H.J. Li, J.Z. Du, X.J. Du, C.F. Xu, C.Y. Sun, H.X. Wang, et al., Stimuli-responsive clustered nanoparticles for improved tumor penetration and therapeutic efficacy, *Proc. Natl. Acad. Sci. U. S. A.* 113 (2016) 4164–4169.

30. K. Han, W.Y. Zhang, J. Zhang, Q. Lei, S.B. Wang, J.W. Liu, et al., Acidity-triggered tumor-targeted chimeric peptide for enhanced intra-nuclear photodynamic therapy, *Adv. Funct. Mater.* 26 (2016) 4351–4361.

31. D.W. Zheng, J.L. Chen, J.Y. Zhu, L. Rong, B. Li, Q. Lei, et al., Highly integrated nano-platform for breaking the barrier between chemotherapy and immunotherapy, *Nano Lett.* 16 (2016) 4341–4347.

32. J.J. Hu, D. Xiao, X.Z. Zhang, Advances in peptide functionalization on mesoporous silica nanoparticles for controlled drug release, *Small* 12 (2016) 3344–3359.

33. D. Trachootham, J. Alexandre, P. Huang, Targeting cancer cells by ROS mediated mechanisms: a radical therapeutic approach? *Nat. Rev. Drug Discov.* 8 (2009) 579–591.

34. Y. Kuang, K. Balakrishnan, V. Gandhi, X. Peng, Hydrogen peroxide inducible DNA cross-linking agents: targeted anticancer prodrugs, *J. Am. Chem. Soc.* 133 (2011) 19278–19281.

35. C. Tapeinos, A. Pandit, Physical, chemical, and biological structures based on ROS-sensitive moieties that are able to respond to oxidative microenvironments, *Adv. Mater.* 28 (2016) 5553–5585.

36. X. Liu, J. Xiang, D. Zhu, L. Jiang, Z. Zhou, J. Tang, et al., Fusogenic reactive oxygen species triggered charge-reversal vector for effective gene delivery, *Adv. Mater.* 28 (2016) 1743–1752.

37. M. Wang, S. Sun, C.I. Neufeld, B.P. Ramirez, Q. Xu, Reactive oxygen species responsive protein modification and its intracellular delivery for targeted cancer therapy, *Angew. Chem. Int. Ed.* 53 (2014) 13444–13448.

38. W.H. Chen, G.F. Luo, W.X. Qiu, Q. Lei, S. Hong, S.B. Wang, et al., Programmed nanococktail for intracellular cascade reaction regulating self-synergistic tumor targeting therapy, *Small* 12 (2016) 733–744.

39. M.S. Shim, Y. Xia, A reactive oxygen species (ROS)-responsive polymer for safe, efficient, and targeted gene delivery in cancer cells, *Angew. Chem. Int. Ed.* 52 (2013) 6926–6929.

40. C. de Gracia Lux, S. Joshi-Barr, T. Nguyen, E. Mahmoud, E. Schopf, N. Fomina, et al., Biocompatible polymeric nanoparticles degrade and release cargo in response to biologically relevant levels of hydrogen peroxide, *J. Am. Chem. Soc.* 134 (2012) 15758–15764.

41. M.F. Chung, W.T. Chia, W.L. Wan, Y.J. Lin, H.W. Sung, Controlled release of an anti-inflammatory drug using an ultrasensitive ROS-responsive gas-generating carrier for localized inflammation inhibition, *J. Am. Chem. Soc.* 137 (2015) 12462–12465.

42. K. Han, J.Y. Zhu, S.B. Wang, Z.H. Li, S.X. Cheng, X.Z. Zhang, Tumor targeted gold nanoparticles for FRET-based tumor imaging and light responsive on-demand drug release, *J. Mater. Chem. B* 3 (2015) 8065–8069.

43. J. Lee, J. Park, K. Singha, W.J. Kim, Mesoporous silica nanoparticle facilitated drug release through cascade photosensitizer activation and cleavage of singlet oxygen sensitive linker, *Chem. Commun.* 49 (2013) 1545–1547.

44. G. Yang, X. Sun, J. Liu, L. Feng, Z. Liu, Light-responsive, singlet oxygen triggered on-demand drug release from photosensitizer-doped mesoporous silica nanorods for cancer combination therapy, *Adv. Funct. Mater.* 26 (2016) 4722–4732.

45. Y. Yuan, J. Liu, B. Liu, Conjugated-polyelectrolyte-based polyprodrug: targeted and image-guided photodynamic and chemotherapy with on-demand drug release upon irradiation with a single light source, *Angew. Chem. Int. Ed.* 53 (2014) 7163–7168.

46. Q. He, J. Shi, MSN Anti-cancer nanomedicines: chemotherapy enhancement, overcoming of drug resistance, and metastasis inhibition, *Adv. Mater.* 26 (2014) 391–411.

47. Z. Li, J.C. Barnes, A. Bosoy, J.F. Stoddart, J.I. Zink, Mesoporous silica nanoparticles in biomedical applications, *Chem. Soc. Rev.* 41 (2012) 2590e2605.

48. P. Yang, S. Gai, J. Lin, Functionalized mesoporous silica materials for controlled drug delivery, *Chem. Soc. Rev.* 41 (2012) 3679–3698.

49. F. Tang, L. Li, D. Chen, Mesoporous silica nanoparticles: synthesis, biocompatibility and drug delivery, *Adv. Mater.* 24 (2012) 1504–1534.

50. L.F. Dong, P. Low, J.C. Dyason, X.F. Wang, L. Prochazka, P.K. Witting, et al., a-Tocopheryl succinate induces apoptosis by targeting ubiquinone-binding sites in mitochondrial respiratory complex II, *Oncogene* 27 (2008) 4324–4335.

51. M. Stapelberg, N. Gellert, E. Swettenham, M. Tomasetti, P.K. Witting, A. Procopio, et al., a-Tocopheryl succinate inhibits malignant mesothelioma by disrupting the fibroblast growth factor autocrine loop Mechanism and the role of oxidative stress, *J. Biol. Chem.* 280 (2005) 25369–25376.

52. Y.H. Kang, E. Lee, M.K. Choi, J.L. Ku, S.H. Kim, Y.G. Park, et al., Role of reactive oxygen species in the induction of apoptosis by a-tocopheryl succinate, *Int. J. Cancer* 112 (2004) 385–392.

53. D.S. Wilson, G. Dalmasso, L. Wang, S.V. Sitaraman, D. Merlin, N. Murthy, Orally delivered thioketal nanoparticles loaded with TNF-a-siRNA target inflammation and inhibit gene expression in the intestines, *Nat. Mater.* 9 (2010) 923–928.

54. L. Pan, Q. He, J. Liu, Y. Chen, M. Ma, L. Zhang, et al., Nuclear-targeted drug delivery of TAT peptide-conjugated monodisperse mesoporous silica nanoparticles, *J. Am. Chem. Soc.* 134 (2012) 5722–5725.

55. J.-J. Hu, Q. Lei, M.-Y. Peng, D.-W. Zheng, Y.-X. Chen, X.-Z. Zhang. A positive feedback strategy for enhanced chemotherapy based on ROS-triggered self-accelerating drug release nanosystem. *Biomaterials* 128 (2017) 136–146.

56. Q. Zhang, X. Wang, P.Z. Li, K.T. Nguyen, X.J. Wang, Z. Luo, et al., Biocompatible, uniform, and redispersible mesoporous silica nanoparticles for cancer targeted drug delivery in vivo, *Adv. Funct. Mater.* 24 (2014) 2450–2461.

57. H.L. Pu, W.L. Chiang, B. Maiti, Z.X. Liao, Y.C. Ho, M.S. Shim, et al., Nanoparticles with dual responses to oxidative stress and reduced pH for drug release and anti-inflammatory applications, *ACS Nano* 8 (2014) 1213–1221.

58. B. Genty, J. Briantais, N. Baker, The relationship between the quantum yield of photosynthetic electron transport and quenching of chlorophyll fluorescence, *Biochem. Biophys. Acta* 990 (1989) 87–92.

59. Bunn PA Jr, Kelly K: New chemotherapeutic agents prolong survival and improve quality of life in non-small cell lung cancer: A review of the literature and future directions, *Clin. Cancer Res.* 4 (1998) 1087–1100.

60. F.A. Shepherd, Treatment of advanced nonsmall cell lung cancer, *Semin. Oncol.* 21 (1994) 7–18.

61. O.S. Breathnach, B. Freidlin, B. Conley, et al., Twenty-two years of phase III trials for patients with advanced non-small-cell lung cancer: Sobering results, *J. Clin. Oncol.* 19 (2001) 1734–1742.

62. D.S. Hsu, B.S. Balakumaran, C.R. Acharya, V. Vlahovic, K.S. Walters, K. Garman, C. Anders, R.F. Riedel, J. Lancaster, D. Harpole, H.K. Dressman, J.R. Nevins, P.G. Febbo, A. Potti. Pharmacogenomic strategies provide a rational approach to the treatment of cisplatin-resistant patients with advanced cancer, *J. Clin. Oncol.* 25(28) (2007) 4350–4357. doi:10.1200/JCO.2007.11.0593. This article was retracted on November 16, 2010.

63. K. Kelly, J. Crowley, P.A. Bunn, et al., Randomized phase III trial of paclitaxel plus carboplatin versus vinorelbine plus cisplatin in the treatment of patients with advanced non-small cell lung cancer: A Southwest Oncology Group trial, *J. Clin. Oncol.* 19 (2001) 3210–3218.

64. J.H. Schiller, D. Harrington, C.P. Belani, et al., Comparison of four chemotherapy regimens for advanced non-small cell lung cancer, *N. Engl. J. Med.* 346 (2002) 92–98.

65. F.V. Fossella, R. DeVore, R.N. Kerr, et al., Randomized Phase III trial of docetaxel versus vinorelbine or ifosamide in patients with non small cell lung cancer previously treated with platinum containing chemotherapy regiments, *J. Clin. Oncol.* 18 (2000) 2354–2362.

66. N. Hanna, F.A. Shepherd, F.V. Fossella, et al., Randomized phase III trial of pemetrexed vs docetaxel in patients with NSCLC previously treated with chemotherapy, *J. Clin. Oncol.* 22 (2004) 1589–1597.

67. F.A. Shepherd, J. Rodrigues Pereira, T. Cieleanu, et al., Erlotinib in previously treated non small cell lung cancer, *N. Engl. J. Med.* 353 (2005) 123–132.

68. T.R. Golub, D.K. Slonim, J. Mesirov, et al., Molecular classification of cancer: Class discovery and class prediction by gene expression profiling, *Science* 286 (1999) 531–537.

69. T.R. Golub, Genome-wide views of cancer, *N. Engl. J. Med.* 344 (2001) 601–602.

70. A. Bild, G. Yao, J.T. Chang, et al., Oncogenic pathways signatures in human cancers as guide to targeted therapies, *Nature* 439 (2006) 353–357.

71. C.M. Perou, T. Sorlie, M.B. Eisen, et al., Molecular portraits of human breast tumors, *Nature* 406 (2000) 747–752.

72. A. Rosenwald, G. Wright, W.C. Chan, et al., The use of molecular profiling to predict survival after chemotherapy for diffuse large B cell lymphoma, *N. Engl. J. Med.* 346 (2002) 1937–1947.

73. M.A. Shipp, K.N. Ross, P. Tamayo, et al., Diffuse large B-cell lymphoma outcome prediction by gene expression profiling and supervised machine learning, *Nat. Med.* 8 (2002) 68–74.

74. M.J. van de Vijver, Y.D. He, L.J. van't Veer, et al., A gene expression signature as a prediction of survival in breast cancer, *N. Engl. J. Med.* 347 (2002) 1999–2009.

75. S. Ramaswamy, K.N. Ross, E.S. Lander, et al., A molecular signature of metastasis in primary solid tumor, *Nat. Genet.* 33 (2003) 49–54.

76. A. Potti, H.K. Dressman, A. Bild, et al., Genomic signatures to guide the use of chemotherapeutics, *Nat. Med.* 12 (2006) 1294–1300.

77. P. Therasse, S.G. Arbuck, E.A. Eisenhauer, et al., New guidelines to evaluate the response to treatment in solid tumors: European Organization for Research and Treatment of Cancer, National Cancer Institute of the US, National Cancer Institute of Canada, *J. Natl. Cancer Inst.* 92 (2000) 205–216.

78. G.J. Rustin, P. Timmers, A. Nelstrop, et al., Comparison of CA-125 and standard definitions of progression of ovarian cancer in the intergroup trial of cisplatin and paclitaxel versus cisplatin and cyclophosphamide, *J. Clin. Oncol.* 24 (2006) 45–51.

79. T. Mosmann, Rapid colorimetric assay for cellular growth and survival: Application to proliferation and cytotoxic assay, *J. Immunol. Meth* 65 (1983) 55–63.

80. M.V. Berridge, A.S. Tan, Characterization of the cellular reduction of 3-(4,5-dimethylthiazol-2-yl)-2,5-diphenyltetrazolium bromide (MTT): Subcellular localization, substrate dependence, and involvement if mitochondrial electron transport in MTT reduction, *Arch. Biochem. Biophys.* 303 (1993) 474–482.

81. B. Györffy, P. Surowiak, O. Kiesslich, et al., Gene expression profiling of 30 cancer cell lines predicts resistance towards 11 anticancer drugs at clinically achieved concentrations, *Int. J. Cancer* 118 (2006) 1699–1712.

82. S. Johnson, R. Perez, A. Godwin, et al., Role of platinum-DNA adduct formation and removal in cisplatin resistance in human ovarian cancer cell lines, *Biochem. Pharmacol.* 47 (1994) 689–697.

83. L. Yen, A. Woo, G. Christopoulopoulos, et al., Enhanced host cell reactivation capacity and expression of DNA repair genes in human breast cancer cells resistant to bi-functional alkylating agents, *Mutat. Res.* 337 (1995) 179–189.

84. L. Paz-Ares, S. Bezares, J. Tabernero, et al., Review of a promising new agent in pemetrexed disodium, *Cancer* 97 (2003) 2056–2063.

85. A. Potti, S. Mukherjee, R. Petersen, et al., A genomic strategy to refine prognosis in early-stage non–small-cell lung cancer, *N. Engl. J. Med.* 355 (2006) 570–580.

86. Loutfy H. Madkour, *Reactive Oxygen Species (ROS), Nanoparticles, and Endoplasmic Reticulum (ER) Stress-Induced Cell Death Mechanisms.* Paperback ISBN: 9780128224816. Imprint: Academic Press Published Date: 1st August 2020. https://www.elsevier.com/books/reactive-oxygen-species-ros-nanoparticles-and-endoplasmic-reticulum-er-stress-induced-cell-death-mechanisms/madkour/978-0-12-822481-6.

87. Loutfy H. Madkour, *Nanoparticles Induce Oxidative and Endoplasmic Reticulum Antioxidant Therapeutic Defenses.* Copyright 2020 Publisher Springer International Publishing. Copyright Holder Springer Nature Switzerland AG eBook ISBN 978-3-030-37297-2 DOI 10.1007/978-3-030-37297-2 Hardcover ISBN 978-3-030-37296-5 Series ISSN 2194–0452 Edition Number 1. https://www.springer.com/gp/book/9783030372965?utm_campaign=3_pier05_buy_print&utm_content=en_08082017&utm_medium=referral&utm_source=google_books#otherversion=9783030372972.

88. Loutfy H. Madkour, *Nucleic Acids as Gene Anticancer Drug Delivery Therapy.* 1st Edition. Publishing house: Elsevier, (2020). Paperback ISBN: 9780128197776 Imprint: Academic Press Published Date: 2nd January 2020 Imprint: Academic Press Copyright: Paperback ISBN: 9780128197776 © Academic Press 2020 Published: 2nd January 2020 Imprint: Academic Press Paperback ISBN: 9780128197776. https://www.elsevier.com/books/nucleic-acids-as-gene-anticancer-drug-deliverytherapy/madkour/978-0-12-819777-6

89. Loutfy H. Madkour, *Nanoelectronic Materials: Fundamentals and Applications (Advanced Structured Materials)* 1st ed. 2019 Edition: https://link.springer.com/book/10.1007%2F978-3-030-21621-4 Series Title Advanced Structured Materials Series Volume 116 Copyright 2019 Publisher Springer International Publishing Copyright Holder Springer Nature Switzerland AG. eBook ISBN 978-3-030-21621-4 DOI 10.1007/978-3-030-21621-4 Hardcover ISBN 978-3-030-21620-7 Series ISSN 1869-8433 Edition Number 1 Number of Pages XLIII, 783 Number of Illustrations 122 b/w illustrations, 494 illustrations in colour Topics. ISBN-10: 3030216209 ISBN-13: 978-3030216207 #117 in Nanotechnology (Books) #725 in Materials Science (Books) #187336 in Textbooks. https://books.google.com.eg/books/about/Nanoelectronic_Materials.html?id=YQXCxAEACAAJ&source=kp_book_description&redir_esc=y; https://www.springer.com/gp/book/9783030216207.

12 Pharmacokinetics, Biodistribution, and Therapeutic Applications of Recently Developed siRNA and DNA Repair Genes Recurrence

12.1 RNAi AS A POTENTIAL THERAPEUTIC

RNA interference (RNAi) is an endogenous post-transcriptional regulation process, which involves small regulatory RNAs such as small-interfering RNAs (siRNAs) or microRNAs (miRNAs) that silence target messenger RNAs in a sequence-specific manner. Ever since the discovery of RNAi in Caenorhabditis elegans [1] and the demonstration of siRNA activity in mammalian cells [2], RNAi has gained significant attention as a potential therapeutic for various diseases including viral infections and cancer, especially for those lacking "druggable" targets. The efforts to develop siRNA therapeutics resulted in the first trial in human [3] in less than a decade since the discovery. However, realizing the clinical potential of siRNA therapeutics has found to be a daunting task, in large part due to the unfavorable pharmacokinetics (PK) and biodistribution (BD) profiles of systemically administered siRNA [4–6]. This challenge has been tackled in various ways, including chemical modification of siRNAs and/or the use of nanoparticulate delivery systems based on lipids, polymers, and inorganic platforms, which aim to protect the siRNAs from serum proteins and renal clearance and help cross target cell membranes. These approaches have improved the bioavailability of siRNA and enabled at least 30 siRNA-based drugs to enter clinical trials [7]. Nevertheless, 70% of them address ocular diseases, where siRNA is administered locally, or target the liver, lung, or kidney, the filtering organs in which the formulations are naturally captured, indicating that the systemic delivery of RNAi therapeutics to other organs remains a critical challenge. To overcome this challenge and translate the broad potential of RNAi therapeutics to clinical benefits, it is important to understand the level of PK and BD control achieved by current delivery approaches. The purpose of this chapter is to provide an overview of the current status of the art in siRNA delivery with respect to the effects of carriers on PK, BD, and pharmacological effects of systemically administered siRNA. Due to the large volume of literature, we mainly discuss the studies published in the past 5 years.

12.2 THERAPEUTIC APPLICATIONS OF siRNA AND TARGET GENES

12.2.1 OCULAR DISEASES

RNAi has been found to be effective in the treatment of ocular diseases [8]. In early studies, local injection of siRNA targeting vascular endothelial growth factor (VEGF) was shown to reduce neovascularization in several animal models of eye injuries, such as laser-induced photocoagulation [9], suture-induced corneal angiogenesis [10], and CpG oligodeoxynucleotide- or herpes simplex virus-induced neovascularization [11]. Neovascularization is a critical pathological event in age-related macular degeneration (AMD) [12] and diabetic retinopathy [13,14]. Therefore, siRNAs suppressing the expression of VEGF, receptors, and/or its regulation have been explored as a potential therapy and tested in human for the treatment of AMD (Bevasiranib silencing VEGF) [15] and diabetic macular edema (PF-04523655 silencing hypoxia inducible gene) [16].

Fibrotic eye diseases are significant complications of eye surgeries. Transforming growth factor β (TGF-β) is identified as a main culprit of postoperative ocular scarring; thus, siRNA targeting TGF-β or its receptor is used to inhibit fibrotic responses to wounding. For example, siRNA targeting type II receptor of TGF-β was shown to reduce inflammatory responses and collagen deposition in a mouse model of subconjunctival inflammation and fibrosis [17]. Similarly, siRNA-mediated downregulation of IκB kinase beta (IKKβ), an activator of NF-κB-mediated inflammation and cell proliferation, reduced subconjunctival scarring in a monkey model of glaucoma filtration surgery [18]. siRNA is also pursued for glaucoma therapy. siRNA targeting β2-adrenoceptors (SYL040012) was shown to reduce the expression of β2 adrenergic receptor and the production of aqueous humor, thereby reducing intraocular pressure [19].

Based on promising preclinical results, several siRNA therapeutics entered clinical trials for ocular disease therapy [8,20]. Due to the accessibility and the blood ocular barrier, most siRNAs targeting ocular diseases are administered via local routes, such as intravitreal injection, subconjunctival injection, or topical instillation [8,20]. Therefore, ocular application of siRNA will not be covered in the following PK/BD discussion.

DOI: 10.1201/9781003229674-12

TABLE 12.1

Target Genes for siRNA Therapeutics in Cancer

Target Genes	Function of Target Genes	Diseases	References
VEGF	Angiogenesis	Lung cancer and metastasis	[31]
VEGFR	Angiogenesis	Lung adenocarcinoma	[32]
c-myc	Cell proliferation	Melanoma cancer	[33]
c-myc, MDM2, VEGF	Cell proliferation; p53 inhibition; angiogenesis	Melanoma cancer	[34]
EphA2	Cell–cell interactions	Ovarian cancer	[35]
Raf-1	RAS/MAPK signaling pathway	Melanoma cancer	[36]
PLK1	Cell division	Renal cell carcinoma	[37]
CDK1	Cell cycle progression	Breast cancer	[38]
Survivin	Drug resistance	Drug-resistant lung cancer and cervical cancer	[39]
MDR-1	Drug resistance	Drug-resistant ovarian tumor	[40]

12.2.2 CANCER

Due to the high selectivity and specificity, siRNA has been widely explored as a new therapeutic agent to replace or supplement traditional cytotoxic chemotherapy [21–23]. Targets often considered for siRNA-based cancer therapy include genes promoting uninhibited cell growth, such as VEGFs [24], c-myc [25], EphA2 [26], Raf-1 [27], polo-like kinase 1 (Plk1) [28], cyclin-dependent kinases (CDKs) [29], and those helping cancer cells survive or resist chemotherapy such as survivin and multi-drug resistance (MDR) genes [30] (Table 12.1).

VEGF and corresponding receptors (VEGFRs) participate in the regulation of blood vessel development during early embryogenesis [41]. Binding of VEGF to VEGFR activates multiple cellular pathways important for angiogenesis, an essential component of tumor growth and metastasis. Therefore, siRNAs targeting VEGF/VEGFR are explored as potential anti-cancer therapeutics. c-myc is an oncogene overexpressed in various human tumors, which promotes cell growth, transformation, and angiogenesis [25]. In particular, c-myc expression in melanoma is indispensable for nucleotide metabolism and proliferation of tumor cells [42]. Downregulation of c-myc inhibits tumor growth and sensitizes cancer cells to chemotherapy, possibly by induction of p53 and inhibition of Bcl-2 proteins, which trigger cell apoptosis [43].

EphA2 is a well-known receptor tyrosine kinase belonging to the Eph family, overexpressed in many cancers including breast cancers and ovarian cancers, implicated in poor clinical outcomes [44]. Contact-dependent cell–cell interactions controlled by Eph receptors and ephrin (ligand of Eph receptors) signaling are tightly regulated in normal embryonic development and maintenance of homeostasis [45]. During oncogenesis, normal EphA2–EphrinA1 signaling is disrupted due to the loss of cell contacts, leading to overexpression of EphA2 and oncogenic signal transduction [45]. This dysregulated signaling is implicated in several critical aspects of oncogenesis such as cytoskeleton modulation, cell adhesion, migration, metastasis, proliferation, and angiogenesis [45]. Plk1, a serine/threonine-protein

kinase, is responsible for cell mitosis in mammalian cells. It is overexpressed in various human cancers as a proto-oncogene, which inactivates tumor suppressor proteins like p53 [46,47]. CDKs are also serine/threonine kinases and essential for the regulation of the cell cycle progression [48]. The abnormal expression or activity of distinct CDK complexes causes cells to escape from a well-controlled cell cycle, resulting in malignant transformation [49–51]. Palbociclib, an inhibitor of CDK4/6, received breakthrough therapy designation from the FDA in April 2013, for the initial treatment of patients with breast cancer [52].

Survivin is an inhibitor of programmed cell death (apoptosis), expressed in various types of malignant tumor cells, especially in drug-resistant cells [53]. Survivin was initially identified as an inhibitor of caspase-9 and also found to be involved in the regulation of the mitotic spindle checkpoint and the promotion of angiogenesis and chemo resistance [54]. Therefore, siRNA targeting survivin is pursued as a way of potentiating the activity of chemotherapeutics. Another main cause of failure in chemotherapy is MDR-related P-glycoprotein (Pgp). Pgp, a typical ATP-binding cassette membrane transporter, causes efflux of a broad range of drugs from a cell, reducing effective accumulation of the drugs in the cell [55]. Overexpression of Pgp, also known as MDR 1 protein 1 (MDR-1), and upregulation of its functional activity in cancer cells lead to reduced sensitivity to chemotherapy, thus making an attractive target for siRNA therapy [56].

12.2.3 LIVER DISEASES

As a filtering organ where most nanoparticulate delivery systems are naturally captured, the liver has been the main target for most siRNA therapeutics currently in clinical evaluation stages [57]. Target diseases include hepatocellular carcinoma (HCC), viral hepatitis, liver fibrosis, and hypercholesterolemia [58].

12.2.3.1 HCC

HCC occurs by cumulative generic mutations, which lead to the dysfunctional regulation of cellular machinery and

TABLE 12.2

Target Genes for siRNA Therapeutics in HCC

Target Genes	Function of Target Genes	References
VEGF	Tumor angiogenesis and pathogenesis	[65]
EGFR	Cell survival, proliferation, and differentiation	[68]
NIK	Cell proliferation	[71]
ApoB	Formation of LDL, metabolism of dietary, and endogenous cholesterol	[72]
Notch-1	Tumorigenesis; epithelial–mesenchymal transition	[73]

proliferation [59]. RNAi therapy has been pursued to modulate the mutated genes involved in the oncogenesis of HCC, such as adenomatous polyposis coli, VEGF-A, fibroblast growth factor substrate 2, and phosphoinositide 3-kinase [60–63] (Table 12.2). These genes play an essential role in signal transduction pathways in HCC pathogenesis, including Wnt/β-catenin, VEGF, FGF, and PI3K/AKT/mTOR pathways [64–67]. For example, HCC is a highly vascularized tumor, where pro-angiogenic factors like VEGF-A, the major VEGF responsible for tumor angiogenesis and pathogenesis, are frequently overexpressed [65]. Therefore, several studies explored siRNA targeting the VEGF pathway for HCC therapy. The epidermal growth factor receptor (EGFR) signaling pathway is another important target [68], with its overexpression detected in 40%–70% of the tumors in pre-neoplastic HCC [69].

In addition to siRNAs, several miRNAs have been identified as a potential therapy of HCC. For example, miR-122, a liver-specific tumor suppressor miRNA frequently down-regulated in HCC, has drawn increasing attention over the years [70]. Due to the similarity in structure, miRNAs are delivered in similar ways as siRNAs.

12.2.3.2 Hepatic Viral Infections (Table 12.3)

Hepatitis virus infection accounts for most cases of liver infections. When left untreated, patients infected by hepatitis B, C, and D viruses are chronically disturbed and further develop liver cirrhosis and HCC [74]. Currently, 90% hepatitis B vaccine is effective in preventing hepatitis B virus (HBV) infection, but >700,000 deaths still occur worldwide as a consequence of HBV infection [75]. Patients with chronic HBV infection are currently treated with antiviral agents such as tenofovir and entecavir together with

immunomodulators like IFN-α 2b, but side effects and viral resistance limit the effectiveness of these therapies [76]. In this regard, RNAi is considered a potentially attractive treatment for HBV infection. Hepatitis B virion is composed of circular double-stranded DNA, which contains four overlapping open-reading frames (ORFs: S, Pol, X, and C) that encode essential proteins like pre-core protein (also known as HBeAg), core protein (HBcAg), envelope protein (HBsAg), X protein, and viral polymerase [77]. Among them, the X protein, encoded by ORF X gene, was known to regulate transcription and translation by transactivation of viral and cellular promoters, and several studies showed that HBx-specific siRNAs could suppress HBV viral replication [78,79]. ORF C is another valid target. It encodes polyadenylation region that plays important function in all the transcripts [80] and contains sequences that can encode nuclear localization signal needed for transporting covalently closed circular DNA, which serves as the template for viral transcription [81,82].

Hepatitis C virus (HCV) comprises seven different genotypes with more than 50 subtypes and billions of quasispecies [83]. Current treatment by PEGylated interferons and nucleoside inhibitors like ribavirin is effective in 70%–80% of patients with genotype 2 or 3 but less effective in patients with other genotypes [84]. Side effects are also common among patients receiving this combination treatment [84]. HCV genome sequences are highly variable as compared to HBV, but 5′-untranslated region (5′-UTR) contains conserved internal ribosome-entering site (IRES), essential for virus replication, providing a useful target for RNAi therapy [85–88]. Moreover, siRNAs targeting HCV-core gene [89] or E1, E2 [90] resulted in dramatic reduction in virus RNA by interfering with multiple signaling pathways

TABLE 12.3

Target Genes for siRNA Therapeutics in Hepatic Viral Infections

Target Genes	Function of Target Genes	Diseases	References
HBx	Regulates HBV transcription and translation	HBV	[78,93]
Core	Regulates viral DNA replication	HBV	[81,82]
IRES in 5′-UTR	Facilitates RNA translation	HCV	[86–88]
Core	Triggers activation of multiple signaling pathways in HCV	HCV	[89]
E1, E2	Viral attachment to cells	HCV	[90]
L protein, VP24, and VP35	L protein: RNA polymerase activity; VP24/VP35: inhibitory effects on host type 1 interferon response	Ebola virus	[91]

TABLE 12.4

Target Genes for siRNA Therapeutics in Respiratory Diseases

Target Genes	Function of Target Genes	Disease	References
Gα12 & Gα13	Promotes the growth and oncogenic transformation	SCLC	[96]
WT1	Encodes a transcription factor involved in gonadal development	Melanoma lung metastasis	[97]
NP gene	Produces NPs	Influenza infection	[98,99]
P protein	Essential for RNA-dependent RNA polymerase (RdRP) holoenzyme to exit the promoter and to form a closed complex capable of sustained elongation	RSV and PIV	[100]
ENaC	Stimulates sodium and water absorption, counteracting cystic fibrosis transmembrane regulator (CFTR) activity	Cystic fibrosis	[101]
IL-4	Promotes the differentiation and proliferation of Th2 cells and facilitates the antibody class switching of B cells to IgE	Asthma-associated inflammatory reactions	[102]
IL-13	Induces vascular cell adhesion molecule-1, and chemokines (e.g., eotaxin, MIP-1a) to recruit and activate inflammatory cells; directly affects airway smooth muscle	Airway resistance in allergen exposure	[103]

in HCV or inhibiting the viral attachment to the cells. In addition to hepatitis virus infections, the liver is also one of the primary sites for Ebola virus replication, and RNAi has been pursued as a potential treatment [91,92].

12.2.4 Respiratory Diseases

RNAi as a potential treatment of respiratory diseases has been reviewed extensively in recent literature [94,95]. A number of studies have demonstrated the use of siRNAs for the treatment of lung cancer, viral infection, cystic fibrosis, and inflammatory lung diseases (Table 12.4). Knockdown of G proteins (Gα12 and Gα13) was shown to abolish H69 tumorigenicity in mice for the treatment of small-cell lung cancer (SCLC) [96]. Silencing of the Wilms' tumor gene (WT1) was shown to be effective in treating melanoma lung metastases [97]. Administration of siRNAs targeting the conserved regions of influenza virus genes or nucleocapsid protein (NP) gene resulted in prevention and treatment of influenza infection [98,99]. The effectiveness of siRNA was also demonstrated in respiratory syncytial virus (RSV) and parainfluenza virus (PIV) infections [100]. siRNA therapeutics have been pursued for the therapy of cystic fibrosis, a genetic disorder that fatally affects the lung functions. Epithelial sodium channel (ENaC) was identified as a potential target for RNAi therapy of cystic fibrosis [101]. For asthma-associated inflammatory reactions, the knockdown of IL-4 alleviated airway inflammations [102], and siRNA targeting IL-13 reduced airway resistance in allergen-challenged mice [103].

12.3 PHARMACOKINETICS OF siRNA THERAPEUTICS

12.3.1 Preclinical Studies

For systemic delivery of siRNA, it is critical to maintain siRNA stable with a long half-life ($t_{1/2}$) in circulation. To investigate the effect of carriers on the circulation $t_{1/2}$ of siRNA, the siRNA is often labeled with radioactive elements or fluorescent dyes, and the radioactivity or fluorescence intensity of blood is measured at regular time points. siRNA complexed with nanoparticles (NPs) typically shows a longer $t_{1/2}$ (the time required to reduce the plasma concentration of a drug to one half of its initial value), higher area under the curve (AUC) (the overall amount of a drug in the bloodstream after a dose), lower plasma clearance (Cl) (the volume of plasma in the vascular compartment cleared of a drug per unit time), and longer mean retention time (MRT) (the average time a drug molecule stays in the body) than free (naked) siRNA, provided that the complex remains stable in circulation.

Xia et al. used magnetic mesoporous silica NPs (M-MSN) as a carrier of siRNA [31]. Here, siRNA was loaded in mesopores of the carrier, which was capped with polyethyleneimine (PEI) and surface modified with polyethylene glycol (PEG) and a fusogenic peptide. Fluorescence dye (Cy3) was conjugated to the 5′ end of the sense strand for detection of siRNA in blood. The blood level of free Cy3-siRNA was reduced to 1% of the injected dose per gram (ID/g) of blood within 20 min. In contrast, Cy3-siRNA loaded in M-MSN maintained ~5% of the injected dose per gram of blood in the first hour [31]. This difference translated to significantly increased bioavailability of siRNA. Free Cy3-siRNA showed an AUC of 40.13 ± 30.49 min mg/mL, a plasma Cl of 57.96 ± 58.07 mL/min/kg, and a MRT of 70.67 ± 20.39 min, whereas Cy3-siRNA packaged in M-MSN showed AUC, Cl, and MRT of 573.34 ± 145.12 min mg/mL, 2.41 ± 0.51 mL/min/kg, and 310.15 ± 21.68 min, respectively [31].

As with other nanomedicine, surface modification of carriers with PEG helps extend the $t_{1/2}$ and increase the AUC. Kissel et al. developed amphiphilic biodegradable non-viral polymeric siRNA carrier, based on PEI, polycaprolactone (PCL), and PEG [104]. To study PK of siRNA complexed with the polymer, they used ^{111}In-radiolabeled siRNA and measured the radioactivity of the blood samples over time. Upon intravenous (IV) injection, siRNA/PEI-g-PCL-b-PEG complexes showed longer circulation times, less steep α and β elimination phases, and higher AUC values as compared to free siRNA or siRNA/PEI complexes (Figure 12.1) [104].

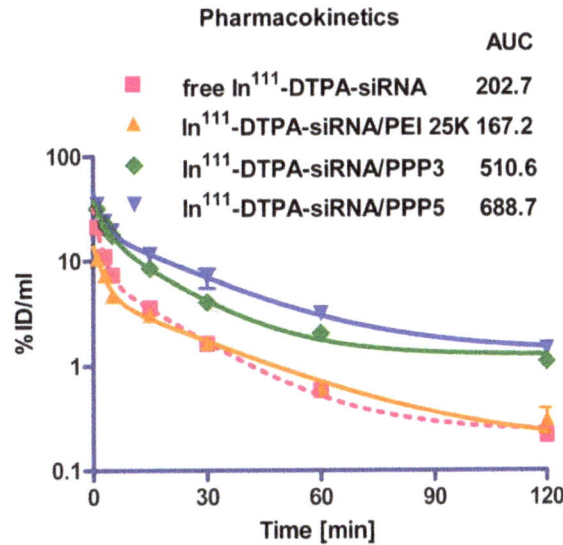

FIGURE 12.1 PK of siRNA polyplexes and free siRNA as measured by gamma scintillation counting of blood samples. PPP indicates PEI-g-(PCL-b-PEG); 3 and 5 indicate graft density of PCLPEG to PEI. (Reprinted with permission from Ref. [104]. Copyright (2012) Elsevier.)

On the other hand, siRNA/PEI complex showed a similar PK as free siRNA due to the instability of the complex (i.e., early dissociation of the complex in blood). Similarly, Harashima et al. compared PK parameters of a liposomal siRNA carrier, called a multi-functional envelope-type nanodevice (MEND), with and without PEGylation, and confirmed the significance of PEG modification [37]. siRNA and lipid envelope were labeled with radioisotopes, ^{32}P and ^{3}H, respectively, and traced in normal mice after IV injection. The siRNA encapsulated in the MEND was eliminated from the bloodstream as rapidly as free siRNA,

suggesting rapid clearance via the mononuclear phagocyte system (MPS) (Figure 12.2). On the other hand, siRNA formulated in the PEGMEND showed a longer $t_{1/2\beta}$ (16.9 vs. 1.35 h of free siRNA) and higher AUC (344 vs. 2.1 μg h of free siRNA). The ^{3}H-labeled lipid component showed a similar blood concentration profile as ^{32}P-labeled siRNA, suggesting that the complex was stable during circulation.

Another approach to increase the stability of siRNA/ carrier complex involves covalent cross-linking of the carrier and introduction of hydrophobic interactions [105]. Kataoka et al. developed a polyion complex micelle system

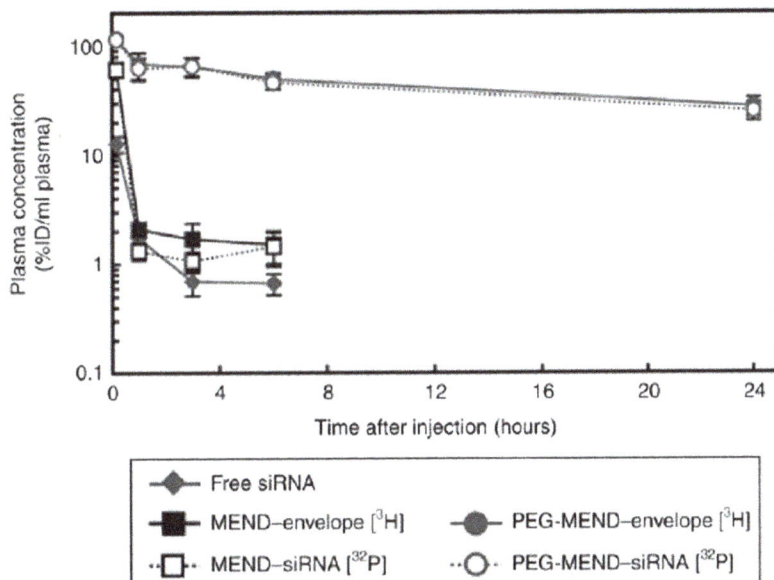

FIGURE 12.2 Blood concentration profile of systemically injected MENDs. The lipid envelope and siRNA were labeled with RIs ^{3}H and ^{32}P, respectively. MENDs and free siRNA were injected via the tail vein of ICR mice, and then at 0.17, 1, 3, 6, and 24 h after injection, the radioactivity in plasma was measured by liquid scintillation counting. The data are represented as the mean±SD (n=3). MEND, multi-functional envelope-type nanodevice; RI, radio isotope. (Reprinted with permission from Ref. [37]. Copyright (2013) Nature Publishing Group.)

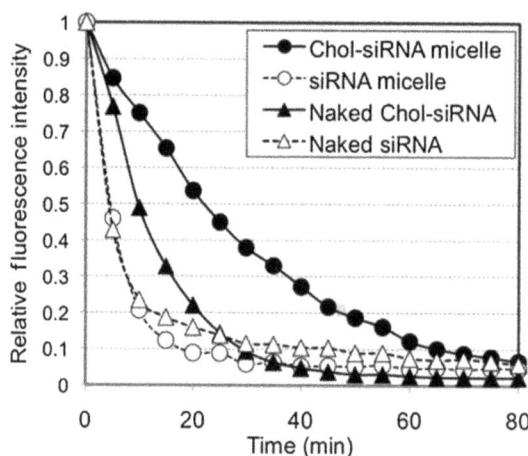

FIGURE 12.3 *In vivo* performance of siRNA encapsulated in PEG-PLL (MPA) micelles. Blood circulation profiles, determined by IVRT-CLSM after IV injection (3.6 nmol siRNA/mouse) into BALB/c nude mice (open triangle: naked Chol-free/Cy5-siRNA, closed triangle: naked Chol/Cy5-siRNA, open circle: Chol-free/Cy5-siRNA micelles, and closed circle: Chol/Cy5-siRNA micelles). Data represent the average value (n = 3). (Reprinted with permission from Ref. [105]. Copyright (2014) Elsevier.)

based on cholesterol-conjugated siRNA (chol-siRNA) and PEG-poly(L-lysine) block-co-polymer (PEG-PLL) modified with 1-(3-mercaptopropyl)amidine (MPA), where the micelles were stabilized by disulfide cross-linking of the polymer and hydrophobic association of cholesterol groups [105]. siRNA was fluorescently labeled by conjugating Cy5 dye to 5′ end of the anti-sense strand, and the blood level of siRNA was measured by intravital real-time confocal laser scanning imaging (IVRT-CLSM) [105,106]. Unmodified siRNA (chol-free siRNA) loaded in PEG-PLL (MPA) micelles was rapidly eliminated from circulation, similar to naked siRNA, with a blood $t_{1/2}$ less than 5 min, indicating that disulfide cross-linking of polymer alone did not stabilize the siRNA/micelle complexes. In contrast, micelles containing chol-siRNA showed a $t_{1/2}$ longer than 20 min, which indicated the contribution of cholesterol to the stability of the complex (Figure 12.3) [105].

One caveat of using labeled siRNA in PK studies is that the labeled siRNA can be catabolized and misrepresent siRNA. Moreover, the labeling can cause structural modification in siRNA and change its PK and BD. For example, siRNA labeled with ^{111}In via conjugation to 3′ end [107] and siRNA labeled with 3H through internal substitution [108] showed different PK and BD profiles. The former showed predominantly high distribution in the kidney and low distribution in the liver compared to other organs, but the latter showed high distribution in the salivary gland, spleen, and liver, in addition to the kidney 1 h after administration [107,108].

To overcome such challenges, the amount of siRNA circulating or accumulating in tissues of interest has been determined by other analytical means such as Northern blotting [109], mass spectrometry, and qRT-PCR [37], which can selectively detect full-length siRNA. Swart et al. compared PK profiles of ³H-labeled siRNA with [110] and without a lipid nanoparticle (LNP) vehicle [108] after IV injection. Both free siRNA and LNP-complexed siRNA

showed a multi-exponential decrease in the concentration of total radiolabeled components with, however, vastly different elimination half-lives: 10 min for free siRNA and 162 h for siRNA/LNP complex [108,110]. Mass spectrometric profiling of metabolites in plasma, urine, and tissues found that free siRNAs were rapidly metabolized and distributed to tissues as low-molecular-weight metabolites [108]. In contrast, when injected as a siRNA/LNP complex, the guide strand of 3H-siRNA was detectable in plasma up to 48 and 168-h post-dose, as measured by LC–MS – radioactivity (RA) and RTqPCR, respectively, with a C_{max} of 1.04 µM (LC–MS–RA) or 2.56 µM (RT-qPCR) after 1 h [110]. LC–MS–RA analysis found siRNA degradation products (14–18 mers) as the predominant component of total radioactivity in plasma but did not detect complete degradation products, which indicates the LNP formulation protected siRNA from metabolism at least partly [110].

12.3.2 CLINICAL STUDIES

QPI-1002 was the first siRNA therapeutic systemically delivered to human [111]. QPI-1002 was a siRNA targeting proapoptotic protein p53, developed for the prevention of delayed graft function in patients receiving kidney transplantation. Since the target organ (kidney) was the natural destination of siRNA, it was administered as free siRNA without a carrier [111]. QPI-1002 completed Phase II trials in 2014, but its PK results are not available.

Clinical PK data for siRNA–lipid complex have been reported recently. ALN-VSP was LNPs (also known as SNALPs, stable nucleic acid–lipid particles) containing VEGF-A and kinesin spindle protein siRNAs, with a size of 80–100 nm and a near neutral zeta potential, developed for the treatment of advanced cancer and liver metastases [112]. ALNVSP was administered as 15-min IV infusion, and blood levels of total and unencapsulated siRNA were determined by the hybridization ELISA method and analyzed by non-compartmental method. The C_{max} and AUC were similar for both siRNAs and dose-dependent. Most siRNA circulated as LNP according to the comparison between total and free siRNA, and the level declined to a plateau in 6–7 h [112]. Another lipid-based siRNA tested in human was Atu027, a siRNA targeting protein kinase N3 (PKN3) carried by cationic LNPs, developed for the therapy of primary tumors and metastases [113]. Atu 027 was given as IV infusion for 4 h and analyzed with ELISA detecting single-strand RNA. The blood level increased during the infusion period and declined after the end of infusion. The siRNA level declined more rapidly than lipid components, which suggests potential dissociation of the complex during circulation.

CALAA-01 was the first polymer-based siRNA therapeutic tested in human for cancer therapy [22]. CALAA-01 consisted of two components: siRNA designed to reduce the expression of the M2 subunit of rib nucleotide reductase (RRM2), a well-established target for cancer therapy, and the carrier component made of cationic cyclodextrin-based polymer (CDP), PEG modified with a terminal adamantane group (ADPEG), and AD-PEG conjugated to human transferrin (AD-PEG-Tf). NPs targeted to transferrin receptors were produced by mixing siRNA and CDP, to which the AD-conjugated polymers were attached via inclusion complex formation [114]. PK studies from Phase I clinical trials with 24 patients were recently reported and compared with data obtained from multi-species animal studies [115]. siRNA in plasma was analyzed by the hybridization-ligation assay, which detected the oligonucleotide via hybridization of complementary template and ligation of signaling probe to the template [116]. The plasma concentrations of siRNA component of CALAA-1 rapidly declined to below the detection limit by 30 min after the end of infusion in most patients, with no apparent accumulation upon multiple dosing (Figure 12.4) [115]. There was a good correlation between AUC and C_{max} of siRNA, which increased linearly with the dose (in mg/kg) [115]. Similar trends were observed in preclinical studies with different animal species including mice, rats, dogs, and monkeys. It is worthwhile to note that CALAA-1 was cleared through the kidney [117], unlike other NP-based therapeutics that undergoes accumulation in the MPS. The authors attributed it to disassembly of siRNA/polymer complex at the kidney glomerular basement membrane but excluded the possibility of disassembly in circulation due to the stability demonstrated in the gel mobility shift assay [117].

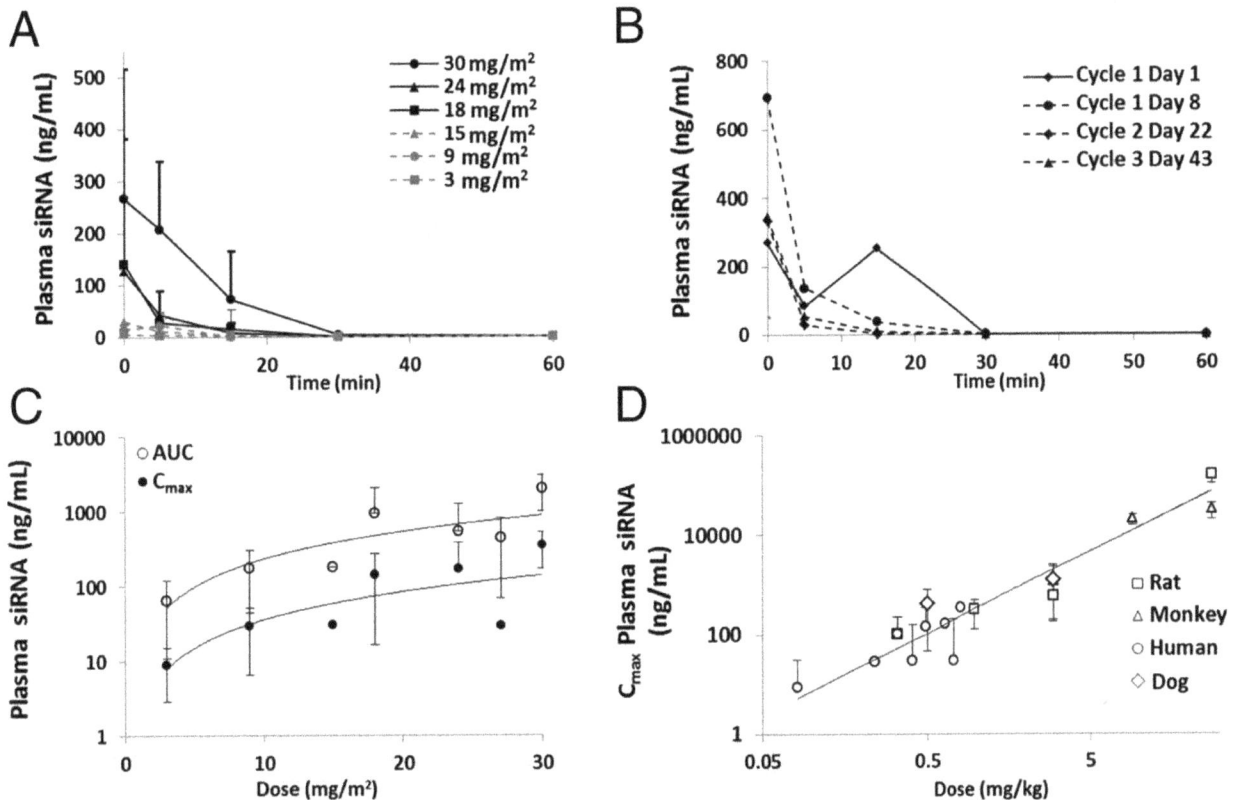

FIGURE 12.4 PK assessment of CALAA-01 in patients and across species. (A) Time course of average plasma concentration of the siRNA component of CALAA-01 following the end of infusion for all dosing cohorts. (B) Time course of plasma CALAA-01 siRNA following the end of infusion from cycles 1–3 of CALAA-01 from one patient who received 30 mg/m² CALAA-01. Plasma concentration curves are similar at each cycle. Lines connecting data points are guides for the eye only. (C) AUC and C_{max} relationship to dose in humans. (D) Scaling of CALAA-01 C_{max} across four different species (Reprinted with permission from Ref. [115].)

12.4 BIODISTRIBUTION OF siRNA THERAPEUTICS

Similar to PK studies, siRNA BD is studied by tracking surrogate signals of fluorescent dyes or radioactive elements incorporated in siRNA or siRNA itself via PCR. Less frequently, NP carriers are tracked in lieu of siRNA under an assumption that the NPs represent the siRNA BD. Many BD studies are performed in animal models with solid xenograft tumors. siRNA stably encapsulated in NPs shows increased tumor accumulation as compared to naked siRNA to some extent, due to the increased circulation $t_{1/2}$ and the enhanced permeability and retention (EPR) effect common in solid tumors. However, the majority of the injected dose ends up in organs where the MPS is located, including the spleen, liver, and lung.

12.4.1 TRACKING siRNA LABELED WITH FLUORESCENT DYES

Huang et al. used a liposome–polycation–hyaluronic acid (LPH) NP system decorated with GC4-single-chain variable fragment (scFv) for systemic delivery of a combination of siRNAs [34]. FITC-labeled siRNA was first complexed with protamine in the presence of hyaluronic acid (HA), combined with cationic liposomes, and injected IV to mice bearing experimental lung metastasis. At 4h after IV injection, major organs were collected and lysed to yield supernatants, of which fluorescence intensity was determined to represent the level of siRNA. With free siRNAs, most fluorescence signals were seen in the liver. siRNA carried by LPH NPs showed similar BD as free siRNA, except for three times stronger intensity in tumors [34]. This group used a similar NP system based on a liposome–polycation–DNA (LPD) with PEGylated Asn-Gly-Arg peptide (PEG-NGR) as a targeting ligand for the delivery of doxorubicin and siRNA combination [118]. At 4-h post-injection, the fluorescent signals of siRNA and doxorubicin delivered as LPD-PEGNGR NPs were mainly detected in tumor, followed by the liver and the kidney, whereas free siRNA was mainly seen in the liver and the kidney and free doxorubicin was broadly seen in the tumor, liver, kidney, spleen, and heart, respectively (Figure 12.5) [118].

A CD44-targeted, inorganic siRNA delivery system was prepared by combining calcium phosphate (CaP)–siRNA complex and 3,4-dihydroxy-L-phenylalanine (dopa)-conjugated HA [119]. This system took advantage of the ability of CaP to co-precipitate with siRNA and form condensed NPs, dopa to bind to the CaP crystals, and HA to prevent the growth of crystal size and to target CD44 and CD168 (also known as Receptor for Hyaluronan Mediated Motility overexpressed in various cancer cells [119]. The CaP/Cy5.5-labeled siRNA/dopa-HA NPs were administered IV in nude mice bearing HT29-luc tumors. *Ex vivo* imaging after 4h showed relatively high accumulation of

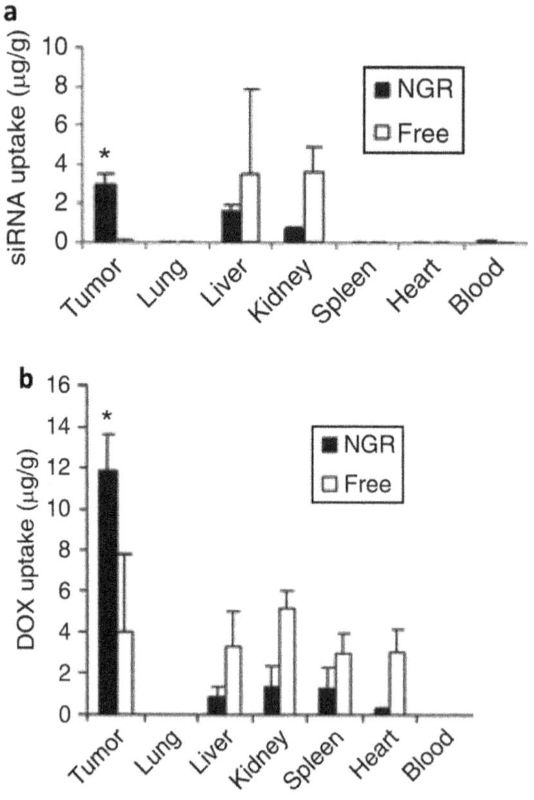

FIGURE 12.5 Tissue distribution of FITC-siRNA (a) and DOX (b) delivered with LPD-PEG-NGR (NGR). Data=mean±SD, n=3. *p<0.05 compared with free siRNA or DOX (Free). (Reprinted with permission from Ref. [118]. Copyright (2010) Nature Publishing Group.)

the NPs in the tumor and the liver but no significant signals in the spleen and the lung (Figure 12.6). The accumulation of CaP/siRNA/dopa-HA in the liver was attributed to the presence of the HA receptor in hepatocytes. Without dopa-HA, CaP/siRNA formed particles as large as N4 μm, which were captured predominantly by the liver, most likely due to the size [119].

CaP was also used to stabilize polymeric micelles [120]. siRNA was first encapsulated in micelles of PEG-conjugated polyaspartamide derivative (poly[N'-[N-(20aminoethyl)-2-aminoethyl]aspartamide]) and stabilized with CaP complexation [120]. BD of siRNA was examined by tracing the fluorescence of Alexa Fluor 647-labeled siRNA in transgenic mice with spontaneous pancreatic tumors. At 6h after injection of the hybrid micelles, 0.9% and 1.5% of the injected siRNA were found in each gram of pancreas/tumor and kidney, respectively, which corresponded to six times (pancreas/tumor) and half (kidney) the levels of naked siRNA, with no significant difference in other organs [120]. The siRNA/micelles accumulated in tumors achieved 61% reporter gene silencing at 24h after injection, whereas scrambled siRNA/micelles had no effect [120].

A hybrid of cationic lipid and polymer NPs was used for the delivery of CDK1 siRNA for the therapy of triple negative breast cancer (TNBC) [38]. siRNA was encapsulated in PLA-PEG block-co-polymer by the double emulsion method. Here, cationic cholesterol derivative was included in the organic phase to help condense siRNA in the NPs. Upon IV administration to SUM149 tumor bearing mice, Cy5-siRNA encapsulated in NPs showed persistent signals in the tumor, liver, spleen, and kidney up to 72-h post-injection, whereas free Cy5-siRNA was barely seen at 12h after injection [38]. At a dose of 2 mg/kg every other day, CDK siRNA/NP system suppressed the growth of SUM149

and BT549 xenograft tumors, an effect comparable to 50 mg/kg dinaciclib (a known CDK1 inhibitor), whereas neither free CDK1 siRNA nor scrambled siRNA in NPs was effective. Real-time PCR and Western blot of tumor tissues found that CDK1 siRNA-loaded NPs suppressed the levels of CDK1 mRNA and CDK1 protein expression levels, respectively, confirming that the tumor suppression was mediated by CDK1 silencing in tumors [38].

To enhance the formation and stability of siRNA–carrier complex, Kim et al. used a polymerized siRNA (poly-siRNA), where several siRNA molecules were linked to one another via disulfide bond, and thiolated human serum albumin (tHSA), which formed a stable complex with the poly-siRNA via intermolecular disulfide cross-linking [121]. The poly-siRNA/tHSA complex was systemically delivered to mice bearing squamous cell carcinoma (SCC7) and human prostatic carcinoma (PC-3) tumors. siRNA was labeled with Cy5.5 fluorescence dye, and the fluorescence intensity of each organ was measured by *ex vivo* imaging [121]. Overall, poly-siRNA/tHSA complex showed a stronger fluorescence signal throughout the whole body than free poly-siRNA, indicating relatively good stability of poly-siRNA/tHSA NPs [121]. *Ex vivo* imaging of organs at 24h after IV injection revealed that animals treated with naked poly-siRNA had relatively high fluorescence intensity in the liver, kidney, and tumor, whereas those treated with poly-siRNA–tHSA complex did predominantly in tumors [121]. Consistently, poly-VEGF siRNA/tHSA showed superior anti-cancer effects to that of a complex containing poly-scrambled siRNA through inhibition of tumor angiogenesis [121]. This group later replaced tHSA with thiolated glycol chitosan (tGC) for the delivery of poly-siRNA and observed a similar pattern—relatively high fluorescence level in tumor as compared to that of naked poly-siRNA [40].

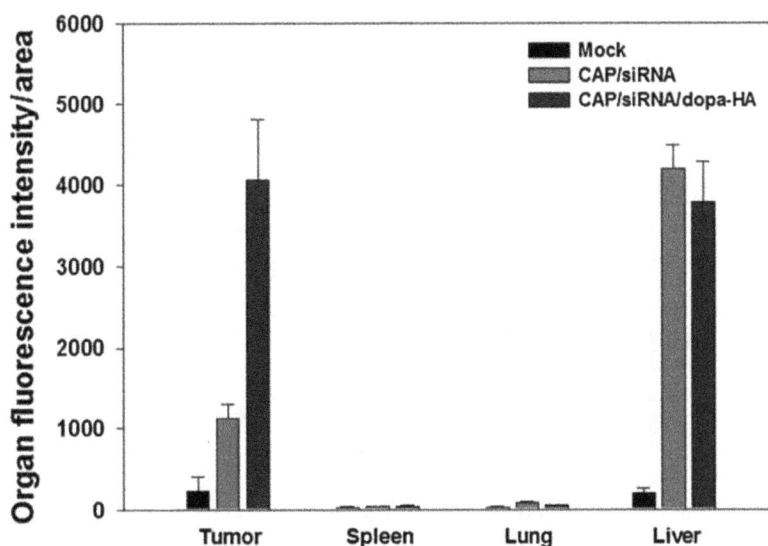

FIGURE 12.6 Normalized organ distribution of Cy5.5-siRNA delivered by CAP/siRNA and CAP/siRNA/dopa-HA. Normalized organ fluorescence intensity was obtained by dividing the fluorescence intensity of the organ by the area of the organ using image analysis software. (Reprinted with permission from Ref. [119]. Copyright (2014) Elsevier.)

12.4.2 TRACKING RADIOLABELED siRNA

BD of the CDP-based siRNA NPs (discussed in Section 12.3.2) was evaluated using siRNA labeled with ^{64}Cu and positron emission tomography (PET)–computer tomography (CT) *in vivo* imaging [114]. Free ^{64}Cu-DOTA-conjugated siRNA showed rapid blood clearance through liver accumulation (23% ID/cm^3 at 60 min) and kidney filtration followed by the bladder accumulation (73% ID/cm^3 at 60 min). ^{64}Cu-DOTAsiRNA packaged in transferrin receptor (TfR)-targeted CDP NPs showed similar BD to

that of naked ^{64}Cu-DOTA-siRNA, except for slightly higher liver accumulation (26% ID/cm^3 at 60 min) and a delayed peak in kidney accumulation [114]. In both cases, percentage injected dose per cm^3 tumor was no higher than 2%.

Swart et al. used 3H-labeled siRNA to study BD of siRNA delivered with LNPs [110]. BD of siRNA/LNPs was estimated by quantitative whole-body autoradiography (QWBA) and matrix-assisted laser desorption ionization mass spectrometry imaging (MALDI-MSI) techniques, where QWBA measured the radiolabeled siRNA and

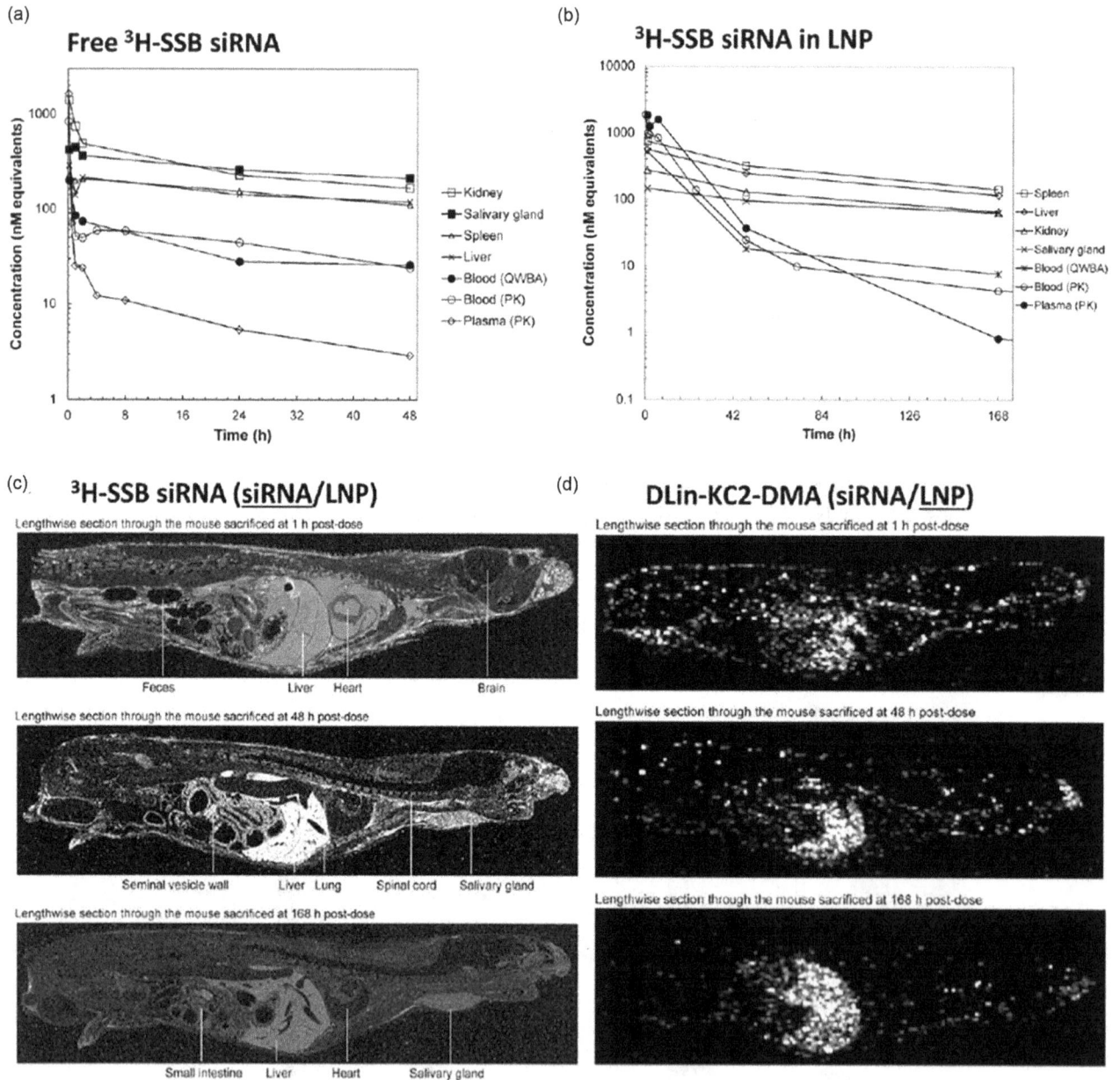

FIGURE 12.7 (a) Concentration–time profiles of radiolabeled naked 3H-SSB siRNA in dried blood, plasma, and selected tissues [108]; (b) concentration–time profiles of radiolabeled ^{3}H-SSB siRNA in LNP in dried blood, plasma, and selected tissues; (c) selected whole-body autoradioluminographs and (d) selected whole-body MALDI-MS images at 1, 48, and 168 h [110] after a single IV administration of free ^{3}H-SSB siRNA (5mg/kg siRNA) or [^{3}H]-SBB siRNA in LNP vehicle (2.5 mg/kg siRNA) to male CD-1 mice. In (c), the whitest area corresponds to the highest concentration of radiolabeled siRNA. In (d), the whitest area corresponds to the highest concentration of DLin-KC2-DMA (one of the main components of the LNP vehicle). (Reprinted from Refs. [108,110]. Copyright (2013, 2014) The American Society for Pharmacology and Experimental Therapeutics.)

MALDI-MSI measured the cationic lipid component. Following a single IV administration, animals treated with free siRNA showed the highest radioactivity in kidney and salivary gland, and the radioactivity in different organs declined in a similar pattern (Figure 12.7a) [108]. In contrast, animals treated with siRNA/LNPs showed the highest radioactivity of siRNA in the spleen and liver, which lasted over 168 h, whereas the blood level radioactivity gradually decreased (Figure 12.7b) [110]. MALDI-MSI found similar distribution of the cationic lipid as that of siRNA radioactivity, suggesting that siRNA and lipid circulated together and co-distributed as a LNP complex (Figure 12.7c and d).

Harashima et al. evaluated the BD of siRNA delivered with MEND by tracking siRNA and the carrier separately [37]. Here, siRNA was labeled with ^{32}P and the carrier with ^{3}H. Both siRNA and the carrier showed significant increase in tumor accumulation with PEGylation of the MEND. According to the radioactivity measurement, the levels of tumor accumulation of siRNA delivered with MEND and PEG-MEND were 3.0% ID/g of tumor and 5.1% ID/g of tumor, respectively. On the other hand, when measured by the stem-loop primer-mediated qRTPCR, which measured full-length siRNA, the values were much lower: 0.0079% ID/g tumor (siRNA by MEND) and 1.9% ID/g tumor (siRNA by PEG-MEND). ^{32}P-labeled siRNA showed differential organ distribution according to the delivery methods (free, MEND, PEG-MEND) (Figure 12.8a). It is worthy to note that the radioactivity of free siRNA was detected in the liver, spleen, kidney, and lung 6 h after injection, but the stem-loop qRT-PCR did not detect siRNA in any of these organs (Figure 12.8b). This discrepancy strongly suggests that the radioactivity measurement may have overestimated the amount of siRNA by counting catabolites of the labeled siRNA as well. BD of siRNA indeed coincided better with that of carriers when measured with the stem-loop qRT-PCR [37].

12.4.3 Tracking siRNA Itself

With the notion that the labeled siRNA may be degraded to inactive catabolizes, alternative methods are used to detect siRNA itself instead of labels. For example, Northern blotting was used to determine the integrity of siRNA and complement quantitative measurement based on radioactivity

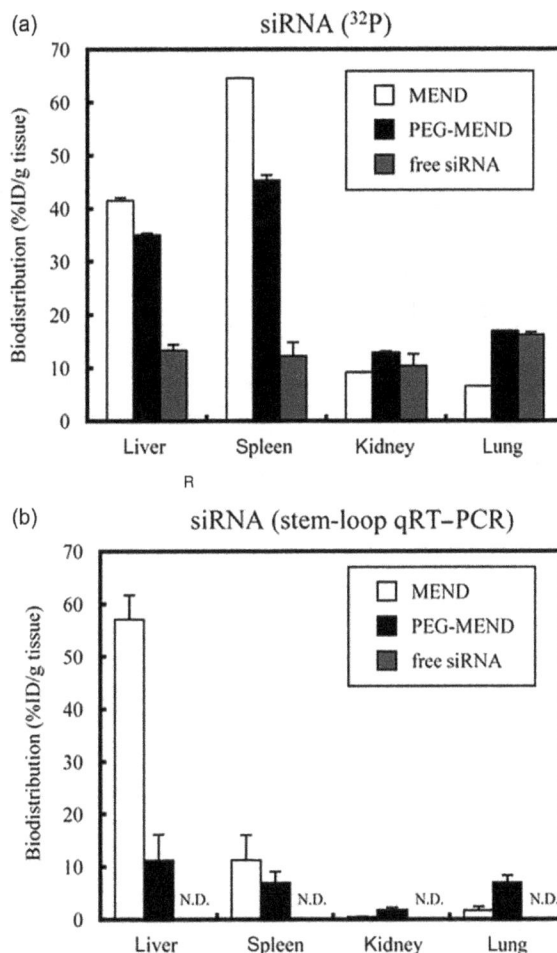

FIGURE 12.8 Comparison of the methodology between radioisotope and stem-loop qRT-PCR methods. Accumulations in liver, spleen, kidney, and lung 6 h after injection were measured by the two methodologies. Free siRNA and formulated siRNA in these organs were determined by using radioisotope (a) and stem-loop qRT-PCR method (b). N.D.: not detected. (Reprinted from Ref. [37]. Copyright (2013) Nature Publishing Group.)

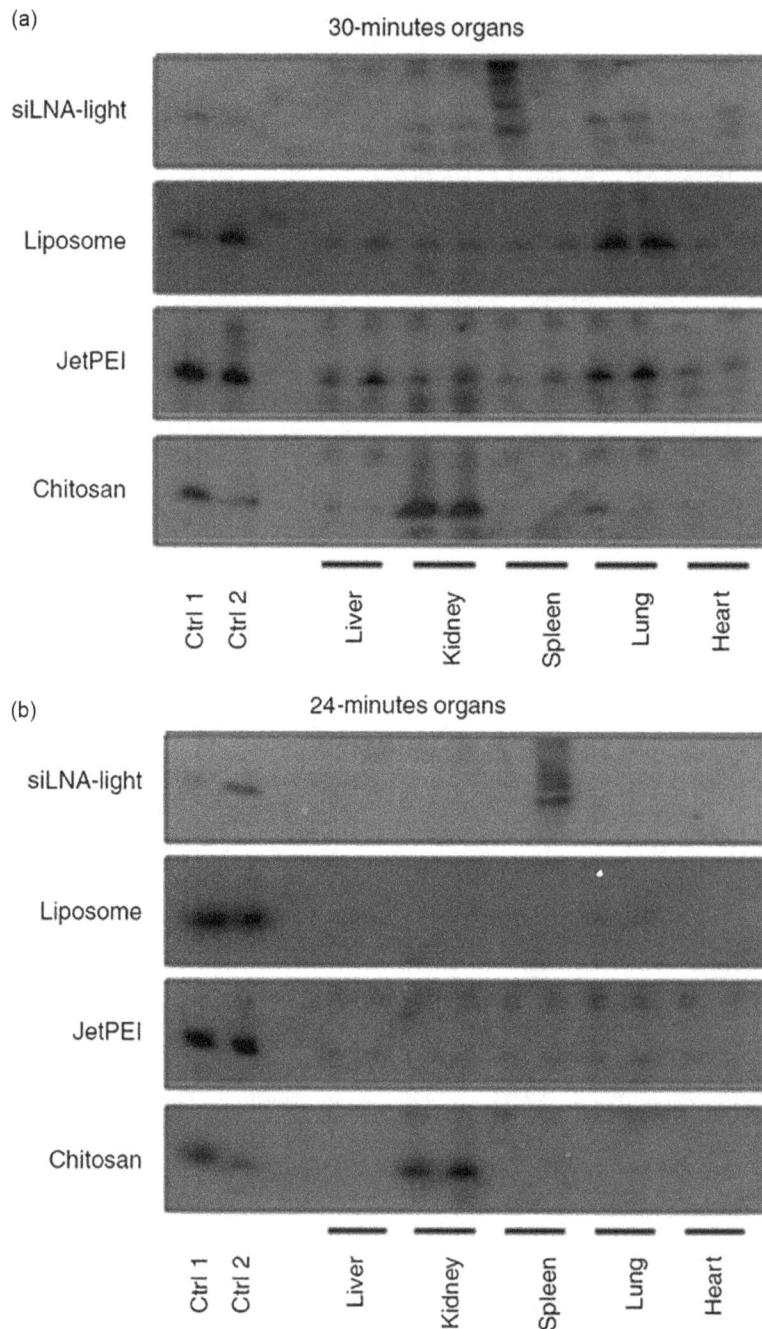

FIGURE 12.9 Organ distribution of siRNA delivered with different carriers at 30 min (a) or 24 h (b) after IV injection, analyzed with Northern blotting. Lane 1: 1.5-ng duplexes (Ctrl 1); lane 2: 1-ng siRNA/NP complex (Ctrl 2); lane 3: blank; lanes 4–13: duplexes or siRNA/NP complex in organs. Ctrl, control; LNA, locked nucleic acid; siLNA, LNA-modified siRNA; siLNA-light, lightly LNA-modified siRNA. (Reprinted with permission from Ref. [109]. Copyright (2009) Nature Publishing Group.)

counting [109]. Various formulations including chitosan, liposome, or JetPEI NPs were injected intravenously into mice as complexes with ^{32}P-labeled siRNA. The radioactivity measurement found that liposomal formulation increased the accumulation of siRNA in the lung five- to ten-fold higher than other organs (Figure 12.9a), with 5% of 30-min levels still present at 24 h (Figure 12.9b). Similarly, JetPEI/siRNA complex showed greater levels in the lung (two- to ten-fold) than in the other organs (Figure 12.9a). On the other hand, chitosan/siRNA complex showed different

organ distribution patterns with pronounced accumulation in the kidney (Figure 12.9a). The Northern blotting analysis with total RNA extracted from tissues showed consistent patterns over 24 h, confirming the validity of radioactive label as a marker of intact siRNA [109].

Alternatively, qPCR was employed to study BD of siRNA delivered with LNP [122]. Seven organs of interest were collected at different time points, and the level of siRNA was measured with the stem-loop qPCR. At 0.5 and 2-h post-IV injection, the siRNA levels were highest in the liver, followed by the spleen and kidney, with little in the lung and heart, and almost none in the duodenum and brain. Reflecting the siRNA distribution, the greatest level of target mRNA knockdown was observed in the liver (85%) and spleen (25%), with no detectable knockdown in the lung, kidney, heart, duodenum, or brain [122].

12.4.4 Tracking Carriers

Carrier concentrations in tissues are sometimes measured as an indirect measure of siRNA distribution. Chen et al. developed a new carrier of siRNA based on HA, hydrophobically modified for self-assembly formation, conjugated with a phosphate receptor Zn (II)-dipicolylamine (DPA/Zn) for RNA binding, and stabilized with CaP surface layer [123]. BD of the siRNA/carrier assembly (CaP-HDz/siLuc-NFs) was studied by tracking Cy5.5-labeled carriers in a human colon cancer (HCT116) xenograft mouse model. From 3-h post-administration, tumors showed strong fluorescence,

which reached the maximum at 6-h and lasted until 48-h post-injection (Figure 12.10a). *Ex vivo* images exhibited consistently strong fluorescence intensities in tumors. Noticeable fluorescence signal was also found in the liver, lung, and kidney at 48h after injection (Figure 12.10b). As an indirect measure of the siRNA integrity, a model siRNA silencing the luciferase-expressing gene (siLuc) was delivered with the CaP-HDz carrier, showing 79.4% reduction of luminescence signal in tumor (Figure 12.10c and d).

Mirkin et al. developed spherical nucleic acid (SNA) gold NP conjugates as a carrier of siRNA, where siRNA duplexes were conjugated to an inorganic gold NP core via thiol–gold bond, forming densely packed, highly oriented nucleic acid corona around the core [124]. BD of SNA particles was evaluated in glioblastoma multi-forme (GBM)-bearing mice based on the level of Au in the tissue by ICP-MS. Similar to other siRNA delivery systems, most Au was detected in the liver and spleen after 24h, and 1% of the total SNA injected was found in the brain tumor. The

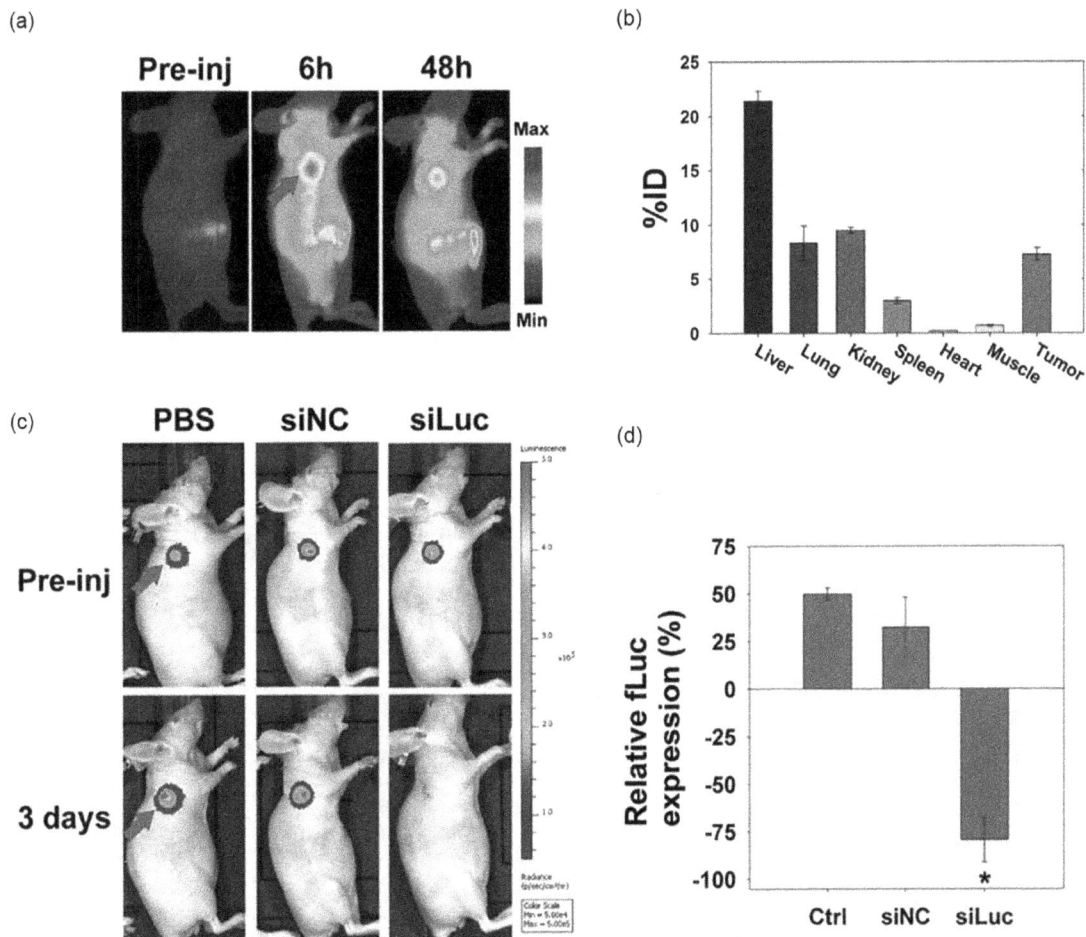

FIGURE 12.10 *In vivo* monitoring of tumor-targeting and gene silencing effect of CaP-HDz/siRNA-NFs. (a) *In vivo* near-infrared fluorescence (NIRF) imaging of HCT116 tumor-bearing mice systemically administered with CaP-HDz/siLuc-NFs labeled with Cy5.5. (b) Quantitative analysis of fluorescence intensities at the major organs and tumor tissues of mice treated with CaP-HDz/siLuc-NFs labeled with Cy5.5 48h after IV injection. (c) *In vivo* bioluminescence imaging (BLI) of fLuc gene expression in fLuc-expressing HCT116 tumor-bearing mice intravenously injected with PBS, free siLuc, or CaP-HDz/siLuc-NFs (280μL; RNA=700pmol). (d) Quantitative analysis of fLuc expression at tumors after IV injection of CaPHDz/siLuc-NFs into the fLuc-expressing HCT116 tumor mice (n=4). Red arrow indicates tumor site; *p<0.005 vs. control or siNC. (Reprinted with permission from Ref. [123].)

delivery of intact siRNA was confirmed by evaluating the silencing effect of siRNA targeting Bcl2Like12 (Bcl2L12) oncogene and survival of GBM-bearing mice [124].

BD of M-MSN (discussed in Section 12.3.1), containing iron in the core, was studied by measuring the iron level in organs by atomic absorption analysis [31]. M-MSN NPs loaded with siRNA were injected to A549 lung cancer

bearing mice. One day after injection, 10% of the total administered NPs accumulated in the tumor, and ~4% remained after 3 days. The highest iron concentration was found in the liver (~27% ID/g), followed by the lung (~15% ID/g), spleen (~14% ID/g), and kidney (~4% ID/g) after 24 h (Figure 12.11a). Separate tracking of the fluorescently labeled siRNA loaded in M-MSN revealed that the

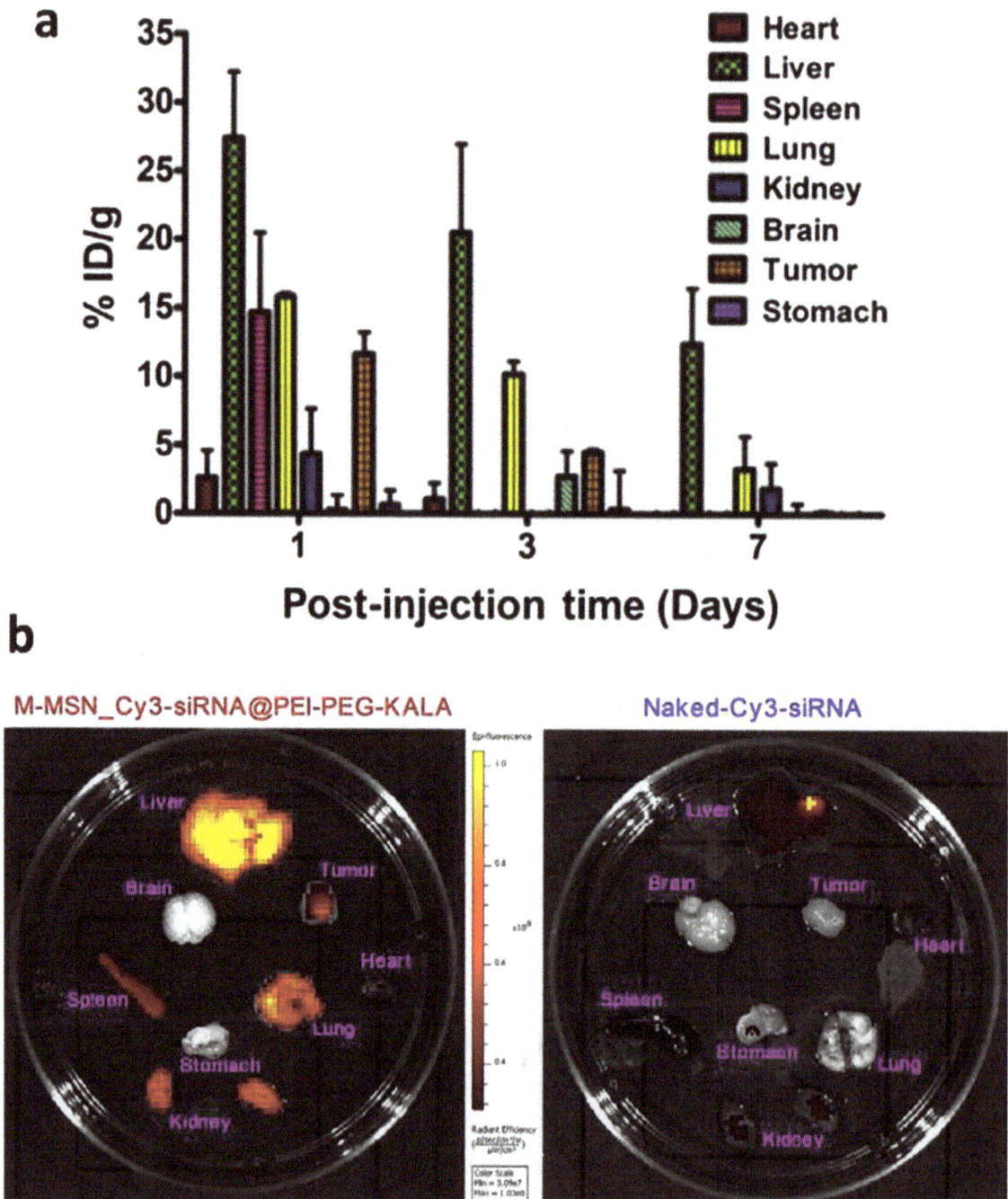

FIGURE 12.11 (a) Distribution profile of M-MSN_NC siRNA@PEI-PEG-KALA in tumor and various organs of tumor-bearing mice after tail vein administration. The % of NP distribution was determined from measurement of Fe element content at different time points (1, 3, 7 days after particle injection), subtracting the basal Fe content of tumor bearing mice without particle injection (n=3). (b) Fluorescence images of excised mouse organs (heart, liver, spleen, lung, kidney, brain, tumor, and stomach) 24 h after injection of M-MSN_Cy3-siRNA@ PEI-PEG-KALA (left), naked-Cy3-siRNA (right) using an IVIS spectrum with excitation and emission wavelengths of 554/568 nm. (Reprinted with permission from Ref. [31]. Copyright (2014) Elsevier.)

carrier distribution was consistent with siRNA distribution, which was significantly higher than that of free siRNA. Fluorescence images of excised mouse organs (brain, tumor, spleen, lung, kidney, heart, stomach, and liver) obtained 24h after injection of the NPs showed relatively high siRNA accumulation in the liver, lung, spleen, kidney as well as in tumor. In contrast, organs from the animals receiving free siRNA showed little fluorescence except for the liver and kidney (Figure 12.11b) [31].

Tracking carriers may serve as a surrogate of siRNA in a BD study if siRNA and carriers remain stable in circulation, but this may not be always a valid assumption. Escriou et al. tracked carriers and siRNA, separately labeled with distinct fluorescent dyes, and found different BD patterns [125]. They used liposomes containing cationic lipid (DOPE) and an anionic polymer (polyglutamate, PG) as a complexation aid and studied the effect of PG on BD of the complexes in

the lung and liver. The tissue level of lipid remained constant irrespective of the presence of PG (Figure 12.12a). However, siRNA level increased by two- to three-folds with PG (Figure 12.12b), which was interpreted as a consequence of the enhanced stability of the PG-containing complexes [125]. The conclusion would have been different if they measured the level of carriers only.

12.4.5 TARGETED VS. NON-TARGETED

One notable trend observed with the so-called targeted gene carriers is that the targeting ligands seemed to play a minimal role in changing initial BD of siRNA. The dual-stabilized polymeric micelles, discussed in Section 12.3.1, were further decorated with cyclic RGD (cRGD) peptide ligands for tumor-targeting [105]. *Ex vivo* organ imaging at 4h after IV injection found that BD of Cy5-labeled siRNA

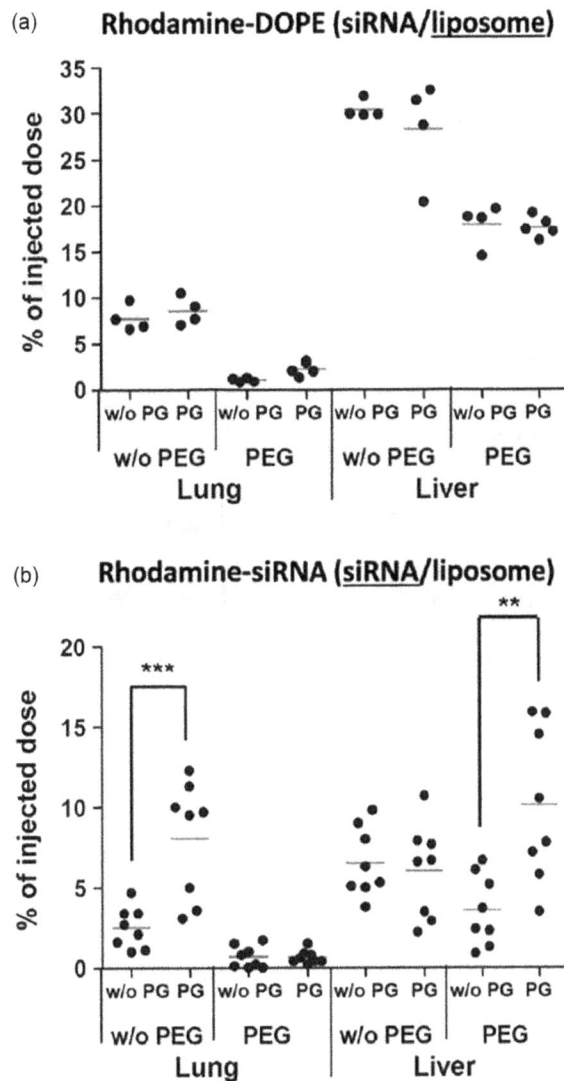

FIGURE 12.12 Lipoplexes recovery after IV injection. siRNA lipoplexes, formed with or without PG at a charge ratio of 8, were labeled with fluorescent lipid (a, 5% rhodamine-DOPE incorporated in cationic liposome) or with fluorescent siRNA (b, 5′ rhodamine-labeled siRNA used to form siRNA lipoplexes) and IV injected (10 μg siRNA/mouse). Two hours post-injection, lung and liver were removed and fluorescent lipid (a) or fluorescent siRNA (b) was extracted and quantified; n=4 (a) or n=8 (b), **p<0.005; ***p<0.002. (Reprinted with permission from Ref. [125]. Copyright (2011) Elsevier.)

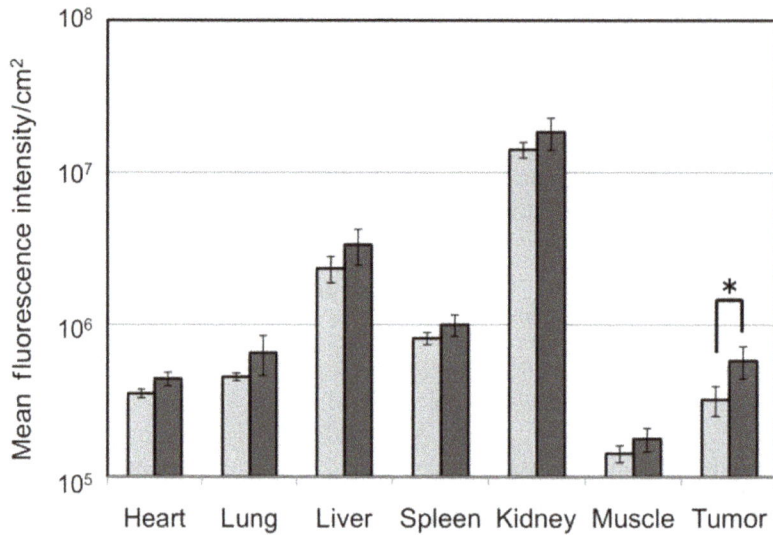

FIGURE 12.13   BD of non-targeted (gray bars) or actively targeted (black bars) Chol/Cy5-siRNA micelles (1.8 nmol siRNA/mouse) at 4 h after IV injection via tail vein of BALB/c nude mice. (Reprinted with permission from Ref. [105]. Copyright (2014) Elsevier.)

fluorescence was similar between non-targeted and targeted micelles, with the majority of signals found in the kidney and liver. A difference attributable to cRGD was seen as slight increase in tumor accumulation (Figure 12.13) [105].

A comparable observation was made in an earlier study with TfR-targeted CDP-based NPs (discussed in Section 12.3.2), where both non-targeted and targeted NPs showed similar BD and tumor localization of siRNA (Figure 12.14)

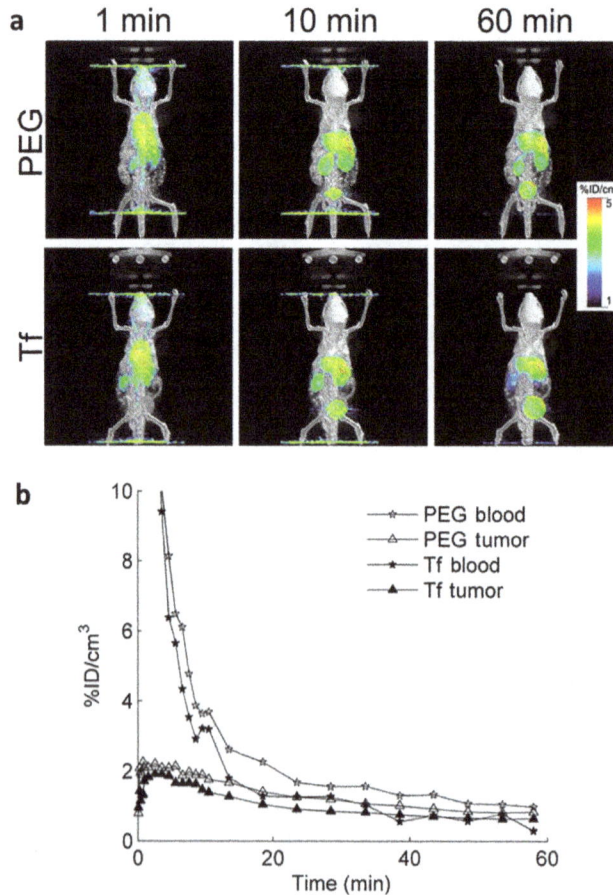

FIGURE 12.14   Tissue distribution of ^{64}Cu-DOTA-siRNA delivered by targeted (Tf) and non-targeted (PEG) NPs. (a) Fused micro-PET/CT images of mice at 1, 10, and 60 min after injection. (b) Blood clearance and tumor localization of Tf-targeted and non-targeted siRNA NPs. (Reprinted with permission from Ref. [114]. Copyright (2007) National Academy of Sciences, USA.)

[114]. Despite the similarity in BD, siRNA delivered with TfR-targeted NPs showed 50% greater gene silencing effect than non-targeted NPs, indicating more efficient entry of the targeted NPs into tumor cells [114]. This study suggests that the contribution of a targeting molecule is to facilitate cellular uptake of the NPs rather than to actively guide the NPs to the target tissues as the name implies [114]. On the other hand, other studies show the increase in overall tumor localization of targeted NPs [126,127]. In interpreting those studies, it will be worthwhile to consider that the increased tumor accumulation is likely a net result of the EPR-driven extravasation of NPs (initial BD: targeted ≈ non-targeted) and efficient cellular uptake and retention at target cells (targeted > non-targeted).

12.5 PHARMACOLOGICAL EFFECTS OF siRNA THERAPEUTICS

Due to the favorable BD of siRNA delivery systems, the liver and lung are among the primary targets of siRNA therapeutics. This section provides a brief overview of recent preclinical studies on pharmacological effects of siRNA therapeutics in liver and lung diseases.

12.5.1 LIVER DISEASES

12.5.1.1 HCC

Initial efforts to treat HCC with siRNA involved free siRNA injection. siRNA targeting VEGF expression in hepatoma and endothelial cells with no specific carrier system was tested in a murine orthotopic hepatoma model [61]. Animals were injected with 200 µg/kg of siRNAVEGF intraperitoneally, every 2 days for 14 days starting from 24 h prior to tumor cell inoculation. When determined terminally, tumor burden was reduced by 63% [61]. The anti-tumor efficacy was attributed to the inhibition of tumor angiogenesis, corresponding to intratumoral microvessel density [61]. Similarly, siRNA targeting anti-apoptotic protein heme oxygenase 1 (HO-1) was intraperitoneally injected to immune-competent mice bearing HO-1+ Hepa129 tumors in the liver and reduced tumor growth by 50% with no damages in normal organs [128]. The authors [129] attributed this effect to proapoptotic and possibly anti-angiogenic activity of siHO-1 [128].

For improving siRNA delivery to the liver and HCC, NPs based on cationic lipid such as 1,2-dioleyloxy-3-trimethylammonium propane (DOTAP) are widely used as a carrier of siRNA. Schmitz et al. made a complex of VEGF-targeting siRNA with DOTAP and injected the complex intraperitoneally multiple times to mice with pre-existing liver fibrosis as well as orthotopic HCC (Hepa129 cells injected to the left liver lobe) [130]. The VEGF-siRNA/DOTAP complexes resulted in significant reduction in the number of HCC satellites in the liver (82% mice had < 30 satellites), whereas free VEGF-siRNA and control siRNA had a minimal effect (22.1% and 12.5% mice

with < 30 satellites, respectively). DOTAP helped VEGF-siRNA enter HCC satellites and silence VEGF expression in hepatic tissues. However, the effect of the internalized VEGF-siRNA–DOTAP complex on tumors was more likely through immune activation via interferon-1 upregulation than VEGF silencing [130]. In fact, intratumoral VEGF expression was not reduced by VEGF-siRNA/DOTAP complexes but rather increased [130]. More recently, Shen et al. screened several lipid NPs for optimal siRNA delivery to HCC and identified a combination of lipids that showed significant anti-tumor effect with cancer-targeting siRNAs [131]. An interesting note in this study is that good *in vitro* transfection efficiency did not necessarily translate to good *in vivo* silencing effect in orthotopic HCC tumors, which indicates the significance of circulation stability of gene–carrier complexes [131].

To further improve cell specificity of siRNA delivery, cell-interactive ligands have been added to the carrier. For example, a model siRNA was encapsulated in PEGylated DOTAP-based immunoliposomes decorated with anti-EGFR Fab' [132]. A BD study in an orthotopic mouse model of HCC showed that the immunoliposomes accumulated in the liver and were taken up by HCC cells to greater extents than non-targeted liposomes, achieving higher silencing effect on the model luciferase gene expression [132]. This system was later used for the co-delivery of doxorubicin and siRNA targeting RRM2, a gene important for DNA synthesis and repair and highly expressed in HCC [126]. The siRNA and drug delivered with immunoliposomes showed 50%–60% ID/g in the HCC tumors, compared to 20%–30% ID/g of non-targeted liposomes, 8 h after injection. Accordingly, animals treated with siRNA-RRM2 and doxorubicin in immunoliposomes showed the most significant retardation of tumor growth, compared to those receiving each treatment or dual loads in non-targeted liposomes [126].

12.5.1.2 Liver Infections

Due to the preferable BD in the liver, hepatitis infections like HBV and HCV were one of the earliest targets of siRNA therapeutics. For example, siRNA targeting the S region of HBV RNA was delivered with SNALPs based on a mixture of cationic and fusogenic lipids [133,134]. Here, 2'-OH of siRNA was chemically modified to increase the resistance against nucleases [133]. IV-injected SNALP particles were accumulated predominantly in the liver (28%) with minimal accumulation in other organs (8.2% in spleen and 0.3% in the lung, respectively) 24 h after injection [133]. Reflecting the high liver accumulation, siRNA delivered with SNALPs achieved a significant reduction of the level of HBV DNA copies and HBsAg proteins for 7 days after dosing [133]. In another case, siRNAs targeting HBV transcript sites 1407 or 1794 were delivered with lipid assemblies based on three different lipids, including one conjugated to PEG2000 by oxime linkages, which could be cleaved at pH lower than 5.5 [78]. A BD study with the radiolabeled assemblies found that regardless of the PEG concentration in the formulation, most of the dose (>50%) was detected in the liver after 1-h post-injection, and other organs such as spleen, kidney, blood, and lung showed minimal accumulation of the particles. Accordingly, HBV transgenic mice receiving the siRNA-lipid assemblies showed significant reduction in HBV replication, indicated by the reduced levels of HBV mRNA and HBeAg proteins in the liver and HBsAg in serum, equivalent to daily intra-peritoneal treatment of Lamivudine, a licensed drug for HBV treatment [78]. Later, this group introduced a new cationic lipid DODAG (N′, N′-dioctadecyl-N-4,8-diaza-10-aminodecanoyl-glycylamide) and achieved a similarly effective knockdown of HBV infection [135].

siRNA targeting 5′-UTR of HCV genome was encapsulated in liposomes composed of a cationic lipid, phosphatidylcholine (PC), and lactosylated phosphatidylethanol, which targeted the asialoglycoprotein receptor on hepatocytes [86]. A BD study with a fluorescently labeled (Alexa-568) siRNA in BALB/c mice showed preferential accumulation of siRNA in the liver in 30 min after injection with the lactosylated liposomes, whereas those delivered with non-lactosylated liposomes showed equally strong signals in the spleen and liver [86]. In a pharmacodynamics study with an HCV transgenic mouse model, siRNA targeting 325–344 nucleotides of HCV genome, delivered with the lactosylated liposomes, efficiently suppressed HCV protein expression in a dose-dependent manner 48 h after a single treatment [86]. Similarly, siRNA was incorporated in cationic liposomes (DTC-apo) composed of DOTAP and cholesterol decorated with apolipoprotein A-1, the protein component of high-density lipoprotein (HDL) targeting hepatocytes. A BD study using fluorescently labeled 21-mer dsDNA encapsulated in DTC-apo showed relatively high fluorescence intensity in the liver compared to other organs like kidney, lung, and spleen [89]. Without the apolipoprotein ligand, fluorescence was preferentially seen in the lung and spleen [89]. *In vivo* silencing effect was tested in a HCV mouse model created with hydrodynamic injection of plasmid DNA-expressing viral structural proteins. HCV-specific siRNA/DTC-apo complex inhibited viral gene expression by 65% in the liver at 2 mg/kg siRNA on Day 2 post-administration. The extent and duration of siRNA were further improved by 2′-O-methylmodification of siRNA [89]. Apolipoprotein A-1 was later replaced with a recombinant form of apolipoprotein (rhApo) derived from Escherichia coli to avoid the safety concern (e.g., pathogen contamination) related to the origin (plasma) [136]. In addition to siRNA, synthetic shRNA targeting the IRES of the HCV genome was incorporated in a mixture of lipids to form lipid NPs, showing long-lasting potent efficacy against HCV in mice with minimal toxicity [87].

More recently, it was demonstrated that simple co-injection of a hepatocyte-targeted peptide could help deliver siRNA targeting conserved HBV sequences to the liver [77]. The peptide consisted of N-acetylgalactosamine (NAG), a ligand with high affinity for asialoglycoprotein receptors

highly expressed on the hepatocytes, and melittin-like peptide (MLP), an endosomolytic agent to facilitate endolysosomal escape of siRNA [77]. A co-injection of NAG-MLP with liver-tropic cholesterol-conjugated siRNA increased the hepatic gene silencing effect in a dose-dependent manner, resulting in multi-log repression of viral RNA, proteins, and viral DNA with long duration of effect in mouse models of HBV infection. This formulation is unique in that it does not require pre-formulation of the complex like typical siRNA delivery systems, thus reducing the complexity in large-scale manufacturing. It has recently entered Phase IIa clinical trial for the treatment of chronic HBV infection (NCT02065336) [137].

As one of the primary sites for Ebola virus replication, the liver also serves as a valid target for siRNA therapy of Ebola virus infection. siRNA targeting individual regions of Zaire Ebola virus (ZEBOV) L gene was delivered with SNALPs [92]. Despite the evidence suggesting premature release of siRNA in circulation (differential BD of labeled SNALPs and siRNA), siRNA/SNALPs provided post-exposure protection to guinea pig challenged with a lethal Ebola virus. Animals challenged with ZEBOV received siRNA treatment at 1, 24, 48, 72, 96, 120, and 144 h after the infection. On Day 30, 100% survival rate (n=5) was observed in the group treated with the siRNA/SNALP formulation, while the control group treated with scrambled siRNA/SNALPs presented 20% survival rate. Consistently, the plague titer analysis on day 7 showed a significantly reduced blood level in animals treated with siRNA/SNALPs compared to the control group. Later, this group encapsulated a cocktail of three siRNAs that each targeted L protein, VP24, and VP35 genes in ZEBOV in SNALPs and showed complete post-exposure protection against ZEBOV in monkeys [91]. Tekmira Pharmaceuticals commenced a Phase I clinical trial for the cocktail siRNA–SNALP formulation (TKM-100802) in January 2014 (NCT02041715) [138]. Two patients transported from West Africa to the United States during the 2014 outbreak of Ebola virus disease were treated with TKM-100802 and other supportive measures and recovered without serious long-term sequelae, although the actual role the siRNA formulation played in the recovery of these patients remains to be investigated [139].

12.5.2 Respiratory Diseases

For systemic delivery of siRNA to the lung, cationic polymers such as PEI are frequently used as carriers [140]. In an early study by Klibanov et al. deacylated PEI was used as a carrier of siRNA to the lung [99]. Here, deacylation increased the number of protonatable nitrogens of PEI, thereby facilitating complexation with siRNA and transfection of target cells. Luc-siRNA-deacylated PEI complexes were administered to mice transfected with luciferase-encoding DNA by retro-obrital injection, and the luciferase activities in different tissues were measured at 24 h after the treatment. The Luc-siRNA/polymer complexes showed 77% or 93% suppression of the gene expression in the lung, depending on the molecular weight of the polymer. Consistently, siRNA targeting influenza viral genes, as complexed with deacylated PEI, led to significant reduction in the virus titer in the lung of influenza-infected mice 24 h after injection [99]. More recently, Bolcato-Bellemin et al. used PEI as a carrier of siRNA with sticky overhangs (ssiRNA) targeting cyclin B1 or survivin to suppress tumor progression in a lung metastasis model [141]. Here, ssiRNA formed a larger linear nucleic acid structure via hybridization of the complementary overhangs and made a more stable complex with PEI, which survived better than a classic siRNA/PEI complex in circulation [142].

Cationic liposomes tend to accumulate in the liver and hence are popular in the delivery to the liver, but they are also used for lung delivery. McMillan et al. used cationic liposomes containing DOTAP and DOPE as a carrier of siRNA targeting lung endothelium [143]. A BD study with the liposomes labeled with a non-covalently incorporated fluorescent dye found the highest fluorescence intensity was found in the liver, followed by lung and spleen. The liposomes transfected various cell populations in the lung, including CD146+ endothelial cells and CD326+ epithelial cells. Accordingly, mice treated with lamin A/C-specific siRNA-liposomes (2 mg/kg siRNA) showed 80% knockdown of lamin A/C in the lung at 48 h after a single IV injection, with the majority silencing occurring in the endothelial and epithelial cells [143]. A new choice of cationic lipids and combinations improved lung-specific BD of liposomes [144]. Kaufmann et al. used "DACC" liposomes containing AtuFECT01 (β-L-arginyl-2,3-L-diaminopropionic acid-N-palmityl-Noleyl-amide trihydrochloride) as a cationic lipid for systemic administration of siRNA. When combined with cholesterol and mPEG2000-DSPE in optimal ratios, DACC liposomes delivered the most siRNA to the lung tissues at 1 h after systemic application, followed by the spleen and liver. On the other hand, other liposomes containing AtuFECT01 and different co-lipids and/or PEG-lipids showed typical BD pattern of cationic liposomes (high liver and spleen distribution) [144]. In accordance with the BD profile, DACC lipoplexes with siRNA specific for Tie-2 gene showed over 80% reduction in Tie-2 mRNA in lung tissue of mice but no significant Tie-2 knockdown in liver, kidney, and heart tissues after three daily injections of 2.8 mg siRNA/kg [144]. DACC lipoplexes also helped deliver siRNAs targeting other genes in the lung vasculature including CD31, responsible for multiple processes of tumorigenesis, increasing the survival rate in an experimental lung metastasis mouse model [144]. Geick et al. also found BD favorable for lung delivery of siRNA with a lipopolyamine called staramine [145]. siRNA level in each tissue was measured by the stem-loop qRT PCR over 96-h post-IV injection. Liver accumulation was dominant immediately after the injection, but lung accumulation occurred over time, exceeding the levels in the liver, spleen, and kidney in 24 h. Consistently, siRNA/staramine complexes showed ~60% reduction of target mRNA in the lung over 96 h after a single administration,

whereas the level of target mRNA in the liver was not significantly different from the one treated with control siRNA [145]. The siRNA retention in the lung was attributed to the affinity of nanocomplexes for the endothelial lining in the capillary bed and relatively low exposure to phagocytic cells [145].

Other types of siRNA carriers to the lung include hybrids of lipid and polymer or lipid and inorganic components. Polymeric NPs made of conjugates of low-molecular-weight polycation (PEI) and lipids were used for delivery of siRNA to lung endothelial cells [146]. Unlike lipid-based carriers, the lipid–polymer hybrid NPs achieved the gene silencing effect at a dose that did not affect hepatocytes or immune cells. The biological effects of siRNAs delivered with the NPs were confirmed in the lung, as an inducer of an emphysema-like phenotype (by silencing VEGFR-2 gene) or a suppressor of primary and metastatic Lewis lung carcinoma (by silencing VEGFR-1 and Dll4) [146].

In addition to systemic administration, siRNA has been directly delivered to the lung as an aerosol (intratracheal or intranasal administration in experimental studies). One of the advantages of airway delivery is the potential to achieve high local concentration of siRNA in the lung without going through blood circulation, which can compromise the stability of the siRNA/carrier complexes or siRNA itself and subject them to distribution in other MPS organs. Minko et al. administered siRNA/cationic liposome complexes via IV injection or intratracheal instillation to mice bearing tumors in the lung to compare the BD [147]. At 24-h post-administration, both the carrier and the siRNA showed substantially high peak concentrations and long retentions in the lung compared to other organs after intratracheal administration. On the other hand, IV injection resulted in broad distribution in other organs with relatively low levels of liposomes and siRNA in the lung [147]. Kissel et al. also delivered siRNA with PEI or PEG-grafted PEI (PEG-PEI) as carriers via intratracheal instillation and observed the BD of siRNA and the polymer by single-photon emission computed tomography (SPECT) and radioactivity counting of organs [148]. Both siRNA and PEG-PEI were detectable in the lung at 48 h after instillation. Without PEG, siRNA/PEI complexes showed differential lung accumulation of each component: negligible level of siRNA and high level of PEI (even higher than that of PEG-PEI), which suggested dissociation of the complex in the lung and preferential association of PEI with mucus and cell membranes [148]. The locally delivered EGFP-specific siRNA/PEG-PEI complexes reached bronchial cells and alveolar cells and knocked down the EGFP expression in the lung by 42% after 5-day post-instillation [148]. Airway administration is potentially a promising way of delivering siRNA to the lung; however, studies to date suggest remaining challenges in airway delivery of siRNA, including the destructive interaction with anionic components in the lung [148] and local irritation that can lead to inflammatory consequences [149].

12.5.3 Potential Toxicity of siRNA Therapeutics

siRNA with suboptimal potency can result in unintended side effects such as downregulation of off-target genes or activation of innate immune responses [150]. Efforts to mitigate these off-target effects include chemical modification of siRNA, redesign of the sequence, and the use of siRNA cocktails [150–152]. Toxicity may also come from the delivery systems. For example, intravenously injected lipoplexes have shown to induce the production of pro-inflammatory cytokines with signs of hepatocyte injury [153,154]. These pro-inflammatory effects were initially attributed to the polynucleotide part of the complex rather than the carrier [153,154]; however, later studies have reported intrinsic pro-inflammatory properties of some cationic lipids [155–157]. PEI, the most commonly used polymeric gene carrier, shows molecular weight, structure, and dose-dependent toxicity [158]. This challenge is currently tackled by developing degradable polycations, which can be degraded into less toxic small molecules [159].

12.6 DNA RECURRENCE-ASSOCIATED GENES

It is important to identify systemically recurrence-associated genes using The Cancer Genome Atlas (TCGA) RNA sequencing database [160]. Recurrence of papillary thyroid cancer is not uncommon, but incorporating clinicopathologic parameters to predict recurrence is suboptimal. It has been found that [160] 1807 genes were associated with recurrence-free survival. There were 676 genes of which high expression was associated with a greater risk of recurrence. These genes were enriched in pathways involved in cell cycle regulation and DNA repair. Among 1131 genes of which low expression was associated with recurrence, Kyoto Encyclopedia of Genes and Genomes–annotated functions were metabolism, calcium signaling, glycan biosynthesis, and the Notch signaling pathway. Canonical pathways identified by Ingenuity Pathway Analysis included RXR function, nitric oxide signaling, interleukin-8 signaling, and nutrient sensing. In addition, low expression of the majority of thyroid differentiation genes was associated with a significantly less recurrence-free survival.

The incidence of thyroid cancer, particularly papillary thyroid cancer, has been increasing rapidly in recent decades [161]. Papillary thyroid cancer tends to be biologically indolent and has an excellent prognosis. Nonetheless, more than one-quarter of patients may experience disease recurrence during long-term follow-up [162]. Several schemes, including clarification of the staging classification of the American Joint Committee on Cancer, have been developed to predict risk for death but not the risk for recurrence.

In 2009, the American Thyroid Association (ATA) first proposed a three-level, initial risk-stratification system to predict disease recurrence and/or persistence [163]; however, the proportion of variance explained by the ATA system for risk of recurrence is suboptimal, ranging from 19% to 34% [164]. Although a new, dynamic, risk-stratification system has been developed, the information required for stratification is available mainly during the follow-up period. This situation indicates a need for early identification of additional factors associated with disease recurrence.

Genetic and molecular approaches are being used increasingly for recognizing important biologic processes in oncology. The most frequent genetic alteration seen in papillary thyroid cancer is a point mutation at codon 600 of the BRAF gene (BRAF^{V600E}) [165]. It remains debatable whether this information concerning this mutation added predictive value for disease-specific mortality or risk of recurrence beyond the current clinicopathologic information collected for tumor staging [166].

In recent years, the prognostic importance of the TERT promoter mutations in thyroid cancer has attracted much attention; nonetheless, the frequency of the TERT promoter mutations in papillary thyroid cancer is considerably less than that in poorly differentiated or anaplastic cancer [167]. Given the biologic complexity of cancer, it is unlikely to find a single target accounting for disease recurrence. A systemic approach is required to identify a gene expression signature associated with recurrent disease.

TCGA project is meant to produce a comprehensive atlas of cancer genomes to accelerate our understanding of the molecular basis of cancer and improve cancer prevention, detection, and therapy. The TCGA study of papillary thyroid cancer analyzed a large cohort of tumor tissue and matched normal tissues across multiple sequencing platforms [168]; however, the follow-up data were not available at the time of initial TCGA publication. In this study [160], it has been employed as a systematic approach for characterizing recurrence-associated genes and their relevant functional networks using the updated TCGA data.

12.6.1 Functional Enrichment Analyses

Recurrence-associated genes were subjected to functional enrichment analyses [160], which were conducted using three software packages separately: Web-based Gene Set Analysis Toolkit (WebGestalt), [169] Database for Annotation, Visualization, and Integration Discovery (DAVID), [170] and Ingenuity Pathway Analysis (Qiagen, Redwood City, CA) [171]. WebGestalt and DAVID analyses were focused mainly on the Kyoto Encyclopedia of Genes and Genomes (KEGG) annotation database [172,173]. In WebGestalt, the minimum number of genes for enrichment was set at 5, and the significance analysis was performed using the hypergeometric test with the significance level set at $P=0.01$. In DAVID, the parameters were set to their default values.

Using the TCGA thyroid cancer database, 504 patients with data for both clinical and gene expression were analyzed. Pathologic stages I, II, III, and IV comprised 56%, 10%, 22%, and 11%, respectively. The median follow-up

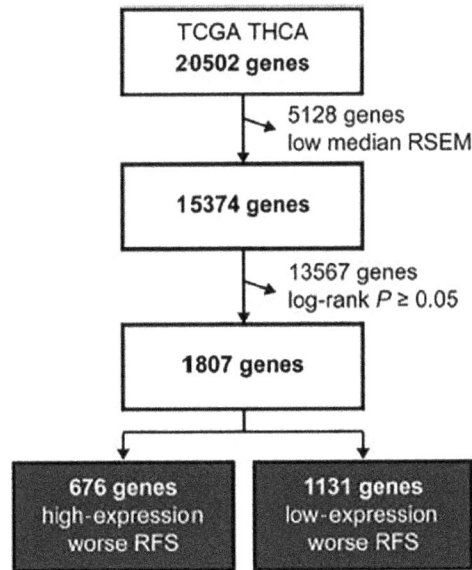

FIGURE 12.15 Study flowchart. RFS, recurrence-free survival; RSEM, RNA-Seq by expectation maximization; TCGA, The Cancer Genome Atlas; THCA, thyroid cancer.

duration was 29.9 months (mean, 37.7±32.1; range, 0.2–180.8 months). During follow-up, 16 (3%) patients were deceased at 39.0±24.5 months. Recurrence was observed in 47 (9%) patients. The median time from initial treatment to recurrence was 16.1 months (mean, 19.6±14.7; range, 0.2–59.5 months). As expected, an advanced pathologic stage was associated with a greater likelihood of recurrence [160].

Among 20,502 genes analyzed, the distribution of median RSEM values was significantly skewed (median, 187.0; interquartile range, 4.1–800.0). To avoid variation caused by low-level expressions, genes with a median RSEM value of less than 4.1 were excluded from analysis. A total of 15,374 (75%) genes were applicable to the analysis of the difference in RFS between high- and low-expression groups defined by median splits. A study flowchart is detailed in Figure 12.15.

There were 676 genes of which high expression was associated with a significantly lesser RFS [160]. The overlapping KEGG-enriched pathways were determined at the significance levels of P<0.01 in WebGestalt and P<0.1 in DAVID, respectively. Of the 10 enriched pathways, most were biologic processes involved in cell cycle regulation and DNA repair [160]. The Kaplan–Meier estimates of RFS of several representative genes are shown in Figure 12.16.

Good concordance was observed between the enriched functional pathways identified by the KEGG module and Ingenuity Pathway Analysis (Figure 12.17a). The top tox lists of Ingenuity Pathway Analysis were "Cell Cycle: G2/M DNA Damage Checkpoint Regulation," "Increases Liver Hyperplasia/Hyperproliferation," "Cell Cycle: G1/S Checkpoint Regulation," "RAR Activation," and "p53 Signaling." Consistent with a recent report [174], it has been

found that expression of BRAF mRNA was not associated with RFS (logrank P=0.76).

In addition, we found 1131 genes for which low expression was associated with a significantly less RFS. The complete list of these genes is reported in [160]. The nine significantly enriched KEGG pathways identified by WebGestalt and DAVID were related to metabolism, calcium signaling, glycan biosynthesis, and the Notch signaling pathway [160]. The results appeared partially consistent with canonical pathways identified by Ingenuity Pathway Analysis (Figure 12.17b). The top tox lists were "LPS/IL-1 Mediated Inhibition of RXR Function," "Cardiac Hypertrophy," "Xenobiotic Metabolism Signaling," "Increases Glomerular Injury," and "NRF2-mediated Oxidative Stress Response."

Initial TCGA global analysis proposed that the differentiation status of thyroid cancer can be determined by a set of genes involved in thyroid metabolism and function and was designated the thyroid differentiation score (TDS) [168]. The TDS comprises expression data of 13 mRNAs and 3 miRNAs. Interestingly, we found that the expression of seven TDS genes was in association with RFS (Figure 12.18). Low expression of these TDS genes was associated typically with a decrease in RFS. The only exception was PVRL4, high expression of which had a greater risk of recurrence. Low expression of TSHR, which encodes thyroid-stimulating hormone receptor, was also associated with a significantly less RFS. The results of the remaining TDS genes has been shown in Supplementary Figure S2 http://dx.doi.org/10.1016/j.surg.2016.12.039 [160]. RFS was not associated with other genes participating in thyroid development, such as NKX2-1 (TTF1, logrank P=0.74), FOXE1 (TTF2, log-rank P=0.75), and PAX8 (log-rank P=0.19).

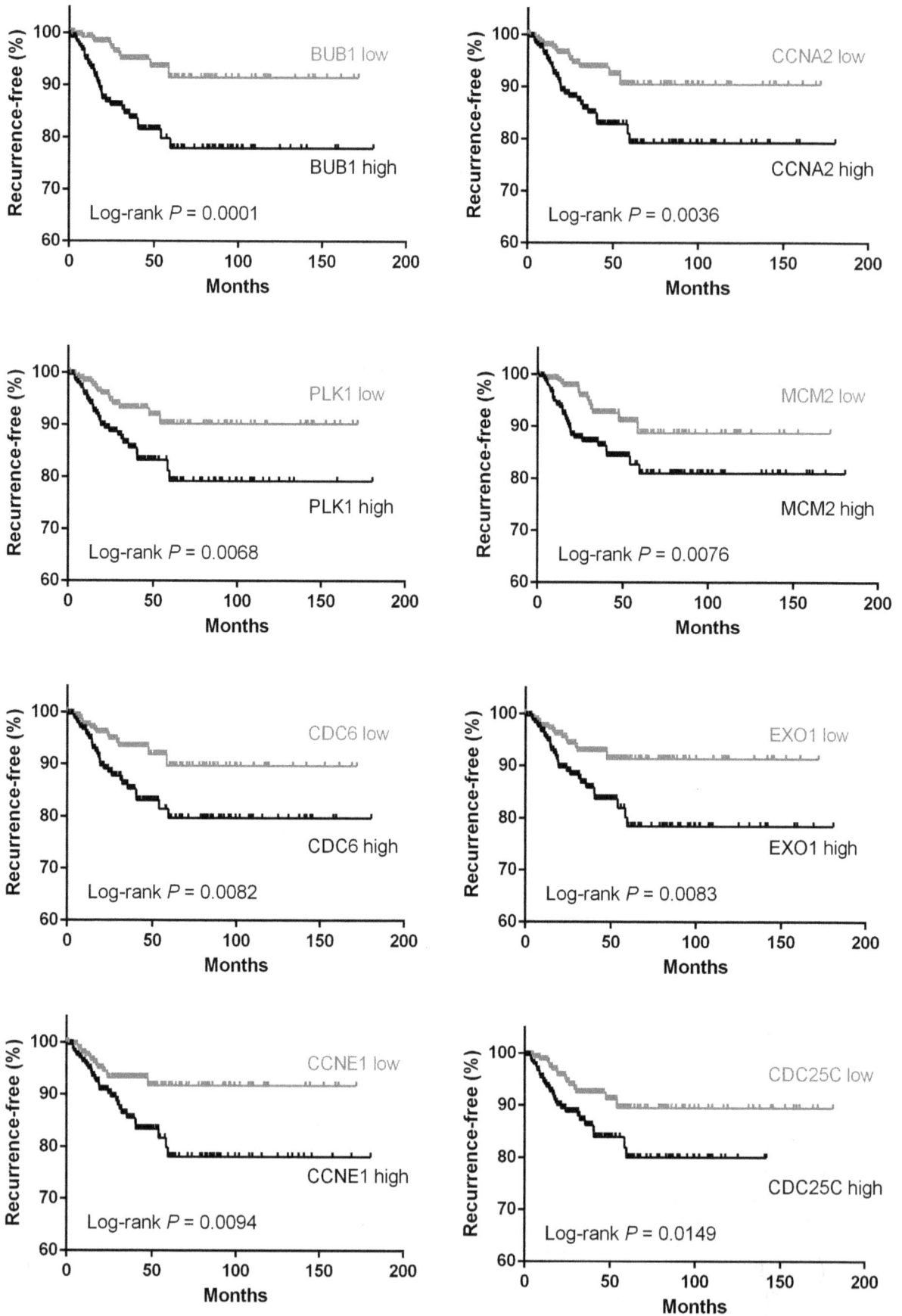

FIGURE 12.16   Kaplan–Meier recurrence-free survival of patients with papillary thyroid cancer (n=504) dichotomized according to genes of which high expression was associated with recurrence.

(a)

(b)

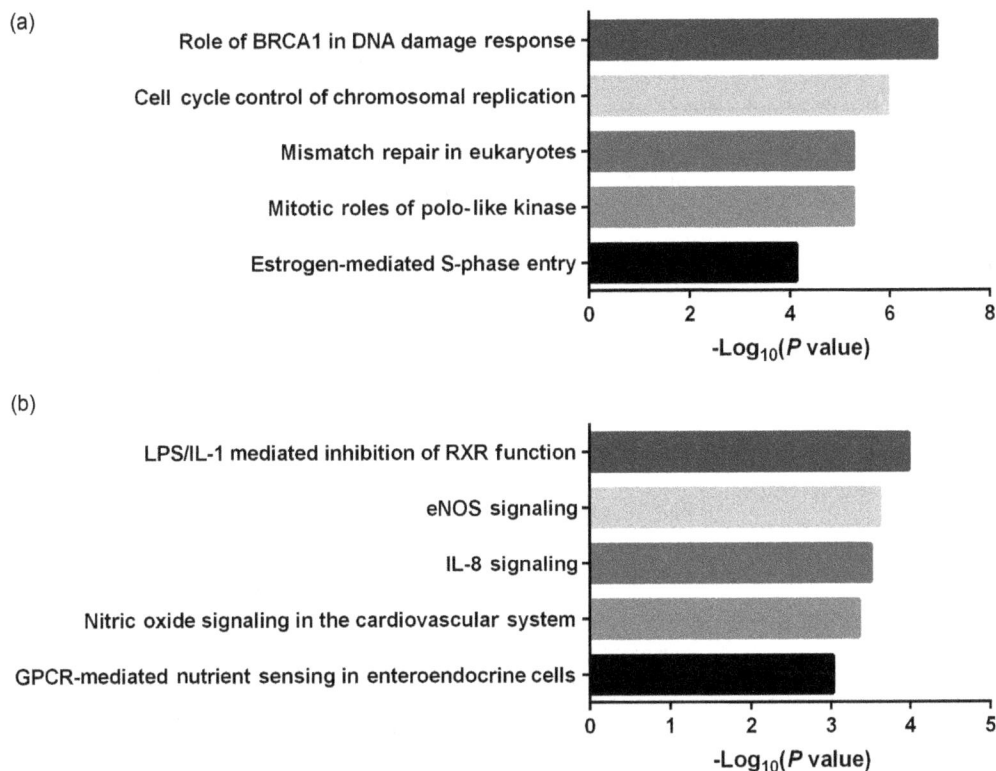

FIGURE 12.17 Ingenuity pathway analysis of genes of which high (a) and low (b) expression was associated with recurrence in papillary thyroid cancer.

12.7 GENOMIC GLOBAL ANALYSIS OF THE TCGA

Initial genomic global analysis of the TCGA of papillary thyroid cancer revealed that papillary thyroid cancers can be separated into two main groups, $BRAF^{V600E}$-like and RAS-like [168]. The classifier design was based on the $BRAF^{V600E}$-RAS score, which highly correlated with the TDS, although the two scores were derived independently and have no genes in common. $BRAF^{V600E}$-like papillary cancers are enriched for the classic and tall cell histology, are less differentiated, and have an increased ERK output or overactivation of the mitogen-activated protein kinase (MAPK) pathway. Conversely, RAS-like cancers are characterized by follicular-variant histology, are associated with younger patients, and have a lesser expression of immune response genes. The two groups are fundamentally different at all genomic levels.

Using the ATA risk of recurrence as a surrogate outcome, the initial analysis found that the risk of recurrence was associated with mutation density and the TDS. The TDS only weakly correlated with tumor purity, indicating that the TDS was not influenced strongly by tumor stromal content or lymphocyte infiltration [168]. The analysis on real events during follow-up is in concordance with the results [160], showing that low expression of thyroid differentiation genes carried a greater risk of recurrence.

In a previous report, histopathologic characterization of radioactive iodine (RAI)-refractory disease suggested that dedifferentiation is not uncommon [175]. Dedifferentiation likely dampens the responses to RAI therapy. At present, patients with an RAI-refractory disease have limited alternative options for treatment and a decreased overall survival, partly because thyroid cancer is poorly responsive to cytotoxic chemotherapy [176].

Cancer is driven by changes in patterns of gene expression due to the accumulation of mutations or epigenetic modifications. The TCGA data support previous observations that RAI-refractory lesions have a greater frequency of $BRAF^{V600E}$ [177,178]. Mutations leading to constitutive activation of the MAPK signaling pathway inhibit the expression of proteins involved in the biosynthesis of thyroid hormones, including sodium iodide symporter SLC5A5 (NIS) [179]. Of note, among the thyroid differentiation genes, it has been found that downregulation of NIS was the strongest predictor of a decreased RFS (Fig 12.18, logrank P=0.0003). Nuclear receptor ligands and epigenetic modifiers have been used to promote tumor redifferentiation, [180] while conventional redifferentiation agents, such as retinoic acid, had no clinically important benefits [181].

A plausible explanation is that pathways involving retinoic acid receptors and/or retinoid X receptors are also downregulated in these neoplasms. In these analyses, low

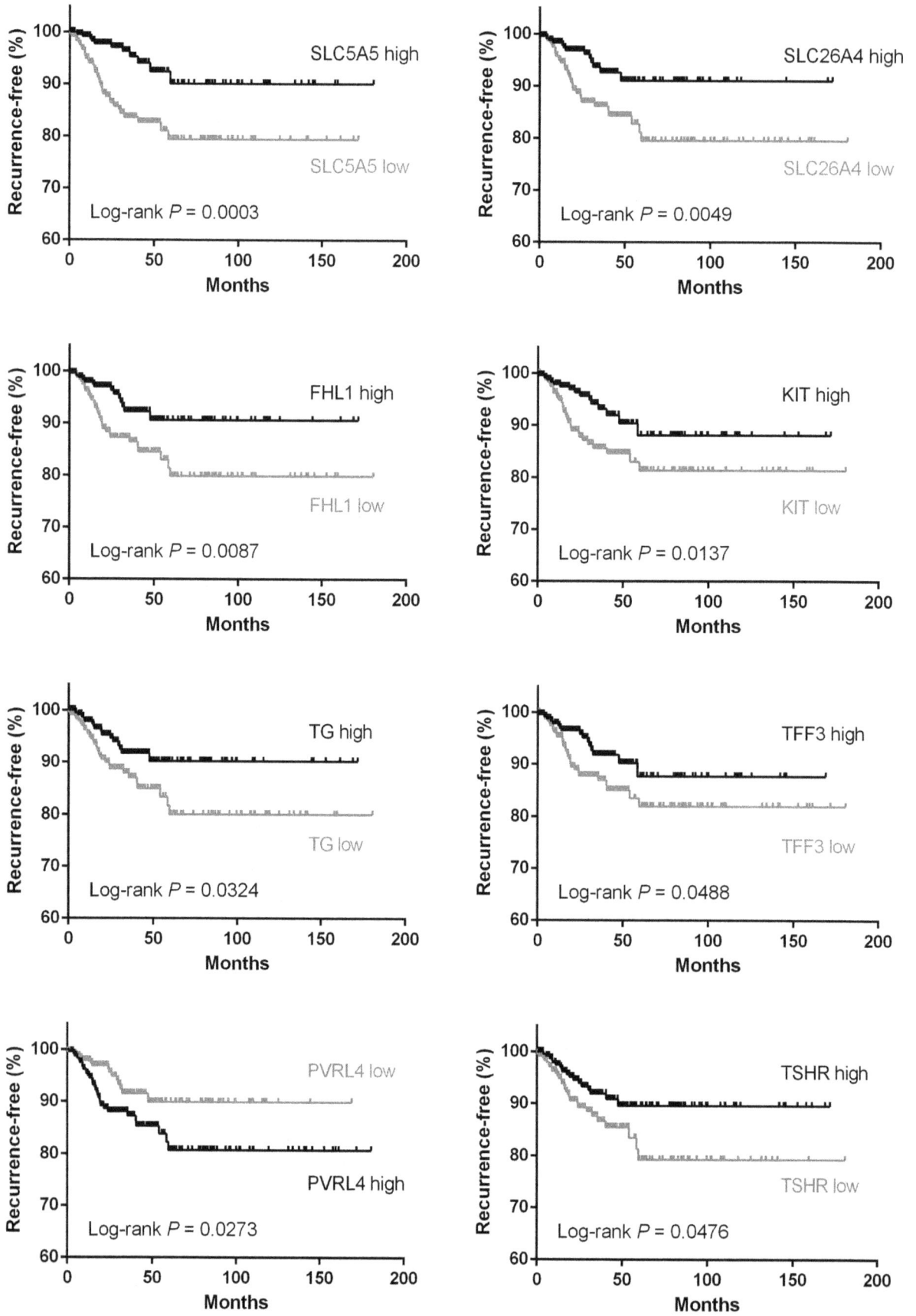

FIGURE 12.18   Kaplan–Meier recurrence-free survival of patients with papillary thyroid cancer (n=504) dichotomized according to genes in association with thyroid differentiation. The sodium iodide symporter (NIS) is encoded by the solute carrier family 5 member 5 (SLC5A5).

expression of retinoic acid receptor beta (RARB) was associated with a significantly lesser RFS (log-rank P=0.03). Consistent with this observation, recent studies demonstrated that RARB expression was downregulated in papillary thyroid cancer and RARB silencing increased cell viability, decreased expression of NIS, and suppressed iodine uptake in thyroid cancer cells [182,183]. A more promising strategy may be targeting the MAPK signaling pathway. Accumulating evidence suggests that MAPK inhibition may provide better results in terms of iodine uptake and tumor response [184–186]. Further research is necessary to provide a more personalized approach, tailored to specific molecular alterations in individual patient tumors.

A novel finding in the present study [160] is that high expression of cell-cycle-regulating and DNA repair genes was associated with recurrence. Alterations in cell-cycle-regulating genes promote transition through the cell cycle and ultimately drive tumor proliferation. Although prior studies suggest that Ki-67/MIB-1 stain positivity confers a greater risk of recurrence, [187] differentiated thyroid cancer has long been considered as a quiescent, chemotherapy-resistant neoplasm. It is arguable whether modern drugs offer better effectiveness with fewer adverse events [188].

The findings [160] do not imply that cytotoxic agents possess high therapeutic potential in papillary thyroid cancer. Transcriptome analysis across 12 TCGA cancer types indicates that papillary thyroid cancer is poorly overlapped with other cancers in terms of differentially expressed genes [189]. Instead, it has been speculated that a proliferation signature may be used as a prognostic marker.

DNA repair machinery maintains a balance between genomic integrity and cell death. Previous work mainly focused on the association between polymorphisms of DNA repair genes and the risk of developing thyroid cancer [190]. Upregulation of DNA repair genes may render tumor cells less vulnerable to DNA damage and more resistant to treatment. It has been found that high expression of DNA repair genes was associated with an increased risk of recurrence. It may reflect genomic instability of more aggressive cancer; an alternative explanation is that tumors equipped with better repair capacity would more likely survive from RAI therapy.

The TCGA analysis showed that two significantly mutated genes related to DNA repair (PPM1D and CHEK2) occurred concomitantly with driver mutations in the MAPK pathway [168]. Interestingly, MAPK inhibition may result in radiosensitization by suppressing DNA repair pathways [191]. Combination or sequential treatments with RAI therapy and inhibition of the DNA-damage response may represent a new concept for the management of papillary thyroid cancer.

Limitations of this study [160] include the relatively short follow-up periods and not controlling for histologic variants or tumor stage of the papillary thyroid cancers studied. Additionally, in the present study, patients were divided into dichotomous groups for each gene analyzed. The underlying pathology is more likely to be "continuous" rather than categorical, and such groupings may not be meaningful biologically [192].

A recent analysis of the TCGA data by Stanford University used clinicopathologic characteristics to define good and poor prognosis [193]. The authors [160] reported individual potential targets and proposed a Prediction Analysis of Microarrays classifier. This study aimed at identifying recurrence-associated genes instead of developing a validated prognostic index. It has been hypothesized that using pathway analysis would provide a better mechanistic understanding of the biologic processes involved in tumor recurrence.

12.8 CONCLUSIONS

We discussed several siRNA delivery approaches focusing on their contributions to the control of PK and BD of siRNA. Solid tumors are obviously one of the most anticipated targets, and many studies show PK/BD profiles favorable for siRNA delivery to tumors. Despite the optimism prevalent in the literature, one may recognize that most clinical translations are made in the applications targeting the liver and the lung, where the majority of siRNA/NP systems naturally accumulate. This indicates that systemic delivery of siRNA in a therapeutic dose to tissues other than MPS organs remains suboptimal. Given the discrepancy, some of the current experimental practices may be worth reconsideration. First, many studies rely on labeling siRNA for PK and BD studies. As mentioned earlier, these approaches are valid only when the labeled components represent the full-length, bioactive siRNA; otherwise, inactive catabolites retaining the label may be mistaken for siRNA in target tissues. In addition, one should also consider that structural changes due to labeling may alter the PK/BD profiles of siRNA. To avoid overestimation of siRNA in PK/BD studies, it is desirable to complement with hybridization-based methods that can detect full-length siRNA, such as Northern blot analysis, hybridization-ligation assay, or PCR-based assay. Second, BD of siRNA is often presented as % of injected dose per unit mass of tissue at the final time point of the study. While this presentation offers a useful means to compare the relative concentrations of siRNA in different tissues, it rarely reports the amount of siRNA collected in the feces and urine, making it difficult to judge the fraction of siRNA that was immediately excreted. A caveat of this practice is that relative siRNA distribution in selected tissues can mislead to an overrated optimism for target-specific siRNA delivery, when in reality the absolute amount of siRNA in target tissue may be only a small fraction of the injected dose. Such misinterpretation may be prevented by considering the concentration in each tissue in addition to the relative quantity. Finally, it is not unusual to see studies tracking carriers in lieu of siRNA in PK/BD studies. This approach may be valid when the siRNA/carrier complex remains stable throughout the study, which, however, should not be taken for granted without proof. It is possible that siRNA/carrier complexes disassemble prematurely during circulation but still show favorable pharmacological effects due to other biological events related to the carrier itself. In order to identify actual contribution of carriers to the siRNA delivery, it is desirable to track siRNA and carrier separately through distinct labeling and/or detection techniques.

In conclusion, we identified a set of recurrence-associated genes in papillary thyroid cancer. Pathway analyses indicate that upregulation of cell-cycle-regulating genes and DNA repair genes and downregulation of thyroid differentiation genes carried a high risk of recurrence. Further research [194–197] will be required to determine whether pharmacologic measures that target these pathways improve clinical outcomes.

REFERENCES

1. A. Fire, S. Xu, M.K. Montgomery, S.A. Kostas, S.E. Driver, C.C. Mello, Potent and specific genetic interference by double-stranded RNA in Caenorhabditis elegans, *Nature* 391 (1998) 806–811.

2. S.M. Elbashir, J. Harborth, W. Lendeckel, A. Yalcin, K.Weber, T Tuschl, Duplexes of 21-nucleotide RNAs mediate RNA interference in cultured mammalian cells, *Nature* 24 (2001) 494–498.

3. https://clinicaltrials.gov/show/NCT00363714, A dose escalation trial of an intravitreal Injection of Sirna-027 in patients with subfoveal choroidal neovascularization (CNV) secondary to age-related macular degeneration (AMD).

4. D. Haussecker, Current issues of RNAi therapeutics delivery and development, *J. Control. Release* 195 (2014) 49–54.

5. S. Seth, R. Johns, M.V. Templin, Delivery and biodistribution of siRNA for cancer therapy: challenges and future prospects, *Ther. Deliv.* 3 (2012) 245–261.

6. R.Kanasty, J.R.Dorkin, A.Vegas, D. Anderson, Delivery materials for siRNA therapeutics, *Nat. Mater.* 12 (2013) 967–977.

7. https://clinicaltrials.gov/ct2/show/NCT02065336, Study of ARC-520 in patients with chronic hepatitis B virus.

8. A. Guzman-Aranguez, P. Loma, J. Pintor, Small-interfering RNAs (siRNAs) as a promising tool for ocular therapy, *Br. J. Pharmacol.* 170 (2013) 730–747.

9. S.J. Reich, J. Fosnot, A. Kuroki, W. Tang, X. Yang, A.M. Maguire, J. Bennett, M.J. Tolentino, Small interfering RNA (siRNA) targeting VEGF effectively inhibits ocular neovascularization in a mouse model, *Mol. Vis.* 9 (2003) 210–216.

10. M. Murata, T. Takanami, S. Shimizu, Y. Kubota, S. Horiuchi, W. Habano, J.-x. Ma, S. Sato, Inhibition of ocular angiogenesis by diced small interfering RNAs (siRNAs) specific to vascular endothelial growth factor (VEGF), *Curr. Eye Res.* 31 (2006) 171–180.

11. B. Kim, Q. Tang, P.S. Biswas, J. Xu, R.M. Schiffelers, F.Y. Xie, A.M. Ansari, P.V. Scaria, M.C. Woodle, P. Lu, B.T. Rouse, Inhibition of ocular angiogenesis by siRNA targeting vascular endothelial growth factor pathway genes, *Am. J. Pathol.* 165 (2004) 2177–2185.

12. P.K. Kaiser, R.C. Symons, S.M. Shah, E.J. Quinlan, H. Tabandeh, D.V. Do, G. Reisen, J.A. Lockridge, B. Short, R. Guerciolini, Q.D. Nguyen, I. Sirna-027 Study, RNAi-based treatment for neovascular age-related macular degeneration by Sirna-027, *Am J. Ophthalmol.* 150 (2010) 33–39.

13. R.N. Frank, Diabetic retinopathy, *N. Engl. J. Med.* 350 (2004) 48–58.

14. A.P. Adamis, J.W. Miller, M.T. Bernal, D.J. D'Amico, J. Folkman, T.K. Yeo, K.T. Yeo, Increased vascular endothelial growth factor levels in the vitreous of eyes with proliferative diabetic retinopathy, *Am J. Ophthalmol.* 118 (1994) 445–450.

15. A.O. Garba, S.A. Mousa, Bevasiranib for the treatment of wet, age-related macular degeneration, *Ophthalmol. Eye Dis.* 2 (2010) 75–83.

16. Q.D. Nguyen, R.A. Schachar, C.I. Nduaka, M. Sperling, A.S. Basile, K.J. Klamerus, K. Chi-Burris, E. Yan, D.A. Paggiarino, I. Rosenblatt, R. Aitchison, Dose-ranging evaluation of intravitreal siRNA PF-04523655 for diabetic macular edema (the DEGAS study), *Invest. Ophthalmol. Vis. Sci.* 53 (2012) 7666–7674.

17. H. Nakamura, S.S. Siddiqui, X. Shen, A.B. Malik, J.S. Pulido, N.M. Kumar, B.Y. Yue, RNA interference targeting transforming growth factor-beta type II receptor suppresses ocular inflammation and fibrosis, *Mol. Vis.* 10 (2004) 703–711.

18. H. Ye, Y. Qian, M. Lin, Y. Duan, X. Sun, Y. Zhuo, J. Ge, Cationic nano-copolymers mediated IKK beta targeting siRNA to modulate wound healing in a monkey model of glaucoma filtration surgery, *Mol. Vis.* 16 (2010) 2502–2510.

19. T. Martinez, M.V. Gonzalez, I. Roehl, N.Wright, C. Paneda, A.I. Jimenez, In vitro and in vivo efficacy of SYL040012, a novel siRNA compound for treatment of glaucoma, *Mol. Ther.* 22 (2014) 81–91.

20. A. Thakur, S. Fitzpatrick, A. Zaman, K. Kugathasan, B. Muirhead, G. Hortelano, H. Sheardown, Strategies for ocular siRNA delivery: potential and limitations of non-viral nanocarriers, *J. Biol. Eng.* 6 (2012) 7.

21. C. Rodriguez-Aguayo, A. Chavez-Reyes, G. Lopez-Berestein, A.K. Sood, RNAi in cancer therapy, in: K. Cheng, R.I. Mahato (Eds.), *Advanced Delivery and Therapeutic Applications of RNAi*, John Wiley and Sons, Ltd, Chichester (2013), pp. 271–307.

22. M.E. Davis, J.E. Zuckerman, C.H.J. Choi, D. Seligson, A. Tolcher, C.A. Alabi, Y. Yen, J.D. Heidel, A. Ribas, Evidence of RNAi in humans from systemically administered siRNA via targeted nanoparticles, *Nature* 464 (2010) 1067–1070.

23. N.S. Gandhi, R.K. Tekade, M.B. Chougule, Nanocarrier mediated delivery of siRNA/miRNA in combination with chemotherapeutic agents for cancer therapy: current progress and advances, *J. Control. Release* 194 (2014) 238–256.

24. D.R. Senger, S.J. Galli, A.M. Dvorak, C.A. Perruzzi, V.S. Harvey, H.F. Dvorak, Tumor cells secrete a vascular permeability factor that promotes accumulation of ascites fluid, *Science* 219 (1983) 983–985.

25. M.D. Cole, The myc oncogene: its role in transformation and differentiation, *Annu. Rev. Genet.* 20 (1986) 361–384.

26. E.P. Sulman, X.X. Tang, C. Allen, J.A. Biegel, D.E. Pleasure, G.M. Brodeur, N. Ikegaki, ECK, a human EPH-related gene, maps to 1p36.1, a common region of alteration in human cancers, *Genomics* 40 (1997) 371–374.

27. U.R. Rapp, M.D. Goldsborough, G.E. Mark, T.I. Bonner, J. Groffen, F.H. Reynolds Jr., J.R. Stephenson, Structure and biological activity of v-raf, a unique oncogene transduced by a retrovirus, *Proc. Natl. Acad. Sci. U. S. A.* 80 (1983) 4218–4222.

28. U. Holtrich, G.Wolf, A. Brauninger, T. Karn, B. Bohme, H. Rubsamen-Waigmann, K. Strebhardt, Induction and down-regulation of PLK, a human serine/threonine kinase expressed in proliferating cells and tumors, *Proc. Natl. Acad. Sci. U. S. A.* 91 (1994) 1736–1740.

29. M.G. Lee, P. Nurse, Complementation used to clone a human homologue of the fission yeast cell cycle control gene cdc2, *Nature* 327 (1987) 31–35.

30. R.L. Juliano, V. Ling, A surface glycoprotein modulating drug permeability in Chinese hamster ovary cell mutants, *Biochim. Biophys. Acta* 455 (1976) 152–162.

31. Y. Chen, H. Gu, D.S. Zhang, F. Li, T. Liu, W. Xia, Highly effective inhibition of lung cancer growth and metastasis by systemic delivery of siRNA via multimodal mesoporous silica-based nanocarrier, *Biomaterials* 35 (2014) 10058–10069.

32. X. Liu, W. Wang, D. Samarsky, L. Liu, Q. Xu, W. Zhang, G. Zhu, P. Wu, X. Zuo, H. Deng, J. Zhang, Z. Wu, X. Chen, L. Zhao, Z. Qiu, Z. Zhang, Q. Zeng, W. Yang, B. Zhang, A. Ji, Tumor-targeted in vivo gene silencing via systemic delivery of cRGD-conjugated siRNA, *Nucleic Acids Res.* 42 (2015) 11805–11817.

33. Y. Chen, S.R. Bathula, Q. Yang, L. Huang, Targeted nanoparticles deliver siRNA to melanoma, *J. Investig. Dermatol.* 130 (2010) 2790–2798.

34. Y. Chen, X. Zhu, X. Zhang, B. Liu, L. Huang, Nanoparticles modified with tumor targeting scFv deliver siRNA and miRNA for cancer therapy, *Mol. Ther.* 18 (2010) 1650–1656.

35. C.N. Landen Jr., A. Chavez-Reyes, C. Bucana, R. Schmandt, M.T. Deavers, G. Lopez-Berestein, A.K. Sood, Therapeutic EphA2 gene targeting in vivo using neutral liposomal small interfering RNA delivery, *Cancer Res.* 65 (2005) 6910–6918.

36. S.T. Chou, Q. Leng, P. Scaria, J.D. Kahn, L.J. Tricoli, M. Woodle, A.J. Mixson, Surface modified HK: siRNA nanoplexes with enhanced pharmacokinetics and tumor growth inhibition, *Biomacromolecules* 14 (2013) 752–760.

37. Y. Sakurai, H. Hatakeyama, Y. Sato, M. Hyodo, H. Akita, H. Harashima, Gene silencing via RNAi and siRNA quantification in tumor tissue using MEND, a liposomal siRNA delivery system, *Mol. Ther.* 21 (2013) 1195–1203.

38. Y. Liu, Y.H. Zhu, C.Q. Mao, S. Dou, S. Shen, Z.B. Tan, J. Wang, Triple negative breast cancer therapy with CDK1 siRNA delivered by cationic lipid assisted PEG-PLA nanoparticles, *J. Control. Release* 192 (2014) 114–121.

39. L. Zhu, F. Perche, T. Wang, V.P. Torchilin, Matrix metalloproteinase 2-sensitive multifunctional polymeric micelles for tumor-specific co-delivery of siRNA and hydrophobic drugs, *Biomaterials* 35 (2014) 4213–4222.

40. J.Y. Yhee, S. Song, S.J. Lee, S.G. Park, K.S. Kim, M.G. Kim, S. Son, H. Koo, I.C. Kwon, J.H. Jeong, S.Y. Jeong, S.H. Kim, K. Kim, Cancer-targeted MDR-1 siRNA delivery using self-cross-linked glycol chitosan nanoparticles to overcome drug resistance, *J. Control. Release* 198 (2015) 1–9.

41. G. Neufeld, T. Cohen, S. Gengrinovitch, Z. Poltorak, Vascular endothelial growth factor (VEGF) and its receptors, *FASEB J.* 13 (1999) 9–22.

42. D. Zhuang, S. Mannava, V. Grachtchouk, W.H. Tang, S. Patil, J.A. Wawrzyniak, A.E. Berman, T.J. Giordano, E.V. Prochownik, M.S. Soengas, M.A. Nikiforov, C-MYC overexpression is required for continuous suppression of oncogene-induced senescence in melanoma cells, *Oncogene* 27 (2008) 6623–6634.

43. R.W. Johnstone, A.A. Ruefli, S.W. Lowe, Apoptosis: a link between cancer genetics and chemotherapy, *Cell* 108 (2002) 153–164.

44. P.H. Thaker, M. Deavers, J. Celestino, A. Thornton, M.S. Fletcher, C.N. Landen, M.S. Kinch, P.A. Kiener, A.K. Sood, EphA2 expression is associated with aggressive features in ovarian carcinoma, *Clin. Cancer Res.* 10 (2004) 5145–5150.

45. M. Nakamoto, A.D. Bergemann, Diverse roles for the Eph family of receptor tyrosine kinases in carcinogenesis, *Microsc. Res. Tech.* 59 (2002) 58–67.

46. F. Eckerdt, J. Yuan, K. Strebhardt, Polo-like kinases and oncogenesis, *Oncogene* 24 (2005) 267–276.

47. K. Ando, T. Ozaki, H. Yamamoto, K. Furuya, M. Hosoda, S. Hayashi, M. Fukuzawa, A. Nakagawara, Polo-like kinase 1 (Plk1) inhibits p53 function by physical interaction and phosphorylation, *J. Biol. Chem.* 279 (2004) 25549–25561.

48. M. Malumbres, M. Barbacid, Mammalian cyclin-dependent kinases, *Trends Biochem. Sci.* 30 (2005) 630–641.

49. M. Malumbres, M. Barbacid, To cycle or not to cycle: a critical decision in cancer, *Nat. Rev. Cancer* 1 (2001) 222–231.

50. M. Malumbres, Cyclin-dependent kinases, *Genome Biol.* 15 (2014) 122.

51. P. Bonelli, F.M. Tuccillo, A. Borrelli, A. Schiattarella, F.M. Buonaguro, CDK/CCN and CDKI alterations for cancer prognosis and therapeutic predictivity, *Biomed. Res. Int.* 2014 (2014) 361020.

52. http://www.focr.org/breakthrough-therapies, Breakthrough therapies.

53. G. Ambrosini, C. Adida, D.C. Altieri, A novel anti-apoptosis gene, survivin, expressed in cancer and lymphoma, *Nat. Med.* 3 (1997) 917–921.

54. D.C. Altieri, Survivin, versatile modulation of cell division and apoptosis in cancer, *Oncogene* 22 (2003) 8581–8589.

55. G. Bradley, V. Ling, P-glycoprotein, multidrug resistance and tumor progression, *Cancer Metastasis Rev.* 13 (1994) 223–233.

56. M. Abbasi, A. Lavasanifar, H. Uludag, Recent attempts at RNAi-mediated P-glycoprotein downregulation for reversal of multidrug resistance in cancer, *Med. Res. Rev.* 33 (2013) 33–53.

57. C. Lorenzer, M. Dirin, A.M. Winkler, V. Baumann, J. Winkler, Going beyond the liver: progress and challenges of targeted delivery of siRNA therapeutics, *J. Control. Release* 203 (2015) 1–15.

58. P. Arbuthnot, A. Ely, M.S. Weinberg, Hepatic delivery of RNA interference activators for therapeutic application, *Curr. Gene Ther.* 9 (2009) 91–103.

59. A. Erez, O.A. Shchelochkov, S.E. Plon, F. Scaglia, B. Lee, Insights into the pathogenesis and treatment of cancer from inborn errors of metabolism, *Am. J. Hum. Genet.* 88 (2011) 402–421.

60. M.R.S. Alix Scholer-Dahirel, A. Loo, L. Bagdasarian, R. Meyer, R. Guo, S. Woolfenden, J.M. Kristine, K. Yu, K. Killary, D. Sonkin, Y.-M. Yao, M. Warmuth, W.R. Sellers, F.S. Robert Schlegel, R.E. Mosher, M.E. McLaughlin, Maintenance of adenomatous polyposis coli (APC)-mutant colorectal cancer is dependent on Wnt/β-catenin signaling, *Proc. Natl. Acad. Sci. U. S. A.* 108 (2011) 17135–17140.

61. E. Raskopf, A. Vogt, T. Sauerbruch, V. Schmitz, siRNA targeting VEGF inhibits hepatocellular carcinoma growth and tumor angiogenesis in vivo, *J. Hepatol.* 49 (2008) 977–984.

62. K. Zhang, K. Chu, X.Wu, H. Gao, J. Wang, Y.C. Yuan, S. Loera, K. Ho, Y.Wang, W. Chow, F. Un, P. Chu, Y. Yen, Amplification of FRS2 and activation of FGFR/FRS2 signaling pathway in high-grade liposarcoma, *Cancer Res.* 73 (2013) 1298–1307.

63. P.G. Rychahou, L.N. Jackson, S.R. Silva, S. Rajaraman, B.M. Evers, Targeted molecular therapy of the PI3K pathway: therapeutic significance of PI3K subunit targeting in colorectal carcinoma, *Ann. Surg.* 243 (2006) 833–842 (discussion 843–834).

64. H. Clevers, Wnt/beta-catenin signaling in development and disease, *Cell* 127 (2006) 469–480.

65. A.O. Kaseb, A. Hanbali, M. Cotant, M.M. Hassan, I. Wollner, P.A. Philip, Vascular endothelial growth factor in the management of hepatocellular carcinoma: a review of literature, *Cancer* 115 (2009) 4895–4906.

66. V.P. Eswarakumar, I. Lax, J. Schlessinger, Cellular signaling by fibroblast growth factor receptors, *Cytokine Growth Factor Rev.* 16 (2005) 139–149.

67. D.A. Fruman, C. Rommel, PI3K and cancer: lessons, challenges and opportunities, *Nat. Rev. Drug Discov.* 13 (2014) 140–156.

68. P. Huang, X. Xu, L. Wang, B. Zhu, X. Wang, J. Xia, The role of EGF–EGFR signaling pathway in hepatocellular carcinoma inflammatory microenvironment, *J. Cell. Mol. Med.* 18 (2014) 218–230.

69. S. Whittaker, R. Marais, A.X. Zhu, The role of signaling pathways in the development and treatment of hepatocellular carcinoma, *Oncogene* 29 (2010) 4989–5005.

70. G. Szabo, S. Bala, MicroRNAs in liver disease, *Nat. Rev. Gastroenterol. Hepatol.* 10 (2013) 542–552.

71. F. Azam, A. Koulaouzidis, Hepatitis B virus and hepatocarcinogenesis, *Ann. Hepatol.* 7 (2008) 125–129.

72. A.B. Cefalu, J.P. Pirruccello, D. Noto, S. Gabriel, V. Valenti, N. Gupta, R. Spina, P. Tarugi, S. Kathiresan, M.R. Averna, A novel APOB mutation identified by exome sequencing cosegregates with steatosis, liver cancer, and hypocholesterolemia, *Arterioscler. Thromb. Vasc. Biol.* 33 (2013) 2021–2025.

73. X.Q.Wang, W. Zhang, E.L. Lui, Y. Zhu, P. Lu, X. Yu, J. Sun, S. Yang, R.T. Poon, S.T. Fan, Notch1–Snail1–E-cadherin pathway in metastatic hepatocellular carcinoma, *Int. J. Cancer* 131 (2012) E163–E172.

74. M. Riaz, M. Idrees, H. Kanwal, F. Kabir, An overview of triple infection with hepatitis B, C and D viruses, *Virol. J.* 8 (2011) 368.

75. http://www.cdc.gov/hepatitis/B/bFAQ.htm, Hepatitis B information for public.

76. D. Halegoua-De Marzio, H.-W. Hann, Then and now: the progress in hepatitis B treatment over the past 20 years, *World J. Gastroenterol.* 20 (2014) 401–413.

77. C.I.Wooddell, D.B. Rozema, M. Hossbach, M. John, H.L. Hamilton, Q. Chu, J.O. Hegge, J.J. Klein, D.H. Wakefield, C.E. Oropeza, J. Deckert, I. Roehl, K. Jahn-Hofmann, P. Hadwiger, H.-P. Vornlocher, A. McLachlan, D.L. Lewis, Hepatocyte-targeted RNAi therapeutics for the treatment of chronic hepatitis B virus infection, *Mol. Ther.* 21 (2013) 973–985.

78. S. Carmona, M.R. Jorgensen, S. Kolli, C. Crowther, F.H. Salazar, P.L. Marion, M. Fujino, Y. Natori, M. Thanou, P. Arbuthnot, A.D. Miller, Controlling HBV replication in vivo by intravenous administration of triggered PEGylated siRNA-nanoparticles, *Mol. Pharm.* 6 (2009) 706–717.

79. S.I. Kim, D. Shin, T.H. Choi, J.C. Lee, G.-J.Cheon, K.-Y. Kim, M. Park, M. Kim, Systemic and specific delivery of small interfering RNAs to the liver mediated by apolipoprotein A–I, *Mol. Ther.* 15 (2007) 1145–1152.

80. M. Konishi, C.H. Wu, G.Y. Wu, Inhibition of HBV replication by siRNA in a stable HBV-producing cell line, *Hepatology* 38 (2003) 842–850.

81. G. Li, G. Jiang, J. Lu, S. Chen, L. Cui, J. Jiao, Y. Wang, Inhibition of hepatitis B virus cccDNA by siRNA in transgenic mice, *Cell Biochem. Biophys.* 69 (2014) 649–654.

82. G.-Q. Li, H.-X. Gu, D. Li, W.-Z. Xu, Inhibition of hepatitis B virus cccDNA replication by siRNA, *Biochem. Biophys. Res. Commun.* 355 (2007) 404–408.

83. D. Grimm, All for one, one for all: new combinatorial RNAi therapies combat hepatitis C virus evolution, *Mol. Ther.* 20 (2012) 1661–1663.

84. T.J. Liang, M.G. Ghany, Current and future therapies for hepatitis C virus infection, *N. Engl. J. Med.* 368 (2013) 1907–1917.

85. M. Korf, D. Jarczak, C. Beger, M.P. Manns, M. Kruger, Inhibition of hepatitis C virus translation and subgenomic replication by siRNAs directed against highly conserved HCV sequence and cellular HCV cofactors, *J. Hepatol.* 43 (2005) 225–234.

86. T. Watanabe, T. Umehara, F. Yasui, S.-I. Nakagawa, J. Yano, T. Ohgi, S. Sonoke, K. Satoh, K. Inoue, M. Yoshiba, M. Kohara, Liver target delivery of small interfering RNA to the HCV gene by lactosylated cationic liposome, *J. Hepatol.* 47 (2007) 744–750.

87. H. Ma, A. Dallas, H. Ilves, J. Shorenstein, I. MacLachlan, K. Klumpp, B.H. Johnston, Formulated minimal-length synthetic small hairpin RNAs are potent inhibitors of hepatitis C virus in mice with humanized livers, *Gastroenterology* 146 (2014) 63–66.

88. P.K. Chandra, A.K. Kundu, S. Hazari, S. Chandra, L. Bao, T. Ooms, G.F. Morris, T. Wu, T.K. Mandal, S. Dash, Inhibition of hepatitis C virus replication by intracellular delivery of multiple siRNAs by nanosomes, *Mol. Ther.* 20 (2012) 1724–1736.

89. S.I. Kim, D. Shin, H. Lee, B.Y. Ahn, Y. Yoon, M. Kim, Targeted delivery of siRNA against hepatitis C virus by apolipoprotein A–I-bound cationic liposomes, *J. Hepatol.* 50 (2009) 479–488.

90. M. Ansar, U.A. Ashfaq, I. Shahid, M.T. Sarwar, T. Javed, S. Rehman, S. Hassan, S. Riazuddin, Inhibition of full length hepatitis C virus particles of 1a genotype through small interference RNA, *Virol. J.* 8 (2011) 8–203.

91. T.W. Geisbert, A.C.H. Lee, M. Robbins, J.B. Geisbert, A.N. Honko, V. Sood, J.C. Johnson, S. de Jong, I. Tavakoli, A. Judge, L.E. Hensley, I. MacLachlan, Postexposure protection of non-human primates against a lethal Ebola virus challenge with RNA interference: a proof-of-concept study, *Lancet* 375 (2010) 1896–1905.

92. T.W. Geisbert, L.E. Hensley, E. Kagan, E.Z. Yu, J.B. Geisbert, K. Daddario-DiCaprio, E.A. Fritz, P.B. Jahrling, K. McClintock, J.R. Phelps, A.C.H. Lee, A. Judge, L.B. Jeffs, I. MacLachlan, Postexposure protection of guinea pigs against a lethal Ebola virus challenge is conferred by RNA interference, *J. Infect. Dis.* 193 (2006) 1650–1657.

93. A. Shlomai, Y. Shaul, Inhibition of hepatitis B virus expression and replication by RNA interference, *Hepatology* 37 (2003) 764–770.

94. O.M. Merkel, I. Rubinstein, T. Kissel, siRNA delivery to the lung: what's new? *Adv. Drug Deliv. Rev.* 75 (2014) 112–128.

95. C. Kelly, A.B. Yadav, P.J. McKiernan, C.M. Greene, S.A. Cryan, RNAi in respiratory diseases, in: K. Cheng, R.I. Mahato (Eds.), *Advanced Delivery and Therapeutic Applications of RNAi*, John Wiley and Sons, Ltd, Chichester (2013), pp. 391–416.

96. M. Grzelinski, O. Pinkenburg, T. Buch, M. Gold, S. Stohr, H. Kalwa, T. Gudermann, A. Aigner, Critical role of G(alpha)12 and G(alpha)13 for human small cell lung cancer cell proliferation in vitro and tumor growth in vivo, *Clin. Cancer Res.* 16 (2010) 1402–1415.

97. D.E. Zamora-Avila, P. Zapata-Benavides, M.A. Franco-Molina, S. Saavedra- Alonso, L.M. Trejo-Avila, D. Resendez-Perez, J.L. Mendez-Vazquez, J. Isaias-Badillo, C. Rodriguez-Padilla, WT1 gene silencing by aerosol delivery of PEI–RNAi complexes inhibits B16–F10 lung metastases growth, *Cancer Gene Ther.* 16 (2009) 892–899.

98. Q. Ge, L. Filip, A. Bai, T. Nguyen, H.N. Eisen, J. Chen, Inhibition of influenza virus production in virus-infected mice by RNA interference, *Proc. Natl. Acad. Sci. U. S. A.* 101 (2004) 8676–8681.

99. M. Thomas, J.J. Lu, Q. Ge, C. Zhang, J. Chen, A.M. Klibanov, Full deacylation of polyethylenimine dramatically boosts its gene delivery efficiency and specificity to mouse lung, *Proc. Natl. Acad. Sci. U. S. A.* 102 (2005) 5679–5684.

100. V. Bitko, A. Musiyenko, O. Shulyayeva, S. Barik, Inhibition of respiratory viruses by nasally administered siRNA, *Nat. Med.* 11 (2005) 50–55.

101. K.L. Clark, S.A. Hughes, P. Bulsara, J. Coates, K.Moores, J. Parry, M. Carr, R.J.Mayer, P. Wilson, C. Gruenloh, D. Levin, J. Darton, W.M. Weber, K. Sobczak, D.R. Gill, S.C. Hyde, L.A. Davies, I.A. Pringle, S.G. Sumner-Jones, V. Jadhav, S. Jamison, W.R. Strapps, V. Pickering, M.R. Edbrooke, Pharmacological characterization of a novel ENaCalpha siRNA (GSK2225745) with potential for the treatment of cystic fibrosis, *Mol. Ther.-Nucleic Acids* 2 (2013), e65.

102. J.H. Seong, K.M. Lee, S.T. Kim, S.E. Jin, C.K. Kim, Polyethylenimine-based antisense oligodeoxynucleotides of IL-4 suppress the production of IL-4 in a murine model of airway inflammation, *J. Gene. Med.* 8 (2006) 314–323.

103. T.N. Lively, K. Kossen, A. Balhorn, T. Koya, S. Zinnen, K. Takeda, J.J. Lucas, B. Polisky, I.M. Richards, E.W. Gelfand, Effect of chemically modified IL-13 short interfering RNA on development of airway hyperresponsiveness in mice, *J. Allergy Clin. Immunol.* 121 (2008) 88–94.

104. M. Zheng, D. Librizzi, A. Kilic, Y. Liu, H. Renz, O.M. Merkel, T. Kissel, Enhancing in vivo circulation and siRNA delivery with biodegradable polyethylenimine graft-polycaprolactone-block-poly(ethylene glycol) copolymers, *Biomaterials* 33 (2012) 6551–6558.

105. Y. Oe, R.J. Christie, M. Naito, S.A. Low, S. Fukushima, K. Toh, Y.Miura, Y. Matsumoto, N. Nishiyama, K. Miyata, K. Kataoka, Actively-targeted polyion complex micelles stabilized by cholesterol and disulfide cross-linking for systemic delivery of siRNA to solid tumors, *Biomaterials* 35 (2014) 7887–7895.

106. Y. Matsumoto, T. Nomoto, H. Cabral, Y. Matsumoto, S. Watanabe, R.J. Christie, K. Miyata, M. Oba, T. Ogura, Y. Yamasaki, N. Nishiyama, T. Yamasoba, K. Kataoka, Direct and instantaneous observation of intravenously injected substances using intravital confocal micro-videography, *Biomed. Opt. Express* 1 (2010) 1209–1216.

107. F.M. van de Water, O.C. Boerman, A.C. Wouterse, J.G. Peters, F.G. Russel, R. Masereeuw, Intravenously administered short interfering RNA accumulates in the kidney and selectively suppresses gene function in renal proximal tubules, *Drug Metab. Dispos.* 34 (2006) 1393–1397.

108. J. Christensen, K. Litherland, T. Faller, E. van de Kerkhof, F. Natt, J. Hunziker, J. Krauser, P. Swart, Metabolism studies of unformulated internally [3H]-labeled short interfering RNAs in mice, *Drug Metab. Dispos.* 41 (2013) 1211–1219.

109. S. Gao, F. Dagnaes-Hansen, E.J. Nielsen, J. Wengel, F. Besenbacher, K.A. Howard, J. Kjems, The effect of chemical modification and nanoparticle formulation on stability and biodistribution of siRNA in mice, *Mol. Ther.* 17 (2009) 1225–1233.

110. J. Christensen, K. Litherland, T. Faller, E. van de Kerkhof, F. Natt, J. Hunziker, J. Boos, I. Beuvink, K. Bowman, J. Baryza, M. Beverly, C. Vargeese, O. Heudi, M. Stoeckli, J. Krauser, P. Swart, Biodistribution and metabolism studies of lipid nanoparticle formulated internally [3H]-labeled siRNA in mice, *Drug Metab. Dispos.* 42 (2014) 431–440.

111. G. Ozcan, B. Ozpolat, R.L. Coleman, A.K. Sood, G. Lopez-Berestein, Preclinical and clinical development of siRNA-based therapeutics, *Adv. Drug Deliv. Rev.* 87 (2015) 108–119.

112. J. Tabernero, G.I. Shapiro, P.M. LoRusso, A. Cervantes, G.K. Schwartz, G.J. Weiss, L. Paz-Ares, D.C. Cho, J.R. Infante, M. Alsina, M.M. Gounder, R. Falzone, J. Harrop, A.C. White, I. Toudjarska, D. Bumcrot, R.E. Meyers, G. Hinkle, N. Svrzikapa, R.M. Hutabarat, V.A. Clausen, J. Cehelsky, S.V. Nochur, C. Gamba-Vitalo, A.K. Vaishnaw, D.W. Sah, J.A. Gollob, H.A. Burris, First-in-humans trial of an RNA interference therapeutic targeting VEGF and KSP in cancer patients with liver involvement, *Cancer Discov.* 3 (2013) 406–417.

113. B. Schultheis, D. Strumberg, A. Santel, C. Vank, F. Gebhardt, O. Keil, C. Lange, K. Giese, J. Kaufmann, M. Khan, J. Drevs, First-in-human phase I study of the liposomal RNA interference therapeutic Atu027 in patients with advanced solid tumors, *J. Clin. Oncol.* 32 (2014) 4141–4148.

114. D.W. Bartlett, H. Su, I.J. Hildebrandt, W.A. Weber, M.E. Davis, Impact of tumor specific targeting on the biodistribution and efficacy of siRNA nanoparticles measured by multimodality in vivo imaging, *Proc. Natl. Acad. Sci. U. S. A.* 104 (2007) 15549–15554.

115. J.E. Zuckerman, I. Gritli, A. Tolcher, J.D. Heidel, D. Lim, R.Morgan, B. Chmielowski, A. Ribas, M.E. Davis, Y. Yen, Correlating animal and human phase Ia/Ib clinical data with CALAA-01, a targeted, polymer-based nanoparticle containing siRNA, *Proc. Natl. Acad. Sci. U. S. A.* 111 (2014) 11449–11454.

116. R.Z. Yu, B. Baker, A. Chappell, R.S. Geary, E. Cheung, A.A. Levin, Development of an ultrasensitive noncompetitive hybridization-ligation enzyme-linked immunosorbent assay for the determination of phosphorothioate oligodeoxynucleotide in plasma, *Anal. Biochem.* 304 (2002) 19–25.

117. J.E. Zuckerman, C.H. Choi, H. Han, M.E. Davis, Polycation-siRNA nanoparticles can disassemble at the kidney glomerular basement membrane, *Proc. Natl. Acad. Sci. U. S. A.* 109 (2012) 3137–3142.

118. Y. Chen, J.J. Wu, L. Huang, Nanoparticles targeted with NGR motif deliver c-myc siRNA and doxorubicin for anticancer therapy, *Mol. Ther.* 18 (2010) 828–834.

119. M.S. Lee, J.E. Lee, E. Byun, N.W. Kim, K. Lee, H. Lee, S.J. Sim, D.S. Lee, J.H. Jeong, Target-specific delivery of siRNA by stabilized calcium phosphate nanoparticles using dopa-hyaluronic acid conjugate, *J. Control. Release* 192 (2014) 122–130.

120. F. Pittella, H. Cabral, Y. Maeda, P. Mi, S. Watanabe, H. Takemoto, H.J. Kim, N. Nishiyama, K. Miyata, K. Kataoka, Systemic siRNA delivery to a spontaneous pancreatic tumor model in transgenic mice by PEGylated calcium phosphate hybrid micelles, *J. Control. Release* 178 (2014) 18–24.

121. S. Son, S. Song, S.J. Lee, S.Min, S.A. Kim, J.Y. Yhee, M.S. Huh, I. Chan Kwon, S.Y. Jeong, Y. Byun, S.H. Kim, K. Kim, Self-crosslinked human serum albumin nanocarriers for systemic delivery of polymerized siRNA to tumors, *Biomaterials* 34 (2013) 9475–9485.

122. B. Shi, E. Keough, A. Matter, K. Leander, S. Young, E. Carlini, A.B. Sachs, W. Tao, M. Abrams, B. Howell, L. Sepp-Lorenzino, Biodistribution of small interfering RNA at the organ and cellular levels after lipid nanoparticle-mediated delivery, *J. Histochem. Cytochem.* 59 (2011) 727–740.

123. K.Y. Choi, O.F. Silvestre, X. Huang, K.H. Min, G.P. Howard, N. Hida, A.J. Jin, N. Carvajal, S.W. Lee, J.I. Hong, X. Chen, Versatile RNA interference nanoplatform for systemic delivery of RNAs, *ACS Nano.* 8 (2014) 4559–4570.

124. S.A. Jensen, E.S. Day, C.H. Ko, L.A. Hurley, J.P. Luciano, F.M. Kouri, T.J. Merkel, A.J. Luthi, P.C. Patel, J.I. Cutler, W.L. Daniel, A.W. Scott, M.W. Rotz, T.J. Meade, D.A. Giljohann, C.A. Mirkin, A.H. Stegh, Spherical nucleic acid nanoparticle conjugates as an RNAi-based therapy for glioblastoma, *Sci. Transl. Med.* 5 (2013) 209ra152.

125. A. Schlegel, C. Largeau, P. Bigey, M. Bessodes, K. Lebozec, D. Scherman, V. Escriou, Anionic polymers for decreased toxicity and enhanced in vivo delivery of siRNA complexed with cationic liposomes, *J. Control. Release* 152 (2011) 393–401.

126. J. Gao, H. Chen, Y. Yu, J. Song, H. Song, X. Su, W. Li, X. Tong, W. Qian, H. Wang, J. Dai, Y. Guo, Inhibition of hepatocellular carcinoma growth using immunoliposomes for co-delivery of adriamycin and ribonucleotide reductase M2 siRNA, *Biomaterials* 34 (2013) 10084–10098.

127. X.B. Xiong, A. Lavasanifar, Traceable multifunctional micellar nanocarriers for cancer-targeted co-delivery of MDR-1 siRNA and doxorubicin, *ACS Nano.* 5 (2011) 5202–5213.

128. G. Sass, P. Leukel, V. Schmitz, E. Raskopf, M. Ocker, D. Neureiter, M. Meissnitzer, E. Tasika, A. Tannapfel, G. Tiegs, Inhibition of heme oxygenase 1 expression by small interfering RNA decreases orthotopic tumor growth in livers of mice, *Int. J. Cancer* 123 (2008) 1269–1277.

129. J. Park, J. Park, Y. Pei, J. Xu, Y. Yeo, Pharmacokinetics and biodistribution of recently-developed siRNA nanomedicines. *Adv. Drug Deliv. Rev.* 104 (2016) 93–109.

130. M. Kornek, V. Lukacs-Kornek, A. Limmer, E. Raskopf, U. Becker, M. Klockner, T. Sauerbruch, V. Schmitz, 1,2-Dioleoyl-3-trimethylammonium-propane (DOTAP)-formulated, immune-stimulatory vascular endothelial growth factor a small interfering RNA (siRNA) increases antitumoral efficacy in murine orthotopic hepatocellular carcinoma with liver fibrosis, *Mol. Med.* 14 (2008) 365–373.

131. L. Li, R.Wang, D.Wilcox, A. Sarthy, X. Lin, X. Huang, L. Tian, P. Dande, R.D. Hubbard, T.M. Hansen, C.Wada, X. Zhao, W.M. Kohlbrenner, S.W. Fesik, Y. Shen, Developing lipid nanoparticle-based siRNA therapeutics for hepatocellular carcinoma using an integrated approach, *Mol. Cancer Ther.* 12 (2013) 2308–2318.

132. J. Gao, Y. Yu, Y. Zhang, J. Song, H. Chen, W. Li, W. Qian, L. Deng, G. Kou, J. Chen, Y. Guo, EGFR-specific PEGylated immunoliposomes for active siRNA delivery in hepatocellular carcinoma, *Biomaterials* 33 (2012) 270–282.

133. D.V. Morrissey, J.A. Lockridge, L. Shaw, K. Blanchard, K. Jensen, W. Breen, K. Hartsough, L. Machemer, S. Radka, V. Jadhav, N. Vaish, S. Zinnen, C. Vargeese, K. Bowman,

C.S. Shaffer, L.B. Jeffs, A. Judge, I. MacLachlan, B. Polisky, Potent and persistent in vivo anti-HBV activity of chemically modified siRNAs, *Nat. Biotechnol.* 23 (2005) 1002–1007.

134. D.V. Morrissey, K. Blanchard, L. Shaw, K. Jensen, J.A. Lockridge, B. Dickinson, J.A. McSwiggen, C. Vargeese, K. Bowman, C.S. Shaffer, B.A. Polisky, S. Zinnen, Activity of stabilized short interfering RNA in a mouse model of hepatitis B virus replication, *Hepatology* 41 (2005) 1349–1356.

135. M. Mével, N. Kamaly, S. Carmona, M.H. Oliver, M.R. Jorgensen, C. Crowther, F.H. Salazar, P.L. Marion, M. Fujino, Y. Natori, M. Thanou, P. Arbuthnot, J.-J. Yaouanc, P.A. Jaffrès, A.D. Miller, DODAG; a versatile new cationic lipid that mediates efficient delivery of pDNA and siRNA, *J. Control. Release* 143 (2010) 222–232.

136. H. Lee, S.I. Kim, D. Shin, Y. Yoon, T.H. Choi, G.-J. Cheon, M. Kim, Hepatic siRNA delivery using recombinant human apolipoprotein A–I in mice, *Biochem. Biophys. Res. Commun.* 378 (2009) 192–196.

137. https://clinicaltrials.gov/show/NCT02065336, Study of ARC-520 in patients with chronic hepatitis B virus.

138. https://clinicaltrials.gov/show/NCT02041715, Safety, tolerability and pharmacokinetic first in human (FIH) study for intravenous (IV) TKM-100802.

139. C.S. Kraft, A.L. Hewlett, S. Koepsell, A.M. Winkler, C.J. Kratochvil, L. Larson, J.B. Varkey, A.K. Mehta, G.M. Lyon, R.J. Friedman-Moraco, V.C. Marconi, C.E. Hill, J.N. Sullivan, D.W. Johnson, S.J. Lisco, M.J. Mulligan, T.M. Uyeki, A.K. McElroy, T. Sealy, S. Campbell, C. Spiropoulou, U. Stroher, I. Crozier, R. Sacra, M.J. Connor Jr., V. Sueblinvong, H.A. Franch, P.W. Smith, B.S. Ribner, The use of TKM-100802 and convalescent plasma in 2 patients with Ebola virus disease in the United States, *Clin. Infect. Dis.* 61 (2015) 496–502.

140. M. Gunther, J. Lipka, A. Malek, D. Gutsch, W. Kreyling, A. Aigner, Polyethylenimines for RNAi-mediated gene targeting in vivo and siRNA delivery to the lung, *Eur. J. Pharm. Biopharm.* 77 (2011) 438–449.

141. M.E. Bonnet, J.B. Gossart, E. Benoit, M. Messmer, O. Zounib, V. Moreau, J.P. Behr, N. Lenne-Samuel, V. Kedinger, A. Meulle, P. Erbacher, A.L. Bolcato-Bellemin, Systemic delivery of sticky siRNAs targeting the cell cycle for lung tumor metastasis inhibition, *J. Control. Release* 170 (2013) 183–190.

142. A.-L. Bolcato-Bellemin, M.-E. Bonnet, G. Creusat, P. Erbacher, J.-P. Behr, Sticky overhangs enhance siRNA-mediated gene silencing, *Proc. Natl. Acad. Sci. U. S. A.* 104 (2007) 16050–16055.

143. J. McCaskill, R. Singhania, M. Burgess, R. Allavena, S. Wu, A. Blumenthal, N.A. McMillan, Efficient biodistribution and gene silencing in the lung epithelium via intravenous liposomal delivery of siRNA, *Mol. Ther. Nucleic Acids* 2 (2013) e96.

144. V. Fehring, U. Schaeper, K. Ahrens, A. Santel, O. Keil, M. Eisermann, K. Giese, J. Kaufmann, Delivery of therapeutic siRNA to the lung endothelium via novel lipoplex formulation DACC, *Mol. Ther.* 22 (2014) 811–820.

145. K.J. Polach, M. Matar, J. Rice, G. Slobodkin, J. Sparks, R. Congo, A. Rea-Ramsey, D. McClure, E. Brunhoeber, M. Krampert, A. Schuster, K. Jahn-Hofmann, M. John, H.P. Vornlocher, J.G. Fewell, K. Anwer, A. Geick, Delivery of siRNA to the mouse lung via a functionalized lipopolyamine, *Mol. Ther.* 20 (2012) 91–100.

146. J.E. Dahlman, C. Barnes, O.F. Khan, A. Thiriot, S. Jhunjunwala, T.E. Shaw, Y. Xing, H.B. Sager, G. Sahay, L. Speciner, A. Bader, R.L. Bogorad, H. Yin, T. Racie, Y. Dong, S. Jiang, D. Seedorf, A. Dave, K. Singh Sandhu, M.J. Webber, T. Novobrantseva, V.M. Ruda, A.K. Lytton-Jean, C.G. Levins, B. Kalish, D.K. Mudge, M. Perez, L. Abezgauz, P. Dutta, L. Smith, K. Charisse, M.W. Kieran, K. Fitzgerald, M. Nahrendorf, D. Danino, R.M. Tuder, U.H. von Andrian, A. Akinc, D. Panigrahy, A. Schroeder, V. Koteliansky, R. Langer, D.G. Anderson, In vivo endothelial siRNA delivery using polymeric nanoparticles with low molecular weight, Nat. Nanotechnol. 9 (2014) 648–655.

147. O.B. Garbuzenko, M. Saad, S. Betigeri, M. Zhang, A.A. Vetcher, V.A. Soldatenkov, D.C. Reimer, V.P. Pozharov, T. Minko, Intratracheal versus intravenous liposomal delivery of siRNA, antisense oligonucleotides and anticancer drug, Pharm. Res. 26 (2009) 382–394.

148. O.M. Merkel, A. Beyerle, D. Librizzi, A. Pfestroff, T.M. Behr, B. Sproat, P.J. Barth, T. Kissel, Nonviral siRNA delivery to the lung: investigation of PEG-PEI polyplexes and their in vivo performance, Mol. Pharm. 6 (2009) 1246–1260.

149. B. Gutbier, S.M. Kube, K. Reppe, A. Santel, C. Lange, J. Kaufmann, N. Suttorp, M. Witzenrath, RNAi-mediated suppression of constitutive pulmonary gene expression by small interfering RNA in mice, Pulm. Pharmacol. Ther. 23 (2010) 334–344.

150. A. Wittrup, J. Lieberman, Knocking down disease: a progress report on siRNA therapeutics, Nat. Rev. Genet. 16 (2015) 543–552.

151. A.L. Jackson, J. Burchard, D. Leake, A. Reynolds, J. Schelter, J. Guo, J.M. Johnson, L. Lim, J. Karpilow, K. Nichols, W. Marshall, A. Khvorova, P.S. Linsley, Position specific chemical modification of siRNAs reduces "off-target" transcript silencing. RNA 12 (2006) 1197–1205.

152. L. Huang, J. Jin, P. Deighan, E. Kiner, L. McReynolds, J. Lieberman, Efficient and specific gene knockdown by small interfering RNAs produced in bacteria, Nat. Biotechnol. 31 (2013) 350–356.

153. S. Loisel, C. Le Gall, L. Doucet, C. Ferec, V. Floch, Contribution of plasmid DNA to hepatotoxicity after systemic administration of lipoplexes, Hum. Gene Ther. 12 (2001) 685–696.

154. J.D. Tousignant, A.L. Gates, L.A. Ingram, C.L. Johnson, J.B. Nietupski, S.H. Cheng, S.J. Eastman, R.K. Scheule, Comprehensive analysis of the acute toxicities induced by systemic administration of cationic lipid:plasmid DNA complexes in mice, Hum. Gene Ther. 11 (2000) 2493–2513.

155. W. Yan, W. Chen, L. Huang, Mechanism of adjuvant activity of cationic liposome: phosphorylation of a MAP kinase, ERK and induction of chemokines, Mol. Immunol. 44 (2007) 3672–3681.

156. D.P. Vangasseri, Z. Cui, W. Chen, D.A. Hokey, L.D. Falo Jr., L. Huang, Immunostimulation of dendritic cells by cationic liposomes, Mol. Membr. Biol. 23 (2006) 385–395.

157. T. Tanaka, A. Legat, E. Adam, J. Steuve, J.S. Gatot, M. Vandenbranden, L. Ulianov, C. Lonez, J.M. Ruysschaert, E. Muraille, M. Tuynder, M. Goldman, A. Jacquet, DiC14-amidine cationic liposomes stimulate myeloid dendritic cells through Toll-like receptor 4, Eur. J. Immunol. 38 (2008) 1351–1357.

158. D. Fischer, T. Bieber, Y. Li, H.-P. Elsässer, T. Kissel, A novel non-viral vector for DNA delivery based on low molecular weight, branched polyethylenimine: effect of molecular weight on transfection efficiency and cytotoxicity, Pharm. Res. 16 (1999) 1273–1279.

159. M.A. Islam, T.E. Park, B. Singh, S.Maharjan, J. Firdous, M.H. Cho, S.K. Kang, C.H. Yun, Y.J. Choi, C.S. Cho, Major degradable polycations as carriers for DNA and siRNA, J. Control. Release 193 (2014) 74–89.

160. M.-N. Chien, P.-S. Yang, J.-J. Lee, T.-Y. Wang, Y.-C. Hsu, S.-P. Cheng, Recurrence-associated genes in papillary thyroid cancer: an analysis of data from the cancer genome atlas. Surgery 161 (2017) 1642–1650.

161. Y. Mao, M. Xing, Recent incidences and differential trends of thyroid cancer in the USA. Endocr. Relat. Cancer 23 (2016) 313–322.

162. R.H. Grogan, S.P. Kaplan, H. Cao, R.E. Weiss, L.J. Degroot, C.A. Simon, et al., A study of recurrence and death from papillary thyroid cancer with 27 years of median follow-up. Surgery 154 (2013) 1436–1446.

163. American Thyroid Association (ATA) Guidelines Taskforce on Thyroid Nodules and Differentiated Thyroid Cancer, D.S. Cooper, G.M. Doherty, B.R. Haugen, R.T. Kloos, S.L. Lee, S.J. Mandel, et al., Revised American Thyroid Association management guidelines for patients with thyroid nodules and differentiated thyroid cancer. Thyroid 19 (2009) 1167–1214.

164. B.R. Haugen, E.K. Alexander, K.C. Bible, G.M. Doherty, S.J. Mandel, Y.E. Nikiforov, et al., 2015 American Thyroid Association management guidelines for adult patients with thyroid nodules and differentiated thyroid cancer: the American Thyroid Association guidelines task force on thyroid nodules and differentiated thyroid cancer. Thyroid 26 (2016) 1–133.

165. S.P. Cheng, Y.C. Hsu, C.L. Liu, T.P. Liu, M.N. Chien, T.Y. Wang, et al., Significance of allelic percentage of BRAF c. 1799T A (V600E) mutation in papillary thyroid carcinoma. Ann. Surg. Oncol. 21 (2014) S619–S626.

166. G. Gandolfi, V. Sancisi, S. Piana, A. Ciarrocchi, Time to reconsider the meaning of BRAF V600E mutation in papillary thyroid carcinoma. Int. J. Cancer 137 (2015) 1001–1111.

167. R. Liu, M. Xing, TERT promoter mutations in thyroid cancer. Endocr. Relat. Cancer 23 (2016) R143–R155.

168. Cancer Genome Atlas Research Network, Integrated genomic characterization of papillary thyroid carcinoma. Cell 159 (2014) 676–690.

169. J. Wang, D. Duncan, Z. Shi, B. Zhang, WEB-based gene set analysis toolkit (WebGestalt): update 2013. Nucleic Acids Res. 41 (2013) W77–W83.

170. D.W. Huang, B.T. Sherman, R.A. Lempicki, Systematic and integrative analysis of large gene lists using DAVID bioinformatics resources. Nat. Protoc. 4 (2009) 44–57.

171. Y.C. Chang, Y.C. Hsu, C.L. Liu, S.Y. Huang, M.C. Hu, S.P. Cheng, Local anesthetics induce apoptosis in human thyroid cancer cells through the mitogen-activated protein kinase pathway. PLoS One 9 (2014) e89563.

172. M. Kanehisa, Y. Sato, M. Kawashima, M. Furumichi, M. Tanabe, KEGG as a reference resource for gene and protein annotation. Nucleic Acids Res. 44 (2016) D457–D462.

173. F. Lee, J.J. Lee, W.C. Jan, C.J. Wu, H.H. Chen, S.P. Cheng, Molecular pathways associated with transcriptional alterations in hyperparathyroidism. Oncol. Lett. 12 (2016) 621–626.

174. Y.J. Chai, J.W. Yi, H.G. Jee, Y.A. Kim, J.H. Kim, M. Xing, et al., Significance of the BRAF mRNA expression level in papillary thyroid carcinoma: an analysis of the cancer genome atlas data. PLoS One 11 (2016) e0159235.

175. M. Rivera, R.A. Ghossein, H. Schoder, D. Gomez, S.M. Larson, R.M. Tuttle, Histopathologic characterization of radioactive iodine-refractory fluorodeoxyglucose-positron emission tomography-positive thyroid carcinoma. *Cancer* 113 (2008) 48–56.

176. D. Viola, L. Valerio, E. Molinaro, L. Agate, V. Bottici, A. Biagini, et al., Treatment of advanced thyroid cancer with targeted therapies: ten years of experience. *Endocr. Relat. Cancer* 23 (2016) R185–R205.

177. C. Mian, S. Barollo, G. Pennelli, N. Pavan, M. Rugge, M.R. Pelizzo, et al., Molecular characteristics in papillary thyroid cancers (PTCs) with no 131I uptake. *Clin. Endocrinol.* 68 (2008) 108–116.

178. M.M. Sabra, J.M. Dominguez, R.K. Grewal, S.M. Larson, R.A. Ghossein, R.M. Tuttle, et al., Clinical outcomes and molecular profile of differentiated thyroid cancers with radioiodine-avid distant metastases. *J. Clin. Endocrinol. Metab.* 98 (2013) E829–E836.

179. C. Portulano, M. Paroder-Belenitsky, N. Carrasco, The Na$^+$/I$^-$ symporter (NIS): mechanism and medical impact. *Endocr. Rev.* 35 (2014) 106–149.

180. C. Spitzweg, K.C. Bible, L.C. Hofbauer, J.C. Morris, Advanced radioiodine-refractory differentiated thyroid cancer: the sodium iodide symporter and other emerging therapeutic targets. *Lancet Diabetes Endocrinol.* 2 (2014) 830–842.

181. D. Handkiewicz-Junak, J. Roskosz, K. Hasse-Lazar, S. Szpak-Ulczok, Z. Puch, A. Kukulska, et al., 13-cis-retinoic acid redifferentiation therapy and recombinant human thyrotropin-aided radioiodine treatment of non-functional metastatic thyroid cancer: a single-center, 53-patient phase 2 study. *Thyroid Res.* 2 (2009) 8.

182. A.A. Czajka, A. Wojcicka, A. Kubiak, M. Kotlarek, E. Bakula-Zalewska, L. Koperski, et al., Family of microRNA-146 regulates RARb in papillary thyroid carcinoma. *PLoS One* 11 (2016) e0151968.

183. C.T. Shen, Z.L. Qiu, H.J. Song, W.J. Wei, Q.Y. Luo, miRNA-106a directly targeting RARB associates with the expression of Na(+)/I(−) symporter in thyroid cancer by regulating MAPK signaling pathway. *J. Exp. Clin. Cancer Res.* 35 (2016) 101.

184. A.L. Ho, R.K. Grewal, R. Leboeuf, E.J. Sherman, D.G. Pfister, D. Deandreis, et al., Selumetinib-enhanced radioiodine uptake in advanced thyroid cancer. *N. Engl. J. Med.* 368 (2013) 623–632.

185. S.M. Rothenberg, D.G. McFadden, E.L. Palmer, G.H. Daniels, L.J. Wirth, Redifferentiation of iodine-refractory BRAF V600E-mutant metastatic papillary thyroid cancer with dabrafenib. *Clin. Cancer Res.* 21 (2015) 1028–1035.

186. M.S. Brose, M.E. Cabanillas, E.E. Cohen, L.J. Wirth, T. Riehl, H. Yue, et al., Vemurafenib in patients with BRAF(V600E)-positive metastatic or unresectable papillary thyroid cancer refractory to radioactive iodine: a non-randomised, multicentre, open-label, phase 2 trial. *Lancet Oncol.* 17 (2016) 1272–1282.

187. N. Ranjbari, F. Rahim, The Ki-67/MIB-1 index level and recurrence of papillary thyroid carcinoma. *Med. Hypotheses* 80 (2013) 311–314.

188. A. Albero, J.E. Lopez, A. Torres, L. de la Cruz, T. Martin, Effectiveness of chemotherapy in advanced differentiated thyroid cancer: a systematic review. *Endocr. Relat. Cancer* 23 (2016) R71–R84.

189. L. Peng, X.W. Bian, D.K. Li, C. Xu, G.M. Wang, Q.Y. Xia, et al., Large-scale RNA-seq transcriptome analysis of 4043 cancers and 548 normal tissue controls across 12 TCGA cancer types. *Sci. Rep.* 5 (2015) 13413.

190. E. Gatzidou, C. Michailidi, S. Tseleni-Balafouta, S. Theocharis, An epitome of DNA repair related genes and mechanisms in thyroid carcinoma. *Cancer Lett.* 290 (2010) 139–147.

191. A. Estrada-Bernal, M. Chatterjee, S.J. Haque, L. Yang, M.A. Morgan, S. Kotian, et al., MEK inhibitor GSK1120212-mediated radiosensitization of pancreatic cancer cells involves inhibition of DNA double-strand break repair pathways. *Cell Cycle* 14 (2015) 3713–3724.

192. H.M. Bovelstad, S. Nygard, H.L. Storvold, M. Aldrin, O. Borgan, A. Frigessi, et al., Predicting survival from micro-array data – a comparative study. *Bioinformatics* 23 (2007) 2080–2087.

193. K. Brennan, C. Holsinger, C. Dosiou, J.B. Sunwoo, H. Akatsu, R. Haile, et al., Development of prognostic signatures for intermediate-risk papillary thyroid cancer. *BMC Cancer* 16 (2016) 736.

194. Loutfy H. Madkour, *Reactive Oxygen Species (ROS), Nanoparticles, and Endoplasmic Reticulum (ER) Stress-Induced Cell Death Mechanisms* (2020). Paperback ISBN: 9780128224816 Imprint: Academic Press. Published Date: 1st August 2020. https://www.elsevier.com/books/reactive-oxygen-species-ros-nanoparticles-and-endoplasmic-reticulum-er-stress-induced-cell-death-mechanisms/madkour/978-0-12-822481-6

195. Loutfy H. Madkour, *Nanoparticles Induce Oxidative and Endoplasmic Reticulum Antioxidant Therapeutic Defenses* (2020). Copyright 2020 Publisher Springer International Publishing Copyright Holder Springer Nature Switzerland AG eBook ISBN 978-3-030-37297-2. doi:10.1007/978-3-030-37297-2. Hardcover ISBN 978-3-030-37296-5. Series ISSN 2194-0452. Edition Number 1. https://www.springer.com/gp/book/9783030372965?utm_campaign=3_pier05_buy_print&utm_content=en_08082017&utm_medium=referral&utm_source=google_books#otherversion=9783030372972

196. Loutfy H. Madkour, *Nucleic Acids as Gene Anticancer Drug Delivery Therapy*. 1st Edition. Publishing House: Elsevier (2020). Paperback ISBN: 9780128197776. Imprint: Academic Press Published Date: 2nd January 2020 Imprint: Academic Press Copyright: Paperback ISBN: 9780128197776. © Academic Press 2020 Published: 2nd January 2020. Imprint: Academic Press Paperback ISBN: 9780128197776. https://www.elsevier.com/books/nucleic-acids-as-gene-anticancer-drug-delivery therapy/madkour/978-0-12-819777-6

197. Loutfy H. Madkour, *Nanoelectronic Materials: Fundamentals and Applications (Advanced Structured Materials)* 1st Edition. 2019 Edition. https://link.springer.com/book/10.1007%2F978-3-030-21621-4. Series Title: Advanced Structured Materials Series Volume 116. Copyright 2019 Publisher. Springer International Publishing Copyright Holder Springer Nature Switzerland AG. eBook ISBN 978-3-030-21621-4. doi:10.1007/978-3-030-21621-4. Hardcover ISBN 978-3-030-21620-7. Series ISSN 1869-8433. Edition Number 1. Number of Pages XLIII, 783 Number of Illustrations 122 b/w illustrations, 494 illustrations in colour Topics. ISBN-10: 3030216209. ISBN-13: 978-3030216207 #117 in Nanotechnology (Books) #725 in Materials Science (Books) #187336 in Textbooks. https://books.google.com.eg/books/about/Nanoelectronic_Materials.html?id=YQXCxAEACAAJ&source=kp_book_description&redir_esc=y

13 Nanotechnologies Assemblies of siRNA and Chemotherapeutic Drugs Codelivered for Cancer Therapeutic Applications

13.1 DOUBLE-STRANDED RNA (dsRNA)

The discovery that dsRNA can trigger catalytic degradation of messenger RNA (mRNA) has inspired more than two decades of research aimed at understanding and harnessing this mechanism. Because well-designed RNA interference (RNAi) therapeutics can potently and specifically suppress translation of any gene, including intracellular targets traditionally considered "undruggable," they have been heavily studied as a potential new class of pharmaceutics that can modulate drug targets that are inaccessible by conventional small-molecule inhibitors and antibody drugs. In particular, synthetic, double-stranded small-interfering RNA (siRNA) has emerged as a leading candidate for the development of gene silencing therapeutics [1,2]. siRNA is potentially advantageous in comparison to other RNAi approaches because it can directly load into the RNA-induced silencing complex (RISC) machinery, simplifying dosing control and circumventing the requirement for delivery into the nucleus (e.g., as required with shRNA-encoding vectors) [3,4]. However, emergence of clinically approved siRNA therapies has remained slow, with the primary challenge being the formidable anatomical and physiological barriers that must be overcome to deliver siRNA to its intracellular site of action in target cell types [5].

To date, systemic delivery of siRNA therapeutics to targets in the liver has been most extensively tested in clinical trials; this approach is motivated by the ability to exploit the liver's physiological function as a filtration and clearance system [6–8]. Through strategic targeting of relevant hepatic genes, multiple siRNA therapeutics have proven efficacious in preclinical and clinical trials [7,9,10]. One of the most advanced along the regulatory pathway is a therapeutic by Alnylam currently in Phase III trials that target the transthyretin gene for treatment of transthyretin amyloidosis [7,11]. However, development of systemically delivered siRNA therapeutics that target tissues other than the liver has proven more challenging [8].

Local delivery systems offer a potentially more translatable alternative, as they confer the advantages of reducing off-target side effects and enable higher gene silencing at the target site [8]. For these reasons, many of the first therapeutic applications of siRNA tested clinically involved local delivery (primarily topical or injection-based).

However, initial clinical trials involving local siRNA delivery were largely disappointing and did not meet the high expectations of the scientific and medical communities [12,13]. These studies revealed unexpected concerns regarding siRNA safety (e.g., therapies based on naked siRNA-triggered immune responses) and pharmacokinetics [8,12–15]. The advancement of siRNA molecular design principles and improved delivery systems has increased the number of candidate siRNA therapeutics entering the clinical pipeline, but there is currently a dearth of locally delivered siRNA therapeutics in testing relative to systemically delivered formulations [8,12]. This chapter will focus on recent technologies that leverage the significant advantages of local siRNA delivery and have made progress toward overcoming the barriers that have thus far limited these applications.

13.2 siRNA MECHANISM

The molecular phenomenon of RNAi-based post-transcriptional gene silencing, first termed "reversible cosuppression," was unraveled following the unexpected observation by Napoli et al. in 1990 that introduction of a transgene intended to overexpress chalcone synthase (CHS, a gene for flower pigmentation) yielded more white flowers and was associated with a 50-fold reduction of CHS mRNA [16]. The gene silencing capability of antisense oligodeoxynucleotides (ODNs) was first elucidated, but it was discovered soon thereafter that dsRNAs are capable of achieving 100- to 1000-fold more potent gene suppression than ODNs [17]. The delivery of dsRNA of varying lengths, siRNA, short-hairpin RNA (shRNA), and plasmids expressing shRNA can trigger gene-specific silencing, which is optimal when there is full complementarity between the guide strand and the target mRNA sequence [2,18]. These synthetic dsRNA molecules are more effective than ODNs because they "hijack" the catalytically active gene silencing machinery that is integral to endogenous, negative-feedback pathways utilized by naturally expressed microRNA (miRNA) [2,19,20]. When larger dsRNAs are delivered to the cellular cytoplasm, they are cleaved by the enzyme dicer into siRNA, which are 19–21 nucleotides in length and characterized by 3′ nucleotide overhangs. The siRNA strands are

DOI: 10.1201/9781003229674-13

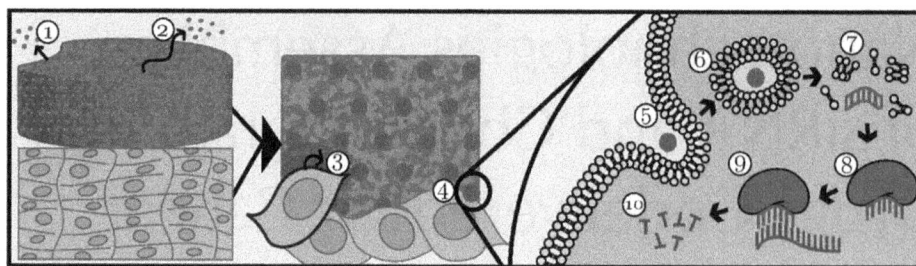

FIGURE 13.1 Schematic of local delivery and mechanism of action of siRNA. The green circle represents siRNA packaged into a carrier. A local delivery reservoir releases siRNA via (1) degradation of the reservoir and/or (2) diffusion. The reservoir, shown in direct contact with host tissue, can also facilitate (3) cell migration into the reservoir and (4) substrate-mediated siRNA uptake through (5) endocytosis. If the siRNA avoids (6) degradation by the endo-lysosomal system and (7) reaches the cytoplasm, its guide strand can be (8) incorporated into the activated RISC complex, which (9) binds to complementary mRNA and (10) initiates its degradation.

then separated, and the antisense or guide strand, recognized by a less stable 5′ end, is incorporated into the RISC [21]. The activated RISC loaded with the siRNA guide strand binds to complementary mRNA and initiates its degradation (Figure 13.1). Importantly, the activated RISC has enzymatic activity, enabling a single siRNA to elicit the degradation of multiple mRNAs [22]. In contrast, synthetic microRNA (miRNA) often modulates multiple mRNA targets with partial complementarity and thus can influence larger systems of genes [23]. While the coordinated control of multiple, related genes through miRNA therapeutics is a powerful strategy, properly designed siRNA-based therapeutics are desirable because they offer more predictable functional effects based on modulation of specific genes.

13.3 siRNA DELIVERY CHALLENGES

13.3.1 General Delivery Barriers

While discovery and development of small-molecule drugs for clinical use remains an enormous challenge, the translation of siRNA therapeutics is comparatively unchartered. Thus, in addition to traditional drug development challenges, the "normal" pipeline for development of an siRNA drug for FDA clearance has yet to be established [8,12]. The major difficulty faced when designing siRNA therapeutics is that of delivery to its site of action; synthetic dsRNA or siRNA molecules have relatively poor pharmacokinetic properties and thus face more formidable extracellular and intracellular delivery challenges relative to small-molecule drugs. Oral bioavailability of siRNA molecules is very poor because they are relatively large, hydrophilic, and susceptible to degradation, and systemic, intravenous delivery of siRNA results in rapid renal filtration and clearance through the urine [24]. siRNA also has a short half-life *in vivo* and can be degraded by nucleases, especially if optimized chemical modifications are not incorporated onto the siRNA molecule [25]. Furthermore, siRNA does not readily translocate lipid bilayers, such as those that constitute the outer cellular membrane and the endo-lysosomal intracellular vesicles. The latter can cause siRNA that has been internalized by target cells to be degraded within lysosomes

or exocytosed, rather than becoming bioavailable for interaction with the RISC machinery in the cytosol [24,26,27]. For example, only 1%–2% of the siRNA delivered by lipid nanoparticles is believed to be released into the cytosol and to be bioavailable for RISC loading and target gene silencing [27]. While it is not the focus of the current review, there are a variety of delivery systems under development for overcoming these systemic and general delivery barriers [24].

Utilization of siRNA therapeutically is also complicated by the potential for toxicity and immunogenicity of both the siRNA molecules and the carriers used. siRNA molecules can activate Toll-like receptors (TLRs), which are a part of the innate immune system that recognizes and mounts an immune response against microbial invaders [28–32]. Additionally, siRNA can elicit off-target effects due to partial sequence complementarity to unintended genes or by saturating the cell's RISC machinery, altering endogenous miRNA gene regulatory processes [31,33,34]. Furthermore, systems used to deliver siRNA can induce toxic and immunogenic consequences [24]. These inadvertent effects can override therapeutic benefits and confound interpretation of experiments designed to test the functional significance of siRNA therapeutics [14].

13.3.2 Local Delivery Considerations

Localized siRNA delivery obviates many of the systemic delivery barriers but also raises unique challenges. In topical strategies, the skin, the mucosal membranes, and the epithelial cells can act as delivery barriers to target cells [35]. For example, siRNA delivery to cervicovaginal or gastrointestinal tissues requires transversing a superficial mucosal layer [36–38]. However, in most depot systems, direct contact exists between the local delivery reservoir and the target cells (Figure 13.2). In this scenario, a primary design concern is to control the kinetics of siRNA release such that duration of gene silencing can be temporally controlled and/or sustained without repeated treatments. Without a mechanism for controlled release from the delivery system, siRNA activity has a finite half-life

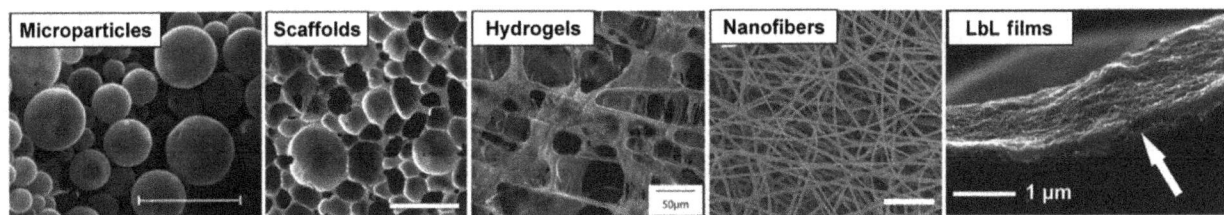

FIGURE 13.2 Scanning electron microscopy images of commonly employed constructs for local siRNA delivery [39,50,56–58].

and will diminish over time. This is especially important in applications where the siRNA dose cannot be easily reapplied, including delivery from the surface of an implanted device, delivery to sites that are not easily accessible and/or would require assistance from a healthcare professional, or delivery from depots that also serve as biodegradable tissue engineering scaffolds [39]. At sites of tissue repair, there is the added challenge of rapid cellular turnover and proliferation as the different phases of regeneration proceed; when transfected cells undergo mitosis, the siRNA dose is diluted among the daughter cells. In this challenging environment, siRNA gene suppression has been shown to be maximal at approximately 2 days post-transfection and to disappear almost entirely after one week [5,40]. By creating delivery platforms with tunable release profiles, gene silencing can be customized for specific therapeutic applications and for sustained effect in tissues that are remodeling and/or regenerating.

Local siRNA delivery systems and their degradation products must also be noncytotoxic and should not interfere with the desired therapeutic response. Materials that degrade into biocompatible, resorbable by-products eliminate the need for physical removal of the delivery system. For some systems, the rate at which the material degrades can be used to tune the temporal release profile of the siRNA [41,42]. Altering the kinetics for diffusion-based release is also possible, for example, by regulating the delivery system's cross-linking density and/or porosity via synthesis techniques [43–45]. Of particular interest for regenerative medicine and tissue engineering are multifunctional, porous biomaterials that enable controlled siRNA release, support cellular ingrowth, and degrade at rates that match *de novo* tissue formation [46–49]. Therefore, many delivery systems are fabricated using materials with inherent *in vivo* degradation mechanisms; for example, scaffold and microparticle systems are commonly based on hydrolytically degradable polyesters such as poly(lactic-co-glycolic acid) (PLGA) [43,44,48,50]. However, the degradation products of PLGA acidify the local environment and can result in inflammation, creating impetus for the exploration of other biodegradable systems [51,52]. Environmentally responsive systems that respond to cellular stimuli like proteases or reactive oxygen species (ROS) offer a promising alternative. For instance, biomaterials incorporating polythioketal cross-linkers confer ROS-dependent degradation that produces nonacidic, cytocompatible by-products [53,54]. The material choice for a local delivery depot determines not only the degradation rate but also the adherence of cells, their viability, and their phenotype. In addition, the affinity of an siRNA therapeutic for the material influences release and cellular uptake characteristics [42]. All of these concerns should be considered, with the goal of designing a system in which the reservoir and siRNA therapeutic work synergistically to elicit the desired cellular response.

Another approach to engineering delivery systems for spatially confined, efficient cellular uptake is to leverage the phenomenon of substrate-mediated uptake [49,55]. Substrate-mediated uptake or "reverse transfection" occurs when nucleic acids immobilized on a material surface are internalized by cells adherent to that surface rather than being internalized via solution phase endocytosis or pinocytosis (Figure 13.2). Substrate-mediated delivery concentrates the therapeutic at the cell–material interface and can enhance transfection efficiency by 10- to 100-fold [42,49,55]. This reduces diffusion of the siRNA away from the target site and is also especially relevant for tissue regenerative applications where cells adhere and grow within a biomaterial that possesses dual functions as a delivery depot and tissue template.

While local delivery presents novel challenges, it also has inherent advantages over systemic delivery that make it a logical focus for translation of siRNA therapies to a broader range of clinical applications. Systemic delivery systems elicit greater concerns regarding off-site toxicity, often cannot achieve sufficient doses within the tissue of interest, and must overcome the rapid renal clearance of siRNA which leads to low bioavailability [35]. Although many disease states will necessitate systemic delivery (e.g., metastatic carcinomas, systemic infections), local delivery may be a superior strategy for a subset of pathologies [37].

13.4 siRNA MODIFICATIONS AND CARRIERS

Though local siRNA delivery avoids many of the challenges associated with systemic injection, it does require measures to prevent siRNA degradation and to overcome cell membrane/endo-lysosomal barriers following depot injection/implantation *in vivo*. A variety of chemical modifications, conjugation strategies, and lipid/polymer carriers have been identified to address the challenges inherent to siRNA therapies. As these strategies have previously been reviewed comprehensively [24], this aspect of the literature will not be exhaustively overviewed herein.

A commonly utilized chemical modification to siRNA molecules is replacement of phosphodiester linkages with phosphorothioate linkages at select locations on the backbone, which confers improved resistance of siRNA to nuclease degradation [25,59,60]. Further, modifications to the siRNA backbone at the 2′ position, such as 2′-O-methyl (2OME), endow siRNA molecules with greater stability and eliminate the TLR-driven immune response without impacting silencing efficacy [25,59,61,62]. Careful siRNA sequence selection can also aid in avoiding modulation of nontargeted genes and enhance the activity at the targeted gene. Systematic, computer-aided optimization of siRNA sequence and design has become standard practice and accelerates identification of siRNA sequences likely to exhibit high target gene silencing with minimal off-target effects and immunogenicity [25,31].

Direct conjugation to molecules such as polymers, peptides, lipids, antibodies, and aptamers has also been explored for improving siRNA pharmacokinetic properties [63–65]. Lipid-like moieties such as cholesterol, α-tocopherol, and palmitic acid improve siRNA stability, cellular uptake, and gene silencing ability [66–68]. Alternatively, conjugation of targeting ligands to siRNA has shown promise as a means to facilitate receptor-mediated, cell-specific uptake. For example, Alnylam demonstrated the *in vivo* silencing efficacy of triantennary and trivalent N-acetylgalactosamine siRNA conjugates and showed hepatocyte-specific uptake when delivering the conjugates carrier-free [69,70]. The conjugation of cell integrin-binding peptides such as RGD and cell-penetrating peptides (CPPs) has also been explored for modifying siRNA molecules as well as carrier systems [71,72]. CPPs have emerged as potent cellular membrane translocators, but they are also associated with concerns regarding cytotoxicity and immunogenicity [73,74].

While optimization of siRNA sequence and chemical modifications can improve upon safety and efficacy, siRNA activity benefits from delivery via a carrier system in most applications. These carriers typically improve stability against nucleases and enhance cellular penetration capacity and/or endosomal escape; thus, siRNA formulation into nanocarriers is often utilized synergistically with systems for localized, sustained delivery [24]. siRNA carriers vary widely but commonly consist of lipids/liposomes, polymers, or viral constructs [24,63,65,75,76]. Transfection with lipids/liposomes is the most broadly utilized technique, with a variety of commercial reagents available that can facilitate fusion with and transport across cellular membranes [24,63,77]. Similarly, cationic polymers and dendrimers are conventionally used for siRNA packaging, protection, and delivery. Synthetic polymers, such as linear or branched polyethyleneimine (PEI), poly(L-lysine), poly(amidoamine) (PAMAM) dendrimers, poly(β-amino esters) (PBAEs), poly(dimethylaminoethylmethacrylate) (pDMAEMA), and histidine and/or imidazole-containing copolymers, as well as natural polymers like atelocollagen and chitosan, are among the most extensively utilized [24,78–84]. These cationic polymers electrostatically package/protect siRNA and,

in some cases, contain secondary and tertiary amines that enable endosomal escape via the proton sponge effect [78]. Other polymers have also been developed that have active membrane-disruptive behavior triggered by the slightly acidic pH of the endo-lysosomal pathway. These polymer-based systems have been utilized primarily to form siRNA nanoformulations with actively endosomolytic cores and have been combined with a variety of micelle/polyplex surface chemistries [84–88]. Several of these systems leverage a poly(DMAEMA-co-butyl methacrylate-co-propylacrylic acid (PAA) polymer block that is approximately charge-neutral and forms a stable micelle core at physiologic pH. When exposed to a more acidic pH, the DMAEMA and PAA monomers become concurrently more protonated, yielding a net cationic state that triggers micelle destabilization and endo-lysosomal membrane interaction/disruption [84].

Cationic lipids and polymers have a number of short-comings that are gradually being addressed through both rational design and high-throughput synthesis/screening approaches. Traditional cationic transfection reagents generally cause cytotoxicity, especially at high concentrations, and are disposed to aggregation and loss of activity in serum- and salt-containing environments. Additionally, while the nanocarrier should remain stable in the extracellular environment, the siRNA must be released from the packaging system intracellularly in order to ensure efficient incorporation into the RISC complex [24,89]. Recent and ongoing research addresses these concerns; bioreducible, biodegradable, and environmentally responsive polymers and PEGylation strategies can be utilized both to reduce cytotoxicity and to incorporate mechanisms of siRNA release [24,80,88,90,91].

13.5 LOCAL DELIVERY STRATEGIES

Local delivery of siRNA has been pursued to direct cellular responses in applications ranging from tissue engineering and regenerative medicine to treatment of carcinomas and infections. This section reviews some of the most promising local, reservoir-based siRNA delivery strategies reported to date [92].

13.5.1 Microparticles

Microparticles were the earliest explored delivery strategy for localized, sustained delivery of siRNA. Microparticles are generally formed using a double-emulsion technique (water/oil/water) followed by solvent extraction/evaporation. The initial aqueous phase, containing the oligonucleotide (often prepackaged into a carrier), is added to the oil phase, containing the polymer that will comprise the matrix of the microparticles. This emulsion is added to a final aqueous phase containing a surfactant, allowing stable microparticle formation. The particles are then isolated through evaporative removal of the volatile, nonpolar solvent. Microparticles can be tuned to possess optimal size for a combination of injectability and tissue retention and have proven effective at protecting loaded nucleic acids from degradation [44,93–96].

Exploration into the loading and release characteristics of microparticles has elucidated the effects of dose of nucleic acid loaded, polymer molecular weight, and particle size. Early reports revealed that smaller PLGA microspheres (1–2 μm) released loaded oligonucleotide more rapidly than larger microspheres (10–20 μm) [95]. While the small microspheres exhibited a typical burst release profile over several days, followed by a slower rate of release over two months, larger microspheres released ODN in a triphasic profile, with a less substantial initial stage of burst release followed by sustained release for about a month, at which point the remaining ODN was quickly released. This final phase of release was due to degradation of the microspheres and could therefore be modulated by modifying the molecular weight of PLGA used to form the microparticles; for example, slower release after 25 days was seen in microspheres of 30,000 MW PLGA than in microspheres of 3,000 MW PLGA [95]. It was additionally shown that loading efficiency using the double-emulsion, solvent evaporation technique was approximately doubled with the large microspheres in comparison to the small microspheres (60%–70% vs. 30% encapsulation efficiency) [95,96].

Another key concern when designing microparticle systems is the release characteristics of the loaded nucleic acid. Changes in pH, for example, that occur in ischemic environments, in endosomal compartments, or due to release of degradation products, can significantly impact release kinetics and particle behavior. The impact of pH extremes on PLGA microparticle release of loaded ODN was investigated in a study comparing PLGA microparticles with 0%, 5%, and 10% PEG composition [93]. At physiological pH, all microparticle compositions exhibited >85% release of the total loaded ODN in a sustained, triphasic manner over 28 days. However, at a pH of 5 and 10, PLGA microparticles with no PEG content achieved < 50% total ODN release due to microparticle aggregation. Inhibiting this aggregation through the incorporation of PEG accomplished greater total ODN release at pH extremes while maintaining a similar release profile to 100% PLGA microparticles at physiological pH. However, in all cases, a higher degree of burst release was still observed at the pH extremes [93]. This study also investigated the impact of quantity of oligonucleotide loaded on release rate, revealing that higher loading was associated with a greater burst release. The capacity to modulate release kinetics by varying composition, loading density, and size is central to microparticle utility in nucleic acid delivery applications [94,97].

The application of PLGA microparticles for sustained nucleic acid delivery was first demonstrated with encapsulated ODN. In in vitro studies with RAW 264.7 macrophage-like cells, a 4-h exposure to microparticles loaded with an ODN designed to silence the transcription factor nuclear factor kappa-light-chain-enhancer of activated

B cells (NFκ-β) reduced protein expression of NFκ-β by approximately half and reduced downstream inflammatory cytokine production. Sustained release of ODN from the microspheres was shown for approximately one month in vitro, but the capacity of the microparticles to elicit long-term silencing was not investigated [50]. These ODN-loaded microparticles established a precedent for using microparticles to deliver siRNA, an application that is discussed in more detail in the following sections [94,97–99].

13.5.2 SCAFFOLDS

The use of polymer scaffolds to facilitate sustained release of siRNA is a potentially transformative strategy to influence local cellular behavior in tissue regenerative applications. An extensive array of polymers and polymer combinations have been explored for scaffold fabrication. Naturally derived polymers, such as physiological extracellular matrix (ECM) components and polysaccharides (commonly anionic alginate, agarose, dextran, and hyaluronic acid (HA) and cationic chitosan), are often utilized because they have inherent cell-adhesion and degradation mechanisms. Collagen is a particularly popular ECM biomaterial because it is a fibrous ECM component that is enzymatically degradable [100]. One of the earliest studies that investigated scaffold-mediated delivery as a means to control siRNA release kinetics utilized collagen scaffolds loaded with siRNA formulated with PAMAM dendrimers [101]. These scaffolds achieved greater than 50% gene silencing at 7 days (using a 200-nM siRNA dose) in in vitro studies with fibroblasts, demonstrating the potential for sustained silencing via scaffold-based local delivery.

While natural polymers offer advantages in terms of host cell recognition, using synthetic materials enables greater control over a range of scaffold properties, including the pore structure, degradation mechanism/rate, and mechanical stiffness/strength. PLGA offers the distinct advantage of highly tunable degradation rates, and PLGA scaffolds have been shown to promote cellular ingrowth and produce localized and long-term nucleic acid transfection in numerous applications [49,102]. Poly(ester urethane) (PEUR) scaffolds formed from nontoxic isocyanates, such as lysine triisocyanate (LTI), have also been successfully adapted for the sustained delivery of a variety of biomacromolecules [103–105].

For all scaffold-based delivery applications, it is vital that the siRNA intracellular delivery technology can be readily incorporated into the bulk delivery depot without significant loss of gene silencing activity. Lyophilization of siRNA-loaded poly- and lipoplexes can reduce their activity, primarily because extensive particle aggregation occurs at high concentrations. Several stabilization strategies have been developed to maintain gene silencing efficacy post-fabrication into local delivery systems [39,106–108]. For example, siRNA nanoparticles were shown to have a 50% activity loss when directly incorporated into PEUR scaffolds. However, when the natural sugar trehalose was used as a stabilizing agent, nanoparticle size and activity were retained relative to fresh siRNA formulations [39,109]. Additionally, siRNA complexed with either chitosan or TransIT TKO transfection reagent and lyophilized onto the surface of tissue culture plates maintained transfection efficiency only when sucrose was utilized as a lyoprotectant [107]. Sucrose stabilization showed similar efficacy as a lyoprotectant of polyplexes of DNA and PEI [108]. These results demonstrate the necessity of carefully optimizing the integration of the siRNA intracellular delivery system with the bulk scaffold/depot fabrication method and chemistry.

13.5.3 ELECTROSPUN FIBERS

Electrospun fibers are another strategy for localized, reservoir-based delivery. Electrospinning enables the formation of nanoscale fibrous structures (biomimetic of those present in natural ECM) using polymers [48]. These fibers are often used in scaffold-like coatings or dressings but merit discussion independent of the generalized scaffold discussion above. While adsorption of siRNA onto electrospun fibers can mediate gene silencing, a more powerful strategy for controlled release is encapsulation of siRNA into these fibers. For example, siRNA complexed with chitosan and encapsulated into PLGA nanofibers demonstrated sustained siRNA release dictated by PLGA degradation for more than 30 days [43]. It was also shown that the fibers mediated transfection superior to that of the standard forward transfection method; specifically, 48 h after seeding green fluorescent protein (GFP)-expressing human lung carcinoma cells onto the PLGA fibers in vitro, maximum silencing of about 60% was observed. Given the controlled release profile shown, there is a strong impetus to further explore the capacity of this system to achieve sustained silencing.

Electrospun fibers formed from polycaprolactone (PCL), a synthetic polymer with a slower hydrolytic degradation mechanism than PLGA, have also been investigated as a means to control the release of siRNA [48]. The Chew group loaded naked siRNA into PCL nanofibers but showed minimal (3%) release of siRNA over 28 days [57]. The incorporation of poly(ethylene glycol) (PEG), a hydrophilic polymer, increased the release of the encapsulated siRNA (up to 30%) by acting as a porogen. While this modification showed promise as a way to tune siRNA release kinetics from the fibers, a full and sustained release profile was not achieved. Additionally, the combination PCL-PEG nanofiber scaffolds proved less cytocompatible than PCL scaffolds when the cells were seeded onto them. The PCL-PEG system produced in vitro silencing in cells seeded upon the scaffolds, of approximately 20% when naked siRNA was encapsulated and about 80% when siRNA-TKO complexes were incorporated. Surprisingly, there was no effect of scaffold composition (0%, 20%, and 60% PEG were investigated) on gene silencing [57]. The Chew group subsequently improved upon the siRNA release through

copolymerization of ethyl ethylene phosphate with PCL [110]. siRNA–TKO complexes or naked siRNA loaded into these nanofibers demonstrated scaffold-mediated silencing of fibroblasts in vitro (approximately 40% with the siRNA–TKO complexes and 20% with naked siRNA). In all cases, the most effective nanofiber-mediated silencing was achieved when siRNA was packaged into commercial transfection reagents prior to nanofiber incorporation. However, these agents were also associated with significant cytotoxicity. Nevertheless, these nanofiber-based delivery systems establish silencing efficacy in model gene targets and motivate further development of matrix biomimetic electrospun constructs for controlled siRNA release.

13.5.4 HYDROGELS

Hydrogels are a subclass of swellable, highly hydrated scaffolds that can also be composed of natural or synthetic polymers. Strong proof-of concept work from the Alsberg group has proven siRNA-based silencing of model genes from a variety of natural hydrogel systems. In particular, they investigated collagen, alginate, and dextran injectable hydrogels using calcium- and photo-cross-linking techniques, with the goal of identifying differences in siRNA release rates and silencing efficacy from these systems. A study comparing calcium-cross-linked alginate, photo-cross-linked alginate, and collagen revealed that each of these hydrogels, when loaded with 13.3 µg of naked siRNA per 100 µL gel, achieved greater than 90% gene silencing of encapsulated HEK293 cells in vitro [111]. More recently, this group demonstrated tunable and sustained siRNA release using photo-crosslinked hydrogels comprising dextran (8% or 12% w/w) and linear PEI incorporated at varying concentrations (0, 5, or 10 µg/100 µL gel) [112]. Both a higher concentration of PEI and a higher mass percentage dextran composition corresponded to slower release kinetics and less burst release, with sustained release achieved out to 8 days.

Hybrid delivery systems comprising combinations of natural and synthetic polymers can leverage the advantages of each (e.g., cytocompatibility of natural materials and tunability of synthetic materials). In a recent study, hydrogels synthesized with a combination of alginate, HA, and hydroxyethylcellulose were 3-dimensionally coprinted with PCL and loaded with Lipofectamine-complexed siRNAs in defined spatial patterns [56]. This system allowed gene silencing of GFP-expressing mesenchymal stem cells seeded upon the hydrogels, with the strongest silencing effects localized to the areas patterned with siRNA against the GFP gene. This proof-of-concept work could be modified for long-term gene silencing by optimizing the selection of siRNA carrier and/or hydrogel composition to allow for controlled release. The authors' application of a novel fabrication technique to achieve spatial and temporal control of gene silencing activity is particularly exciting for engineering of multicomponent or gradient tissue architectures [42].

Another subset of hydrogels that is promising for use in local delivery is environmentally responsive hydrogels that undergo stimuli-dependent gelation. For instance, poly(N-isopropylacrylamide) (pNIPAAM) is a well-characterized thermoresponsive polymer with an ideal transition temperature from sol to gel that occurs between room and physiologic temperature. pNIPAAM-based hydrogels have been proven to support cellular growth and infiltration, and the random or block copolymerization with other monomers can be used to tune its transition temperature, degradability, and other characteristics [113–116]. Hydrogels based upon pNIPAAM and other thermoresponsive polymers have been pursued as injectable systems that form a reservoir confining siRNA to the site of injection. For example, a copolymer of NIPAAM and acrylamide (AAM) has been investigated for application as an injectable depot when loaded with gold nanoshell-encapsulated DNA [117]. Additional work has described an injectable hydrogel composed of NIPAAM and layered double hydroxides (LDHs; either MgAl or MgFe), where the LDHs were utilized to electrostatically incorporate siRNA [118]. The combination pNIPAAM-LDH gel elicited >80% silencing in osteoarthritic chondrocytes in vitro at 6 days of a model gene. This promising result provides strong motivation for exploration of this system and other pNIPAAM-based injectable options in conjunction with functional gene targets and in vivo models.

While pNIPAAM remains a strong option for injectable systems, many other approaches have shown promise. Recent work by Ishii et al. produced a redox-active injectable gel comprised of polyion complexes of a triblock cationic polymer PMNT-PEG-PMNT (PMNT=poly[4-(2,2,6,6-tetramethylpiperidine-N-oxyl) aminomethylstyrene]) and poly acrylic acid (PAAc) [119]. Sustained release of PAAc from the gel was shown over 28 days, with negligible burst characteristics and a release of about 30% at last measure. This system would be of interest particularly in treatment of inflammatory conditions, as PMNT contains a TEMPO nitroxide radical, known for its capacity to scavenge ROS. While this gel has not been investigated for nucleic acid delivery, it may be amenable to incorporation of siRNA (in replacement of PAAc) and merits further investigation in therapeutic applications. Another injectable system that has demonstrated promise is a liquid crystalline formulation composed of monoglycerides, PEI, propylene glycol, and Tris buffer [120]. PEI functions to package siRNA and in vitro studies showed 44% of total loaded siRNA–PEI complexes were released over 72-h in vitro. Subcutaneous implantation of the gels in mice revealed gel degradation over 30 days but also indicated an immune response upon implantation. However, despite this drawback, the capacity to load and release siRNA complexes motivates investigation of gene silencing capabilities. While the injectable strategies discussed above have not yet progressed to functional gene targets, similar systems incorporating prepackaged oligonucleotide have been investigated in cancer therapies, and these applications are discussed further below [117,121].

13.5.5 Surface Coatings

Coatings onto devices or other biomaterials, such as wound dressings, have also been pursued for local siRNA delivery; coating types include hydrogels as well as single- or multilayer-surface coatings. The simplest version of a coating for local delivery is a single-layer adsorbed or deposited onto a surface. In these adsorbed coatings, control over the release kinetics is limited, but this approach has helped to elucidate the benefit of substrate-mediated transfection [48]. For example, complexes of plasmid DNA (pDNA) and PEI adsorbed onto nanographene oxide substrates exhibited sustained release (over 7 days) and resulted in both a higher transfection efficacy and a lower cytotoxicity than complexes delivered in solution [122]. This approach capitalized on efficient, substrate-mediated transfection and also facilitated gene delivery localized to patterns on the nanographene oxide, enabling spatial control of therapeutic delivery.

Multilayer coatings, many of which are assembled through layer-by-layer (LbL) processes, have been one of the most promising approaches to surface-mediated siRNA release. LbL films are typically formed by alternating deposition of materials of opposing charge, with the layers bound together by electrostatic forces. Relative to other systems, LbL coatings offer a high degree of control over release kinetics of a loaded therapeutic. By altering the number of layers and the composition of the layers, it is possible to tune the release rate of loaded molecules and to achieve sustained release [123–125]. The Hammond group has extensively characterized LbL assembly, utilizing this approach to coat a variety of devices and biomaterials. They investigated several LbL systems for coating siRNA onto a woven nylon surgical dressing. Each LbL system used protamine sulfate (PrS) as the cationic layering agent, while the anionic layers comprised calcium phosphate (CaPh) siRNA nanoparticles, dextran sulfate, and/or laponite (LaP) silicate clay [126]. The most promising candidate was composed of PrS/CaP/PrS/LaP; these films demonstrated a siRNA loading capacity of 19 μg/cm^2 and an approximately linear release profile for about 6 days (release leveled off at 10 days with a third of the siRNA unreleased). These films achieved target gene silencing in fibroblasts seeded upon them, with peak silencing of 64% observed at 7 days. The highly tunable release from LbL systems makes them among the most exciting options under investigation for local siRNA delivery, and there is a strong need to investigate these systems in treatment of disease states.

13.6 THERAPEUTIC APPLICATIONS

Due to the flexibility to design siRNA against any gene target and the tunability of delivery reservoirs, localized RNAi is a broadly applicable therapeutic approach with potential applications in tissue engineering, regenerative medicine, medical device implants, cancer, infections, and immunomodulation. The prospective applications

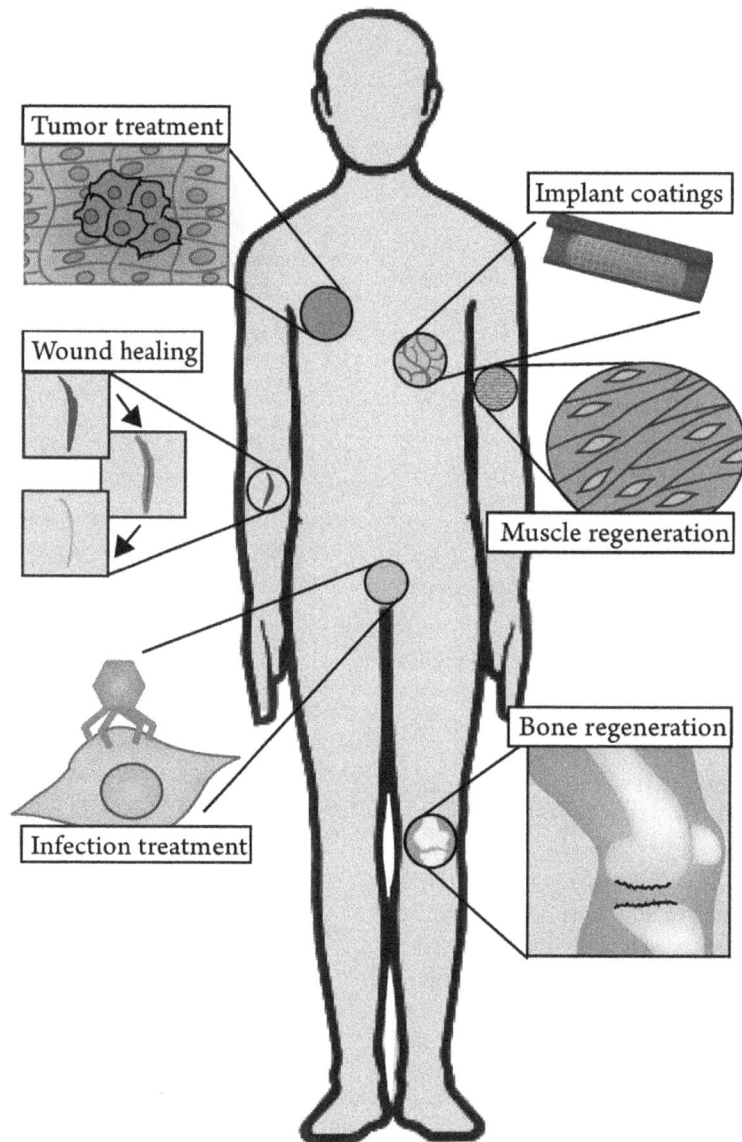

FIGURE 13.3 Schematic demonstrating the breadth of potential applications for local, reservoir-based delivery of siRNA therapeutics. Pictured: tumor treatment, wound healing (e.g., concerning fibrosis and angiogenesis), infection treatment (e.g., sexually transmitted diseases), implant coatings (e.g., stents), muscle/tendon regeneration, and bone repair.

(Figure 13.3) amenable to local reservoir-based delivery will be discussed briefly in general and specifically as they relate to promising therapeutic targets that have been most extensively explored [92].

13.6.1 TISSUE REGENERATION

Application of siRNA against other osteogenesis-related genes such as osteopontin and osteocalcin has also been explored as a means to regulate bone mineralization. An LbL film composed of alternating layers of CaPh shRNA nanoparticles and PLL achieved a sustained silencing effect (at 21 days) in human osteoblasts grown on the films, superior to that of the nanoparticles delivered in solution [127]. The strategy of alternately depositing nucleic acid nanoparticles and polymer layers, coupled with the long-term

silencing effect shown, suggests the potential for LbL to achieve timed release of siRNA against multiple targets by loading of different siRNAs at different "depths" within the LbL film. However, the gene silencing effect was only assessed at 21 days, and the release characteristics of the system have not yet been elucidated.

Regeneration of muscle and connective tissue is also a primary interest in tissue engineering, especially as a treatment for genetic diseases such as muscular dystrophy. siRNA against myostatin, a gene that impedes muscle growth, delivered at a dose of 0.5 nmols from atelocollagen nanoparticles was shown to increase muscle growth, size, and activity in a mouse model of muscular dystrophy [128,129]. The results [92] were achieved via a local injection into mouse masseter muscle; however, the proven impact of myostatin siRNA on muscle growth motivates its further exploration in controlled delivery depots to regenerate weak or otherwise compromised muscle tissue. The use of siRNA to promote functional tendon regeneration has also been examined using siRNA against the collagen V α1 (Col5α1) chain. The ratio of collagen V to collagen I is important for tendon fibrillogenesis, and overexpression of Col5α1 negatively impacts fibril diameter. By silencing Col5α1 mRNA in cultured tenocytes using Lipofectamine-complexed siRNA and thereafter combining the transfected cells with normal tenocytes at an optimized ratio, fibrils of a larger diameter (closer to that of a healthy tendon) were generated *in vitro* [130]. This study and those involving bone and muscle restoration establish the utility of siRNA therapeutics as a means to stimulate functional musculoskeletal tissue regeneration at sites of pathology or injury.

13.6.2 DIRECTING CELLULAR DIFFERENTIATION

The therapies described above demonstrate the potential value of RNAi in functional tissue regeneration by modulating cellular behavior. A related strategy involves using siRNA to drive cellular differentiation to that of a desired tissue type.

In another study aiming to modulate cellular differentiation, embryonic stem cells (ESCs) were seeded onto PLGA/PLA scaffolds loaded with siRNA/lipidoid complexes against a type III tyrosine kinase insert domain receptor (KDR) [131]. The goal was to drive differentiation of ESCs toward a particular germ layer. For tissue engineering and regenerative medicine applications, it is often desirable to work with cells of a specific lineage; however, ESCs naturally differentiate into a mixture of the three germ layers (endoderm, mesoderm, and ectoderm), and techniques to induce differentiation toward a single layer are complicated and incompletely effective. KDR expression occurs early in embryonic development; due to its role as a receptor for VEGF, KDR is critical in development of the cardiovascular system and is associated with development of the endoderm germ layer. Therefore, it was hypothesized that KDR silencing would block endodermic differentiation of ESCs. 70% knockdown of KDR was achieved in hESCs seeded on scaffolds loaded with 0.01 ng/cell siRNA, leading to a pronounced influence on hESC differentiation; a 60%–90% downregulation of genes characteristic of the endoderm and a corresponding upregulation of genes characteristic of the mesoderm were observed [131]. The long-term silencing capacity of the system as well as its capacity to fully direct embryogenesis remains to be investigated.

13.6.3 BONE PATHOLOGIES

Several strategies to promote bone regeneration are discussed above; however, distinct from these approaches is the application of RNAi to treat bone and cartilage pathologies (e.g., osteoarthritis and osteonecrosis). One genetic target explored for treatment of osteoarthritis is NF-κβ. NF-κβ is a transcription factor that impacts myriad cellular processes; one pathological implication of NF-κβ is that its upregulation contributes to local inflammation and tissue damage associated with osteoarthritis.

Often, siRNA-based treatments of bone pathologies (i.e., osteoarthritis or steroid-associated osteonecrosis) are based upon repeated local injections at the site of bone repair and lack a mechanism for sustained release and prolonged silencing [131–135]. While these can be useful options, controlling the temporal gene silencing profile would enable greater convenience and, potentially, efficacy. Testing of these therapeutically validated targets with technologies for local, sustained release is justified and may enable development of superior, translatable treatments for bone disorders.

13.6.4 ANGIOGENESIS AND WOUND HEALING

Several functional targets for stimulation of angiogenesis via genetic repression have been identified, among them prolyl hydroxylase domain 2 (PHD2). PHD2 is an endogenous negative regulator of the transcription factor hypoxia-inducible factor-1α (HIF-1α), and its inhibition promotes expression of genes controlled by HIF-1α, including VEGF, stromal-cell-derived factor 1 (SDF-1), and additional pro-angiogenic factors [136–138]. PHD2 deficiency stimulates both formation and maturation of blood vessels, and silencing its expression is therefore of interest both in broad tissue engineering applications and in chronic skin wounds [139].

To prove the therapeutic utility of this system, siRNA against PHD2 was investigated in scaffolds utilizing LTI and 5% trehalose. At 14 days, 80% silencing of PHD2 was observed, resulting in greater than twofold upregulation of downstream pro-angiogenic markers VEGF and fibroblast growth factor. Silencing PHD2 also increased vascular volume within the scaffolds by more than twofold and increased mean vascular thickness, suggesting that PHD2 silencing may support both angiogenesis and vessel enlargement and maturation (Figure 13.4) [39]. This approach to local PHD2 siRNA delivery shows promise as a means of promoting angiogenesis in wound healing and tissue regeneration applications. Additionally, the sustained and controllable release from the PEUR scaffolds provides motivation to investigate this delivery system in other localized pathologies.

13.6.5 FIBROSIS

The modulation of the immune response, typically to reduce inflammation and/or fibrosis, is another area particularly suited for local therapeutic delivery from reservoir systems. Upon tissue injury, an inflammatory response is activated and normally leads to either tissue regeneration or fibrosis and eventual scar formation. Fibrosis, while characteristic of the natural healing process, becomes problematic when the deposition of connective tissue impedes functionality of damaged organs or medical implants. Excessive scar formation can also cause esthetic issues (e.g., keloids) [136].

(a)   (b)

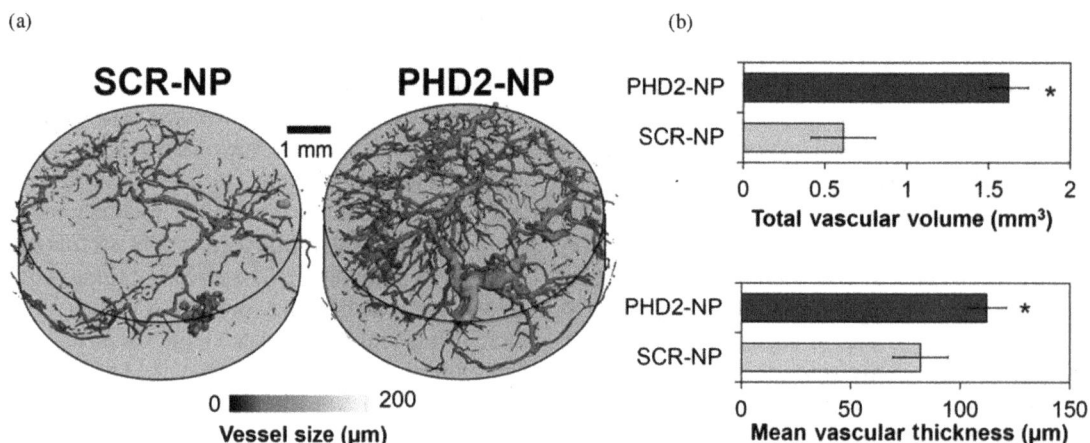

FIGURE 13.4 Sustained silencing of PHD2 increases angiogenesis within PEUR tissue scaffolds. (a) Micro-CT images visually demonstrate the increased vasculature within the PHD2-NP scaffolds. (b) Quantitative analysis of 3D micro-CT vessel images reveals a significant increase in vascular volume within PHD2-NP-loaded scaffolds relative to control scaffolds containing scrambled (SCR) siRNA. *p<0.05 [39].

RNAi shows particular promise to decrease the fibrotic response and improve the quality of regenerated tissue.

In addition to the issues related to excessive scar deposition, fibrosis can also contribute to encapsulation of medical implants and tissue engineering constructs, damaging their functionality by creating a relatively acellular capsule at the cell–material interface. Fibrous capsules are characterized by acellular tissue, primarily collagen, and form due to the physiological foreign body reaction. Fibrosis can impede implant performance by obstructing input/output of devices (relevant to neural electrodes or glucose sensors) and by blocking vascularization and surrounding tissue integration of the implant (relevant to tissue engineering scaffolds). In an attempt to ameliorate the fibrotic response, siRNA designed against mammalian target of rapamycin (mTOR), an effector of cellular proliferation, was complexed with branched PEI and encapsulated by PEG hydrogel coatings on model polymer implants [140]. mTOR inhibition limited fibroblast proliferation as well as decreased fibroblast expression of type I collagen *in vitro*, and sustained release spanning 2 weeks *in vitro* was achieved from the PEG hydrogel system.

13.6.6 INFLAMMATION

Controlled delivery of siRNA is also promising for pathologies characterized by excessive, local inflammation. In a temporomandibular joint inflammation model, siRNA silencing of IgG cell surface Fc receptor (an antibody-binding receptor functional in the immune response) reduced production of inflammatory cytokines IL-6 and IL1-β by ~50% and ~20%, respectively [99].

Vascular inflammation is also implicated in atherosclerosis and the clinical problem of intimal hyperplasia following vascular grafting and stent placement. Intimal hyperplasia is characterized by invasion of the vessel lumen by smooth muscle cells and is a primary cause of graft/stented vessel

stenosis and failure. Therapeutic-eluting stent coatings to modulate the inflammatory response and cell proliferation within the stent can reduce rates of stent failure, and siRNA strategies merit investigation in this application [141].

13.6.7 MICROBIAL INFECTIONS

The use of local siRNA depots to treat infections or their negative consequences is another area of ongoing research. A broadly applicable strategy for treating infections is through the delivery of siRNA targeting the viral genome. siRNA targeting the hepatitis C virus (used as a model infection) and delivered from multilayer films was shown to inhibit viral replication and infection in *in vitro* experiments [41]. siRNA complexed to PEI was adsorbed onto films of PLL and PGA, and, building from this starter layer, PEI-siRNA, HA, and chitosan were used to form the successive layers of the film. Increasing the number of layers (from 1 to 3 to 5) was shown to improve transfection efficacy, and siRNA delivered from films exhibited prolonged inhibition of hepatitis C viral replication (over 12 days) *in vitro*. These films are promising for reducing viral infections and merit future investigation in an *in vivo* model.

Additionally, siRNA therapies have been tested as a prophylactic in viral sexually transmitted infections (STIs) such as herpes simplex virus 2 (HSV2). siRNA against genes crucial to HSV2, at a dose of 500 pmol complexed with Oligofectamine, protected mice from developing HSV2 when applied as a topical microbicide intravaginally within hours of HSV2 infection [142].

13.6.8 CLINICAL PROSPECTS

The only siRNA delivery depot in the clinical pipeline is the siG12D LODER therapeutic, developed by Silenseed Ltd., to combat nonresectable pancreatic ductal adenocarcinoma (PDA) [143]. A mutation in the KRAS oncogene is a typical characteristic of PDA, and a particularly common mutation is a substitution of the glycine at codon 12 with aspartate (G12D).

In *in vivo* studies, the siG12D LODER matrix (loaded such that the final siRNA dose was 0.32 mg/kg) was stitched to tumors to ensure localized release over time. Testing was done in immunocompetent mice with Panc02 mouse pancreatic cancer cell subcutaneous tumors as well as in immunocompromised mice with Panc1 tumors. siG12D LODER implantation onto the tumors resulted in development of a large necrotic area (> 60% of total tumor area for the Panc02-derived tumors). In the Panc1-derived tumors, the treatment also caused a reduction in tumor volume and increased mouse survival time. siG12D LODER was additionally evaluated in an orthotopic tumor model using Panc1 cells, and the therapy was also effective in this setting, inhibiting tumor growth and lengthening survival time (Figure 13.5). These promising results *in vivo* in a relevant disease model set siG12D LODER apart in the realm of local, controlled-release siRNA therapeutics. To date, siG12D LODER has successfully undergone Phase I clinical trials; although the journey to clinical application is by no means complete, this therapeutic exhibits great potential. Importantly, clinical translation of siG12D LODER could also help to spur more broad interest in translational development of systems for sustained, localized, siRNA delivery.

13.6.9 CANCER

While RNAi therapeutics have been investigated extensively for the treatment of cancers via systemic delivery, some carcinomas are well-suited to local delivery strategies. siRNA injected intratumorally has been shown to inhibit tumor growth, providing motivation for approaches using injectable depot-like systems, especially in cases where primary tumors may be inoperable [82]. A widely investigated strategy involves the injection of a hydrogel or a hydrogel precursor at the local tumor site. In work by Sood and authors, a chitosan hydrogel was loaded with chitosan–siRNA complexes [144]. siRNA was targeted to tissue transglutaminase, a gene critical to carcinoma growth and chemoresistance. The hydrogels were injected intratumorally and shown to inhibit tumor growth in both melanoma and breast tumor models in mice. The system shows promise to localize cancer treatment at a tumor site; however, as described, it required multiple injections over several weeks and was not designed for sustained release.

Another study investigated local, hydrogel-based delivery of siRNA for treatment of breast cancer. The hydrogel, comprised of PAMAM dendrimers cross-linked with dextran aldehyde, was loaded with siRNA encapsulated by PBAE nanoparticles [145]. The study investigated the degradation characteristics of the nanoparticles alone in PBS (60% degraded at 7h and completely degraded at 24h) as well as nanoparticles loaded into the hydrogel. The gel was shown to protect the nanoparticles from rapid degradation. The hydrogel-loaded nanoparticles exhibited a phase of rapid degradation (about 50%) over 24h followed by a second and sustained phase of degradation reaching completion at 12days. siRNA–PBAE complexes loaded into the hydrogels also exhibited sustained release over 6days (30% of the siRNA was released after 24h, followed by slower release) which was associated with hydrogel degradation. The first phase of degradation was found to correspond to burst release of physically entrapped nanoparticles, with the remaining sustained release being due to release of nanoparticles chemically linked to the hydrogel (via a covalent bond between aldehydes on the dextran component and amines on the surface of the PBAE nanoparticles) [145]. When 10 μg of siRNA was loaded into this system and injected intratumorally into a mouse tumor model, 70% silencing of the model gene luciferase was achieved at 6days (as opposed to a maximum of 20% knockdown achieved using an injection of siRNA–PBAE complexes without the hydrogel). The comprehensive investigation of the release kinetics of this system as well as the sustained silencing shown provides impetus for application of this and similar systems to functional genetic targets.

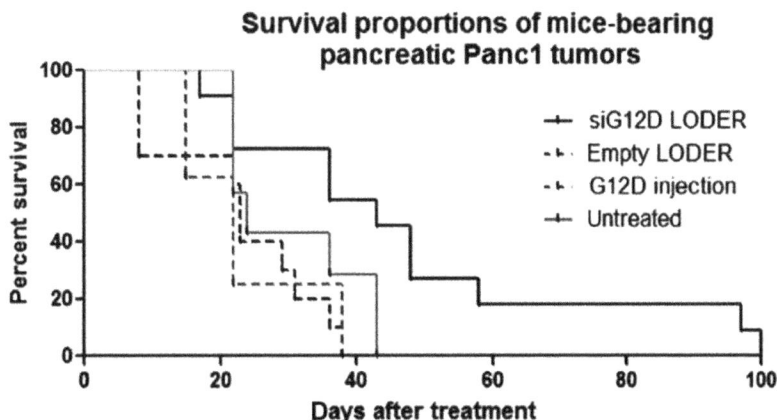

Survival proportions of mice-bearing pancreatic Panc1 tumors

FIGURE 13.5   Treatment with siG12D LODER significantly improves mean survival time of mice with orthotopic Panc1 tumors.

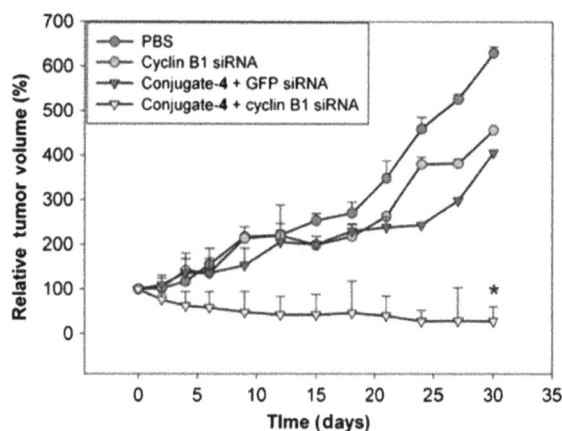

FIGURE 13.6 Cyclin B1 siRNA delivered via PEI-poly(organophosphazene) hydrogels inhibits tumor growth in a mouse tumor xenograft model. Conjugate 4 corresponds to poly(organophosphazene) conjugated to linear PEI of MW800. *p <0.001 vs. PBS-injected group.

Hydrogels comprised of NIPAAM-co-AAM have also been investigated for application in intratumoral injections. This polymer exhibits thermoresponsive gelation at 40°C and was loaded with silica gold nanoshells encapsulating an anticancer drug and DNA duplexes [117]. The release of therapeutic (e.g., DNA, used as a model for siRNA) from the nanoshells was shown to be optically triggered by irradiation with a specific wavelength of light, as evaluated at room temperature with nanoshells in polymer solution. Controlled, optically triggered release of DNA from the nanoshells was established, with delivery localized to the site of tumors by the hydrogel system. However, the cellular uptake of the released DNA has yet to be investigated. PEI-conjugated poly(organophosphazene) is another thermally responsive polymer used in injectable hydrogel applications; it was shown to encapsulate siRNA and gel upon transition to body temperature. siRNA against cyclin B1 (critical to cell division) and VEGF (significant in tumor angiogenesis) were investigated in separate applications of this hydrogel delivery system [121,146]. This system has the potential to translate to various local, long-term gene delivery applications, as it exhibited sustained release for a week *in vivo* and N60% protein expression inhibition in a mouse tumor model at 30 days (using a 50-μg dose of cyclin B1 siRNA) (Figure 13.6) [146]. The *in vitro* transfection of the system was improved upon by conjugating a CPP to poly(organophosphazene) via a degradable linker (> 90% VEGF protein-level inhibition), but the *in vivo* tumor inhibition remained similar to the previous hydrogel system lacking a CPP [121,146].

13.7   siRNA FOR COLORECTAL CANCER THERAPY

Colorectal cancer is one of the main causes of death worldwide, and its incidence is increasing as its prognosis remains poor. In addition to the primary surgical procedure, which removes primary and regional tumors and lymph nodes by open surgical resection, colorectal cancer therapy also includes chemotherapy, local ablation by radiation therapy, and targeted therapy, especially for patients with hepatic metastasis or recurrent colon cancer. Currently, different multidrug combinations that combine agents with proven anticancer activity, such as 5-fluorouracil, irinotecan, oxaliplatin, and capecitabine, have been used for colorectal cancer therapy in the clinic [147–150]. As a biologically active metabolite derived from the irinotecan hydrochloride (CPT-11), SN-38 (7-ethyl-10- hydroxycamptothecin) exhibits approximately 1000-fold higher cytotoxicity against various cancer cells compared with CPT-11 [151]. However, the clinical application of SN-38 is limited by its poor solubility in pharmaceutically acceptable media. To overcome this problem, several drug delivery systems (DDSs) have been designed for efficient delivery of SN-38, such as nanoparticles [152,153], liposomes [154], carbon nanotubes [155], and polymeric micelles [156,157].

For targeted therapy, in addition to monoclonal antibodies used in the clinic, such as bevacizumab (Avastin®) and ziv-aflibercept (Zaltrap®) [158,159] that binding to vascular endothelial growth factor (VEGF) and inhibiting tumor angiogenesis, anti-VEGF siRNA exhibits great potential for inhibition of angiogenesis [160,161]. siRNAs are specifically short dsRNA fragments of 19–25 base-pairs that can incorporate into an RISC to silence a target mRNA in a sequence-specific manner. However, many critical hurdles remain for *in vivo* application of siRNA as a feasible therapeutic, including poor biostability, poor cellular uptake, and activation of the immune response. In particular, if siRNA is exposed to the plasma or other protein-rich biological media, it becomes very unstable and is quickly degraded by nucleases, leading to poor transfection efficiency. To enhance the efficiency of *in vivo* siRNA delivery, delivery systems, including viral and nonviral vectors, have been developed. Viral vectors can achieve highly efficient gene transfer but have the risk of causing undesired immune stimulation [162]. In contrast, nonviral vectors such as cationic polymer- or micelle-based carriers ("polyplexes" or "micelleplexes") [163] and liposomes have been reported as good siRNA carriers that can suppress expression of target genes with very little immunotoxicity [164]. And polymers such as polyethylene glycol (PEG) can be conjugated to siRNA to further improve its stability and prolong its blood circulation time after intravenous (i.v) administration [165,166].

Among the different types of metallic nanoparticles, iron oxide nanoparticles have shown great potential for clinical translation because of their diverse applications, including in drug delivery [167–169], tumor destruction via hyperthermia [170], and magnetic resonance imaging (MRI) [171,172]. Iron oxide nanoparticles with superparamagnetic properties are often used as negative MRI contrast agents in T2-weighted imaging. Several magnetic nanoparticle formulations have also combined nanocarriers and iron oxide nanoparticles for applications in biotechnology and medical fields [173–175].

The utilization of biocompatible nanocarriers allows integration of multiple functions, including drug loading, tumor-specific targeting delivery, and gene delivery. In this study, we developed a multifunctional nanoconstruct that utilizes PDMA-block-poly(ε-caprolactone) (PDMA-b-PCL) micelles as a nanoplatform (Scheme 13.1). The amphiphilic

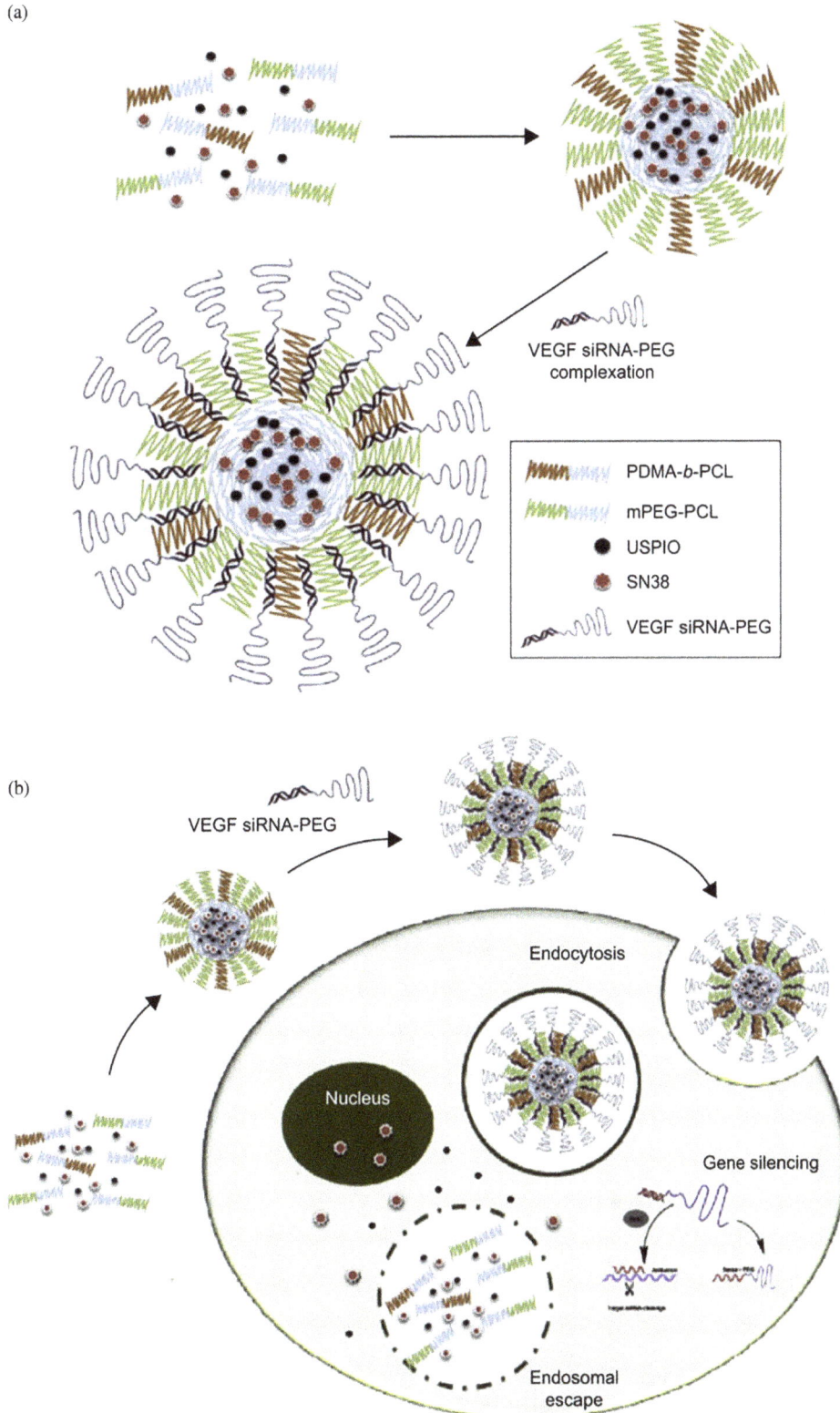

SCHEME 13.1 (a) Multifunctional SN-38/USPIO-loaded siRNA-PEG micelleplexes. (b) Schematic of the synthesis process and the intracellular therapeutic mechanism of the multifunctional SN-38/USPIO-loaded siRNA-PEG micelleplexes.

PDMA-b-PCL diblock copolymer was synthesized by free-radical polymerization and ring-opening polymerization prior to encapsulation of the chemotherapeutic drug SN-38 and ultra-small superparamagnetic iron oxide (USPIO) nanoparticles. The SN-38/USPIO-loaded micelles were then complexed with VEGF siRNA-PEG, and micelleplexes formed via electrostatic attraction between the anionic moiety of the siRNA and the cationic moiety of the PDMA-b-PCL micelles. The cytotoxicity and VEGF silencing efficiency of SN-38/USPIO-loaded micelleplexes were subsequently evaluated in the human colon cancer cell line LS174T, and a xenograft LS174T tumor-bearing mouse model was used to investigate the *in vivo* biodistribution, antitumor efficacy, and MRI applicability. By preparing the mixed micelles using PDMA-b-PCL and methoxy PEG-PCL (mPEG-PCL) copolymers, we further improved the *in vivo* biostability and biosafety of the micelleplexes. These SN-38/USPIO-loaded siRNA-PEG-mixed micelleplexes efficiently accumulated in the tumor via the enhanced permeability and retention (EPR) effect. The SN-38 and VEGF siRNA specifically exhibited dual anticancer effects, and the USPIO provided the option of use in MRI, allowing this nanomedicine to exhibit both therapeutic and diagnostic capabilities and to provide novel opportunities for future colorectal cancer therapy.

13.8 NANOASSEMBLIES FOR COMBINATORIAL DELIVERY OF siRNA

To date, a growing number of studies have shown the therapeutic promise of siRNA interference in treating a variety of diseases such as cancer and viral infection [176–178]. Despite the great potential, an efficient delivery is essential for the applications of the siRNA technique [179]. Currently, a common method for siRNA delivery is the use of nonviral systems including cationic polymers and lipids (e.g., Lipofectamine) which were also commonly used to transport pDNA [180]. In comparison, polymer-based nonviral vectors have great advantages over cationic lipids with respect to safety, convenient large-scale production, and physiological stability. Up to now, a variety of synthetic and natural cationic polymers have been investigated as gene or siRNA carriers, including poly(ethylene imine) (PEI) [181], poly(L-lysine) [182], chitosan [183], and polyamidoamine (PAMAM) dendrimers [184]. Among them, PEI has been considered as the most effective carrier since it provides stable pDNA or siRNA complexation and exhibits a unique "proton sponge effect" for endosomal release of the nanocomplexes into cytosol [185]. To address the toxicity issue of high-molecular-weight PEI, biodegradable PEI was synthesized through coupling small-molecular-weight PEI with biodegradable structures containing biodegradable disulfide [186] or ester bond [187]. In addition, PEG modification has been reported as an effective method in reducing toxicity and improving the stability of the nanocomplex with DNA [188].

On the other hand, although a large amount of small-molecular drugs such as paclitaxel and doxorubicin (DOX) have demonstrated their anticancer potency, their clinical applications are facing tremendous challenges, including low water solubility, lack of targeting leading to acute toxicity to normal tissues, and multi-drug resistance. Over the past two decades, polymeric micelles based on amphiphilic block copolymers which may potentially overcome these challenges have been extensively studied, resulting in the successful development of polymer-based micellar systems entering clinical trials [189,190] or receiving clinical approval (i.e., Genexol in Korea).

A recent advance in nanomedicine-mediated cancer therapy is the development of multifunctional carriers for jointly delivering a chemotherapeutic drug and a genetic material such as pDNA or siRNA [191]. So far, several promising systems for such codelivery purpose have been developed based on polymeric [192,193], liposomal [194,195], and silica-based [196,197] cationic nanoparticles. PEGylation was generally conducted via covalent linkage to improve the stability and meanwhile decrease the toxicity of the nanocomplex by shielding the positive charge. Among various studies, joint delivery of an anticancer drug and a reporter gene has been succeeded *in vitro* with amphiphilic copolymers of PCL and PEI [198]. A relatively high positive charge of the nanocomplex was needed in order to maintain stability in aqueous solution. On the other hand, PEG conjugation to the copolymer of polyester and PEI was found to hinder the DNA complexation to some extent, depending on the copolymer composition [188,199]. Enlightened by these reports, we herein developed a multifunctional delivery system based on PEG, PCL, and PEI for the joint delivery of siRNA and anticancer drug, using a hierarchical assembly strategy. Because PEG modification was conducted after siRNA has been complexed in our strategy, the advantage of PEGylation can be retained while its disadvantage (i.e., hindering siRNA or pDNA complexation) can be avoided. The delivery capability of this multifunctional carrier was assessed through codelivering DOX and siRNA against the BCL-2 gene, which is a key apoptosis inhibitor overexpressed in many malignant tumors. Small-molecular drugs such as DOX mostly act as cytotoxic agents inducing cancer cell apoptosis. However, the cancer cells may develop several mechanisms to escape apoptosis via overexpression of antiapoptotic genes such as BCL-2 gene [200]. Recently, downregulation of BCL-2 gene expression by siRNA targeting BCL-2 mRNA was reported to sensitize the cancer cells such as breast MCF-7 and hepatoblastoma HepG2 to DOX [201,202]. Furthermore, codelivery of DOX and siRNA or antisense oligonucleotide targeting BCL-2 has demonstrated great potential in enhancing the efficacy of chemotherapy [195–197,203]. Different from our delivery system, silica nanoparticle or liposomes were applied for the codelivery in these reports.

To facilitate the internalization of the nanocomplex into cancer cells, it has been incorporated folic acid (FA) into the multifunctional delivery system through the PEG spacer. Previous studies have shown that expression of the folate receptors was higher in many epithelial tumors and FA bound to the FA receptors (FRs) on the cancer cell surfaces with high affinity [204,205], which make FA an ideal candidate to direct the delivery of nanocomplexes into the targeted tumor cells. Herein, we assayed the folate-targeted delivery of the multifunctional delivery vector to the human hepatoma Bel-7402 cells overexpressing FR.

13.8.1 Synthesis and Characterization of Block Copolymers

Two block copolymers PEI-PCL and FA-PEG-PGA were synthesized [206] for preparing the hierarchical assemblies for codelivery of siRNA and anticancer drug DOX (Figure 13.7). PEI-PCL was synthesized by conjugating the NHS-activated PCL chains onto linear PEI with primary amino terminals (lPEI-NH$_2$). Low-molecular-weight lPEI was selected as a building block in consideration that it has low toxicity [207,208] and the inter-molecularly linked PEI upon PCL assembly may resemble high-molecular PEI in terms of siRNA complexation efficiency. Another block copolymer allyl-PEG-PGA (abbreviated as PEG-PGA) with negatively charged PGA blocks at neutral pH was synthesized by ring-opening polymerization of g-benzyl L-glutamate N-carboxyanhydride monomer using

primary amine-terminated PEG as a macroinitiator, followed by removing the benzyl protection group. The block copolymer bearing tumor-targeting molecule FA, that is, FA-PEG-PGA, was synthesized by conjugating FA to NH$_2$-PEG-PGA which was converted from allyl-PEG-PGA by radical addition reaction of cysteamine hydrochloride using AIBN as an initiator [206]. The chemical structures of the above copolymers were characterized by ^{1}H NMR, FTIR, and GPC measurements, which strongly demonstrated the successful synthesis [206]. The molecular weight characteristics of PEI-PCL, FA-PEG-PGA, and their prepolymers are listed in Table 13.1.

13.8.2 Study on Cell Uptake

FA receptor-mediated cell uptake of the hierarchical nanocomplex D-PCE/FITC/FA (N/P=30; C/N=1/10; DOX in D-PCE 6.56%) was evaluated using flow cytometry and laser confocal microscopy in FR-enriched human hepatoma Bel-7402 cells. FITC-labeled scrambled siRNA, that is, SCR-FITC, was used in order to visualize the cell uptake of siRNA. As shown in Figure 13.8 [206], after 4 h of incubation, cells incubated with D-PCE/FITC/FA showed much stronger DOX (red) and siRNA (green) fluorescences in comparison with cells incubated with the nontargeting D-PCE/FITC/NFA. According to the quantitative

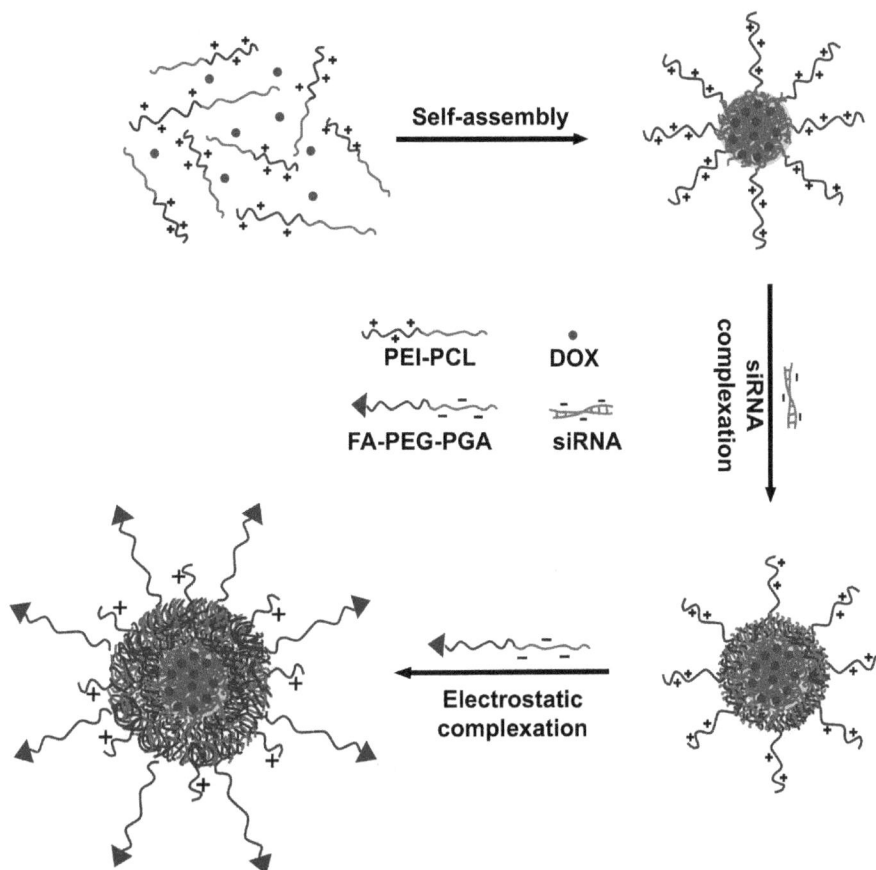

FIGURE 13.7 Formation of hierarchical nanoassemblies for combinatorial delivery of siRNA and anticancer drugs.

TABLE 13.1
Characteristics of Polymer Molecular Weight

Sample	Mn[a]	Mn	Mw	Mw/Mn
PCL-OH	1500	1644[b]	1748[b]	1.06[b]
PEI-PCL	3600	4080[b]	4943[b]	1.21[b]
Allyl-PEG-OH	3700	3996[c]	4124[c]	1.03[c]
Allyl-PEG-PBLG	9300	10,197[c]	12,981[c]	1.27[c]
FA-PEG-PGA	7100	8865[d]	11,409[d]	1.29[d]

[a] Determined by ^{1}H NMR.
[b] Determined by GPC using $CHCl_3$ as the eluent.
[c] Determined by GPC using DMF as the eluent.
[d] Determined by aqueous GPC.

flow cytometric analysis, percentage of FITC-positive cells increased by about twofold when incubating the cells with D-PCE/FITC/FA in comparison to incubating cells with D-PCE/FITC/NFA (78.3%±5.1% vs. 42.8%±3.5%) (Figure 13.8b). Flow cytometric measurement of DOX-positive cells received similar results. Apparently, DOX and siRNA were much more efficiently transferred into cells using the targeting nanocomplex rather than the non-targeting one. Moreover, regardless of the difference in fluorescence intensities of DOX and siRNA, distributions of DOX-fluorescent cells and siRNA-fluorescent cells are identical in the low-magnification confocal images [206], and high-magnification confocal images further revealed the identical intracellular distributions of DOX and siRNA fluorescences in the cytoplasm and periphery of nuclei (Figure 13.8a). Overlapping of red and green fluorescences of cells transfected with D-PCE/FITC/FA generates yellow stains in the merged image (Figure 13.8a, marked with arrowhead). The results [206] strongly demonstrated that siRNA and DOX were codelivered into the Bel-7402 cells by the hierarchical nanoassembly. As shown in Figure 13.8, cell transfection with D-PCE/FITC/FA in the presence of an excessive amount of free FA (1 mg/L) resulted in the significantly decreased intracellular fluorescences of DOX and siRNA. Quantitative flow cytometric analysis showed that the percentage of FITC-positive cells was significantly lowered to a close level (44.0%±2.9% vs. 42.8%±3.5%) for cells treated with D-PCE/FITC/NFA, and similar results were received for DOX-positive cells. These data strongly imply the FR-mediated pathway of D-PCE/siRNA/FA internalization into the FR-enriched Bel-7402 cells.

Codelivery of small-molecular drug and siRNA into the same cells is a key for achieving synergistic effect in combined drug and siRNA therapy of cancer. This is especially important when the siRNA was jointly used to improve the drug potency, like in our case that BCL-2 siRNA was used to improve the cell susceptibility to DOX-inducible apoptosis. The above study indicates that the proposed hierarchical nanoassembling approach provides an ideal platform for codelivery of siRNA and hydrophobic drugs and a facile way to introduce ligand-directed specific cell transfection.

This notion is supported by further biological studies reported in [206].

13.9 LIPOSOMES AND siRNA DELIVERY FOR MELANOMA THERAPY

Melanoma is the most malignant form of skin cancer and is a lead cause for the majority of skin cancer deaths worldwide. Over the past decades, some progress has been made in the treatment of melanoma using immunotherapy, chemotherapy, and radiotherapy [209]; however, these conventional treatment methods have produced limited success due to significant immune-related toxicities, frequent development of drug resistance, and poor drug tissue distribution. Therefore, there is a significant need for alternative approaches of drug delivery to the melanoma cells.

One recent successful treatment approach includes the localized drug delivery to melanoma cells via the topical route [210,211]. For melanoma therapy, delivery of therapeutics to upper layers of the dermis is critical as melanocytes reside in the basal epidermis and on the top of dermis [212]. Therefore, drug molecules need to pass not only through the stratum corneum but also across the viable epidermis in order to reach the melanocytes. Due to the small pore sizes, the stratum corneum is a significant barrier especially for the delivery of macromolecules such as siRNA and pDNA [213]. In the past decade, a few studies have shown progress in delivering macromolecules such as siRNA to the upper epidermis by using lipids [210,214]. However, none of the lipid-based systems has been able to provide a direct evidence to show the effective permeation through stratum corneum and deposition of macromolecules deep in the basal epidermis. For example, Geusens et al. (2009) [210] developed the so-called ultradeformable liposomes for siRNA delivery to melanoma cells which could efficiently transfect cells [210]. However, the ability of the developed liposomal system in permeating skin layers was not demonstrated. Later, the same group in 2010 demonstrated that the developed ultradeformable liposomal system can penetrate stratum corneum and deposit siRNA at the upper epidermis but did not reach lower epidermis/upper dermis where

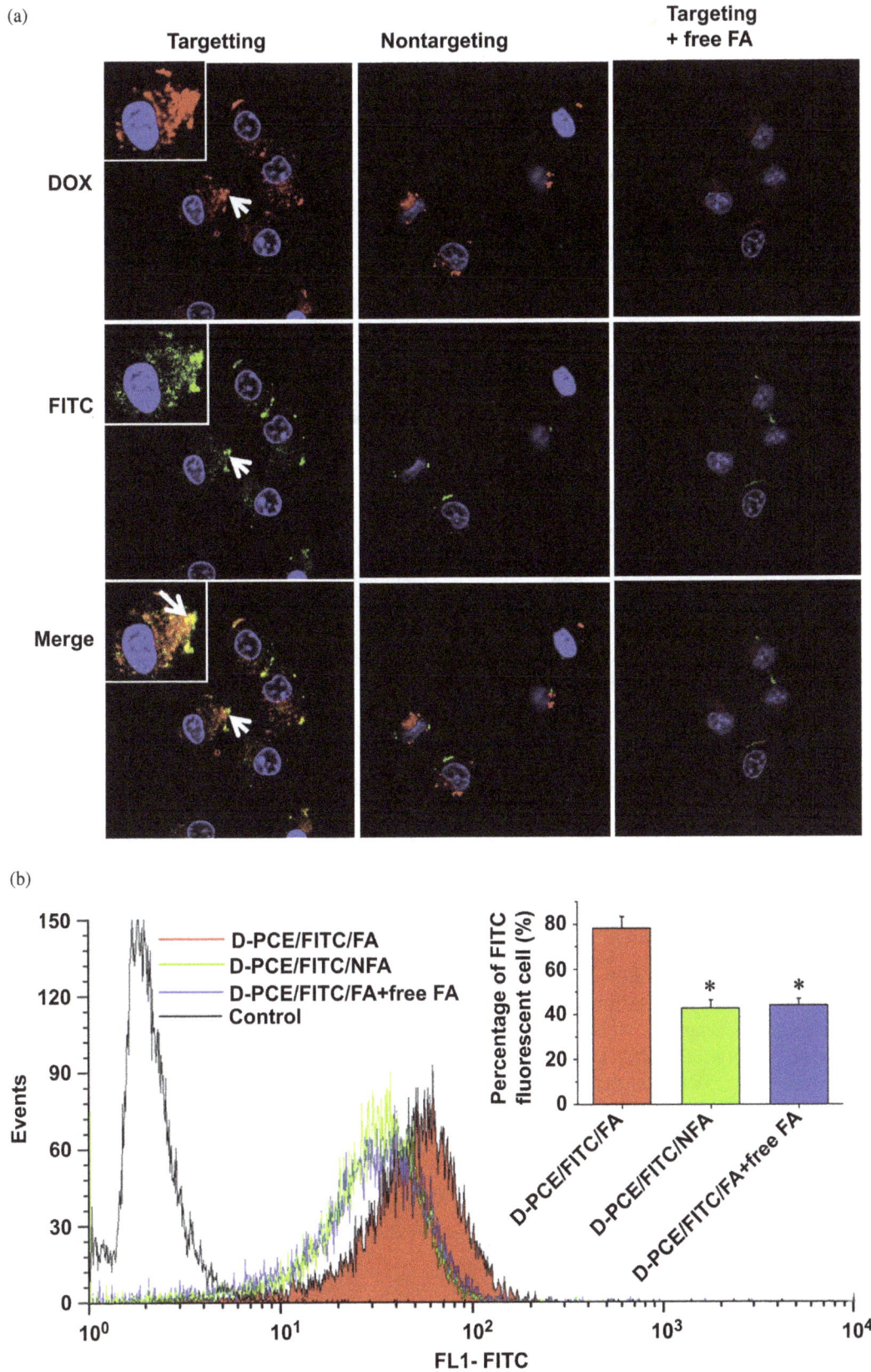

FIGURE 13.8   (a) High-magnification (x100) laser confocal microscopic images of Bel-7402 cells incubated with D-PCE/FITC/FA (targeting), D-PCE/FITC/NFA (nontargeting), and D-PCE/FITC/FA in the presence of 1 mg/L FA (targeting+FA). (b) Quantitative determination of FITC-positive cells by flow cytometry (n=3; *P<0.05, compared with D-PCE/FITC/FA). Incubation time: 4h. Dose: 20nM siRNA. N/P=30; C/N=1/10; DOX in D-PCE: 6.56%. Nuclei: stained blue with Hoechest 33342 (Aldrich); red florescence: DOX; green fluorescence: siRNA-FITC.

melanocytes reside [214]. This prompted us to take upon this task and develop a liposomal system that can effectively reach and deposit siRNA at lower epidermis/upper dermis.

Delivery of macromolecules such as siRNA into cells that reside in the basal epidermis of the skin is a major challenge due to the transport barriers that need to be overcome. siRNAs have potential therapeutic applications in various dermatological diseases such as psoriasis, atopic dermatitis, and cancer. Unfortunately, a low permeability of siRNA through the stratum corneum and epidermis has significantly limited its use for topical application. The objective of this section was to develop a topical siRNA delivery system that can permeate through the stratum corneum and viable epidermis and efficiently deposit therapeutic levels of siRNA to the basal epidermis/upper dermis where melanoma cells reside. To achieve this objective, a series of liposome compositions that contained various concentrations of edge activator in their structures were prepared and then complexed with siRNA at different ratios to generate a small library of liposome–siRNA complexes (lipoplexes) with different physicochemical properties [215]. In that study, it has used melanoma as a disease model. Through use of quantitative imaging analysis, it has been identified the necessary design parameters for effective permeation of lipoplexes through the skin layers and deposition at the upper dermis. The ability of the formulated lipoplexes to internalize into melanoma cells, knock down the expression of the BRAF protein, and induce cell death in melanoma cells was studied by fluorescent microscopy, in-cell immunofluorescence assay, and WST-1 cell proliferation assay. By providing direct quantitative and qualitative microscopy evidence, the results of this study [215] demonstrate for the first time that the passive delivery of an edge-activated liposomal formulation can effectively carry siRNA through the stratum corneum and deposit it at the lower epidermis/upper dermis.

Therefore, the objective of this section study was to develop a topical siRNA delivery system that can permeate through the stratum corneum and viable epidermis and efficiently deliver BRAF-targeted siRNA to the basal epidermis where melanoma cells reside. The study [215] has been focused on designing a delivery system for topical administration of BRAF-siRNA (v-Raf murine sarcoma viral oncogene homolog B). Molecular analysis of melanoma cells from patients has shown that the majority of the melanocytes contain a mutation in the gene that encodes BRAF protein. Among BRAF mutations, 90% involves a single-point mutation that substitutes thymine with adenine at nucleotide 1799 [216]. This mutation in the gene-encoding BRAF protein activates the downstream signals of the mitogen-activated protein kinase pathway and ultimately causes an oncogenic increase of melanocytes proliferation and division [217]. Due to the high incidence of mutation in BRAF gene in melanoma cells and increased risk of mortality, we selected the BRAF-siRNA as the model therapeutic for delivery.

The authors [215,218–221] have been previously shown that cationic moieties should be present in a molecule to

effectively permeate through the stratum corneum and deposit in the skin [222]. Therefore, to achieve the objective and in an attempt to overcome the stratum corneum barrier, it has been first prepared a series of cationic liposomal formulations equipped with sodium cholate (NaChol) as an edge activator. While other edge activators such as ethanol, sodium deoxycholate, and Tween exist, it has been utilized NaChol due to its higher activity [214,223]. NaChol is a surfactant that is known for its ability to open pores in stratum corneum accelerating permeation of nanoparticles through the skin. This molecule has a pKa of 5.5 which is close to the pH of skin. It has been suggested that at this pH, NaChol protonation occurs in the lipid complex. This protonation tends to be strongly exothermic, and this may modulate the skin barrier in favor of the lipoplex permeation [214]. Next, through the use of quantitative imaging analysis, we identified the necessary design parameters for effective permeation of liposome–siRNA complexes (lipoplexes) through the skin layers and deposition in the upper dermis. The liposomal formulations were then examined in terms of their ability to internalize into melanoma cells by quantitative fluorescent microscopy and effective knockdown of BRAF expression by in-cell immunofluorescence assay. Finally, the ability of the lipoplexes to kill melanoma cells was studied by using WST-1 cell proliferation assay.

13.9.1 Intracellular Localization of the Lipoplexes and Protein Expression Knockdown

In the next part of the study, it has been examined the ability of lipoplexes to internalize into human melanoma cells as they are the ultimate target for the developed siRNA delivery system. For this purpose, green fluorescent-labeled DOTAP:Nachol liposomes were complexed with siGLO at different ratios and used to transfect UACC-903 melanoma cells. The results demonstrated that all lipoplexes could effectively internalize into melanoma cells, most likely due their positive surface charges. For example, Figure 13.9 shows the ability of the DOTAP:Nachol liposomes (8:1) in complex with siGLO at 16:1 ratio to internalize and localize in the cytoplasm of UACC 903 melanoma cells, thereby raising the possibility of effective protein expression knockdown in these cells. This particular formulation of lipoplexes was chosen based on the previous experiments that showed the highest rate of permeation through the skin layers.

To examine whether the lipoplexes could release the siRNA inside the cytoplasm which in turn would result in protein expression knockdown, it has been performed the next set of studies using therapeutic BRAF siRNA.

13.10 TARGETED DELIVERY: MECHANISTIC PATHWAY

Target-specific deliveries of therapeutic agents [224] are based on stimuli-responsive factors induced by either

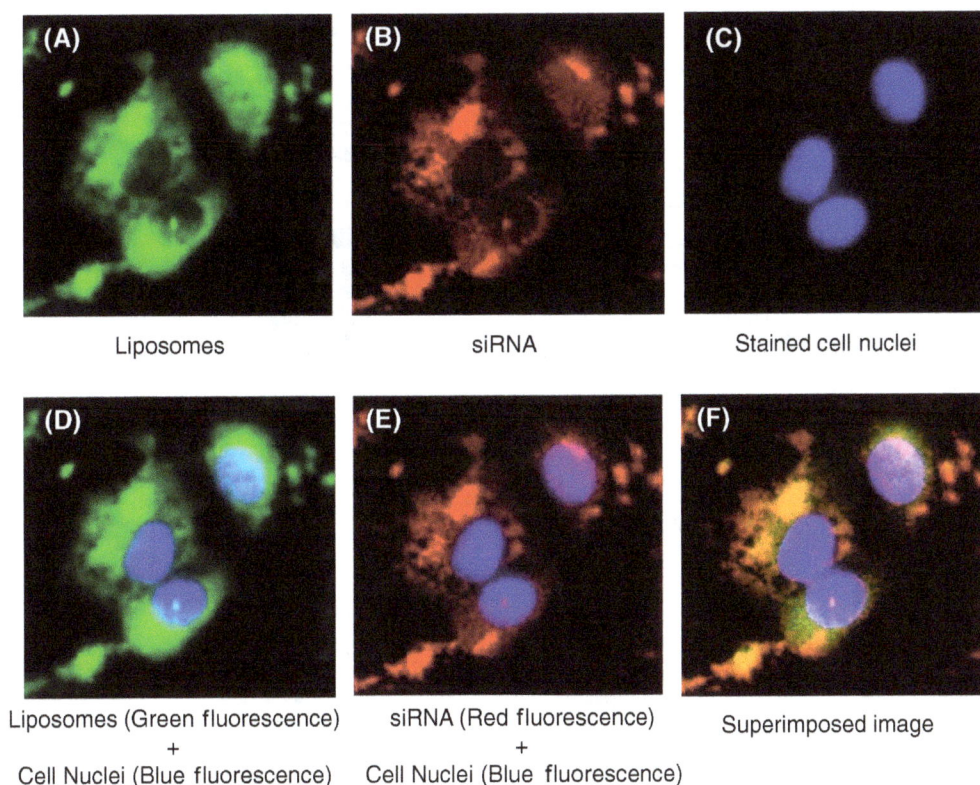

FIGURE 13.9 (a–f) Intracellular localization of liposomes and siRNA. Typical images of human UACC 903 melanoma cells incubated for 1 h with liposomes (green fluorescence) in complex with siGLO (red fluorescence). Cell nuclei were stained with nuclear-specific dye DAPI (blue fluorescence). Superimposed image shows colocalization of liposomes and siRNA.

endogenous (pH, redox, enzyme) or exogenous stimuli (temperature, acoustic, light) as shown in Figure 13.10a [225,226]. pH-sensitive chitosan-based supramolecular gel is used for oral drug delivery of insulin. The pH sensitivity of the nanogel protects insulin while it is in the stomach, and the bioadhesivity of chitosan enables prolonged contact with the intestinal mucosae to increase the absorption of insulin [227]. The drug delivery platform based on mechanized silica nanoparticles (MSNPs), which consists of MSNs vehicles, acid-cleavage intermediate linkages, and reversible supramolecular nanovalves, was devised to achieve multimodal controlled release of two drugs, gemcitabine (GEM) and DOX, by arranging the order of stimuli in sequence. The release time and dosage of GEM are precisely controlled via external voltage, whereas subsequent acid treatment triggers the release of DOX, which is attributed to breakage of the intermediate linkages containing ketal groups [228]. Dynamic cross-linked supramolecular networks of poly(glycidyl methacrylate) derivative chains on mesoporous silica nanoparticles respond well against the dual stimuli of pH and glutathione-(GSH-) linkage, which control the release of anticancer drug DOX hydrochloride under a simulated tumor intracellular environment (pH=5.0, CGSH=2~10mM). Disassembly of the cross-linked polymer network occurs by lowering the pH, and cleavage of disulfide bonds efficiently promotes drug release kinetics (Figure 13.10b) [229]. Glutathione disulfide

(GSSG) is the oxidized form of glutathione (GSH), which is the major endogenous antioxidant. Glutathione protects biological systems from oxidizing factors, such as ROS, by terminating them; GSH is oxidized to GSSG, and then, it is reduced back to GSH by glutathione reductase (GR). The unique antimetastatic mechanism of glutathione disulfide (GSSG)-based liposomes completely prevents cell detachment and migration, significantly inhibits cancer cell invasion, and has been confirmed as a potential treatment for cancer metastasis [230]. Temperature-sensitive liposomes with temperature-sensitive amphiphilic polymer poly(EOEOVE)-OD4 are used for tumor-specific chemotherapy. DOX-encapsulated liposomes are administered intravenously into tumor-bearing mice, and tumor growth is significantly suppressed only when the tumor site is heated to 45°C for 10min after 6–12h of injection (Figure 13.10c) [231]. Biocompatible poly(N-(2- hydroxypropyl-methacrylamide) (PHPMA)-functionalized cyclodextrin (CD) is the building block that houses two guests, for example, poly(N, N-dimethylacrylamide) (PDMAAm) and poly(N, N-diethylacrylamide) (PDEAAm), prepared via reversible addition–fragmentation chain transfer (RAFT) polymerization and can form a well-defined supramolecular ABA triblock copolymer responsive to UV light and temperature. CD-based host/guest complexes show thermoresponsivity due to the negative enthalpy of complex formation. The application of these stimuli leads

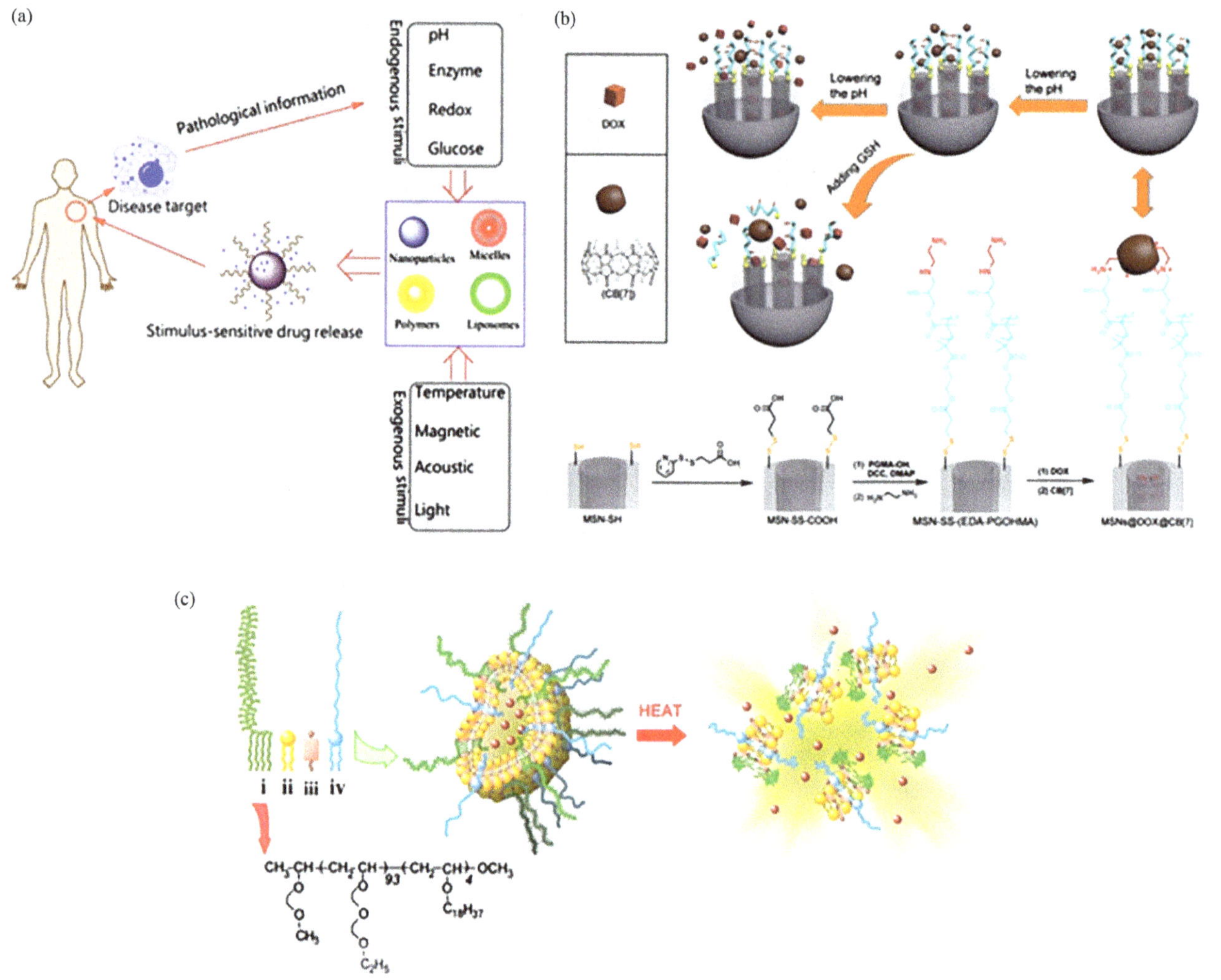

FIGURE 13.10 Stimuli-responsive targeted delivery of therapeutic agents. (a) Schematic illustration of stimuli-responsive DDS [225]; (b) schematic diagram of pH and GSH dual-responsive dynamic cross-linked supramolecular network on MSN-SS-(EDA-PGOHMA); (c) and synthetic route with CB7 assembly [227]. Design of temperature-sensitive liposomes composed of thermosensitive poly(EOEOVE)-OD4 (i), membrane-forming EYPC (ii), membrane-stabilizing cholesterol (iii), and highly hydrophilic and nontoxic PEG-lipid (iv). Heat-triggered release of DOX from liposomes is illustrated with the structure of poly(EOEOVE)-OD4 [229].

to the disassembly of the triblock copolymer, which has been shown to be reversible, and is ultimately responsible for regulated delivery. In case of PDEAAm, temperature-induced aggregation is observed after heating above the cloud point of the PDEAAm block [232]. Tripeptide Lys–Phe–Gly (KFG), a biologically important tripeptide, is spontaneously self-assembled into well-defined nanostructures in aqueous media, showing an exciting phenomenon of reversible and concentration-dependent switching of nanostructures between nanovesicles and nanotubes as evidenced by dynamic light scattering, transmission electron microscopy, and atomic force microscopy studies. The tripeptide vesicles have inner aqueous compartments and are stable at pH 7.4, but they rupture rapidly at pH 6. The pH-sensitive response of the vesicles is exploited for delivery of a chemotherapeutic anticancer drug (DOX), resulting in enhanced cytotoxicity for both drug-sensitive and drug-resistant cells. The absence of the KFG sequence in the receptor polypeptide chain of tyrosine kinase nerve growth factor (Trk NGF) strongly affects the activation of signaling cascades. Efficient intracellular release of the drug is confirmed by fluorescence-activated cell sorting analysis, fluorescence microscopy, and confocal microscopy [233]. A combination of an aptamer for target recognition and enzyme phosphatidylcholine 2-acetylhydrolase (PLA2) for rupture of lipid bilayer of liposomes containing uranin and gadopentetic acid (GdDTPA) as signaling agents have been investigated for fluorescence and MRI detection. Thus, aptamer–PLA2 triggers the release mechanism via the target-responsive liposome system for signal transduction and selective recognition of biological molecules [234].

13.11 MAGNETIC FIELD FOR CANCER TREATMENT

Magnetic (micro- or nanoparticles) materials were explored a couple of decades ago as potential carriers for specific drug targeting. External magnetic fields can be used as a responsive DDS to transport drugs to tumor sites. Recently, superparamagnetic Fe_3O_4 magnetic nanoparticles have been synthesized through grafting using four-armed pentaerythritol poly(ε-caprolactone) in the form of micelles for magnetically targeted controlled drug (DOX) delivery (Figure 13.11a) [235]. The loading of DOX into the nanoparticle and its release under the influence of high-frequency alternating magnetic fields (HFAMFs) is schematically shown in Figure 13.11b. The release profiles at the two different temperatures are not remarkable, whereas drug release is considerable (51.5%) under the influence of a magnetic field for 1 h (Figure 13.11c) as the self-assembled structure ruptures under a strong magnetic field. This form of magnetically controlled DOX release is quite advanced in magnetically active polymeric micelles and is superior from a patient compliance viewpoint compared to other conventional methods used for drug delivery (diffusion, pH, thermal response, etc.). The efficacy of magnetic fields for

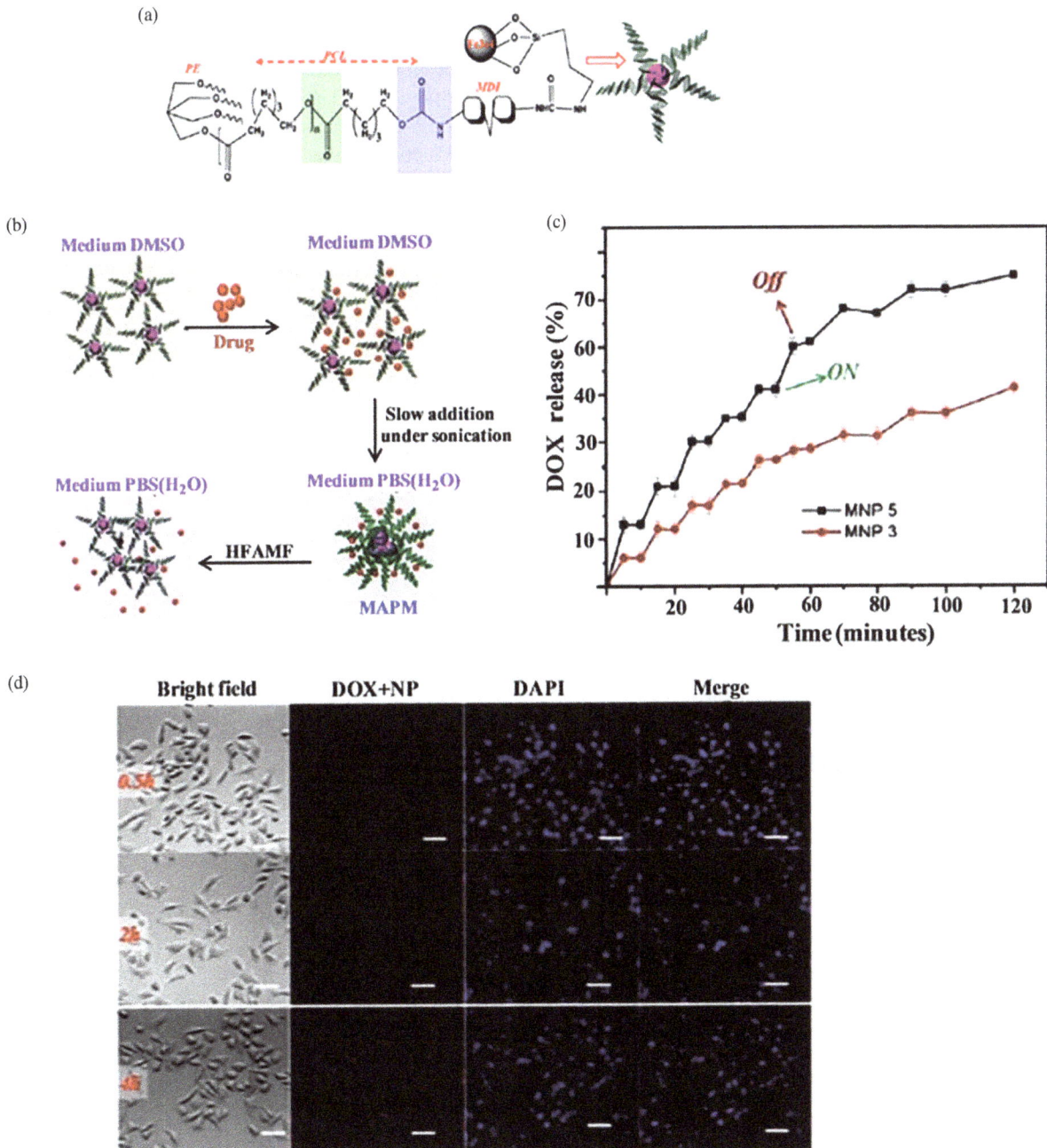

FIGURE 13.11 Release and cellular uptake of drug using magnetic nanoparticles under magnetic field. (a) Schematic representation of a four-armed PE–PCL immobilized magnetic nanoparticle (MNP); (b) schematic representation of DOX-loaded MNP and DOX release under the influence of HFAMF; (c) the release kinetics of MNP 3 (particle size of 3 nm) and MNP 5 (particle size of 5 nm) under the influence of HFAMF at 37°C; and (d) cellular uptake study of DOX-loaded MAPM on HeLa cell in the presence of a static magnetic field where the nucleus was stained by DAPI (blue) [233]. The scale bar is 40 μm.

drug release is indicated by effective intercellular uptake after only 0.5 h of incubation in the presence of a magnetic field with no incorporation of the drug in absence of the field (Figure 13.11d). A magnetically driven paclitaxel delivery system has been designed by incorporating iron oxide and a drug in a palmitoyl chitosan matrix through a nanoprecipitation method for controlled drug delivery under magnetic field [236]. Enhanced cell (MCF-7) death occurs due to the hyperthermic effects of magnetic nanoparticles in the presence of an external magnetic field, resulting in a biocompatible and biodegradable carrier for the precise delivery of powerful cytotoxic anticancer agents. A dramatic change in the amount of drug release is found when the remote magnetic field is switched "on" and "off" using silica magnetic nanocapsules containing camptothecin (hydrophobic) and DOX (hydrophilic) in drug-enriched areas near mouse breast tumors, and the nanocapsules are effective at reducing tumor cell growth [237]. Magnetic carriers for drug delivery using superparamagnetic nickel ferrite nanoparticles functionalized with poly(vinyl alcohol), poly(ethylene oxide), and poly(methacrylic acid) (PMAA) and subsequently conjugated with DOX anticancer drug have significantly enhanced the release rate under magnetic fields by creating mechanical deformation, which generates compressive and tensile stresses to eject drug molecules [238].

13.12   ELECTRIC FIELD FOR CANCER THERAPY

Attention is being given to stimuli-responsive or "smart" biomaterials in the fields of biotechnology and biomedicine [239–243]. Stimuli-responsive materials, which respond to heat [244,245], pH [246,247], light [248,249], enzymes [250,251], and magnetic fields [252,253], are widely used in the biomedical arena. Electrical signals are easier to generate and control than other stimuli. Electric stimuli have successfully been utilized to trigger the release of molecules via conductive polymeric bulk materials or implantable electronic delivery devices. Drug release systems based on conductive polymers have successfully been utilized, as they offer the possibility of drug administration through electrical stimulation. Ge et al. [254] designed an electric-field-responsive DDS using nanoparticles of the conductive polymer polypyrrole. Polypyrrole nanoparticles serve as a drug reservoir for electric-field-triggered release when they are embedded in biocompatible and biodegradable hydrogels of poly[(D, L-lactic acid)-co-(glycolic acid)]-b-poly(ethylene oxide)-b-poly-[(D, L-lactic acid)-co-(glycolicacid)] (PLGA-PEG-PLGA) (Figure 13.12a). This gel is injectable (solution at low temperature but converts into a gel at body temperature), and upon application of an external DC electric field, it releases the drug from the nanogel, allowing the drug to diffuse into the surroundings

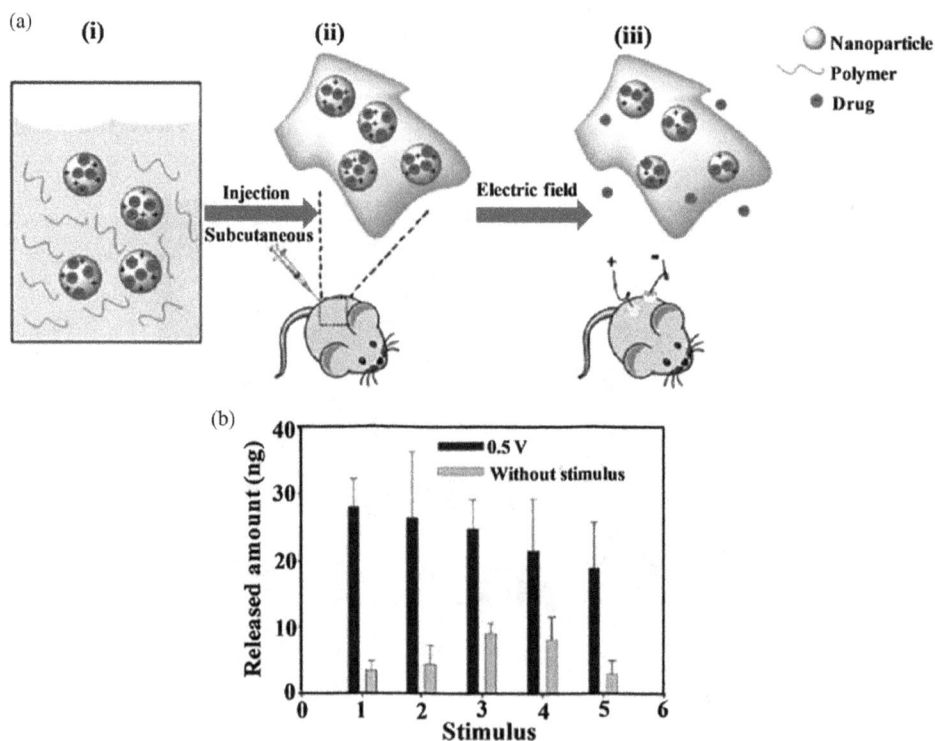

FIGURE 13.12   Electric-field-guided control release of drug. (a) General scheme for the application of this system: (i) the nanoparticle–polymer solution is (ii) subcutaneously injected into a mouse, followed by (iii) application of a DC electric field to induce the release of drug cargo inside the nanoparticles; (b) released amount of daunorubicin in PBS (pH 7.2) following an applied voltage (0.5 V) duration of 10 s, repeated every 5 min [252].

from the hydrogel. Each electric stimulus releases ~25 ng of drug into the solution (Figure 13.12b) with minimal release in the absence of an electric field, indicating undesired release from the hydrogel. This type of delivery system has great advantages over conventional sustained drug release because the released dose of this drug can be roughly controlled by either the strength or the duration of the electric field. Electrically controlled drug delivery has been demonstrated by Weaver et al. [255], who used a graphene oxide composite with a polypyrrole scaffold that had a linear release profile under the influence of voltage stimulation, and dosages were adjusted by altering the magnitude of the stimulation, proving on-demand drug delivery. Carbon nanotubes (CNTs) can act as drug nanoreservoirs by holding drug molecules within their inner cavity, releasing them in bioactive form under electrical stimulations [256]. A polypyrrole coating over CNT drug nanoreservoirs seals the ends of the CNTs, effectively loading the drug, which allows electrical triggering to release the drug with the application of voltage [257]. A dual-stimuli (electric field and pH) responsive system of chitosan–gold

nanocomposites (CGNCs) has been designed for site-specific controlled delivery of the anticancer drug 5-FU at the reduced pH of cancer cell environments [258].

13.13 THERMAL TREATMENT FOR CANCER THERAPY

Photodynamic therapy is an advanced approach that offers control of drug delivery through the use of an external photon source to provide active therapeutic release to a targeted area. Chitosan-functionalized MoS_2 (MoS_2-CS) nanosheets can act as a chemotherapeutic drug nanocarrier for near-infrared (NIR) photothermal-triggered DDSs, facilitating the combination of chemotherapy and photothermal treatment for cancer therapy [259]. The synthesis procedure of single-layer MoS_2 nanosheets and NIR-triggered drug release from MoS_2 nanocarriers for cancer therapy are shown in Figure 13.13a. Drug release profiles show a sharp increase upon irradiation with NIR laser followed by power-dependent release and show nonsignificant release in the absence of irradiation (Figure 13.13b). MoS2-CS plays

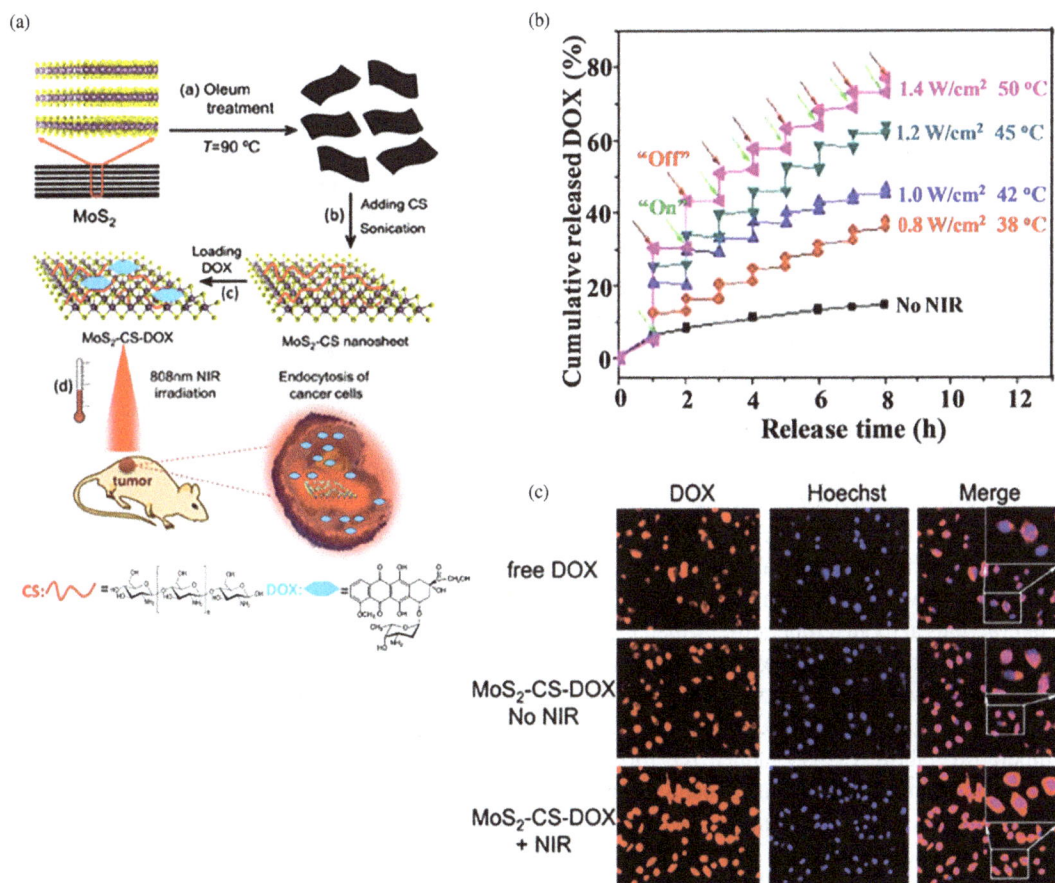

FIGURE 13.13 Laser-guided control drug delivery using MoS2 for cancer treatment. (a) Schematic illustration of high-throughput synthesis of MoS2-CS nanosheets as an NIR photothermal-triggered DDS for efficient cancer therapy. (i, ii) Oleum treatment exfoliation process to produce single-layer MoS2 nanosheets that are then modified with CS, (iii) DOX loading process, and (iv) NIR photothermal-triggered drug delivery of the MoS2 nanosheets to the tumor site. (b) Release profile of DOX in PBS buffer (pH 5.00) in the absence and presence of an 808-nm NIR laser. (c) Fluorescence images of KB cells treated with free DOX, MoS2-CS-DOX, and MoS2-CS-DOX under 808-nm NIR irradiation (inset: high magnification of the rectangle area) [257].

an important role in regulating the release of DOX molecules and enhances their nuclear accumulation under NIR irradiation (Figure 13.13c).

Effective treatment of pancreatic cancer *in vivo* under NIR irradiation has been carried out, confirming the synergistic efficacy of hyperthermia and chemotherapy. This kind of nanocarrier offers a new possibility for better "on-demand" DDSs that can enhance antitumor efficacy. Dual-in-dual synergistic therapy based on the use of dual anticancer drug-loaded graphene oxide (GO) stabilized with poloxamer 188 has been developed to generate heat and deliver drugs to kill cancer cells under NIR laser irradiation [260]. Dual drug (DOX and irinotecan)-loaded GO (GO-DI) in combination with laser irradiation caused higher cytotoxicity than that caused by the administration of a free single drug or a combination of drugs and blank GO in various cancer cells, especially in MDA-MB-231-resistant breast cancer cells, suggesting that GO-DI is a powerful tool for drug delivery and can achieve improved therapeutic efficacy and overcome drug resistance in combined chemophotothermal therapy. A photoactivatable o-nitrobenzyl (ONB) derivative of 5-fluorouracil (5-FU) attached to the surface of upconverting nanoparticles served as a photocaging nanocarrier that absorbed NIR radiation with upconversion in the UV range, which triggers cleavage of the bonds between ONB and FU at the nanoparticle interface to release chemotherapeutic 5-fluorouracil (5-FU) [261]. The efficiency of triggered release is sufficiently high (77%) for the total ONB–FU conjugate, whereas the rate of drug release can be tuned with laser power output. The development of this type of UCNP provides a valuable platform for targeted chemotherapy. Thermoresponsive micelles using an amphiphilic diblock copolymer, poly{γ-2-[2-(2-methoxyethoxy)-ethoxy]ethoxy-ε-caprolactone}-b-poly(γ-octyloxy-ε-caprolactone), display a low critical solution temperature (LCST) of 38°C and can release the therapeutic agent in a controlled fashion [262]. When the anticancer drug DOX is loaded into the micelle, the micelles exhibit statistically higher cytotoxicity against MCF-7 cells at temperatures above the LCST. β-cyclodextrin-poly(N-isopropylacrylamide) star polymer is able to form a supramolecular self-assembled inclusion complex with PTX via host–guest interactions at room temperature, which is below the lower critical solution temperature of the star polymer and significantly improves the solubilization of PTX [263]. Phase transitions of poly(N-isopropylacrylamide) segments at body temperature (above LCST) induce the formation of nanoparticles, which greatly enhance cellular uptake of the polymer–drug complex, resulting in efficient thermoresponsive delivery of PTX. Dual pH/light-responsive cross-linked polymeric micelles (CPMs), prepared by the self-assembly of amphiphilic glycol chitosan-o-nitrobenzyl succinate conjugates (GC-NBSCs) and then cross-linked using glutaraldehyde (GA), are used as a drug carrier that can release drugs quickly at low pH under light irradiation [264]. Thus, GC-NBSC CPMs provide a favorable platform

to construct dual pH/light-responsive smart DDS for cancer therapy. Biodegradable plasmon resonant liposome gold nanoparticles, which are synthesized using 1,2-distearoyl-sn-glycero-3-phosphocholine (DSPC)-cholesterol coating with gold nanoparticles, are capable of killing cancer cells through photothermal therapy.

13.14 DIFFERENTIAL DRUG DELIVERY TO TISSUES, A GOAL OF DDS

DDSs are exploited to alter the pharmacokinetic and biodistribution of a drug [265,266]. Their aim is usually to provide a sustained drug release profile, restrict the drug delivery to nontarget tissues, enhance the drug dose at the target tissue, and increase the drug assimilation by the target cells. In the design and selection of the type of a lipid-based drug delivery carrier, different factors should be taken into account to achieve a successful therapeutic outcome in the body. These could be classified into the factors related to the drug chemical and therapeutic characteristics, the factors related to the carrier physicochemical properties, and the factors related to the histological and cellular features of the target tissue and cells. A thorough review of these factors and their role in drug delivery is presented in the opinion paper of Allen and Cullis [266], and I just briefly explain them from a different perspective.

With respect to the drug chemical structure, the therapeutic and toxic dose of the drug for the potentially accessible different tissues/cells, the drug hydrophilicity/lipophilicity, and the carrier physical structure are the factors that should be considered [266,267]. For instance, for chemotherapeutic agents that affect a broad spectrum of the body tissues and cells, drug delivery carriers that could restrict out-of target drug release in the circulation and patrol therapeutic dose of the drug to the pathological site such as solid tumors are suitable carriers [268–270]. In this regard, for instance, liposomes are not a good candidate for the delivery of nonpotent, large, hydrophobic drugs as they would fail to accommodate therapeutic dose of the drug in the limited spaces of the liposome membrane [271,272]. They also fail to protect them from interaction with various blood cells and tissues as they travel in the circulation to reach tumor microenvironment. As a result, a substantially lower dose of the drug would reach cancer cells to pose a therapeutic effect. Instead, lipid emulsions or liposomes with drug-entrapping agents in their interior would be a more appropriate candidate for the delivery of these drugs as they could accommodate higher content of the drug in their structure [272,273]. For highly potent drugs, like some immunoconjugates with selective interaction with the target cells, stable large copolymer/lipid mixed micelles could enhance the circulation half-life of the drug and penetrate to deep areas of the target tissue due to their small sizes and natural tendency for cell assimilation [266,274]. A small proportion of these carriers are imagined to be taken up by the cells, especially by different blood cells, hepatic and nephrotic cells, predicted not to be accompanied by serious consequences, as the dose of the drug agent would be negligible. However, it is highly recommended to examine their toxicity for hyperactivity reactions and accumulative dose through repeated doses [275].

If the point is to decrease the level of cellular drug delivery and enhance the drug circulation half-life, highly stable liposomal structures of average size 100 nm, for example, PEGylated stealth liposomes, are recommended as these drug carrier systems could be stable in blood for days and could be accumulated to a high level in tumor 1 to 3 days post-injection [266,276]. These liposomes are shown to be accumulated in the tumor through the EPR effect, in which the exclusively leaky vasculature of the tumor allows the extravasation of these nanoparticulated lipid assemblies to the interstitial spaces of cancer cells [276]. The lack of a lymphatic system in tumor blocks their drainage, leading the drug retention in the tumor tissue, whereas non-PEGylated liposomes could be exploited when the point is to deliver the drug to mononuclear phagocyte system for therapeutic purposes, for example, antileishmanial drugs against the parasite that is resident within macrophages [266].

Besides the factors that are explained above, the differential tissue and cellular features of the pathological site are already exploited for the "triggered-delivery of the drug." These include the difference in pH [277], enzymatic activity [278], and cell receptor between a pathological tissue and normal tissue [279]. However, there are critical obstacles for their exploitation that must be taken into account. For instance, pH-sensitive DDSs are designed based on the fact that the tumor interstitial space is more acidic than the surrounding normal tissues and such a difference could be exploited by the design of a pH-sensitive lipid–drug carrier [277]. In this regard, pH-sensitive PEGylated liposomes in which a PEG lipid with a pH-sensitive hydrolyzable bond is used could lose their PEG chains upon PEG-lipid hydrolysis in acidic pH in vitro. However, an acidic region in a tumor is out of reach of tumor vessels with packed cells. These cells and interstitial areas have low nutrient and gas communication with blood vessels, and for these reasons, they are also out of reach of liposomes with large sizes [280]. For the liposome to become a practical pH-sensitive delivery system, it must first pass the mentioned barrier, which is pretty bleak. With respect to the enzymatic activity and cell-receptor difference, these are more appropriate factors as they could break the thermodynamic barrier of the lipid assembly for cell assimilation [268]. For instance, use of lipid species that could be converted to the emulsifier-like species upon the enzymatic activity of the target tissue could result in the disintegration of the lipid assembly, triggered-release of drug, and cellular uptake of the carrier. Similarly, multi-epitope, lipid-based drug delivery might enhance the cellular uptake of the carrier and drug, in a cell population that overexpresses multiple receptors [279,281–283].

13.15 FUTURE CHALLENGES IN CANCER THERAPY

Novel DDSs promise a bright future for cancer treatment in the next decade or so; they might become major arsenal for safer and more efficient treatments by ensuring proper drug localization at the site of action in a controlled manner. The enhanced therapeutic efficacy of targeted nanocarriers has been established in cancer treatment using multiple animal models that target tumors and deliver drugs for targeted radiotherapy, imaging-guided radiotherapy, and precision medicine [284,285]. Although major advances have been made by current DDSs in the treatment of most cancers, much work lies ahead to monitor the mortality rate due to cancer. Most of these carriers have been designed and tested in small animal models, achieving great therapeutic results; however, the translation of animal results into clinical success has been limited. More clinical data are needed to fully understand the advantages and disadvantages of these vehicles. Now, we have entered into an era of molecular targeting of cancer that may further improve the chemotherapeutic index by detecting malignant cells (active targeting moiety), tracking their location in the body (real-time in vivo imaging), killing cancer cells while producing minimal adverse side effects by sparing normal cells (active targeting and controlled drug release or hyperthermia ablation), and monitoring the study in real time. Ion beam therapy seems to be a promising tool for oncologists to treat cancer in near the future instead of high-risk surgery, widespread damage from other forms of radiation therapy, such as X-rays, or collateral damage induced by chemotherapeutic drugs. Classic radiation treatment involves mainly X-rays, which lose energy all along their path through the body and thereby damage healthy cells in their path. The beams of protons or heavier ions, such as carbon and neon, can be accelerated precisely with calculated energy to accurately target tumor cells, sparing healthy tissue above and below the targeted site. The main advantage of employing ion beam radiation for cancer treatment is that it has the potential to precisely target any type or form of tumor, which may be very small or large and may be dangerously shaped or positioned surrounding the spinal cord, in the center of the brain, or close to the optic nerves. Even though proton therapy is commonly used at present, heavier carbon ions deposit more energy in tumor tissues. Therefore, carbon or other heavier elements are considerably more destructive toward the tumor, and hence, they require a fewer number of doses for treatment. For example, liver cancer requires 30 days of treatment using proton therapy, whereas only just four days of treatment is sufficient for carbon therapy. Carbon therapy provides the highest linear energy transfer of any currently available form of clinical radiation. This high energy irradiation to tumor cells results in the destruction of most double-stranded DNA; this extensive destruction is very difficult for other conventional radiation therapies to accomplish, as they predominantly break single-stranded DNA. Recent technological advancements in the fields of accelerator engineering, beam delivery, treatment planning, and tumor visualization have transferred ion beam therapy from physics laboratories to clinics.

REFERENCES

1. R.W. Carthew, E.J. Sontheimer, Origins and mechanisms of miRNAs and siRNAs, *Cell* 136 (2009) 642–655.
2. Y. Yao, C. Wang, R.R. Varshney, D.A. Wang, Antisense makes sense in engineered regenerative medicine, *Pharm. Res.* 26 (2009) 263–275.
3. K. Sliva, B.S. Schnierle, Selective gene silencing by viral delivery of short hairpin RNA, *Virology* 7 (2010) 248.
4. D.W. Bartlett, M.E. Davis, Insights into the kinetics of siRNA-mediated gene silencing from live-cell and live-animal bioluminescent imaging, *Nucleic Acids Res.* 34 (2006) 322–333.
5. D.M. Dykxhoorn, D. Palliser, J. Lieberman, The silent treatment: SiRNAs as small molecule drugs, *Gene Ther.* 13 (2006) 541–552.
6. H. Yin, R.L. Kanasty, A.A. Eltoukhy, A.J. Vegas, J.R. Dorkin, D.G. Anderson, Non-viral vectors for gene-based therapy, *Nat. Rev. Gen.* 15 (2014) 541–555.
7. T. Coelho, D. Adams, A. Silva, P. Lozeron, P.N. Hawkins, T.Mant, J. Perez, J. Chiesa, S. Warrington, E. Tranter, M. Munisamy, R. Falzone, J. Harrop, J. Cehelsky, B.R. Bettencourt, M. Geissler, J.S. Butler, A. Sehgal, R.E. Meyers, Q. Chen, T. Borland, R.M. Hutabarat, V.A. Clausen, R. Alvarez, K. Fitzgerald, C. Gamba-Vitalo, S.V. Nochur, A.K. Vaishnaw, D.W. Sah, J.A. Gollob, O.B. Suhr, Safety and efficacy of RNAi therapy for transthyretin amyloidosis, *New Engl. J. Med.* 369 (2013) 819–829.
8. D. Haussecker, Current issues of RNAi therapeutics delivery and development, *J. Control Release* 195 (2014) 49–54.
9. J.E. Zuckerman, T. Hsueh, R.C. Koya, M.E. Davis, A. Ribas, SiRNA knockdown of ribonucleotide reductase inhibits melanoma cell line proliferation alone or synergistically with temozolomide, *J. Invest. Dermatol.* 131 (2011) 453–460.
10. M. Yasuda, L. Gan, B. Chen, S. Kadirvel, C. Yu, J.D. Phillips, M.I. New, A. Liebow, K. Fitzgerald, W. Querbes, R.J. Desnick, RNAi-mediated silencing of hepatic ALAS1 effectively prevents and treats the induced acute attacks in acute intermittent porphyria mice, *Proc. Natl. Acad. Sci. U. S. A.* 111 (2014) 7777–7782.
11. Alnylam RNAi roundtable: conjugate delivery, 2012.
12. D. Haussecker, The business of RNAi therapeutics in 2012, *Mol. Ther. Nucleic Acids* 1 (2012) e8.
13. H.Y. Xue, S. Liu, H.L. Wong, Nanotoxicity: a key obstacle to clinical translation of siRNA-based nanomedicine, *Nanomedicine* 9 (2014) 295–312.
14. M.E. Kleinman, K. Yamada, A. Takeda, V. Chandrasekaran, M. Nozaki, J.Z. Baffi, R.J. Albuquerque, S. Yamasaki, M. Itaya, Y. Pan, B. Appukuttan, D. Gibbs, Z. Yang, K. Kariko, B.K. Ambati, T.A. Wilgus, L.A. DiPietro, E. Sakurai, K. Zhang, J.R. Smith, E.W. Taylor, J. Ambati, Sequence- and target-independent angiogenesis suppression by siRNA via TLR3, *Nature* 452 (2008) 591–597.
15. T. Inoue, M. Sugimoto, T. Sakurai, R. Saito, N. Futaki, Y. Hashimoto, Y. Honma, I. Arai, S. Nakaike, Modulation of scratching behavior by silencing an endogenous cyclooxygenase-1 gene in the skin through the administration of siRNA, *J. Gene. Med.* 9 (2007) 994–1001.
16. C. Napoli, C. Lemieux, R. Jorgensen, Introduction of a chimeric chalcone synthase gene into petunia results in reversible co-suppression of homologous genes ín trans, *Plant Cell* 2 (1990) 279–289.
17. J. Bertrand, M. Pottier, A. Vekris, P. Opolon, A. Maksimenko, C. Malvy, Comparison of antisense oligonucleotides and siRNAs in cell culture and in vivo, *Biochem. Biophys. Res. Commun.* 296 (2002) 1000–1004.
18. D.H. Kim, M.A. Behlke, S.D. Rose, M.S. Chang, S. Choi, J.J. Rossi, Synthetic dsRNA dicer substrates enhance RNAi potency and efficacy, *Nat. Biotechnol.* 23 (2005) 222–226.
19. B.F. Baker, 2′-O-(2-methoxy)ethyl-modified anti-intercellular adhesion molecule 1 (ICAM-1) oligonucleotides selectively increase the ICAM-1 mRNA level and inhibit formation of the ICAM-1 translation initiation complex in human umbilical vein endothelial cells, *J. Biol. Chem.* 272 (1997) 11994–12000.
20. S.M. Hammond, E. Bernstein, D. Beach, G.J. Hannon, An RNA-directed nuclease mediates post-transcriptional gene silencing in drosophila cells, *Nature* 404 (2000) 293–296.
21. E. Bernstein, A.A. Caudy, S.M. Hammond, G.J. Hannon, Role for a bidentate ribonuclease in the initiation step of RNA interference, *Nature* 409 (2001) 363–366.
22. B. Haley, P.D. Zamore, Kinetic analysis of the RNAi enzyme complex, *Nat. Struct. Biol.* 11 (2004) 599–606.
23. K.R. Beavers, C.E. Nelson, C.L. Duvall, MiRNA inhibition in tissue engineering and regenerative medicine, *Adv. Drug Deliv. Rev.* 88 (2014) 123–137.
24. K.A. Whitehead, R. Langer, D.G. Anderson, Knocking down barriers: advances in siRNA delivery, *Nat. Rev. Drug Discov.* 8 (2009) 129–138.
25. M.A. Behlke, Chemical modification of siRNAs for in vivo use, *Oligonucleotides* 18 (2008) 305–319.
26. J. Martinez, A. Patkaniowska, H. Urlaub, R. Luhrmann, T. Tuschl, Single-stranded antisense siRNAs guide target RNA cleavage in RNAi, *Cell* 110 (2004) 563–574.
27. J. Gilleron, W. Querbes, A. Zeigerer, A. Borodovsky, G. Marsico, U. Schubert, K. Manygoats, S. Seifert, C. Andree, M. Stoter, H. Epstein-Barash, L. Zhang, V. Koteliansky, K. Fitzgerald, E. Fava, M. Bickle, Y. Kalaidzidis, A. Akinc, M. Maier, M. Zerial, Image-based analysis of lipid nanoparticle-mediated siRNA delivery, intracellular trafficking and endosomal escape, *Nat. Biotechnol.* 31 (2013) 638–646.
28. S.M. Elbashir, J. Harborth, W. Lendeckel, A. Yalcin, K. Weber, T. Tuschl, Duplexes of 21-nucleotide RNAs mediate RNA interference in cultured mammalian cells, *Nature* 411 (2001) 494–498.
29. K. Kariko, P. Bhuyan, J. Capodici, D. Weissman, Small interfering RNAs mediate sequence independent gene suppression and induce immune activation by signaling through toll-like receptor 3, *J. Immunol.* 172 (2004) 6545–6549.
30. F. Heil, H. Hemmi, H. Hochrein, F. Ampenberger, C. Kirschning, S. Akira, G. Lipford, H. Wagner, S. Bauer, Species-specific recognition of single-stranded RNA via Toll-like receptor 7 and 8, *Science* 303 (2004) 1526–1529.
31. A.L. Jackson, P.S. Linsley, Recognizing and avoiding siRNA off-target effects for target identification and therapeutic application, *Nat. Rev. Drug Discov.* 9 (2010) 57–67.
32. J.E. Zuckerman, I. Gritli, A. Tolcher, J.D. Heidel, D. Lim, R.Morgan, B. Chmielowski, A. Ribas, M.E. Davis, Y. Yen, Correlating animal and human phase IA/IB clinical data with CALAA-01, a targeted, polymer-based nanoparticle containing siRNA, *Proc. Natl. Acad. Sci. U. S. A.* 111 (2014) 11449–11454.

33. R. Yi, B.P. Doehle, Y. Qin, I.G. Macara, B.R. Cullen, Overexpression of exportin 5 enhances RNA interference mediated by short hairpin RNAs and microRNAs, *RNA* 11 (2005) 220–226.

34. A.L. Jackson, S.R. Bartz, J. Schelter, S.V. Kobayashi, J. Burchard, M. Mao, B. Li, G. Cavet, P.S. Linsley, Expression profiling reveals off-target gene regulation by RNAi, *Nat. Biotechnol.* 21 (2003) 635–637.

35. F.T. Vicentini, L.N. Borgheti-Cardoso, L.V. Depieri, M.D. de Macedo, T.F. Abelha, R. Petrilli, M.V. Bentley, Delivery systems and local administration routes for therapeutic siRNA, *Pharm. Res.* 30 (2013) 915–931.

36. A. Sadio, J.K. Gustafsson, B. Pereira, C.P. Gomes, G.C. Hansson, L. David, A.P. Pego, R. Almeida, Modified-chitosan/siRNA nanoparticles downregulate cellular cdx2 expression and cross the gastric mucus barrier, *PLoS One* 9 (2014) e99449.

37. J.R. Weiser, W.M. Saltzman, Controlled release for local delivery of drugs: barriers and models, *J. Control Release* 190 (2014) 664–673.

38. L.A. Wheeler, V. Vrbanac, R. Trifonova, M.A. Brehm, A. Gilboa-Geffen, S. Tanno, D.L. Greiner, A.D. Luster, A.M. Tager, J. Lieberman, Durable knockdown and protection from HIV transmission in humanized mice treated with gel-formulated CD4 aptamer-siRNA chimeras, *Mol. Ther.* 21 (2013) 1378–1389.

39. C.E. Nelson, A.J. Kim, E.J. Adolph, M.K. Gupta, F. Yu, K.M. Hocking, J.M. Davidson, S.A. Guelcher, C.L. Duvall, Tunable delivery of siRNA from a biodegradable scaffold to promote angiogenesis in vivo, *Adv. Mat.* 26 (2014) 607–614.

40. J.M. Layzer, In vivo activity of nuclease-resistant siRNAs, *RNA* 10 (2004) 766–771.

41. M. Dimitrova, C. Affolter, F. Meyer, I. Nguyen, D.G. Richard, C. Schuster, R. Bartenschlager, J.C. Voegel, J. Ogier, T.F. Baumert, Sustained delivery of siRNAs targeting viral infection by cell-degradable multilayered polyelectrolyte films, *Proc. Natl. Acad. Sci. U. S. A.* 105 (2008) 16320–16325.

42. L.D. Laporte, L.D. Shea, Matrices and scaffolds for DNA delivery in tissue engineering, *Adv. Drug Deliv. Rev.* 59 (2007) 292–307.

43. M. Chen, S. Gao, M. Dong, J. Song, C. Yang, K.A. Howard, J. Kjems, F. Besenbacher, Chitosan/siRNA nanoparticles encapsulated in PLGA nanofibers for siRNA delivery, *ACS Nano* 6 (2012) 4835–4844.

44. D. Klose, F. Siepmann, K. Elkharraz, S. Krenzlin, J. Siepmann, How porosity and size affect the drug release mechanisms from PLGA-based microparticles, *Int. J. Pharm.* 314 (2006) 198–206.

45. H.H.D. Tai, S. Takae, W. Wang, T. Vermonden, E.W. Hennink, P.S. Stayton, A.S. Hoffman, A. Endruweit, C. Alexander, S.M. Howdle, K.M. Shakesheff, Photo-crosslinked hydrogels from thermoresponsive PEGMEMA-PPGMA-EGDMA copolymers containing multiple methacrylate groups: mechanical property, swelling, protein release, cytotoxicity, *Biomacromolecules* 10 (2009) 2895–2903.

46. B.K.G.A. Mann, A.T. Tsai, R.H. Schmelen, J.L. West, Smooth muscle cell growth in photopolymerized hydrogels with cell adhesive and proteolytically degradable domains: synthetic ECM analogs for tissue engineering, *Biomaterials* 22 (2001) 3045–3051.

47. J.L. West, J.A. Hubbell, Polymeric biomaterials with degradation sites for proteases involved in cell migration, *Macromolecules* 32 (1999) 241–244.

48. P.X. Ma, Biomimetic materials for tissue engineering, *Adv. Drug. Deliv. Rev.* 60 (2008) 184–198.

49. L.D. Shea, E. Smiley, J. Bonadio, D.J. Mooney, DNA delivery from polymer matrices for tissue engineering, *Nat. Biotechnol.* 17 (1999) 551–554.

50. G. De Rosa, M.C. Maiuri, F. Ungaro, D. De Stefano, F. Quaglia, M.I. La Rotonda, R. Carnuccio, Enhanced intracellular uptake and inhibition of NF-κβ activation by decoy oligonucleotide released from PLGA microspheres, *J. Gene Med.* 7 (2005) 771–781.

51. T. Estey, J. Kang, S.P. Schwendeman, J.F. Carpenter, BSA degradation under acidic conditions: a model for protein instability during release from PLGA delivery systems, *J. Pharm. Sci.* 95 (2006) 1626–1639.

52. R.P. Felix Lanao, S.C. Leeuwenburgh, J.G. Wolke, J.A. Jansen, In vitro degradation rate of apatitic calcium phosphate cement with incorporated PLGA microspheres, *Acta Biomater.* 7 (2011) 3459–3468.

53. J.R. Martin, M.K. Gupta, J.M. Page, F. Yu, J.M. Davidson, S.A. Guelcher, C.L. Duvall, A porous tissue engineering scaffold selectively degraded by cell-generated reactive oxygen species, *Biomaterials* 35 (2014) 3766–3776.

54. D.S. Wilson, G. Dalmasso, L. Wang, S.V. Sitaraman, D. Merlin, N. Murthy, Orally delivered thioketal nanoparticles loaded with TNF-α–siRNA target inflammation and inhibit gene expression in the intestines, *Nat. Mater.* 9 (2010) 923–928.

55. T. Segura, L.D. Shea, Surface-tethered DNA complexes for enhanced gene delivery, *Bioconjug. Chem.* 13 (2002) 621–629.

56. M.Ø. Andersen, D.Q.S. Le, M. Chen, J.V. Nygaard, M. Kassem, C. Bünger, J. Kjems, Spatially controlled delivery of siRNAs to stem cells in implants generated by multi-component additive manufacturing, *Adv. Funct. Mater.* 23 (2013) 5599–5607.

57. H. Cao, X. Jiang, C. Chai, S.Y. Chew, RNA interference by nanofiber-based siRNA delivery system, *J. Control Release* 144 (2010) 203–212.

58. S.W.K.B. Lee, S. Chen, Y. Shao-Horn, P.T. Hammond, Layer-by-layer assembly of all carbon nanotube ultrathin films for electrochemical applications, *J. Am. Chem. Soc.* 131 (2008) 671–679.

59. M. Amarzguioui, T. Holen, E. Babaie, H. Prydz, Tolerance for mutations and chemical modifications in a siRNA, *Nucleic Acids Res.* 31 (2003) 589–595.

60. D.A. Braasch, S. Jensen, Y. Liu, K. Kaur, K. Arar, M.A. White, D.R. Corey, RNA interference in mammalian cells by chemically-modified RNA, *Biochemistry* 42 (2003) 7967–7975.

61. A. Judge, I. MacLachlan, Overcoming the innate immune response to small interfering RNA, *Hum. Gene Ther.* 19 (2008) 111–124.

62. Y.L. Chiu, SiRNA function in RNAi: a chemical modification analysis, *RNA* 9 (2003) 1034–1048.

63. J. Wang, Z. Lu, M.G. Wientjes, J.L. Au, Delivery of siRNA therapeutics: barriers and carriers, *AAPS J.* 12 (2010) 492–503.

64. J.H. Jeong, H. Mok, Y. Oh, T.G. Park, SiRNA conjugate delivery systems, *Bioconjug. Chem.* 20 (2009) 5–14.

65. R. Kanasty, J.R. Dorkin, A. Vegas, D. Anderson, Delivery materials for siRNA therapeutics, *Nat. Mater.* 12 (2013) 967–977.

66. T. Kubo, Y. Takei, K. Mihara, K. Yanagihara, T. Seyama, Amino-modified and lipid conjugated dicer-substrate siRNA enhances RNAi efficacy, *Bioconjug. Chem.* 23 (2012) 164–173.

67. K. Nishina, T. Unno, Y. Uno, T. Kubodera, T. Kanouchi, H. Mizusawa, T. Yokota, Efficient in vivo delivery of siRNA to the liver by conjugation of alpha-tocopherol, *Mol. Ther.* 16 (2008) 734–740.

68. S.Y. Wu, N.A. McMillan, Lipidic systems for in vivo siRNA delivery, *AAPS J.* 11 (2009) 639–652.

69. K.G. Rajeev, J.K. Nair, M. Jayaraman, K. Charisse, N. Taneja, J. O'Shea, J.L.Willoughby, K. Yucius, T. Nguyen, S. Shulga-Morskaya, S. Milstein, A. Liebow, W. Querbes, A. Borodovsky, K. Fitzgerald, M.A. Maier, M. Manoharan, Hepatocyte-specific delivery of siRNAs conjugated to novel non-nucleosidic trivalent N-acetylgalactosamine elicits robust gene silencing in vivo, *ChemBioChem* 16 (2015) 903–908.

70. S. Matsuda, K. Keiser, J.K. Nair, K. Charisse, R.M. Manoharan, P. Kretschmer, C.G. Peng, A. VKi, P. Kandasamy, J.L. Willoughby, A. Liebow, W. Querbes, K. Yucius, T. Nguyen, S. Milstein, M.A. Maier, K.G. Rajeev, M. Manoharan, SiRNA conjugates carrying sequentially assembled trivalent N-acetylgalactosamine linked through nucleosides elicit robust gene silencing in vivo in hepatocytes, *ACS Chem. Biol.* 10 (2015) 1181–1187.

71. M.R. Alam, X. Ming, M. Fisher, J.G. Lackey, K.G. Rajeev, M. Manoharan, R.L. Juliano, Multivalent cyclic RGD conjugates for targeted delivery of small interfering RNA, *Bioconjug. Chem.* 22 (2011) 1673–1681.

72. L.N. Patel, J.L. Zaro, W.C. Shen, Cell penetrating peptides: intracellular pathways and pharmaceutical perspectives, *Pharm. Res.* 24 (2007) 1977–1992.

73. C. De Coupade, A. Fittipaldi, V. Chagnas, M. Michel, S. Carlier, E. Tasciotti, A. Darmon, D. Ravel, J. Kearsey, M. Giacca, F. Cailler, Novel human-derived cell penetrating peptides for specific subcellular delivery of therapeutic biomolecules, *Biochem. J.* 390 (2005) 407–418.

74. T. Holm, H. Raagel, S.E. Andaloussi, M. Hein, M. Mae, M. Pooga, U. Langel, Retroinversion of certain cell-penetrating peptides causes severe cellular toxicity, *Biochim. Biophys. Acta* 2011 (1808) 1544–1551.

75. H.L.-J.A. Lee, Y. Chen, K.T. Love, A.I. Park, E.D. Karagiannis, A. Sehgal, W. Querbes, C.S. Zurenko, M. Jayaraman, C.G. Peng, K. Charisse, A. Borodovsky, M. Manoharan, J.S. Donahoe, J. Truelove, M. Nahrendorf, R. Langer, D.G. Anderson, Molecularly self-assembled nucleic acid nanoparticles for targeted in vivo siRNA delivery, *Nat. Nanotechnol.* 7 (2012) 389–393.

76. C. Shen, A.K. Buck, X. Liu, M. Winkler, S.N. Reske, Gene silencing by adenovirus delivered siRNA, *FEBS Lett.* 539 (2003) 111–114.

77. A. de Fougerolles, H. Vornlocher, J. Maraganore, J. Lieberman, Interfering with disease: a progress report on siRNA therapeutics, *Nat. Rev. Drug Discov.* 6 (2007).

78. A. Akinc, M. Thomas, A.M. Klibanov, R. Langer, Exploring polyethylenimine mediated DNA transfection and the proton sponge hypothesis, *J. Gene Med.* 7 (2005) 657–663.

79. C. Pichon, C. Goncalves, P. Midoux, Histidine-rich peptides and polymers for nucleic acids delivery, *Adv. Drug Deliv. Rev.* 53 (2001).

80. R.E. Vandenbroucke, B.G. De Geest, S. Bonne, M. Vinken, T. Van Haecke, H. Heimberg, E. Wagner, V. Rogiers, S.C. De Smedt, J. Demeester, N.N. Sanders, Prolonged gene silencing in hepatoma cells and primary hepatocytes after small interfering RNA delivery with biodegradable poly(beta-amino esters), *J. Gene Med.* 10 (2008) 783–794.

81. W. Zauner, M. Ogris, E. Wagner, Polylysine-based transfection systems utilizing receptor mediated delivery, *Adv. Drug Deliv. Rev.* 30 (1998) 97–113.

82. S.M. Noh, S.E. Han, G. Shim, K.E. Lee, C.W. Kim, S.S. Han, Y. Choi, Y.K. Kim, W.K. Kim, Y.K. Oh, Tocopheryl oligochitosan-based self-assembling oligomersomes for siRNA delivery, *Biomaterials* 32 (2011) 849–857.

83. F. Takeshita, Y. Minakuchi, S. Nagahara, K. Honma, H. Sasaki, K. Hirai, T. Teratani, N. Namatame, Y. Yamamoto, K. Hanai, T. Kato, A. Sano, T. Ochiya, Efficient delivery of small interfering RNA to bone-metastatic tumors by using atelocollagen in vivo, *Proc. Natl. Acad. Sci. U. S. A.* 102 (2005) 12177–12182.

84. A.J. Convertine, D.S. Benoit, C.L. Duvall, A.S. Hoffman, P.S. Stayton, Development of a novel endosomolytic diblock copolymer for siRNA delivery, *J. Control Release* 133 (2009) 221–229.

85. H. Li, S.S. Yu, M. Miteva, C.E. Nelson, T. Werfel, T.D. Giorgio, C.L. Duvall, Matrix metalloproteinase responsive, proximity-activated polymeric nanoparticles for siRNA delivery, *Adv. Funct. Mater.* 23 (2013) 3040–3052.

86. C.E. Nelson, R.J. Kintzing, A. Hanna, J.M. Shannon, M.K. Gupta, C.L. Duvall, Balancing cationic and hydrophobic content of PEGylated siRNA polyplexes enhances endosome escape, stability, blood circulation time, and bioactivity in vivo, *ACS Nano* 7 (2013) 8870–8880.

87. H. Li, M. Miteva, K.C. Kirkbride, M.J. Cheng, C.E. Nelson, E.M. Simpson, M.K. Gupta, C.L. Duvall, T.D. Giorgio, Dual mmp7-proximity-activated and folate receptor targeted nanoparticles for siRNA delivery, *Biomacromolecules* 16 (2015) 192–201.

88. M. Miteva, K.C. Kirkbride, K.V. Kilchrist, T.A. Werfel, H. Li, C.E. Nelson, M.K. Gupta, T.D. Giorgio, C.L. Duvall, Tuning PEGylation of mixed micelles to overcome intracellular and systemic siRNA delivery barriers, *Biomaterials* 38 (2015) 97–107.

89. B. Ozpolat, A.K. Sood, G. Lopez-Berestein, Liposomal siRNA nanocarriers for cancer therapy, *Adv. Drug. Deliv. Rev.* 66 (2014) 110–116.

90. M.D. Green, A.A. Foster, C.T. Greco, R. Roy, R.M. Lehr, T.H. Epps III, M.O. Sullivan, Catch and release: photocleavable cationic diblock copolymers as a potential platform for nucleic acid delivery, *Polym. Chem.* 5 (2014) 5535–5541.

91. K.L. Kozielski, S.Y. Tzeng, B.A. Hurtado DeMendoza, J.J. Green, Bioreducible cationic polymer-based nanoparticles for efficient and environmentally triggered cytoplasmic siRNA delivery to primary human brain cancer cells, *ACS Nano* 8 (2015) 3232–3241.

92. S.M. Sarett, C.E. Nelson, C.L. Duvall, Technologies for controlled, local delivery of siRNA, *J. Control. Release* 218 (2015) 94–113.

93. X. Zhu, L. Lu, B.L. Currier, A.J. Windebank, M.J. Yaszemski, Controlled release of NFκβ decoy oligonucleotides from biodegradable polymer microparticles, *Biomaterials* 23 (2002) 2683–2692.

94. P.M. Mountziaris, D.C. Sing, S.A. Chew, S.N. Tzouanas, E.D. Lehman, F.K. Kasper, A.G. Mikos, Controlled release of anti-inflammatory siRNA from biodegradable polymeric microparticles intended for intra-articular delivery to the temporomandibular joint, *Pharm. Res.* 28 (2011) 1370–1384.

95. S.J. Lewis, W.J. Irwin, S. Akhtar, Development of a sustained-release biodegradable polymer delivery system for site-specific delivery of oligonucleotides: characterization of p(LA-GA) copolymer microspheres in vitro, *J. Drug Targets* 5 (1998) 291–302.

96. S. Akhtar, K.J. Lewis, Antisense oligonucleotide delivery to cultured macrophages is improved by incorporation into sustained-release biodegradable polymer microspheres, *Int. J. Pharm.* 151 (1997) 57–67.

97. P. Pradhan, H. Qin, J.A. Leleux, D. Gwak, I. Sakamaki, L.W. Kwak, K. Roy, The effect of combined IL10 siRNA and CPG ODN as pathogen-mimicking microparticles on TH1/TH2 cytokine balance in dendritic cells and protective immunity against B cell lymphoma, *Biomaterials* 35 (2014) 5491–5504.

98. A. Singh, S. Suri, K. Roy, *In-situ* crosslinking hydrogels for combinatorial delivery of chemokines and siRNA-DNA carrying microparticles to dendritic cells, *Biomaterials* 30 (2009) 5187–5200.

99. P.M. Mountziaris, S.N. Tzouanas, D.C. Sing, P.R. Kramer, F.K. Kasper, A.G. Mikos, Intra-articular controlled release of anti-inflammatory siRNA with biodegradable polymer microparticles ameliorates temporomandibular joint inflammation, *Acta Biomater.* 8 (2012) 3552–3560.

100. E.S. Place, N.D. Evans, M.M. Stevens, Complexity in biomaterials for tissue engineering, *Nat. Mater.* 8 (2009) 457–470.

101. R. Vinas-Castells, C. Holladay, A. di Luca, V.M. Diaz, A. Pandit, Snail1 downregulation using small interfering RNA complexes delivered through collagen scaffolds, *Bioconjug. Chem.* 20 (2009) 2262–2269.

102. D.M. Salvay, M. Zelivyanskaya, L.D. Shea, Gene delivery by surface immobilization of plasmid to tissue-engineering scaffolds, *Gene Ther.* 17 (2010) 1134–1141.

103. S.A. Guelcher, Biodegradable polyurethanes: synthesis and applications in regenerative medicine, *Tissue Eng. Part B Rev.* 14 (2008) 3–17.

104. A.E. Hafeman, B. Li, T. Yoshii, K. Zienkiewicz, J.M. Davidson, S.A. Guelcher, Injectable biodegradable polyurethane scaffolds with release of platelet-derived growth factor for tissue repair and regeneration, *Pharm. Res.* 25 (2008) 2387–2399.

105. B. Li, K.V. Brown, J.C. Wenke, S.A. Guelcher, Sustained release of vancomycin from polyurethane scaffolds inhibits infection of bone wounds in a rat femoral segmental defect model, *J. Control. Release* 145 (2010) 221–230.

106. Y. Lei, M. Rahim, Q. Ng, T. Segura, Hyaluronic acid and fibrin hydrogels with concentrated DNA/PEI polyplexes for local gene delivery, *J. Control. Release* 153 (2011) 255–261.

107. M.O. Andersen, K.A. Howard, S.R. Paludan, F. Besenbacher, J. Kjems, Delivery of siRNA from lyophilized polymeric surfaces, *Biomaterials* 29 (2008) 506–512.

108. Y. Lei, S. Huang, P. Sharif-Kashani, Y. Chen, P. Kavehpour, T. Segura, Incorporation of active DNA/cationic polymer polyplexes into hydrogel scaffolds, *Biomaterials* 31 (2010) 9106–9116.

109. C.E. Nelson, M.K. Gupta, E.J. Adolph, J.M. Shannon, S.A. Guelcher, C.L. Duvall, Sustained local delivery of siRNA from an injectable scaffold, *Biomaterials* 33 (2012) 1154–1161.

110. P.O. Rujitanaroj, Y.C. Wang, J. Wang, S.Y. Chew, Nanofiber-mediated controlled release of siRNA complexes for long term gene-silencing applications, *Biomaterials* 32 (2011) 5915–5923.

111. M.D. Krebs, O. Jeon, E. Alsberg, Localized and sustained delivery of silencing RNA from macroscopic biopolymer hydrogels, *J. Am. Chem. Soc.* 131 (2009) 9204–9206.

112. K. Nguyen, P.N. Dang, E. Alsberg, Functionalized, biodegradable hydrogels for control over sustained and localized siRNA delivery to incorporated and surrounding cells, *Acta Biomater.* 9 (2013) 4487–4495.

113. A. Galperin, T.J. Long, S. Garty, B.D. Ratner, Synthesis and fabrication of a degradable poly(n-isopropyl acrylamide) scaffold for tissue engineering applications, *J. Biomed. Mater. Res. A.* 101 (2013) 775–786.

114. M.K. Gupta, J.R. Martin, T.A. Werfel, T. Shen, J.M. Page, C.L. Duvall, Cell protective, ABC triblock polymer-based thermoresponsive hydrogels with ROS-triggered degradation and drug release, *J. Am. Chem. Soc.* 136 (2014) 14896–14902.

115. R.V. Joshi, C.E. Nelson, K.M. Poole, M.C. Skala, C.L. Duvall, Dual pH- and temperature-responsive microparticles for protein delivery to ischemic tissues, *Acta Biomater.* 9 (2013) 6526–6534.

116. Z. Ma, D.M. Nelson, Y. Hong, W.R. Wagner, Thermally responsive injectable hydrogel incorporating methacrylate-polylactide for hydrolytic lability, *Biomacromolecules* 11 (2010) 1873–1881.

117. L.E. Strong, S.N. Dahotre, J.L. West, Hydrogel-nanoparticle composites for optically modulated cancer therapeutic delivery, *J. Control. Release* 178 (2014) 63–68.

118. H.Y. Yang, R.J. van Ee, K. Timmer, E.G. Craenmehr, J.H. Huang, F.C. Oner, W.J. Dhert, A.H. Kragten, N. Willems, G.C. Grinwis, M.A. Tryfonidou, N.E. Papen-Botterhuis, L.B. Creemers, A novel injectable thermoresponsive and cytocompatible gel of poly(n-isopropylacrylamide) with layered double hydroxides facilitates siRNA delivery into chondrocytes in 3d culture, *Acta Biomater.* 23 (2015) 214–228.

119. S. Ishii, J. Kaneko, Y. Nagasaki, Dual stimuli-responsive redox-active injectable gel by polyion complex based flower micelles for biomedical applications, *Macromolecules* 48 (2015) 3088–3094.

120. L.N. Borgheti-Cardoso, L.V. Depieri, S.A. Kooijmans, H. Diniz, R.A. Calzzani, F.T. Vicentini, R. van derMeel, M.C. Fantini, M.M. Iyomasa, R.M. Schiffelers, M.V. Bentley, An in situ gelling liquid crystalline system based on monoglycerides and polyethylenimine for local delivery of siRNAs, *Eur. J. Pharm. Sci.* 74 (2015) 103–117.

121. Y.M. Kim, M.R. Park, S.C. Song, An injectable cell penetrable nano-polyplex hydrogel for localized siRNA delivery, *Biomaterials* 34 (2013) 4493–4500.

122. K. Li, L. Feng, J. Shen, Q. Zhang, Z. Liu, S.T. Lee, J. Liu, Patterned substrates of nanographene oxide mediating highly localized and efficient gene delivery, *ACS Appl. Mater. Int.* 6 (2014) 5900–5907.

123. J. Min, R.D. Braatz, P.T. Hammond, Tunable staged release of therapeutics from layer-by-layer coatings with clay interlayer barrier, *Biomaterials* 35 (2014) 2507–2517.

124. B.S. Kim, R.C. Smith, Z. Poon, P.T. Hammond, MAD (multiagent delivery) nanolayer: delivering multiple therapeutics from hierarchically assembled surface coatings, *Langmuir* 25 (2009) 14086–14092.

125. J.S.N. Hong, A.C. Drake, P.C. DeMuth, J.B. Lee, J. Chen, P.T. Hammond, Graphene multilayers as gates for multi-week sequential release of proteins from surfaces, *ACS Nano* 6 (2012) 81–88.

126. S. Castleberry, M. Wang, P.T. Hammond, Nanolayered siRNA dressing for sustained localized knockdown, *ACS Nano* 7 (2013) 5251–5261.

127. X. Zhang, A. Kovtun, C. Mendoza-Palomares, M. Oulad-Abdelghani, F. Fioretti, S. Rinckenbach, D. Mainard, M. Epple, N. Benkirane-Jessel, SiRNA-loaded multi-shell nanoparticles incorporated into a multilayered film as a reservoir for gene silencing, *Biomaterials* 31 (2010) 6013–6018.

128. N. Kinouchi, Y. Ohsawa, N. Ishimaru, H. Ohuchi, Y. Sunada, Y. Hayashi, Y. Tanimoto, K. Moriyama, S. Noji, Atelocollagen-mediated local and systemic applications of myostatin-targeting siRNA increase skeletal muscle mass, *Gene Ther.* 15 (2008) 1126–1130.

129. E. Kawakami, N. Kawai, N. Kinouchi, H. Mori, Y. Ohsawa, N. Ishimaru, Y. Sunada, S. Noji, E. Tanaka, Local applications of myostatin-siRNA with atelocollagen increase skeletal muscle mass and recovery of muscle function, *PLoS One* 8 (2013) e64719.

130. P. Lu, G.R. Zhang, X.H. Song, X.H. Zou, L.L. Wang, H.W. Ouyang, Col V siRNA engineered tenocytes for tendon tissue engineering, *PLoS One* 6 (2011) e21154.

131. J. Zoldan, A.K. Lytton-Jean, E.D. Karagiannis, K. Deiorio-Haggar, L.M. Bellan, R. Langer, D.G. Anderson, Directing human embryonic stem cell differentiation by non-viral delivery of siRNA in 3D culture, *Biomaterials* 32 (2011) 7793–7800.

132. L.X. Chen, L. Lin, H.J. Wang, X.L. Wei, X. Fu, J.Y. Zhang, C.L. Yu, Suppression of early experimental osteoarthritis by in vivo delivery of the adenoviral vector-mediated nf-kappabp65-specific siRNA, *Osteoarthr. Cartilage* 16 (2008) 174–184.

133. L.C.H. Zheng, S. Chen, T. Tang, W. Fu, L. Huang, D. Ho, K. Chow, Y. Wang, J.F. Griffith, W. He, H. Zhou, D. Zhao, G. Zhang, X. Wang, L. Qin, Blockage of Src by specific siRNA as a novel therapeutic strategy to prevent destructive repair in steroid-associated osteonecrosis in rabbits, *J. Bone Miner. Res.* 30 (2015) 2044–2057.

134. X. Chu, H. You, X. Yuan, W. Zhao, W. Li, X. Guo, Protective effect of lentivirus mediated siRNA targeting ADAMTS-5 on cartilage degradation in a rat model of osteoarthritis, *Int. J. Mol. Med.* 31 (2013) 1222–1228.

135. Y. Pi, X. Zhang, Z. Shao, F. Zhao, X. Hu, Y. Ao, Intra-articular delivery of anti-HIF-2alpha siRNA by chondrocyte-homing nanoparticles to prevent cartilage degeneration in arthritic mice, *Gene Ther.* 22 (2015) 439–448.

136. S.K. Cheema, E. Chen, L.D. Shea, A.B. Mathur, Regulation and guidance of cell behavior for tissue regeneration via the siRNA mechanism, *Wound Repair Regen.* 15 (2007) 286–295.

137. G.L. Semenza, Regulation of oxygen homeostasis by hypoxia-inducible factor 1, *Physiology* 24 (2009) 97–106.

138. H. Agis, G. Watzek, R. Gruber, Prolyl hydroxylase inhibitors increase the production of vascular endothelial growth factor by periodontal fibroblasts, *J. Periodontal Res.* 47 (2012) 165–173.

139. M. Mazzone, D. Dettori, R. Leite de Oliveira, S. Loges, T. Schmidt, B. Jonckx, Y.M. Tian, A.A. Lanahan, P. Pollard, C. Ruiz de Almodovar, F. De Smet, S. Vinckier, J. Aragones, K. Debackere, A. Luttun, S. Wyns, B. Jordan, A. Pisacane, B. Gallez, M.G. Lampugnani, E. Dejana, M. Simons, P. Ratcliffe, P. Maxwell, P. Carmeliet, Heterozygous deficiency of phd2 restores tumor oxygenation and inhibits metastasis via endothelial normalization, *Cell* 136 (2009) 839–851.

140. H. Takahashi, Y. Wang, D.W. Grainger, Device-based local delivery of siRNA against mammalian target of rapamycin (mTOR) in a murine subcutaneous implant model to inhibit fibrous encapsulation, *J. Control. Release* 147 (2010) 400–407.

141. S. Goldman, K. Zadina, T. Moritz, T. Ovitt, G. Sethi, J.G. Copeland, L. Thottapurathu, B. Krasnicka, N. Ellis, R.J. Anderson, W. Henderson, V.A.C.S. Group, Long-term patency of saphenous vein and left internal mammary artery grafts after coronary artery bypass surgery: results from a department of veterans affairs cooperative study, *J. Am. Coll. Cardiol.* 44 (2004) 2149–2156.

142. D. Palliser, D. Chowdhury, Q.Y. Wang, S.J. Lee, R.T. Bronson, D.M. Knipe, J. Lieberman, An siRNA-based microbicide protects mice from lethal herpes simplex virus 2 infection, *Nature* 439 (2006) 89–94.

143. E.Z. Khvalevsky, R. Gabai, I.H. Rachmut, E. Horwitz, Z. Brunschwig, A. Orbach, A. Shemi, T. Golan, A.J. Domb, E. Yavin, H. Giladi, L. Rivkin, A. Simerzin, R. Eliakim, A. Khalaileh, A. Hubert, M. Lahav, Y. Kopelman, E. Goldin, A. Dancour, Y. Hants, S. Arbel-Alon, R. Abramovitch, A. Shemi, E. Galun, Mutant KRAS is a druggable target for pancreatic cancer, *Proc. Natl. Acad. Sci. U. S. A.* 110 (2013) 20723–20728.

144. H.D. Han, E.M. Mora, J.W. Roh, M. Nishimura, S.J. Lee, R.L. Stone, M. Bar-Eli, G. Lopez-Berestein, A.K. Sood, Chitosan hydrogel for localized gene silencing, *Cancer Biol. Ther.* 11 (2011) 839–845.

145. N. Segovia, M. Pont, N. Oliva, V. Ramos, S. Borros, N. Artzi, Hydrogel doped with nanoparticles for local sustained release of siRNA in breast cancer, *Adv. Healthc Mater.* 4 (2015) 271–280.

146. Y. Kim, M. Park, S. Song, Injectable polyplex hydrogel for localized and long-term delivery of siRNA, *ACS Nano* 6 (2012) 5757–5766.

147. J.A. Meyerhardt, R.J. Mayer, Systemic therapy for colorectal cancer, *N. Engl. J. Med.* 352 (2005) 476–487, doi: 10.1056/NEJMra040958.

148. F. Loupakis, C. Cremolini, G. Masi, S. Lonardi, V. Zagonel, L. Salvatore, et al., Initial therapy with FOLFOXIRI and bevacizumab for metastatic colorectal cancer, *N. Engl. J. Med.* 371 (2014) 1609–1618, doi: 10.1056/NEJMoa1403108.

149. E. Van Cutsem, C.-H. K€ohne, E. Hitre, J. Zaluski, C.-R. Chang Chien, A. Makhson, et al., Cetuximab and chemotherapy as initial treatment for metastatic colorectal cancer, *N. Engl. J. Med.* 360 (2009) 1408–1417, doi: 10.1056/NEJMoa0805019.

150. J. Tol, M. Koopman, A. Cats, C.J. Rodenburg, G.J.M. Creemers, J.G. Schrama, et al., Chemotherapy, bevacizumab, and cetuximab in metastatic colorectal cancer, *N. Engl. J. Med.* 360 (2009) 563–572, doi: 10.1056/NEJMoa0808268.

151. C.H. Takimoto, S.G. Arbuck, Topoisomerase I Targeting Agents: the Camptothecins. *Cancer Chemotherapy and Biotherapy: Principles and Practice*, third ed., Lippincott Williams Wilkins, Philadelphia, 2001, pp. 579–646.

152. E. Sayari, M. Dinarvand, M. Amini, M. Azhdarzadeh, E. Mollarazi, Z. Ghasemi, et al., MUC1 aptamer conjugated to chitosan nanoparticles, an efficient targeted carrier designed for anticancer SN38 delivery, *Int. J. Pharm.* 473 (2014) 304–315, doi: 10.1016/j.ijpharm.2014.05.041.

153. C.-L. Peng, H.-M. Tsai, S.-J. Yang, T.-Y. Luo, C.-F. Lin, W.-J. Lin, et al., Development of thermosensitive poly(n-isopropylacrylamide-co-((2-dimethylamino) ethyl methacrylate))-based nanoparticles for controlled drug release, *Nanotechnology* 22 (2011) 265608, doi: 10.1088/0957-4484/22/26/265608.

154. A. Pal, S. Khan, Y.F. Wang, N. Kamath, A.K. Sarkar, A. Ahmad, et al., Preclinical safety, pharmacokinetics and antitumor efficacy profile of liposome entrapped SN-38 formulation, *Anticancer Res.* 25 (2005) 331–341.

155. P.-C. Lee, Y.-C. Chiou, J.-M. Wong, C.-L. Peng, M.-J. Shieh, Targeting colorectal cancer cells with single-walled carbon nanotubes conjugated to anticancer agent SN-38 and EGFR antibody, *Biomaterials* 34 (2013) 8756–8765, doi: 10.1016/j.biomaterials.2013.07.067.

156. Y. Matsumura, Preclinical and clinical studies of NK012, an SN-38-incorporating polymeric micelles, which is designed based on EPR effect, *Adv. Drug Deliv. Rev.* 63 (2011) 184–192, doi: 10.1016/j.addr.2010.05.008.

157. C.L. Peng, P.S. Lai, F.H. Lin, Wu S. Yueh-Hsiu, M.J. Shieh, Dual chemotherapy and photodynamic therapy in an HT-29 human colon cancer xenograft model using SN-38-loaded chlorin-core star block copolymer micelles, *Biomaterials* 30 (2009) 3614–3625, doi: 10.1016/j.biomaterials.2009.03.048.

158. N. Ferrara, K.J. Hillan, W. Novotny, Bevacizumab (Avastin), a humanized anti-VEGF monoclonal antibody for cancer therapy, *Biochem. Biophys. Res. Commun.* 333 (2005) 328–335, doi: 10.1016/j.bbrc.2005.05.132.

159. K.K. Ciombor, J. Berlin, E. Chan, Aflibercept, *Clin. Cancer Res.* 19 (2013) 1920–1925, doi: 10.1158/1078-0432.CCR-12-2911.

160. D.J. Pieramici, M.D. Rabena, Anti-VEGF therapy: comparison of current and future agents, *Eye (Lond)* 22 (2008) 1330–1336, doi: 10.1038/eye.2008.88.

161. D. Castanotto, J.J. Rossi, The promises and pitfalls of RNA-interference-based therapeutics, *Nature* 457 (2009) 426–433, doi: 10.1038/nature07758.

162. R.S. Tomar, H. Matta, P.M. Chaudhary, Use of adeno-associated viral vector for delivery of small interfering RNA, *Oncogene* 22 (2003) 5712–5715, doi: 10.1038/sj.onc.1206733.

163. D.J. Gary, H. Lee, R. Sharma, J.-S. Lee, Y. Kim, Z.Y. Cui, et al., Influence of nanocarrier architecture on in vitro siRNA delivery performance and in vivo biodistribution: polyplexes vs micelleplexes, *ACS Nano* 5 (2011) 3493–3505, doi: 10.1021/nn102540y.

164. Y. Chen, L. Huang, Tumor-targeted delivery of siRNA by non-viral vector: safe and effective cancer therapy, *Expert Opin. Drug Deliv.* 5 (2008) 1301–1311, doi: 10.1517/17425240802568505.

165. S.H. Kim, J.H. Jeong, S.H. Lee, S.W. Kim, T.G. Park, PEG conjugated VEGF siRNA for anti-angiogenic gene therapy, *J. Control. Release* 116 (2006) 123–129, doi: 10.1016/j.jconrel.2006.05.023.

166. S.-Y. Lee, C.-Y. Yang, C.-L. Peng, M.-F. Wei, K.-C. Chen, C.-J. Yao, M.-J. Shieh. A theranostic micelleplex co-delivering SN-38 and VEGF siRNA for colorectal cancer therapy. *Biomaterials* 86 (2016) 92–105.

167. M.K. Yu, J. Park, S. Jon, Targeting strategies for multifunctional nanoparticles in cancer imaging and therapy, *Theranostics* 2 (2012) 3–44, doi: 10.7150/thno.3463.

168. J.-M. Shen, F.-Y. Gao, T. Yin, H.-X. Zhang, M. Ma, Y.-J. Yang, et al., cRGD functionalized polymeric magnetic nanoparticles as a dual-drug delivery system for safe targeted cancer therapy, *Pharmacol. Res.* 70 (2013) 102–115, doi: 10.1016/j.phrs.2013.01.009.

169. O. Veiseh, J.W. Gunn, M. Zhang, Design and fabrication of magnetic nanoparticles for targeted drug delivery and imaging, *Adv. Drug Deliv. Rev.* 62 (2010) 284–304, doi: 10.1016/j.addr.2009.11.002.

170. A.A.M. Elsherbini, M. Saber, M. Aggag, A. El-Shahawy, H.A.A. Shokier, Magnetic nanoparticle-induced hyperthermia treatment under magnetic resonance imaging, *Magn. Reson Imaging* 29 (2011) 272–280, doi: 10.1016/j.mri.2010.08.010.

171. W. Choi Il, J.-Y. Kim, S.U. Heo, Y.Y. Jeong, Y.H. Kim, G. Tae, The effect of mechanical properties of iron oxide nanoparticle-loaded functional nano-carrier on tumor targeting and imaging, *J. Control. Release* 162 (2012) 267–275, doi: 10.1016/j.jconrel.2012.07.020.

172. M. Colombo, S. Carregal-Romero, M.F. Casula, L. Gut_errez, M.P. Morales, I.B. B€ohm, et al., Biological applications of magnetic nanoparticles, *Chem. Soc. Rev.* 41 (2012) 4306–4334, doi: 10.1039/c2cs15337h.

173. X. Zheng, J. Lu, L. Deng, Y. Xiong, J. Chen, Preparation and characterization of magnetic cationic liposome in gene delivery, *Int. J. Pharm.* 366 (2009) 211–217, doi: 10.1016/j.ijpharm.2008.09.019.

174. J. Zhang, X. Li, J.M. Rosenholm, H. Gu, Synthesis and characterization of pore size-tunable magnetic mesoporous silica nanoparticles, *J. Colloid Interface Sci.* 361 (2011) 16–24, doi: 10.1016/j.jcis.2011.05.038.

175. G.H. Gao, J.W. Lee, M.K. Nguyen, G.H. Im, J. Yang, H. Heo, et al., pH-responsive polymeric micelle based on PEG-poly(b-amino ester)/(amido amine) as intelligent vehicle for magnetic resonance imaging in detection of cerebral ischemic area, *J. Control. Release* 155 (2011) 11–17, doi: 10.1016/j.jconrel.2010.09.012.

176. D. Dykxhoorn, Novina C, Sharp P., Killing the messenger: short RNAs that silence gene expression, *Nat. Rev. Mol. Cell Biol.* 4 (2003) 457–467.

177. A. Fire, S.Q. Xu, M. Montgomery, S. Kostas, S. Driver, C. Mello, Potent and specific genetic interference by double-stranded RNA in Caenorhabditis elegans, *Nature* 391 (1998) 806–811.

178. B. Li, Q. Tang, D. Cheng, C. Qin, Y. Xie, Q. Wei, et al., Using siRNA in prophylactic and therapeutic regimens against SARS coronavirus in Rhesus macaque, *Nat. Med.* 11 (2005) 944–951.

179. T.S. Zimmermann, A.C.H. Lee, A. Akinc, B. Bramlage, D. Bumcrot, M.N. Fedoruk, et al., RNAi-mediated gene silencing in non-human primates, *Nature* 441 (2006) 111–114.

180. A. Akinc, A. Zumbuehl, M. Goldberg, E. Leshchiner, V. Busini, N. Hossain, et al., A combinatorial library of lipid-like materials for delivery of RNAi therapeutics, *Nat. Biotechnol.* 26 (2008) 561–569.

181. T. Merdan, J. Kopecek, T. Kissel, Prospects for cationic polymers in gene and oligonucleotide therapy against cancer, *Adv. Drug Deliv. Rev.* 54 (2002) 715–758.

182. K. Miyata, Y. Kakizawa, N. Nishiyama, Y. Yamasaki, T. Watanabe, M. Kohara, et al., Freeze-dried formulations for in vivo gene delivery of PEGylated polyplex micelles with disulfide crosslinked cores to the liver, *J. Control. Release* 109 (2005) 15–23.

183. F. Maclaughlin, R. Mumper, J. Wang, J. Tagliaferri, I. Gill, M. Hichicliffe, et al., Chitosan and depolymerized chitosan oligomers as condensing carriers for in vivo plasmid delivery, *J. Control. Release* 56 (1998) 259–272.

184. K. Wood, S. Little, R. Langer, P. Hammond, A family of hierarchically self-assembling linear-dendritic hybrid polymers for highly efficient targeted gene delivery, *Angew. Chem. Int. Ed. Engl.* 44 (2005) 6407–6408.

185. O. Boussif, F. Lezoualc'h, M. Zanta, M. Mergny, D. Scherman, B. Demeneix, et al., A versatile vector for gene and oligonucleotide transfer into cells in culture and in vivo: polyethylenimine, *Proc. Natl. Acad. Sci. U. S. A.* 92 (1995) 7297–7301.

186. M. Breunig, C. Hozsa, U. Lungwitz, K. Watanabe, I. Umeda, H. Kato, et al., Mechanistic investigation of poly(ethylene imine)-based siRNA delivery: disulfide bonds boost intracellular release of the cargo, *J. Control. Release* 130 (2008) 57–63.

187. H. Tian, C. Deng, H. Lin, J. Sun, M. Deng, X. Chen, et al., Biodegradable cationic PEG-PEI-PBLG hyperbranched block copolymer: synthesis and micelle characterization, *Biomaterials* 26 (2005) 4209–4217.

188. X. Shuai, T. Merdan, F. Unger, M. Wittmar, T. Kissel, Novel biodegradable ternary copolymers hy-PEI-g-PCL-b-PEG: synthesis, characterization, and potential as efficient nonviral gene delivery vectors, *Macromolecules* 36 (2003) 5751–5759.

189. T. Yap, C. Carden, S. Kaye, Beyond chemotherapy: targeted therapies in ovarian cancer, *Nat. Rev. Cancer* 9 (2009) 167–181.

190. V. Moebus, C. Jackisch, H. Lueck, A. Bois, C. Thomssen, C. Kurbacher, et al., Intense dose-dense sequential chemotherapy with epirubicin, paclitaxel, and cyclophosphamide compared with conventionally scheduled chemotherapy in high-risk primary breast cancer: mature results of an AGO phase III study, *J. Clin. Oncol.* 28 (2010) 2874–2880.

191. Y. Wang, S. Gao, W. Ye, H. Yoon, Y. Yang, Co-delivery of drugs and DNA from cationic core-shell nanoparticles self-assembled from a biodegradable copolymer, *Nat. Mater.* 5 (2006) 791–796.

192. C. Zhu, S. Jung, S. Luo, F. Meng, X. Zhu, T. Park, et al., Co-delivery of siRNA and paclitaxel into cancer cells by biodegradable cationic micelles based on PDMAEMA-PCL-PDMAEMA triblock copolymers, *Biomaterials* 31 (2010) 2408–2416.

193. C. Beh, W. Seow, Y. Wang, Y. Zhang, Z. Ong, P. Ee, et al., Efficient delivery of bcl-2- targeted siRNA using cationic polymer nanoparticles: downregulating mRNA expression level and sensitizing cancer cells to anticancer drug, *Biomacromolecules* 10 (2009) 41–48.

194. Z. Xu, Z. Zhang, Y. Chen, L. Chen, L. Lin, Y. Li, The characteristics and performance of a multifunctional nanoassembly system for the co-delivery of docetaxel and iSur-pDNA in a mouse hepatocellular carcinoma model, *Biomaterials* 31 (2010) 916–922.

195. M. Saad, O. Garbuzenko, T. Minko, Co-delivery of siRNA and an anticancer drug for treatment of multidrug-resistant cancer, *Nanomedicine* 3 (2008) 761–776.

196. H. Meng, M. Liong, T. Xia, Z. Li, Z. Ji, J. Zink, et al., Engineered design of mesoporous silica nanoparticles to deliver doxorubicin and P-glycoprotein siRNA to overcome drug resistance in a cancer cell line, *ACS Nano* 4 (2010) 4539–4550.

197. A. Chen, M. Zhang, D. Wei, D. Stueber, O. Taratula, T. Minko, et al., Co-delivery of doxorubicin and bcl-2 siRNA by mesoporous silica nanoparticles enhances the efficacy of chemotherapy in multidrug-resistant cancer cells, *Small* 5 (2009) 2673–2677.

198. L.Y. Qiu, Y.H. Bae, Self-assembled polyethylenimine-graft-poly(e-caprolactone) micelles as potential dual carriers of genes and anticancer drugs, *Biomaterials* 28 (2007) 4132–4142.

199. Y. Liu, T. Steele, T. Kissel, Degradation of hyper-branched poly(ethylenimine)-graft poly(caprolactone)-block-monomethoxy-poly(ethylene glycol) as a potential gene delivery vector, *Macromol. Rapid Commun.* 31 (2010) 1509–1515.

200. F. Igney, P. Krammer, Death and anti-death: tumour resistance to apoptosis, *Nat. Rev. Cancer* 2 (2002) 277–288.

201. R. Lima, L. Martins, J. Guimarães, C. Sambade, M. Vasconcelos, Specific downregulation of bcl-2 and xIAP by RNAi enhances the effects of chemotherapeutic agents in MCF-7 human breast cancer cells, *Cancer Gene Ther.* 11 (2004) 309–316.

202. X. Lei, M. Zhong, L. Feng, B. Zhu, S. Tang, D. Liao, siRNA-mediated bcl-2 and bcl-xl gene silencing sensitizes human hepatoblastoma cells to chemotherapeutic drugs, *Clin. Exp. Pharmacol. Physiol.* 34 (2007) 450–456.

203. R. Pakunlu, Y. Wang, W. Tsao, V. Pozharov, T. Cook, T. Minko, Enhancement of the efficacy of chemotherapy for lung cancer by simultaneous suppression of multidrug resistance and antiapoptotic cellular defense: novel multicomponent delivery system, *Cancer Res.* 64 (2004) 6214–6224.

204. B.A.J. Sudimach, R.J. Lee, Targeted drug delivery via the folate receptor, *Adv. Drug. Deliv. Rev.* 41 (2000) 147–162.

205. P. Low, W. Henne, D. Doorneweerd, Discovery and development of folic-acid based receptor targeting for imaging and therapy of cancer and inflammatory diseases, *Acc. Chem. Res.* 41 (2008) 120–129.

206. N. Cao, D. Cheng, S. Zou, H. Ai, J. Gao, X. Shuai, The synergistic effect of hierarchical assemblies of siRNA and chemotherapeutic drugs co-delivered into hepatic cancer cells, *Biomaterials* 32 (2011) 2222–2232.

207. D. Fischer, Y. Li, B. Ahlemeyer, J. Krieglstein, T. Kissel, In vitro cytotoxicity testing of polycations: influence of polymer structure on cell viability and hemolysis, *Biomaterials* 24 (2003) 1121–1131.

208. M. Neu, D. Fischer, T. Kissel, Recent advances in rational gene transfer vector design based on poly(ethylene imine) and its derivatives, *J. Gene Med.* 7 (2005) 992–1009.

209. S.J. O'Day, C.J. Kim, D.S. Reintgen, Metastatic melanoma: chemotherapy to biochemotherapy, *Cancer Control* 9 (2002) 31–38.

210. B. Geusens, J. Lambert, S.C. De Smedt, K. Buyens, N.N. Sanders, M. Van Gele, Ultradeformable cationic liposomes for delivery of small interfering RNA (siRNA) into human primary melanocytes, *J. Control. Release* 133 (2009) 214–220.

211. A. Kim, E.H. Lee, S.H. Choi, C.K. Kim, In vitro and in vivo transfection efficiency of a novel ultradeformable cationic liposome, *Biomaterials* 25 (2004) 305–313.

212. E. McLafferty, C. Hendry, F. Alistair, The integumentary system: anatomy, physiology and function of skin, *Nurs. Stand.* 27 (2012) 35–42.

213. Y. Itoh, A. Shimazu, Y. Sadzuka, T. Sonobe, S. Itai, Novel method for stratum corneum pore size determination using positron annihilation lifetime spectroscopy, *Int. J. Pharm.* 358 (2008) 91–95.

214. B. Geusens, M. Van Gele, S. Braat, S.C. De Smedt, M.C.A. Stuart, T.W. Prow, W. Sanchez, M.S. Roberts, N.N. Sanders, J. Lambert, Flexible nanosomes (SECosomes) enable efficient siRNA delivery in cultured primary skin cells and in the viable epidermis of ex vivo human skin, *Adv. Funct. Mater.* 20 (2010) 4077–4090.

215. M. Dorrani, O.B. Garbuzenko, T. Minko, B. Michniak-Kohn. Development of edge-activated liposomes for siRNA delivery to human basal epidermis for melanoma therapy. *J. Control. Release* 228 (2016) 150–158.

216. S. Jang, M.B. Atkins, Treatment of BRAF-mutant melanoma: the role of vemurafenib and other therapies, *Clin. Pharmacol. Ther.* 95 (2014) 24–31.

217. T. Huang, J. Zhuge, W.W. Zhang, Sensitive detection of BRAF V600E mutation by amplification refractory mutation system (ARMS)-PCR, *Biomark. Res.* 1 (2013) 3.

218. Loutfy H. Madkour, *Reactive Oxygen Species (ROS), Nanoparticles, and Endoplasmic Reticulum (ER) Stress-Induced Cell Death Mechanisms.* Paperback ISBN: 9780128224816. Imprint: Academic Press Published Date: 1st August 2020. https://www.elsevier.com/books/

reactive-oxygen-species-ros-nanoparticles-and-endoplas-mic-reticulum-er-stress-induced-cell-death-mechanisms/madkour/978-0-12-822481-6.

219. Loutfy H. Madkour, *Nanoparticles Induce Oxidative and Endoplasmic Reticulum Antioxidant Therapeutic Defenses*. Copyright 2020 Publisher Springer International Publishing. Copyright Holder Springer Nature Switzerland AG eBook ISBN 978-3-030-37297-2 DOI 10.1007/978-3-030-37297-2 Hardcover ISBN 978-3-030-37296-5 Series ISSN 2194–0452 Edition Number 1. https://www.springer.com/gp/book/9783030372965?utm_campaign=3_pier05_buy_print&utm_content=en_08082017&utm_medium=referral&utm_source=google_books#otherversion=9783030372972.

220. Loutfy H. Madkour, *Nucleic Acids as Gene Anticancer Drug Delivery Therapy*. 1st Edition. Publishing house: Elsevier, (2020). Paperback ISBN: 9780128197776 Imprint: Academic Press Published Date: 2nd January 2020 Imprint: Academic Press Copyright: Paperback ISBN: 9780128197776 © Academic Press 2020 Published: 2nd January 2020 Imprint: Academic Press Paperback ISBN: 9780128197776. https://www.elsevier.com/books/nucleic-acids-as-gene-anticancer-drug-deliverytherapy/madkour/978-0-12-819777-6.

221. Loutfy H. Madkour, *Nanoelectronic Materials: Fundamentals and Applications (Advanced Structured Materials)* 1st ed. 2019 Edition: https://link.springer.com/book/10.1007%2F978-3-030-21621-4 Series Title Advanced Structured Materials Series Volume 116 Copyright 2019 Publisher Springer International Publishing Copyright Holder Springer Nature Switzerland AG. eBook ISBN 978-3-030-21621-4 DOI 10.1007/978-3-030-21621-4 Hardcover ISBN 978-3-030-21620-7 Series ISSN 1869-8433 Edition Number 1 Number of Pages XLIII, 783 Number of Illustrations 122 b/w illustrations, 494 illustrations in colour Topics. ISBN-10: 3030216209 ISBN-13: 978-3030216207 #117 in Nanotechnology (Books) #725 in Materials Science (Books) #187336 in Textbooks. https://books.google.com.eg/books/about/Nanoelectronic_Materials.html?id=YQXCxAEACAAJ&source=kp_book_description&redir_esc=y; https://www.springer.com/gp/book/9783030216207.

222. M. Dorrani, M. Kaul, A. Parhi, E.J. LaVoie, D.S. Pilch, B. Michniak-Kohn, TXA497 as a topical antibacterial agent: comparative antistaphylococcal, skin deposition, and skin permeation studies with mupirocin, *Int. J. Pharm.* 476 (2014) 199–204.

223. E.H. Lee, A. Kim, Y.K. Oh, C.K. Kim, Effect of edge activators on the formation and transfection efficiency of ultra-deformable liposomes, *Biomaterials* 26 (2005) 205–210.

224. S. Senapati, A.K. Mahanta, S. Kumar, P. Maiti, Controlled drug delivery vehicles for cancer treatment and their performance, *Signal Transduct. Target. Ther.* 3 (2018) 1–19, doi: 10.1038/s41392-017-0004-3.

225. S. Rasouli, S. Davaran, F. Rasouli, M. Mahkam, R. Salehi, Synthesis, characterization and pH-controllable methotrexate release from biocompatible polymer/silica nanocomposite for anticancer drug delivery, *Drug Deliv.* 21 (2014) 155–163.

226. D. Liu, F. Yang, F. Xiong, N. Gu, The smart drug delivery system and its clinical potential, *Theranostics* 6 (2016) 1306–1323.

227. M. Saboktakin, A. Maharramov, M. Ramazanov, pH sensitive chitosan-based supramolecular gel for oral drug delivery of insulin, *J. Mol. Genet. Med.* 9 (2015) 170.

228. T. Wang, G. Sun, M. Wang, B. Zhou, J. Fu, Voltage/pH-driven mechanized silica nanoparticles for the multimodal controlled release of drugs, *ACS Appl. Mater. Interfaces* 7 (2015) , 21295–21304.

229. Q.-L. Li, et al., pH and glutathione dual-responsive dynamic cross-linked supramolecular network on mesoporous silica nanoparticles for controlled anticancer drug release, *ACS Appl. Mater. Interfaces* 7 (2015) 28656–28664.

230. S.S. Sadhu, et al., In vitro and in vivo antimetastatic effect of glutathione disulfide liposomes, *Cancer Growth Metastas.* 10 (2017) 117906441769525.

231. K. Kono, et al., Highly temperature-sensitive liposomes based on a thermosensitive block copolymer for tumor-specific chemotherapy, *Biomaterials* 31 (2010) 7096–7105.

232. B.V.K.J. Schmidt, M. Hetzer, H. Ritter, C. Barner-Kowollik, UV Light and temperature responsive supramolecular ABA triblock copolymers via reversible cyclodextrin complexation, *Macromolecules* 46 (2013) 1054–1065.

233. P. Moitra, K. Kumar, P. Kondaiah, S. Bhattacharya, Efficacious anticancer drug delivery mediated by a pH-sensitive self-assembly of a conserved tripeptide derived from tyrosine kinase NGF receptor, *Angew. Chem. Int. Ed. Engl.* 53 (2014) 1113–1117.

234. H. Xing, et al., Multimodal detection of a small molecule target using stimuli responsive liposome triggered by aptamer–enzyme conjugate, *Anal. Chem.* 88 (2016) 1506–1510.

235. S. Panja, S. Maji, T.K. Maiti, S. Chattopadhyay, A smart magnetically active nanovehicle for on-demand targeted drug delivery: where van der Waals force balances the magnetic interaction, *ACS Appl. Mater. Interfaces* 7 (2015) 24229–24241.

236. M. Mansouri, M.H. Nazarpak, A. Solouk, S. Akbari, M.M. Hasani-Sadrabadi, Magnetic responsive of paclitaxel delivery system based on SPION and palmitoyl chitosan, *J. Magn. Magn. Mater.* 421 (2017) 316–325.

237. S.D. Kong, et al. Magnetically vectored nanocapsules for tumor penetration and remotely switchable on-demand drug release, *Nano. Lett.* 10 (2010) 5088–5092.

238. S. Rana, A. Gallo, R.S. Srivastava, R.D.K. Misra, On the suitability of nanocrystalline ferrites as a magnetic carrier for drug delivery: functionalization, conjugation and drug release kinetics. *Acta Biomater.* 3 (2007) 233–242.

239. D.G. Anderson, Materials science: smart biomaterials, *Science* 305 (2004) 1923–1924.

240. M.A.C. Stuart, et al., Emerging applications of stimuli-responsive polymer materials, *Nat. Mater.* 9 (2010) 101–113.

241. X. Guo, F.C. Szoka, Chemical approaches to triggerable lipid vesicles for drug and gene delivery, *Acc. Chem. Res.* 36 (2003) 335–341.

242. D.A. LaVan, T. McGuire, R. Langer, Small-scale systems for in vivo drug delivery, *Nat. Biotechnol.* 21 (2003) 1184–1191.

243. A.C.R. Grayson, et al., Multi-pulse drug delivery from a resorbable polymeric microchip device. *Nat. Mater.* 2 (2003) 767–772.

244. M.S. Yavuz, et al., Gold nanocages covered by smart polymers for controlled release with near-infrared light, *Nat. Mater.* 8 (2009) 935–939.

245. S.-W. Choi, Y. Zhang, Y. Xia, A temperature-sensitive drug release system based on phase-change materials, *Angew. Chem. Int. Ed. Engl.* 49 (2010) 7904–7908.

246. E.R. Gillies, T.B. Jonsson, J.M.J. Fréchet, Stimuli-responsive supramolecular assemblies of linear-dendritic copolymers, *J. Am. Chem. Soc.* 126 (2004) 11936–11943.

247. K.T. Kim, J.J.L.M. Cornelissen, R.J.M. Nolte, J.C.M. van Hest, A Polymersome nanoreactor with controllable permeability induced by stimuli-responsive block copolymers, *Adv. Mater.* 21 (2009) 2787–2791.

248. M.A. Kasyutich, O. Cornelissen, J.J.L.M., Nolte, R.J.M. Self-assembly and optically triggered disassembly of hierarchical dendron–virus complexes, *Nat. Chem.* 2 (2010) 394–399.

249. T. Dvir, M.R. Banghart, B.P. Timko, R. Langer, D.S. Kohane, Photo-targeted nanoparticles. *Nano. Lett.* 10 (2010) 250–254.

250. M.A. Azagarsamy, P. Sokkalingam, S. Thayumanavan, Enzyme-triggered disassembly of dendrimer-based amphiphilic nanocontainers. *J. Am. Chem. Soc.* 131 (2009) 14184–14185.

251. P.D. Thornton, A. Heise, Highly specific dual enzyme-mediated payload release from peptide-coated silica particles, *J. Am. Chem. Soc.* 132 (2010) 2024–2028.

252. Y. Namiki, et al., A novel magnetic crystal–lipid nanostructure for magnetically guided in vivo gene delivery, *Nat. Nanotechnol.* 4 (2009) 598–606.

253. P. Dames, et al., Targeted delivery of magnetic aerosol droplets to the lung, *Nat. Nanotechnol.* 2 (2007) 495–499.

254. J. Ge, E. Neofytou, T.J. Cahill, R.E. Beygui, R.N. Zare, Drug release from electric-field-responsive nanoparticles, *ACS Nano* 6 (2012) 227–233.

255. C.L. Weaver, J.M. LaRosa, X. Luo, X.T. Cui, Electrically controlled drug delivery from graphene oxide nanocomposite films. *ACS Nano* 8 (2014) 1834–1843.

256. X. Luo, C. Matranga, S. Tan, N. Alba, X.T. Cui, Carbon nanotube nanoreservior for controlled release of anti-inflammatory dexamethasone, *Biomaterials* 32 (2011) 6316–6323.

257. R. Wadhwa, C.F. Lagenaur, X.T. Cui, Electrochemically controlled release of dexamethasone from conducting polymer polypyrrole coated electrode, *J. Control. Release* 110 (2006) 531–541.

258. P.R. Chandran, N. Sandhyarani, An electric field responsive drug delivery system based on chitosan–gold nanocomposites for site specific and controlled delivery of 5-fluorouracil, *RSC Adv.* 4 (2014) 44922–44929.

259. W. Yin, et al., High-throughput synthesis of single-layer MoS2 nanosheets as a near-infrared photothermal-triggered drug delivery for effective cancer therapy, *ACS Nano* 8, 6922–6933 (2014).

260. T.H. Tran, et al., Development of a graphene oxide nanocarrier for dual-drug chemo-phototherapy to overcome drug resistance in cancer. *ACS Appl. Mater. Interfaces* 7 (2015) 28647–28655.

261. L.L. Fedoryshin, A.J. Tavares, E. Petryayeva, S. Doughan, U.J. Krull, Near-infrared-triggered anticancer drug release from upconverting nanoparticles. *ACS Appl. Mater. Interfaces* 6 (2014) 13600–13606.

262. Y. Cheng, et al., Thermally controlled release of anticancer drug from self-assembled γ-substituted amphiphilic poly(ε-caprolactone) micellar nanoparticles, *Biomacromolecules* 13 (2012) 2163–2173.

263. X. Song, et al., Thermoresponsive delivery of paclitaxel by β-cyclodextrin-based poly(N-isopropylacrylamide) star polymer via inclusion complexation, *Biomacromolecules* 17 (2016) 3957–3963.

264. L. Meng, et al., Chitosan-based nanocarriers with pH and light dual response for anticancer drug delivery, Biomacromolecules 14, 2601–2610 (2013).

265. M. Teymouri, M. Mashreghi, E. Saburi, A. Hejazi, A.R. Nikpoor, The trip of a drug inside the body: From a lipid-based nanocarrier to a target cell, *J. Control. Release* 309 (2019) 59–71.

266. T.M. Allen, P.R. Cullis, Drug delivery systems: entering the mainstream, *Science* 303 (2004) 1818–1822.

267. T. Harner, D. Mackay, Measurement of octanol-air partition coefficients for chlorobenzenes, PCBs, and DDT, *Environ. Sci. Technol.* 29 (1995) 1599–1606.

268. V. Torchilin, Liposomes in drug delivery, in: *Fundamentals and Applications of Controlled Release Drug Delivery*, Springer, 2012, pp. 289–328.

269. A. Akbarzadeh, R. Rezaei-Sadabady, S. Davaran, S.W. Joo, N. Zarghami, Y. Hanifehpour, M. Samiei, M. Kouhi, K. Nejati-Koshki, Liposome: classification, preparation, and applications, *Nanoscale Res. Lett.* 8 (2013) 102.

270. S.D. Li, L. Huang, Nanoparticles evading the reticuloendothelial system: role of the supported bilayer, *Biochim. Biophys. Acta* 1788 (2009) 2259–2266.

271. S. Kulkarni, G. Betageri, M. Singh, Factors affecting microencapsulation of drugs in liposomes, *J. Microencapsul.* 12 (1995) 229–246.

272. J. Chen, W.-L. Lu, W. Gu, S.-S. Lu, Z.-P. Chen, B.-C. Cai, X.-X. Yang, Drug-in-cyclodextrin- in-liposomes: a promising delivery system for hydrophobic drugs, *Expert Opin. Drug Deliv.* 11 (2014) 565–577.

273. N.R. Desai, E.C. Shinal, M. Ganesan, E.A. Carpentier, Emulsion Compositions for Administration of Sparingly Water Soluble Ionizable Hydrophobic Drugs, in, Google Patents (1989).

274. K. Kataoka, A. Harada, Y. Nagasaki, Block copolymer micelles for drug delivery: design, characterization and biological significance, *Adv. Drug Deliv. Rev.* 47 (2001) 113–131.

275. J. Szebeni, P. Bedőcs, Z. Rozsnyay, Z. Weiszhár, R. Urbanics, L. Rosivall, R. Cohen, O. Garbuzenko, G. Báthori, M. Tóth, Liposome-induced complement activation and related cardiopulmonary distress in pigs: factors promoting reactogenicity of Doxil and AmBisome, *Nanomedicine* 8 (2012) 176–184.

276. M. Teymouri, H. Farzaneh, A. Badiee, S. Golmohammadzadeh, K. Sadri, M.R. Jaafari, Investigation of Hexadecylphosphocholine (miltefosine) usage in PEGylated liposomal doxorubicin as a synergistic ingredient: in vitro and in vivo evaluation in mice bearing C26 colon carcinoma and B16F0 melanoma, *Eur. J. Pharm. Sci.* 80 (2015) 66–73.

277. V.P. Torchilin, F. Zhou, L. Huang, pH-sensitive liposomes, *J. Liposome Res.* 3 (1993) 201–255.

278. T. Terada, M. Iwai, S. Kawakami, F. Yamashita, M. Hashida, Novel PEG-matrix metalloproteinase-2 cleavable peptide-lipid containing galactosylated liposomes for hepatocellular carcinoma-selective targeting, *J. Control. Release* 111 (2006) 333–342.

279. J. Akhtari, S.M. Rezayat, M. Teymouri, S.H. Alavizadeh, F. Gheybi, A. Badiee, M.R. Jaafari, Targeting, bio distributive and tumor growth inhibiting characterization of anti-HER2 affibody coupling to liposomal doxorubicin using BALB/c mice bearing TUBO tumors, *Int. J. Pharm.* 505 (2016) 89–95.

280. O. Trédan, C.M. Galmarini, K. Patel, I.F. Tannock, Drug resistance and the solid tumor microenvironment, *J. Natl. Cancer Inst.* 99 (2007) 1441–1454.

281. R.B. Hamanaka, N.S. Chandel, Targeting glucose metabolism for cancer therapy, *J. Exp. Med.* 209 (2012) 211–215.

282. X. Duan, X. Yang, C. Li, L. Song, Highly water-soluble methotrexate-Polyethyleneglycol-rhodamine prodrug micelle for high tumor inhibition activity, *AAPS PharmSciTech* 20 (2019) 245.

283. G.A. Gonzalez-Conchas, L. Rodriguez-Romo, D. Hernandez-Barajas, J.F. Gonzalez- Guerrero, I.A. Rodriguez-Fernandez, A. Verdines-Perez, A.J. Templeton, A. Ocana, B. Seruga, I.F. Tannock, E. Amir, F.E. Vera-Badillo, Epidermal growth factor receptor overexpression and outcomes in early breast cancer: a systematic review and a meta-analysis, *Cancer Treat. Rev.* 62 (2018) 1–8.

284. P. Mi, et al., Hybrid calcium phosphate-polymeric micelles incorporating gadolinium chelates for imaging-guided gadolinium neutron capture tumor therapy, *ACS Nano* 9 (2015) 5913–5921.

285. P. Mi, et al., Block copolymer-boron cluster conjugate for effective boron neutron capture therapy of solid tumors, *J. Control. Release* 254 (2017) 1–9.

14 Targeted Systemic Combinatorial Delivery of siRNA Polyplexes– Functional Quantum Dot-siRNA Nanoplexes

14.1 TARGETED SYSTEMIC DELIVERY OF siRNA TO CERVICAL CANCER MODEL

For systemic delivery of small interfering RNA (siRNA) to solid tumors, it has been developed an actively targeted unimer polyion complex-assembled gold nanoparticle (uPIC-AuNP) [1] by a two-step assembling process. First is the monodispersed uPIC formation from the single molecules of therapeutic siRNA and the block catiomer, cyclic RGD (cRGD) peptide-installed poly(ethylene glycol)-block-poly(L-lysine) modified with lipoic acid (LA) at the ω-end (cRGD-PEG-PLL-LA). Second is the surface decoration of a 20-nm-sized AuNP with uPICs. The cRGD-installed uPIC-AuNPs (cRGD-uPIC-AuNP) provided the targetability for selective binding to the cancer and cancer-related endothelial cellular surface, while regulating their size b50 nm with a quite narrow distribution. The targeting efficacy of the cRGD-uPIC-AuNP was confirmed by *in vitro* cellular uptake in cultured cervical cancer (HeLa) cells and *in vivo* tumor accumulation in a subcutaneous HeLa model after systemic administration, compared with a non-targeted control uPIC-AuNP. Due to the targetability of the ligand, the cRGD-uPIC-AuNP achieved the significantly enhanced gene silencing ability in the subcutaneous HeLa tumor. Ultimately, the systemic delivery of siRNA targeted for papilloma virus-derived E6 oncogene by cRGD-uPIC-AuNP significantly inhibited the growth of subcutaneous HeLa tumor.

The siRNA has attracted much attention as a potential therapeutic agent for cancer because it can elicit the sequence-specific degradation of messenger RNAs (mRNAs) coding cancer-related proteins in mammalian cells [2–4]. So far, a variety of siRNA delivery vehicles, including polymers [5–8], lipids [9–11], and inorganic nanoparticles [12–17], have been developed for systemic siRNA delivery to solid tumors. Nevertheless, the poor bioavailability of siRNA, which is mainly due to the rapid enzymatic degradation and renal clearance after systemic administration, still remains to be major issues in the drug delivery field [18].

PEGylated nanoparticles have demonstrated the strong potential for cancer-targeted drug delivery. They can passively accumulate in solid tumors through the leaky tumor vasculature as well as immature lymphatic drainage [19–21]. In this regard, several recent studies reported that sub-50 nm nanoparticles could deeply penetrate even in thick fibrotic tumor models and metastatic tumor models [22–24]. These findings motivated us to precisely construct an siRNA-loaded sub-50 nm nanoparticle for efficient accumulation and penetration in a wide variety of solid tumors. To this end, it has been challenged a bottom-up approach using monodispersed building blocks, highlighting a unimer polyion complex (uPIC), which can be selectively prepared from the single molecules of siRNA and PEG-block-poly(L-lysine) (PEG-PLL) through their charge-matched ion-pairing as well as the steric repulsive effect of PEG [25–27]. The siRNA-loaded uPICs were further assembled onto monodispersed gold nanoparticles (AuNPs) with a size of 20 nm for fabrication of sub-50 nm-sized nanocarriers with a quite narrow size distribution [26]. The obtained nanocarrier, uPIC-AuNP, showed the prolonged blood circulation and enhanced accumulation in a subcutaneous cervical cancer model, demonstrating the platform utility for further development toward cancer targeting.

In this chapter, we describe various strategies that have been developed for ligand-siRNA therapeutics to increase their selectivity toward tumors (Scheme 14.1). "Decorating" the NP with the ligand together with PEG shell, however, does not adequately describe how ligand molecules may affect stability of the core particle. As investigators have reported, ligand molecules and their specific linkages to the NP may significantly influence release of siRNA and their efficacy

Another important criterion in targeted drug delivery is the active mechanism based on ligand-receptor interaction. Cancer-targeting ligand-installed nanocarriers permit their preferable binding to cancer and cancer-related cellular surface in tumor tissues [28–31]. Thus, the present study aimed to newly develop a ligand-installed uPIC-AuNP for enhanced targetability to solid tumors. To construct the active targeting formulation, a cyclic Arg-Gly-Asp (cRGD) peptide ligand was installed at the PEG terminus in PEG-PLL, as shown in Figure 14.1 [1].

DOI: 10.1201/9781003229674-14

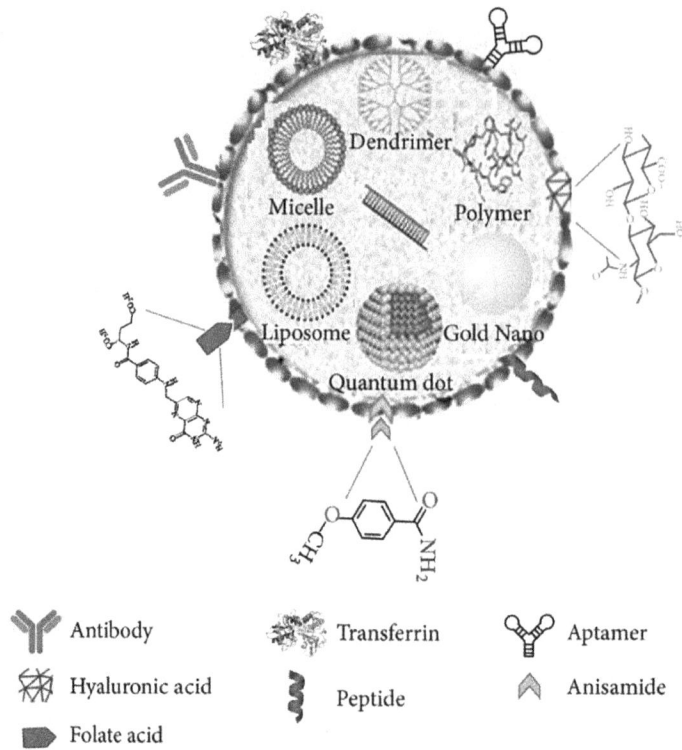

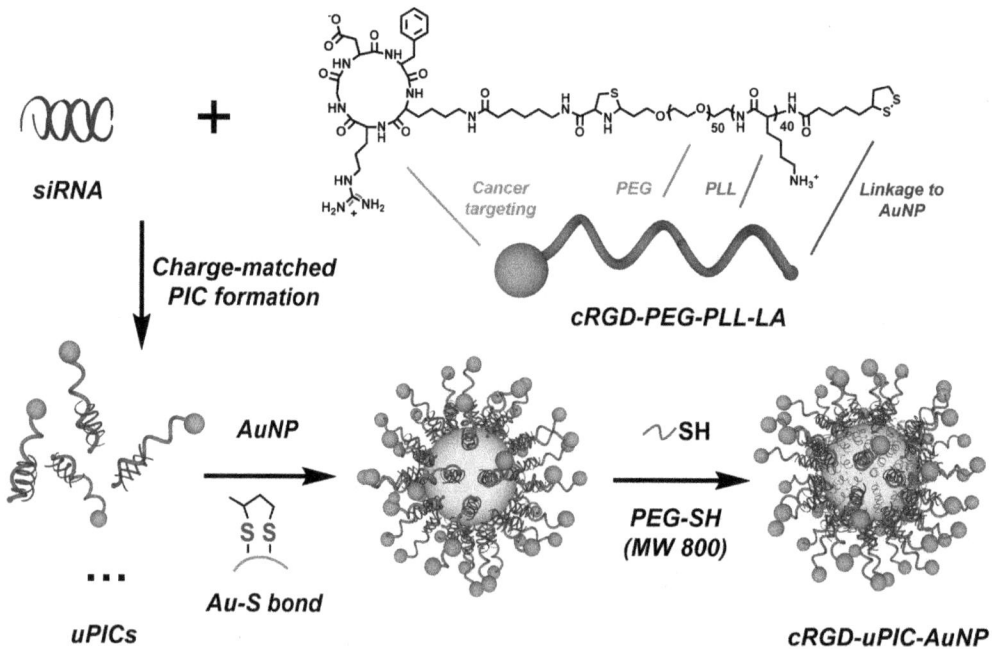

FIGURE 14.1 Schematic illustration of cRGD-uPIC-AuNP preparation. First, the monodispersed cRGD-installed uPICs were formed by a single pair of siRNA and cRGD-PEG-PLL modified with lipoic acid (LA) at the ω-end (cRGD-PEG-PLL-LA), where cRGD and LA moieties were utilized for cancer targeting and AuNP conjugation, respectively. Second, the uPICs were conjugated onto a 20 nm AuNP core through double Au–S bonds, followed by grafting of short PEG for construction of monodispersed 40-nm-sized cRGD-uPIC-AuNP.

The cRGD peptide is able to specifically bind to $\alpha_v\beta_3/\alpha_v\beta_5$ integrins, which are overexpressed on various cancer cell and tumoral endothelial cell surface [32], thereby successfully used for cancer-targeted drug delivery [33–35]. To estimate

the potential of targeted uPIC-AuNP for human cervical cancer treatment, E6 oncogene derived from human papilloma virus (HPV) was selected as a silencing target, because E6 protein is known to inactivate a tumor suppressor protein, p53, and is a cause of >70% of cervical cancer patients [36]. Thus, the silencing of E6 oncogene is a promising strategy for human cervical cancer therapy with minimal adverse side effects to normal organs [37]. Herein, it has been validated the targeting efficacy of cRGD peptide-installed uPIC-AuNPs (cRGD-uPIC-AuNPs) in terms of cellular uptake and tumor accumulation, demonstrating the significant E6 oncogene silencing and antitumor activity in cervical cancer models via intravenous administration. This section demonstrates that the bottom-up construction of nanocarriers using monodispersed building blocks can be employed as delivery platforms for RNA interference-based cancer therapy [1].

14.1.1 PREPARATION AND PHYSICOCHEMICAL CHARACTERIZATIONS OF TARGETED uPIC-AuNP

Monodispersed cRGD-uPIC-AuNP was prepared by a two-step procedure, i.e., uPIC formation and uPIC conjugation with AuNP. First, varying concentrations of the block copolymers were mixed with siRNA in 10 mM HEPES buffer (pH 7.2) to evaluate the effect of mixing ratios on their PIC formation. The PIC formation was evaluated by FCS in terms of the change in diffusion coefficient of Alexa647-siRNA. The diffusion coefficient of Alexa647-siRNA progressively decreased with an increase in [polymer]/[siRNA] from 0 to 1 and leveled off at [polymer]/[siRNA] = 1 [1], indicating that siRNA was bound to cRGD-PEGPLL-LA at [polymer]/[siRNA] b 1 and the binding was saturated at [polymer]/[siRNA] = 1. Thus, the complex solution prepared at [polymer]/[siRNA] = 1 was further analyzed by AUC to determine the MW of siRNA/cRGD-PEG-PLL-LA complexes [1]. The obtained MW (23.1 kDa) is apparently comparable to the sum of MWs of siRNA (13.3 kDa) and cRGD-PEG-PLL-LA (8.5 kDa), demonstrating the selective formation of uPIC. Of note, MeO-PEG-PLL-LA without cRGD peptide was also confirmed to form the uPIC with a single molecule of siRNA, as previously reported [26], Table S1.

Second, the uPIC prepared at [polymer]/[siRNA] =1 was conjugated on the AuNP with a diameter of 20 nm through double Au–S bonds. The capping amount of uPIC per AuNP was estimated by the fluorescence-based quantification using Alexa647-siRNA and divided by the

concentration of AuNPs [12]. Regardless of MeO and cRGD, the capping amount increased progressively with the increase in the feeding molar ratio of uPIC to AuNP ([uPIC]/[AuNP]) and leveled off at [uPIC]/[AuNP] = 1000:1 [1], allowing the maximum capping amount of approximately 100. Thus, the siRNA density on AuNP surface was calculated to be 0.09 siRNA/nm^2 from diving the amount of uPICs by the surface area of 18 nm AuNP, which is comparable to that of 0.06 siRNA/nm^2 reported for siRNA-conjugated AuNPs (33 siRNA/13 nm AuNP) [12]. Considering both the high capping amount of uPICs and the economical uses of polymer and siRNA, we selected the uPIC-AuNP prepared at [uPIC]/[AuNP] = 500:1, i.e., the capping amount of uPIC = ~90, for all the following experiments. Of note, the capping amount derived from MeO-PEG-PLL-LA was significantly higher than that of the previous formulation prepared from MeO-PEG-PLL with a single thiol moiety at ω-end (MeO-PEG-PLL-SH, capping number of uPIC = ~20 [26]) [1], presumably due to higher affinity of LA moiety to AuNP. Evidences have demonstrated that higher PEG density on AuNP results in lower serum protein adsorption [38] and longer blood circulation property [39,40]. Thus, short PEG chains with MW 800 were further grafted onto the uPIC-AuNP to improve the coverage of PEG [41–43]. An excess amount of PEG-SH was added to saturate the uncovered AuNP surface, and the conjugation amount of PEG-SH was determined to be approximately 2300 per AuNP using Ellman's assay [38]. The resulting uPIC-AuNPs exhibited more neutral zeta-potential without obvious changes in size, PDI, and uPIC capping amount, compared with the precursor without PEG-SH conjugation [1].

The successful construction of uPIC-AuNP (decorated with the short PEG-SH) was further verified by UV–Vis spectroscopy, DLS, and TEM (Figure 14.2 and Table 14.1). In the UV–Vis absorbance spectra, red shifts from 520 nm to 528 nm were observed for MeO- and cRGDuPIC-AuNPs (Figure 14.2a), indicating the change in SPR of AuNPs due to the conjugation of uPICs without aggregate formation. The hydrodynamic diameter increased from 20 nm for bare AuNPs to approximately 40 nm for MeO-, cRAD-, and cRGD-uPIC-AuNPs with narrow size distributions (PDI in DLS b 0.13, Figure 14.2 b and Table 14.1).

TABLE 14.1
Physicochemical Properties of Bare AuNPs and MeO/cRAD/cRGD-uPIC-AuNPs

Sample	Hydrodynamic Diameter (nm)[a]	PDI	Zeta-Potential (mV)[b]	siRNA Capping Amount	Grafted PEG amount[c]
Bare AuNP	20	0.02	−30.4±1.0	0	0
MeO	40	0.07	−11.3±1.2	90±4	2322±322
cRAD	42	0.12	−11.9±0.9	88±5	2284±303
cRGD	42	0.10	−11.6±1.1	92±4	2334±178

[a] The hydrodynamic diameter was determined by DLS.
[b] The zeta-potential was measured in the 10 mM HEPES buffer (pH 7.2) without NaCl.
[c] The grafted amount of short PEG chains was determined using Ellman's reagent.

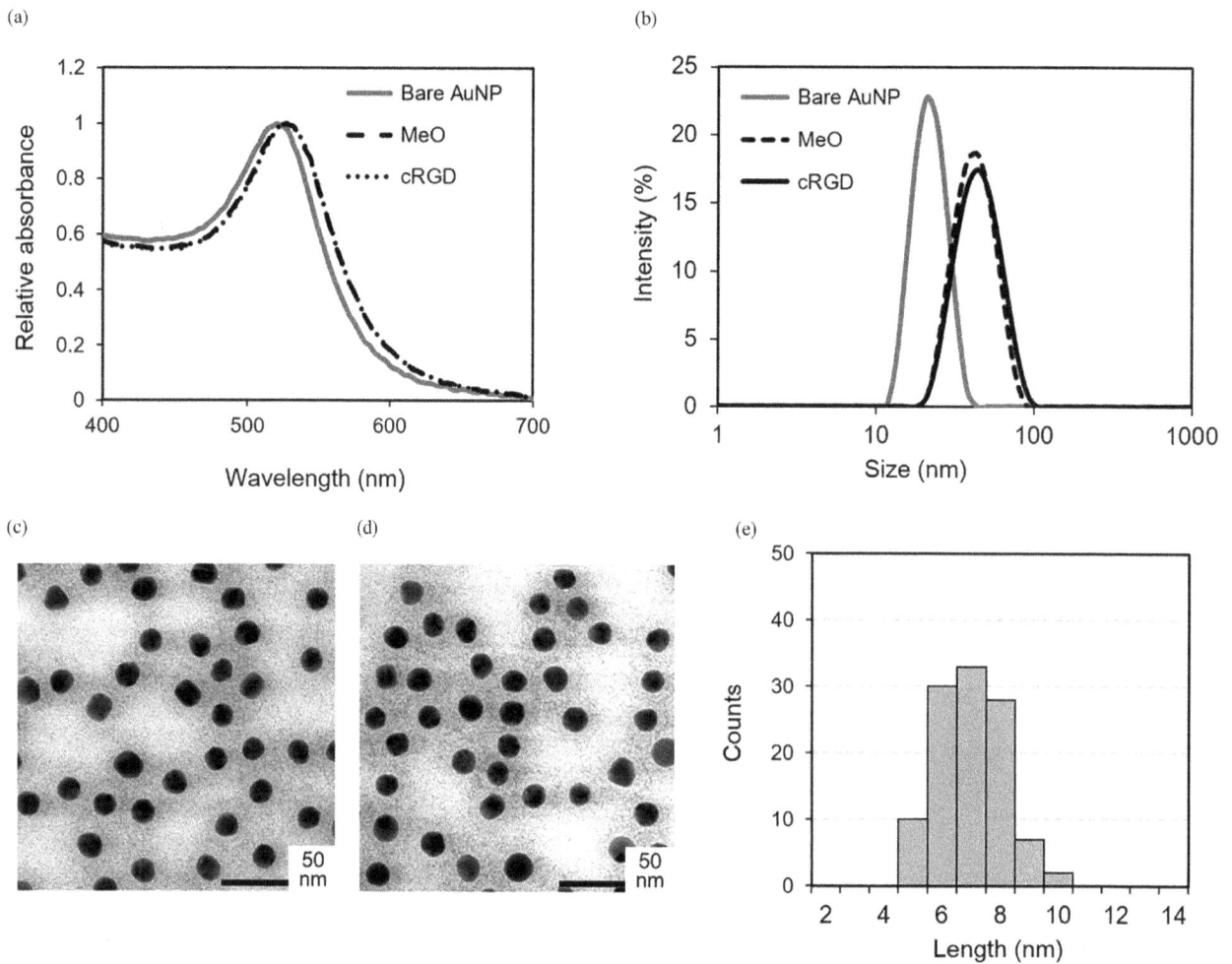

FIGURE 14.2 (a) UV–Vis absorbance of bare AuNPs and MeO/cRGD-uPIC-AuNPs. (b) Intensity-based histograms of bare AuNPs and MeO/cRGD-uPIC-AuNPs. (c and d) TEM images of MeO-uPIC-AuNP (c) and cRGD-uPIC-AuNP (d) (scale bar: 50 nm). (e) Thickness of uPIC layer on cRGD-uPIC-AuNPs calculated from TEM images (n=100).

Also, the zeta-potential was significantly changed from −30 mV for bare AuNPs to −11 mV for MeO-, cRAD-, and cRGD-uPIC-AuNPs (Table 14.1). These changes in size and surface charge were apparently consistent with the decoration of AuNP with uPICs. The thickness of uPIC layer was further analyzed in terms of the distance from the periphery of AuNP to the stained border of the uPIC-AuNP in the TEM images (Figure 14.2c and d). The calculated thickness (~8 nm) (Figure 14.2e) was comparable to the size of uPIC, indicating the single-layer formation of uPICs on AuNP.

Next, the stability of the uPIC-AuNPs was evaluated in terms of their size change in 10% FBS-containing PBS at 37°C by DLS measurements. Both MeO- and cRGD-uPIC-AuNPs did not display obvious changes in size and PDI during 8 h of incubation (Figure 14.3a), indicating that neither aggregation nor dissociation occurred in the serum-containing media. On the other hand, the present uPIC-AuNP formulation was designed to preferentially release uPICs within the reductive cytoplasmic condition through the replacement of S–Au bonds with a high concentration of reduced glutathione [26,44]. Under the reductive condition (10 mM DTT, 37°C) mimicking the cytoplasmic

environment, the release amount of uPICs from the uPIC-AuNP was monitored from the fluorescence intensity of Alexa647-siRNA (Figure 14.3b). The gradual increase in Alexa647-based fluorescence intensity was clearly observed for several hours, demonstrating the time-dependent release of uPICs from uPIC-AuNP under the reductive condition.

14.1.2 In Vitro siRNA Delivery by Targeted uPIC-AuNP

To validate the targetability of cRGD-uPIC-AuNP, the siRNA delivery efficacy was evaluated against cultured HeLa-luc cells, which are known to overexpress $\alpha_v\beta_5$ integrin as a receptor of cRGD peptide [45,46]. Prior to evaluation of the delivery efficacy, viability of HeLa-luc cells was measured after 48 h of treatment with the nanocarriers. No significant changes in cell viability were observed for both siCont-loaded MeO- and cRGDuPIC-AuNPs at siRNA concentrations of 100, 200, and 400 nM [1], indicating the negligible cytotoxicity of uPIC-AuNPs. Next, in order to clarify the targeting ability for HeLa-luc cells, cellular uptake was compared among MeO-, cRAD-, and

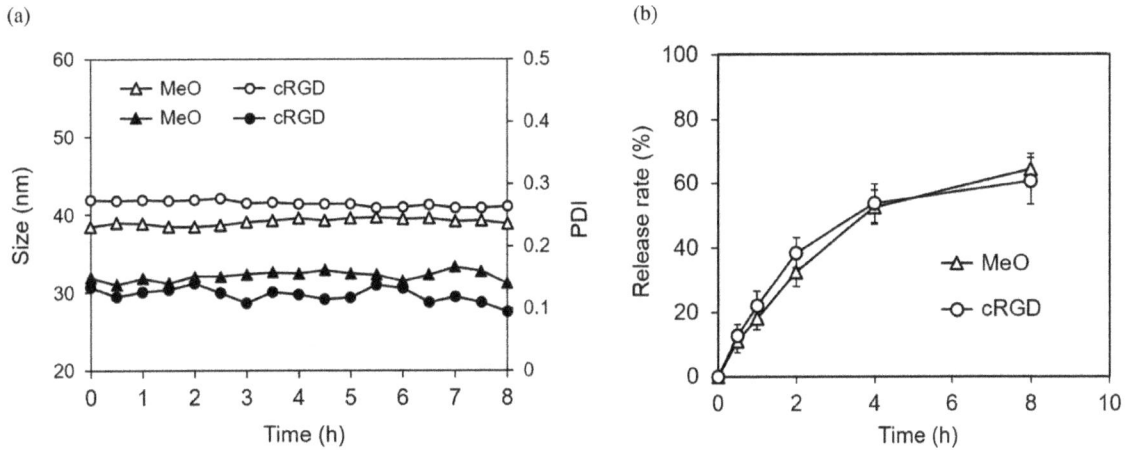

FIGURE 14.3 (a) Change in cumulant diameter (open circle and triangle) and PDI (closed circle and triangle) of MeO- and cRGD-uPIC-AuNPs after incubation in PBS containing 10% FBS at 37°C. (b) Release of siRNA from uPIC-AuNP in PBS containing 10% FBS and 10 mM DTT at 37°C. Results are expressed as mean and standard deviation (n=4).

cRGD-uPIC-AuNPs. After incubation with Alexa647-siRNA-loaded nanocarriers for 2 h and 6 h, HeLa-luc cells were harvested and analyzed by flow cytometry. The mean fluorescence intensity of the cells treated with cRGD-uPIC-AuNP was significantly higher than those treated with MeO-uPIC-AuNP and cRADuPIC-AuNP

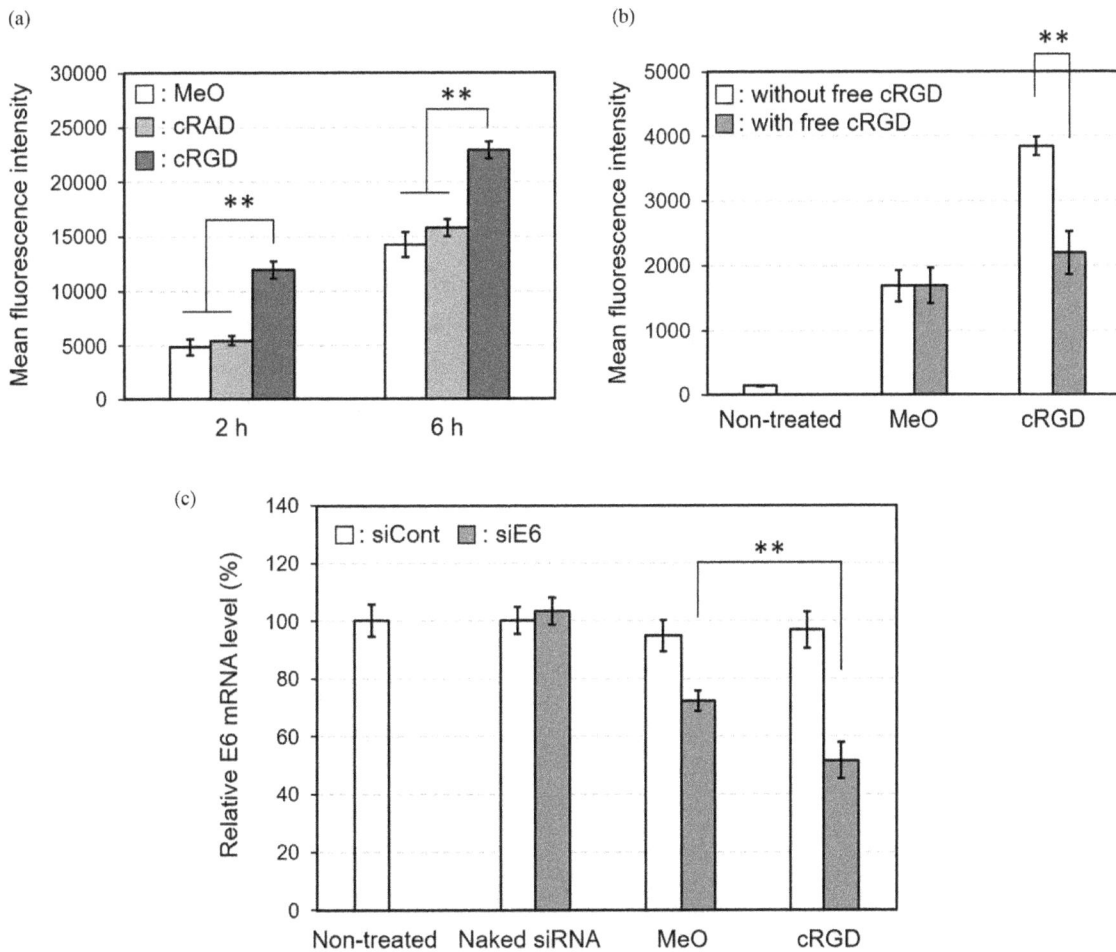

FIGURE 14.4 *In vitro* siRNA delivery efficacy of MeO- and cRGD-uPIC-AuNPs in cultured HeLa-luc cells. (a) Cellular uptake of Alexa647-siRNA determined by flow cytometer. (b) Competition assay on cellular uptake of Alexa647-siRNA by coincubation of uPIC-AuNPs with an excess amount of free cRGD (20 μM). (C) E6 mRNA level in HeLa-luc cells treated with siE6 or siCont-loaded nanocarriers for 48 h. siRNA concentration is 200 nM in all figures. All results are expressed as mean and standard deviation (n=4, **p<0.01).

(Figure 14.4a), demonstrating more efficient cellular uptake of siRNA payloads delivered by the targeted uPIC-AuNP. Particularly, the result that cRAD ligands did not facilitate the cellular uptake of uPIC-AuNP suggests that the enhanced cell internalization was due to the specific recognition between cRGD ligands and αvβ5 integrins rather than nonspecific adsorption mediated by cyclic peptides. This enhanced cellular uptake of cRGD-uPIC-AuNP was also determined by ICP-MS, as shown that higher amount of Au was found in the cells treated with cRGD nanocarriers, compared with MeO control nanocarriers [1]. Note that the enhanced cellular uptake of cRGD-uPIC-AuNPs was affected by the loading amount of cRGD ligands on nanoparticle, as the decrease in the cRGD loading amount apparently compromised the enhanced cellular uptake. The specific recognition of cRGD to $\alpha_v\beta_5$ integrin was further validated by the competition assay, where the nanocarriers were coincubated with an excess amount of free cRGD peptide (20 μM). The cellular uptake of Alexa647-siRNA in the treatment with cRGDuPIC-AuNP significantly reduced to the similar level to the treatment with MeO-uPIC-AuNP (Figure 14.4b), suggesting that the enhanced cellular uptake of the targeted uPIC-AuNP was attributed to the specific binding of cRGD ligands with the integrin receptors. The *in vitro* gene silencing efficacy of cRGD-uPIC-AuNP was evaluated using siRNA targeting E6 oncogene in HPV-18-positive HeLa-luc cells because E6 reduction is able to recover a tumor suppressor protein, p53, for cervical cancer treatment [47]. After incubation with MeO and cRGD-uPIC-AuNPs for 48 h, the E6 mRNA level in HeLa-luc cells was measured by qRT-PCR. It was found that both MeO-uPIC-AuNP and cRGD-uPIC-AuNP elicited the sequence-specific E6 mRNA silencing in a dose-dependent manner (Figure 14.4c). Notably, cRGD-uPIC-AuNP achieved significantly higher gene silencing efficacy compared with the non-targeted control, probably because of the facilitated cellular uptake of cRGD-uPIC-AuNP.

14.1.3   *In Vivo* Tumor Accumulation and Gene Silencing of cRGD-uPIC-AuNP

The targetability of cRGD-uPIC-AuNP was validated in a subcutaneous HeLa-luc tumor model after intravenous administration. The fluorescence intensity of Alexa647 in the tumor tissues was recorded by an IVIS instrument at 2 h, 4 h, and 6 h post-injection of Alexa647-siRNA-loaded MeO-uPIC-AuNP or cRGD-uPIC-AuNP at a dose of 5 μg siRNA/mouse. The obtained result shows the significantly enhanced tumor accumulation of siRNA payloads by cRGD-uPIC-AuNP, compared with MeO-uPIC-AuNP (Figure 14.5a). The Au content in tumor tissues at 4 h post-injection was also significantly higher for cRGD-uPIC-AuNP, as determined by ICP-MS [1]. The targeting ability of cRGD-uPIC-AuNPs was further evaluated by IVCLSM observation (Figure 14.5B). In this experiment, the mixture of Alexa488-siRNA-loaded cRGD-uPIC-AuNP and

Alexa647-siRNA-loaded MeO-uPIC-AuNP was intravenously administered into subcutaneous HeLa-luc tumor model and the fluorescence of each dye was observed simultaneously in the same area of tumor. In the IVCLSM images, Alexa488- and Alexa647-siRNAs were shown in green and red, respectively, and vascular endothelial cells were stained with CD31 antibody shown in blue [48,49]. In the overlay image, the bloodstream appeared to be yellow at 10 min post-injection, indicating that both MeO- and cRGD-uPIC-AuNPs circulated in the tumor vessels. At 4 h post-injection, whereas Alexa647-siRNA fluorescence was hardly detected in the tumor tissue, Alexa488-siRNA fluorescence remains to be observed with some strong fluorescence spots outside of blood vessels, consistent with the enhanced tumor accumulation of cRGD-uPIC-AuNPs.

Next, *in vivo* E6 gene silencing efficacy of uPIC-AuNPs was evaluated in the same tumor model. At 48 h after the last injection (20 μg siRNA/mouse/injection, total three injections), the tumors were excised and E6 mRNA amount was measured by qRT-PCR. Compared with the siCont-loaded nanocarriers that showed no gene silencing effect, both siE6-loaded MeO- and cRGD-uPIC-AuNPs induced significant gene silencing in the tumor tissue (Figure 14.5c). Notably, the cRGD-uPIC-AuNP exhibited higher E6 gene silencing efficacy compared with MeO-uPIC-AuNP, demonstrating more efficient *in vivo* gene silencing efficacy probably due to the enhanced tumor accumulation by cRGD peptide ligands.

14.1.4   *In Vivo* Tumor Growth Inhibition by Intravenous Administration of siE6-Loaded cRGD-uPIC-AuNP

The antitumor efficacy of cRGD-uPIC-AuNP was further evaluated by systemic delivery of siE6 to the subcutaneous HeLa-luc tumor. The siE6-loaded cRGD-uPIC-AuNP, siE6-loaded MeO-uPIC-AuNP, siCont-loaded cRGD-uPIC-AuNP, and saline were injected 6 times into the tail vein of tumor-bearing mice (20 μg siRNA/injection). At day 12, the size of tumors treated with siE6-loaded cRGD-uPIC-AuNP was significantly smaller than those treated with siE6-loaded MeO-uPIC-AuNP, as well as siCont-loaded cRGD-uPIC-AuNP (Figure 14.6a). This result indicates that cRGD ligands significantly enhanced the siE6-mediated antitumor activity of uPIC-AuNPs, consistent with the E6 gene silencing profile in the tumor tissue (Figure 14.5c). Of note, the antitumor activity of cRGD-uPIC-AuNP was significantly higher than that of a commercially available transfection reagent, *in vivo*-jetPEI® [1]. In addition, the systemic administration of cRGD-uPIC-AuNP and MeO-uPIC-AuNP did not cause apparent body weight loss in the treated mice (Figure 14.6b), suggesting that uPIC-AuNPs had negligible systemic toxicity under the tested experimental condition regardless of the presence of cRGD ligands.

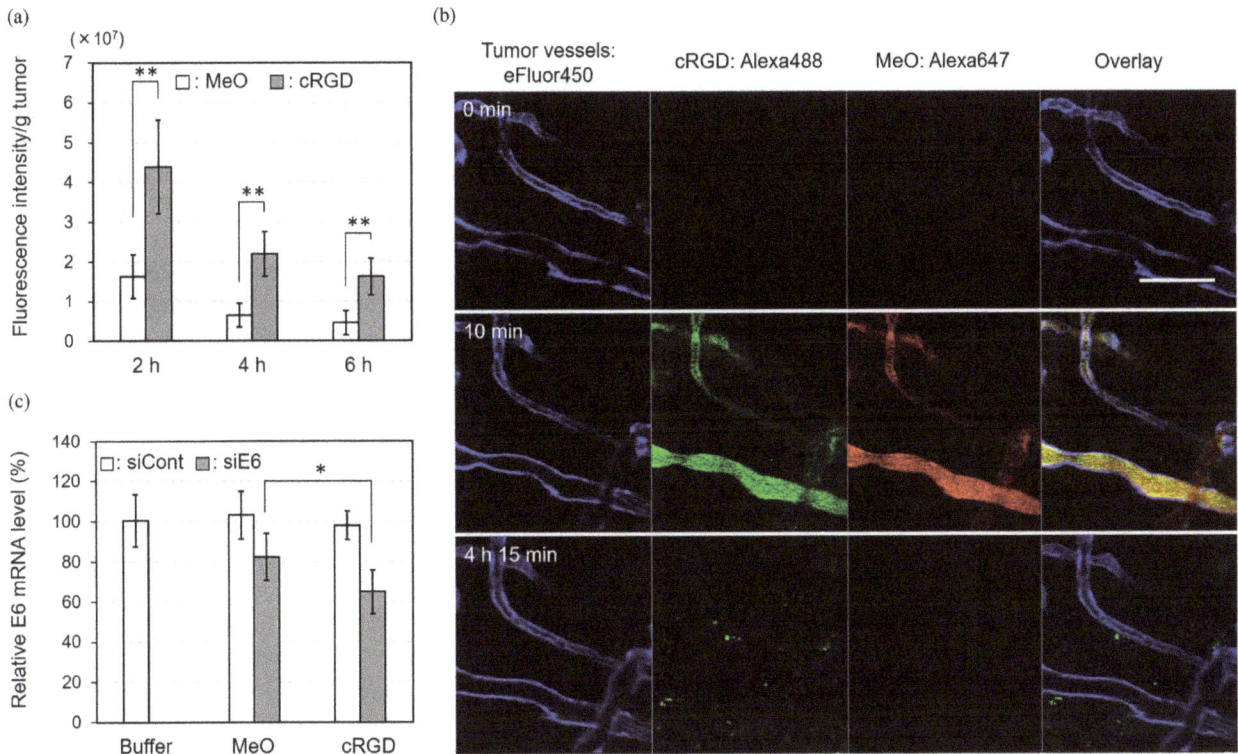

FIGURE 14.5 (a) Tumor accumulation of Alexa647-siRNA delivered by MeO-uPIC-AuNP and cRGD-uPIC-AuNP in subcutaneous HeLa-luc tumor-bearing mice by intravenous administration (5 μg siRNA/mouse). Alexa647-based fluorescence intensity was quantified by IVIS. Results are expressed as mean and standard deviation (n=4, **p<0.01). (b) IVCLSM images of subcutaneous HeLa-luc tumor tissue simultaneously treated with Alexa488-siRNA-loaded cRGD-uPIC-AuNPs (green) and Alexa647-siRNA-loaded MeO-uPIC-AuNPs (red). After preinjection of eFluor450-labeled PECAM-1 for staining tumor vessels (blue), the mixture of MeO- and cRGD-uPIC-AuNPs was intravenously injected into the tail vein at a dose of 5 μg siRNA for each (scale bar: 100 μm). (c) E6 mRNA levels in subcutaneous HeLa-luc tumor tissues after treatment with uPIC-AuNPs. Samples (20 μg siRNA/injection/mouse) were intravenously injected into the mouse tail vein at 48, 60, and 72 h before measurement. Results are expressed as mean and standard deviation (n=5, *p<0.05).

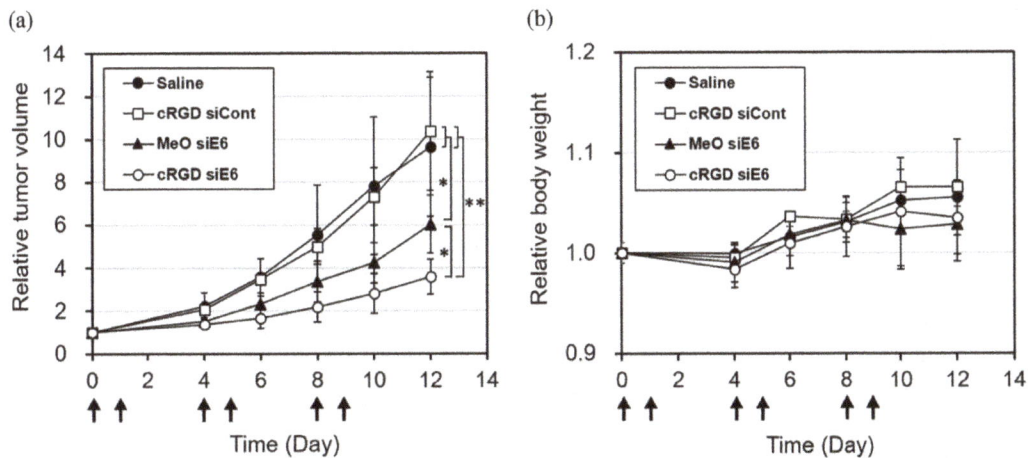

FIGURE 14.6 *In vivo* antitumor efficacy of siE6-loaded cRGD-uPIC-AuNP on subcutaneous HeLa-luc tumor model. (a) Relative tumor sizes in the mice treated with siE6-loaded cRGD-uPIC-AuNP, siE6-loaded MeO-uPIC-AuNP, siCont-loaded cRGD-uPIC-AuNP, or saline. (b) Relative body weights of the mice in the same experiment as (a). Arrows indicate the day for intravenous injection of samples (20 μg siRNA/injection/mouse). All results are expressed as mean and standard deviation (n= 5–6, *p<0.05 and **p<0.01).

14.2 TARGETED COMBINATORIAL siRNA POLYPLEXES

The siRNA promises high efficacy and excellent specificity to silence the target gene expression, which shows potential for cancer treatment. However, systemic delivery of siRNA with selectivity to the tumor site and into the cytosol of tumor cells remains a major limitation. To achieve this, it has been generated oligoaminoamide-based sequence-defined polycationic oligomers by solid-phase-assisted synthesis [50], which can form polyplexes with anionic siRNA by electrostatic interaction to serve as siRNA carrier. Targeting for folate receptor (FR)-overexpressing tumors, it has been optimized the physicochemical properties of polyplexes by combinatorial optimization of PEGylated folate-conjugated oligomer (for FR targeting and shielding of surface charges) and 3-arm oligomer (for size modification and particle stability). For unidirectional fast coupling between the two groups of oligomers, it has been activated [50] the cysteine thiol groups of one of the oligomers with 5,5′-dithio-bis(2-nitrobenzoic acid) to achieve a fast chemical linkage through disulfide formation with the free thiol groups of the other oligomer. These targeted combinatorial polyplexes (TCPs) are homogeneous spherical particles with favorable size and surface charge, which showed strong siRNA binding activity. TCPs were internalized into cells by FR-mediated endocytosis, triggered significant eGFP-luciferase marker gene silencing, and transfection with antitumoral EG5 siRNA suppressed cell proliferation in FR-expressing tumor cells. Moreover, the most promising formulation TCP1 after intravenous administration in tumor-bearing mice exhibited siRNA delivery into the tumor, resulting in EG5 gene silencing at mRNA level. Therefore, by covalent combination of two sequence-defined functional oligomers, it has been developed a siRNA carrier system with optimized size and surface charge for efficient tumor cell-directed gene silencing and cytotoxicity *in vitro* and *in vivo*.

RNA interference (RNAi)-based therapy has been extensively investigated over the past decades, which provides an option to combat many severe diseases including cancer [3]. Attractively, siRNA, as one of the RNAi therapeutics, offers a tremendous potential for sequence-specific suppression of gene expression via mRNA degradation pathways [51]. However, successful applications of RNAi-based cancer therapy require sufficient intracellular delivery of siRNA to the target site and effective knockdown of targeted transcripts. Thus, an ideal siRNA delivery system should possess multifunctionalities to conquer multiple barriers all the way to its site of action [52]. Generally, the siRNA carrier needs to incorporate siRNA into nanoparticles of suitable size to protect siRNA from nucleases and renal clearance and also enables passive targeting to tumor by enhanced permeability and retention (EPR) effect [53]. Surface shielding domains are also essential to limit the interaction with serum proteins during its extracellular transportation. Next, the siRNA delivery vehicle needs

to mediate efficient and selective cellular uptake, which can be achieved through specific targeting ligands. And finally, sufficient intracellular endosomal escape of siRNA is another critical issue. In recent years, great efforts have been made in the development of various siRNA carriers. Polymeric materials [54–66], liposomes [67,68], inorganic platforms [69], and hybrid systems [16,26,70,71] all showed their potential [11]. However, systemic delivery of siRNA directed to the tumor site remains a major limitation.

Derived from the classic gene carrier polyethylenimine (PEI) [72,73], a set of artificial amino acids was developed comprising repeats of the 1,2-diaminoethane motif [74]. The artificial oligoamino acids, such as succinoyl-tetraethylene pentamine (Stp) and succinoyl-pentaethylene hexamine (Sph) [75], in combination with natural α-amino acids, were applied in solid-phase-assisted synthesis to generate sequence-defined cationic oligomers [76]. These oligomers provide excellent nucleic acid binding ability, endosomal buffering capacity, and site-specific positioning of multiple functionalities. Further studies have been undertaken to optimize such cationic carriers by systematic variation of the topology [77]; inclusion of small chemical delivery motifs such as buffering histidines [78], fatty acids [79], tyrosine trimers [59], and disulfide-forming units [80]; targeting ligands [81–88]; and combinations of such elements [89]. Accordingly, this strategy of a step-by-step optimization resulted in a library of >1000 oligomers which included precise siRNA carriers.

Combination of two different oligomers from the library provides an efficient alternative to obtain a multifunctional carrier, which may formulate therapeutic nucleic acids and overcome possible disadvantages of single oligomers. For example, a c-Met targeting PEGylated oligomer, which is deficient in DNA condensation, was combined in a 7/3 ratio with a 3-arm oligomer to facilitate nucleic acid compaction [85]. In the current work section, it has been focused [50] on the targeting of FR-overexpressing tumors. We selected PEGylated folate-conjugated oligomers (for FR targeting and shielding of surface charges) and optimized the physicochemical properties of polyplexes by combination with a 3-arm oligomer (for optimizing particle size and stability) at various molar ratios. For unidirectional fast coupling between the two types of oligomers, we activated the cysteine thiol groups of one of the oligomers with 5,5′-dithio-bis(2-nitrobenzoic acid) (DTNB) to achieve a fast chemical linkage through disulfide formation with the free thiol groups of the other oligomer. These TCPs with favorable particle size and surface charge showed significant tumor cell-specific eGFP-luciferase marker gene silencing and inhibiting tumor growth by EG5 gene knockdown *in vitro*. FR-mediated internalization was monitored by flow cytometry and immuno-TEM. Moreover, after intravenous administration in tumor-bearing mice, the most promising TCP1 generated with a 3-arm Stp oligomer and a TNB-modified 4-arm PEGylated targeted Sph oligomer exhibited siRNA delivery into the tumor and resulted in *in vivo* EG5 gene silencing as demonstrated at the tumoral mRNA level.

	TCP1	TCP3
TNB Oligomer #1	(4-arm *873*) K-(PEG$_{24}$-Folate)-K-[K-(Sph$_4$-C-TNB)$_2$]$_2$ (N/P 11.2)	(3-arm *769*) TNB-C-Stp$_3$-K-(Stp$_3$-C-TNB)$_2$ (N/P 4.8)
Thiol Oligomer #2	(3-arm *386*) C-Stp$_3$-K-(Stp$_3$-C)$_2$ (N/P 4.8)	(4-arm *709*) K-(PEG$_{24}$-Folate)-K-[K-(Sph$_4$-C)$_2$]$_2$ (N/P 11.2)
Combined Structure	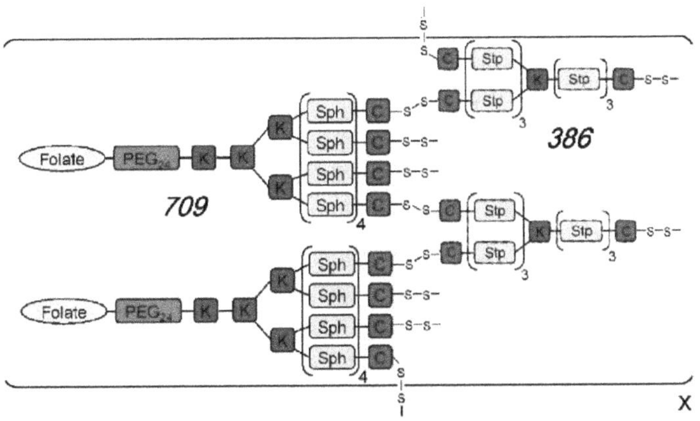 (709-S-S-386-S-S)$_x$	

	TCP2	TCP4
TNB Oligomer #1	(3-arm *770*) TNB-C-H-(Stp-H)$_3$-K-[(H-Stp)$_3$-H-C-TNB]$_2$ (N/P 7.4)	(2-arm *874*) K-(PEG$_{24}$-Folate)-K-(Sph$_4$-Y$_3$-C-TNB)$_2$ (N/P 8.6)
Thiol Oligomer #2	(2-arm *717*) K-(PEG$_{24}$-Folate)-K-(Sph$_4$-Y$_3$-C)$_2$ (N/P 8.6)	(3-arm *689*) C-H-(Stp-H)$_3$-K-[(H-Stp)$_3$-H-C]$_2$ (N/P 7.4)
Combined Structure	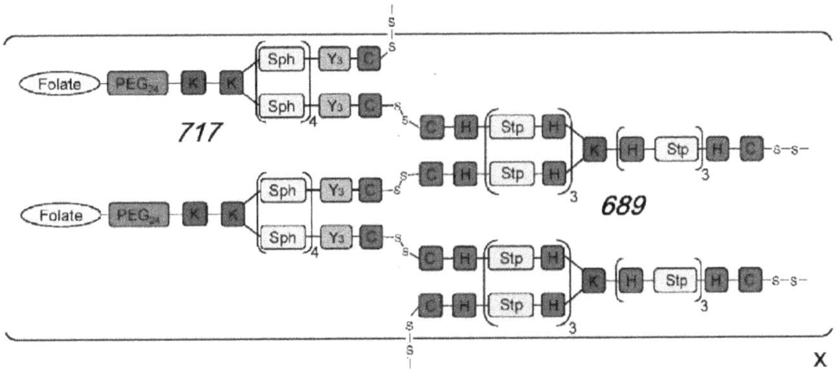 (717-S-S-689-S-S)$_x$	

SCHEME 14.2 Targeted combinatorial polyplex (TCP) formulations. siRNA was co-formulated with TNB-modified oligomers and unmodified thiol-oligomers at various molar ratios to form the TCP carriers. In most experiments, polyplexes were formed at N/P 16 using an equal molar oligomer ratio of 1:1; for these conditions, the individual N/P ratio of each oligomer is presented. The oligomer sequences are indicated (left to right) from C- to N-terminus. C: cysteine; H: histidine; K: lysine; Y: tyrosine; S-S: disulfide crosslinking; PEG24: polyethylene glycol; TNB: 5-thio-2-nitrobenzoic acid; Stp: succinoyl-tetraethylene pentamine; Sph: succinoyl-pentaethylene hexamine. K-(and K-[refer to branching] by α- and ε-amino modification of lysines). x: hypothetic nanogel structures resulting from disulfide crosslinking in three dimensions within the TCP.

14.3 OLIGOMER SYNTHESIS AND FORMATION OF TARGETED COMBINATORIAL POLYPLEXES (TCPs)

Based on the previous studies, it has been selected four oligomers from the library to generate novel combinatorial formulations for targeted siRNA delivery (Scheme 14.2). Three-arm Stp oligomers 386 and 689 were chosen for their strong siRNA binding ability, which provide a highly stable cationic core to compact siRNA [76,79,86,90]. Moreover, PEG-folate-conjugated Sph oligomers (4-arm) 709 and (2-arm) 717 were used for FR targeting and surface shielding [89].

Here, we combined these two types of oligomers, in order to optimize the siRNA polyplexes by co-formulation. All oligomers contain terminal cysteines with free thiol groups for subsequent disulfide formation within siRNA polyplexes. As standard disulfide formation by air oxidation was previously found to be a rather slow and incomplete process, we intended to make this step faster and more specific.

Therefore, we activated the thiol groups of oligomer #1 with 5,5′-dithio-bis(2-nitrobenzoic acid) (DTNB) to produce TNB-modified oligomer (Figure 14.7a). The TNB-modified oligomer forms a binary siRNA polyplex with siRNA, and in the following incubation with the unmodified thiol-oligomer #2, it will undergo a fast unidirectional coupling through disulfide formation with the free thiol groups of thiol-oligomer #2 in three dimensions, resulting in hypothetic nanogel structures (Scheme 14.1). The combination of siRNA with both oligomers thus generates TCPs, which are composed of compact cationic core for siRNA binding, well-shielded PEG layer and folates as targeting ligands (Figure 14.7b). TCPs were optimized by testing different TNB-modified oligomers #1/unmodified thiol oligomers #2 at various molar ratios and evaluating three different siRNA/oligomer #1/oligomer #2 mixing sequences. Preliminary gene silencing experiments demonstrated similar efficiencies of the tested mixing sequences, with the first alternative (preincubated siRNA with the TNB-modified oligomer #1, followed

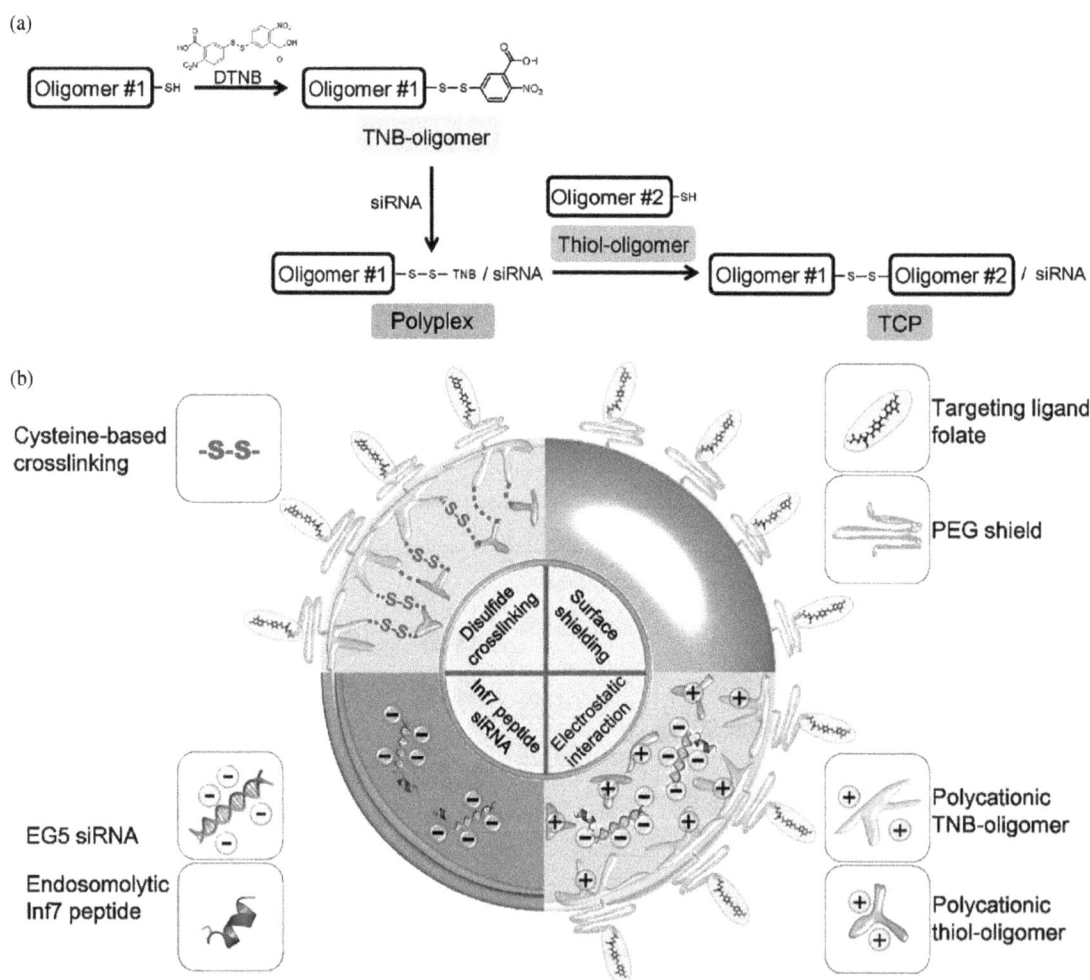

FIGURE 14.7 Targeted combinatorial polyplexes (TCPs) with folate ligand for siRNA delivery. A) TNB-modified oligomer #1 is obtained by reacting the solid-phase-derived thiol precursor oligomer #1 with 10 eq of DTNB for 2 h at room temperature. The incubation of TNB-modified oligomer #1 with siRNA forms a binary polyplex. Addition of thiol-oligomer #2 results in fast unidirectional coupling of TNB-modified oligomer #1 through disulfide formation with the free thiol groups of #2. In this way, siRNA, TNB-modified oligomer, and unmodified thiol-oligomer were formulated to produce a TCP. B) Schematic presentation of key elements of a TCP. Endosomolytic Inf7 peptide was conjugated to siRNA for enhanced endosomal escape [81].

by disulfide exchange reaction with thiol oligomer #2). For practical reasons, all further testing was performed with this mixing sequence. Four combinatorial formulations, TCP1, TCP2, TCP3, and TCP4, were developed (Scheme 14.1). TCP1 and TCP3 share the similar combined structure of **386 + 709** (Scheme 14.1 top); TCP2 and TCP4 share the similar combined structure of **689 + 717** (Scheme 14.1 bottom). Differences rise from the alterative TNB activations of oligomers. After systematic screening and evaluating different molar ratios of oligomers [50], equal molar (1:1) oligomer ratios and an N/P ratio of 16 were determined as most useful for the subsequent TCP studies.

14.4 FUNCTIONAL QUANTUM DOT-siRNA NANOPLEXES

SOX9 plays an important role in mesenchymal condensations during the early development of embryonic skeletons. However, its function in the chondrogenic differentiation of adult mesenchymal stem cells (MSCs) has not been fully investigated because SOX9 RNA interference in adult MSCs has seldom been studied. This study used SOX9 gene as the target gene and the quantum dot (QD)-based nanomaterial QD-NH2 (ZnS shell and polyethylene glycol (PEG) coating) with a fluorescent tracer function as the gene carrier to transfect siSOX9 into MSCs after sulfosuccinimidyl-4-(N-maleimidomethyl) cyclohexane-1-carboxylate (sulfo-SMCC) activation *in vitro* and *in vivo*. The results showed that QD-SMCC could effectively bind and deliver siRNAs into the MSCs, followed by efficient siRNA escape from the endosomes. The siRNAs released from QD-SMCC retained their structural integrity and could effectively inhibit the targeted gene expression, leading to reduced chondrogenic differentiation of MSCs and delayed cartilage repair. QDs were excreted from living cells instead of dead cells, and the ZnS shell and PEG coating layer greatly reduced the cytotoxicity of the QDs. The transfection efficiency of QD-SMCC was superior to that of PEI. In addition, QD-SMCC has an intrinsic signal for noninvasive imaging of siRNA transport. The results indicate that SOX9 is imperative for the chondrogenesis of MSCs and QD-SMCC has great potential for real-time tracking of transfection.

The chondrogenic differentiation of MSCs is regulated by a series of signaling molecules, among which SOX9 plays an important role. This has been verified via an analysis of SOX9 knockout chimeras and conditional knockout mice. In chimeric mice, SOX9_/_ cells are excluded from cartilage primordia throughout embryonic development [91]. During embryogenesis, SOX9 is required for mesenchymal condensation, a prerequisite for limb bud formation, and for the inhibition of precocious hypertrophic conversion of proliferating chondrocytes in the growth plate [91]. SOX9 can bind to type II collagen (col2a1) and aggrecan (acan) enhancer elements [92]. The overexpression of SOX9 promotes the expression of col2a1 and acan and accelerates the differentiation of adult MSCs toward chondrocytes [93]. However, few studies have reported the effect of SOX9 interference on the chondrogenesis of adult MSC.

One of the major challenges in RNA interference is the lack of a safe and efficient gene delivery method. Carriers for RNA include viral and nonviral carriers [94]. Viral carriers enclose RNA sequences in the viral capsid and achieve efficient and stable transfection by taking advantage of the viruses' infection properties [95]. However, using viruses as RNA carriers poses potential risks such as cell mutation and immune responses [96]. Another limitation is the lack of an intrinsic signal for long-term and real-time imaging of siRNA transport and release [97]. Nonviral carriers include liposomes, cationic polymers, and nanomaterials, which can bind with RNA molecules by electrostatic adsorption or covalent coupling [98]. Many nonviral carriers are easy to synthesize and modify. In addition, they are less immunogenic and have been successfully used for delivery of genes to stem cells [99,100]. Overall, there is a critical need for an effective and low-toxic nanocarrier that can not only deliver RNA but also monitor the transport process in real time.

Water-soluble QDs, which are often applied to label biological molecules, may be an excellent choice. QDs exhibit strong fluorescence and can pass through the cell membranes and blood-brain barrier [101]. The toxic effect of CdSe QDs can be improved by modification such as the incorporation of a ZnS shell and polyethylene glycol (PEG) coating [102,103]. Previously, QD-based siRNA delivery was usually achieved by mixing QDs with transfection agents such as PEI or combined with another class of nanomaterial [97,104]. However, the addition of other agents may lead to vulnerability to intracellular degradation or increased cytotoxicity. An alternative is the use of nonselective or selective bioconjugation techniques. Selective bioconjugation can occur without a preceding reduction reaction, thus retaining the integrity of the siRNA [105]. The use of a heterobifunctional crosslinker such as sulfo succinimidyl-4-(N-maleimido methyl)cyclohexane-1-carboxylate (sulfo-SMCC) results in selective bioconjugation toward specific sites on the protein to form a stable thioether bond with a sulfhydryl-exposed antibody [106]. QD-SMCC has been applied in immunohistochemistry only for antibody bioconjugation. The potential for gene delivery, particularly in the study of MSC differentiation, has yet to be sufficiently investigated.

In this study section, it has been developed [107] functional QD nanoplexes by sulfosuccinimidyl-4-(N-maleimidomethyl) cyclohexane-1-carboxylate (sulfo-SMCC) activation of PEG-coated CdSe/ZnS QDs as the gene carrier of siRNA to study the effect of SOX9 RNA interference on the chondrogenic differentiation of MSCs. This study confirmed the importance of SOX9 in chondrogenesis, as evidenced by the findings that SOX9 knockdown significantly inhibited the expression of cartilage-specific markers including acan and col2a1 in MSCs and further delayed cartilage repair. Moreover, QD-SMCC has an intrinsic signal for noninvasive imaging of siRNA transport. The results indicate that SOX9 is imperative for the

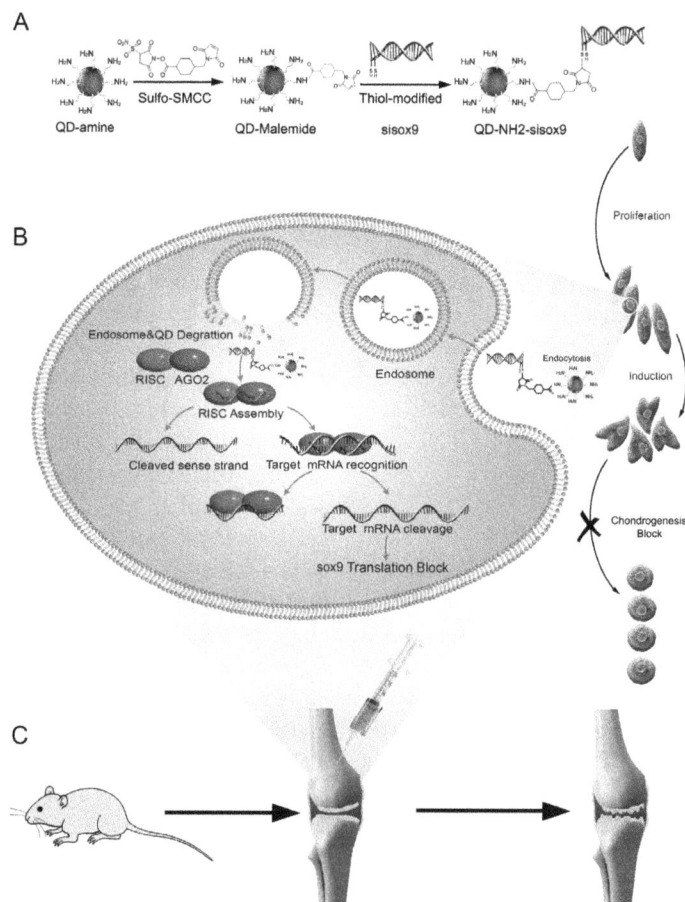

FIGURE 14.8 Schematic diagram of the QD-SMCC-si conjugation process and its *in vitro* and *in vivo* inhibitory effects on the chondrogenic differentiation of MSCs. (A) Aminomodified QDs were conjugated with thiol-modified biomolecules via SMCC. (B) The transfection process and inhibitory effects of QD-SMCC-si *in vitro*. (C) The inhibitory effects of QD-SMCC-si *in vitro* and *in vivo*.

chondrogenesis of MSCs and QD-SMCC has great potential for real-time tracking of transfection.

In this study section, it has been applied PEG-coated CdSe/ZnS QDs that were bioconjugated with SMCC, which are commonly used to label antibodies, for gene transfer to study the effect of SOX9 RNA interference on the chondrogenic differentiation of adult MSCs (Figure 14.8). As a control, PEI was also investigated. The effect of SOX9 knockdown on cartilage regeneration *in vivo* was further studied in a cartilage defective model. This study suggests that QD-SMCC is a promising vector for real-time tracking of transfection.

14.4.1 Characterization of QD-SMCC-siRNA [107]

A transmission electron microscope (TEM) was used to detect the micromorphology of QDs and QD-SMCC-si (Figure 14.9a and b). The DLS measurements showed that the size of the QD particles was 9.6 nm (Figure 14.9c) and that of the QD-SMCC-si complex was 16.7 nm (Figure 14.9d). Zeta-potential measurements revealed that the QD-SMCC complex had a zeta-potential of 16.5 ± 1.6 mV (Figure 14.9e), with a negatively charged siRNA surface (-17.2 ± 2.1 mV). After the siRNA was conjugated to QD-SMCC in a 1:5 ratio,

the complex became positively charged (11.4 ± 1.3 mV). To determine the appropriate QD loads of the siRNAs, the siRNAs were mixed with several concentrations of QD-SMCC at molar ratios of 10:1, 5:1, 1:1, 1:5, and 1:10 (Figure 14.9f). As the ratio of the siRNA/QD-SMCC complex decreased, the fluorescence intensity of the siRNA gradually decreased. When the molar ratio was higher than 1:5, free siRNA was detected on the agarose gel, indicating that the siRNA molecules were not completely complexed with QD-SMCC. When the ratio of the complex was 1:5 or less, the RNA was fully bound to QD-SMCC, and there was no RNA in the complex that would migrate toward the anode.

As shown in Figure 14.9g, cell viability was maintained at approximately 95% for a QD-SMCC concentration range of 20–80 pmol. When the concentration of QD-SMCC was higher than 200 pmol, the cell viability was 63% (Figure 14.9g). In comparison, 25–35 pmol/L of PEI maintained the best cell viability. The cytotoxicity of QDSMCC was lower than that of PEI within a range of 20–120 pmol/L (Figure 14.9g, $P < 0.05$).

As siRNA carriers, QDs have attracted attention regarding the treatment of diseases [108–110]. Most QDs have been modified with other siRNA delivery agents, resulting in greatly increased QD sizes. Li-modified QDs with

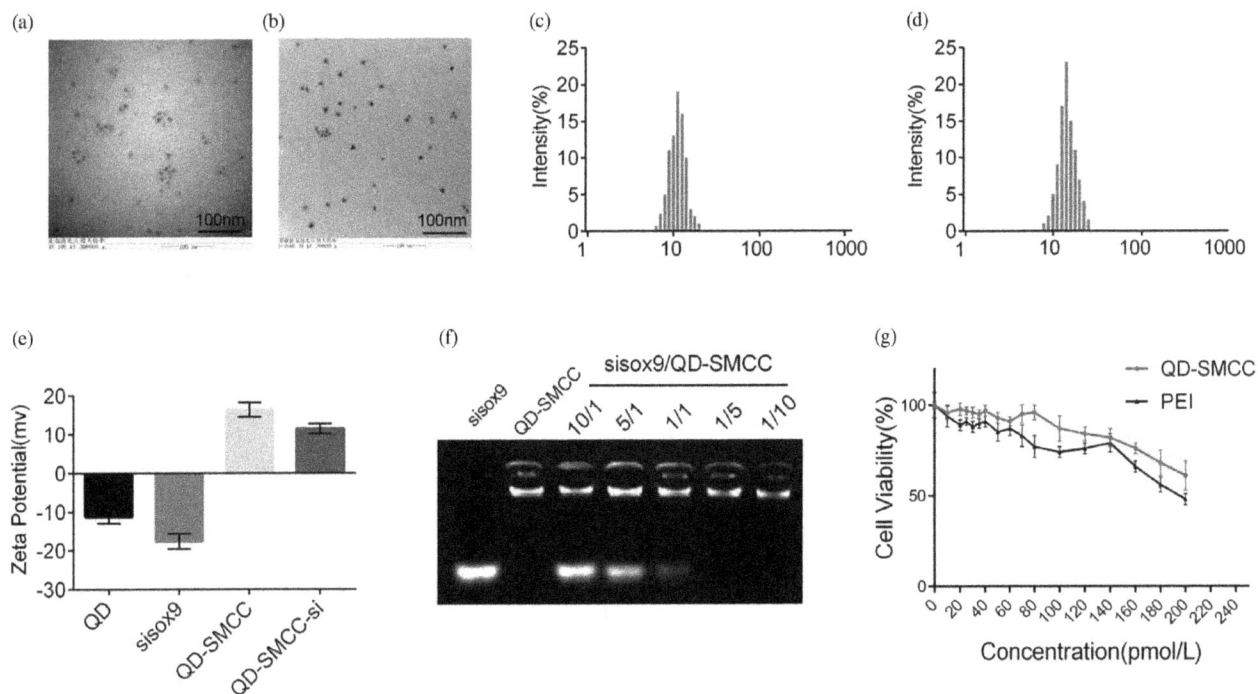

FIGURE 14.9 TEM, DLS, MTT, and zeta-potential analyses of the QD-SMCCs, as well as a gel retardation assay to evaluate the binding between the siRNAs and QD-SMCCs. (a) TEM image of the QDs. (b) TEM image of QD-SMCC-si. (c) DLS image of the QDs. (d) DLS image of QD-SMCC-si. (e) Changes in the surface charge. (f) Effective loading of siRNA on the QD-SMCC, as determined by agarose gel electrophoresis. Lanes 3–7 correspond to siRNA/QD-SMCC ratios of 10:1, 5:1, 1:1, 1:5, and 1:10, respectively. Lanes 1 and 2 correspond to siSOX9 and QD-SMCC. (g) The cytotoxicities of QD-SMCC and PEI were assessed with an MTT viability assay.

PEG, and the QDs' diameter was 84.2 nm after modification. PEI-modified QD605 had a diameter of up to 150 nm [111,112]. Comparatively, QD-peptide conjugates are relatively smaller. In our study, the diameter of the QDSMCC-si complex increased from 9.6 to 16.7 nm after bioconjugation (Figure 14.9c and d). We know that small nanoparticles are clearly advantageous in gene transfection because they can easily pass through capillaries and the tissue space to be ingested by the cells [113]. Our study is unique in that it relies on simple bioconjugation between QD-SMCC and siRNA, leading to effective interference of the MSCs. For the QD-NH$_2$ platform to function as a gene carrier, it must be highly soluble in aqueous solutions and stable under physiological conditions and should not form aggregates. Sulfo-SMCC can form stable amide bonds with QD-NH$_2$. PEG-amino modified on the QDs has a strong proton-absorbing capability inside acidic cellular organelles such as endosomes. The coexistence of PEG-amino and QD is expected to facilitate siRNA release inside cells.

The study [107] also showed that the QD-SMCC nanocomposites were positively charged, with zeta-potentials in the range of 11.4±0.9 mV (Figure 14.9e). The positive charge of QD-SMCC-si may also interact with the negative charge on the surface of MSCs to promote QD-SMCC-si entry into the cells. The TEM results verified that the particles were uniformly distributed after they were covalently bioconjugated to the siRNA. Covalent bioconjugation to the siRNA permits a higher degree of protection against nucleases and ensures that the siRNA is delivered to the cytoplasm, which contributes to the improved gene transfection.

The transfection efficiency of the QD-SMCC-si complexes was 68.6%, which was higher than that of PEI (56.4%).

14.4.2 CELLULAR ULTRASTRUCTURAL RESPONSE TO THE QD-SMCC-siRNAs

To study the ultrastructure of MSCs transfected with QD-SMCC-si, the cells were fixed at different time points and evaluated by TEM. After the QD-SMCC-si was transfected into the MSCs, a large amount of QD-SMCC-si was aggregated onto the surface of the cells (Figure 14.10a). Three hours after transfection, the MSCs extended a large number of filopodia toward a cluster of QD-SMCC-si and enveloped them (Figure 14.10b). Six hours after transfection, the phagocytized QD-SMCC-si gradually moved away from the cell membrane into endosomes wrapped by lipid membranes (Figure 14.10c). Twelve hours later, after some of the endosomes had ruptured, the QD-SMCC-si was released into the cytoplasm (Figure 14.10d).

It has been further observed the QD-SMCC-si transfection process by CLSM. Within the MSCs, green fluorescence represented the FAM-siRNAs, red fluorescence represented the QD-SMCCs, and blue fluorescence represented the Hoechst 33342-labeled nuclei. Furthermore, acidic organelles (including endosomes and lysosomes) were labeled in yellow with LysoTracker™ Yellow. After 3 h of incubation, the red QD-SMCCs and the green FAM-siRNAs gathered around the cell membranes (Figure 14.10e). After 6 h of incubation, the green FAM-siRNAs and the red QD-SMCCs were mainly distributed in the yellow-labeled organelles, suggesting that

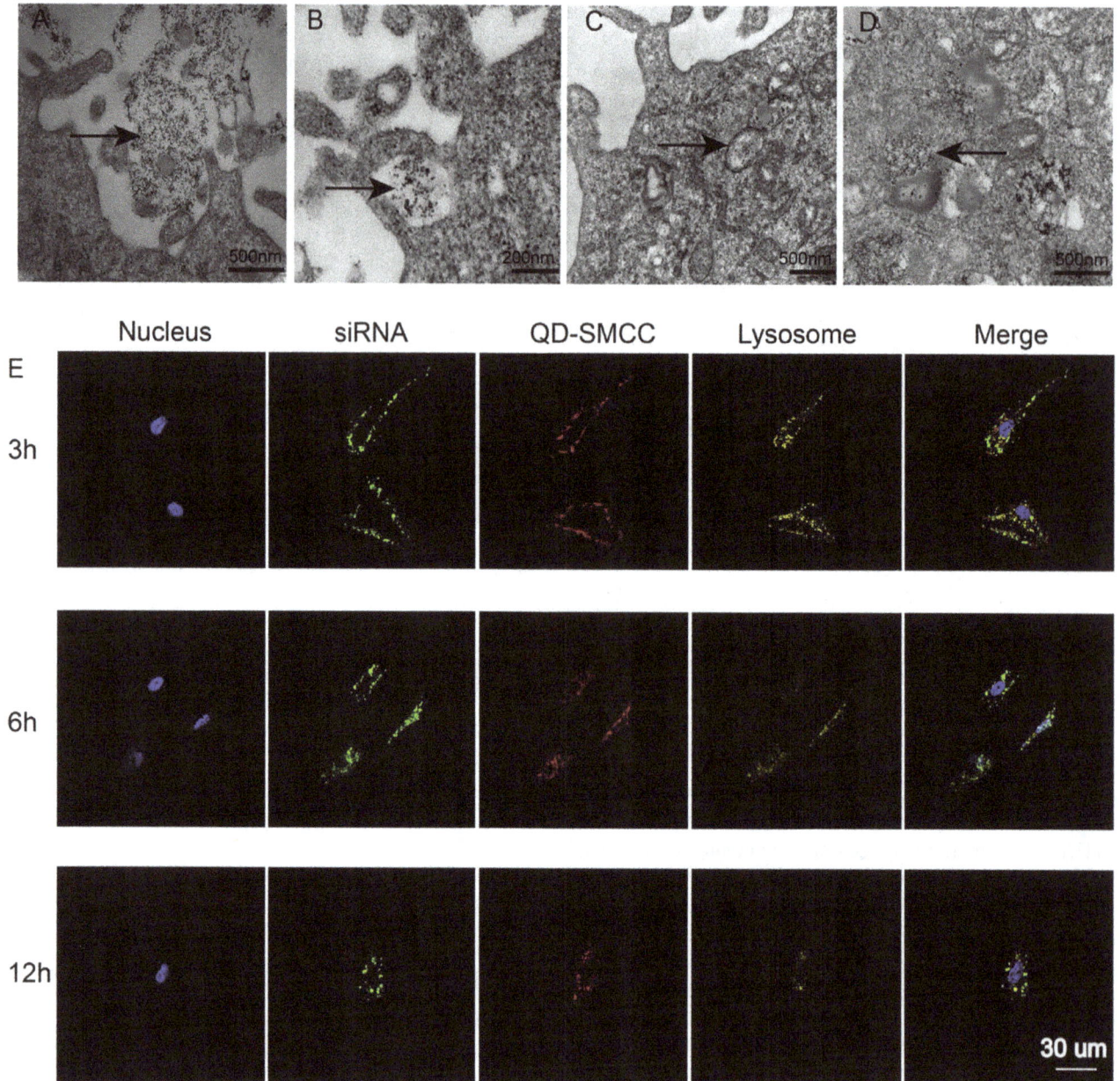

FIGURE 14.10 TEM and confocal laser scanning microscopy images of MSCs following treatment with the QD-SMCC-siRNA. (a) TEM showed that the MSCs extended many filopodia toward a cluster of QD-SMCC-si particles after 2 h of transfection. (b) Three hours after transfection, the QD-SMCC-si clusters were being phagocytized. (c) Six hours after transfection, the early endosomes contained QD-SMCC-si clusters. (d) Twelve hours later, the late endosomes resembled transparent droplets containing the QD-SMCCs and cell debris and were dispersed in the cytoplasm. (E) CLSM showed the transfection process of QD-SMCC-si in MSCs.

the nanoparticles were retained in the endosomes or early lysosomes. Twelve hours later, the green FAM-siRNAs and the red QD-SMCCs were no longer distributed in the yellow-labeled organelles, which escaped from the endosomes. This finding indicates that the QD-SMCCs could effectively deliver the siRNAs into MSCs and enable their escape from endosomes to silence genes in the cytoplasm.

We observed the cell entry process of the QD-SMCC-si by CLSM and found that the cells extended many filopodia toward a cluster of QD-SMCC and simultaneously enveloped them (Figure 14.10). After the endosomes ruptured, QD-SMCC-si was released into the cytoplasm. Some

studies have shown that the QDs were eventually deposited within the cells and caused cytotoxicity due to nonspecific uptake and peroxidation [114,115], but we found that QDs are excreted from living cells rather than dead cells. The elimination rate of QDs decreased over time; in accord with the survey performed by ICP-MS, a portion of the initial QDs were retained in the cells after 48 h. Previous reports indicated that elimination of nanoparticles slowed over time and not all internalized nanoparticles were excreted [116–118]. It is recognized that many types of stem cells with membrane transporters are capable of expelling toxic reagents from the cytoplasm for self-protection [119].

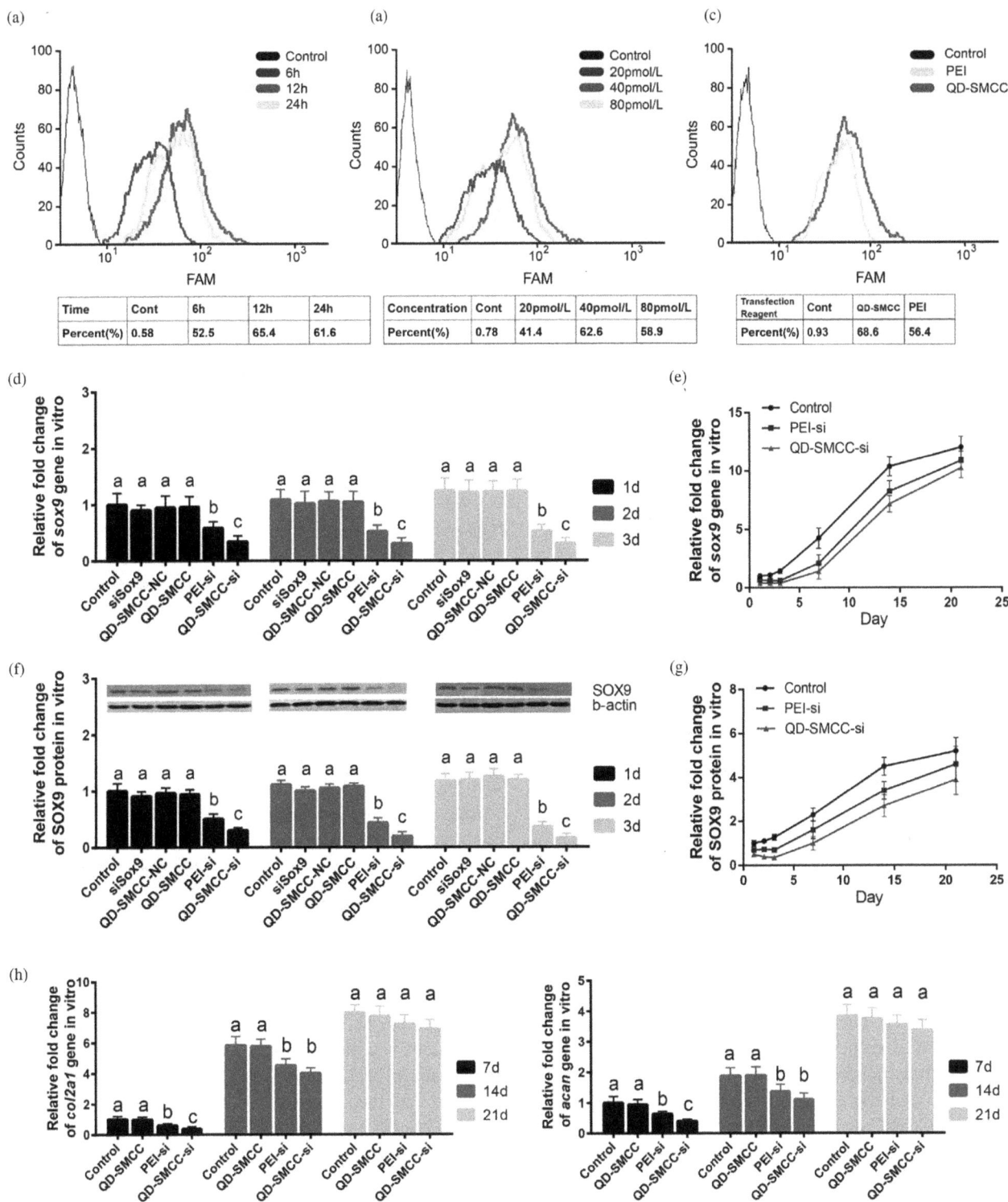

FIGURE 14.11 FACS, RT-PCR, and Western blot analyses of SOX9 expression in MSCs following treatment with the QD-SMCC-si particles for various times. RT-PCR analysis of col2a1 and acan in the MSCs following treatment with the QD-SMCC-si particles *in vitro* for various times. (a) Number of siSOX9-positive MSCs following treatment with the QD-SMCC-si particles for various times. (b) Number of siSOX9-positive MSCs following treatment with various concentrations of the QD-SMCC-si particles. (c) Number of siSOX9-positive MSCs following treatment with the different transfection reagents. (d) RT-PCR analysis of SOX9 mRNA levels in the MSCs following treatment with the different transfection reagents for 1, 2, and 3 days. (e) The levels of the SOX9 mRNA changed from days 1 to 21. (f) Western blot analysis of the SOX9 protein levels in the MSCs following treatment with the different transfection reagents for 1, 2, and 3 days. (g) The levels of the SOX9 protein changed from days 1 to 21. (h) RT-PCR analysis of the col2a1 and acan mRNA levels in the MSCs following treatment with the different transfection reagents for 7, 14, and 21 days. The bars with different letters are significantly different from each other at $P < 0.05$.

However, the mechanism of QD excretion should be studied. Because the toxicity of QDs is related to the release of toxic elements, Seon evaluated the toxicity of Se and Cd. Cadmium is recognized as a toxic material that leads to side effects such as mitochondrial dysfunction, the induction of oxidative stress, the disruption of intracellular calcium signaling, and apoptosis [120]. After evaluating the toxicity of Cd, Peng found that the toxicity of Cd was apparent at concentrations reaching 8.9 mM [121]. In contrast, selenium is an essential element that is toxic when the concentration becomes excessive [122]. We found that QD-SMCC had the highest transfection efficiency at a concentration of 40 pmol. The dose of QDs is far lower than 8.9 mM; therefore, no significant cytotoxic effects were observed in the study. The low cytotoxicity of QD-SMCC may result from the ZnS and PEG coating layer that protects the QDs from being exposed to the intracellular environment, thereby preventing Cd^{2+} release.

14.4.3 Quantification of the Transfection Efficiency of QD-SMCC-si In Vitro

To compare the effects of different transfection times on transfection efficiency, it has been determined the number of FAM-siSOX9-positive transfected MSCs using fluorescence-activated cell sorting (FACS). The FACS analysis [107] showed that 0.58% of the untreated MSCs were positive, whereas 52.5%, 65.4%, and 61.6% of the MSCs were positive following incubation with the QD-SMCC-si complex for 6, 12, and 24 h, respectively (Figure 14.11a). The results indicated that 12 h of transfection could efficiently deliver the siRNA into the cells. The effects of different concentrations on transfection efficiency were further examined by FACS, which showed that QD-SMCC had the highest transfection efficiency (62.6%) at a concentration of 40 pmol/L (Figure 14.11b). Finally, it has been determined the efficiency of different transfection reagents. The FACS analysis showed that 68.6% of the MSCs were positive for QD-SMCC-siSOX9 (Figure 14.11c), whereas 56.4% of the cells were positive for PEI-si (P<0.05). The results obtained [107] indicate that the transfection efficiency of QD-SMCC was higher than that of PEI. After transfection, there were no significant differences between the control, free siRNA, QD-SMCC, and QD-SMCC-siNC groups. As expected, the level of SOX9 was significantly decreased in the QD-SMCC-si and PEI-si groups compared with that of the control (0.34±0.04 and 0.58±0.07, Figure 14.11d). Between the QD-SMCC-si and PEI-si groups, QD-SMCC-si had a relatively higher inhibition efficiency (0.30±0.06) than PEI-si (0.52±0.08) at day 3 (P<0.05, Figure 14.11d). After the cells were treated with a chondrogenic supplement, the reduced SOX9 expression in the QD-SMCC-si and PEI-si groups gradually increased in a time-dependent manner. After 21 days of induction, the level of SOX9 was close to the control (Figure 14.11e), suggesting that QD-SMCC-si inhibited the early stages of chondrogenic differentiation. During chondrogenesis, QD-SMCC-si showed higher transfection efficiency than PEI.

WB showed that SOX9 protein level was the lowest on the third day after transfection, and the expression of SOX9 at the protein level was reduced to 0.16±0.07 by QD-SMCC-si and to 0.36±0.08 by PEI-siSOX9 (Figure 14.11f), indicating that the QDS-transfected siSOX9 played an interference effect within cells. During chondrogenic differentiation, QD-SMCC-si-downregulated SOX9 levels were gradually elevated (Figure 14.11g). Comparatively, QD-SMCC was slightly superior to PEI.

The inhibition of SOX9 clearly downregulated the expression of the col2a1 and acan genes (0.35±0.07 and 0.40±0.06) in the MSCs transfected with QD-SMCC (Figure 14.11h). During the early stage of chondrogenesis, downregulation of the col2a1 and acan genes (0.58±0.05 and 0.63±0.08) was also observed in the PEI-si group. During culture, the expression of cartilage-specific markers, including col2a1 and acan, increased in the control group over time after TGF-b stimulation, demonstrating that chondrogenesis was induced (Figure 14.11h).

We further verified the interference effects of the QD-transfected siSOX9 at the gene and protein levels *in vitro*. We showed that siSOX9 knocked down the expression at both the RNA and protein levels and was superior to PEI (Figure 14.11). The gene silencing effect of SOX9 can significantly reduce the expression of chondrogenic-specific markers, including col2a1 and acan. The results indicated that QD-SMCC did not have detectable adverse effects that limit the differentiation. Using this delivery system, we demonstrated that SOX9 knockdown reduced the expression of col2a1 and acan and delayed the differentiation of adult MSCs into chondrocytes (Figure 14.11). Similarly to chondrogenesis during embryonic development, SOX9 plays key roles in the early stage of chondrogenesis in adult MSCs [100].

14.4.4 In Vivo Fluorescence Imaging and Histological Evaluation

In vivo fluorescence imaging was performed to investigate the potential of QD-SMCC as a promising tool for real-time gene tracking. The significant bioluminescence of the transfected cells was also confirmed *in vivo*, whereas little to no signal above background was found in the rats that were injected with the unlabeled control cells (Figure 14.12a and b, P<0.05). The results [107] suggest that the QD-SMCC exhibited strong fluorescence and offer great potential for imaging and related biomedical applications because deep imaging within tissues has become possible by the introduction of advanced fluorescence microscopy. Based on macroscopic observations after the samples were harvested, severe synovitis, osteophyte formation, or infection was not observed (Figure 14.12c). Histological evaluation staining images of the repaired tissue in cartilage defects are shown in Figure 14.12d. The differences between the control, QD-SMCC, QD-SMCC-si, and PEI-si groups were not as significant as those observed at 2 weeks after surgery. In the QD-SMCC-si group, the surface was irregular and covered with thin, fibrin-like tissue.

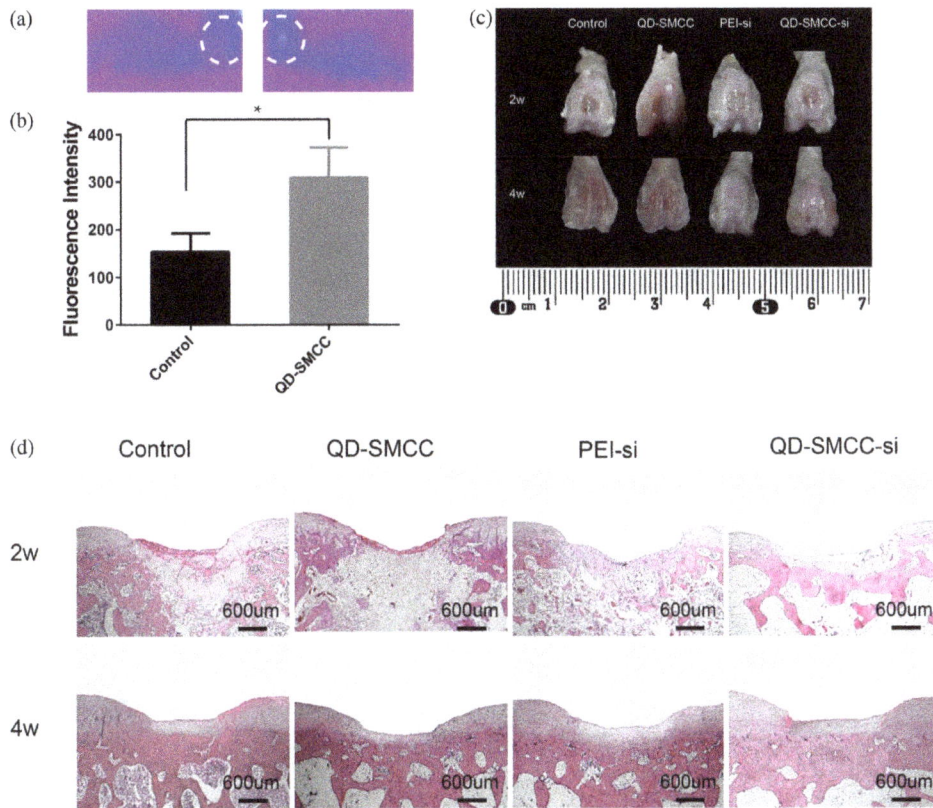

FIGURE 14.12 Macroscopic assessment, *in vivo* fluorescence images, and HE staining of the articular cartilage defects in rat models. (a) *In vivo* optical images and (b) quantitative analysis of the transfected cells. (c) Macroscopic assessment of the repaired tissue at the articular cartilage defects in rat models. (d) HE staining of the repaired tissue at the articular cartilage defect in rat models. * indicates P<0.05.

The histological findings showed that the QD-SMCC-si-transfected MSCs exhibited delayed cartilage regeneration compared with the control, as demonstrated by the presence of more fibrous tissue in the newly formed tissue that loosely interfaced with the surrounding tissue in the early stage (Figure 14.12). The PCR and WB results also agreed with the histological staining and showed a relative decrease in the expression of the cartilage-specific markers. We proved that the silencing of SOX9 delayed cartilage repair. Gene overexpression and knockdown provide useful tools for genetic functional analysis. Insights gained from experimental RNAi use may be useful in identifying potential therapeutic targets. Over time, the interference is weakened and eventually eliminated. The signal in the joint can be tracked using the bioconjugated QD-SMCC (Figure 14.12). The cationic surface of the QD-SMCC effectively binds the gene via bioconjugation, leading to efficient gene delivery *in vitro* and *in vivo* while maintaining the fluorescence properties and high biocompatibility of the QD-SMCC.

14.4.5 Silencing Efficiency of QD-SMCC-si and Suppression of SOX9 In Vivo

To investigate the expression of SOX9 in the cartilage defect model, we used immunohistochemical, RT-PCR and WB analyses. Two weeks after the operation, there was very

little SOX9 staining in the QD-SMCC-si and PEI-si groups. In contrast, there was SOX9-positive staining in the control and QD-SMCC groups (Figure 14.13a). The RT-PCR and WB results further verified that the expression of SOX9 was decreased in the QD-SMCC-si and PEI-si groups compared with that observed for the control and QD-SMCC groups (Figure 14.13b). The mRNA level of SOX9 decreased (0.49±0.07) for QD-SMCC transfected cells 2 weeks after operation (Figure 14.13b), and the WB result (0.55±0.08) was also consistent with the PCR results. The level of SOX9 mRNA and protein expression in MSCs was significantly lower following transfection with QD-SMCC compared with that of PEI. The expression level of SOX9 increased significantly from weeks 2 to 4 for the QD-SMCC and PEI groups during culture. Two weeks postoperatively, the inhibition of SOX9 clearly downregulated the expression of COL2A1 and ACAN protein (0.46±0.09 and 0.56±0.08) in the QD-SMCC-si group (Figure 14.13c).

We further studied the effect of SOX9 interference on neocartilage formation after implanting the MSCs into a cartilage defect model. Articular cartilage is an avascular tissue with very low cell density; it is therefore difficult for the QDs to be translocated to other organs. At first, no significant changes were detected in the tissues. However, QDs accumulated in the liver, kidney, spleen, blood, and bone marrow through time-dependent redistribution. Many

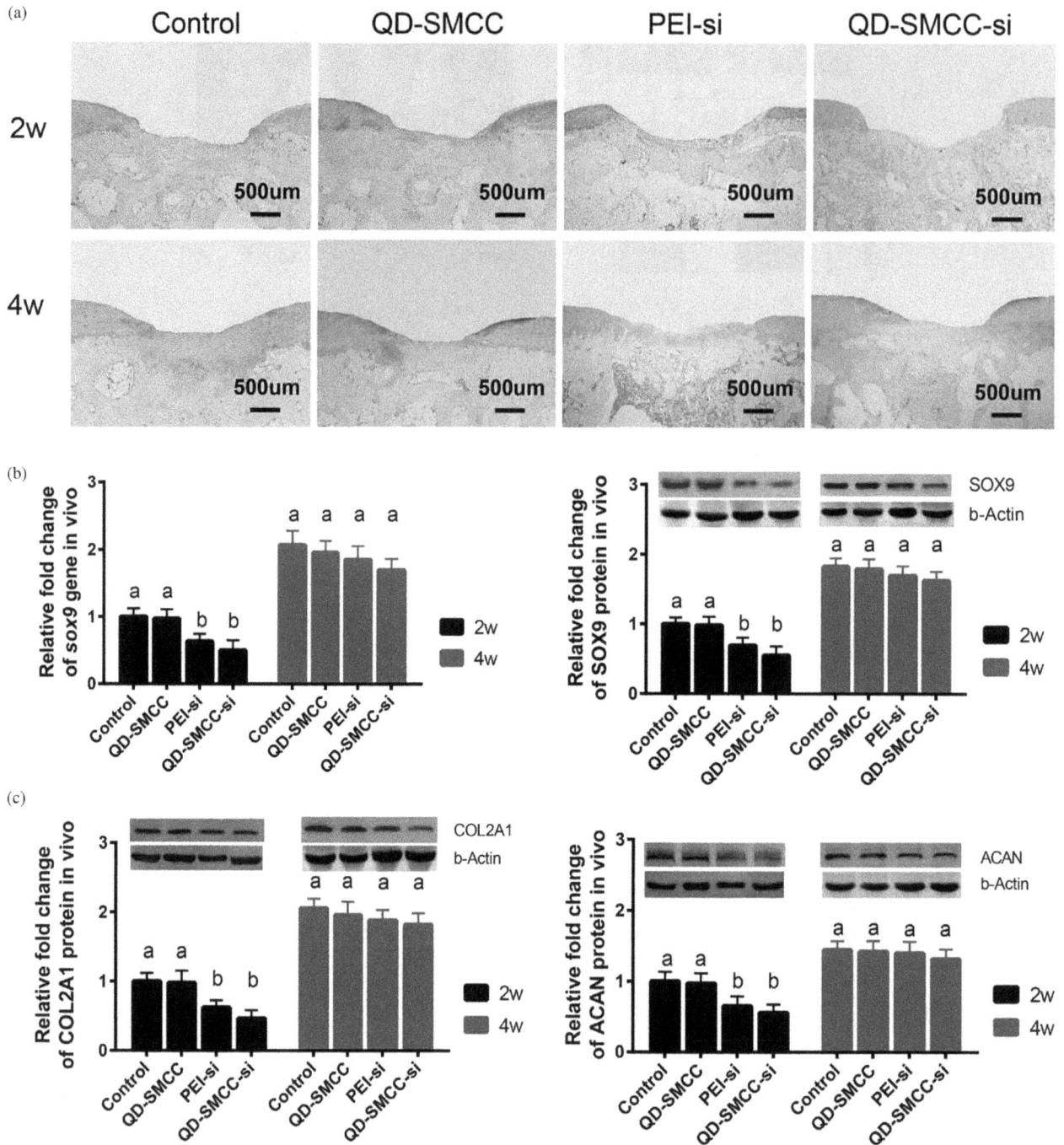

FIGURE 14.13 Sox9, col2a1, and acan expression in the rat cartilage defect sites. (a) Immunohistochemical staining for SOX9 in rat cartilage. (b) RT-PCR and Western blot analysis of the SOX9 levels in the MSCs following treatment with the different transfection reagents for 2 and 4 weeks. (c) COL2A1 and ACAN protein levels in the MSCs following treatment with different transfection reagents for 2 and 4 weeks. The bars with different letters are significantly different from each other at $P < 0.05$.

researchers are convinced that QDs will never be used in clinical practice because of their potential toxicity [123]. The perception that QDs are toxic is derived from *in vitro* studies indicating that cadmium can induce oxidative stress, DNA damage, and apoptosis. However, such a deduction is inappropriate because few toxicity tests based on cells can be adapted to more complex biosystems [123]. ZnS-capped CdSe QDs do not produce ROS, and the ZnS shell is effective in inhibiting the reactivity of QDs [124]. Hauck showed

that ZnS-capped CdSe QDs did no short-term (less than a week) or long-term (more than 80 days) harm on SD rats after implementing a pioneering and comprehensive *in vivo* toxicity test. Moreover, they detected no changes in the weight or behavior of the animals or hematological markers, in contrast to controls. Based on biochemical and histological analyses, no organic damage or inflammation was identified even though QDs or materials degraded from them were found in the kidney, spleen, and liver [125]. Because the amount and structure of nanoparticles [126–129] are in constant flux *in vivo*, only a small portion of injected nanoparticles will interact with cells. Parameters such as size and surface chemistry will be altered as nanoparticles travel through the human body. SOX9 plays an important role in the chondrogenesis of MSCs. The results also showed that transfection with QD-SMCC was superior to that with PEI at 2 weeks after the operation in an *in vivo* study (Figure 14.13). The silencing effect of QD-SMCC-si was confirmed with a single QD-SMCC to preclude the toxicity caused by the inhibition of cartilage repair. However, the delayed neocartilage formation was not as significant for the MSCs transfected with the QD-SMCC and PEI vehicles compared with the control after 4 weeks. The results indicated that nanoparticle-based transfection plays a role in the early stage of chondrogenesis. Unlike a virus vector, QD and PEI are transfection reagents for transient gene expression. In transient transfection, the introduced nucleic acid is inserted into the nucleus of the cell for a certain period and is not integrated into the genome. Transiently transfected siSOX9 is not passed from generation to generation during cell division, and it can be lost by environmental factors or diluted out during cell division.

14.5 CONCLUSIONS

In this chapter, an actively targeted nanocarrier was developed from two monodispersed components of cRGD-installed uPICs and 20-nm-sized AuNP for cancer-targeted systemic siRNA delivery. Uniform cRGD-installed uPICs were generated from a single pair of cRGD peptide-installed block copolymer and siRNA, which were further conjugated on the AuNP with additional short PEG chains to construct the size-regulated nanocarrier. The equipment of cRGD peptide on the surface of the well-defined nanocarrier was able to recognize $\alpha_v\beta_5$ integrin receptors on HeLa-luc cells, allowing the enhanced cellular internalization in cultured cells and higher accumulation of siRNA in the subcutaneous cervical tumor following systemic administration. Ultimately, the targeted nanocarrier induced more efficient E6 oncogene silencing in the cervical cancer model compared with non-targeted control, resulting in the significantly enhanced antitumor efficacy. This study highlights the potential utility of an actively targeted and size-regulated nanocarrier for cervical cancer treatment derived from the oncogene silencing.

In the current study, to formulate siRNA by reacting a DTNB-modified oligomer with a thiol-containing oligomer, we generated folate-bearing TCPs) for FR-directed siRNA delivery. TCP particles were spherical homogenous particles that exhibited compact siRNA binding activity and PEG-shielded nanoparticle surface. Thus, the development of therapeutic TCPs promises substantial FR-responsive tumor targeting and also reveals great potential for a safe and effective delivery system for RNAi-based cancer therapy.

In this study, we developed the nanomaterial QD-NH$_2$ with a fluorescent tracer function as a gene carrier to transfect siSOX9 into MSCs after SMCC activation. The results suggest that SOX9 is crucial for chondrogenic differentiation of MSCs, which may be a potential target for cartilage therapy. QD-SMCC is promising in gene delivery both *in vitro* and *in vivo*. We envision the application of QD-SMCC as imaging-trackable nanocarriers for safe and efficient gene delivery.

REFERENCES

1. Y. Yi, H.J. Kim, P. Mi, M. Zheng, H. Takemoto, K. Toh, B.S. Kim, K. Hayashi, M. Naito, Y. Matsumoto, K. Miyata, K. Kataoka, Targeted systemic delivery of siRNA to cervical cancer model using cyclic RGD-installed unimer polyion complex-assembled gold nanoparticles, *J. Control. Release* 244 (2016) 247–256.
2. S.M. Elbashir, J. Harborth, W. Lendeckel, A. Yalcin, K. Weber, T. Tuschl, Duplexes of 21-nucleotide RNAs mediate RNA interference in cultured mammalian cells, *Nature* 411 (2001) 494–498.
3. L. Aagaard, J.J. Rossi, RNAi therapeutics: principles, prospects and challenges, *Adv. Drug Deliv. Rev.* 59 (2007) 75–86.
4. P. Resnier, T. Montier, V. Mathieu, J.P. Benoit, C. Passirani, A review of the current status of siRNA nanomedicines in the treatment of cancer, *Biomaterials* 34 (2013) 6429–6443.
5. R.J. Christie, K.Miyata, Y. Matsumoto, T. Nomoto, D. Menasco, T.C. Lai, et al., Effect of polymer structure on micelles formed between siRNA and cationic block copolymer comprising thiols and amidines, *Biomacromolecules* 12 (2011) 3174–3185.
6. A. Falamarzian, X. Xiong, H. Uludag, A. Lavasanifar, Polymericmicelles for siRNA delivery, *J. Drug Deliv. Sci. Technol.* 22 (2012) 43–54.
7. X. Liu, C. Sun, X. Yang, J. Wang, Polymeric-micelle-based nanomedicine for siRNA delivery, *Part. Part. Syst. Charact.* 30 (2013) 211–228.
8. A.M. Jhaveri, V.P. Torchilin, Multifunctional polymeric micelles for delivery of drugs and siRNA, *Front. Pharmacol.* 5 (2014) 77.
9. Y.C. Tseng, S. Mozumdar, L. Huang, Lipid-based systemic delivery of siRNA, *Adv. Drug Deliv. Rev.* 61 (2009) 721–731.
10. A. Schroeder, C.G. Levins, C. Cortez, R. Langer, D.G. Anderson, Lipid-based nanotherapeutics for siRNA delivery, *J. Intern. Med.* 267 (2010) 9–21.
11. R. Kanasty, J.R. Dorkin, A. Vegas, D. Anderson, Delivery materials for siRNA therapeutics, *Nat. Mater.* 12 (2013) 967–977.
12. D.A. Giljohann, D.S. Seferos, A.E. Prigodich, P.C. Patel, C.A. Mirkin, Gene regulation with polyvalent siRNA-nanoparticle conjugates, *J. Am. Chem. Soc.* 131 (2009) 2072–2073.
13. A.K. Lytton-Jean, R. Langer, D.G. Anderson, Five years of siRNA delivery: spotlight on gold nanoparticles, *Small* 7 (2011) 1932–1937.
14. J.I. Cutler, E. Auyeung, C.A. Mirkin, Spherical nucleic acids, *J. Am. Chem. Soc.* 134 (2012) 1376–1391.
15. S.H. Ku, K. Kim, K. Choi, S.H. Kim, I.C. Kwon, Tumor-targeting multifunctional nanoparticles for siRNA delivery: recent advances in cancer therapy, *Adv. Healthc. Mater.* 3 (2014) 1182–1193.

16. F. Pittella, H. Cabral, Y. Maeda, P. Mi, S. Watanabe, H. Takemoto, et al., Systemic siRNA delivery to a spontaneous pancreatic tumor model in transgenic mice by PEGylated calcium phosphate hybridmicelles, *J. Control. Release* 178 (2014) 18–24.

17. J. Conde, A. Ambrosone, Y. Hernandez, F. Tian, M. McCully, C.C. Berry, et al., 15 Years on siRNA delivery: beyond the state-of-the-art on inorganic nanoparticles for RNAi therapeutics, *Nano Today* 10 (2015) 421–450.

18. A. Wittrup, J. Lieberman, Knocking down disease: a progress report on siRNA therapeutics, *Nat. Rev. Genet.* 16 (2015) 543–552.

19. Y. Matsumura, H. Maeda, A new concept for macromolecular therapeutics in cancer chemotherapy: mechanism of tumoritropic accumulation of proteins and the antitumor agent smancs, *Cancer Res.* 46 (1986) 6387–6392.

20. K. Kataoka, A. Harada, Y. Nagasaki, Block copolymer micelles for drug delivery: design, characterization and biological significance, *Adv. Drug Deliv. Rev.* 47 (2001) 113–131.

21. Y. Matsumura, K. Kataoka, Preclinical and clinical studies of anticancer agent-incorporating polymer micelles, *Cancer Sci.* 100 (2009) 572–579.

22. H. Cabral, Y. Matsumoto, K. Mizuno, Q. Chen, M. Murakami, M. Kimura, et al., Accumulation of sub-100 nm polymeric micelles in poorly permeable tumours depends on size, *Nat. Nanotechnol.* 6 (2011) 815–823.

23. L. Tang, X. Yang, Q. Yin, K. Cai, H. Wang, I. Chaudhury, et al., Investigating the optimal size of anticancer nanomedicine, *Proc. Natl. Acad. Sci. U. S. A.* 111 (2014) 15344–15349.

24. H. Cabral, J. Makino, Y.Matsumoto, P.Mi, H.Wu, T. Nomoto, et al., Systemic targeting of lymph node metastasis through the blood vascular system by using size-controlled nanocarriers, *ACS Nano* 9 (2015) 4957–4967.

25. Y. Anraku, A. Kishimura, Y. Yamasaki, K. Kataoka, Living unimodal growth of polyion complex vesicles via two-dimensional supramolecular polymerization, *J. Am. Chem. Soc.* 135 (2013) 1423–1429.

26. H.J. Kim, H. Takemoto, Y. Yi, M. Zheng, Y. Maeda, H. Chaya, et al., Precise engineering of siRNA delivery vehicles to tumors using polyion complexes and gold nanoparticles, *ACS Nano* 8 (2014) 8979–8991.

27. K. Hayashi, H. Chaya, S. Fukushima, S.Watanabe, H. Takemoto, K. Osada, et al., Influence of RNA strand rigidity on polyion complex formation with block catiomers, *Macromol. Rapid Commun.* 37 (2016) 486–493.

28. T.M. Allen, Ligand-targeted therapeutics in anticancer therapy, *Nat. Rev. Cancer* 2 (2002) 750–763.

29. O.C. Farokhzad, J. Cheng, B.A. Teply, I. Sherifi, S. Jon, P.W. Kantoff, et al., Targeted nanoparticle-aptamer bioconjugates for cancer chemotherapy in vivo, *Proc. Natl. Acad. Sci. U. S. A.* 103 (2006) 6315–6320.

30. V. Torchilin, Antibody-modified liposomes for cancer chemotherapy, *Expert Opin. Drug Deliv.* 5 (2008) 1003–1025.

31. N. Bertrand, J. Wu, X. Xu, N. Kamaly, O.C. Farokhzad, Cancer nanotechnology: the impact of passive and active targeting in the era of modern cancer biology, *Adv. Drug Deliv. Rev.* 66 (2014) 2–25.

32. F. Danhier, A. Le Breton, V. Preat, RGD-based strategies to target alpha(v) beta(3) integrin in cancer therapy and diagnosis, *Mol. Pharm.* 9 (2012) 2961–2973.

33. W. Arap, R. Pasqualini, E. Ruoslahti, Cancer treatment by targeted drug delivery to tumor vasculature in a mouse model, *Science* 279 (1998) 377–380.

34. R.M. Schiffelers, A. Ansari, J. Xu, Q. Zhou, Q. Tang, G. Storm, et al., Cancer siRNA therapy by tumor selective delivery with ligand-targeted sterically stabilized nanoparticle, *Nucleic Acids Res.* 32 (2004), e149.

35. R.J. Christie, Y. Matsumoto, K. Miyata, T. Nomoto, S. Fukushima, K. Osada, et al., Targeted polymeric micelles for siRNA treatment of experimental cancer by intravenous injection, *ACS Nano* 6 (2012) 5174–5189.

36. J. Doorbar, W. Quint, L. Banks, I.G. Bravo, M. Stoler, T.R. Broker, et al., The biology and life-cycle of human papillomaviruses, *Vaccine* 30S (2012) F55–F70.

37. H. Nishida, Y.Matsumoto, K. Kawana, R.J. Christie, M. Naito, B.S. Kim, Systemic delivery of siRNA by actively targeted polyion complex micelles for silencing the E6 and E7 human papillomavirus oncogenes, *J. Control. Release* 231 (2016) 29–37.

38. C.D. Walkey, J.B. Olsen, H. Guo, A. Emili, W.C. Chan, Nanoparticle size and surface chemistry determine serum protein adsorption and macrophage uptake, *J. Am. Chem. Soc.* 134 (2012) 2139–2147.

39. Q. Yang, S.W. Jones, C.L. Parker, W.C. Zamboni, J.E. Bear, S.K. Lai, Evading immune cell uptake and clearance requires PEG grafting at densities substantially exceeding the minimum for brush conformation, *Mol. Pharm.* 11 (2014) 1250–1258.

40. J.S. Suk, Q. Xu, N. Kim, J. Hanes, L.M. Ensign, PEGylation as a strategy for improving nanoparticle-based drug and gene delivery, *Adv. Drug Deliv. Rev.* 99 (2016) 28–51.

41. K. Uchida, H. Otsuka, M. Kaneko, K. Kataoka, Y. Nagasaki, A reactive poly(ethylene glycol) layer to achieve specific surface plasmon resonance sensing with a high S/N ratio: the substantial role of a short underbrushed PEG layer in minimizing nonspecific adsorption, *Anal. Chem.* 77 (2005) 1075–1080.

42. C.A. Simpson, A.C. Agrawal, A. Balinski, K.M. Harkness, D.E. Cliffel, Short-chain PEG mixed monolayer protected gold clusters increase clearance and red blood cell counts, *ACS Nano* 5 (2011) 3577–3584.

43. T. Ishii, K. Miyata, Y. Anraku, M. Naito, Y. Yi, T. Jinbo, et al., Enhanced target recognition of nanoparticles by cocktail PEGylation with chains of varying lengths, *Chem. Commun.* 52 (2016) 1517–1519.

44. R. Cheng, F. Feng, F. Meng, C. Deng, J. Feijen, Z. Zhong, Glutathione-responsive nanovehicles as a promising platform for targeted intracellular drug and gene delivery, *J. Control. Release* 152 (2011) 2–12.

45. M. Oba, S. Fukushima, N. Kanayama, K. Aoyagi, N. Nishiyama, H. Koyama, et al., Cyclic RGD peptide-conjugated polyplex micelles as a targetable gene delivery system directed to cells possessing alphavbeta3 and alphavbeta5 integrins, *Bioconjug. Chem.* 18 (2007) 1415–1423.

46. D.M. Shayakhmetov, A.M. Eberly, Z. Li, A. Lieber, Deletion of penton RGD motifs affects the efficiency of both the internalization and the endosome escape of viral particles containing adenovirus serotype 5 or 35 fiber knobs, *J. Virol.* 79 (2005) 1053–1061.

47. A.H.S. Hall, K.A. Alexander, RNA interference of human papillomavirus type 18 E6 and E7 induces senescence in HeLa cells, *J. Virol.* 77 (2003) 6066–6069.

48. P.J. Newman, The biology of PECAM-1, *J. Clin. Invest.* 99 (1997) 3–8.

49. W. Kawamura, Y. Miura, D. Kokuryo, K. Toh, N. Yamada, T. Nomoto, et al., Densitytunable conjugation of cyclic RGD ligands with polyion complex vesicles for the neovascular imaging of orthotopic glioblastomas, *Sci. Technol. Adv. Mater.* 16 (2015) 035004.

50. D.-J. Lee, D. He, E. Kessel, K. Padari, S. Kempter, U. Lächelt, J.O. Rädler, M. Pooga, E. Wagner. Tumoral gene silencing by receptor-targeted combinatorial siRNA polyplexes. *J. Control. Release* 244 (2016) 280–291.

51. K.A. Whitehead, R. Langer, D.G. Anderson, Knocking down barriers: advances in siRNA delivery, *Nat. Rev. Drug Discov.* 8 (2009) 129–138.

52. E. Wagner, Biomaterials in RNAi therapeutics: quo vadis? *Biomater. Sci.* 1 (2013) 804–809.

53. H. Maeda, T. Sawa, T. Konno, Mechanism of tumor-targeted delivery of macromolecular drugs, including the EPR effect in solid tumor and clinical overview of the prototype polymeric drug SMANCS, *J. Control. Release* 74 (2001) 47–61.

54. Q. Leng, A.J. Mixson, Small interfering RNA targeting Raf-1 inhibits tumor growth in vitro and in vivo, *Cancer Gene Ther.* 12 (2005) 682–690.

55. K.A. Howard, U.L. Rahbek, X. Liu, C.K. Damgaard, S.Z. Glud, M.O. Andersen, M.B. Hovgaard, A. Schmitz, J.R. Nyengaard, F. Besenbacher, J. Kjems, RNA interference in vitro and in vivo using a novel chitosan/siRNA nanoparticle system, *Mol. Ther.* 14 (2006) 476–484.

56. J. Hoon Jeong, L.V. Christensen, J.W. Yockman, Z. Zhong, J.F. Engbersen, W. Jong Kim, J. Feijen, S. Wan Kim, Reducible poly(amido ethylenimine) directed to enhance RNA interference, *Biomaterials* 28 (2007) 1912–1917.

57. M.E. Davis, The first targeted delivery of siRNA in humans via a self-assembling, cyclodextrin polymer-based nanoparticle: from concept to clinic, *Mol. Pharm.* 6 (2009) 659–668.

58. E. Wagner, Polymers for siRNA delivery: inspired by viruses to be targeted, dynamic, and precise, *Acc. Chem. Res.* 45 (2012) 1005–1013.

59. C. Troiber, D. Edinger, P. Kos, L. Schreiner, R. Kläger, A. Herrmann, E. Wagner, Stabilizing effect of tyrosine trimers on pDNA and siRNA polyplexes, *Biomaterials* 34 (2013) 1624–1633.

60. R.G. Parmar, M. Busuek, E.S. Walsh, K.R. Leander, B.J. Howell, L. Sepp-Lorenzino, E. Kemp, L.S. Crocker, A. Leone, C.J. Kochansky, B.A. Carr, R.M. Garbaccio, S.L. Colletti, W.Wang, Endosomolytic bioreducible poly(amido amine disulfide) polymer conjugates for the in vivo systemic delivery of siRNA therapeutics, *Bioconjug. Chem.* 24 (2013) 640–647.

61. D.J. Lee, E.Wagner, T. Lehto, Sequence-defined oligoaminoamides for the delivery of siRNAs, *Methods Mol. Biol.* 1206 (2015) 15–27.

62. S. Hobel, A. Aigner, Polyethylenimines for siRNA and miRNA delivery in vivo, *Wiley Interdiscip. Rev. Nanomed. Nanobiotechnol.* 5 (2013) 484–501.

63. D. He, E. Wagner, Defined polymeric materials for gene delivery, *Macromol. Biosci.* 15 (2015) 600–612.

64. L. Liu, M. Zheng, D. Librizzi, T. Renette, O.M. Merkel, T. Kissel, Efficient and tumor targeted siRNA delivery mediated by polyethylenimine-graft-polycaprolactoneblock-poly(ethylene glycol)-folate (PEI- PCL-PEG-Fol), *Mol. Pharm.* 13 (2016) 134–143.

65. P.M. Klein, K. Müller, C. Gutmann, P. Kos, A. Krhac Levacic, D. Edinger, M. Höhn, J.C. Leroux, M.A. Gauthier, E. Wagner, Twin disulfides as opportunity for improving stability and transfection efficiency of oligoaminoethane polyplexes, *J. Control. Release* 205 (2015) 109–119.

66. T. Lehto, E. Wagner, Sequence-defined polymers for the delivery of oligonucleotides, *Nanomedicine* 9 (2014) 2843–2859.

67. S. Zhang, D. Zhi, L. Huang, Lipid-based vectors for siRNA delivery, *J. Drug Target.* 20 (2012) 724–735.

68. Y. Sakurai, H. Hatakeyama, Y. Sato, M. Hyodo, H. Akita, H. Harashima, Gene silencing via RNAi and siRNA quantification in tumor tissue using MEND, a liposomal siRNA delivery system, *Mol. Ther.* 21 (2013) 1195–1203.

69. F. Tang, L. Li, D. Chen, Mesoporous silica nanoparticles: synthesis, biocompatibility and drug delivery, *Adv. Mater.* 24 (2012) 1504–1534.

70. K. Möller, K. Müller, H. Engelke, C. Bräuchle, E. Wagner, T. Bein, Highly efficient siRNA delivery from core-shellmesoporous silica nanoparticles with multifunctional polymer caps, *Nanoscale* 8 (2016) 4007–4019.

71. P. Heissig, P.M. Klein, P. Hadwiger, E. Wagner, DNA as tunable adaptor for siRNA polyplex stabilization and functionalization, *Mol. Ther. Nucleic Acids* 5 (2016) e288. doi:10.1038/mtna.2016.1036

72. D. Edinger, E. Wagner, Bioresponsive polymers for the delivery of therapeutic nucleic acids, *Wiley Interdiscip. Rev. Nanomed. Nanobiotechnol.* 3 (2011) 33–46.

73. O. Boussif, F. Lezoualc'h, M.A. Zanta, M.D. Mergny, D. Scherman, B. Demeneix, J.P. Behr, A versatile vector for gene and oligonucleotide transfer into cells in culture and in vivo: polyethylenimine, *Proc. Natl. Acad. Sci. U. S. A.* 92 (1995) 7297–7301.

74. D. Schaffert, N. Badgujar, E. Wagner, Novel Fmoc-polyamino acids for solid-phase synthesis of defined polyamidoamines, *Org. Lett.* 13 (2011) 1586–1589.

75. E.E. Salcher, P. Kos, T. Fröhlich, N. Badgujar, M. Scheible, E. Wagner, Sequence-defined four-arm oligo(ethanamino) amides for pDNA and siRNA delivery: impact of building blocks on efficacy, *J. Control. Release* 164 (2012) 380–386.

76. D. Schaffert, C. Troiber, E.E. Salcher, T. Fröhlich, I.Martin, N. Badgujar, C. Dohmen, D. Edinger, R. Kläger, G. Maiwald, K. Farkasova, S. Seeber, K. Jahn-Hofmann, P. Hadwiger, E. Wagner, Solid-phase synthesis of sequence-defined T-, i-, and U-shape polymers for pDNA and siRNA delivery, *Angew. Chem. Int. Ed.* 50 (2011) 8986–8989.

77. C. Scholz, P. Kos, E. Wagner, Comb-like oligoaminoethane carriers: change in topology improves pDNA delivery, *Bioconjug. Chem.* 25 (2014) 251–261.

78. U. Lächelt, P. Kos, F.M. Mickler, A. Herrmann, E.E. Salcher, W. Rödl, N. Badgujar, C. Bräuchle, E. Wagner, Fine-tuning of proton sponges by precise diaminoethanes and histidines in pDNA polyplexes, *Nanomedicine* 10 (2014) 35–44.

79. T. Fröhlich, D. Edinger, R. Kläger, C. Troiber, E. Salcher, N. Badgujar, I. Martin, D. Schaffert, A. Cengizeroglu, P. Hadwiger, H.P. Vornlocher, E.Wagner, Structure–activity relationships of siRNA carriers based on sequence-defined oligo (ethane amino) amides, *J. Control. Release* 160 (2012) 532–541.

80. P.M. Klein, E. Wagner, Bioreducible polycations as shuttles for therapeutic nucleic acid and protein transfection, *Antioxid. Redox Signal.* 21 (2014) 804–817.

81. C. Dohmen, D. Edinger, T. Fröhlich, L. Schreiner, U. Lächelt, C. Troiber, J. Rädler, P. Hadwiger, H.P. Vornlocher, E. Wagner, Nanosized multifunctional polyplexes for receptor- mediated siRNA delivery, *ACS Nano* 6 (2012) 5198–5208.

82. D.J. Lee, E. Kessel, D. Edinger, D. He, P.M. Klein, L. Voith von Voithenberg, D.C. Lamb, U. Lächelt, T. Lehto, E. Wagner, Dual antitumoral potency of EG5 siRNA nanoplexes armed with cytotoxic bifunctional glutamyl-methotrexate targeting ligand, *Biomaterials* 77 (2016) 98–110.

83. I. Martin, C. Dohmen, C. Mas-Moruno, C. Troiber, P. Kos, D. Schaffert, U. Lächelt, M. Teixido, M. Gunther, H. Kessler, E. Giralt, E. Wagner, Solid-phase-assisted synthesis of targeting peptide-PEG-oligo(ethane amino)amides for receptor-mediated gene delivery, *Org. Biomol. Chem.* 10 (2012) 3258–3268.

84. S. An, D. He, E. Wagner, C. Jiang, Peptide-like polymers exerting effective gliomatargeted siRNA delivery and release for therapeutic application, *Small* 11 (2015) 5142–5150.

85. P. Kos, U. Lächelt, D. He, Y. Nie, Z. Gu, E. Wagner, Dual-targeted polyplexes based on sequence-defined peptide-PEG-oligoamino amides, *J. Pharm. Sci.* 104 (2015) 464–475.

86. P. Kos, U. Lächelt, A. Herrmann, F.M.Mickler, M. Döblinger, D. He, A. Krhac Levacic, S. Morys, C. Bräuchle, E. Wagner, Histidine-rich stabilized polyplexes for cMet-directed tumor-targeted gene transfer, *Nanoscale* 7 (2015) 5350–5362.

87. W. Zhang, W. Rödl, D. He, M. Döblinger, U. Lächelt, E. Wagner, Combination of sequence- defined oligoamino-amides with transferrin-polycation conjugates for receptor-targeted gene delivery, *J. Gene Med.* 17 (2015) 161–172.

88. W. Zhang, K. Müller, E. Kessel, S. Reinhard, D. He, P.M. Klein, M. Höhn, W. Rödl, S. Kempter, E. Wagner, Targeted siRNA delivery using a lipo-oligoaminoamide nanocore with an influenza peptide and transferrin shell, *Adv. Healthc. Mater.* (2016). doi:10.1002/adhm.201600057

89. D.He, K.Müller, A.Krhac Levacic, P.Kos, U.Lächelt, E.Wagner, Combinatorial optimization of sequence-defined oligo(ethanamino)amides for folate receptor targeted pDNA and siRNA delivery, *Bioconjug. Chem.* 27 (3) (2016) 647–659. doi:10.1021/acs.bioconjchem.5b00649

90. D. Edinger, R. Kläger, C. Troiber, C. Dohmen, E. Wagner, Gene silencing and antitumoral effects of Eg5 or Ran siRNA oligoaminoamide polyplexes, *Drug Deliv. Transl. Res.* 4 (2014) 84–95.

91. W. Bi, J.M. Deng, Z. Zhang, R.R. Behringer, B. de Crombrugghe, Sox9 is required for cartilage formation, *Nat. Genet.* 22 (1) (1999) 85–89.

92. I. Sekiya, K. Tsuji, P. Koopman, H. Watanabe, Y. Yamada, K. Shinomiya, A. Nifuji, M. Noda, SOX9 enhances aggrecan gene promoter/enhancer activity and is upregulated by retinoic acid in a cartilage-derived cell line, TC6, *J. Biol. Chem.* 275 (15) (2000) 10738–10744.

93. L.J. Ng, S. Wheatley, G.E. Muscat, J. Conway-Campbell, J. Bowles, E. Wright, D.M. Bell, P.P. Tam, K.S. Cheah, P. Koopman, SOX9 binds DNA, activates transcription, and coexpresses with type II collagen during chondrogenesis in the mouse, *Dev. Biol.* 183 (1) (1997) 108–121.

94. W.B. Tan, S. Jiang, Y. Zhang, Quantum-dot based nanoparticles for targeted silencing of HER2/neu gene via RNA interference, *Biomaterials* 28 (8) (2007) 1565–1571.

95. T.H. Hutson, E. Foster, L.D. Moon, R.J. Yanez-Munoz, Lentiviral vector-mediated RNA silencing in the central nervous system, *Hum. Gene Ther. Methods* 25 (1) (2014) 14–32.

96. B.L. Davidson, P.B. McCray Jr., Current prospects for RNA interference-based therapies, *Nat. Rev. Genet.* 12 (5) (2011) 329–340.

97. L. Qi, X. Gao, Quantum dot-amphipol nanocomplex for intracellular delivery and real-time imaging of siRNA, *ACS Nano* 2 (7) (2008) 1403–1410.

98. J.H. Kim, J.S. Park, H.N. Yang, D.G. Woo, S.Y. Jeon, H.J. Do, H.Y. Lim, J.M. Kim, K.H. Park, The use of biodegradable PLGA nanoparticles to mediate SOX9 gene delivery in human mesenchymal stem cells (hMSCs) and induce chondrogenesis, *Biomaterials* 32 (1) (2011) 268–278.

99. K. Ma, D.D. Wang, Y. Lin, J. Wang, V. Petrenko, C. Mao, Synergetic targeted delivery of sleeping-beauty transposon system to mesenchymal stem cells using LPD nanoparticles modified with a phage-displayed targeting peptide, *Adv. Funct. Mater.* 23 (9) (2013) 1172–1181.

100. S.Y. Jeon, J.S. Park, H.N. Yang, H.J. Lim, S.W. Yi, H. Park, K.H. Park, Co-delivery of Cbfa-1-targeting siRNA and SOX9 protein using PLGA nanoparticles to induce chondrogenesis of human mesenchymal stem cells, *Biomaterials* 35 (28) (2014) 8236–8248.

101. G. Xu, K.T. Yong, I. Roy, S.D. Mahajan, H. Ding, S.A. Schwartz, P.N. Prasad, Bioconjugated quantum rods as targeted probes for efficient transmigration across an in vitro blood-brain barrier, *Bioconjug. Chem.* 19 (6) (2008) 1179–1185.

102. D. Painuly, A. Bhatt, V.K. Krishnan, Physicochemical and in vitro biocompatibility evaluation of water-soluble CdSe/ZnS core/shell, *J. Biomater. Appl.* 28 (8) (2014) 1125–1137.

103. L. Ju, G. Zhang, C. Zhang, L. Sun, Y. Jiang, C. Yan, P.J. Duerksen-Hughes, X. Zhang, X. Zhu, F.F. Chen, J. Yang, Quantum dot-related genotoxicity perturbation can be attenuated by PEG encapsulation, *Mutat. Res.* 753 (1) (2013) 54–64.

104. A.A. Chen, A.M. Derfus, S.R. Khetani, S.N. Bhatia, Quantum dots to monitor RNAi delivery and improve gene silencing, *Nucleic Acids Res.* 33 (22) (2005) e190.

105. M. Pereira, E.P. Lai, Capillary electrophoresis for the characterization of quantum dots after non-selective or selective bioconjugation with antibodies for immunoassay, *J. Nanobiotechnol.* 6 (2008) 10.

106. Y. Xing, Q. Chaudry, C. Shen, K.Y. Kong, H.E. Zhau, L.W. Chung, J.A. Petros, R.M. O'Regan, M.V. Yezhelyev, J.W. Simons, M.D. Wang, S. Nie, Bioconjugated quantum dots for multiplexed and quantitative immunohistochemistry, *Nat. Protoc.* 2 (5) (2007) 1152–1165.

107. Y. Wu, B. Zhou, F. Xu, X. Wang, G. Liu, L. Zheng, J. Zhao, X. Zhang, Functional quantum dot-siRNA nanoplexes to regulate chondrogenic differentiation of mesenchymal stem cells. *Acta Biomaterialia* 46 (2016) 165–176.

108. X. Gao, Y. Cui, R.M. Levenson, L.W. Chung, S. Nie, In vivo cancer targeting and imaging with semiconductor quantum dots, *Nat. Biotechnol.* 22 (8) (2004) 969–976.

109. J.S. Lee, J.J. Green, K.T. Love, J. Sunshine, R. Langer, D.G. Anderson, Gold, poly (beta-amino ester) nanoparticles for small interfering RNA delivery, *Nano Lett.* 9 (6) (2009) 2402–2406.

110. X.Y. Wu, H.J. Liu, J.Q. Liu, K.N. Haley, J.A. Treadway, J.P. Larson, N.F. Ge, F. Peale, M.P. Bruchez, Immunofluorescent labeling of cancer marker Her2 and other cellular targets with semiconductor quantum dots, *Nat. Biotechnol.* 21 (1) (2003) 41–46.

111. S.L.Li, Z.H.Liu, F.T.Ji, Z.J.Xiao, M.J.Wang, Y.J.Peng, Y.L.Zhang, L.Liu, Z.B.Liang, F.Li, Delivery of quantum dot-siRNA nanoplexes in SK-N-SH cells for BACE1 gene silencing and intracellular imaging, *Mol. Ther.Nucl.Acids.* 1 (2012) e20. doi:10.1038/mtna.2012.11

112. H.N. Yang, J.S. Park, S.Y. Jeon, W. Park, K. Na, K.H. Park, The effect of quantum dot size and poly(ethylenimine) coating on the efficiency of gene delivery into human mesenchymal stem cells, *Biomaterials* 35 (29) (2014) 8439–8449.

113. P. van de Wetering, E.E. Moret, N.M. Schuurmans-Nieuwenbroek, M.J. van Steenbergen, W.E. Hennink, Structure-activity relationships of water-soluble cationic methacrylate/methacrylamide polymers for nonviral gene delivery, *Bioconjug. Chem.* 10 (4) (1999) 589–597.

114. J. Lovric, H.S. Bazzi, Y. Cuie, G.R. Fortin, F.M. Winnik, D. Maysinger, Differences in subcellular distribution and toxicity of green and red emitting CdTe quantum dots, *J. Mol. Med.* 83 (5) (2005) 377–385.

115. A. Shiohara, A. Hoshino, K. Hanaki, K. Suzuki, K. Yamamoto, On the cytotoxicity caused by quantum dots, *Microbiol. Immunol.* 48 (9) (2004) 669–675.

116. X. Jiang, C. Rocker, M. Hafner, S. Brandholt, R.M. Dorlich, G.U. Nienhaus, Endoand exocytosis of zwitterionic quantum dot nanoparticles by live HeLa cells, *ACS Nano* 4 (11) (2010) 6787–6797.

117. S. Ohta, S. Inasawa, Y. Yamaguchi, Real time observation and kinetic modeling of the cellular uptake and removal of silicon quantum dots, *Biomaterials* 33 (18) (2012) 4639–4645.

118. B.D. Chithrani, W.C. Chan, Elucidating the mechanism of cellular uptake and removal of protein-coated gold nanoparticles of different sizes and shapes, *Nano Lett.* 7 (6) (2007) 1542–1550.

119. B. Sarkadi, C. Ozvegy-Laczka, K. Nemet, A. Varadi, ABCG2 – a transporter for all seasons, *FEBS Lett.* 567 (1) (2004) 116–120.

120. S.H. Oh, S.C. Lim, A rapid and transient ROS generation by cadmium triggers apoptosis via caspase-dependent pathway in HepG2 cells and this is inhibited through N-acetylcysteine-mediated catalase upregulation, *Toxicol. Appl. Pharmacol.* 212 (3) (2006) 212–223.

121. L. Peng, M. He, B. Chen, Q. Wu, Z. Zhang, D. Pang, Y. Zhu, B. Hu, Cellular uptake, elimination and toxicity of CdSe/ZnS quantum dots in HepG2 cells, *Biomaterials* 34 (37) (2013) 9545–9558.

122. V. Valdiglesias, E. Pasaro, J. Mendez, B. Laffon, In vitro evaluation of selenium genotoxic, cytotoxic, and protective effects: a review, *Arch. Toxicol.* 84 (5) (2010) 337–351.

123. K.M. Tsoi, Q. Dai, B.A. Alman, W.C. Chan, Are quantum dots toxic? Exploring the discrepancy between cell culture and animal studies, *Acc. Chem. Res.* 46 (3) (2013) 662–671.

124. B.I. Ipe, M. Lehnig, C.M. Niemeyer, On the generation of free radical species from quantum dots, *Small* 1 (7) (2005) 706–709.

125. T.S. Hauck, R.E. Anderson, H.C. Fischer, S. Newbigging, W.C. Chan, In vivo quantum-dot toxicity assessment, *Small* 6 (1) (2010) 138–144.

126. Loutfy H. Madkour, *Reactive Oxygen Species (ROS), Nanoparticles, and Endoplasmic Reticulum (ER) Stress-Induced Cell Death Mechanisms* (2020). Paperback ISBN: 9780128224816 Imprint: Academic Press. Published Date: 1st August 2020. https://www.elsevier.com/books/reactive-oxygen-species-ros-nanoparticles-and-endoplasmic-reticulum-er-stress-induced-cell-death-mechanisms/madkour/978-0-12-822481-6

127. Loutfy H. Madkour, *Nanoparticles Induce Oxidative and Endoplasmic Reticulum Antioxidant Therapeutic Defenses* (2020). Copyright 2020 Publisher Springer International Publishing Copyright Holder Springer Nature Switzerland AG eBook ISBN 978-3-030-37297-2. doi:10.1007/978-3-030-37297-2. Hardcover ISBN 978-3-030-37296-5. Series ISSN 2194-0452. Edition Number 1. https://www.springer.com/gp/book/9783030372965?utm_campaign=3_pier05_buy_print&utm_content=en_08082017&utm_medium=referral&utm_source=google_books#otherversion=9783030372972

128. Loutfy H. Madkour, *Nucleic Acids as Gene Anticancer Drug Delivery Therapy.* 1st Edition. Publishing House: Elsevier (2020). Paperback ISBN: 9780128197776. Imprint: Academic Press Published Date: 2nd January 2020 Imprint: Academic Press Copyright: Paperback ISBN: 9780128197776. © Academic Press 2020 Published: 2nd January 2020. Imprint: Academic Press Paperback ISBN: 9780128197776. https://www.elsevier.com/books/nucleic-acids-as-gene-anticancer-drug-delivery therapy/madkour/978-0-12-819777-6

129. Loutfy H. Madkour, *Nanoelectronic Materials: Fundamentals and Applications (Advanced Structured Materials)* 1st Edition. 2019 Edition. https://link.springer.com/book/10.1007%2F978-3-030-21621-4. Series Title: Advanced Structured Materials Series Volume 116. Copyright 2019 Publisher. Springer International Publishing Copyright Holder Springer Nature Switzerland AG. eBook ISBN 978-3-030-21621-4. doi:10.1007/978-3-030-21621-4. Hardcover ISBN 978-3-030-21620-7. Series ISSN 1869-8433. Edition Number 1. Number of Pages XLIII, 783 Number of Illustrations 122 b/w illustrations, 494 illustrations in colour Topics. ISBN-10: 3030216209. ISBN-13: 978-3030216207 #117 in Nanotechnology (Books) #725 in Materials Science (Books) #187336 in Textbooks. https://books.google.com.eg/books/about/Nanoelectronic_Materials.html?id=YQXCxAEACAAJ&source=kp_book_description&redir_esc=y. https://www.springer.com/gp/book/9783030216207

15 Recent Advances of Nanotechnologies for Cancer Immunotherapy Treatment

15.1 BASICS OF IMMUNOTHERAPY AND THE TUMOR MICROENVIRONMENT

Cancer can be regarded as a genetic disease that involves genes with key roles in cell proliferation and differentiation, which gives the cells ability to proliferate out of control and invade regional or distant regions [1] The immune system is also responsible for recognizing and destroying the aberrant cells and prevents the occurrence or development of cancer, which requires the immune cells to have the ability to effectively recognize cancer versus normal cells [2,3]. Mature T lymphocytes and B lymphocytes are actually the remaining cells that have passed the negative clonal selection during their development in thymus and bone marrow, in which lymphocytes expressing high-affinity antigen receptors to self-antigens are eliminated. Although the negative clonal selection process reduces the harm of autoimmunity to the body, it also eliminates the cell clones having the specificity that could potentially target and resist cancer cells. As a result, the minority proteins encoded by chromosomal aberrations or synthesized through altered posttranslational modifications that are exclusively to tumor cells, also named tumor-associated antigens (TAAs), have become the crucial subject for immune cells to recognize cancer cells [4,5]. In some cases, the immunogenic TAAs could be normal self-proteins that are not expressed in differentiated cells or only expressed at a low level, but expressed or overexpressed in cancer cells.

Cancer is the leading cause of premature death worldwide. Although the standard treatments for cancer are chemotherapy, radiation therapy, and surgery, there remains a strong need for a safer and efficacious treatment to improve patient survival and quality of life [6]. It has been demonstrated that the immune system plays a significant role in tumor suppression by inducing apoptosis and phagocytosis of tumor cells. In contrast, the immune system can also facilitate tumor proliferation, vascularization, metastasis, and invasion [7–9]. Therefore, cancer immunotherapy that involves new medications and treatment strategies to provoke the immune system against tumors is attractive and anticipated to improve upon the current cancer therapy.

Cancer immunotherapy is the treatment method that utilizes the host's immune system to fight against tumor cells [10,11]. It has gained increasing interest in clinical trials due to its durable efficacy and low toxicity compared to the traditional antitumor treatments, such as chemotherapy and radiotherapy. Cancer immunotherapy can be categorized into passive and active immunotherapy. Passive immunotherapy refers to the treatment that enhances existing antitumor responses by using monoclonal antibodies, cytokines, and lymphocytes. Active immunotherapy is attributed to the stimulation of immune system to kill tumor cells through targeting TAAs, including tumor vaccines and cell therapy. Moreover, both approaches can be either specific or nonspecific immunotherapy. Among these strategies, antibody therapy is the most effective and successful treatment applied in a variety of cancers, especially solid tumors [12]. More importantly, the emergence of ICB antibodies provides new insight into cancer immunotherapy in recent years.

The immune system acts as the "police force" to protect the organism from foreign invaders including bacteria, germs, viruses, and parasites. The recognition and eradication of the foreign invaders rely on precise cooperation of two components of the immune system: the innate and adaptive immunity. The innate immunity acts as the first line of defense through rapid activation of granulocytes (neutrophils, basophils, eosinophils, and mastocytes) and phagocytes (macrophagocytes and dendritic cells), which recognize general molecular patterns on pathogens or danger signals derived from inflammation, infection, and tissue damage [13,14]. The adaptive immunity functions by recognizing specific antigens (specificity) instead of the general molecular patterns, and it is capable of responding rapidly to pathogens or antigens it has encountered before (memory) [15]. These characteristics are implemented by random rearrangement of massive sequences in gene cassettes encoding the antigen recognition receptor complex that is located on the surface of lymphocytes. Huge variations of T-cell and B-cell receptors (TCR and BCR) for antigens with theoretically limitless specificities of T cells and B cells can be generated by this random rearrangement. The immune system launches a series of essential activities after the initial encounter with pathogens, which include rapid recruitment of non-antigen-specific innate immune cells, activation of humoral immune responses, pathogen processing and presentation by antigen-presenting cells (APCs) to T-cell and B-cell lymphocytes, followed by a more time-consuming and elaborate activation and expansion of antigen-specific lymphocytes, and finally lead to clearance of pathogens [16,17]. The sequential implementation of the innate and adaptive immunity could also leave pools of longeval memory lymphocytes that are specific to the invading antigen that can respond much quicker at the subsequent encounters with the same pathogen.

DOI: 10.1201/9781003229674-15

Immune checkpoints are crucial for maintaining immune homeostasis and preventing autoimmunity as they are regulators of immune system. However, increasing research has identified that in various types of cancer, the intrinsic mechanisms of immune checkpoint are overactivated resulting in escaping immune surveillance on tumor cells. Owning to the overactivation of immune checkpoint, a majority of effector T cells would differentiate into exhausted T cells at late stage of diseases. The inhibitory receptors are normally overexpressed on exhausted T cells, and effector cytokines' secretion is also decreased [18]. Thus, it is vital to recover T cells' effector function and reverse immunosuppressive tumor microenvironment to improve potent antitumor immunity. In many preclinical trials, it has been demonstrated that immune checkpoint inhibitors could release inhibitory mechanisms of T-cell-mediated immunity and promote CTL responses [19]. Immune checkpoint inhibitors, including cytotoxic T-lymphocyte antigen-4 (CTLA-4), programmed cell death protein 1 (PD-1)/programmed cell death-ligand 1 (PD-L1) axis, indoleamine 2,3-dioxygenase (IDO), cluster of differentiation 47 (CD47), cluster of differentiation 40 (CD40), and 4-1BB (CD137), are at the forefront of immunotherapy for a variety of cancers. The expression patterns, intrinsic signaling pathways, and mechanisms of these immune checkpoint inhibitors are quite different from each other despite of some commonalities. The two major kinds of antibodies, CTLA-4 and PD-1/PD-L1 axis, have exhibited significant clinical successes and provided great potential in cancer immunotherapy [20,21].

Rapid growth of tumors is often accompanied by vast tumor cell death due to hypoxia or accumulation of gene mutation, which will lead to the release of damage-associated molecular patterns (DAMPs) and TAAs [22]. The DAMPs can stimulate and recruit phagocytes and APCs, which process and present TAA-derived peptides to tumor-specific lymphocytes through the major histocompatibility complex (MHC). The activated CD8+ cytotoxic T lymphocytes specifically recognize and eliminate the cancer cells through TCR-mediated recognition of TAA epitopes displayed by tumor MHC-I molecules or through the combination of the NKG2D receptor on CD8+ cytotoxic T-lymphocytes and NKG2D ligands expressed on tumor cells. Activated CD4+ T-lymphocytes generate cytokines including tumor necrosis factor (TNF)-α and interferon-γ that are able to inhibit tumor growth while also upregulating MHC-I expression on tumor cells, thus assisting the target recognition by TAA-specific CD-8+ T-lymphocytes [23,24] (Figure 15.1).

Immune system activation toward cancer cells leads to a competition wherein immune cells inhibit fast cellular proliferation and mutation fosters tumor growth, but the formation

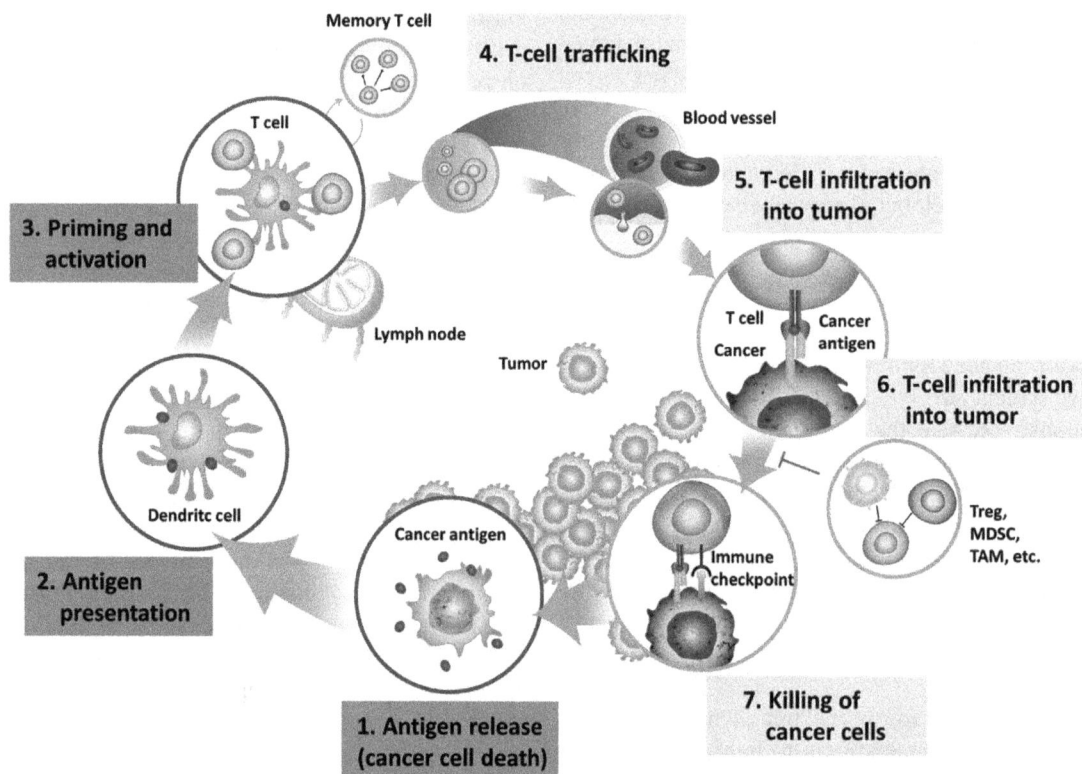

FIGURE 15.1 The cancer-immunity cycle that involves exposure or release of tumor antigens, tumor antigen processing and presentation by APCs, priming and activation of effective immune cells and formation of memory cells, trafficking and infiltration of T cells to tumor tissues, and the recognition and killing of tumor cells. (Reprinted from Ref. [5], Copyright (2019), with permission from Elsevier.)

of a detectable tumor is often the result of the failure of body immunity to tumor cells. If the immunity could not eradicate all the tumor cells at the beginning, it usually forms a selective force to tumor cell clones that can alter the composition of tumors and gradually leave and promote the growth of tumor cell clones with the least immunogenicity. Ultimately, the immunoediting effect often gives rise to the most invasive and uncontrolled tumors formed by the most insensitive cells [25]. Tumor cells have several mechanisms that assist in evading from being detected and eliminated by the immune system:

(1) Downregulation of MHC-I on tumor cells as a consequence of mutations of MHC genes or molecules involved in TAA antigen processing and presentation can reduce immunogenicity of tumor cells and evade cytotoxic T-lymphocyte-mediated lysis [26].

(2) Tumor cells could suppress immunity by expressing programmed death-ligand 1 (PD-L1) that binds to the negative costimulator programmed death (PD)-1 on lymphocyte's membrane, or by secreting immunosuppression cytokines that suppress the activation and differentiation of APCs and lymphocytes, such as transforming growth factor (TGF)-β [27,28].

(3) Tumor cells could resist cytotoxic T-lymphocyte-mediated killing effects by expressing granzyme serine proteases to inhibit the perforin/granzyme pathway that mediates tumor cell lysis, and decoy receptors for cell death including soluble Fas, osteoprotegerin, and decoy receptor-3, 4. In addition, increased expression of oncogenic and antiapoptotic molecules such as the signal transducer and activator of transcription 3 and B-cell lymphoma 2 (Bcl2) also resists T-lymphocyte-mediated lysis [29].

(4) Immunoregulatory cells with immunosuppressive effects, such as myeloid-derived suppressor cells and M2-type tumor-associated macrophages, could be recruited by tumor cells in the tumor microenvironment, which could produce immunosuppressive cytokines and also secrete the vascular endothelial growth factor and matrix metalloproteinases that favor tumor angiogenesis for tumor growth and invasion [30,31].

(5) A physical barrier around the tumor could be generated by tumor cells through secreting a series of molecules such as collagen, thus forming an immune privilege area and preventing the lymphocytes and APCs from entering the tumor area [32].

15.1.1 Nanotechnology in Cancer Immunotherapy

Recent years have witnessed the rise of nanotechnology as a solution to improve these technical weaknesses due to its inherent biophysical properties and multifunctional modifying potential. Nanotechnology has emerged as powerful weapon to promote multidisciplinary corporation [33].

It has been demonstrated that poly(lactic-cohydroxymethyl-glycolic-acid)polymeric particles could be engineered to load antibody with high efficiency and the antibody could be released in different kinetics [34]. It has exhibited many advantages, such as protecting the payload from degradation *in vivo*, realizing the controlled release of contents, prolonging the therapeutic effect, enhancing the targeting delivery, and reducing the side effects. [35]. Increasing evidences have shown that the incorporation of nanoparticle delivery system into immunotherapy could improve the accumulation and retention of antibodies in the target cells [36]. The encapsulation of immune checkpoint inhibitors into nanoparticles could not only elevate the immunotherapeutic responses but also decrease off-target effects [37]. Furthermore, nanoparticles are identified to be a versatile delivery platform that could encapsulate vaccine or drugs for chemotherapy, photothermal therapy, and so on. Combining immune checkpoint inhibitors with nanoparticles encapsulating different kinds of drugs could significantly enhance the antitumor effect compared to immune checkpoint antibody alone [38]. Strikingly, nanoparticles can also act as a nonviral gene delivery system. Targeting delivery of siRNA to the immune inhibitory pathways could also efficiently boost antitumor immune responses compared to antibodies, and the side effects could be reduced to some extent [39]. Therefore, the incorporation of nanoparticle delivery system with cancer immune checkpoint therapy could provide a promising strategy for antitumor treatment.

On the basis of the above mechanisms, numerous novel molecular drugs aiming to enhance immunity against tumor cells have been rising in the past decade and exhibited considerable progress in both lab experiments and clinical treatments [40–42]. However, only a limited portion of the immunotherapeutic molecules could encounter and interact with the targets, as the majority will be eliminated by renal clearance, impeded by metabolism during the blood circulation or cannot penetrate biological barriers and successfully reach the target site [43,44]. Under the circumstance, nanoparticles are utilized as suitable vehicles for immunotherapeutic molecules to counteract the pharmacokinetic shortages. Due to their inherent properties, nanoparticles could passively enrich within tumor tissue because of the immature tumor vasculature and damaged lymphatic drainage, which is also known as the enhanced permeation and retention (EPR) effect [45]. The first-generation nanoparticles principally depended on the EPR effect to enrich in tumor tissues, but the treatment effects varied among different types of cancer mainly because of variances in the tumor vascular structure and permeability [46]. Similarly, effects of the passive enriched nanoparticles on metastatic tumor lesions were often insufficient also due to the different vascular beds of metastatic lesions [47]. To overcome this limitation, positive target ability is equipped through modification of the nanoparticles with tumor-specific antibodies, and cellular uptake is also intensified, thus enhancing treatment efficacy and lowering off-target side effects [48].

Appropriate selection and construction of the nanoparticle structure in the aspects of size, shape, coated ligands, loading method, zeta potential, hydrophilicity, elasticity, and biocompatibility lead to suitable nano-vehicles for immunotherapeutic molecules, which generally ought to have a prolonged biological half-life period, protect payloads during circulation, penetrate through barriers or have target effects, controllably release payloads under specific microenvironments, and have low biotoxicity. Nanoparticles less than 5nm in diameter tend to be excreted through renal filtration, and nanoparticles with diameter larger than 200nm could be rapidly eliminated in spleen due to the size of inter-endothelial slits; [49] thus, the diameter in the range from 5 to 200nm is the optimal size for nanoparticles. The shape of nanoparticles should also be elaborated as different shapes process different characteristics. For instance, worm-like nanoparticles exhibit preferable fluid dynamics compared with rod-shaped, fingerprint-shaped, or spherical nanoparticles; [50] spherical nanoparticles are less likely to be accumulated in spleen, but flat cylindrical nanoparticles had the most retention in the liver, lung, and spleen organs [51]. Nanoparticles with slight negative charge had significantly lower retention in organs and had a prolonged circulation half-life time, but positive surface charge could assist the adherence to the anionic cellular membrane and is more advantageous in inducing cellular internalization [52,53]. Structural stability in blood circulation is another critical aspect, which is needed to exercise caution especially for nanoparticles like polymeric micelles, as they are often not able to maintain the structural integrity well in the rapid bloodstream and will cause declines in delivery efficiency [54]. Special designs including intensified structure stability or the environment-triggered releasing strategy are needed for these nanoparticles to achieve preferable transportation ability. Collectively, appropriate design of nanoparticles in accordance with the experimental purposes facilitates in optimizing the delivery efficiency and therapeutic effects of payloads.

Nanoparticles have been widely researched to be incorporated into tumor immunotherapy in recent years based on their inherent biophysical properties and multitudinous modifying potential, with tremendous progress made in preclinical and clinical trials. However, there are few reviews summarizing the advances in the fast-updating research area. In this chapter, we summarized and discussed the current status of nanoparticle-enhanced cancer immunotherapy strategies in the aspects of intensified delivery of tumor vaccines and immune adjuvants, ICI vehicles, targeting capacity to tumor-draining lymph nodes and immune cells, triggered releasing and regulating specific tumor microenvironments, and adoptive cell therapy enhancement effects.

15.2 DELIVERY OF TUMOR VACCINES BY NANOPARTICLES FOR TUMOR IMMUNOTHERAPY

Immune escape is often caused by the loss of valid TAA processing and presentation by immune cells; hence, the additional provision of specific tumor antigens to immune cells could stimulate and enhance the antitumor immune process [55,56]. Traditionally, most of the antigens are purified cytomembrane proteins, peptides, polysaccharides, or the DNA or RNA encoding these tumor antigens, which have medium reactogenicity but generally weak immunogenicity due to insufficient exogenous immune-provoking components. The emergence of whole-cell antitumor vaccines not only imported multiple tumor-specific antigens but also enhanced the antitumor immunoreaction. Accompanied by advanced delivery methods of nanoparticles that could precisely load the antitumor vaccines to targeted lymph nodes or immunocytes, the effects have been amplified in recent years. The basic characteristics of recent studies focusing on the antitumor vaccine delivery by nanoparticles and the therapeutic effects are listed in [24,57–70]. By the form of payloads, it could be classified into three categories: tumor-specific antigen delivery, immune bio-adjuvant delivery, and co-delivery of antigens and adjuvants. In order to generate antitumor immunity in experiments, ovalbumin (OVA) was mostly selected as the model tumor antigen due to its exogeneity, easy feasibility, and suitable immunogenicity. OVA was conjugated as a payload to various types of nanoparticles, including silica nanoparticles [57], liposomes [61,66,68], gold nanoparticles [60], alginate nanoparticles [62], and polymeric nanoparticles [65], and injected into mice bearing OVA-expressing melanoma, lymphoma, or thymoma-bearing animal models. Compared with single delivery of antigens, conjugated delivery of antigen–nanoparticle compounds induced significantly stronger antigen-specific antibody responses and CD8+ cytotoxic T-lymphocyte responses accompanied by increased levels of antigen-specific IgG, interferon-γ, and specific types of interleukins, inhibiting tumor growth and prolonging survival of mice [24]. On the other hand, delivery of multiple antigens instead of only single OVA may further enhance the antitumor immunoreaction. Zhang et al. conjugated two tumor-specific peptides and one immunoadjuvant with layered double hydroxide nanoparticles and found a significantly stronger inhibition effect to melanoma compared with single antigen-delivering nanoparticles [59].

Genetic antigens could also be the payload of nanoparticles to stimulate immunity against cancer. After delivered intracellularly, tumor-specific antigens or immune adjuvants encoded by the genetic vaccine could be formed through transcription and translation and continuously stimulate the immune system to generate long-term immunity [68] (Figure 15.2).

They also have the advantages of easy manufacture, preserving, strong cellular immunity stimulation, being cross-immunity inducing, and promising immunogenicity. Recent studies showed efficiency of the antitumor genetic vaccines in inducing both the antigen-specific cytotoxic T-lymphocyte response, and humoral immune response and tumor suppression effects [60,64,66,68,69]. However, their safety concerns should still be noted for the possibility of genomic instability caused by the integration into the genome of the host cell, and the immunologic tolerance of

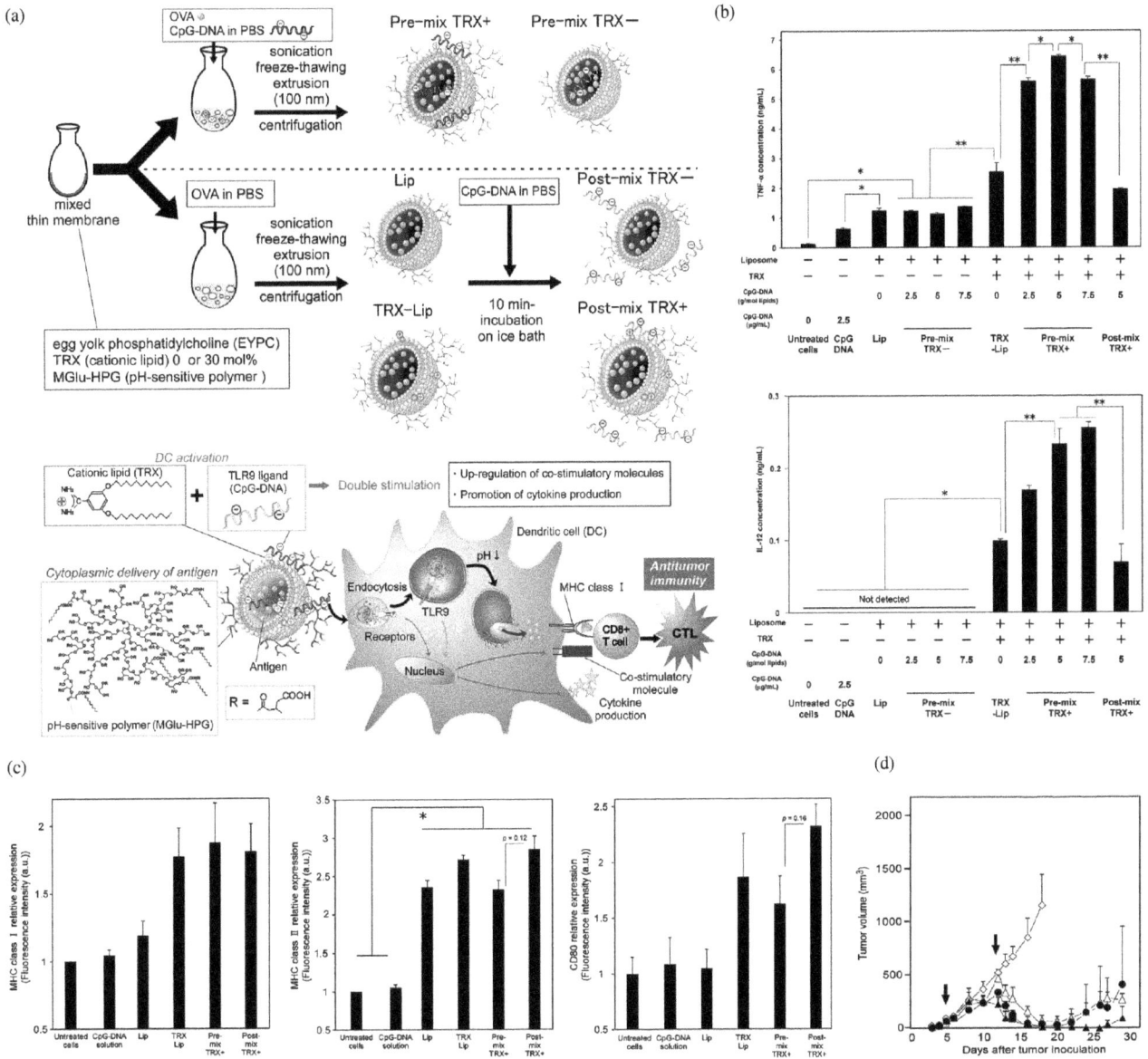

FIGURE 15.2 Genetic tumor nanovaccine enhanced immunotherapy. (A) Synthesis process and working mechanism of the nanoliposome. (B) Enhanced secretion of TNF-α and IL-12 after treatment. (C) Increased MHC-I, MHC-II, and CD80 expression after treatment. (D) *In vivo* antitumor effects of the genetic liposome nanovaccine. (Reprinted from Ref. [68], Copyright (2017), with permission from Elsevier.)

the immune system after long-term overexpression of the encoded antigens.

Bio-adjuvants of cancer vaccine are usually ligands to pattern recognition receptors, including the toll-like receptor (TLR), C-type lectin receptor, NOD-like receptor, and RIG-like receptor, which could assist the innate immune response, facilitate polarization of naive T lymphocytes to T helper cells, and accordingly induce the adaptive immunity [71–73]. TCR agonists are the most studied immune adjuvant integrated into nanoparticles, and they showed significantly higher immune activation effects than the free soluble form. The co-delivery of adjuvants with antigens within the same nano-system achieved even better results, mainly through mechanisms of enhancing the immunogenicity

of weak antigens, reducing the required amount of antigen for effective immune stimulation, and preserving payloads from biolysis. Among the studies, several types of TLR agonists (for example, CpG (TLR9 agonist) and MPLA (TLR4 agonist)) were usually simultaneously conjugated to nanoparticles accompanied by another TAA to realize stronger effects, as multiple TLRs were generally required to be stimulated by pathogens to further increase the levels of inflammatory chemokines and cytokines [74]. In addition, the co-delivery of immune bio-adjuvants with immunosuppressive pathway inhibitors could also significantly suppress the proliferation of immunosuppressive cells and synergistically enhance the tumor-specific cellular immune response [75] (Figure 15.3).

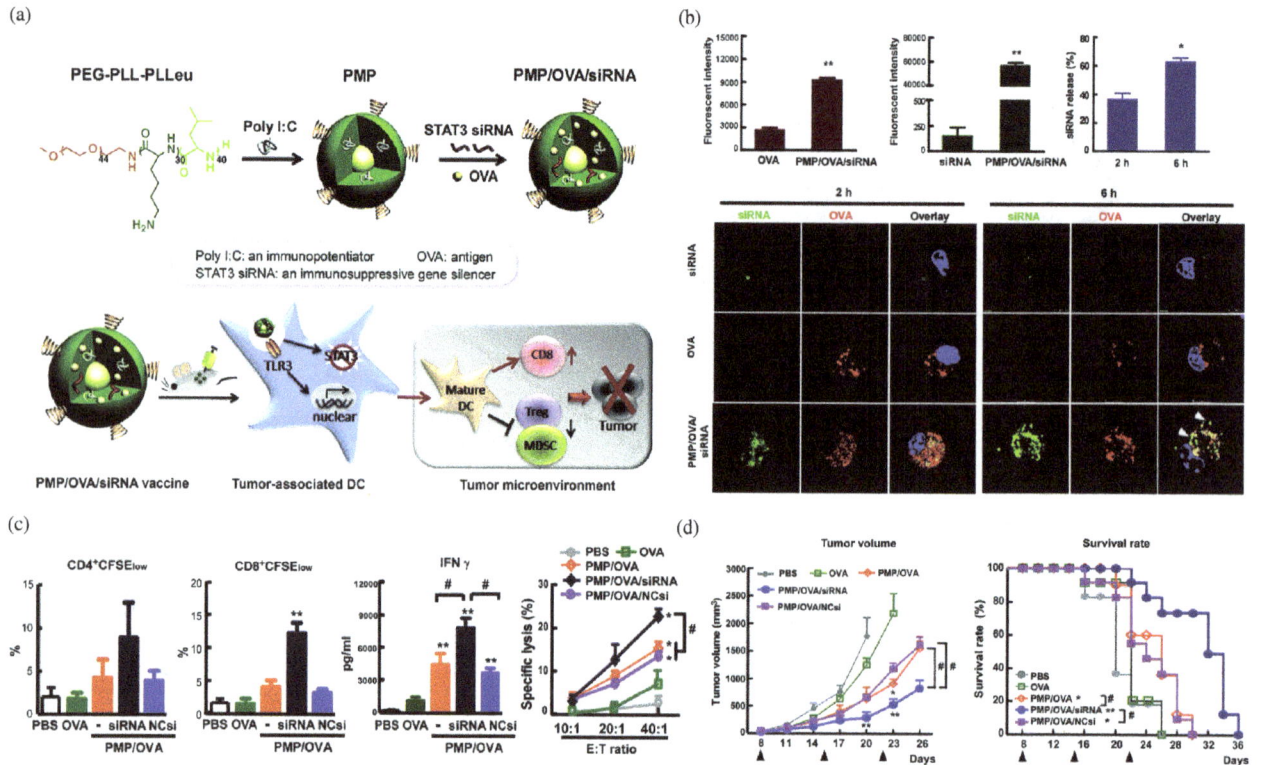

FIGURE 15.3 Tumor-specific cellular immune response induced by tumor nanovaccine co-delivering the bio-adjuvant and immunosuppressive pathway inhibitor. (A) Synthesis and working mechanism of the co-delivery nanovaccine. (B) Enhanced cellular uptake and intracellular localization of siRNA and tumor antigen (OVA) in mouse bone marrow dendritic cells. (C) Increased tumor antigen-specific CD4+ and CD8+ T-cell proliferation, IFN-γ production, and CTL response by the nanovaccine. (D) The antitumor effects of the co-delivery nanovaccine and survival curves of tumor-bearing mice. (Reprinted from Ref. [75], Copyright (2015), with permission from Elsevier.)

The whole-cell antitumor vaccine is mainly generated from two sources, whole tumor cell membrane or tumor cell lysates. Different from individual tumor-specific antigens, the whole-cell antitumor vaccine contains a full range of epitopes and could induce a multivalent immune response [76,77]. Several groups fabricated core-shell PLGA nanostructures coated with cancer cell membrane antigens and formed a robust platform toward multi-antigenic immune responses. In addition, clay nanoparticles with antigens loaded were found to be able to form subcutaneous nodules with a loose structure at the site of injection, which acted as a depot for sustained antigen release and immune cell recruit, and induced continuous immune stimulation and memory T-cell proliferation for up to 35 days [78]. Another strategy to develop a whole-cell antitumor vaccine by nanoparticles is to generate the TAAs *in situ*, which means the generation of tumor cell lysates from damaged or dying cancer cells. It has been proved that the TAAs could be generated *in situ* after chemotherapy [79] or radiotherapy, [80] and more importantly, combined with photothermal therapy (PTT) or photodynamic therapy (PDT), specific nanoparticle platforms developed by Chen [81] and Xu et al. [82] were shown to have the ability to significantly further enhance the therapeutic efficacy of PTT and PDT and reinforce tumor cell destruction and the subsequent TAA generation *in situ*, thus inducing strong antitumor immunity to inhibit the development of original and metastatic tumor lesions.

15.3 ANTIGENIC PEPTIDE-BASED NANOVACCINES

Nanocarrier-based drug delivery systems have been studied extensively for cancer diagnosis and therapy. Nanoparticles can deliver therapeutic compounds to specific cells (either tumor cells or immune cells), thereby improving the efficacy and reducing the toxicity [83,84]. Some types of nanocarriers, such as polysaccharide-based nanogels and mesoporous silica nanoparticles, even exhibit intrinsic immunostimulating activity [85]. Simultaneous delivery of multiple immunotherapeutic compounds can be achieved using nanoparticles to boost anticancer immune response [37]. In fact, nanovaccines (vaccines formulated in nanoparticles) can provide an improvement in immunotherapy compared to free antigens and immunomodulators. Among different strategies of nanomedicine-based cancer immunotherapy, co-delivery of a tumor antigen and an immunostimulating agent to DCs has been the most extensively studied. Various delivery systems, including polymeric nanocarriers, lipid-based, metallic, and inorganic nanostructures, have been developed for this purpose [86].

Free-form antigens are often internalized by DCs through endocytosis and accumulated in the lysosomes. In this mechanism, antigens will be presented at the DC surface via MHC II, which consequently facilitates activation of CD4+ T cells (Th) [87,88]. As for cancer immunotherapy, enhanced CD8+ T-cell immunoresponses are required to eliminate tumor cells, and therefore, increased delivery of antigens and immunoadjuvants to DCs is needed [85,89]. In the following section, various nanoparticle systems developed within the last 5 years for the delivery of peptide-based vaccines and adjuvants for cancer therapy (summarized in [90]) have been discussed.

15.3.1 Polymeric Nanocarriers

Due to the highly flexible properties of polymers, polymeric nanoparticles are widely studied for peptide vaccine delivery. They can be prepared in various sizes and morphologies and conjugated with a ligand for active targeting to specific immune cells. Polymeric nanoparticles can protect the encapsulated antigen and adjuvant from enzymatic degradation, establish a sustained and tunable release profile for the entrapped payload, and, therefore, enhance the immune response in comparison with the antigen and adjuvant delivered in the free form.

15.3.1.1 PLGA Nanoparticles

PLGA (poly(lactic-co-glycolic acid)) is a biocompatible and biodegradable copolymer that undergoes hydrolytic degradation by esterases. The rate of degradation of the copolymer can be tuned by adjusting the ratio of glycolic acid to lactic acid. This copolymer is widely used for preparation of particulate drug delivery systems [91,92]. Since these particles exhibit a similar size to pathogens (i.e., 100–1000 nm), PLGA solid core nanoparticles naturally target DCs, are internalized by phagocytosis, and exhibit 100 times more uptake by DCs compared to the free antigen [93]. Tumor antigens encapsulated in PLGA nanoparticles induce antigen presentation with both MHC I and MHC II, leading to activation of both CTL (CD8+) and Th (CD4+) immune responses [94,95].

Zhang et al. [96] reported the development of PLGA nanoparticles encapsulating murine melanoma antigenic peptides, either from hgp100 (KVPRNQDWL) or tyrosine-related protein II (TRP2, SVYDFFVWL), along with monophosphoryl lipid A (MPLA), a TLR agonist. After 24 h of incubation with the bone marrow–derived dendritic cells (BMDCs), the nanoparticles were internalized. Rosalia et al. [88] modified a PLGA nanoparticle surface with a monoclonal antibody (mAb) that targeted CD40 overexpressed on DCs. The targeted formulation containing OVA as the protein antigen along with Pam3Csk4 (TLR 1/2 agonist) and poly (I:C) (TLR 3 agonist) displayed sixfold increased DC binding and internalization relative to the non-targeted formulation in preclinical study on an animal model. This led to increased IFN-γ production, enhanced OVA-specific CD4+ activation, and, consequently, reduced tumor growth in the B16/OVA tumor model. Despite their success in boosting the immunoresponses in animal models, the clinical efficiency of PLGA nanovaccines is disappointing. After *in vivo* administration, plain PLGA nanoparticles may adsorb proteins in the body fluids (e.g., albumin), forming a protein corona around the particles, which reduces the colloidal stability and facilitates the clearance by macrophages [97]. Surface modification with methoxy-PEG (mPEG) increases the stability and reduces the macrophage uptake, but the anti-PEG immunity induced by multiple injections must be carefully studied. The clinical efficiency of PLGA nanovaccines may be enhanced by combination therapy with immune checkpoint inhibitors and other immunostimulants

15.3.1.2 Micellar Nanocarriers

Micelles exhibit a core-shell structure wherein the hydrophobic moieties of an amphiphilic polymer form the inner core, while an outer shell is established by the hydrophilic residues [98,99]. They are often used to load poorly soluble compounds into the core, and the hydrophilic segment can be functionalized for cell targeting. The major limitation for both PLGA nanoparticles and polymeric micelles is that they are most suitable for delivering hydrophobic antigens and adjuvants. However, many potent antigens and adjuvants are protein-based, and therefore, alternative methods are needed. Additionally, majority of the nanovaccine preclinical studies were based on an artificial antigen such as OVA, which is not clinically relevant. The effectiveness of these nanovaccines might be overestimated. In fact, tumor antigen selection remains the major hurdle for clinical development of tumor vaccines.

15.3.1.3 Hydrogel Nanoparticles

Hydrogels are made of three-dimensional polymeric networks, which can establish hydrogen bonds with water molecules, and are able to absorb water to swell to a high extent [100]. Polysaccharide-based hydrogel nanoparticles are particularly attractive for antigen delivery due to their natural immunostimulating activities [101] and their ability to entrap hydrophilic macromolecules such as proteins. In order to study the effects of nanogel surface modification on DC targeting and internalization, Thomann-Harwood et al. [102] loaded OVA into chitosan nanogels, which were coated with either alginate (alg) or mannosylated alginate (alg-man). Confocal microscopy revealed receptor-mediated endocytosis, caveola-mediated endocytosis, and to a less extent *macropinocytosis* as the mechanisms for DC uptake of the algman-coated nanogels, which accumulated in the lysosomes. Following *in vitro* incubation of nanogels with DCs, Alg-man coated nanogels enhanced the immunostimulating effects by increasing the production of OVA-specific IFN-γ and the expression of CD86. However, *in vivo* efficiency of the prepared hydrogels on reduction of tumor progression is unknown.

Delivery of immunostimulating cytokines to cancer cells is another effective approach for immunotherapy. However, major obstacles for cytokine therapy include short *in vivo*

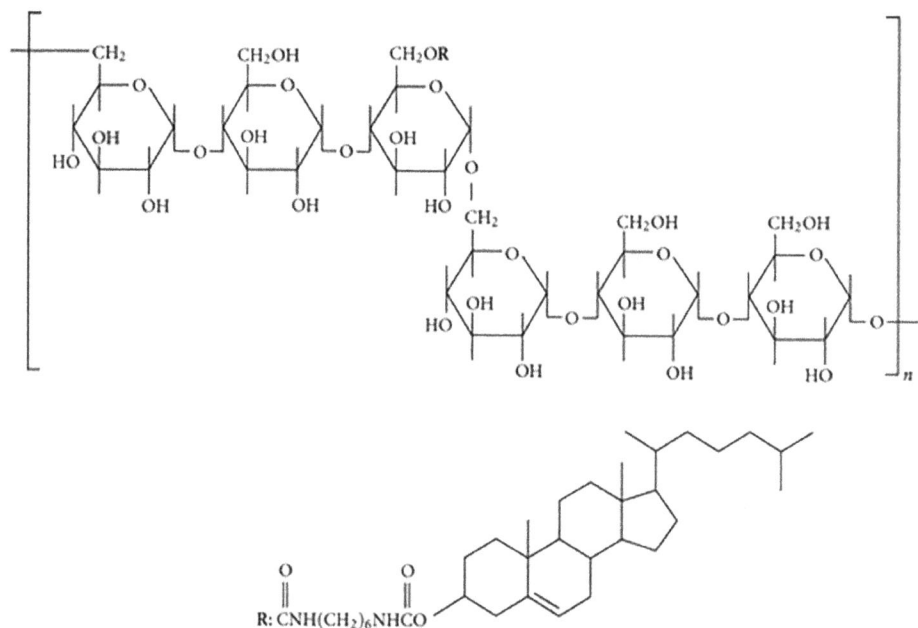

FIGURE 15.4   The chemical structure of cholesterol-bearing pullulan.

half-life and systemic toxicity when administered at high doses. Park et al. [103] prepared a novel delivery vehicle known as nanolipogels (nLGs), simultaneously encapsulating a TGF-β receptor I inhibitor (SB505124) and IL-2 for therapy against melanoma. Both SB505124 and IL-2 were encapsulated in the nanogels composed of PLA-PEG-PGA, which were then coated with lipids, including PC, DSPE-PEG, and cholesterol. nLGs increased the blood circulation half-life of the immunoadjuvants by tenfold compared to the free drugs after *i.v.* injection in animal models. It was demonstrated that nLG enhanced the activation of CD8+ cells in the tumor by threefold, resulting in improved CTL immune response and antitumor efficacy against B16 melanoma. Likewise, Shimizu et al. [104] encapsulated IL-12 into cholesterol-bearing pullulan (CHP)-based hydrogel nanoparticles, creating a slow release formulation for IL-12. The chemical structure of cholesterol-bearing pullulan is shown in Figure 15.4 [90]. After *s.c* injection of the formulation, an increased serum level of IFN-γ and decreased tumor growth were measured compared with free IL-12. However, there was little effect of this nanogel formulation after *i.v.* injection due to elimination by the macrophages in the liver and spleen.

Kitano et al. [105] conducted a clinical study to investigate the safety and efficacy of CHP-based nanogels in human patients suffering from HER-2-positive solid tumors. In this study, truncated HER2 protein I-146 (146 HER2) was loaded into the CHP-based nanogels and the formulation was *s.c* administered biweekly for 6 weeks and for a total of three doses. The treatment exhibited good tolerability and only caused grade 1–2 erythema-like reactions at the site of injection (8/9 patients), which resolved within 48 h. Five out of 9 patients showed significant CD4+ and CD8+ immune responses after the nanogel treatment.

Despite the aforementioned promising results, the current nanogel systems display a burst release profile that is mainly triggered by the large pore size. A technology that can better control the payload release from hydrogels is needed to produce a formulation with prolonged activity [106].

15.3.2 LIPOSOMES

Tumor antigens and immunoadjuvants can be incorporated into liposomes by various methods, including covalent conjugation or complexation (e.g., avidin-biotin, nitrilotriacetic acid-hexahistidine) to the liposomal surface, passive encapsulation, or surface adsorption through electrostatic interactions [107]. These methods are illustrated in Figure 15.5 [90].

Following administration to mice, surface decoration of antigen at the liposomal surface was shown to increase antibody production, activation of CD4+ and CD8+ immunoresponses, and IFN-γ secretion compared to antigens encapsulated inside the liposomes [108,109]. Cationic liposomes interacted with, and protected anionic antigens from degradation, and their positive surface charge facilitated the uptake and internalization by DCs. Cationic liposomes also interacted with the endosomal membrane to trigger cytosolic release of antigens [110]. With efficient cytosolic delivery, the antigen could be expressed on MHC I, stimulating CTL by induction of CD8+ T-cell differentiation [111]. Moreover, cationic liposomes exhibited immunostimulating effects. Cationic liposomes nonspecifically stimulated CD80 and CD86, involved in maturation of T cells, and induced secretion of chemokines such as CCL2, CCL-3, and CCL-4 to activate the CD8+ immune response [112]. They also activated extracellular-signal-regulated

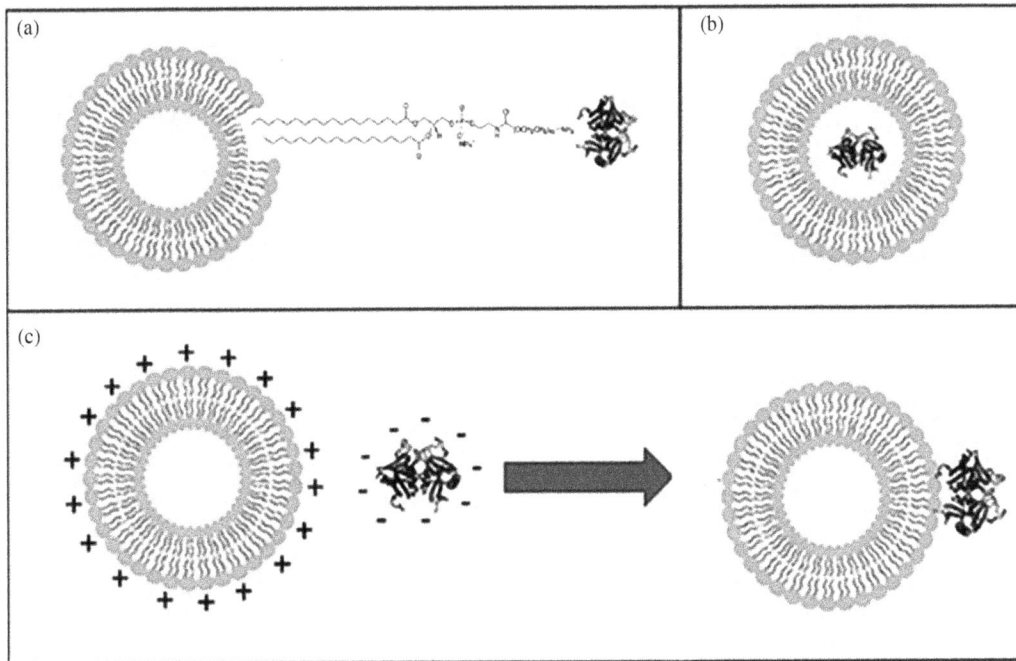

FIGURE 15.5 Various methods used for incorporation of a peptide antigen into a liposome. (A) Covalent conjugation of the antigen to the surface of a liposome by a linker; (B) Passive encapsulation of the antigen into the aqueous interior of a liposome; (C) Surface adsorption of the negatively charged antigen to a cationic liposome through electrostatic interactions.

kinase (ERK) via the generation of reactive oxygen species (ROS), which also played a key role in DC–T-cell signaling [113]. Vangasseri et al. [114] proposed the existence of a cationic lipid receptor, either on the surface or inside the DCs, for recognizing cationic lipids and enhancing the activation of costimulatory molecules. In addition to liposomes and archaeosomes, other lipid-based nanocarriers including ethosomes, a lipid vesicular system that contains a high concentration of ethanol, and solid lipid nanoparticles (SLNs) were demonstrated to activate DCs [115]. However, only a limited number of these delivery systems have been reported, and their application for immunotherapy is yet to be established.

15.3.3 EXOSOMES

Exosomes are nanoscale vesicles (50–100 nm) released from cells that contain cellular components. They can fuse with the membrane of adjacent cells for cell–cell communication [116]. The process for biogenesis of exosomes is illustrated in Figure 15.6 [90].

Exosomes can be released by various cell types including tumor cells, DCs, T cells, and B cells and are intrinsically surface-modified with specific transmembrane markers including CD9, CD63, CD81, heat shock proteins (Hsp60, Hsp70, Hsp90), MHC I, MHC II, intercellular adhesion molecule-1 (ICAM-1), and some endosome-originated peptides (ALIX, TSG-101) [117,118]. DC-derived exosomes (DEXs) can transfer MHC-peptide complexes from DCs to T cells, presenting

their antigens and therefore stimulating tumor-specific CD8+ and CD4+ immunoresponses. Surface expression of CD80 and CD86 as the costimulatory molecules plays a key role in immunogenicity of the DEXs, enhancing maturation of T cells [119–122].

Despite several successful preclinical studies, TEXs exhibited low therapeutic efficacy in clinical trials. Genetic modification of cancer cells can be used as a strategy to improve the delivery efficiency of TEXs. L1210 leukemia cells were genetically modified by a lentiviral vector to downregulate TGF-β1, an immunosuppressor. TEXs derived from the engineered L1210 cells were s.c injected to DBA/2 mice and were taken up by DCs, leading to a twofold increase in production of TNF- α, IL-12p70, IFN-γ, and IL-12; a threefold decrease in TGF-β1; and a fourfold decrease in tumor growth in comparison with TEXs isolated from the parent culture [123]. Relative to many reported nanovaccines that incorporate an artificial tumor antigens, TEXs contain real human tumor antigens and, therefore, exhibit better potential for clinical translation. However, the current biogenesis method of exosomes is costly and poorly reproducible with significant hurdles for scale-up manufacturing. Moreover, the lack of standards for quality control could result in inconsistent quality of exosomes that will negatively affect the clinical translation. It remains challenging to effectively tune the physicochemical properties of exosomes for targeted delivery. Innovative approaches to modulate exosome properties and stability must be developed to leverage the full potential for tumor antigen delivery.

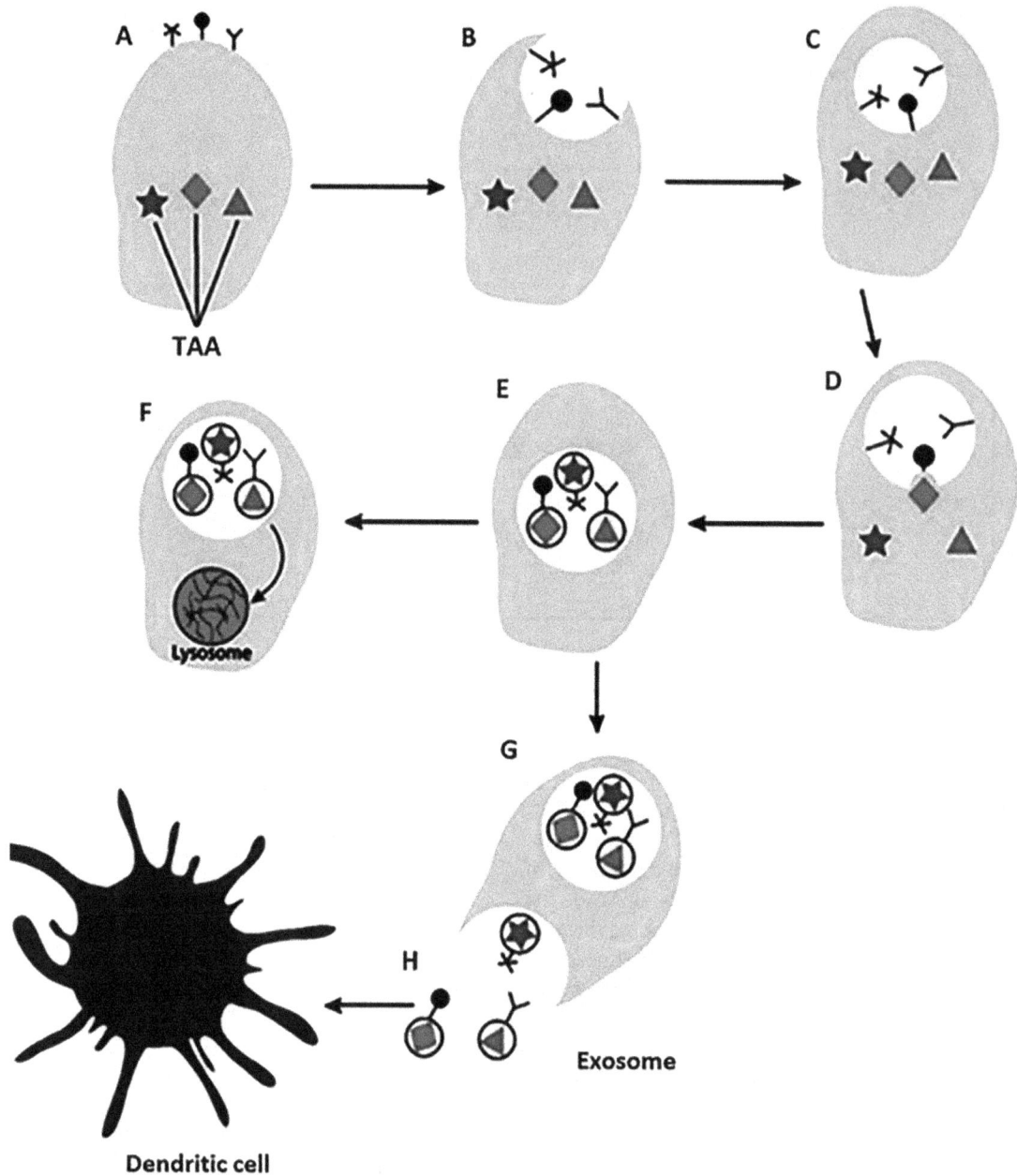

FIGURE 15.6 Schematic illustration of biogenesis of exosomes in a tumor cell. (A–C) Formation of the multivesicular bodies (MVBs) by invagination of the plasma membrane. Note that surface receptors at the plasma membrane are located inside the MVBs; (D and E) Formation of internal vesicles (inside the MVBs) for entrapping TAAs; The MVBs can be (F) digested through the lysosomal compartment or (G and H) fused with the plasma membrane to release the exosomes, which are taken up by DCs.

15.3.4 GOLD NANOPARTICLES

Among all the metallic nanoparticles, gold nanoparticles (AuNPs) have been the most extensively studied for cancer immunotherapy. Their versatile surface chemistry and tunable size and shape make them a good carrier in delivering tumor antigens and immunoadjuvants [124]. AuNPs exhibit significant tendency to interact with DCs [125], leading to secretion of immunostimulating cytokines (IL-1, IL-6, IL-12, and TNF-α) [126] and downregulation of immunosuppressive chemokines (TGF-β1 and IL-10) [127]. Activation of DCs by AuNPs is also evidenced by increased phagocytic activity of DCs and subsequent enhanced maturation of T cells and CD4+ and CD8+ immunoresponses [128]. Therefore, besides their capability as a delivery vehicle for antigens to DCs, AuNPs can serve as an adjuvant in boosting the immunoresponse. Antigenic peptides and adjuvants can be incorporated to AuNPs surface by either chemical conjugation via covalent bonding or surface adsorption (via electrostatic interaction) [129,130]. The clinical application of AuNPs is mostly hampered by the safety issues. AuNPs exhibit high affinity for nucleic acids [131] and may affect regular gene expression. Furthermore, the long-term accumulation of AuNPs in the body remains

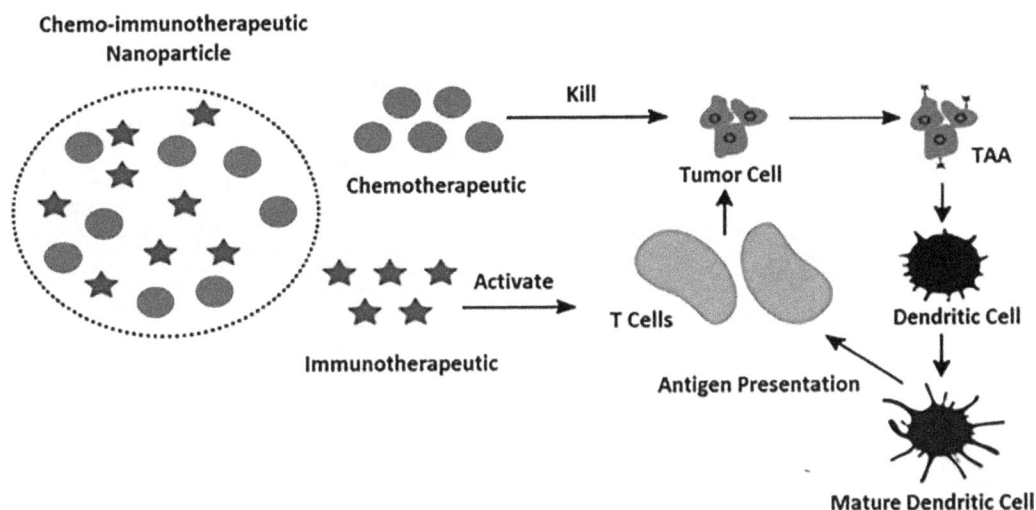

FIGURE 15.7 The schematic representation of the chemoimmunotherapy mediated by nanoparticle drug delivery.

a concern and it has been reported that AuNPs induce oxidative stress via generation of free radicals [132].

15.3.5 Mesoporous Silica Nanoparticles (MSNs)

MSNs also exhibit potent immunostimulating activity by increasing the expression of CD80 and CD86 in DCs, and inducing the secretion of immunostimulating cytokines such as IL-12, IL-2, IL-4, TNF-α, and IFN-γ, which subsequently enhanced CD4+ and CD 8+ immune responses and improved NK cell activation [133]. These effects alone (without antigen) were sufficient to inhibit tumor growth and increase survival of tumor-bearing mice. The 3D scaffold of MSNs allows loading of protein antigens and adjuvants. Kim et al. [134] reported that *s.c* injection of the MSNs loaded with OVA and GM-CSF effectively inhibited the OVA-tumor growth compared to the free formulation. In a recent study performed by Kong et al. [135], biodegradable lipid-coated MSNs containing doxorubicin (a chemotherapeutic drug), all-trans retinoic acid (ATRA, a DC activator) and IL-2 (a T-cell and NK-cell activator) were prepared for chemoimmunotherapy. The mechanisms involved in the chemoimmunotherapy are illustrated in Figure 15.7 [90].

15.3.6 Carbon Nanotubes (CNTs)

Carbon nanotubes (CNTs) are elongated and hollow cylindrical nanostructures made from carbon. They are categorized as single-walled nanotubes (SWNTs) or multi-walled nanotubes (MWNTs). Their surface can be functionalized by covalent or non-covalent (hydrophobic interaction) attachment of a therapeutic molecule and a targeting ligand. In comparison with free antigens, carbon nanotubes exhibit increased internalization by DCs and therefore can be used to deliver tumor antigens and adjuvants for cancer immunotherapy [136]. CNT containing tumor adjuvants and antigens were shown to effectively accumulate in the lymph node following *s.c* or footpad injection, inducing enhanced

CD8+ and CD4+ immune responses [137,138]. mAb can be conjugated to the surface of CNTs to target a specific population of immune cells.

15.4 NANOPARTICLES DELIVERING IMMUNE CHECKPOINT INHIBITORS

Immune checkpoint inhibitors have emerged as the hot spot in tumor immunotherapy recently. PD-1 is one of the most important immune checkpoint molecules and is overexpressed on activated T lymphocytes and has a tight correlation with tumor-associated immune suppression. In a normal situation, combination of PD-1 and PD-L1 can transmit inhibitory signals and reduce the proliferation of CD8+ T cells in lymph nodes, and PD-1 can also control the accumulation of antigen-specific T cells in lymph nodes by regulating the bcl-2 gene, thus protecting normal tissue from attacking under autoimmunity [139–141]. However, tumor cells could also escape from immune attack by overexpressing the PD-L1. Similarly, CTLA-4 could induce T lymphocytes to be nonreactive and negatively regulate the immune response after its incorporation with B7 expressed on activated APCs [142,143]. The immune checkpoint inhibitors including anti-CTLA4 and anti-PD-1/PD-L1 antibodies have entered into clinical treatments and showed impressive curative effects; however, the efficacy is still limited by the relatively low rate of the treatment response and high incidence of side effects. Therefore, nanoparticles are considered for the delivery of these drugs in a targeted and sustainable-releasing pattern, thus reducing the treatment dose and decreasing side effects.

Among the studies developing nanoparticles for the delivery of immune checkpoint inhibitors, although a variance in the nanoparticle types and sizes existed, the conjugation could enhance the immune response against tumors and decrease side effects of immune checkpoint inhibitors, [144–150] which is mainly due to the accumulation of nanoparticles and the sustained release of inhibitors in

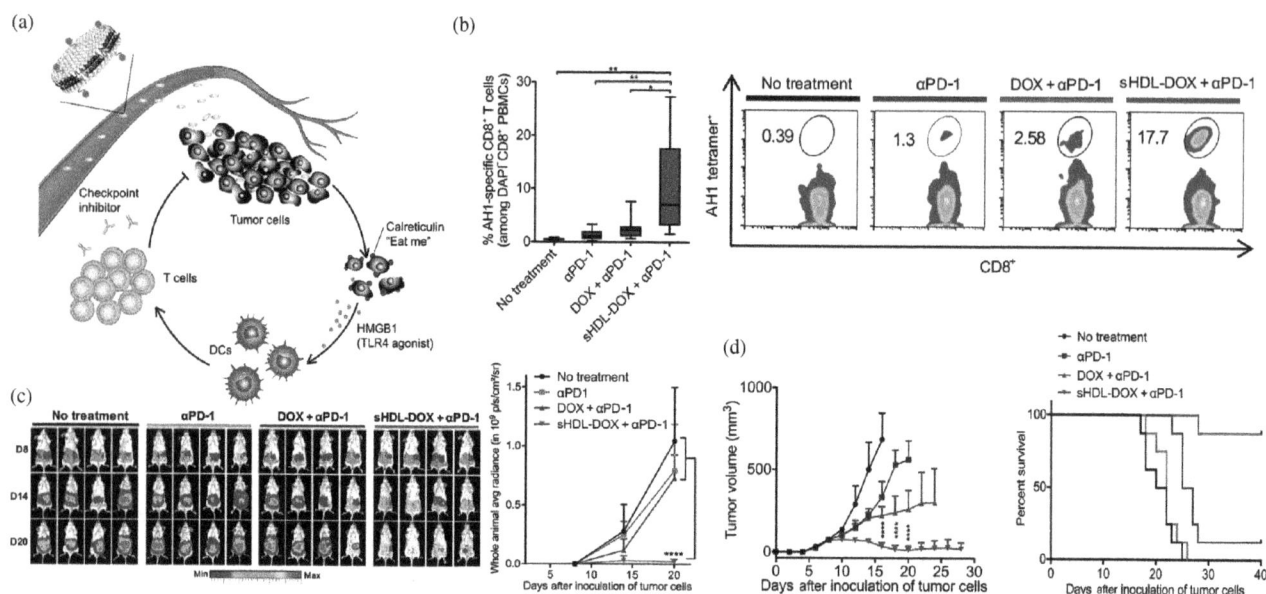

FIGURE 15.8 Elimination of tumors by chemoimmunotherapy with immune checkpoint inhibitor-conjugated nanoparticles. (A) Schematic of immune checkpoint inhibitor-combined nanoparticles for chemoimmunotherapy. (B) Percentage of tumor antigen-specific CD8+ T cells after treatment and the corresponding scatterplots. (C) Whole-animal *in vivo* imaging of tumors after treatment and quantification of the bioluminescence signal. (D) Tumor growth and survival curves after treatment. (Reprinted from Ref. [153], © The Authors, some rights reserved; exclusive licensee American Association for the Advancement of Science. Distributed under a Creative Commons Attribution NonCommercial License 4.0 (CC BY-NC), http://creativecommons.org/licenses/by-nc/4.0/.)

the tumor tissue, as proven by Meir et al. that the amount of inhibitor accumulation within tumor tissues was linearly correlated with the intensity of the immune response against cancer [151]. Furthermore, as the anti-PD-L1 and anti-CTLA4 treatments have been proven to have a synergistic treatment effect due to the different mechanisms, Chae et al. constructed a nano-system delivering both the inhibitors and found a significantly slower tumor growth rate and longer survival of mice in the combined treatment group than either of the individual drug groups [152].

In addition, there are studies combining the nanoparticle-conjugated immune checkpoint inhibitors with other treatment methods to further intensify therapeutic effects. Kuai et al. integrated lipid-doxorubicin (DOX) and anti-PD-1 antibody with synthetic high-density lipoprotein (sHDL) to form pH-responsive nanoparticles [153]. The prolonged circulation enables adequate intratumoral delivery, followed by internalization by tumor cells and pH-related release of payloads in the endosomes and lysosomes. Released DOX killed tumor cells and induced immunogenic cell death and release of danger signals, recruiting APCs to phagocytose the immunogenically dying tumor cells. The immune response would be further enhanced accompanied by the anti-PD-1 antibodies, leading to elimination of tumors and prevention of tumor relapse. As a result, the sHDL-DOX+anti-PD-1 nanoparticles significantly induced an antigen-specific cytotoxic T-cell response, suppressed tumor growth, and prolonged survival than the free DOX+anti-PD-1 treatment or the single anti-PD-1 treatment (Figure 15.8). Similar results were also found by Wang et al. when PD-L1 siRNA-coated nanoparticles were

integrated with a photosensitizer for photodynamic therapy that the combined nanosystem efficiently stimulated the immune response and silenced immune resistance, inhibiting tumor growth and preventing recurrence [154].

Another established negative feedback protein that suppresses the immune response and assists tumor cell proliferation is IDO, which mediates the degradation of tryptophan to kynurenine and other metabolites, thus leading to intracellular accumulation, inducing cell cycle arrest and death of effector T lymphocytes, and promoting regulatory T-cell proliferation with the immunosuppressive effects [155,156]. Sun et al. coated the IDO inhibitor NLG919 and DOX with a redox-responsive immunostimulatory polymeric prodrug carrier. The nanosystem generated greater accumulation of NLG and DOX in tumor tissue than other organs, promoted apoptosis of breast and prostate cancer cells, and formed more significant immunoactivation effects compared with free DOX, liposomal DOX, or free NLG groups [157]. Other similar studies are also consistent with the reported results [158,159].

15.5 THE BASIC MECHANISM OF CYTOTOXIC T LYMPHOCYTE ANTIGEN-4 (CTLA-4)

The basic mechanisms of different ICB will be elucidated. And newly research results about the combination of nanoparticle delivery system with ICB in cancer immunotherapy will be outlined. Furthermore, we will also discuss the underexplored potential in applying nanotechnology to improve the antitumor efficacy of ICB and conquer the limits of immune checkpoint inhibitors (Scheme 15.1) [10].

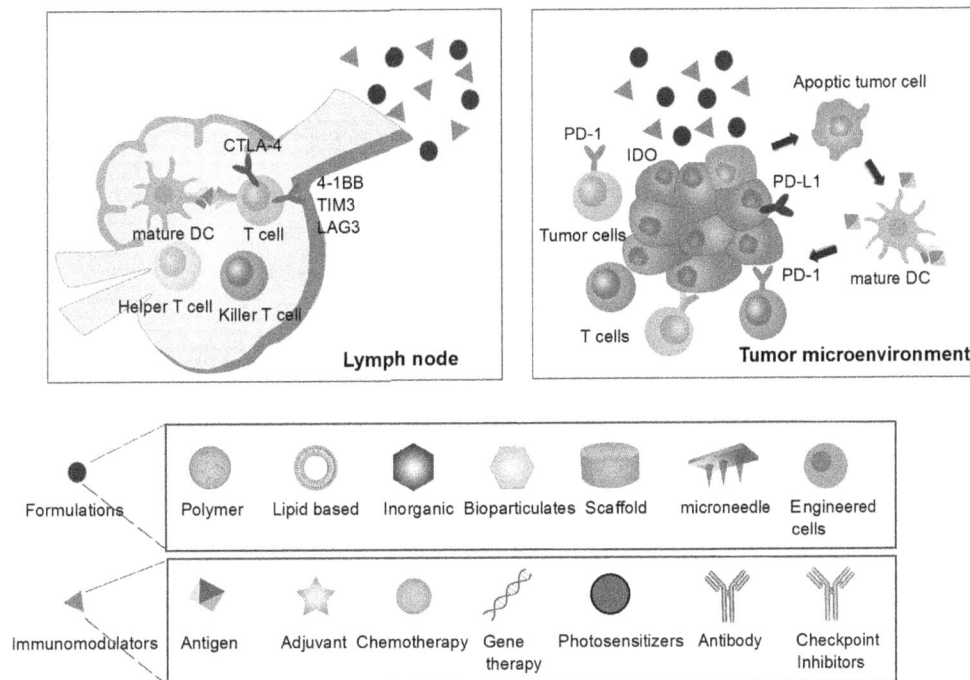

SCHEME 15.1 Schematic illustration of combining drug delivery system with ICB therapy, including therapeutic delivery to lymph nodes and tumor microenvironment.

CTLA-4, a member of immunoglobulin superfamily, was firstly identified by Pierre Golstein in 1987 [160]. It is demonstrated that the protein sequences of CTLA-4 are highly homology to CD28, especially for the extracellular domain. Moreover, its locus is closely linked to CD28. The expression of CTLA-4 can be only induced after T-cell activation. The two ligands of CTLA-4 are CD80 (B7-1) and CD86 (B7-2) [11]. Therefore, CTLA-4 immune checkpoint inhibitor is regarded as primarily acting in secondary lymphoid organs rather than tumor microenvironment. However, the specific mechanism of CTLA-4 signaling pathway is still underexplored. Increasing researches suggested that the activation of two molecules, Src homology phosphotyrosyl phosphatase 2 (SHP2) and protein phosphatase 2A (PP2A), is essential for counteracting kinase signals which are induced by TCR and CD28 [161] (Figure 15.9).

In addition, CTLA-4 can regulate the function of regulatory T cells (Tregs) which are identified to locally suppress antitumor immunity in tumor microenvironment. Since CTLA-4 is known as mainly expressed on CD4+ helper rather than CD8+ T cells, the "braking" function of CTLA-4 antibody is considered as relevant to the enhancement of helper T cells and down-modulation of Tregs immunosuppressive activity, leading to promotion of CTL responses and tumor cells killing [163,164].

15.5.1 Antibodies Blocking CTLA-4

The first human CTLA-4 monoclonal antibodies applied in clinical treatment are ipilimumab and tremelimumab [10]. Ipilimumab is a fully human IgG1 monoclonal antibody that is approved by FDA for melanoma in 2011 [165]. Application of CTLA-4 antibodies in lung cancer, prostate cancer, and various types of cancer in clinical trials is also undergoing. Tremelimumab is a fully human IgG2 monoclonal antibody which is also applied in clinical trials of melanoma, mesothelioma, and NSCLC. However, severe adverse effects can be observed during the clinical treatment especially for ipilimumab. Due to the overactivation and proliferation of T cells, severe or even fatal side effects can be detected in a minority of patients who received ipilimumab treatment. Besides, other gastrointestinal tract–associated side effects (diarrhea, bloating, stomach pain, etc.), colitis, hypophysitis, and breathing problems also can be seen [166].

15.5.2 Combination Therapies Based on CTLA-4 Blockade

To increase the therapeutic efficacy, immune checkpoint therapy is recently combined with other therapeutic modalities for synergistic antitumor effects. They are usually combined with nanotechnology. Utilizing nanoparticles to load antibodies, vaccines, photosensitizers, siRNA, and other types of therapeutic agents has shown improved therapeutic efficiency. Moreover, the monoclonal antibodies loaded in nanoparticles could reduce the off-target toxicity of the antibodies to health tissues. And incorporating checkpoint blockade into various treatment strategies is expected to elicit additional therapeutic benefits in antitumor treatment [167].

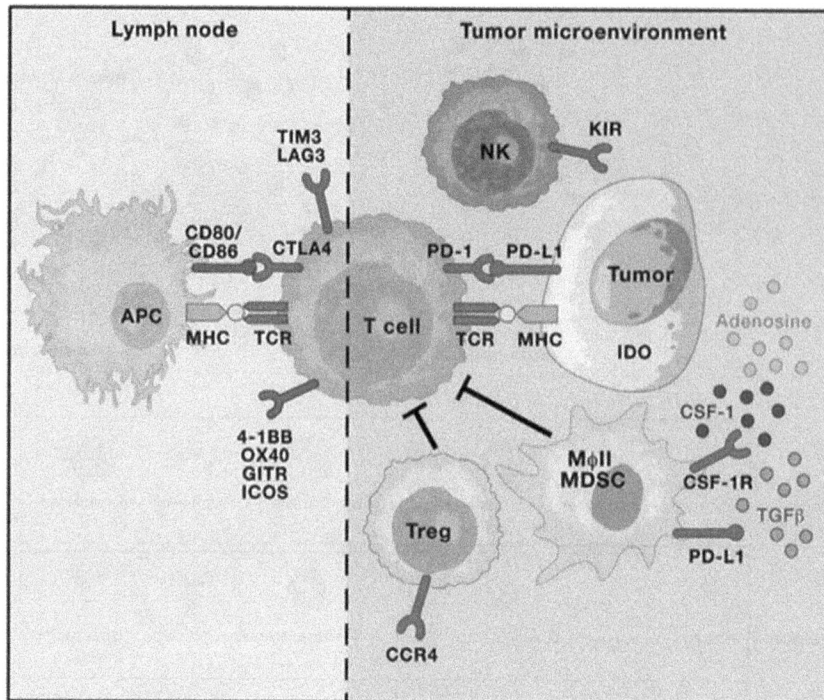

FIGURE 15.9 Basic mechanism of immune checkpoint blockade, including CTLA-4, PD-1/PD-L1 axis, IDO, 4-1BB, and other immune checkpoints. (Reprinted with permission from [162]. Copyright 2017 Elsevier Inc.)

15.5.2.1 Synergistic Effects by Combining Drug-Loaded Nanoparticles with Immune Checkpoint Inhibitors

Photodynamic therapy (PDT) could trigger antitumor immune responses to some extent but with limited penetration depth, and thus, it is not powerful enough to eradicate cancer. Multitasking upconversion nanoparticles (UNCPs) that contained photosensitizer Chlorin e6 (Ce6) and R387 were formulated as UCNP-Ce6-R837. After near-infrared irradiation, the tumor tissues could be destructed with enhanced penetration by producing reactive oxygen species (ROS) under PDT and releasing TAAs which could stimulate DCs' maturation simultaneously for consequently enhanced antitumor immunity. Furthermore, after combining with CTLA-4 checkpoint inhibitor, it showed strong antitumor effects on tumors with enhanced population of effector T cells and inhibited activity of suppressive Tregs. Moreover, tumor reoccurrence could be prevented because of the immune memory effect [168] (Figure 15.10A–C).

15.5.3 siRNA Targeting CTLA-4 Immune Checkpoint

Besides using the immune checkpoint antibodies, small interfering RNA (siRNA) targeting the CTLA-4 immune inhibitory pathways can be efficiently delivered by nanoparticles. The siCTLA-4 nanoparticles were evidenced to downregulate the expression of CTLA-4 in about 4%–6% activated T cells by systematic administration in B16F10 tumor-bearing mice. The antitumor efficacy was thus significantly enhanced and survival time was prolonged by

regulating effector T cells and decreasing the number of Tregs. This research [10] provided new strategy of the nanoparticle-based gene delivery for cancer immunotherapy [169] (Figure 15.10D–F). Although the therapeutic efficacy was improved by the combination of CTLA-4 inhibitors with photosensitizer-loaded nanoparticles for PTT or PDT, it still remains to be underexplored to study the synergistic effects, appropriate dosage schedule, and intrinsic mechanisms. Up to now, the combinational therapy is still limited on PTT/PDT or vaccine. It may be explored to other therapeutic modalities in future.

15.6 THE BASIC MECHANISM OF PD-1/PD-L1 AXIS

PD-1 expression is induced only after TCR engagement that is similar to CTLA-4, while PD-1 is mainly expressed on tumor-infiltrating lymphocytes (TILs) including activated T cells, B cells, and macrophages that is more widely than CTLA-4 [170]. Normally, it takes 6–12 h of transcription activation for PD-1 expression.

PD-L1 (B7-H1, CD274) and PD-L2 (B7-DC, CD273) are the two ligands of PD-1. Even though they have 37% sequence homology, their regulation is quite different. First, PD-L1 is predominantly induced by IFN-γ that is mainly secreted by activated T cells or NK cells, while PDL2 prefers to be induced by IL-4 rather than IFN-γ. Second, PD-L1 is mainly expressed on endothelial cells and activated hematopoietic cells, and PD-L2 is predominantly expressed on activated DCs and macrophages [171–174]. Moreover, PD-1/PD-L1 pathway is much more complicated compared

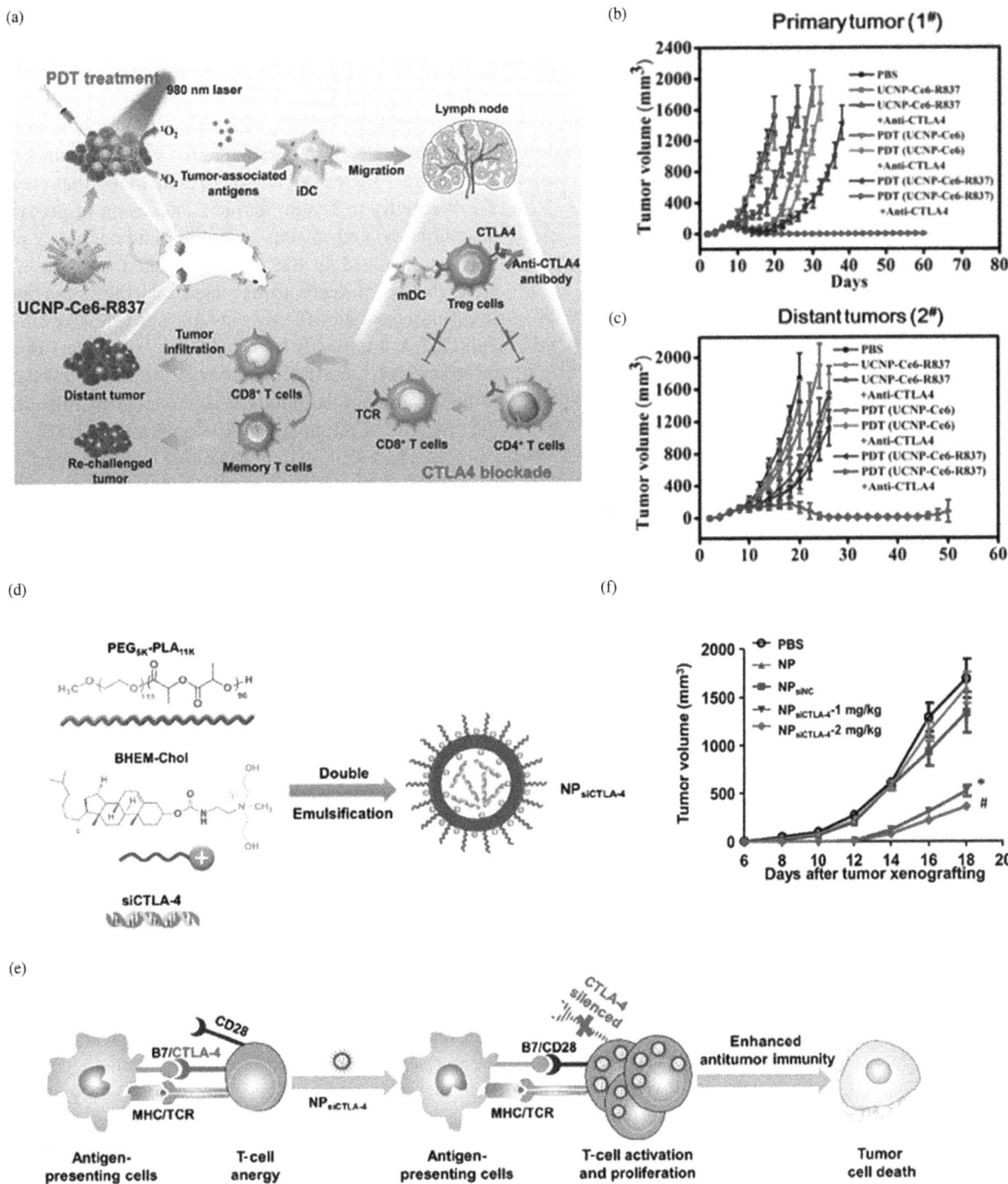

FIGURE 15.10 (A) The mechanisms of combining UCNP-Ce6-R837 nanoparticles and anti-CTLA-4 antibody that enables to induce powerful antitumor efficacy. (B and C) Tumor growth of primary (B) and distant tumors (C) in CT26 after different treatments. (Reprinted with permission from [168]. Copyright 2017 American Chemical Society.) (D) Fabrication of nanoparticles loaded with siCTLA-4. (E) Enhanced antitumor immunity mediated by nanoparticles silencing CTLA-4. (F) Tumor growth after siCTLA-4 treatment in melanoma. (Reprinted with permission from [169]. Copyright 2016 Elsevier Inc.)

to CTLA-4. PD-L1 is identified to be able to engage with CD80 molecules on T cells. PD-L2 is evidenced to bind T-cell-expressed RGMb [175]. The action mechanisms of interaction and regulation patterns of expression among PD-1 and its ligands still need to be defined. These could suggest new targets of ICB for cancer [176,177]. Normally, this process occurs at the tumor margins where the tumor cells and T cells interact with each other leading to the blockade on antitumor responses. The adaptive resistance represents the loss of sensitivity to inflammatory tumor microenvironment for tumor cells (Figure 15.9).

Therefore, due to these immune resistance mechanisms, tumors could evade immune surveillance and form a suitable tumor microenvironment for further proliferation. Hence, several changes could be performed in tumor microenvironment by the resistant mechanisms. First, PD-1 could impact apoptotic genes leading to elevated apoptosis of activated T cells. Second, chronic inflammation in tumor microenvironment can result in T-cell anergy and exhaustion. Third, PD-L1 could induce the generation of Tregs. In addition, PD-1 and PD-L1 engagement also decreases long-term immune memory that is essential for protection against tumor metastasis [178].

15.6.1 Antibodies Blocking PD-1/PD-L1 Pathway

In murine models, the PD-1/PD-L1 blocking antibodies exhibit enhanced tumor selectivity compared to CTLA-4. Currently, immune checkpoint inhibitors blocking PD-1/PD-L1 pathway approved by FDA are mainly nivolumab, pembrolizumab, atezolizumab, avelumab, and durvalumab [10]. Increasing clinical trials are ongoing because of the reproducible and durable antitumor responses of these drugs. Nivolumab, the first monoclonal antibody targeting PD-1, is identified to have powerful impact on a variety of cancers in human clinical trials, including epithelial cancers, melanoma, NSCLC, kidney cancer, and colorectal cancer [179]. Importantly, nivolumab exhibits distinct advantages in chemotherapy-refractory squamous NSCLC. And in the recent phase III clinical trials of advanced melanoma, it shows higher performance than standard chemotherapy [180].

In phase II clinical trial of pembrolizumab, first-line therapy with pembrolizumab is systemically delivered at a dose of 2 mg/kg in 26 patients with advanced Merkel-cell carcinoma. It showed that the objective response rate was 56% (95% confidence interval [CI], 35–76) and the rate of progression-free survival at 6 months was 67% (95% CI, 49–86) [181]. Similar results about the metastases of various solid tumors were also published in clinical trials [172]. In the research, colorectal cancers with 12 different tumor types were treated with anti-PD-1 antibodies to evaluate clinical efficacy in patients. 53% of patients were observed with objective radiographic responses, and 21% of patients achieved complete responses. Moreover, *in vivo* functional analysis showed that increasing infiltration of neoantigen-specific T cells was found in tumors regardless of the cancer tissue origination.

The significant clinical outcomes of PD-1 immune checkpoint inhibitors promote the development of a series of PD-L1 blockade antibodies, and these antibodies are all applied in clinical trials now. Their clinical treatment activity has been identified in melanoma, NSCLC, renal cell carcinoma, etc. [182–185]. Especially, the Fc domain of MPDL3208A (atezolizumab) has been modified to avoid the antibody-dependent cytotoxicity. It is reported that in NSCLC patients, the clinical efficacy of MPDL3208A is correlated with expression level of TILs, not tumor cells. PD-1 immune checkpoint inhibitors have shown their distinct advantages of enhancing antitumor responses in chemotherapy refractory bladder cancer and Hodgkin's lymphoma [186,187].

However, immune-related adverse effects can be observed during the clinical treatment that normally occurs in the first few weeks to months among a minority of patients. The mechanisms of the adverse events still need to be elucidated. Genetic heterogeneity and host microbiota composition were speculated to correlate with the risk. Clinical researches in patients demonstrated that elevating T-cell activity in healthy tissues, increasing of preexisting autoantibody, and raising level of inflammatory cytokines may be involved in the immune-related adverse effects. Nevertheless, it needs to be noted that the organ-specific toxic effects of anti-PD therapy are much less severe than anti-CTLA-4 antibodies. Except the toxic effects in endocrine systems, most of these adverse effects can be reversed. Multidisciplinary corporation is expected to fully realize the potential of immune checkpoint treatment [188].

15.6.2 Combination Therapies Based on PD-1/PD-L1 Pathway Blockade

15.6.2.1 Enhanced Antitumor Effect by Combination of Therapeutic Agents and Immune Checkpoint Inhibitors

Due to the limited therapeutic efficacy of ICB alone, various types of therapeutic agents were applied in combination with immune checkpoint inhibitors. Some molecules that target immunogenic and tumorigenic signaling pathways are involved in combinational cancer therapy. Ibrutinib, a covalent inhibitor for both BTK and ITK, can regulate B-cell receptor pathway and balance the Th1/Th2 T cells for antitumor treatment. After incorporating with anti-PD-L1 antibody, it could effectively suppress tumor growth of lymphoma which was insensitive to single ibrutinib therapy. These preclinical results provided convincing evidence for hematologic malignancies' treatment. Moreover, this combination therapy could also be extended to treat solid tumors in future [189].

Tumor angiogenesis is essential for cancer growth and progression. It is demonstrated that pathological angiogenesis inside tumor might limit the efficacy of cancer immunotherapy [190–192]. Preclinical researches showed that antiangiogenic therapy and anti-PD-L1 therapy could interact with each other to boost cancer immunotherapy. Anti-PD-L1 therapy could make the tumors sensible to antiangiogenic therapy and also prolong its efficacy.

Similar research showed that a bispecific antibody (A2V) that blockaded both angiopoietin-2 (ANGPT2) and vascular endothelial growth factor A (VEGFA) could induce intratumoral blood vessel normalization and promote tumor necrosis. Moreover, it could elicit activation of CD8+ T cells which could upregulate endothelial PD-L1 expression by releasing IFN-γ. They identified that PD-1 blockade combined with A2V could improve antitumor efficacy in melanoma, pancreatic neuroendocrine tumor, and metastatic breast cancer. These researches provide strong evidence for co-targeting angiogenesis and immune checkpoints in antitumor treatment [193].

15.6.2.2 Synergistic Effects by Combining Drug-Loaded Nanoparticles with Immune Checkpoint Inhibitors

PDT is an invasiveness therapeutic procedure that has already been clinically applied for antitumor treatment. Lin's group focused on the combination of PDT and ICB. In their study, it was elucidated that prior PDT could improve the sensitivity of tumors to checkpoint blockade by increasing the tumor immunogenicity. Therefore, Zn-pyrophosphate (ZnP) nanoparticles encapsulating the photosensitizer pyrolipid (ZnP@ pyro) were developed and combined with anti-PD-L1 antibody for metastatic breast cancer treatment. Importantly, the results showed this combination therapy could not only effectively eradicate primary tumor growth but also prevent lung metastasis [194] (Figure 15.11A–C).

Another kind of polymer core-shell nanoparticles was also generated for effective PDT that carries oxaliplatin and photosensitizer pyropheophorbide-lipid (NCP@pyrolipid) [195]. Strikingly, after further combining with anti-PD-L1 antibody, it can effectively inhibit the distant tumors in the murine models of CT26 and MC38 by eliciting increased CD4+ and CD8+ T-cell infiltration (Figure 15.11D and E).

15.6.2.3 Combination Therapy with Immune Checkpoint Inhibitors Loaded Nanoparticles

Various delivery systems were explored to facilitate delivery of anti-PD antibodies. A self-degradable microneedle (MN) patch was formulated for efficient anti-PD-1 antibody delivery in vivo [196]. This microneedle containing nanoparticles that encapsulated both anti-PD-1 and glucose-specific enzyme could facilitate the release of anti-PD-1 after nanoparticles' dissociation. It was demonstrated that the MN path could elicit strong immune responses in murine melanoma model. In addition, anti-PD-1 antibody and 1-methyl-DL-tryptophan (1-MT) were loaded to form m-HA nanoparticles. Utilizing the microneedle for transcutaneous delivery, self-assembled m-HA nanoparticles could achieve significant antitumor efficacy in melanoma model. The microneedle patch provided a promising strategy for checkpoint inhibitor delivery either alone or in combination with two kinds of blockade antibody. It could avoid the systematic side effects at the mean time [197] (Figure 15.12A).

Wang et al. [198] fabricated a DNA "nano-cocoons" to responsively release anti-PD-1 antibody (aPD1) and TLR9 agonist CpG ODNs in tumor resection bed. Compared with free CpG and aPD1, the co-delivery system could significantly improve the antitumor immunity with removing the remained tumor after surgery and preventing metastasis (Figure 15.12B).

Moreover, they developed engineered platelets to facilitate the delivery of anti-PD-L1 antibody. Platelets showed distinct advantages among cell-based delivery system. They could help to accumulate at lesion sites and be also identified to enhance inflammatory conditions. Thus, utilizing the platelet-based anti-PD-L1 delivery system, the immune checkpoint inhibitors could be guided to the surgical bed and target circulating tumor cells in the bloodstream. The results showed that anti-PD-L1 antibody was effectively released as platelet activation. Importantly, prolonged overall survival and inhibition of metastasis were observed after surgery by platelet-bound anti-PD-L1 antibody compared to anti-PD-L1 alone [199] (Figure 15.13A).

Normally, single ICB therapy exhibited poor response for low immunogenic tumors. It was demonstrated that combination chemotherapy with immunotherapy could elevate antitumor efficacy for low immunogenic tumors to some extent. A ROS-responsive gel scaffold was engineered to load gemcitabine and anti-PD-L1 antibody for in situ antitumor treatment. The results showed that gemcitabine could promote the low immunogenic tumor into immunogenic tumor, thus enhancing the sensitivity of tumors to ICB. Moreover, in both melanoma and breast cancer models, inhibition of tumor recurrence after resection could be observed by this combination therapy [200] (Figure 15.13B).

15.6.3 siRNA Targeting PD-1/PD-L1 Immune Checkpoint

With the aid of nanotechnology, gene therapy has been widely applied for a variety of tumors, and it revealed promising efficacy in preliminary clinical trials [201,202]. More and more researches focus on gene therapy mediated by nanosized materials that targets the immune regulatory pathways. An acid-activatable micelleplex was designed by integrating photosensitizer and siRNA targeting PD-L1. The versatile micelleplexes were formulated by two components. One was a pH-sensitive diblock copolymer PEG-b-P(DPA-co-HEA) (PDPA) conjugated with a PS of pheophorbide A (PPa). The other was 1,2-epoxytetradecane alkylated oligoethylenimine (OEIeC14). Thus, the micelleplexes had strong affinity to siRNA and was only activated in endocytic vesicles of tumor cells. The results demonstrated that antitumor immune responses were elevated obviously by the combination treatment of PTT and PD-L1 blockade. Remarkably, it firstly evidenced that the enhanced antitumor immune responses could be elicited by combining siRNA-mediated PDL1 blockade and PTT [203] (Figure 15.13C).

More and more researches are developing the combination modalities on anti-PD therapy. Among them, nanotechnology application in antibody or siRNA delivery exhibited promising strategies and may be further combined with other therapeutic drug-loaded nanoparticles for superior antitumor efficacy to realize the complete tumor eradication. It also needs further understanding on the tumor microenvironment. Moreover, it may also be combined with intrinsic signal pathways and epigenetics to achieve more promising progress. The application of nanotechnology with anti-PD therapy may need to focus on tumor microenvironment.

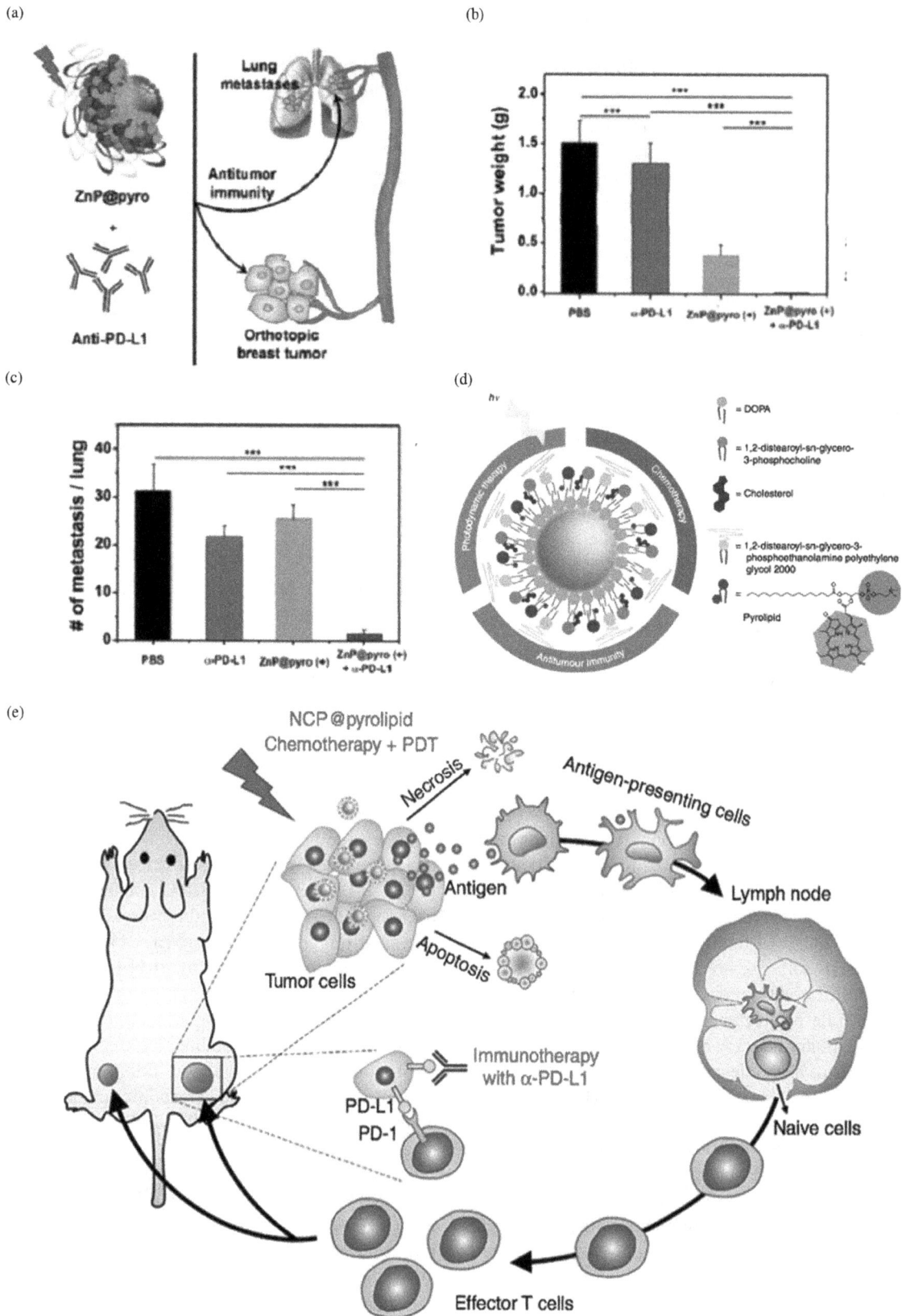

FIGURE 15.11 (A) Combination of Znp@pyro and anti-PD-L1 antibody to eradicate orthotopic breast cancer and inhibit lung metastasis. (B) Tumor weight represented the eradication of breast cancer and (C) tumor nodules in lungs after combining Znp@pyro and anti-PD-L1 antibody treatment. (Reprinted with permission from [194]. Copyright 2016 American Chemical Society.) (D) Synthesis of NCP@pyrolipid and its combined therapeutic modalities. (E) Combination of oxaliplatin and photosensitizer loaded in NCP@pyrolipid with anti-PD-L1 antibody to enhance systemic antitumor immunity. (Reprinted with permission from [195]. Copyright 2016 Nature Publishing Group.)

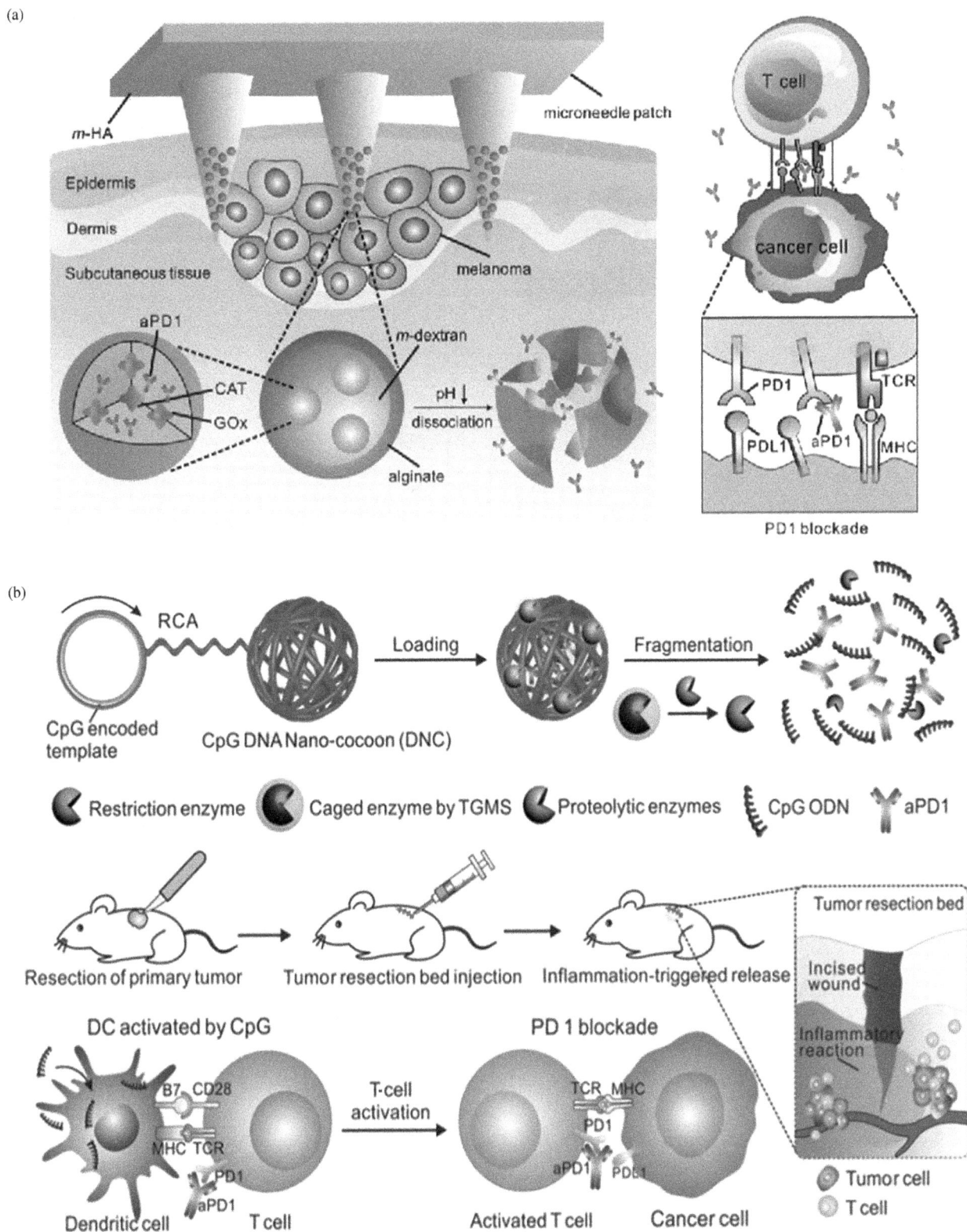

FIGURE 15.12 (A) Delivery of anti-PD-1 antibody utilizing MN patch. Anti-PD-1 antibody could be released when the nanoparticles dissociated by the enzyme, and subsequently, it relieved the PD-1/PD-L1 blockade. (Reprinted with permission from [197]. Copyright 2016 American Chemical Society.) (B) A DNA nanococoon (DNC) was fabricated to load CpG, anti-PD-1 antibody, and restriction enzyme. When the DNC was injected to tumor resection bed, the inflammation condition triggered the restriction enzyme and released the CpG and anti-PD-1 by breaking the DNC. Hence, DCs were activated by CpG and PD-1 was blockaded. (Reprinted with permission from [198]. Copyright 2016 WILEY-VCH Verlag GmbH & Co. KGaA, Weinheim.)

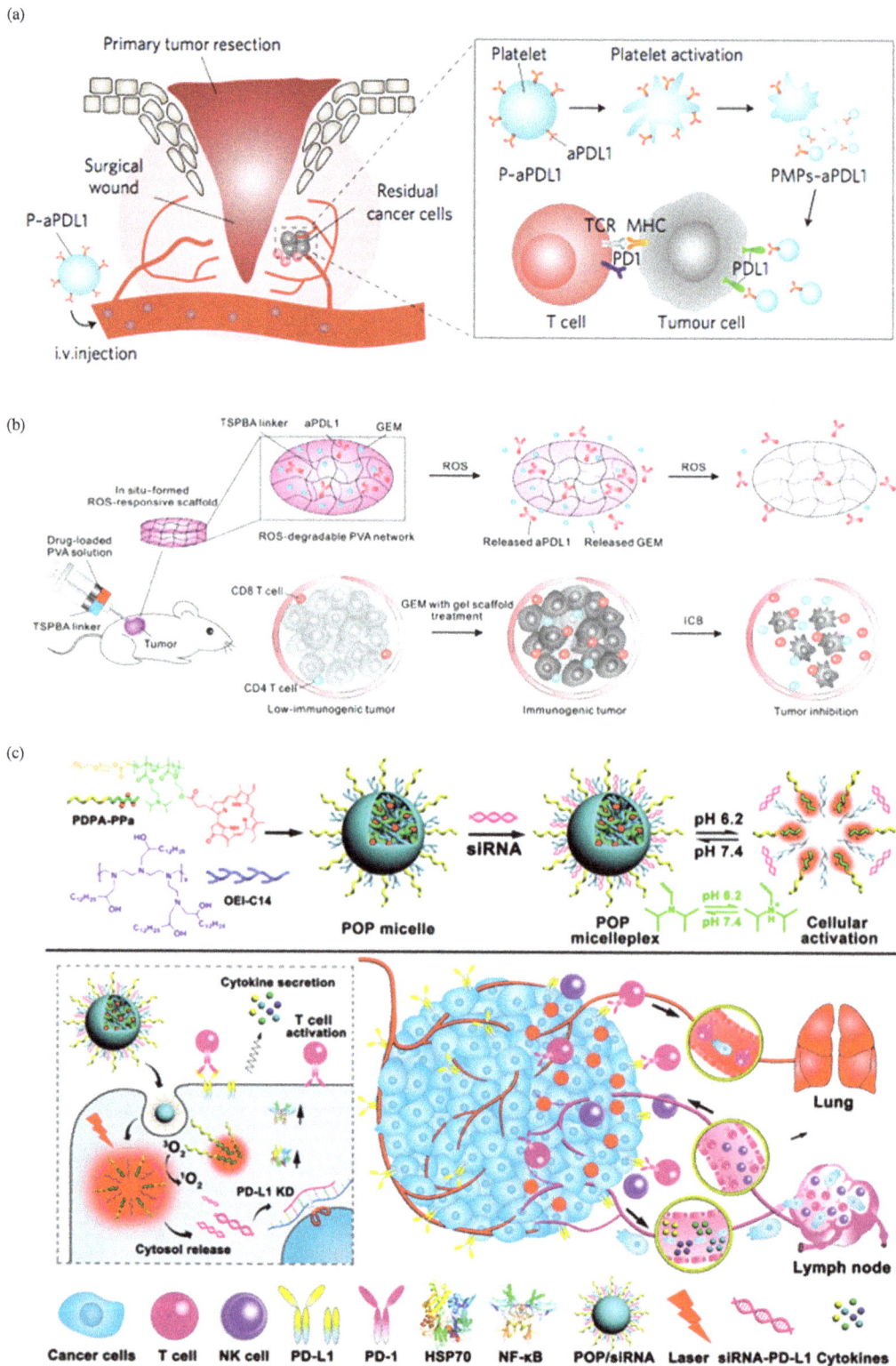

FIGURE 15.13 (A) Platelet-mediated anti-PD-L1 antibody delivery to surgical residual sites. The PD-1/PD-L1ICB was released by anti-PD-L1 antibody. (Reprinted with permission from [199]. Copyright 2017 Nature Publishing Group.) (B) Gemcitabine and anti-PD-L1 were loaded in ROS-degradable hydrogel scaffold and delivered into tumor microenvironment to convert low-immunogenic tumor to immunogenic tumor phenotype. (Reprinted with permission from [200]. Copyright 2018 American Association for the Advancement of Science.) (C) The POP micelleplex was dissociated in an acid microenvironment to release siRNA targeting PD-L1 and photosensitizer. Combining PDT and siPD-L1, the cytokine secretion was increased and more tumor-infiltrating T cells were observed. Hence, the combination therapy efficiently suppressed tumor growth and inhibited lung metastasis in B16F10 model. (Reprinted with permission from [203]. Copyright 2015 American Chemical Society.)

15.7 THE BASIC MECHANISM OF IDO

IDO, an intracellular heme-containing enzyme encoded by IDO1 gene, can regulate the degradation of tryptophan (Trp) into kynurenine (Kyn), which is regarded as the first and rate-limiting step in kynurenine pathway [204]. IDO enzymes contain IDO1 and IDO2. IDO1 is widely distributed in human body, mainly in lymphoid organs and scattered in placenta, anterior chamber, and gastrointestinal mucosa. The expression of IDO1 is highest in APCs, such as DCs and macrophages [205,206]. While the expression of IDO2 is much narrower than IDO1, IDO2 is only expressed in DCs and some of the tissues which also express IDO1 [207]. Most importantly, tryptophan is crucial for maintaining survival and effector functions of T cells. Tryptophan deficiency mediated by IDO could induce naïve CD4+ T cells differentiating into Tregs [208].

Increasing researches identified the immunosuppressive role of IDO. It can help to regulate the host's antitumor immunity, induce inflammatory tumor microenvironment, and stimulate tumor angiogenesis [209]. The expression level of IDO is correlated with the clinical phases, prognosis, and metastasis of various malignant tumors [210]. In preclinical trials, combination of IDO with immunotherapy, chemotherapy, or radiotherapy exhibited satisfied outcomes in antitumor treatment. Therefore, IDO will be a potent therapeutic target for cancer immunotherapy.

15.7.1 INHIBITORS BLOCKING IDO

There are several kinds of IDO inhibitors being explored in clinical trials. First, specific IDO1 inhibitors include NLG919, PF-06840003, INCB024360, and its analogues. Second, specific IDO2 inhibitor represents indoximod. Third, inhibitors both targeting IDO1 and IDO2 contain norharmane and 1-methyl-DL-trytophan (1-MT). 1-MT is extensively investigated among IDO inhibitors. Two isomers of 1-MT, D and L-, are potent inhibitor of IDO2 and IDO1, respectively. Moreover, the IDO inhibitors D-1MT, INCB024360, NLG919 have already been applied in clinical trials and are more applicable for clinical treatment [211,212].

INCB024360 is an orally administrated IDO inhibitor. The first phase I study of this IDO inhibitor was reported in 2013 [213]. Increasing clinical trials of this inhibitor were investigated afterward by using either INCB024360 monotherapy or combination therapy. In a phase Ib/II trial, it is identified that incorporation of INCB024360 and ipilimumab could elicit enhanced antitumor response in advanced melanoma patients than ipilimumab monotherapy (NCT01604889) [214]. NLG919 is also developed as orally bioavailable IDO inhibitor. It is demonstrated that when combined with chemoradiation therapy, NLG919 could effectively prolong the survival of mice with glioblastoma [215]. However, there exists raising questions about the future of IDO inhibitors. In the latest phase III study (NCT02752074), over 700 patients were randomly divided into two groups, Keytruda in combination with Epacadostat or placebo. The results demonstrated that combining Keytruda and Epacadostat failed to prolong overall survival for unresectable or metastatic melanoma compared to Keytruda alone [216]. Further investigations of the Keytruda-Epacadostat combo therapy on other tumor types, such as NSCLC, bladder cancer, and renal cancer, are being studied.

15.7.2 COMBINATION THERAPIES BASED ON IDO BLOCKADE

PDT has shown high efficacy in local tumor treatment but not yet efficient to tumor metastasis suppression. By applying a nanoscale metal-organic framework (nMOF) to entrap IDO inhibitor, the combinational PDT and anti-IDO immunotherapy showed significantly synergistic effects on eliminating local and distant tumors. It may be attributed to increased TILs via IDO inhibitor and induced immunogenic cell death (ICD) effect from the generated ROS by PDT treatment. Moreover, neutrophils and B cells played an important role in antigen presentation for enhanced antitumor immunity after PDT treatment. There is significant increase of infiltrated NK cells in tumor microenvironment for effective tumor therapy [217]. In addition, a hafnium-based nMOF also enabled radiodynamic therapy and local tumors could be eradicated by given low doses of X-ray irradiation. Combining a small molecular IDOi (INCB024360) and radiotherapy, distal tumors could be rejected in CT26 colorectal cancer and breast cancer. Importantly, the population of CD8+ T cells, CD45+ leukocytes, and CD4+ T cells were significantly increased not only in primary but also in distant tumors to elicit systemic antitumor immunity [218] (Figure 15.14A).

NLG919 is a nontoxic IDO-1-selective inhibitor which can enhance tumor regression in preclinical models. A redox-responsive polymeric prodrug of IDO inhibitor NLG919 was developed for co-delivery of anticancer drug DOX. The prodrug can self-assemble into micelles with DOX for combinational immunochemotherapy. As presented, the micelles exhibited effective tumor inhibition against breast cancer 4 T1.2-bearing mice with extended overall survival time and enhanced antitumor immunity. The prodrug micelles exhibited enhanced effector T cells and reduced immunosuppressive cells including T_{reg} and myeloid-derived suppressor cells (MDSCs) in comparison with free DOX or liposomal Doxil® [219] (Figure 15.14B).

15.7.3 siRNA TARGETING IDO IMMUNE CHECKPOINT

By co-delivery of indoleamine 2,3-dioxygenase siRNA (siIDO) and tumor-associated antigen TRP2, inorganic layered double hydroxide nanoparticle-based vaccine exhibited DCs uptaken and endo/lysosome escape for efficient antigen presentation. The nanovaccine exhibited significant melanoma suppression through inducing antitumor

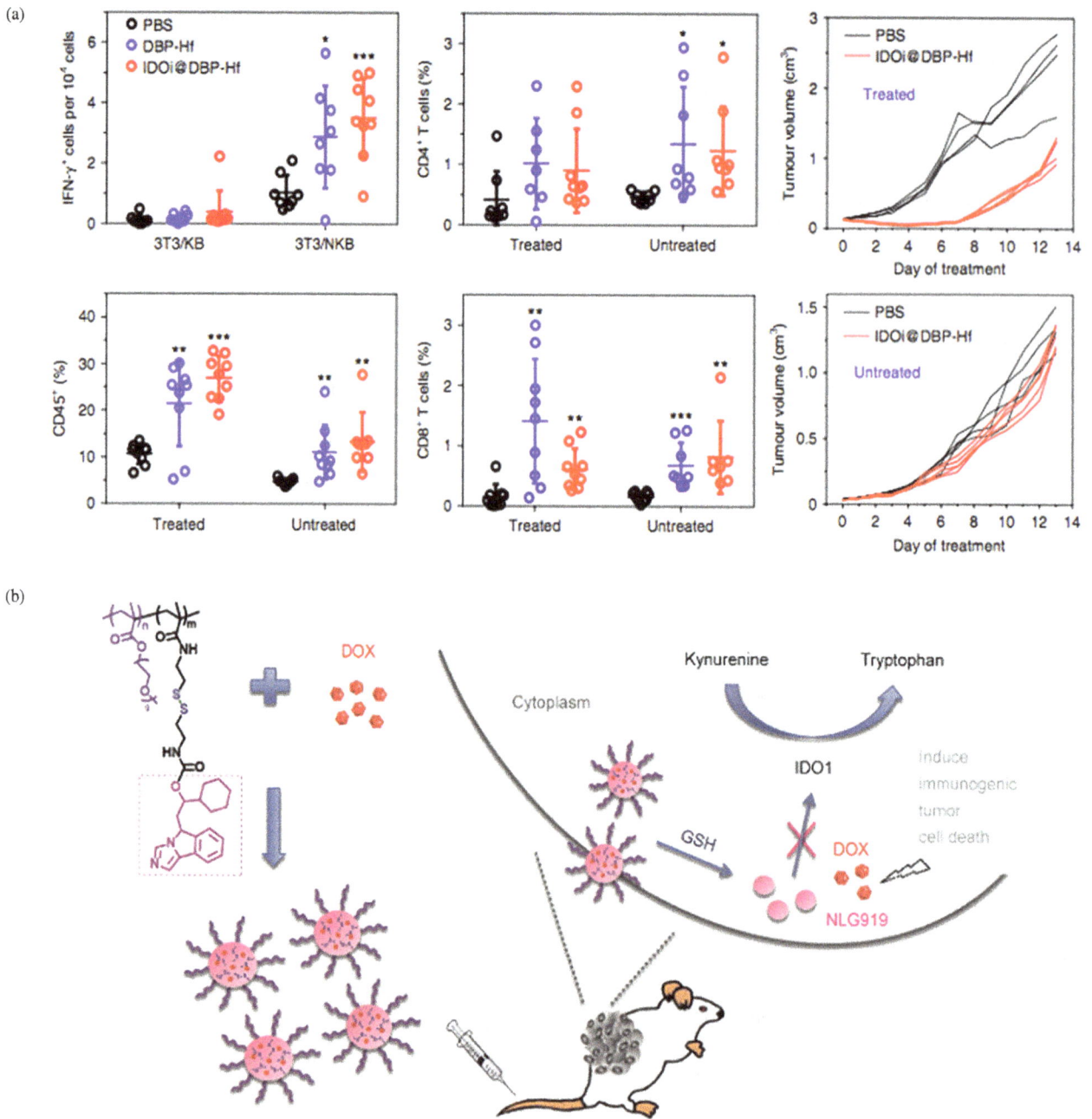

FIGURE 15.14 (A) Tumor growth and antitumor immunity of combination therapy with IDOi@DBP-Hf and radiotherapy. The population of CD8+ T cells, CD45+ leukocytes, and CD4+ T cells were significantly elevated in both primary and distant tumors. (Reprinted with permission from [218]. Copyright 2018 Nature Publishing Group.) (B) Nano-sized micelles were formulated by co-loading NLG919 and DOX into PSSN10 prodrug polymers. Inhibition of IDO pathway suppressed the degradation of Trp into Kyn and promoted therapeutic efficacy of chemotherapy. (Reprinted with permission from [219]. Copyright 2017 Nature Publishing Group.)

immunity and silencing IDO-mediated immunosuppression [220]. Although IDO inhibitors have been incorporated in nanoparticles and developed in combination therapy with PDT, chemotherapy, and vaccine, the efficiency is still under consideration. Especially, there is still not enough evidence to demonstrate the improved therapeutic efficacy after combining with other immunotherapy in clinical trials yet.

15.8 CD47, CD40, AND 4-1BB

CD47 is a transmembrane protein, and it could produce integrin-associated protein that transmits "don't eat me" signal to immune system [221]. By binding to the ligand signal regulatory protein alpha (SIRPα), it can suppress phagocytosis. CD47 is expressed ubiquitously in various kinds of human cells, and increasing evidence has shown that CD47 is overexpressed in a variety of tumor cells. Owing to the

CD47/ SIRPα interaction, tumor cells could avoid clearance by phagocytic cells resulting in immune evasion [222]. Recently, it is demonstrated that anti-CD47 antibody could turn off "don't eat me" signal and promote phagocytosis of tumor cells by macrophages. Moreover, it can initiate antitumor immune response [223]. Hence, human anti-CD47 monoclonal antibodies are being evaluated for malignant tumor treatment. Although tumor-associated myeloid cells are thought to be related to metastasis and drug resistance, some of them, such as macrophages and DCs, play an essential role in antigen presentation and subsequent antitumor immunity of cytotoxic T cells. By using antibody KWAR23 to block SIRPα, the antitumor immunity of myeloid cells in human Burkitt's lymphoma xenograft model could be significantly enhanced by promoting the infiltration of neutrophils and macrophages. It might benefit a number of patients by eliciting durable responses [224]. In addition, CD47 blockade also promoted the phagocytosis of DCs on tumor cells and triggered consequent antitumor immune responses for eliminating immunogenic tumors. It provided combination strategy with chemotherapy against tumor relapse [225].

CD40 is a member of tumor necrosis factor receptor (TNFR) family. Similarly to CD47, CD40 is broadly expressed on normal cells, APCs, and various tumor cells, including lymphomas and solid tumors [226]. One study reported that local delivery of anti-CD40 agonistic antibody with Montanide ISA-51 exhibited significantly extended overall survival with good safety in comparison with systemically administered antibody [227]. Moreover, anti-CD40 antibody could modulate the antitumor immunity by activating APCs and inducing CTLs. Co-delivery of bufalin and anti-CD40 antibody by liposomes showed synergistic therapeutic efficacy in melanoma treatment [228].

4-1BB (CD137) is also a costimulatory member of TNFR family. Researchers reported that the expression of 4-1BB is primarily on activated CD4$^+$ and CD8$^+$ T cells. 4-1BB is crucial for maintaining T-cell effector function and generating immune memory [229]. Co-administration of anti-4-1BB antibody and HPV E6/E7 peptide vaccine is demonstrated to elicit 100% of long-term immune response in the HPV$^+$ TC-1 tumor model, while HPV vaccine alone could only retard disease progression. It was illustrated that anti-4-1BB antibody was an effective T cells' costimulatory antibody that could significantly enhance the therapeutic responses [230]. The application of nanotechnology with CD40, CD47, or 4-1BB remains underexplored, and it may need further investigation with other therapeutic modalities for enhanced antitumor efficacy.

Besides these, many other immune checkpoint molecules are being investigated, including LAG3 (lymphocyte activation gene 3), TIM-3 (T-cell immunoglobulin domain and Mucin domain 3), KIR (killer-cell immunoglobulin-like receptor), B7-H3 (CD276), VISTA (V-domain Ig suppressor of T-cell activation), and so on. Recently, TIGIT (T-cell Ig and ITIM domain) was exploited that it can function as an immune checkpoint that mainly expressed on NK cell and T cells. When it binds to its ligand CD155 on APCs or target cells, the immune responses initiated by NK cells were significantly suppressed. The research demonstrated that blockade of TIGIT could restore the activity of tumor-infiltrating NK cells and enhance antitumor therapeutic effects. Furthermore, it can be incorporated with other ICB, such as PD-1 or PD-L1 to provide promising antitumor immunotherapy in future [231].

15.9 OPPORTUNITIES FOR IMPROVING EFFICACY OF IMMUNE CHECKPOINT INHIBITORS

Despite the significant successes of immune checkpoint inhibitors in clinical trials for a wide range of cancer, some limits for expanding the applicability of antibodies remain to be overcome. In preclinical research, only a fraction of patients exhibited satisfied outcome to the ICB antibodies due to the individual heterogeneity and intrinsic mechanisms of tumorigenesis [232]. Moreover, the off-target side effects could cause severe autoimmune disorders of these antibodies, such as inflammation of endocrine organs, lungs, and other organs [233]. A proportion of patients exhibited drug resistance, even tumor recurrence in the long-term immunotherapy [234,235]. Taking these severe factors into account, personalized, combinational, and alternative therapies of ICB are in urgent demand to improve the therapeutic efficacy.

Recently, more and more researches are attempting to figure out the biomarkers and intrinsic pathways of ICB in order to provide guidelines for treatment and improve the antitumor efficacy for benefiting a majority of patients. Based on these researches, the tumor microenvironment is classified into an immunogenic (hot) and a non-immunogenic (cold) tumor microenvironment. The major differences between them are the components of infiltrating T cells, enriched cytokines, number of functional APCs, and biological characteristics [232]. By detecting PD-L1 expression level of tumor cells, the clinical responses to anti-PD therapy might be predicted somehow. Therefore, combination therapies of immune checkpoint inhibitors can be guided by these biomarkers.

Furthermore, as the nanoparticles could provide versatile drug delivery platform, combination therapies will not only limit in the synergistic immune checkpoint modulators but also combine with vaccine, TAA, immune adjuvant, and so on.

A biomimetic, cancer cell membrane–enveloped polymeric nanovaccine could realize the co-delivery of autologous TAA and immune adjuvant, TLR agonist CpG. The elicited antitumor immune responses of nanovaccine provided significant prophylactic efficacy with remarkable extended overall survival in melanoma model. After further combination with ICB of anti-CTLA-4 and anti-PD-1 cocktail, the nanovaccine exhibited promising applicability in melanoma therapy [236] (Figure 15.15A and B).

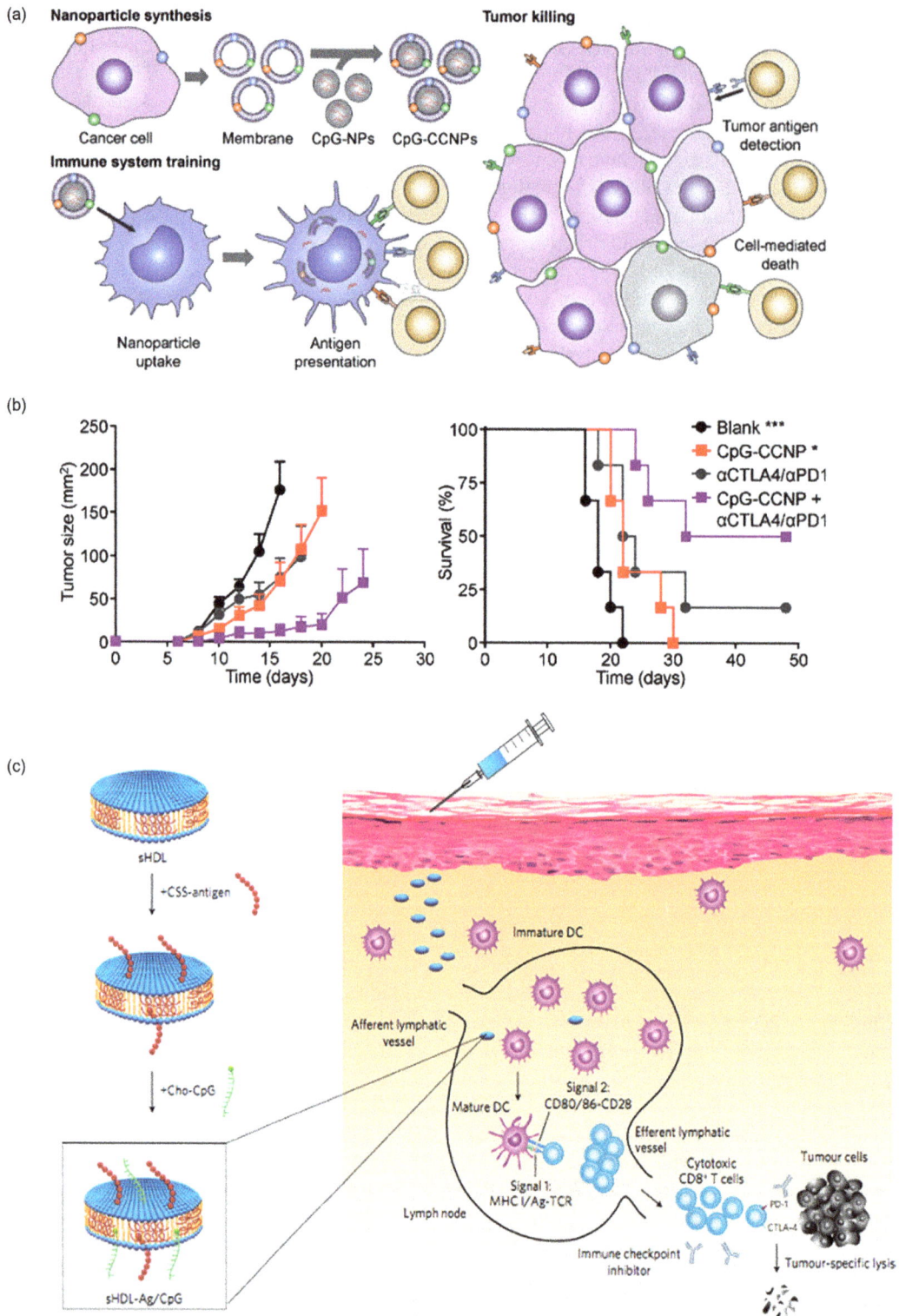

FIGURE 15.15 (A) Cancer cell membrane-derived nanoparticles loading CpG adjuvant (CpG-CCNPs) triggered activation of T cells resulting in tumor cells' killing. (B) After further incorporating anti-CTLA-4 and anti-PD-1 antibody into CpG-CCNPs, smaller tumor size and prolonged overall survival were observed compared to CpGCCNPs alone. (Reprinted with permission from [236]. Copyright 2017 WILEY-VCH Verlag GmbH & Co. KGaA, Weinheim.) (C) The synthetic high-density lipoprotein (sHDL) nanodiscs were utilized to co-deliver antigen peptides and cholesterol CpG (Cho-CpG) adjuvant to induce personalized cancer vaccines. After administration of the nanodiscs, anti-CTLA-4 and anti-PD-1 antibody, CTL responses were significantly enhanced in both MC-38 and B16F10 tumors by promoting antigen presentation and inducing DC maturation. Moreover, eradication of established tumors was also detected. (Reprinted with permission from [237]. Copyright 2017 Nature Publishing Group.)

In addition, a new kind of nanodiscs was developed for co-delivering antigenic peptide mixture and adjuvant with significantly enhanced antigen-specific T-cell responses. The neoantigens were conjugated with high-density lipoprotein mimetic nanodiscs, and the nanovaccine exhibited the robust induction of multi-epitope immune responses for broad-spectrum antitumor immunity. With further combination with anti-PD-1 and anti-CTLA-4 treatment, this nanovaccine could promote removal on established tumors in MC-38 and B16F10 cancers' treatment. It also provided good tendency on developing personal nanomedicine in future [237] (Figure 15.15C).

As the complex immunological pathways are investigated in tumor progression, small molecules targeting diverse intrinsic signaling pathways are also involved in antitumor immunotherapies. Combination of other kinds of immune checkpoint inhibitors was also explored. Poly(lactic-co-hydroxymethylglycolic acid) (pLHMGA) microparticles were formulated to deliver anti-CTLA-4 antibody and CD40 agonistic antibody simultaneously. Treating the MC-38 tumor model with these biodegradable microparticles, improved antitumor efficacy could be observed [34]. OX40 (CD134) is a member of TNFR family. Combination anti-OX40/anti-CTLA-4 antibodies and tumor antigen-specific vaccine could elevate the effector function of T cells, thus destruct tumors and prolong overall survival in prostate adenocarcinoma [238].

15.10 PROSPECTS FOR IMMUNE CHECKPOINT BLOCKADE

To achieve high-target specificity and limit side effects of immune checkpoint monoclonal antibodies, genetic interventions are explored in combinational immunotherapies. With the aid of nanoparticle delivery system, siRNA-based therapy could specifically silence a wide range of target gene that is essential for immune inhibitory pathways. However, the siRNA-based therapy has limited efficacy in inhibiting the expression of target gene and is unlikely to cure the diseases [239].

Novel genome engineering techniques, such as CRISPR-Cas9 genome editing system, are rapidly developed. Target genes that involved in the immune modulatory pathways can be persistently, specifically knocked out utilizing these newly emerging technologies, hence boosting antitumor immune responses and reversing the tumor-suppressive microenvironment. Taking advantages of CRISPR-Cas9 system for knocking out gene in tumor cells, it may promote identification of specific genes that mediate the resistance or sensitivity to ICB for eventually changing the treatment and prognosis in cancer treatment [240]. Therefore, combination nanotechnology with CRISPR-Cas9 system would expand new prospect and provide potent strategy for cancer immunotherapy.

In addition, besides targeting the immune modulatory pathways, increasing researches focus on the epigenetic modification on immune checkpoint. A small molecule BET inhibitor JQ1 was discovered with PD-L1 expression suppression and could inhibit ovarian cancer growth. JQ1 exhibited great potential in augmenting the antitumor immunity as demonstrated suppression of PD-L1 not only on tumor cells but also on tumor-associated macrophages and DCs [241]. Based on this discovery, a personalized cancer vaccine (PVAX) based on 4 T1 breast cancer cells was developed to encapsulate JQ1 and ICG into a hydrogel matrix for postsurgical treatment. ICG could significantly increase the temperature under 808 nm NIR laser irradiation leading to the release of JQ1 and tumor-specific antigens. Therefore, PD-L1 expression was effectively blocked by JQ1 and the host's specific immune response was triggered by tumor-specific antigens. The PVAX treatment could significantly suppress tumor recurrence and inhibit lung metastasis in 4 T1 postsurgical tumor model. Moreover, it could elicit long-term memory of immune response that CD11b+CD8+CD44+CD62L– T cells were obviously increased in immune organs, including spleen, lymph nodes, and bone marrows. Therefore, the investigation on combing epigenetics and ICB will surely be the forefront for cancer immunotherapy in future [242].

Besides genome editing and epigenetic modification of the ICB-related pathway, some other alternative approaches were also investigated. Cellular nanocarriers, such as nanovesicles and microparticles, showed distinct advantages for drug delivery in biomedicine [243]. As it was evidenced that cellular nanocarriers could carry same protein with parent cells [244], some latest researches focused on how to exploit functional cellular nanocarriers with specific therapeutic protein through engineering the parent cells. Cellular vesicles, which were fabricated by a serial extrusion from engineered HEK 293 T cells with PD-1 stably expression, displayed new options to disrupt PD-1/PDL1 axis. Owing to the expression of PD-1 receptor on these cellular vesicles, they could engage to PD-L1 on tumor cells and promote immune responses. Small molecules of IDO inhibitor were further loaded into the PD-1 blockade cellular vesicles to assess synergistic antitumor efficacy, leading to significant reduction of tumor growth, elevated infiltration of CD8+ T cells, and decreased CD4+ FoxP3+ T cells in tumor microenvironment [245]. Similarly, megakaryocyte (MK) progenitor cells were transfected with lentivirus encoding PD-1 receptor and subsequently generated mature PD-1–expressing platelet. The PD-1 platelet could carry low dose of cyclophosphamide to improve antitumor immunity and efficiently target surgery wound to form platelet microparticles (PMPs) after activation. It was demonstrated that the PMPs could obviously eradicate residual melanoma by eliminating Tregs and enhancing the population of CD8+Ki67+GzmB+ lymphocytes [246]. These cellular nanocarriers on PD-1 blockade provide powerful platform and broaden the horizon for immunotherapy. More kinds of cellular nanocarriers with various target proteins for ICB, such as PD-L1, TIGIT, and TIM3, will also be developed.

15.11 TARGETED DELIVERY OF NANOPARTICLES TO LYMPH NODES AND IMMUNE CELLS

Tumor-draining lymph nodes (TDLNs), which majorly constitute tumor-specific T lymphocytes, B lymphocytes, and APCs, are located along the tumor-draining lymphatic channels [247,248]. TDLNs play a crucial role in cellular and humoral immunity against cancer as they are antigen-encountered through drainage of TAAs, but they are often immune-suppressed [249–251]. As nanoparticles have the potential for efficient draining and retention in TDLNs because of their size and particular structure which resembles that of pathogens, their potential effects to intensify activation and proliferation of APCs in TDLNs as the immuno-stimulatory agents have been studied by recent experiments. Jeanbart et al. coated both the adjuvant and TAA to form a nanosystem and delivered it to the TDLN and non-TDLN of tumor-bearing mice [252]. They found that the nanosystem delivered to the TDLN induced a substantially stronger cytotoxic CD8+ T-lymphocyte response both locally and systemically than the non-TDLN group, leading to tumor regression and a longer survival period. Nanoparticle coupling of both the adjuvant and antigen is necessary for the effective TDLN stimulation, and this delivering method could dramatically enhance the antigen presentation process of TDLN APCs, thus increasing the therapeutic efficacy. Similar results were also found by Kang et al. that nanoparticles co-delivering tumor membrane antigens, DAMP signal-augmenting element α-helix HSP70 functional peptide (αHSP70p) and CpG exhibited efficient TDLN trafficking, inducing not only the tumor-specific T-lymphocyte response, but also natural killer cells' immune stimulation and effector memory T cells' proliferation (Figure 15.16) [253]. The distinction between the metastatic TDLN, the TDLN that has been colonized by metastatic tumor cells, and nonmetastatic TDLN is very important for surgical resection and prognosis evaluation, and Cao et al. found that folate receptor-targeted trimodal polymer nanoparticles were efficient for the rapid and precise diagnosis of lymph node metastasis *in vivo* [254]. The folate-functionalized nanoparticles were coated with PFBT, NIR775, and DTPA-BSA (Gd) for the near-infrared, photoacoustic, and magnetic resonance imaging. The results showed that the nanoparticles rapidly accumulated in metastatic lymph nodes, which could effectively detect and distinguish metastatic lymph nodes at 1 h post-injection, and had excellent potential in real-time image-guided surgery.

Besides the TDLN, nanoparticles are also designed to target different types of immune cells, among which the DC is the most targeted cell because of its prominent role in antigen processing and presentation. The DC target is implemented by integrating ligands that combine with the membrane receptors on DCs, including the mannose, CD40, CD11c, DEC205, and DC-SIGN receptors. Studies found that the DC-targeted nanosystem could reinforce the endocytosis of DCs compared with the free form without

nanoparticles [255–259]. Wang et al. conjugated mannose on the lipid–calcium–phosphate nanoparticles and found improved DC engulfment in the targeting-delivered group [260]. As a result, the co-encapsulated PD-L1 siRNA resulted in downregulation of PD-L1 in DCs that presented tumor antigens, further significantly prompted T-cell activation and proliferation, and exhibited profound inhibitory effects on tumor growth and metastasis. Similar results were reported in another study by Liu et al. [261]. In addition, targeting different molecules on the DC seemed to have different DC stimulation efficacy.

He et al. developed a macrophage dual-targeted CpG-loading nanoparticle realized by mannosylated carboxymethyl chitosan (MCMC) and hyaluronan (HA), which resulted in a considerable shift of macrophages to activated M1 types and a significantly enhanced secretion of proinflammatory cytokines [262]. Besides, the nanosystem also activated NF-κB and phosphoinositide 3-kinase/Akt signal pathways and induced Fas/FasL-mediated apoptosis in breast cancer models (Figure 15.17). Cross-linking of B-lymphocyte receptors is the initiation of B-cell proliferation and differentiation to plasma cells secreting specific antibodies. In another study, biodegradable calcium phosphate nanoparticles decorated with model antigen hen egg lysozyme were preferentially bound and internalized by the tumor antigen-specific B lymphocytes, subsequently enhanced the surface expression of B-cell activation markers, and induced high humoral immunity, which was found to be approximately 100-fold more efficient in the activation of B cells than the soluble form of tumor antigens [263].

15.12 NANOPARTICLES INFLUENCING THE TUMOR MICROENVIRONMENT FOR IMMUNOTHERAPY ENHANCEMENT

The tumor microenvironment refers to the surrounding complex scaffold around tumor cells, which is composed of the extracellular matrix, various signaling molecules, blood vessels, immune cells, fibroblasts, and bone marrow–derived inflammatory cells [264]. Tumor cells were closely related to the surrounding microenvironment, by releasing cellular signaling molecules and interacting with immune and other related cells; tumors can influence the microenvironment to further promote the angiogenesis and induce immune tolerance [265,266]. It has been reported that the extracellular matrix within the tumor microenvironment could play inhibitory roles to the adaptive antitumor immune response by inhibiting tumor-specific T-lymphocyte proliferation through type I collagen ligation of LAIR receptors, and T-lymphocyte activation from its naive state [267]. In addition, the abnormal tumor microenvironment could also provide critical biochemical and biomechanical cues to direct tumor cell growth, survival, proliferation, and migration and suppress the antitumor immunity function through suppressive cytokine release, cellular interaction,

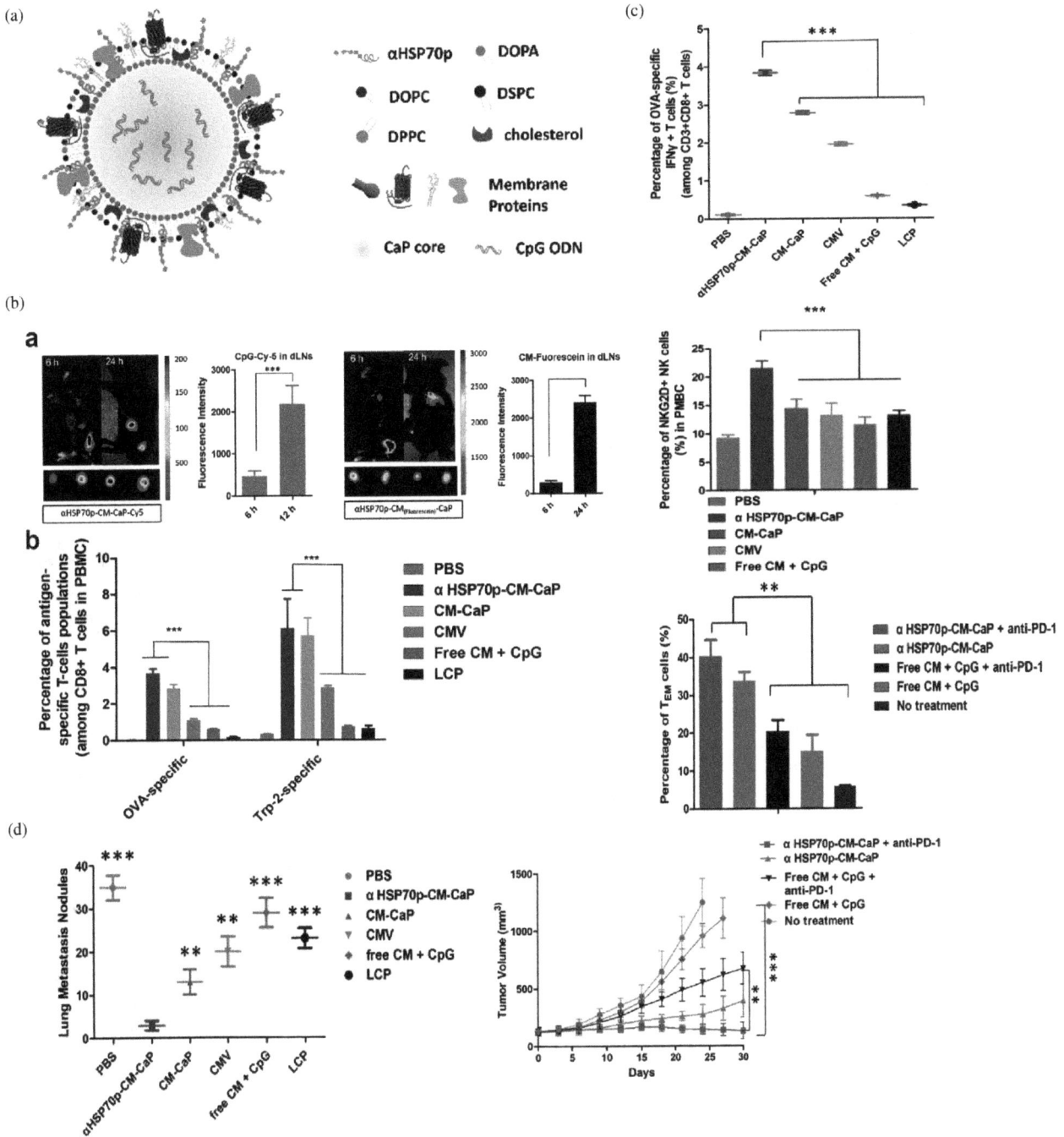

FIGURE 15.16 Tumor-draining lymph node (TDLN)-targeted nanoparticles boost the tumor-specific T-lymphocyte response, natural killer cells' immune stimulation, and effector memory T cells' proliferation. (A) Structure of the TDLN-targeted nanoparticle that enables co-delivery of three elements including tumor cell membrane proteins, adjuvant CpG, and an a-helix peptide modified HSP70p. (B) Prolonged antigen delivery in TDLNs and multiepitope T cells priming *in vivo*: a. fluorescence showing nanoparticle accumulation in the TDLNs and the corresponding fluorescence intensity; b. quantitative analysis of the frequency of the nanoparticle positive CD8α+ T cells in the TDLNs after treatment. (C) The nanoparticle activated antigen-specific CD8+ T cells, NKG2D+ NK cells, and induced effector memory T-cell proliferation *in vivo*. (D) Elimination of primary and secondary tumors by the nanoparticle. (Reprinted from Ref. [253], Copyright (2018), with permission from Elsevier.)

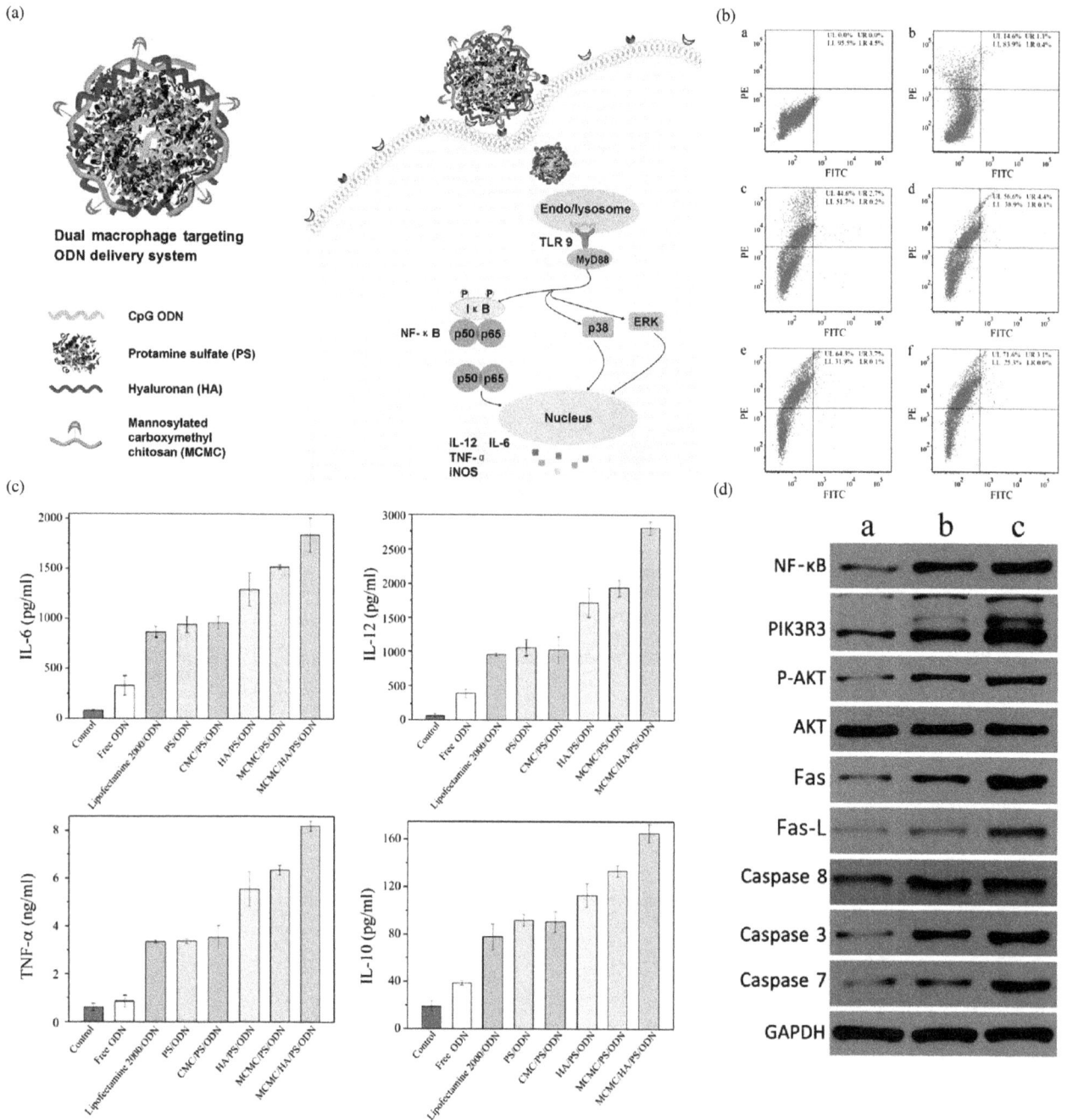

FIGURE 15.17 Macrophage dual-targeted nanoparticle for overcoming cancer-associated immunosuppression. (A) Structure of the dual-targeting delivery system inducing immunological stimulation in macrophages. (B) Flow cytometry showing the shift of the macrophage to activated M1 type that marked by CD80 (a. without treatment, and treated by b. naked nanoparticle, c. nontargeting system, d. mono-targeting system with HA, e. mono-targeting system with MCMC, and f. dual-targeting system with HA and MCMC). (C) Enhanced cytokine secretion of the macrophage after being treated. (D) Western blot analysis showing activated NF-κB, PI3 K/Akt, and Fas/FasL signaling pathways after treatment (a. without treatment, b. treated by naked nanoparticles, and c. treated by the dual-targeting system). Reprinted with permission from Ref. [262]. Copyright (2017) American Chemical Society.

hypoxia condition, and hemodynamic obstruction of immunocytes [268,269]. Thus, the regulation of the abnormal tumor microenvironment could largely relieve the inhibitory effects on the antitumor immunity and further increase therapeutic effects of immunotherapy. On the other hand, the tumor-specific stimuli in the abnormal tumor microenvironment including hypoxia, specific protease or proteins, and abnormal extracellular pH conditions could also be utilized to give nanoparticles the special conditions to accumulate and for orienting release of payloads, thus achieving the regulation of the tumor microenvironment and enhancement of immunotherapy effects.

Hypoxia was a commonly utilized tumor-specific condition for nanoparticle design with hypoxia-responsive chemical constructs coated, as the hypoxia is tightly associated with the immunosuppressive tumor microenvironment and it is also a rare condition in normal tissues [270–272]. The hypoxia environment could induce the polarization of macrophages from the immunosupportive M1 type to immunosuppressive M2 type and was also responsible for recruitment of abundant regulatory T cells and release of immunosuppressive cytokines [273,274]. Im et al. developed a photodynamic agent Chlorin e6 (Ce6)-loaded mesoporous silica nanoparticle with azobenzene used as the hypoxia-sensitive feasible cross-linker, which is also coated with the CpG/GC complex as the immune adjuvants [275]. When the nanoparticles reached a hypoxic region within tumor tissue, the azobenzene cross-linkers were cleaved, and the silica core and the CpG/GC complex were released, leading to delivery of CpG for DC engulfment and activation. The authors also generate photodynamic therapy to induce both tumor cell death and recruit DCs to facilitate the release of TAAs and the uptake of DCs (Figure 15.18). The nanoparticles combined with photodynamic therapy significantly enhanced the antitumor immune response and inhibited tumor growth *in vivo*. Yang et al. produced hollow manganese dioxide nanoparticles coated with PEG, Ce6, and DOX, which could be dissociated under the reduced pH microenvironment, hence releasing therapeutic drugs and meanwhile causing degradation of endogenous hydrogen peroxide to relieve intratumoral hypoxia [276]. A remarkable synergistic effect of the nanoparticle with photodynamic therapy was achieved through intensifying the antitumor immune responses. Moreover, the additional combination of the therapy with immune checkpoint inhibitors led to the ablation of distant tumor metastasis.

The abnormal tumor vasculature featuring a heterogeneous vessel diameter, tortuosity and distribution, and insufficient blood and oxygen supply is closely correlated with hypoxia, reduced pH, and immunosuppressive features within the tumor microenvironment [277]. As a result, normalization of tumor vasculature could be a way to enhance antitumor immunity [278]. Accompanied by oral treatment of erlotinib, an inhibitor of epidermal growth factor

receptor (EGFR), Chen et al. found that the tumor uptake of immunostimulatory drug-loaded nanoparticles was significantly increased, and the combined therapy dramatically relieved the hypoxia status and altered the immunosuppressive tumor microenvironment into immunosupportive in three types of tumor models [279]. The combined treatment also increased the tumor retention of anti-PD-L1 antibody, thus further inhibiting tumor growth and enhancing the treatment efficacy of anti-PD-L1 immunotherapy. On the other hand, the inhibition of copper trafficking could also have antiangiogenesis effects, as copper was required for the secretion of several angiogenic factors and stimulation of endothelial cell proliferation [280,281]. Zhou et al. used a copper-chelating coil-comb block copolymer, which has strong copper-chelating ability, to compose nanoparticles and conjugated it with TLR7/8 agonists and an immunomodulator resiquimod [282]. The nanoparticle exhibited accelerated releases in a reduced pH tumor microenvironment, displayed targeting ability, and dramatically suppressed tumor growth in primary breast tumor and lung metastasis lesions, demonstrating considerable antitumor immune enhancement effects.

The relevant microenvironmental characteristics to differentiate malignancy from normal tissues also included specific enzymes such as matrix metalloproteinase (MMP), which functioned in degrading the extracellular matrix and assisted in carcinogenesis, tumor progression, and metastasis, and its level is also found to be proportional to the malignancy of cancer [283–285]. As a result, MMPs were harnessed as the key to trigger fragmentation of nanostructures and the release of payloads. Shin et al. used a MMP9-cleavable linker to trigger the detachment of the PEG corona in the tumor tissue, and this method significantly enhanced CD44 receptor-mediated endocytosis of nanoparticles, facilitated antigen presentation, and inhibited tumor growth [286] (Figure 15.19).

In addition, the redox-sensitive-based delivery strategy was often utilized as an effective way for controlled release of drugs into the tumor microenvironment. Generally, the nanoparticles contained redox-responsive disulfide bonds that could be degraded by intracellular glutathione. Along with reduction of the disulfide bonds, antigens could be released from the nanoparticle carrier and be cross-presented to induce cellular immunity [287,288]. Wang et al. combined cell-penetrating peptides and redox-responsive disulfide bond cross-linking to design peptide carriers to form antigen delivery nanoparticles [289]. The results showed that the redox-responsive nanoparticles could significantly induce the antigen-specific immune response by significantly increasing IgG titer and levels of cytokines including INF-γ, IL-12, IL-4, and IL-10, stimulating splenocyte proliferation and APC maturation, and could also enhance the immune memory function.

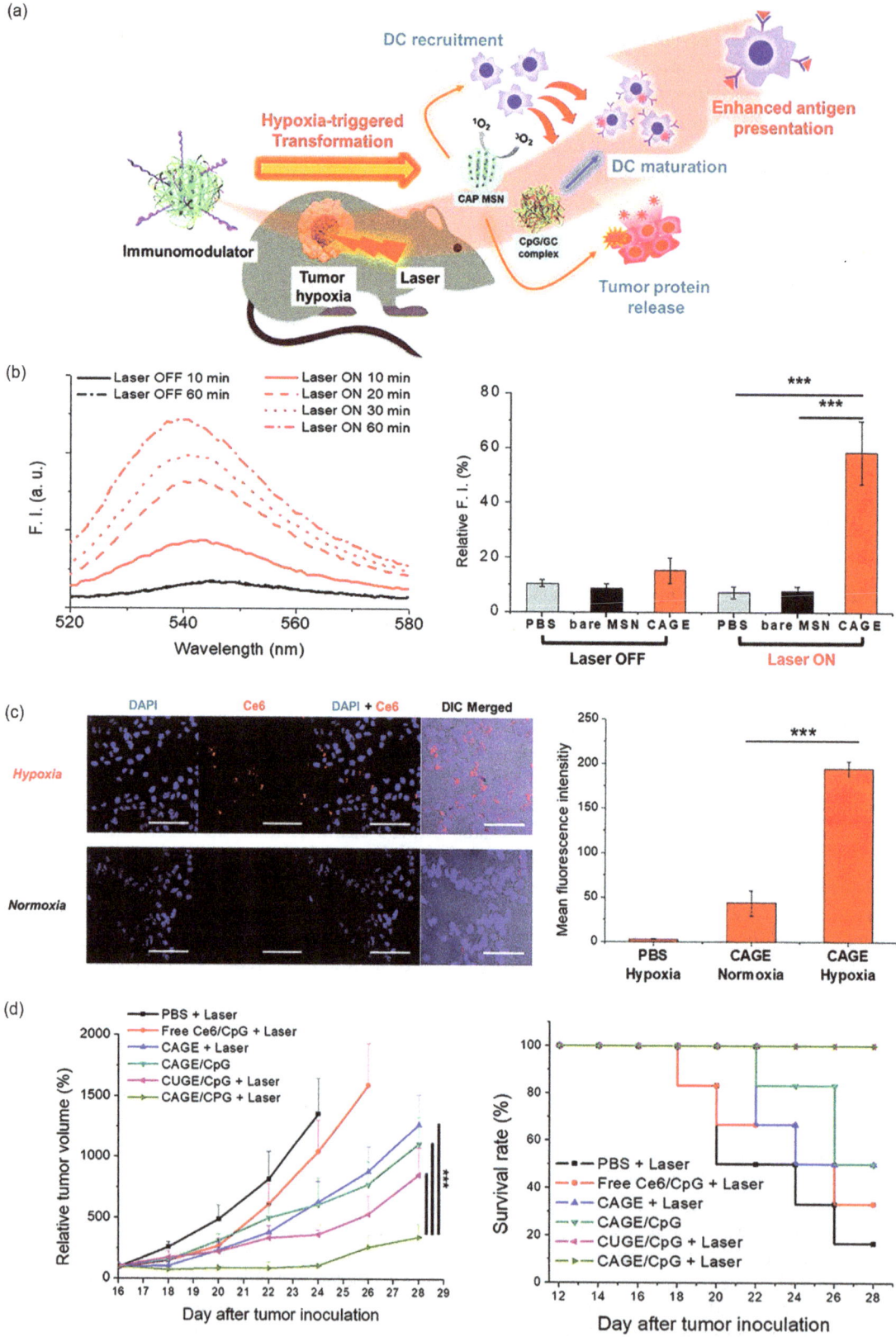

FIGURE 15.18 Hypoxia microenvironment-triggered transforming nanoparticles for cancer immunotherapy via photodynamically enhanced antigen presentation. (A) Schematic illustration of the working mechanism of the hypoxia-triggered transforming nanoparticle combined with photodynamic therapy. (B) Photoresponsive generation of singlet oxygen and the release profile of tumor proteins. (C) Hypoxia-responsive internalization of the nanoparticles into cells under hypoxic or normoxic conditions and the corresponding fluorescence intensity. (D) *In vivo* inhibition of tumor growth by the nanosystem and the survival curves. (Reprinted with permission from Ref. [275]. Copyright (2019) American Chemical Society.)

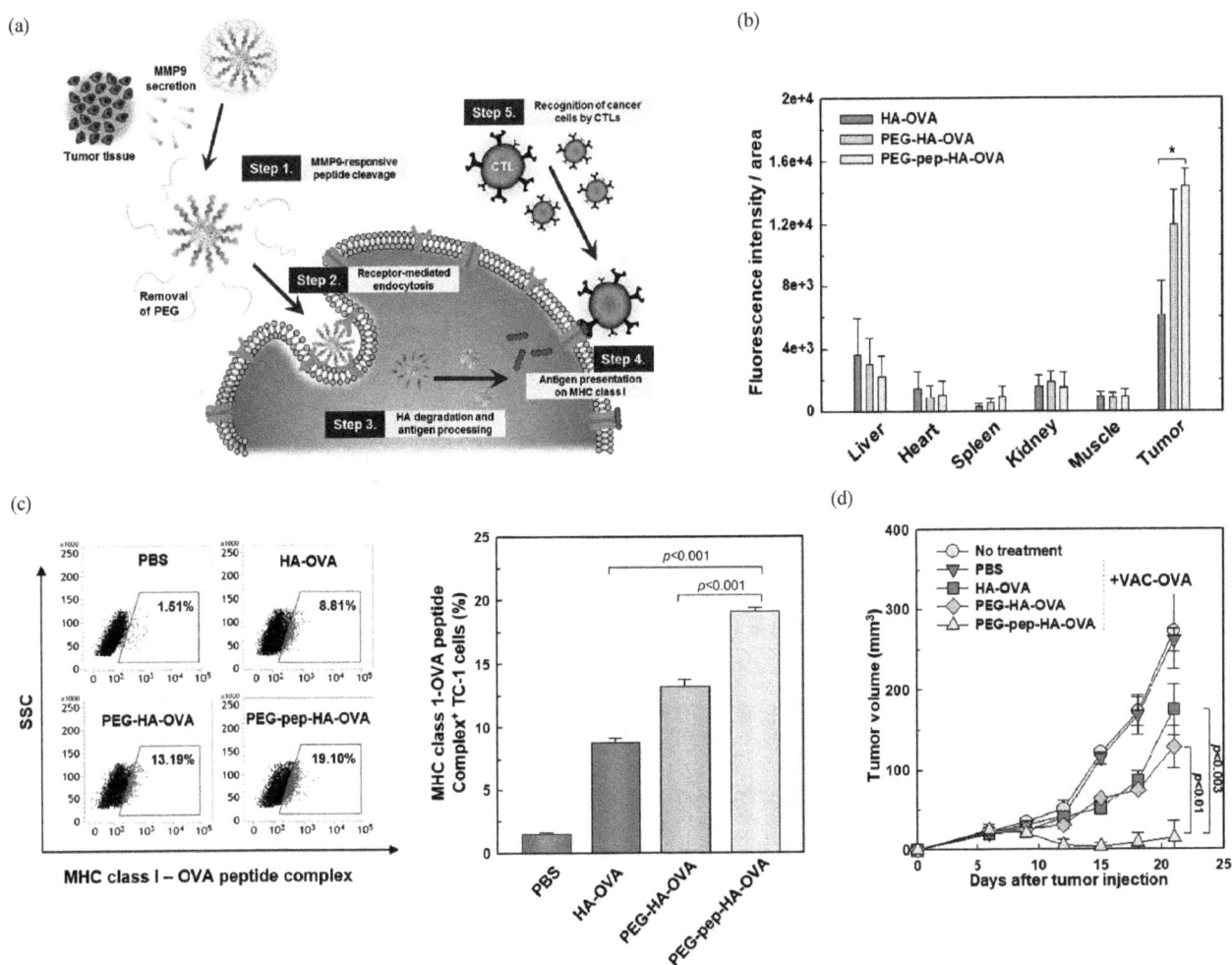

FIGURE 15.19 MMP9-responsive nanoparticle in enhancing cancer immunotherapy. (A) Schematic illustration depicting the working mechanism of the MMP9-responsive polymeric nanoparticle. (B) MMP9-responsive polymeric nanoparticle effectively accumulated in tumor tissue after systemic administration. (C) *In vivo* OVA antigen presentation in tumor cells after nanoparticle treatment. (D) *In vivo* therapeutic efficacy of the nanoparticle in tumor-bearing mice. (Reprinted from Ref. [286], Copyright (2017), with permission from Elsevier.)

15.13 NANOPARTICLES IN ENHANCING ADOPTIVE CELL THERAPY

Adoptive cell therapy (ACT) is a crucial part of cancer immunotherapy, in which tumor-specific lymphocytes are isolated either from peripheral blood or tumor biopsies in patients, and then selected to recognize specific tumor antigens, or alternatively, polyclonal peripheral T cells are artificially gene modified to process desired tumor-targeting ligands. Then, the cells are stimulated and expanded *ex vivo* and finally infused back into patients [290–292]. However, the therapeutic effects of ACT are impaired by insufficient *ex vivo* proliferation, inefficient trafficking of infused lymphocytes, and inadequate T-cell activity in the immunosuppressive tumor microenvironment due to immunosuppressive chemokines and abnormal tumor vasculature [293,294]. Accompanied by specific designed nanoparticles, these limitations of ACT could be significantly altered.

Targeting the lymphocytes with nanoliposomes conjugated with the inhibitor of TGF-β, an important immunosuppressive chemokine, prior to adoptive therapy could dramatically activate T-cell proliferation *ex vivo* and induce tumor regression after refusion [295]. Stephan et al. developed poly-alginate microporous scaffolds which were loaded with proliferated T cells and VEGF antibody. After placing the scaffolds in tumor resection sites or close to inoperable tumors, the polymer could act as a reservoir for T-cell propagation and release, and the VEGF antibody could normalize tumor vasculature, assisting in T-cell infiltration and altering the immunosuppressive microenvironment. As a result, the polymer successively supported tumor-targeting T lymphocytes throughout tumor resection beds and the draining lymph nodes and inhibited tumor relapse, whereas the conventional delivery modalities or injection of tumor-targeting lymphocytes have limited therapeutic effects [296] (Figure 15.20).

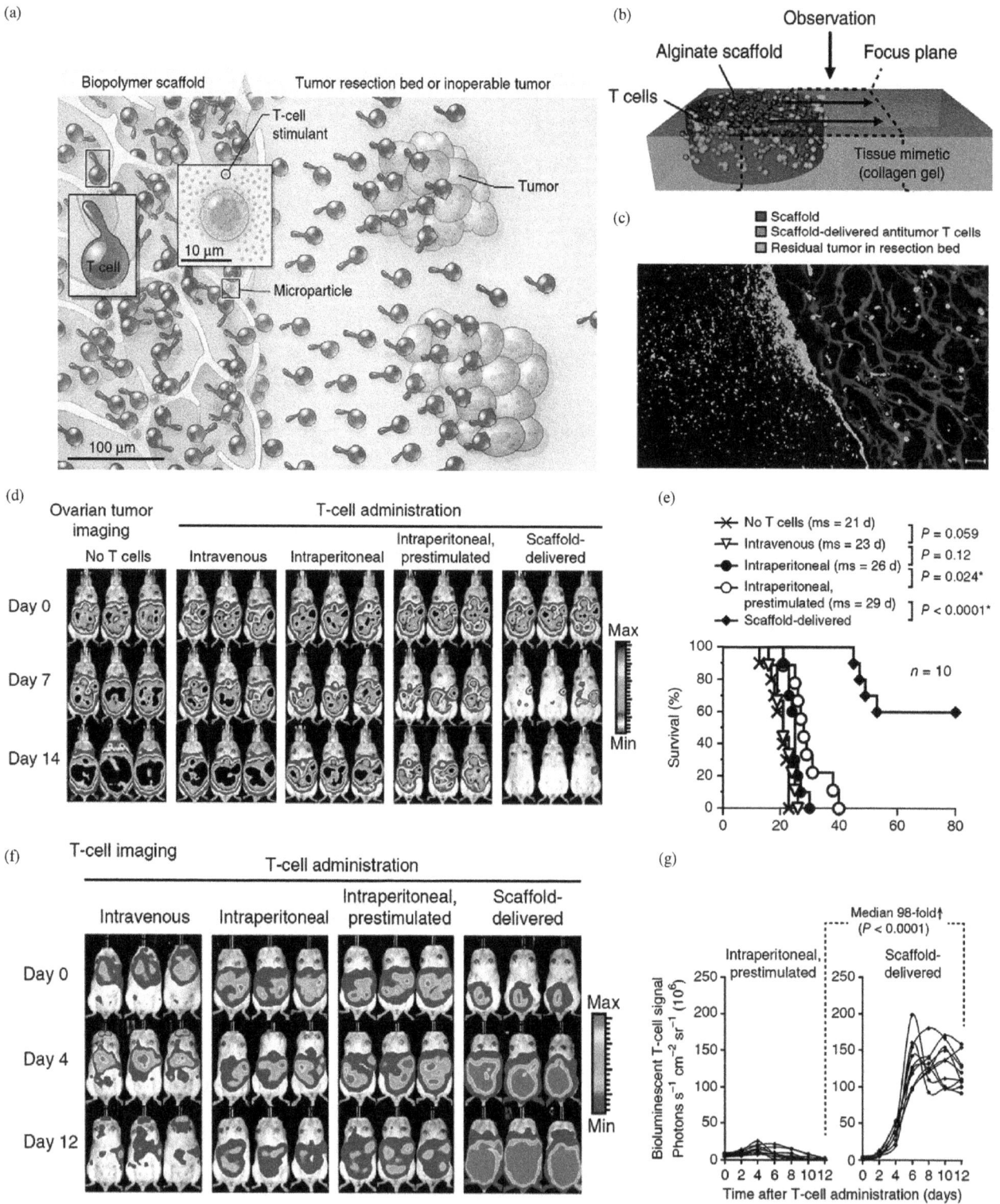

FIGURE 15.20 Nanostructured polyporous scaffold implants enhanced the efficacy of adoptive T-cell therapy. (A and B) Schematic diagram of the T cell-loaded scaffold surgically situated at a tumor site. Stimulatory microspheres incorporated into the device triggered cell expansion and promoted their egress into surrounding tissue. (C) Histological analysis of the scaffold and surrounding tissue 3 days after tumor-specific T cells (orange) was embedded in the scaffold (purple) and implanted into the tumor resection cavity. (D) Serial *in vivo* bioluminescence imaging of tumors. (E) Survival curves of tumor bearing mice following T-cell adoptive therapy. (F) *In vivo* bioluminescent imaging of T cells expressing luciferase. (G) Luciferase signal intensities after T-cell transfer, every line represented one animal and each dot reflected the whole animal photon count. (Reprinted with permission from Springer Nature: Nature Biotechnology, Ref. [296], Copyright (2014).)

Nanoparticles could also act on the *ex vivo* T-cell proliferation to the required quality and reduce the time interval between cell acquirement and infusion. Integrin of T lymphocytes played a crucial role in sustaining the immunological synapse with APCs through its binding to intercellular adhesion molecule-1, and the formation of immunological synapse led to reorganization of the cytoskeleton, which facilitated clustering and prevented migration of T cells [297–299]. Guasch et al. created a nanoparticle that cross-linked with peptides derived from fibronectin, an integrin signaling activator, and found that it was significantly more efficient in stimulating T-cell proliferation and increasing the expansion rate compared with nonfunctionalized nanoparticles [300]. Perica et al. integrated paramagnetic iron-dextran nanoparticles with the MHC-Ig dimer as signal 1 and CD28 antibody as signal 2 to form an artificial APC [301]. The nano-artificial APCs could selectively bind to antigen-specific T-lymphocyte rare naive precursors and be retained in a magnetic column, thus achieving cell enrichment, followed by activation of the selected T cells leading to rapid proliferation and expansion. The enrichment and expansion processes resulted in greater than 1000-fold proliferation of mouse and human antigen-specific T lymphocytes in 1 week. The nano-artificial APCs could not only enhance T-cell proliferation *in vivo* culture but also after adoptive transfer, leading to a robust T-cell response (Figure.15.21).

15.14 NUCLEIC ACID-BASED NANOVACCINES

15.14.1 POLYMERIC NANOPARTICLES

Encapsulation of nucleic acids into polymeric nanoparticles for targeted delivery to DCs and other APCs represents the most popular strategy for promoting cancer immunotherapy [302,303]. Nucleic acids can act as an immune-booster (e.g., CpG ODN, poly I:C, and pDNA), an agent to silence an immunosuppressive molecule (e.g., siRNA) or express a tumor antigen or an immunoadjuvant (e.g., mRNA and pDNA). Mahjub et al. [90] summarize various nanostructures used for preparation of nucleic acid-based cancer immunotherapy.

15.14.1.1 siRNA Polymeric Nanoparticles

siRNA can be delivered using polymeric nanoparticles to silence an immunoinhibitory molecule and subsequently boost the antitumor immune response. For example, CD73 (ecto-5′-nucleotidase), which is overexpressed in tumor and immune cells, catalyzes the production of adenosine from AMP. Adenosine binds to the A2A adenosine receptors (A2AR) at the surface of T cells, resulting in decreased T-cell proliferation, reduced production of costimulatory cytokines such as IFN-γ and TNF-α, suppressed NK cell activity, and impaired secretion of cytolytic molecules such as perforin and FasL. In tumor cells, CD73 is involved in

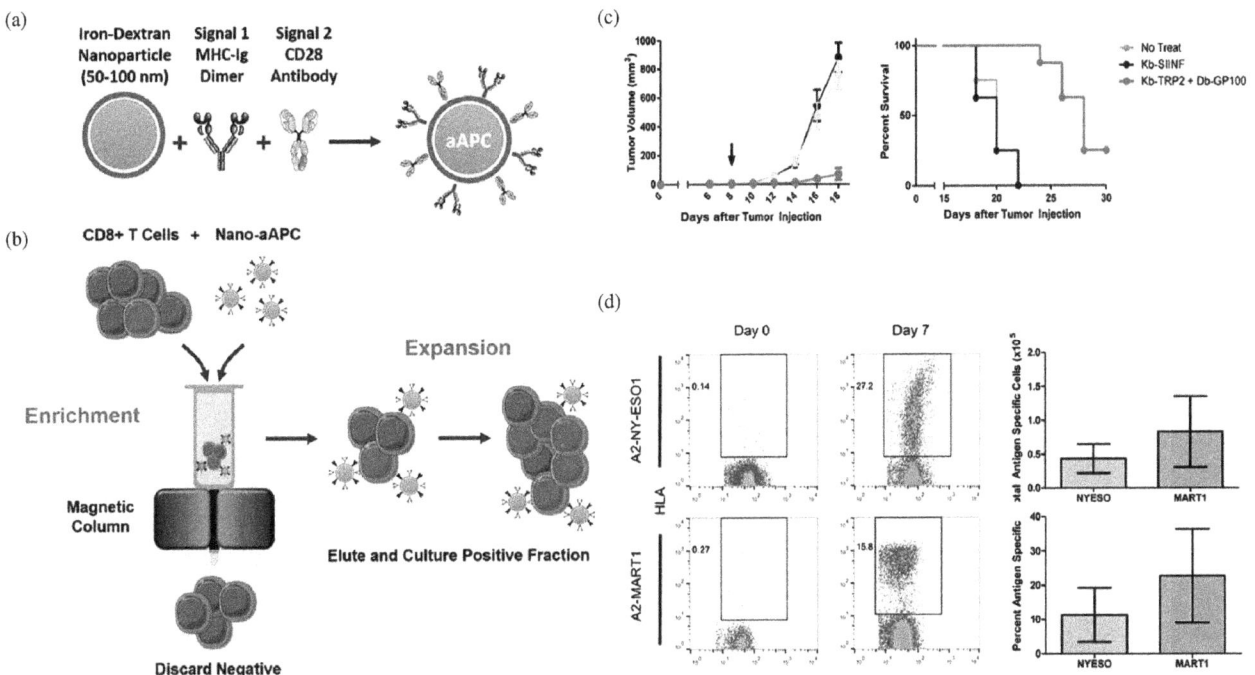

FIGURE 15.21 Enrichment and expansion with nano-artificial APCs for adoptive cell immunotherapy. (A) Nano-artificial APCs are synthesized by coupling the MHC-Ig dimer (signal 1) and anti-CD28 antibody (signal 2) to a 50–100nm iron-dextran nanoparticle. (B) Schematic of magnetic enrichment. Antigen-specific CD8+ T cells (blue) bound to the nano-artificial APC are retained in a magnetic column in the enrichment step, while non-cognate (orange) cells are less likely to bind. Enriched T cells are then activated by the nano-artificial APC and proliferate in the expansion step. (C) Nano-artificial APC enriched and expanded lymphocytes inhibited melanoma growth after adoptive transfer. (D) Enrichment and expansion with the nano-artificial APC functionalized with human HLA-A2 and induced robust expansion against the tumor antigens. (Reprinted with permission from Ref. [301]. Copyright (2015) American Chemical Society.)

tumor neovascularization, metastasis, and invasion [304]. Jadidi-Niaragh et al. [305] loaded CD73 siRNA into chitosan nanoparticles (~100 nm) through ionic gelation using tripolyphosphate (TPP). Following *i.v.* administration to 4T1 breast cancer-bearing mice, the nanoparticles accumulated in the tumor, causing CD73 downregulation in tumor-associated immune cells, including DCs, Treg, and MDSCs. This led to the reduction of inhibitory cytokine IL-10 and increased secretion of immunostimulatory cytokines (IL-17 and IFN-γ). Subsequently, the growth of the primary tumor was thus decreased with reduced lung metastases, while free siRNA and saline-treated mice showed no efficacy. In cancer cells, over-activation of STAT3 is correlated with increased secretion of immunosuppressive factors such as IL-10 and VEGF [306,307], which inhibit activation of DCs and suppress the immune response against tumors [308,309]. Luo et al. [310] prepared a polyplex formulation containing poly(ethylene glycol)-b-poly(llysine)-b-poly(l-leucine) (PEG-PLL-PLLeu) and poly I:C (a TLR 3 agonist immunoadjuvant), which was then mixed with OVA and an siRNA against STAT3. *S.c* administration of the polyplex (~142 nm) to C57BL/6J mice bearing B16 OVA tumor resulted in significant uptake by DCs in the draining lymph node. STAT3 level in the DCs was reduced, leading to increased expression of CD40 and CD86. This treatment also decreased the number of immunosuppressive cells in the lymph node, including T_{reg} and MDSCs, resulting in enhanced antitumor efficacy compared to the formulation without siRNA. It was shown that the polyplex was mostly taken up through the lipid raft mechanism rather than the clathrin-mediated endocytosis and, therefore, could result in an increased cytosolic delivery [311–313]. Although cationic polymeric micelles exhibited increased interaction with negatively charged siRNA and were effective in cytosolic delivery to DC, the positively charged surface displayed poor colloidal stability in physiological fluids and cellular selectivity. Other studies associated with the development of siRNA polymeric nanoparticles for downregulation of various immunosuppressors are summarized in [90].

15.14.1.2 Oligodeoxynucleotide (ODN) Polymeric Nanoparticles

Liang et al. [314] loaded galunisertib (LY2157299, a TGF-β inhibitor) into the hydrophobic core of PEGylated carboxyl-poly (styrene/acrylamide) nanoparticles, which were then surface coated with polyethyleneimine (PEI) to form complexes with CpG1826 ODN. Intratumoral (*i.t*) injection of the complexes to H22 liver-tumor–bearing BALB/c mice induced an increase of splenic CD8+ T cells and a reduction in tumor volume compared to the PBS control, CpG only complexes and LY2157299 only complexes. This formulation was prepared using layer-by-layer (LBL) ionic complexation, and its stability in physiological conditions (i.e., plasma and interstitial fluid) remains to be determined. Therefore, its application might be limited to *i.t.* only. Moreover, the reported fabrication technique appears to

be complicated, time-consuming, and poorly reproducible. Significant barriers are anticipated for scale-up manufacturing. In another study, CpG ODN and IL-10 siRNA were first complexed with polylysine and then co-loaded into the PLGA nanoparticles using a double-emulsion method. The PLGA nanoparticles were intratumorally co-administered with a chemo-drug paclitaxel (PTX) to B16-F10 melanoma-bearing mice. Co-delivery of the CpG ODN, siRNA, and PTX resulted in a reduced IL-10 level and increased production of stimulating cytokines (TNF-α, IL-6, and IL-12) in the DCs in the draining lymph node, inducing enhanced antitumor efficacy compared to PTX only and the PBS control groups [315].

In order to enhance the cytosolic delivery of ODNs, Wilson et al. [83] developed a pH-sensitive diblock-copolymeric micelle (~30 nm) containing components of a cationic moiety (DMAEMA), disulfide and propyl acrylic acid for nucleic acid complexation, chemical conjugation with a peptide antigen, and pH-dependent conformation change, respectively. CpG ODN and an OVA peptide could be co-loaded with this polymeric micelle. Intradermal injection of the formulation displayed enhanced DC uptake through macropinocytosis, caveolae- and clathrin-mediated endocytosis, resulting in increased MHC I antigen cross-presentation and enhanced IFN-γ production compared to co-delivery of free OVA and CpG. Increased DC delivery could be achieved by surface coating of nanoparticles with mannose [316,317] or mAb targeting DCSIGN [318], DC 205 [319], LOX1 [320], Dectin-1 [321], MACI [322], CD40 [323], CD11c, and CD 18 receptors [324]. Many studies involving CpG delivery using polymers for cancer immunotherapy have been reported previously [325–329].

15.14.1.3 pDNA Polymeric Nanoparticles

Plasmid DNA (pDNA) is a more versatile nucleic acid for immunotherapy compared to CpG ODN and siRNA, as it can be recognized by TLR9 as an immunoadjuvant and encoded with a tumor antigen or an immunostimulating molecule. In a study performed by Shukla et al. [330], pDNA encoding TNF-α was condensed with a cationic histidine and cysteine–modified polyarginine (HCR) peptide, followed by encapsulation into the PLA-PEG nanoparticles via a double-emulsion method. The HCR peptide has been shown to facilitate cytosolic delivery and nuclear translocation of pDNA. After intratumoral delivery, significant expression of TNF-α was measured with increased tumor cell apoptosis.

Due to a large number of APCs such as keratinocytes, Langerhans' cells, and dermal DCs located in the dermal region, intradermal pDNA delivery using microneedles induced elevated immunoresponses in comparison with *i.m* or *s.c* [331–333]. A pDNA encoded with HPV-16 E6 and E7 was first complexed with a cationic RALA peptide (a 30 amino acid peptide containing repeated units of arginine–alanine–leucine–alanine) and delivered to the dermal compartment using a PVP microneedle. Significant expression of E6/E7 was detected with elevated levels of dermal IgG and

TNF-α secreted by DCs, leading to improved antitumor efficacy compared to the *i.m* delivery [334]. Nasal mucosal delivery is an alternative route for DNA vaccine. pDNA encoding gastrin-releasing peptide (pGRP) as a tumor antigen was complexed with mannose-modified chitosan and delivered intranasally [335] to mice bearing RM-1 prostate tumor. Significant levels of serum anti-GRP antibody and IFN-γ were measured with enhanced antitumor efficacy. Despite the effectiveness of using mannose as a ligand to target DCs, increased production of IL-10, a potent immunosuppressor, is associated with mannose receptor activation [336].

Oral delivery is the most preferred route for vaccine administration but presents various barriers, including a harsh acidic environment, endogenous nucleolytic enzymes, a mucus layer, and microbial flora [337]. It was shown that vascular endothelial growth factor-A (VEGFA), produced in a high level in the tumor microenvironment, enhanced maturation of inhibitory cells (TAMs and Treg) along with reduced tumor infiltration of lymphocytes. Particularly, Treg proliferation was mediated through VEGF-A binding to its receptor VEGFR-II that was overexpressed in Treg [338,339]. Therefore, blockage of the VEGF-A/VEGFR-II signaling pathway is anticipated to reverse the immunosuppression in tumors [340]. Hu et al. [341] coated the bacteria, *Salmonellae*, with polyplex composed of PEI and pDNA encoding mAb against VEGFR-II. The interaction with PEI increased the viability of this organism in the GI system, and it was shown that *Salmonellae* could be engulfed by DCs located in the Peyer's patches, resulting in improved transfection of pDNA. This oral treatment induced expression of mAb against VEGFR-II, enhanced production of TNF-α and IFN-γ as well as increased population of both CD4+ and CD8+ T cells in spleen, and improved antitumor efficacy. Other proteins that have been encoded in pDNA for cancer immunotherapy include immunostimulatory cytokines IL-12 [342], CD40L [343], and interferon-γ-inducible protein-10 (IP-10) [344] as well as tumor antigens TRP-2 [343] and OVA [345]. Although the system induced immunoresponses through oral route, the safety of bacteria-coated polyplexes should be further evaluated. Moreover, due to significant inter-subject variations in human GI such as microbial flora, bowel motility, and permeability of intestinal epithelium cells, the response to therapy is anticipated to be highly variant among patients.

Zhu et al. [346] explored the possibility of combined delivery of a peptide antigen, a CpG ODN and a short hairpin RNA (shRNA) for simultaneous delivery of an antigen, activation of an immunostimulating pathway, and suppression of an immunoinhibitory molecule in the DCs. An intertwining hybrid DNA-RNA nanocapsule (iDR-NC) containing CpG 1826 (a TLR9 agonist) and a shRNA for silencing STAT3 (an immunoinhibitory gene) were prepared. The iDR-NCs (252 nm) were formed by condensing the self-assembled hybrid CpG-shRNA microflowers (MFs, 1272 nm) through electrostatic interactions with a cationic PEG-grafted polypeptide (PPT-g-PEG). Furthermore,

a tumor-specific peptide neoantigen (CSIINFEKL) was loaded in the nanocapsules via hydrophobic interactions. The molecular design of this system suggested that in the acidic environment of the lysosomes after iDR-NC internalization by DCs, PEG would shed off through cleavage of the acid-liable linkage in PPT-g-PEG, exposing the ionizable cationic PPT component for enhanced cytosolic delivery through the proton sponge effect. *S.c* administration of the iDR-NCs to colon adenocarcinoma-bearing mice caused increased production of TNF-α, IL-6, and IL-12 and ultimately decreased tumor growth.

Nucleic acid-based nanovaccine is an attractive strategy for cancer immunotherapy as it is flexible in introducing a wide range of biomolecules to modulate the immune system, including antigens, immunostimulating molecules, and inhibitors for immunosuppression. Recent efforts have been focused on gene delivery to immune cells, and positively charged lipoplex and polyplex are the major delivery systems utilized. However, their poor serum stability and cellular selectivity are to be resolved for improved efficacy. To ensure efficient gene delivery, the payload must be protected from nuclease-mediated degradation and deliver the payload to the target cell cytosol or nucleus. Chemical modifications of ODNs by phosphorothioate, amidates, and 2′-methyl residues can significantly improve their resistance to nucleases [347]. Cationic materials increase the interaction with cell membrane and improve endosomal escape and cytosolic delivery of nucleic acids. Yet, in contrast cationic carriers also mediate strong interaction with blood components, leading to aggregation of the complexes [348]. Surface modification of lipoplex and polyplex with PEG has been shown to reduce their interaction with plasma components, but also reduces their affinity with cell membrane. A common solution to this is to attach a targeting ligand to the distal end of PEG to trigger internalization by the target cell.

15.14.2 Lipid-Based Nanoparticles (LNPs)

LNPs are among the most studied nonviral delivery systems for nucleic acids. Cationic lipids or ionizable cationic lipids are often used in LNPs to interact and load negatively charged nucleic acids to overcome the delivery barriers, including nuclease-mediated degradation, nonspecific tissue distribution, rapid clearance, and poor cellular uptake [349–351].

15.14.2.1 siRNA LNPs

Qian et al. [352] developed a dual-targeted lipoplex loaded with siRNA for silencing colony-stimulating factor-1 receptor (CSF-1R) in TAMs. A fused targeting peptide consisting of α-peptide targeting scavenger receptor B type 1 (SR-B1) and M2pep (a M2 macrophage binding peptide) was labeled at the lipoplex surface for TAM targeting. After *i.v.* administration to the tumor-bearing mice, the dual-targeted lipoplex exhibited four- to five-fold increased TAM uptake compared to lipoplex modified with either α-peptide or

M2pep alone. This treatment led to decrease in inhibitory cytokines such as IL-10 and TGF-β as well as downregulation of co-inhibitory receptors including PD-1 and T-cell immunoglobulin and mucin-domain containing-3 (Tim-3) in the tumor microenvironment, resulting in improved antitumor efficacy. Other ligands such as folic acid and mannose were also used for targeting TAMs [353–355]. Akita et al. [356] reported increased endosomal escape and enhanced cytosolic delivery of siRNA against suppressor of cytokine signaling 1 (SOCS1) to inhibit the immunosuppressing STAT pathway using a pH-sensitive and cell-penetrating lipoplex formulation, which contained a GALA peptide and a R8 peptide at the surface. Upon *s.c* administration of this lipoplex, SOCS1 expression in DCs was significantly reduced, leading to increased secretion of IFN-γ and IL-6, and ultimately enhanced antitumor effect. Alternative to the lipoplex formulation, the SNALP (stable nucleic acid lipid nanoparticle) technology was developed to deliver siRNA and mRNA with improved biocompatibility and cell selectivity due to their neutral surface charge and improved stability in physiological conditions. An ionizable cationic lipid, 2,2-dilinoleyl-4-(2-dimethylaminoethyl)-[1,3]-dioxolane (DLin-KC2-DMA, Figure 15.22), was synthesized and used together with neutral lipids and a diffusible PEG-lipid to form complexes with siRNA. A siRNA for knocking down programmed death ligand-1 and 2 (PD-L1/ PD-L2, co-inhibitory molecules that reduce DC maturation) and an mRNA encoded with MiHA tumor antigen were loaded into the SNALPs. Following *ex vivo* incubation of the SNALPs with DCs, significant silence of PD-L1/ PD-L2 was measured, and after *i.v.* delivery of the DCs to mice, increased CD8+ T infiltration in the tumor was demonstrated. The control SNALP formulation without siRNA displayed reduced activity in promoting CD8+ maturation [357]. siRNA against CTLA-4, an immune checkpoint inhibitor that inhibits T-cell–DC interaction, was mixed with a cationic lipid BHEM-Chol to form hydrophobic complexes, which were then loaded inside the PEG-PLA polymeric micelles (~140 nm) [169]. Following *i.v.* administration to B-16 melanoma-bearing mice, the formulation reduced CTLA-4 expression in T cells, leading to increased tumor infiltration of CD4+ and CD8+ T cells and a reduced T_{reg} population compared to the formulation containing control siRNA.

In addition to siRNA delivery for silencing immunoinhibitory molecules, immunostimulatory RNAs (isR-NAs, 19-bp dsRNAs) could be incorporated with lipoplex to activate TLR 3/7/8 [355,358], retinoic acid-inducible gene-1-like helicase (R1G1), and double-stranded RNA-activated protein kinase (PKR) in DCs [359,360]. *I.p* injection of the isRNA-lipoplex to B16 melanoma-bearing mice induced increased production of IFN-γ and enhanced antitumor and anti-metastatic activity.

15.14.2.2 Oligonucleotides LNPs

Xu et al. [317] prepared mannose-modified lipid-calcium phosphate (LCP) nanoparticles (~30 nm) for targeting DCs. Phosphorylated Trp2 peptide (p-Trp2) and CpG ODN were co-precipitated by Ca^{2+} to form the LCP core, which was then coated with lipids. *S.c* injection of the LCP to B16F10 melanoma-bearing mice resulted in high accumulation of the nanoparticles in the lymph nodes (~35% of the injected dose), increased DC uptake, and enhanced IFN-γ secretion, leading to tumor growth inhibition. In a study performed by Liu et al. [361], CpG ODN was loaded into PEGylated cationic liposomes, which were surface modified with an IL-4Rα RNA aptamer for targeting MDSCs to reverse their immunoinhibitory phenotype. After *s.c* administration of the formulation to BALB/c mice, significantly reduced tumor angiogenesis and tumor growth were determined. Nevertheless, PEGylation reduced the cellular internalization of the delivery system and the efficacy was only moderate. As discussed earlier, a ligand can be labeled at the distal end of PEG to improve the intracellular delivery.

Besides CpG ODN, bacteria-derived cyclic dinucleotides can also act as an immunoadjuvant. Cyclic di-GMP (c-di-GMP) showed high-affinity binding with cytosolic ATP-dependent RNA helicase DDX41, forming stable complexes to stimulate an interferon gene protein STING, which activated a TANK binding kinase1-interferon regulatory factor 3 (TBK1-IRF3) pathway and promoted the production of IFNs [362–364]. In a study performed by Miyabe et al. [362], the negatively charged c-di-GMP was complexed with a cationic pH-sensitive liposome for improved cytosolic delivery. *S.c* administration of the lipoplex to OVA melanoma-bearing mice promoted secretion of IFN-β from macrophages and enhanced the antitumor activity.

15.14.2.3 pDNA LNPs

pDNA encoding an antigen or immunostimulating cytokine can be delivered using lipoplex to induce antitumor immunity. Lipoplex containing IFN-γ pDNA was shown to improve the antitumor efficacy after *s.c* injection with a peptide antigen [365]. Garu et al. [366] fabricated cationic liposomes composed of lipids containing shikimoyl- and quinoyl- head groups (Figure 15.23) which are structurally

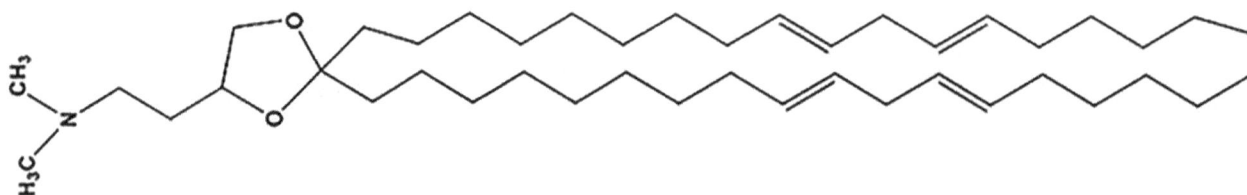

FIGURE 15.22 The chemical structure of Dlin-KC2-DMA.

(a)

(b)

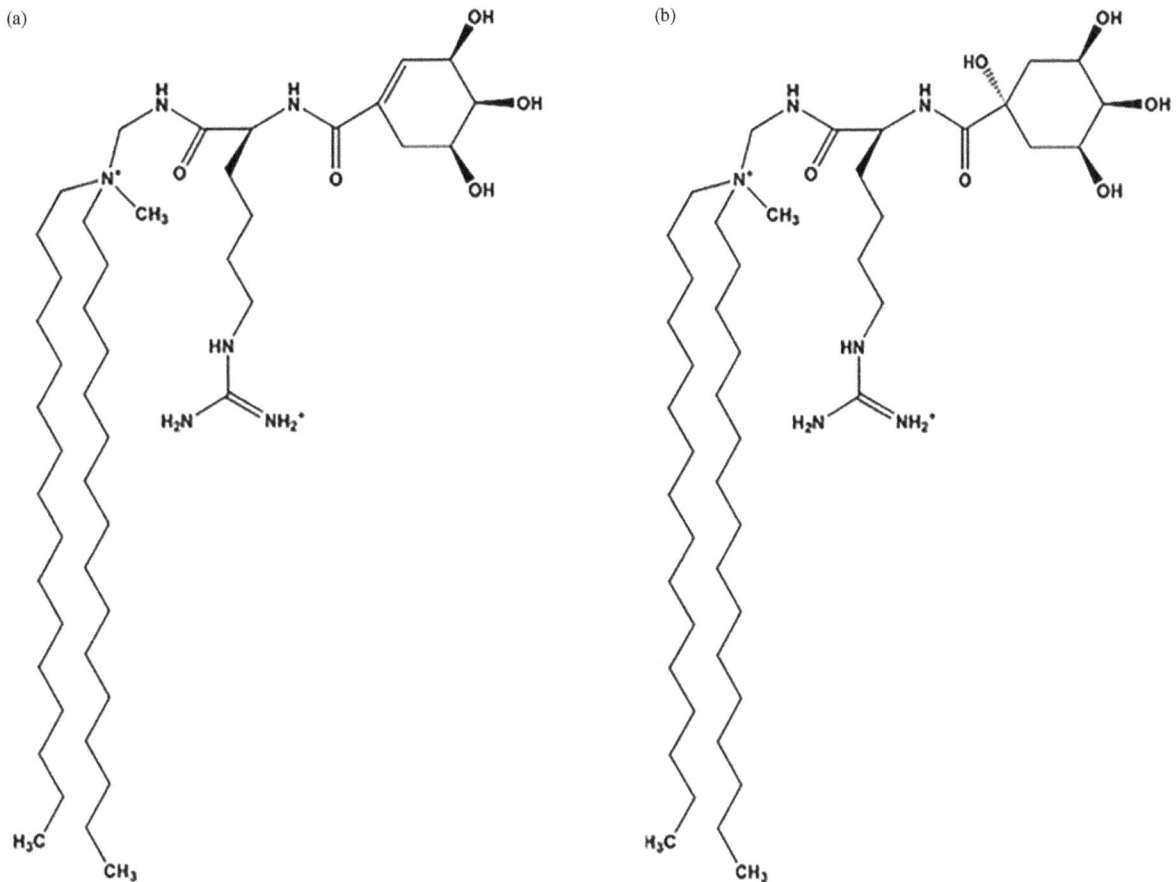

FIGURE 15.23 Chemical structures of the cationic lipid containing either a shikimoyl- (A) or quinoyl- (B) head group.

similar to mannose. Lipoplex was prepared by mixing the cationic liposomes with a melanoma antigen encoding pDNA (pCMV-MART1), and *s.c* delivered to mice. Selective uptake of the lipoplex by DCs in the draining lymph node was shown, leading to an increase in secretion of immunostimulating cytokines (IL-12, IL-6, IL-4, IFN-γ, TNF-α) and reduced tumor growth in comparison with administration of lipoplexes labeled with mannose. In another study, a pDNA encoding telomerase reverse transcriptase (TERT, a tumor antigen) and a pDNA expressing chemokine ligand 21 (CCL21, an immunoadjuvant that enhances DC maturation) were incorporated into lipoplex, which was then mixed with UV inactivated hemagglutinating virus of Japan (HVJ) for improved gene delivery. The HVJ-lipoplex was intramuscularly injected to TS/A breast cancer-bearing mice and induced secretion of immunostimulating cytokines and slowed tumor growth [367]. The viral components in this delivery system introduce significant concerns in safety.

15.14.2.4 mRNA LNPs

mRNA-based nanovaccine has recently emerged as a new strategy for cancer immunotherapy [369,369]. LNP delivery of mRNA is nonintegrating and non-infectious and can be used to express a variety of proteins in both non-dividing and dividing cells [370–372]. *S.c* administration of lipopolyplex

containing OVA mRNA resulted in significant DC uptake through macropinocytosis. Increased production of costimulatory cytokines, including IL-12, IFN-β/γ, and TNF-α, was measured with enhanced antitumor efficacy compared to a lipid polymer formulation loaded with an OVA peptide [368]. In another study, Sayour et al. [373] prepared a DOTAP cationic lipoplex (~100nm) incorporating mRNA expressing OVA. They showed that the lipoplex with a ratio of mRNA:DOTAP (1:15) was highly effective in transfection of the DCs. Following *i.v.* injection of the lipoplex to C57BL/6 melanoma-bearing mice, increases in numbers of the antigen-specific CD8+ T cells in both lymph nodes and splenocytes, the IFN-γ level, and the MHC-I antigen cross-presentation were measured, resulting in decreased tumor growth in comparison with the OVA peptide vaccine formulated in complete Freund's adjuvant (CFA). mRNA vaccines were also developed to prevent viral infections. Pardi et al. [370] developed a lipid nanoparticle (~80 nm) encapsulating an mRNA vaccine encoding pre-membrane and enveloped (prM-E) glycoprotein of ZIKA [H/PF/2013 strain] to elicit high mAb responses through low-dose intradermal immunization against the virus in both mice and non-human primate models. The mRNA was encapsulated into the LNPs using a microfluidic self-assembly process by rapid mixing an mRNA aqueous solution with an ethanol solution containing an ionizable cationic lipid, phosphatidylcholine, cholesterol, and a PEG-lipid. Following administration to mice, the ZIKA mRNA-LNPs conferred protection against the ZIKA virus for at least 5 months, and the mAb titers rose to levels 50–100 times higher than those induced by an immunization with purified inactivated virus or the pDNA vaccine. In rhesus macaques, the mAb levels induced by this ZIKA mRNA-LNPs vaccine were maintained stable for up to 12 weeks. Moreover, the mAb titers induced by a single immunization with 50 μg mRNA LNPs were 50 and 2 times higher than those elicited by either single or double immunizations with 1 mg of naked prM-E pDNA vaccine, respectively. Moreover, Richner et al. [374] generated a versatile ZIKA vaccine platform, in which modified mRNA encoding wild-type (WT) or a variant of ZIKA structural gene encoding prM-E was encapsulated into the LNPs. Among them, the Japanese encephalitis virus (JEV$_{sig}$-prM-E) mRNA LNPs induced the highest neutralizing titers in most animals, conferring sterilizing immunity.

Systemic *i.v.* administration of mRNA-incorporated lipoplex is suggested to mediate activation of APCs in the reticuloendothelial system for inducing overexpression of MHC I/II and enhanced systemic immunoresponse. Kranz et al. [375] prepared a lipoplex formulation composed of cationic liposomes (DOTAP/DOTMA/DOPE) and mRNA encoding various antigenic peptides (OVA, gp70, TRP-1, or oncogene E6/E7 HPV-16). They demonstrated that, following *i.v.* injection in mice, the lipoplex with a low ratio of lipid:mRNA (i.e., 1:5) effectively accumulated in spleen while the counterpart formulation with a high lipid:mRNA ratio (i.e., 5:1) was mostly taken by in the lungs. Within the spleen, the lipoplex was highly localized in DCs rather than other APCs through macropinocytosis and caused increased secretion of IFN-α and upregulation of CD40 and CD86, which are involved in maturation of CD4+ and CD8+ cells, respectively. These immunostimulatory effects were mediated by TLR9, CD11c, and IFN-α receptor 1 (IFNAR1), which were shown to have a pivotal role in production of IFN-γ and TNF-α. The lipoplex was tested clinically in three patients, and an efficient CD8+ T-cell-mediated immunity that resulted in reduced tumor size and metastatic nodules was reported in all three individuals. The side effects included mild flu-like symptoms.

Despite significant challenges for clinical translation, several nucleic acid-based nanovaccines have been evaluated in cancer patients. Recently, a ready-to-use RNA-lipoplex formulation composed of DOTMA and DOPE incorporating various melanoma antigen mRNAs such as NY ESO-1, MAGE-A3, tyrosinase, and TPTE was developed. After *i.v.* administration, the nanovaccine was well-tolerated and only a mild flu-like symptom related to immunostimulation was observed in some patients. The vaccine was shown to be clinically effective in inducing a dose-dependent increase of serum IFN-α [376]. The antitumor immunity is yet to be shown. In another clinical study, MelQbG10, a virus-like nanoparticle (VLP, ~30 nm), derived from bacteriophage Qβ, loaded with CpG ODN and surface-coupled with a peptide antigen Melan-A/MART1,

was evaluated in 22 malignant melanoma patients via *s.c* injection. Patients developed adverse effects such as myalgia, arthralgia, flu-like symptoms, nausea, and vomiting, although ~68% of these effects were mild. Only 7 out of 22 patients displayed partial response to the therapy [377]. Combining other immunoadjuvants (*s.c* montanide ISA-51, an incomplete Freund's adjuvant (IFA) and topical administration of imiquimod, a TLR-7 agonist) increased T-cell infiltration in the lymph nodes, and therefore, enhanced Melan-A/MART1-specific T-cell-mediated immunoresponse in all patients was observed [377].

15.15 MONOCLONAL ANTIBODY (MAB)

mAb belonging to the IgG class has been widely studied for cancer immunotherapy [378]. mAb mediates tumor cell depletion by binding to a specific surface antigen at the cancer cells, triggering antigen-dependent cellular cytotoxicity (ADCC) and complement-dependent cytotoxicity (CDC), which are both dependent on the host immune system. mAb targeting the immune checkpoint has been developed to improve the antitumor immune response [379]. For example, Ipilimumab (Yervoy®) and Tremelimumab (CP-675,206) bind to CTLA-4 receptor in T cells and block the inhibitory function against the costimulatory receptor CD28, thereby enhancing the T cell-DC interaction and reducing the number of T$_{reg}$ [165,180,380]. Nivolumab (Opdivo®), Pidilizumab (C-011), and Pembrolizumab (Keytruda®) target the programmed death signal-1(PD-1) receptor, another negative regulator on the T-cell surface that reduces the interaction with TAAs. Blocking the PD-1 receptor results in enhanced activation of T cells and decreased Treg infiltration to the tumor [381]. Among other immune mAbs, Daclizumab (Zinbryta®), an anti-CD25 mAb [382]; Dacetuzumab, an anti-CD40 mAb [383]; and Durvalumab (Imfinzi®) [384] and Avelumab (Bavencio®) [385], as anti-PD-L1 mAbs, are currently approved or in last stages of clinical trials for cancer immunotherapy.

Despite the success, the response rate of monotherapy with these mAb for advanced cancers is below 30%, and the therapy requires frequent and long-term parenteral dosages [234]. One advantage of applying nanotechnology for mAb delivery is to prolong the efficacy. Nanoparticles incorporating mAbs are summarized in [90].

Wang et al. [196] reported the preparation of hyaluronan-based microneedles (MN) filled with a pH-responsive and alginate-coated ethoxypropene-modified dextran nanoparticle (~ 250 nm) that encapsulated a PD-1 mAb, a glucose oxidase (GOx) and a catalase (CAT). GOx and CAT converted glucose to gluconic acid and reduced the pH in normoglycemic epidermis to ~4.5, which facilitated the nanoparticle degradation and sustained release of the mAb for 3 days. Following application of the MN-skin patch to B16 melanoma-bearing mice, prolonged antitumor response was determined compared to intratumoral administration of the PD-1 mAb. Furthermore, co-delivery of a CTLA-4 mAb with the PD-1 mAb via the MN synergistically enhanced the effect. However, the mAb stability at a low pH and the side effects of low dermal pH need to be studied [386,387]. Gdowski et al. [388] prepared PLGA core-shell nanoparticles (~250 nm) through w/o/w double emulsification and a solvent evaporation method, encapsulating a monoclonal antibody against annexinA2 (AnxA2), as a calcium-dependent phospholipid binding protein expressed on the surface of various tumor cells. The nanoparticles could passively target the tumor region via the EPR effect and exhibited a sustained release profile for the mAb (30% release in 12 days), inducing prolonged antitumor effect.

The immunotherapy of mAb may be further improved when combined with nanovaccines. Kuai et al. [237,389] developed a synthetic high-density lipoprotein (sHDL) nanodisc (~10 nm) composed of lipids and an apolipoprotein A1 (ApoA1) mimic peptide, and the nanodisc was surface conjugated with a tumor neoantigen (i.e., CSSIINFEKL or Adgpk) and CpG ODN. It was shown that combining i.v. administration of either CTLA-4 or PD-1 mAb with s.c injection of the nanodiscs enhanced the antigen presentation by DCs, increased specific activation of CD8+ cells, and increased the antitumor activity compared to mAb alone. In another study, s.c administration of MUC1 mRNA (a tumor antigen) formulated in a cationic and mannose-modified LCP nanoparticle (~60 nm) increased the antitumor effect of CTLA-4 mAb compared to mAb alone. The combination also induced an increased number of CD8+ cells and enhanced the secretion of IFN-γ [390]. The anti-CTLA-4 mAb was also employed to augment nanoparticle-based photodynamic therapy (PDT). The PDT-triggering Prussian blue nanoparticles (PBNPs) composed of $FeCl_3$ and $K_4Fe (CN)_6$ were intratumorally injected into neuroblastoma tumor-bearing mice that were also treated with i.v. anti-CTLA-4 mAb. The combination therapy reduced the tumor growth and prolonged the animal survival [391]. Following NIR irradiation, PDT could destroy the tumor cells by (i) induction of hyperthermia [392,393] and/or (ii) generation of reactive oxygen species (ROS) [394], mediating release of the tumor antigens along with some intrinsic immunoadjuvants such as heat shock proteins [395,396] that stimulate DCs and promote systemic immunoresponses [397]. Other PDT-triggering nanoparticles, including chlorin e6/lanthanide containing upconversion nanoparticles [168] and indocyanine green loaded PLGA nanoparticles [398], were also combined with the anti-CTLA-4 mAb to enhance their antitumor efficacy. A TLR agonist could be incorporated in those PDT nanoparticles to help trigger further enhanced antitumor immunity [168,398].

Recently, an immune checkpoint mAb was used to target nanoparticles containing an immunomodulator to T cells, which then migrated to and activated the tumor microenvironment. Schmid et al. [399] loaded resiquimod (TLR 7/8 agonist) or SD-208 (TGF-β receptor I kinase inhibitor) into PLGA nanoparticles labeled with an anti-PD-1 Fab for binding with T cells. The T cells then brought the drug-loaded nanoparticles, infiltrated the tumor, and slowly released the immunomodulating drugs in the tumor microenvironment. The treatment recruited increased CD8+ T cells in the tumor and extended the survival of tumor-bearing mice compared to free drug. In addition, this tumor microenvironment activation therapy augmented the antitumor efficacy of an anti-PD-1 mAb.

15.16 SMALL MOLECULE NANOMEDICINES

Immunogenic small molecules exhibiting the ability for either stimulating the immunoresponses or inhibiting immunosuppression have also been incorporated in nanoparticles for cancer immunotherapy [90]. Shetab Boushehri et al. [400] prepared matrix PLGA nanoparticles (~150 nm), which were surface decorated with lipopolysaccharide (LPS, a TLR4 agonist). The peritumorally injected nanoparticles to C26 colorectal tumor-bearing BALB/c mice were significantly taken up by both DCs and macrophages, leading to increased production of TNF-α and IL-6. Necrosis at the injection site was significantly decreased relative to free LPS. Yang et al. [401] loaded imiquimod (R837, an imidazoquinoline-derived TLR-7 agonist) into PLGA nanoparticles (~160 nm), which were then coated with OVA as a tumor-specific antigen as well as mannose for DC targeting. Following intradermal administration to OVA-melanoma-bearing mice, the targeted nanoparticles were highly localized in the lymph nodes to promote DC maturation with increased secretion of IL-12 and TNF-α, leading to tumor growth inhibition. PLGA nanoparticles (~100 nm) co-loaded with imiquimod and indocyanine green (ICG, a photothermal agent) were developed to perform combined photothermal and immunotherapy for cancer. Following intratumoral delivery of the nanoparticles and NIR irradiation, the tumor temperature was increased, followed by enhanced DC maturation (overexpression of CD 80 and CD86) and increased levels of CTL-mediated immunostimulatory cytokines, including IL-12, IL-6, and TNF-α [398]. Recently, resiquimod (R848, another imidazoquinoline-derived TLR7/8 agonist) was entrapped into polymeric nanoparticles (~270 nm) composed of mPEGPLA or PLGA/mPEG-PLA and s.c delivered to C57BL/6 mice for activation of DCs (overexpression of CD11b and CD86) with enhanced production of IL-6 [402]. However, the antitumor efficiency was not reported. In the study performed by Seth et al. [403], Gardiquimod (TLR7 agonist) and vadimezan (a vascular disrupting agent) were entrapped into PLGA nanoparticles (194 nm) for intratumoral delivery into melanoma-bearing mice. Increased production of immunostimulatory cytokines including TNF-α, IL-6, IL-12, and IL-1β as well as overexpression of CD40 and CD86 and reduced tumor growth were reported [403]. These small molecule immunostimulating agents are largely restricted to local delivery, as systemic delivery of them has been shown to trigger severe systemic immunotoxicity [404]. This limitation has restricted the clinical translation of these therapeutics.

Some small molecules exhibit potency for suppressing immunoinhibitory cells including Treg and MDSCs. For example, tyrosine kinase inhibitors (TKIs) that inhibit STAT3 were shown to suppress T_{reg} and MDCSCs [405–407]. Huo et al. [408] reported the fabrication of an anisamide analogue modified PLA-PEG polymeric micelles (~73 nm) encapsulating sunitinib. The anisamide ligand targeted the sigma receptor overexpressed on B16F10 melanoma cells. Following *i.v.* administration to B16F10 melanoma-bearing mice, the nanoparticles were highly accumulated in the tumor region, causing decreased tumor infiltration of T_{reg} and MDSCs and increased infiltration of CD8+ T cells. Moreover, enhanced production of Th1-mediating cytokines (IFN-γ and IL-2) and reduced secretion of Th2-mediated cytokines (CCL2, IL-6, IL-10, TGF-β, and TNF-α) were reported with significantly reduced tumor growth inhibition. However, it remains unclear whether the reduced infiltration of T_{reg} and MDSCs was due to direct delivery of sunitinib into immune cells, or passive uptake of sunitinib by immune cells after drug release from the nanoparticles, or modulation of B16F10 cells by sunitinib for their ability of immune cell recruitment and education.

Recently, Ou et al. [409] developed hybrid nanoparticles (117 nm) containing a PLGA core loaded with imatinib (a STAT3 inhibitor), which was coated with a lipid DPPC. For active targeting to neurophilin-1 (Nrp1) receptor which is overexpressed in Treg cells, the surface of nanoparticles was decorated with the tLyp1 peptide. It was shown that the targeted hybrid nanoparticles exhibited enhanced uptake and enhanced cytotoxicity in T_{reg} cells, but not to the other immune cells such as DCs and macrophages. Following *i.v.* injection to tumor-bearing C57BL/6 mice, high accumulation of the nanoparticles in the tumor was reported. When combined with anti-CTLA-4 mAb therapy, the nanoparticle induced enhanced CD8+ activity, increased production of IFN-γ, and improved antitumor efficacy.

Jeanbert et al. [410] reported the synthesis of block-copolymeric micelles composed of polyethylene glycol (PEG)-b-poly (propylene sulfide) conjugated to 6-thioguanine for targeted killing of MDSCs in the lymph node and spleen. The drug-conjugated micelles were more effective in depleting MDSCs in B16-F10 melanoma-bearing mice in comparison with free 6-thioguanine. Following intradermal administration, the micelles enhanced cancer-specific CD4+ and CD8+ immune responses, resulting in increased antitumor efficacy. Garg et al. [411] loaded JSI-124 (cucurbitacin I, a potent STAT3 inhibitor) into poly (ethylene oxide)-*block*-poly (α-carboxylate-ε-caprolactone) (PEOb-PCCL) micelles and discovered that this formulation decreased the STAT3 activity in the bone morrow-derived dendritic cells (BMDCs), leading to increased secretion of IL-12, IL-2, and IFN-γ and reduced production of TGF-β, compared to free JSI-124. However, whether this effect could be replicated *in vivo* remains unknown.

Although nanoparticles incorporating small immunomodulatory compounds have shown efficiency in preclinical models, their clinical application is limited due to the lack of potency. To induce potent immunoresponse for effective anticancer therapy, these immunomodulatory small molecules may need to combine with other agents. Additionally, their delivery needs to be targeted or localized to minimize the side effects and improve the efficacy.

15.17 CONCLUSION, CHALLENGES, AND PERSPECTIVE

Nanoparticle-combined immunotherapy is at the initial stage of exploitation, but tremendous potential of the approach could be clearly witnessed. Compound nanoparticles have been developed in research studies as vehicles for concerted delivery of tumor antigens as vaccination and/or immune stimulatory adjuvants to DCs or other professional APCs. Nanoparticles carrying whole-cell tumor vaccines have multiple antigen immunity and could potentially stimulate cellular and humoral immune responses. Generally, in comparison with the traditional, non-nanoparticle combined tumor antigen vaccines, the nanoparticle-loaded approaches could induce significantly stronger antigen-specific antibody responses and CD8+ cytotoxic T-lymphocyte responses against cancer cells and efficaciously inhibited tumor growth. Based on the inherent physical properties of nanoparticles or the conjugation with targeted ligands, targeting transportation of tumor antigens or adjuvants to TDLNs or specific immune cells such as DCs, T lymphocytes, and macrophages could be realized, thus further enhancing the immune stimulatory effects. In addition, combination of the compound nanoparticles with molecules of immune checkpoint inhibitors or photodynamic therapy could complement each other and more efficiently suppress tumor proliferation at the primary and metastatic sites. Nanoparticles with specific features could also control the release of payloads in response to typical conditions in the tumor microenvironment including hypoxia, specific protease, and decreased pH condition and further alter the immunosuppressive microenvironment into immunosupportive features. Adoptive cell therapy could also be supported by nanoparticle approaches in the aspects of enhancing *ex vivo* T-cell proliferation, recovering the abnormal microenvironment, and intensifying the trafficking and activity of infused lymphocytes.

Despite the impressive benefits of nanoparticles in cancer immunotherapy, there are still challenges that need to be treated with caution and investigated in future studies. First, the delivery ability of nanoparticles to the intended tissues or organs still needs to be strengthened. Currently, nanoparticles can only deliver a small portion of the administered payloads to the intended locations even with targeted ligands coated, which leads to the loss of delivered drugs and systemic cytotoxicity due to normal cell uptake of the nanoparticles. According to the study of Harrington et al. which included 17 patients with different types of locally advanced cancers, only less than 4% of the total administered dose could be accumulated in tumor tissues using pegylated liposome as the delivery method [47]. In addition, considerable heterogeneity of uptake both between different tumor types and between different patients with the same tumor type was also observed, mainly caused by the various tumor vascular conditions [47]. Similarly, because of the poor vascularization, nanoparticle accumulation is often insufficient in small metastatic lesions and the core of large tumors where usually exist risky dormant cancer cells. Other nanoparticles taken up by normal cells can cause toxicity including oxidative stress, pulmonary inflammation, and dysfunction of cells and organs through mechanisms of redox cycling, free radical formation, and hydrophobic interaction [412,413].

For the nanoparticles delivering payloads to the immune organs and cells, as they need to be transported in blood circulation and lymph vessels before reaching the targeted sites, the structural and colloidal stability is crucial to guarantee their final drainage into the immune organs and present payloads to immune cells [59]. Unstable nanoparticles may form micrometer-sized aggregates that could plug the capillary bed of distal organs and cause serious complications to patients. Another challenge is how to efficiently regulate components within the whole immune system by the nanoparticles to optimize the enhancement effects on antitumor immunity. The innate and adaptive immune system works in a network, but currently, little is known about how the other immune components in the immune network are affected to influence the whole antitumor immunity when the intended component is regulated by the administered nanoparticles. Future efforts are still needed to investigate the inter-regulation mechanisms of immune components to maximize treatment effects of the nanoparticles.

Potential immunogenicity of nanoparticles is another crucial concern toward progress in clinical translations. In fact, the utilization of nanoparticles in cancer immunotherapy is based on the immunogenicity or the immune adjuvant effects of nanoparticles or the attached peptides, proteins, or antibody fragments, but it could be detrimental if the immune response against unintended components is activated. Nanoparticles can be antigenic themselves, and if the nanoparticles are recognized as foreign substances and opsonized by plasma protein, the complement pathway will be activated, resulting in rapid phagocytosis and clearance in liver and spleen. Complete activation of the immune response against nanoparticles may lead to serious complications including allergic reactions, hemolysis, thrombogenesis, and even disseminated intravascular coagulation (DIC) [414,415]. More importantly, when nanoparticles are applied for enhancing antitumor immunity, immune checkpoint inhibitors are often conjugated to the nanoparticles or systematically administered to form syncretistic treatment effects. However, one major risk of the immune checkpoint inhibitors is that the drugs can induce serious autoimmune diseases. As a consequence, the simultaneously administered nanoparticles for future clinical translations should be developed in weak antigenicity with the use of a strictly controlled dose, and the patients should be observed with caution as they are theoretically at higher risk of complications.

Collectively, clinical application of the nanoparticles combined with immunotherapy needs the optimization of nanostructures to overcome the several existing disadvantages including the insufficient targeted delivery capacity, systemic cytotoxicity due to normal cell's engulfment, and the potential immunogenicity, and it will be crucial to ascertain the optimal physical and chemical properties of the nanoparticles in future investigations. It has been shown that the diameter of nanoparticles less than 100 nm displayed the most suitable surface chemistries, which could enable long-distance transportation within immune organs, strengthening internalization by immune cells, but other characteristics including the surface charge, shape, elasticity, hydrophilicity, ligands, and loading methods of encapsulating or conjugating payloads still need to be researched and determined to further improve the pharmacokinetics, toxicity, biocompatibility, and biodistribution of the nanoparticles. Only a small proportion of patients could achieve satisfactory survival after receiving one modality of immunotherapy, and there is a growing common view that combination of tumor vaccines with immune checkpoint inhibitors, adoptive T-cell therapy, or tumor microenvironment regulatory treatments could form synergistic effects on inhibiting primary and abscopal tumor lesions. As a consequence, developing pluripotent nanoparticles that integrate the multiple immunotherapy ingredients with targeted delivering and triggered releasing ability may could potentially attain comprehensive antitumor immunity enhancement and improved treatment effects. With further advances of nanotechnology and deeper understanding of interactions between the nanomaterials and immune system, the nanomedicine-combined immunotherapy could be further consummated to achieve more effective therapeutic benefits.

The main goal of cancer immunotherapy is provoking the immune system for eradication of tumor cells through tumor-specific CTL responses or blockage of the inhibitory cells (such as Treg and MDSCs), immunosuppressive pathways, and associated cytokines. Due to the capabilities of nanoparticles for targeting immune cells and tumor cells with prolonged retention in the lymph node, nanoparticulate systems have been extensively studied for delivering a wide range of antigens and adjuvants to boost the antitumor immunity. Various antigens and adjuvants (small molecule, peptide, protein, or nucleic acid) could be incorporated into nanoparticles or attached to the nanoparticle surface via hydrophobic interaction, charge–charge interaction, passive loading, and chemical modification, depending on their physicochemical properties. Many examples have been generated with encouraging *in vivo* results over the past 5 years and are comprehensively reviewed in this chapter.

Although many *in vivo* studies revealed encouraging antitumor efficacy, the clinical translation of nanoparticles for immunotherapy is still in its infancy and has encountered significant challenges. The current animal tumor models are overly simplified and do not exhibit the complicated human tumor microenvironment that is immunosuppressed. Nanoparticles that show encouraging results in animal models often do not induce comparable efficacy in human patients. The induced antitumor immunoresponse is often insignificant or short termed accompanied with high toxicity. These disappointing outcomes could be due to poor targeting of the nanovaccines to specific immune cells. Nonspecific activation of immune cells could induce uncontrolled immunoresponses such as cytokine storm and hypersensitivity reactions that cause significant clinical toxicity. To improve the efficacy of current nanovaccines, their payload release and pharmacokinetic profiles need to be optimized to boost significant and durable immunoresponses. Burst release is often reported with hydrophobic small molecules passively encapsulated in the hydrophobic compartment of nanoparticles as well as peptides/proteins incorporated in hydrogels. Improving the retention of these payloads in the nanoparticles may lead to enhanced and prolonged immunoresponse. In addition, tolerance of the patients' immune system to frequent vaccinations against certain antigens due to CD8+ T-cell depletion serves as another major obstacle for clinical application of nanovaccines [416].

The ideal nanocarrier for cancer immunotherapy should be able to: (i) provide colloidal stability against aggregation and undesirable interaction with blood components; (ii) protect their cargo during blood circulation; (iii) specifically target immune cells; and (iv) load a wide range of immunomodulating agent to effectively remodel the tumor microenvironment [417]. This means that multiple components need to be incorporated into the nanocarriers for multiple functions mentioned above, and fabricating such multifunctional nanoparticles is of challenge. Therefore, more efforts must be put on to resolve the scale-up manufacturing hurdles for nanoparticles to produce large batches of products with consistent quality to fulfill clinical requirements. Furthermore, high heterogeneity in tumor microenvironment among human patients will result in variable therapeutic outcomes upon immunotherapy. Biomarkers must be developed to stratify patients or monitor their therapeutic results to provide personalized care. Safety of nanoparticle immunotherapy must also be carefully assessed as nanoparticles are known to preferentially accumulate in certain tissues, such as liver and spleen, and their increased interaction with blood components could also enhance the systemic immunotoxicity [418]. Some nanoparticles are even capable of crossing the blood-brain barrier (BBB), causing neurotoxicity [419].

Furthermore, preclinical studies with nanovaccines are mostly focused on using artificial model antigens that are clinically irrelevant and the promising preclinical results often do not translate clinically. To address the issue, antigen-capturing nanoparticles (AC-NP) that are capable of adsorbing tumor-derived protein antigens (TDPA) released from radiation-treated cells were recently developed. AC-NPs were shown to deliver to DCs and other immune cells to enhance the antitumor immunity [165,183,381]. It was reported that PLGA nanoparticles adsorbed peptide antigens through various mechanisms including hydrophobic-hydrophobic interactions, ionic interactions, and formation of covalent thioether bonds through the maleimide group at the PLGA nanoparticle surface [420]. In a study performed by Min et al. [421], it was reported that upon incubation with irradiated B16F10 melanoma cells, PLGA nanoparticles captured tumor antigens and immunostimulant molecules effectively, such as Actn4, Ap3d1, Dag 1, Eef2, Tubb3, and DAMP proteins DAMP. It was showed that following PD-1 mAb therapy, the intratumorally delivered PLGA AC-NPs highly accumulated in the tumor-draining lymph nodes, leading to enhanced CD8+ infiltration and reduced Treg in the tumor microenvironment. The therapy also resulted in efficient abscopal effect, defined as an ability for induction of systemic therapeutic effects by local treatment.

To improve drug targeting, ligand decoration at the particle surface is often employed to facilitate specific recognition of the nanoparticles by the target cell. This strategy has been shown to improve the efficacy while reducing the toxicity in preclinical models. However, its clinical translation is yet to be established. As discussed previously by us [422], ligand nanoparticles suffered from several limitations, including inconsistent chemistry, increased immunogenicity (mAb and peptide ligands), reduced tumor penetration, and non-superior tumor delivery compared to their non-targeted counterparts. Nevertheless, the ligand-targeted strategy may exhibit significant advantages for targeting blood-borne targets, such as immune cells.

The Li lab recently developed a solvent-assisted active loading technology that could incorporate poorly soluble drugs into the liposomal aqueous core to provide enhanced loading efficiency and drug retention [423–425]. The Liotta group created a nanocage technology that contained small molecule-based affinity bait inside the nanogels for effective capture and retention of proteins [426]. These two methods may be used to improve the nanovaccine formulations. In hypoxic regions of the tumors, the maturation of immunoinhibitory cells such as Treg cells would be disrupted and therefore could be suggested as the target site for immunostimulation. Development of innovative strategies to enhance penetration of nanoparticles to these poorly permeable and accessible areas in the tumor microenvironment could result in a dramatic increase in efficacy. Developing nanoparticles that show high specificity for a subset of immune cells will greatly enhance the efficacy of the treatment and reduce the side effects. Specific ligands derived from mAb, peptides, and aptamers may be attached to the nanoparticle surface to increase their specificity. New technologies to enhance endosomal escape and cytosolic delivery of nanoparticle payloads must be developed to improve delivery of antigens and certain immunoboosters for enhanced MHC I antigen cross-presentation that will lead to increased CTL activity. For example, nanoparticles harnessing caveolae-mediated internalization have been shown to avoid lysosomal degradation with increased cytosolic delivery. In addition to improving the design of nanovaccines to enhance their efficacy, clinical conditions in each patient need to be considered. Many cancer patients are under chemotherapy with a compromised immune system. Their immune response may not be activated by the vaccination. Treatment schedule should be personalized and optimized to maximize the vaccination effect. The recent trend in this field is to incorporate multiple components in a nanoparticle to target multiple mechanisms in the immune cells for enhanced immunoactivation. Although promising, this may increase the difficulty in scale-up production of these complicated multifunctional nanovaccines, and the possibility of successful large-scale manufacturing must be considered when designing the nanoparticle formulation.

Immune checkpoint therapy is regarded to start a revolution in cancer immunotherapy. Nowadays, a growing number of immune checkpoint inhibitors have been applied in preclinical trials. Even though the successful outcome of immune checkpoint blockers in advanced cancer, further development is still needed to achieve better therapeutic efficacy and minimize the unwanted side effects. By engineering the nanoparticles, it could provide potent and multifunctional platform for drug delivery to enhance the therapeutic efficacy of ICB [10]. Nevertheless, several drawbacks of current nanotechnology still exist. The targeting ability of nanoparticles is limited due to the heterogeneity and biology of tumor. Novel enhanced permeability and retention effect (EPR)-imaging technologies should be developed to investigate the active and passive targeting approach and provide promising evidence for nanoparticle designation. In addition, the scalability and reproducibility of nanotechnology still limit the development and clinical application of nanomedicine. Although there are thousands of papers published on nanoparticle delivery system, only few of nanomaterials can be translated into clinical treatment. It may be due to insufficient exact evidence on the EPR effect in clinic which could hinder the application and efficacy of nanoparticles. It is demonstrated that there is only a tiny amount of delivered drug distributed at tumor sites, and it thus significantly restricts the therapeutic efficacy of nanomedicine [427]. Besides these, preclinical animal models that could highly mimic the physiological environment of human remain to be improved and standardized. The more predictive animal models could facilitate the development of nanotechnology in translational medicine. Finally, to increase the chance of applying nanoparticle-based immune checkpoint therapy into clinical trials, the biomarkers and intrinsic biology of tumors need to be further explored.

The engineered nanoparticles incorporating ICB are considered as a rapid expansion for antitumor treatment. Applying nanoparticles in cancer immunotherapy could promote the multidisciplinary researches to combat tumor, including genome editing, epigenetic modification, biology, photodynamic therapy, and so on. Combination of immune checkpoint therapy and nanotechnology will stand on the threshold of great advances for cancer immunotherapy in future.

15.18 FUTURE DIRECTIONS

Although nanomedicine is a relatively new branch of science, its translation into clinical care has been rapid. The unique properties of nanoparticle drug carriers make them well suited for oncology applications. Nanoparticle chemotherapeutics are composed to influence the treatment of most cancers. However, there are still limited clinical data and a limited number of nanotherapeutics approved for clinical use. To fully understand the advantages and disadvantages of nanoparticle therapeutics, more clinical data are needed it can also help in identifying the best applications for nanochemotherapeutics. Thus, it is crucial to develop and carry out well-designed clinical trials to further the development of these drugs. Clinical investigators should fully understand the particular nanoparticles they are investigating and design trials that take advantage of nanoparticle properties. More complex targeted systems, which can release nanochemotherapeutics at a target site when exposed to external stimuli such as light and temperature, are also under development. Another potential is to develop more nanoparticles capable of delivering combination chemotherapeutics. CPX-351, a liposomal formulation of cytarabine and daunorubicin, showed promising results in its first human study [428]. Together with the progression of nanoscale drug delivery systems, advances in nanoscale imaging suggest the potential for the development of multifunctional "smart" nanoparticles that may facilitate the realization of individualized cancer therapy. Almost all types of nanoparticles including polymeric nanoparticles [429], nanocrystals [430], polymeric micelles [431], dendrimers [432], and carbon nanotubes [433] have been evaluated for their suitability as multifunctional nanoparticles that can be applied for simultaneous *in vivo* imaging and treatment of cancers. Eventually, multiplex nanoparticles may be capable of detecting malignant cells (active targeting moiety), visualizing their location in the body (real-time *in vivo* imaging), killing the cancer cells with minimal side effects by sparing normal cells (active targeting and controlled drug release or photothermal ablation), and monitoring treatment effects in real time.

Recently in 2021, protective immune response against P32 oncogenic peptide-pulsed PBMCs in mouse models of breast cancer has been studied [434]. High expression of p32 in certain tumors makes it a potential target for immunotherapy. In that study [434], the first goal was to design multi-epitope peptides from the P32 protein and the second goal was to compare the prophylactic effects of DC- and PBMC-based vaccines by pulsing them with designed peptides. For these purposes, 160 BALB/c mice were vaccinated in 5 different subgroups of each 4 peptides using PBS (F1–4a), F peptides alone (F1–4b), F peptides with CpG-ODN (F1–4c), F peptides with CpGODN and DCs (F1–4d), and F peptides with CpG-ODN and PBMCs (F1–4e). It was found a significantly higher interferon-γ (IFN-γ) and granzyme B levels in T cells of F4d and F4e subgroups compared to control ($p \leq 0.05$). The result of challenging spleen PBMCs of vaccinated mice with 4T1 cells showed significant up- and downregulation of Fas ligand (FasL) and forkhead box P3 (Foxp3) gene expression between F4d and F4e subgroups with control, respectively. In addition, a significant change was seen in Caspase 3 gene expression of F4d subgroup compared to control (p ≤ 0.05). Supernatant levels of IFN-γ and perforin were significantly increased in F4d and F4e subgroups compared to control. Consequently, significantly lower tumor sizes and prolonged survival time were detected in F4d and F4e subgroups compared to control after challenging mice with 4T1 cells. Accordingly, these results [434] demonstrated that PBMCs pulsed F4 peptide-based vaccine could induce a protective immune response while it is a simple and less expensive vaccine.

Finally, the areas that future serum miRNA studies need to focus on are as follows: (i) recruiting larger cohorts of patients with different ethnicities, (ii) astutely recording patients' HCC etiology and the need to include it into the analysis, (iii) correlating serum miRNA level to other clinical parameters, and lastly, (iv) the use and comparison of standardized internal references.

These strategies necessitate the interaction of hematologists with fundamental cell biologists, immunologists, and material scientists to focus on better understanding current pathology and potential opportunities to develop novel therapies based on receptor expression and biology. Finally, recent advances in nucleic acid nanoparticle systems for efficient siRNA and miRNA delivery are highlighted.

REFERENCES

1. D. Hanahan, R. A. Weinberg, Hallmarks of cancer: the next generation, *Cell* 144 (5) (2011) 646–674.
2. I. Marquez-Rodas, M. A. Aznar, A. Calles, I. Melero, For whom the cell tolls? Intratumoral treatment links innate and adaptive immunity, *Clin. Cancer Res.* 25 (4) (2019) 1127–1129.
3. Y. Wang, C. Yao, L. Ding, C. Li, J. Wang, M. Wu, Y. Lei, Enhancement of the immune function by titanium dioxide nanorods and their application in cancer immunotherapy, *J. Biomed. Nanotechnol.* 13 (4) (2017) 367–380.
4. T. Kieber-Emmons, B. Monzavi-Karbassi, L. F. Hutchins, A. Pennisi, I. Makhoul, Harnessing benefit from targeting tumor associated carbohydrate antigens, *Hum. Vaccines Immunother.* 13 (2) (2017) 323–331.
5. Y. Yang, G.H. Nam, G.B. Kim, Y.K. Kim, I.S. Kim, Intrinsic cancer vaccination, *Adv. Drug Delivery Rev.* 2019 151–152 2–22. doi:10.1016/j.addr.2019.05.007
6. T.-H. Tran, G. Mattheolabakis, H. Aldawsari, M. Amiji, Exosomes as nanocarriers for immunotherapy of cancer and inflammatory diseases, *Clin. Immunol.* 160 (1) (2015) 46–58. doi:10.1016/j.clim.2015.03.021
7. L.E. Paulis, S. Mandal, M. Kreutz, C.G. Figdor, Dendritic cell-based nanovaccines for cancer immunotherapy, *Curr. Opin. Immunol.* 25 (3) (2013) 389–395. doi:10.1016/j.coi.2013.03.001
8. J.M. Silva, M. Videira, R. Gaspar, V. Preat, H.F. Florindo, Immune system targeting by biodegradable nanoparticles for cancer vaccines, *J. Control. Release* 168 (2) (2013) 179–199. doi:10.1016/j.jconrel.2013.03.010
9. J. Begley, A. Ribas, Targeted therapies to improve tumor immunotherapy, *Clin. Cancer Res.* 14 (14) (2008) 4385–4391. doi:10.1158/1078-0432.CCR-07-4804
10. H. Deng, Z. Zhang, The application of nanotechnology in immune checkpoint blockade for cancer treatment, *J. Control. Release* 290 (2018) 28–45.
11. N.L. Syn, M.W.L. Teng, T.S.K. Mok, R.A. Soo, De-novo and acquired resistance to immune checkpoint targeting, *Lancet Oncol.* 18 (12) (2017) e731–e741.
12. K.V. Korneev, K.N. Atretkhany, M.S. Drutskaya, S.I. Grivennikov, D.V. Kuprash, S.A. Nedospasov, TLR-signaling and proinflammatory cytokines as drivers of tumorigenesis, *Cytokine* 89 (2017) 127–135.
13. J. Mora, C. Mertens, J.K. Meier, D.C. Fuhrmann, B. Brune, M. Jung, Strategies to interfere with tumor metabolism through the interplay of innate and adaptive immunity, *Cells*, 8 (5) (2019) 445. doi:10.3390/cells8050445
14. M.D. Vesely, M.H. Kershaw, R.D. Schreiber, M.J. Smyth, Natural innate and adaptive immunity to cancer, *Annu. Rev. Immunol.* 29 (2011) 235–271. doi:10.1146/annurev-immunol-031210-101324
15. H.J. Smith, T.R. McCaw, A.I. Londono, A.A. Katre, S. Meza-Perez, E.S. Yang, A. Forero, D. J. Buchsbaum, T.D. Randall, J.M. Straughn Jr., L.A. Norian, R.C. Arend, The antitumor effects of entinostat in ovarian cancer require adaptive immunity, *Cancer* 124 (24) (2018) 4657–4666. doi:10.1002/cncr.31761
16. E.S. Nakasone, S.A. Hurvitz, K.E. McCann, Harnessing the immune system in the battle against breast cancer, *Drugs Context* 7 (2018) 212520.
17. M. Dougan, G. Dranoff, Immune therapy for cancer, *Annu. Rev. Immunol.* 27 (2009) 83–117.
18. Y. Jiang, Y. Li, B. Zhu, T-cell exhaustion in the tumor microenvironment, *Cell. Death Dis.* 6 (6) (2015) e1792.
19. M.J. Selby, J.J. Engelhardt, M. Quigley, K.A. Henning, T. Chen, M. Srinivasan, A.J. Korman, Anti-CTLA-4 antibodies of IgG2a isotype enhance antitumor activity through reduction of intratumoral regulatory T cells, *Cancer Immunol. Res.* 1 (1) (2013) 32–42.
20. H.O. Alsaab, S. Sau, R. Alzhrani, K. Tatiparti, K. Bhise, S.K. Kashaw, A.K. Lyer, PD-1 and PD-L1 checkpoint signaling inhibition for cancer immunotherapy: mechanism, combinations, and clinical outcome, *Front. Pharmacol.* 8 (2017) 561.
21. Y. Iwai, J. Hamanishi, K. Chamoto, T. Honjo, Cancer immunotherapies targeting the PD-1 signaling pathway, *J. Biomed. Sci.* 24 (1) (2017) 26.
22. R. Lotfi, J. Eisenbacher, G. Solgi, K. Fuchs, T. Yildiz, C. Nienhaus, M. T. Rojewski, H. Schrezenmeier, Human mesenchymal stem cells respond to native but not oxidized damage associated molecular pattern molecules from necrotic (tumor) material, *Eur. J. Immunol.* 41 (7) (2011) 2021–2028.
23. D.S. Chen, I. Mellman, Oncology meets immunology: the cancer-immunity cycle, *Immunity* 39 (1) (2013) 1–10.
24. Y. Li, C. Ayala-Orozco, P.R. Rauta, S. Krishnan. The application of nanotechnology in enhancing immunotherapy for cancer treatment: current effects and perspective. *Nanoscale* 11 (5) (2019) 17157–17178.
25. L.A. Tashireva, V.M. Perelmuter, V.N. Manskikh, E.V. Denisov, O.E. Savelieva, E.V. Kaygorodova, M.V. Zavyalova, Types of immune-inflammatory responses as a reflection of cell-cell interactions under conditions of tissue regeneration and tumor growth, *Biochemistry* 82 (5) (2017) 542–555.
26. A. Tarafdar, L.E. Hopcroft, P. Gallipoli, F. Pellicano, J. Cassels, A. Hair, K. Korfi, H.G. Jorgensen, D. Vetrie, T.L. Holyoake, A.M. Michie, CML cells actively evade host immune surveillance through cytokine-mediated downregulation of MHC-II expression, *Blood*, 129 (2017) 199–208.

27. H.M. Guirgis, The impact of PD-L1 on survival and value of the immune check point inhibitors in non-small-cell lung cancer; proposal, policies and perspective, *J. Immunother. Cancer* 6 (15) (2018) 15.

28. J.F. Jacobs, A.J. Idema, K.F. Bol, S. Nierkens, O.M. Grauer, P. Wesseling, J.A. Grotenhuis, P.M. Hoogerbrugge, I.J. de Vries, G.J. Adema, Regulatory T cells and the PD-L1/PD-1 pathway mediate immune suppression in malignant human brain tumors, *Neuro Oncol.* 11 (4) (2009) 394–402.

29. P. Sinha, V.K. Clements, S. Miller, S. Ostrand-Rosenberg, Tumor immunity: a balancing act between T cell activation, macrophage activation and tumor-induced immune suppression, *Cancer Immunol. Immunother.* 54 (11) (2005) 1137–1142.

30. D.I. Gabrilovich, S. Nagaraj, Myeloid-derived suppressor cells as regulators of the immune system, *Nat. Rev. Immunol.* 9 (2009) 162–174. doi:10.1038/nri2506

31. K.K. Goswami, T. Ghosh, S. Ghosh, M. Sarkar, A. Bose, R. Baral, Tumor promoting role of anti-tumor macrophages in tumor microenvironment, *Cell. Immunol.* 316 (2017) 1–10. doi:10.1016/j.cellimm.2017.04.005

32. M.W. Pickup, J.K. Mouw, V.M. Weaver, The extracellular matrix modulates the hallmarks of cancer, *EMBO Rep.* 15 (12) (2014) 1243–1253.

33. M. Ferrari, Cancer nanotechnology: opportunities and challenges, *Nat. Rev. Cancer* 5 (3) (2005) 161–171.

34. S. Rahimian, M.F. Fransen, J.W. Kleinovink, M. Amidi, F. Ossendorp, W.E. Hennink, Polymeric microparticles for sustained and local delivery of antiCD40 and antiCTLA-4 in immunotherapy of cancer, *Biomaterials* 61 (2015) 33–40.

35. D. Peer, J.M. Karp, S. Hong, O.C. Farokhzad, R. Margalit, R. Langer, Nanocarriers as an emerging platform for cancer therapy, *Nat. Nanotechnol.* 2 (2007) 751–760.

36. H. Maeda, The enhanced permeability and retention (EPR) effect in tumor vasculature: the key role of tumor-selective macromolecular drug targeting, *Adv. Enzym. Regul.* 41 (2001) 189–207.

37. T. Randall, R. Krishnendu, Engineering nanoparticles to overcome barriers to immunotherapy, *Bioeng. Transl. Med.* 1 (1) (2016) 47–62. doi:10.1002/btm2.10005

38. C. Pfirschke, C. Engblom, S. Rickelt, V. Cortez-Retamozo, C. Garris, F. Pucci, T. Yamazaki, V. Poirer-Colame, A. Newton, Y. Redouane, Y.J. Lin, G. Wojtkiewicz, Y. Iwanmoto, M. Mino-Kenudson, T.G. Huynh, R.O. Hynes, G.J. Freeman, G. Kroemer, L. Zitvogel, R. Weissieder, M.J. Pittet, Immunogenic chemotherapy sensitizes tumors to checkpoint blockade therapy, *Immunity* 44 (2) (2016) 343–354.

39. D. Peer, E.J. Park, Y. Morishita, C.V. Carman, M. Shimaoka, Systemic leukocyte directed siRNA delivery revealing cyclin D1 as an anti-inflammatory target, *Science* 319 (2008) 627–630.

40. P.A. Ott, F.S. Hodi, C. Robert, CTLA-4 and PD-1/PD-L1 blockade: new immunotherapeutic modalities with durable clinical benefit in melanoma patients, *Clin. Cancer Res.* 19 (19) (2013) 5300–5309. doi:10.1158/1078-0432. CCR-13-0143

41. S. Baxi, A. Yang, R.L. Gennarelli, N. Khan, Z. Wang, L. Boyce, D. Korenstein, Immune-related adverse events for anti-PD-1 and anti-PD-L1 drugs: systematic review and meta-analysis, *Br. Med. J.* 360 (2018) k793. doi:10.1136/bmj.k793

42. R. Wu, M.A. Forget, J. Chacon, C. Bernatchez, C. Haymaker, J.Q. Chen, P. Hwu, L.G. Radvanyi, Adoptive T-cell therapy using autologous tumor-infiltrating

43. lymphocytes for metastatic melanoma: current status and future outlook, *Cancer J.* 18 (2) (2012) 160–175. doi:10.1097/PPO.0b013e31824d4465

43. N. Mitsuiki, C. Schwab, B. Grimbacher, What did we learn from CTLA-4 insufficiency on the human immune system?, *Immunol. Rev.* 287 (2019) 33–49. doi:10.1111/imr.12721

44. A. Ribas, J.D. Wolchok, Cancer immunotherapy using checkpoint blockade, *Science* 359 (6382) (2018) 1350–1355. doi:10.1126/science.aar4060

45. J.M. Cha, D.G. You, E.J. Choi, S.J. Park, W. Um, J. Jeon, K. Kim, I.C. Kwon, J.C. Park, H.R. Kim, J.H. Park, Improvement of antitumor efficacy by combination of thermosensitive liposome with high-intensity focused ultrasound, *J. Biomed. Nanotechnol.* 12 (9) (2016) 1724–1733. doi:10.1166/jbn.2016.2272

46. H. Hashizume, P. Baluk, S. Morikawa, J.W. McLean, G. Thurston, S. Roberge, R.K. Jain, D.M. McDonald, Openings between defective endothelial cells explain tumor vessel leakiness, *Am. J. Pathol.* 156 (4) (2000) 1363–1380. doi:10.1016/S0002-9440(10)65006-7

47. K.J. Harrington, S. Mohammadtaghi, P.S. Uster, D. Glass, A.M. Peters, R.G. Vile, J.S. Stewart, Effective targeting of solid tumors in patients with locally advanced cancers by radiolabeled pegylated liposomes, *Clin. Cancer Res.* 7 (2) (2001) 243–254.

48. J.K. Vasir, V. Labhasetwar, Targeted drug delivery in cancer therapy, *Technol. Cancer Res. Treat.* 4 (4) (2005) 363–374. doi:10.1177/153303460500400405

49. R.A. Petros, J.M. DeSimone, Strategies in the design of nanoparticles for therapeutic applications, *Nat. Rev. Drug Discov.* 9 (2010) 615–627.

50. Y. Wang, D. Wang, Q. Fu, D. Liu, Y. Ma, K. Racette, Z. He, F. Liu, Shape-controlled paclitaxel nanoparticles with multiple morphologies: rod-shaped, worm-like, spherical, and fingerprint-like, *Mol. Pharm.* 11 (10) (2014) 3766–3771. doi:10.1021/mp500436p

51. E. Blanco, H. Shen, M. Ferrari, Principles of nanoparticle design for overcoming biological barriers to drug delivery, *Nat. Biotechnol.* 33 (2015) 941–951. doi:10.1038/nbt.3330

52. R.V. Benjaminsen, M.A. Mattebjerg, J.R. Henriksen, S.M. Moghimi, T.L. Andresen, The possible "proton sponge" effect of polyethylenimine (PEI) does not include change in lysosomal pH, *Mol. Ther.* 21 (1) (2013) 149–157. doi:10.1038/mt.2012.185

53. Y.Y. Yuan, C.Q. Mao, X.J. Du, J.Z. Du, F. Wang, J. Wang, Surface charge switchable nanoparticles based on zwitterionic polymer for enhanced drug delivery to tumor, *Adv. Mater.* 24 (40) (2012) 5476–5480. doi:10.1002/adma.201202296

54. J. Lu, S.C. Owen, M.S. Shoichet, Stability of self-assembled polymeric micelles in serum, *Macromolecules* 44 (15) (2011) 6002–6008. doi:10.1021/ma200675w

55. S. Terry, P. Savagner, S. Ortiz-Cuaran, L. Mahjoubi, P. Saintigny, J. Thiery, S. Chouaib, New insights into the role of EMT in tumor immune escape, *Mol. Oncol.* 11 (7) (2017) 824–846. doi:10.1002/1878-0261.12093

56. G. Beatty, W. Gladney, Immune escape mechanisms as a guide for cancer immunotherapy, *Clin. Cancer Res.* 21 (4) (2015) 687–692. doi:10.1158/1078-0432.CCR-14-1860

57. Y. Lu, Y. Yang, Z. Gu, J. Zhang, H. Song, G. Xiang, C. Yu, Glutathione-depletion mesoporous organosilica nanoparticles as a self-adjuvant and co-delivery platform for enhanced cancer immunotherapy, *Biomaterials* 175 (2018) 82–92. doi:10.1016/j.biomaterials.2018.05.025

58. S. Yan, W. Gu, B. Zhang, B.E. Rolfe, Z.P. Xu, High adjuvant activity of layered double hydroxide nanoparticles and nanosheets in anti-tumour vaccine formulations, *Dalton Trans.* 47 (2018) 2956–2964. doi:10.1039/C7DT03725B

59. L.X. Zhang, X.X. Xie, D.Q. Liu, Z.P. Xu, R.T. Liu, Efficient co-delivery of neo-epitopes using dispersion-stable layered double hydroxide nanoparticles for enhanced melanoma immunotherapy, *Biomaterials* 174 (2018) 54–66. doi:10.1016/j.biomaterials.2018.05.015

60. T. Yata, Y. Takahashi, M. Tan, H. Nakatsuji, S. Ohtsuki, T. Murakami, H. Imahori, Y. Umeki, T. Shiomi, Y. Takakura, M. Nishikawa, DNA nanotechnology-based composite-type gold nanoparticle-immunostimulatory DNA hydrogel for tumor photothermal immunotherapy, *Biomaterials* 146 (2017) 136–145. doi:10.1016/j.biomaterials.2017.09.014

61. T. Courant, E. Bayon, H.L. Reynaud-Dougier, C. Villiers, M. Menneteau, P.N. Marche, F.P. Navarro, Tailoring nanostructured lipid carriers for the delivery of protein antigens: Physicochemical properties versus immunogenicity studies, *Biomaterials* 136 (2017) 29–42. doi:10.1016/j.biomaterials.2017.05.001

62. C. Zhang, G. Shi, J. Zhang, H. Song, J. Niu, S. Shi, P. Huang, Y. Wang, W. Wang, C. Li and D. Kong, Targeted antigen delivery to dendritic cell via functionalized alginate nanoparticles for cancer immunotherapy, *J. Controlled Release*, 2017, 256, 170–181. doi:10.1016/j.jconrel.2017.04.020

63. V. Sokolova, Z. Shi, S. Huang, Y. Du, M. Kopp, A. Frede, T. Knuschke, J. Buer, D. Yang, J. Wu, A.M. Westendorf, M. Epple, Delivery of the TLR ligand poly(I:C) to liver cells in vitro and in vivo by calcium phosphate nanoparticles leads to a pronounced immunostimulation, *Acta Biomater.* 64 (2017) 401–410. doi:10.1016/j.actbio.2017.09.037

64. L. Liu, Y. Wang, L. Miao, Q. Liu, S. Musetti, J. Li and L. Huang, Combination immunotherapy of MUC1 mRNA nanovaccine and CTLA-4 blockade effectively inhibits growth of triple negative breast cancer, *Mol. Ther.* 26 (1) (2018) 45–55.

65. R.M. Pearson, L.M. Casey, K.R. Hughes, L.Z. Wang, M.G. North, D.R. Getts, S.D. Miller, L.D. Shea, Controlled delivery of single or multiple antigens in tolerogenic nanoparticles using peptide-polymer bioconjugates, *Mol. Ther.* 25 (7) (2017) 1655–1664. doi:10.1016/j.ymthe.2017.04.015

66. R. Verbeke, I. Lentacker, L. Wayteck, K. Breckpot, M. Van Bockstal, B. Descamps, C. Vanhove, S.C. De Smedt, H. Dewitte, Co-delivery of nucleoside-modified mRNA and TLR agonists for cancer immunotherapy: Restoring the immunogenicity of immunosilent mRNA, *J. Controlled Release* 266 (2017) 287–300. doi:10.1016/j.jconrel.2017.09.041

67. H. Takahashi, K. Misato, T. Aoshi, Y. Yamamoto, Y. Kubota, X. Wu, E. Kuroda, K.J. Ishii, H. Yamamoto, Y. Yoshioka, Carbonate apatite nanoparticles act as potent vaccine adjuvant delivery vehicles by enhancing cytokine production induced by encapsulated cytosine-phosphate-guanine oligodeoxynucleotides, *Front. Immunol.* 9 (2018) 783. doi:10.3389/fimmu.2018.00783

68. Y. Yoshizaki, E. Yuba, N. Sakaguchi, K. Koiwai, A. Harada, K. Kono, pH-sensitive polymer-modified liposome-based immunity-inducing system: effects of inclusion of cationic lipid and CpG-DNA, *Biomaterials* 141 (2017) 272–283. doi:10.1016/j.biomaterials.2017.07.001

69. X. Liang, J. Duan, X. Li, X. Zhu, Y. Chen, X. Wang, H. Sun, D. Kong, C. Li, J. Yang, Improved vaccine-induced immune responses via a ROS-triggered nanoparticle-based antigen delivery system, *Nanoscale* 10 (2018) 9489–9503. doi:10.1039/C8NR00355F

70. M. Xu, Y. Chen, P. Banerjee, L. Zong, L. Jiang, Dendritic cells targeting and pH-responsive multi-layered nanocomplexes for smart delivery of DNA vaccines, *AAPS PharmSciTech.* 18 (2017) 2618–2625. doi:10.1208/s12249-017-0741-1

71. W. Long, J. Wang, J. Yang, H. Wu, J. Wang, X. Mu, H. He, Q. Liu, Y. M. Sun, H. Wang, X. D. Zhang, Naturally-derived PHA-L protein nanoparticle as a radioprotector through activation of Toll-like receptor 5, *J. Biomed. Nanotechnol.* 15 (1) (2019) 62–76.

72. G. Zom, M. Willems, S. Khan, T. van der Sluis, J. Kleinovink, M. Camps, G. van der Marel, D. Filippov, C. Melief, F. Ossendorp, Novel TLR2-binding adjuvant induces enhanced T cell responses and tumor eradication, *J. Immunother. Cancer* 6 (2018) 146. doi:10.1186/s40425-018-0455-2

73. B. Seliger, C. Massa, B. Rini, J. Ko, J. Finke, Antitumour and immune-adjuvant activities of protein-tyrosine kinase inhibitors, *Trends Mol. Med.* 16 (4) (2010) 184–192. doi:10.1016/j.molmed.2010.02.001

74. M. Ebrahimian, M. Hashemi, M. Maleki, G. Hashemitabar, K. Abnous, M. Ramezani, A. Haghparast, Co-delivery of dual Toll-like receptor agonists and antigen in poly(lactic-co-glycolic) acid/polyethylenimine cationic hybrid nanoparticles promote efficient in vivo immune responses, *Front. Immunol.* 8 (2017) 1077. doi:10.3389/fimmu.2017.01077

75. Z. Luo, C. Wang, H. Yi, P. Li, H. Pan, L. Liu, L. Cai, Y. Ma, Nanovaccine loaded with poly I:C and STAT3 siRNA robustly elicits anti-tumor immune responses through modulating tumor-associated dendritic cells in vivo, *Biomaterials* 38 (2015) 50–60. doi:10.1016/j.biomaterials.2014.10.050

76. A.N. Alexander, M.K. Huelsmeyer, A. Mitzey, R.R. Dubielzig, I.D. Kurzman, E.G. Macewen, D.M. Vail, Development of an allogeneic whole-cell tumor vaccine expressing xenogeneic gp100 and its implementation in a phase II clinical trial in canine patients with malignant melanoma, *Cancer Immunol. Immunother.* 55 (2006) 433–442. doi:10.1007/s00262-005-0025-6.

77. M. Chen, R. Xiang, Y. Wen, G. Xu, C. Wang, S. Luo, T. Yin, X. Wei, B. Shao, N. Liu, F. Guo, M. Li, S. Zhang, M. Li, K. Ren, Y. Wang, Y. Wei, A whole-cell tumor vaccine modified to express fibroblast activation protein induces antitumor immunity against both tumor cells and cancer-associated fibroblasts, *Sci. Rep.* 5 (2015) 14421. doi:10.1038/srep14421

78. W. Chen, H. Zuo, B. Li, C. Duan, B. Rolfe, B. Zhang, T.J. Mahony, Z.P. Xu, Clay nanoparticles elicit long-term immune responses by forming biodegradable depots for sustained antigen stimulation, *Small* 14 (19) (2018) e1704465. doi:10.1002/smll.201704465

79. J.W. Hodge, C.T. Garnett, B. Farsaci, C. Palena, K.Y. Tsang, S. Ferrone, S.R. Gameiro, Chemotherapy-induced immunogenic modulation of tumor cells enhances killing by cytotoxic T lymphocytes and is distinct from immunogenic cell death, *Int. J. Cancer* 133 (3) (2013) 624–636. doi:10.1002/ijc.28070

80. S.C. Formenti, S. Demaria, Radiotherapy to convert the tumor into an in situ vaccine, *Int. J. Radiat. Oncol. Biol. Phys.* 84 (4) (2012) 879–880. doi:10.1016/j.ijrobp.2012.06.020

81. Q. Chen, L. Xu, C. Liang, C. Wang, R. Peng, Z. Liu, Photothermal therapy with immune-adjuvant nanoparticles together with checkpoint blockade for effective cancer immunotherapy, *Nat. Commun.* 7 (2016) 13193. doi:10.1038/ncomms13193

82. J. Xu, L. Xu, C. Wang, R. Yang, Q. Zhuang, X. Han, Z. Dong, W. Zhu, R. Peng, Z. Liu, Near-infrared-triggered photodynamic therapy with multitasking upconversion

nanoparticles in combination with checkpoint blockade for immunotherapy of colorectal cancer, *ACS Nano* 11 (5) (2017) 4463–4474. doi:10.1021/acsnano.7b00715

83. J.T. Wilson, S. Keller, M.J. Manganiello, C. Cheng, C.-C. Lee, C. Opara, et al., pH Responsive nanoparticle vaccines for dual-delivery of antigens and immunostimulatory oligonucleotides, *ACS Nano* 7 (5) (2013) 3912–3925. doi:10.1021/nn305466z

84. S. Flanary, A.S. Hoffman, P.S. Stayton, Antigen delivery with poly (propylacrylic acid) conjugation enhances MHC-1 presentation and T-cell activation, *Bioconjug. Chem.* 20 (2) (2009) 241–248. doi:10.1021/bc800317a

85. X. Zang, X. Zhao, H. Hu, M. Qiao, Y. Deng, D. Chen, Nanoparticles for tumor immunotherapy, *Eur. J. Pharm. Biopharm.* 115 (2017) 243–256. doi:10.1016/j.ejpb.2017.03.013

86. B. Bahrami, M. Hojjat-Farsangi, H. Mohammadi, E. Anvari, G. Ghalamfarsa, M. Yousefi, et al., Nanoparticles and targeted drug delivery in cancer therapy, *Immunol. Lett.* 190 (2017) 64–83. doi:10.1016/j.imlet.2017.07.015

87. S. Hirosue, I.C. Kourtis, A.J. van der Vlies, J.A. Hubbell, M.A. Swartz, Antigen delivery to dendritic cells by poly (propylene sulfide) nanoparticles with disulfide conjugated peptides: cross-presentation and T cell activation, *Vaccine* 28 (50) (2010) 7897–7906. doi:10.1016/j.vaccine.2010.09.077.

88. R.A. Rosalia, L.J. Cruz, S. van Duikeren, A.T. Tromp, A.L. Silva, W. Jiskoot, et al., CD40-targeted dendritic cell delivery of PLGA-nanoparticle vaccines induce potent anti-tumor responses, *Biomaterials* 40 (2015) 88–97. doi:10.1016/j.biomaterials.2014.10.053

89. S. De Koker, B.N. Lambrecht, M.A. Willart, Y. Van Kooyk, J. Grooten, C. Vervaet, et al., Designing polymeric particles for antigen delivery, *Chem. Soc. Rev.* 40 (1) (2011) 320–339. doi:10.1039/b914943k

90. R. Mahjub, S. Jatana, S.E. Lee, Z. Qin, G. Pauli, M. Soleimani, S. Madadi, S.-D. Li. Recent advances in applying nanotechnologies for cancer immunotherapy. *J. Control. Release* 288 (2018) 239–263

91. L.J. Cruz, P.J. Tacken, I.S. Zeelenberg, M. Srinivas, F. Bonetto, B. Weigelin, et al., Tracking targeted bimodal nanovaccines: immune responses and routing in cells, tissue, and whole organism, *Mol. Pharm.* 11 (12) (2014) 4299–4313. doi:10.1021/mp400717r

92. M. Rowdo, F. Paula, A. Baron, M. Urrutia, J. Mordoh, Immunotherapy in cancer: a combat between tumors and the immune system; you win some, you lose some, *Front. Immunol.* 6 (2015) 127. doi:10.3389/fimmu.2015.00127

93. H.L. Kaufman, M.L. Disis, Immune system versus tumor: shifting the balance in favor of DCs and effective immunity, *J. Clin. Invest.* 113 (5) (2004) 664–667. doi:10.1172/JCI21148

94. A. Pashine, N.M. Valiante, J.B. Ulmer, Targeting the innate immune response with improved vaccine adjuvants, *Nat. Med.* 11 (4s) (2005) S63. doi:10.1038/nm1210

95. Y. Waeckerle-Men, M. Groettrup, PLGA microspheres for improved antigen delivery to dendritic cells as cellular vaccines, *Adv. Drug Deliv. Rev.* 57 (3) (2005) 475–482. doi:10.1016/j.addr.2004.09.007

96. Z. Zhang, S. Tongchusak, Y. Mizukami, Y.J. Kang, T. Ioji, M. Touma, et al., Induction of anti-tumor cytotoxic T cell responses through PLGA-nanoparticle mediated antigen delivery, *Biomaterials* 32 (14) (2011) 3666–3678. doi:10.1016/j.biomaterials.2011.01.067

97. C.L. Oliveira, F. Veiga, C. Varela, F. Roleira, E. Tavares, I. Silveira, et al., Characterization of polymeric nanoparticles for intraveounos delivery: focus on stability, *Colloids Surf. B Biointerf.* 150 (2017) 326–333. doi:10.1016/j.colsurfb.2016.10.046

98. M.-C. Jones, J.-C. Leroux, Polymeric micelles – a new generation of colloidal drug carriers, *Eur. J. Pharm. Biopharm.* 48 (2) (1999) 101–111. doi:10.1016/S0939-6411(99)00039-9

99. O.S. Muddineti, B. Ghosh, S. Biswas, Current trends in the use of vitamin E-based micellar nanocarriers for anticancer drug delivery, *Expert. Opin. Drug Deliv.* 14 (6) (2017) 715–726. doi:10.1080/17425247.2016.1229300

100. S. Shahsavari, G. Bagheri, R. Mahjub, B. Bagheri, M. Radmehr, M. Rafiee-Tehrani, et al., Application of artificial neural networks for optimization of preparation of insulin nanoparticles composed of quaternized aromatic derivatives of chitosan, *Drug Res.* 64 (3) (2014) 151–158. doi:10.1055/s-0033-1354372

101. P. Li, Z. Luo, P. Liu, N. Gao, Y. Zhang, H. Pan, et al., Bioreducible alginate-poly (ethylenimine) nanogels as an antigen-delivery system robustly enhance vaccineelicited humoral and cellular immune responses, *J. Control. Release* 168 (3) (2013) 271–279. doi:10.1016/j.jconrel.2013.03.025

102] L. Thomann-Harwood, P. Kaeuper, N. Rossi, P. Milona, B. Herrmann, K. McCullough, Nanogel vaccines targeting dendritic cells: contributions of the surface decoration and vaccine cargo on cell targeting and activation, *J. Control. Release* 166 (2) (2013) 95–105. doi:10.1016/j.jconrel.2012.11.015

103. J. Park, S.H. Wrzesinski, E. Stern, M. Look, J. Criscione, R. Ragheb, et al., Combination delivery of TGF-β inhibitor and IL-2 by nanoscale liposomal polymeric gels enhances tumour immunotherapy, *Nat. Mater.* 11 (10) (2012) 895. doi:10.1038/nmat3355

104. T. Shimizu, T. Kishida, U. Hasegawa, Y. Ueda, J. Imanishi, H. Yamagishi, et al., Nanogel DDS enables sustained release of IL-12 for tumor immunotherapy, *Biochem. Biophys. Res. Commun.* 367 (2) (2008) 330–335. doi:10.1016/j.bbrc.2007.12.112

105. S. Kitano, S. Kageyama, Y. Nagata, Y. Miyahara, A. Hiasa, H. Naota, et al., HER2-specific T-cell immune responses in patients vaccinated with truncated HER2 protein complexed with nanogels of cholesteryl pullulan, *Clin. Cancer Res.* 12 (24) (2006) 7397–7405. doi:10.1158/1078-0432. CCR-06-1546

106. T.R. Hoare, D.S. Kohane, Hydrogels in drug delivery: progress and challenges, *Polymer* 49 (8) (2008) 1993–2007. doi:10.1016/j.polymer.2008.01.027

107. D.S. Watson, A.N. Endsley, L. Huang, Design considerations for liposomal vaccines: influence of formulation parameters on antibody and cell-mediated immune responses to liposome associated antigens, *Vaccine* 30 (13) (2012) 2256–2272. doi:10.1016/j.vaccine.2012.01.070

108. D. Davis, G. Gregoriadis, Liposomes as adjuvants with immunopurified tetanus toxoid: influence of liposomal characteristics, *Immunology* 61 (2) (1987) 229.

109. E. Shahum, H.-M. Therien, Liposomal adjuvanticity: effect of encapsulation and surface-linkage on antibody production and proliferative response, *Int. J. Immunopharmacol.* 17 (1) (1995) 9–20. doi:10.1016/0192-0561(94)00082-Y

110. E. Yuba, Liposome-based immunity-inducing systems for cancer immunotherapy, *Mol. Immunol.* (2017). doi:10.1016/j.molimm.2017.11.001

111. J. Gao, L.J. Ochyl, E. Yang, J.J. Moon, Cationic liposomes promote antigen crosspresentation in dendritic cells by alkalizing the lysosomal pH and limiting the degradation of antigens, *Int. J. Nanomed.* 12 (2017) 1251. doi:10.2147/IJN.S125866

112. W. Yan, W. Chen, L. Huang, Mechanism of adjuvant activity of cationic liposome: phosphorylation of a MAP kinase, ERK and induction of chemokines, *Mol. Immunol.* 44 (15) (2007) 3672–3681. doi:10.1016/j.molimm.2007.04.009

113. W. Yan, W. Chen, L. Huang, Reactive oxygen species play a central role in the activity of cationic liposome based cancer vaccine, *J. Control. Release* 130 (1) (2008) 22–28. doi:10.1016/j.jconrel.2008.05.005

114. D.P. Vangasseri, Z. Cui, W. Chen, D.A. Hokey, L.D. Falo Jr., L. Huang, Immunostimulation of dendritic cells by cationic liposomes, *Mol. Membr. Biol.* 23 (5) (2006) 385–395. doi:10.1080/09687860600790537

115. A. Bhargava, D.K. Mishra, S.K. Jain, R.K. Srivastava, N.K. Lohiya, P.K. Mishra, Comparative assessment of lipid based nano-carrier systems for dendritic cell based targeting of tumor re-initiating cells in gynecological cancers, *Mol. Immunol.* 79 (2016) 98–112. doi:10.1016/j.molimm.2016.10.003

116. A. Aryani, B. Denecke, Exosomes as a nanodelivery system: a key to the future of neuromedicine? *Mol. Neurobiol.* 53 (2) (2016) 818–834. doi:10.1007/s12035-014-9054-5

117. H. Liu, L. Chen, Y. Peng, S. Yu, J. Liu, L. Wu, et al., Dendritic cells loaded with tumor derived exosomes for cancer immunotherapy, *Oncotarget* 9 (2) (2018)2887.

118. C. Moore, U. Kosgodage, S. Lange, J.M. Inal, The emerging role of exosome and microvesicle-(EMV-) based cancer therapeutics and immunotherapy, *Int. J. Cancer* 141 (3) (2017) 428–436. doi:10.1002/ijc.30672

119. C. Thery, M. Boussac, P. Veron, P. Ricciardi-Castagnoli, G. Raposo, J. Garin, et al., Proteomic analysis of dendritic cell-derived exosomes: a secreted subcellular compartment distinct from apoptotic vesicles, *J. Immunol.* 166 (12) (2001) 7309–7318. doi:10.4049/jimmunol.166.12.7309

120. C. Thery, A. Regnault, J. Garin, J. Wolfers, L. Zitvogel, P. Ricciardi-Castagnoli, et al., Molecular characterization of dendritic cell-derived exosomes: selective accumulation of the heat shock protein hsc73, *J. Cell Biol.* 147 (3) (1999) 599–610. doi:10.1083/jcb.147.3.599

121. C. Thery, M. Ostrowski, E. Segura, Membrane vesicles as conveyors of immune responses, *Nat. Rev. Immunol.* 9 (8) (2009) 581. doi:10.1038/nri2567

122. S. Utsugi-Kobukai, H. Fujimaki, C. Hotta, M. Nakazawa, M. Minami, MHC class I mediated exogenous antigen presentation by exosomes secreted from immature and mature bone marrow derived dendritic cells, *Immunol. Lett.* 89 (2–3) (2003) 125–131. doi:10.1016/S0165-2478(03)00128-7

123. F. Huang, J. Wan, S. Hao, X. Deng, L. Chen, L. Ma, TGF-β1-silenced leukemia cellderived exosomes target dendritic cells to induce potent anti-leukemic immunity in a mouse model, *Cancer Immunol. Immunother.* 66 (10) (2017) 1321–1331. doi:10.1007/s00262-017-2028-5

124. J.P.M. Almeida, E.R. Figueroa, R.A. Drezek, Gold nanoparticle mediated cancer immunotherapy, *Nanomedicine* 10 (3) (2014) 503–514. doi:10.1016/j.nano.2013.09.011

125. J.P.M. Almeida, A.Y. Lin, R.J. Langsner, P. Eckels, A.E. Foster, R.A. Drezek, In vivo immune cell distribution Fof gold nanoparticles in naive and tumor bearing mice, *Small* 10 (4) (2014) 812–819. doi:10.1002/smll.201301998

126. H.J. Yen, Sh. Hsu, C.L. Tsai, Cytotoxicity and immunological response of gold and silver nanoparticles of different sizes, *Small* 5 (13) (2009) 1553–1561. doi:10.1002/smll.200900126

127. Y.S. Tsai, Y.H. Chen, P.C. Cheng, H.T. Tsai, A.L. Shiau, T.S. Tzai, et al., TGF-β1 Conjugated to gold nanoparticles results in protein conformational changes and attenuates the biological function, *Small* 9 (12) (2013) 2119–2128. doi:10.1002/smll.201202755

128. L. Dykman, N. Khlebtsov, Gold nanoparticles in biology and medicine: recent advances and prospects, *Acta Naturae* 3 (2) (2011) 34–55. doi:10.1039/C1CS15166E

129. Y. Krishnamachari, S.M. Geary, C.D. Lemke, A.K. Salem, Nanoparticle delivery systems in cancer vaccines, *Pharm. Res.* 28 (2) (2011) 215–236. doi:10.1007/s11095-010-0241-4

130. I. Saleem, M. Vordermeier, J. Barralet, A. Coombes, Improving peptide-based assays to differentiate between vaccination and Mycobacterium bovis infection in cattle using nanoparticle carriers for adsorbed antigens, *J. Control Release.* 102 (3) (2005) 551–561. doi:10.1016/j.jconrel.2004.10.034

131. H.A. Havel, Where are the nanodrugs? An industry perspective on development of drug products containing nanomaterials, *AAPS J.* 18 (6) (2016) 1351–1353. doi:10.1208/s12248-016-9970-6

132. X. Zhang, Gold nanoparticles: Recent advances in the biomedical applications, *Cell Biochem. Biophys.* 7 (2015) 771–775. doi:10.1007/s12013-015-0529-4

133. H.-C. Guo, X.-M. Feng, S.-Q. Sun, Y.-Q. Wei, D.-H. Sun, X.-T. Liu, et al., Immunization of mice by hollow mesoporous silica nanoparticles as carriers of porcine circovirus type 2 ORF2 protein, *Virol. J.* 9 (1) (2012) 108. doi:10.1186/1743-422X-9-108

134. J. Kim, W.A. Li, Y. Choi, S.A. Lewin, C.S. Verbeke, G. Dranoff, et al., Injectable, spontaneously assembling, inorganic scaffolds modulate immune cells in vivo and increase vaccine efficacy, *Nat. Biotechnol.* 33 (1) (2015) 64. doi:10.1038/nbt.3071

135. M. Kong, J. Tang, Q. Qiao, T. Wu, Y. Qi, S. Tan, et al., Biodegradable hollow mesoporous silica nanoparticles for regulating tumor microenvironment and enhancing antitumor efficiency, *Theranostics* 7 (13) (2017) 3276. doi:10.7150/thno.19987

136. H.A. Hassan, L. Smyth, N. Rubio, K. Ratnasothy, J.T.-W. Wang, S.S. Bansal, et al., Carbon nanotubes' surface chemistry determines their potency as vaccine nanocarriers in vitro and in vivo, *J. Control. Release* 225 (2016) 205–216. doi:10.1016/j.jconrel.2016.01.030

137. H.A. Hassan, L. Smyth, J.T.-W. Wang, P.M. Costa, K. Ratnasothy, S.S. Diebold, et al., Dual stimulation of antigen presenting cells using carbon nanotube-based vaccine delivery system for cancer immunotherapy, *Biomaterials* 104 (2016) 310–322. doi:10.1016/j.biomaterials.2016.07.005

138. J. Meng, J. Meng, J. Duan, H. Kong, L. Li, C. Wang, et al., Carbon nanotubes conjugated to tumor lysate protein enhance the efficacy of an antitumor immunotherapy, *Small* 4 (9) (2008) 1364–1370. doi:10.1002/smll.200701059

139. V.A. Boussiotis, Molecular and biochemical aspects of the PD-1 checkpoint pathway, *N. Engl. J. Med.* 375 (16) (2016) 1767–1778. doi:10.1056/NEJMra1514296

140. J. M. Kim, D.S. Chen, Immune escape to PD-L1/PD-1 blockade: seven steps to success (or failure), *Ann. Oncol.* 27 (8) (2016) 1492–1504. doi:10.1093/annonc/mdw217

141. F.C. Santini, M.D. Hellmann, PD-1/PD-L1 axis in lung cancer, *Cancer J.* 24 (1) (2018) 15–19. doi:10.1097/PPO.0000000000000300

142. Y. Liu, P. Zheng, How does an anti-CTLA-4 antibody promote cancer immunity?, *Trends Immunol.* 39 (12) (2018) 953–956. doi:10.1016/j.it.2018.10.009

143. M.K. Callahan, J.D. Wolchok, Clinical activity, toxicity, biomarkers, and future development of CTLA-4 checkpoint antagonists, *Semin. Oncol.* 42 (4) (2015) 573–586. doi:10.1053/j.seminoncol.2015.05.008

144. N. Cheng, R. Watkins-Schulz, R.D. Junkins, C.N. David, B.M. Johnson, S.A. Montgomery, K.J. Peine, D.B. Darr, H. Yuan, K.P. McKinnon, Q. Liu, L. Miao, L. Huang, E.M. Bachelder, K.M. Ainslie, J.P. Ting, A nanoparticle-incorporated STING activator enhances antitumor immunity in PD-L1-insensitive models of triple-negative breast cancer, *JCI Insight* 3 (22) (2018) e120638. doi:10.1172/jci.insight.120638

145. W. Yu, Y. Wang, J. Zhu, L. Jin, B. Liu, K. Xia, J. Wang, J. Gao, C. Liang, H. Tao, Autophagy inhibitor enhance ZnPc/BSA nanoparticle induced photodynamic therapy by suppressing PD-L1 expression in osteosarcoma immunotherapy, *Biomaterials* 192 (2019) 128–139. doi:10.1016/j.biomaterials.2018.11.019

146. Y. Wu, W. Gu, L. Li, C. Chen, Z.P. Xu, Enhancing PD-1 gene silence in T lymphocytes by comparing the delivery performance of two inorganic nanoparticle platforms, *Nanomaterials* 9 (2) (2019) 159. doi:10.3390/nano9020159

147. Y. Wu, W. Gu, J. Li, C. Chen, Z.P. Xu, Silencing PD-1 and PD-L1 with nanoparticle-delivered small interfering RNA increases cytoxicity of tumor-infiltrating lymphocytes, *Nanomedicine* 14 (8) (2019) 955–967. doi:10.2217/nnm-2018-0237

148. C. Wang, Y. Ye, G.M. Hochu, H. Sadeghifar, Z. Gu, Enhanced cancer immunotherapy by microneedle patch-assisted delivery of anti-PD1 antibody, *Nano Lett.* 16 (4) (2016), 2334–2340. doi:10.1021/acs.nanolett.5b05030

149. Y. Li, M. Fang, J. Zhang, J. Wang, Y. Song, J. Shi, W. Li, G. Wu, J. Ren, Z. Wang, W. Zou, L. Wang, Hydrogel dual delivered celecoxib and anti-PD-1 synergistically improve antitumor immunity, *OncoImmunology* 5 (2) (2016) e1074374. doi:10.1080/2162402X.2015.1074374

150. P. Zhao, D. Atanackovic, S. Dong, H. Yagita, X. He, M. Chen, An anti-programmed death-1 antibody (αPD-1) fusion protein that self-assembles into a multivalent and functional αPD-1 nanoparticle, *Mol. Pharm.* 14 (5) (2017) 1494–1500. doi:10.1021/acs.molpharmaceut.6b01021

151. R. Meir, K. Shamalov, T. Sadan, M. Motiei, G. Yaari, C. J. Cohen, R. Popovtzer, Fast image-guided stratification using anti-programmed death ligand 1 gold nanoparticles for cancer immunotherapy, *ACS Nano* 11 (11) (2017) 11127–11134. doi:10.1021/acsnano.7b05299

152. Y.K. Chae, A. Arya, W. Iams, M.R. Cruz, S. Chandra, J. Choi, F. Giles, Current landscape and future of dual anti-CTLA4 and PD-1/PD-L1 blockade immunotherapy in cancer; lessons learned from clinical trials with melanoma and non-small cell lung cancer (NSCLC), *J. Immunother. Cancer* 6 (1) (2018) 39. doi:10.1186/s40425-018-0349-3

153. R. Kuai, W.M. Yuan, S. Son, J. Nam, Y. Xu, Y.C. Fan, A. Schwendeman, J.J. Moon, Elimination of established tumors with nanodisc-based combination chemoimmunotherapy, *Sci. Adv.* 4 (4) (2018) eaao1736. doi:10.1126/sciadv.aao1736

154. D. Wang, T. Wang, J. Liu, H. Yu, S. Jiao, B. Feng, F. Zhou, Y. Fu, Q. Yin, P. Zhang, Z. Zhang, Z. Zhou, Y. Li, Acid-activatable versatile micelleplexes for PD-L1 blockade-enhanced cancer photodynamic immunotherapy, *Nano Lett.* 16 (9) (2016) 5503–5513. doi:10.1021/acs.nanolett.6b01994

155. S. Lob, A. Konigsrainer, H. G. Rammensee, G. Opelz, P. Terness, Inhibitors of indoleamine-2,3-dioxygenase for cancer therapy: can we see the wood for the trees?, *Nat. Rev. Cancer* 9 (6) (2009) 445–452. doi:10.1038/nrc2639

156. C. Sheridan, IDO inhibitors move center stage in immuno-oncology, *Nat. Biotechnol.* 33 (2015) 321–322. doi:10.1038/nbt0415-321

157. J.J. Sun, Y.C. Chen, Y.X. Huang, W.C. Zhao, Y.H. Liu, R. Venkataramanan, B.F. Lu, S. Li, Programmable co-delivery of the immune checkpoint inhibitor NLG919 and chemotherapeutic doxorubicin via a redox-responsive immunostimulatory polymeric prodrug carrier, *Acta Pharmacol. Sin.* 38 (6) (2017) 823–834. doi:10.1038/aps.2017.44

158. N. Wang, Z. Wang, Z. Xu, X. Chen, G. Zhu, A cisplatin-loaded immunochemotherapeutic nanohybrid bearing immune checkpoint inhibitors for enhanced cervical cancer therapy, *Angew. Chem. Int. Ed.* 57 (13) (2018) 3426–3430. doi:10.1002/anie.201800422

159. Y. Chen, R. Xia, Y. Huang, W. Zhao, J. Li, X. Zhang, P. Wang, R. Venkataramanan, J. Fan, W. Xie, X. Ma, B. Lu, S. Li, An immunostimulatory dual-functional nanocarrier that improves cancer immunochemotherapy, *Nat. Commun.* 7 (2016) 13443. doi:10.1038/ncomms13443

160. J.F. Brunet, F. Denizot, M.F. Luciani, M. Roux-Dosseto, M. Suzan, M.G. Mattei, P. Golstein, A new member of the immunoglobulin superfamily–CTLA-4, *Nature* 328 (6127) (1987) 267–270.

161. C.E. Rudd, A. Taylor, H. Schneider, CD28 and CTLA-4 co-receptor expression and signal transduction, *Immunol. Rev.* 229 (1) (2009) 12–26.

162. P. Sharma, S. Hu-Lieskovan, J.A. Wargo, A. Ribas, Primary, adaptive, and acquired resistance to cancer immunotherapy, *Cell* 168 (4) (2017) 707–723.

163. W. Kajsa, O. Yasushi, P.M. Paz, Y. Tomoyuki, M. Makoto, F. Zoltan, N. Takashi, S. Shimon, CTLA-4 control over Foxp3+ regulatory T cell function, *Science* 322 (5899) (2008) 271–275.

164. K.S. Peggs, S.A. Quezada, C.A. Chambers, A.J. Korman, J.P. Allison, Blockade of CTLA-4 on both effector and regulatory T cell compartments contributes to the antitumor activity of anti-CTLA-4 antibodies, *J. Exp. Med.* 206 (8) (2009) 1717–1725.

165. F.S. Hodi, S.J. O'Day, D.F. McDermott, R.W. Weber, J.A. Sosman, J.B. Haanen, R. Gonzalez, C. Robert, D. Schadendorf, J.C. Hassel, W. Akerley, A.J. van den Eertwegh, J. Lutzky, P. Lorigan, J.M. Vaubel, G.P. Linette, D. Hogg, C.H. Ottensmeier, C. Lebbe, C. Peschel, I. Quirt, J.I. Clark, J.D. Wolchok, J.S. Weber, J. Tian, M.J. Yellin, G.M. Nichol, A. Hoos, W.J. Urba, Improved survival with ipilimumab in patients with metastastic melanoma, *N. Engl. J. Med.* 363 (8) (2010) 711–723. doi:10.1056/NEJMoa1003466

166. FDA Rubber-Stamps Bristol-Myers Squibb's melanoma mAb, *Genetic Engineering & Biotechnology News* (2011). Accessed: March. https://www.genengnews.com/topics/drug-discovery/fda-rubber-stamps-bristol-myers-squibbs-melanoma-mab/

167. M. Vanneman, G. Dranoff, Combining immunotherapy and targeted therapies in cancer treatment, *Nat. Rev. Cancer* 12 (2012) 237–251.

168. J. Xu, L. Xu, C. Wang, R. Yang, Q. Zhuang, X. Han, Z. Dong, W. Zhu, R. Peng, Z. Liu, Near-infrared-triggered photodynamic therapy with multitasking upconversion nanoparticles in combination with checkpoint blockade for immunotherapy of colorectal cancer, *ACS Nano* 11 (2017) 4463–4474. doi:10.1021/acsnano.7b00715

169. S.Y. Li, Y. Liu, C.F. Xu, S. Shen, R. Sun, X.J. Du, J.X. Xia, Y.H. Zhu, J. Wang, Restoring anti-tumor functions of T cells via nanoparticle-mediated immune checkpoint modulation, *J. Control. Release* 231 (2016) 17–28. doi:10.1016/j.jconrel.2016.01.044

170. Y. Agata, A. Kawasaki, H. Nishimura, Y. Ishida, T. Tsubata, H. Yagita, T. Honjo, Expression of the PD-1 antigen on the surface of stimulated mouse T and B lymphocytes, *Int. Immunol.* 8 (5) (1996) 765–772.

171. C.L. Day, D.E. Kaufmann, P. Kiepiela, J.A. Brown, E.S. Moodley, S. Reddy, E.W. Mackey, J.D. Miller, A.J. Leslie, C. Depierres, Z. Mncube, J. Duraiswamy, B. Zhu, Q. Eichbaum, M. Altfeld, E.J. Wherry, H.M. Coovadia, P.J. Goulder, P. Klenerman, R. Ahmed, G.J. Freeman, B.D. Walker, PD-1 expression on HIVspecific T cells is associated with T-cell exhaustion and disease progression, *Nature* 443 (7109) (2006) 350–354.

172. D.T. Le, J.N. Durham, K.N. Smith, H. Wang, B.R. Bartlett, L.K. Aulakh, S. Lu, H. Kemberling, C. Wilt, B.S. Luber, F. Wong, N.S. Azad, A.A. Rucki, D. Laheru, R. Donehower, A. Zaheer, G.A. Fisher, T.S. Crocenzi, J.J. Lee, T.F. Greten, A.G. Duffy, K.K. Ciombor, A.D. Eyring, B.H. Lam, A. Joe, S.P. Kang, M. Holdhoff, L. Danilova, L. Cope, C. Meyer, S. Zhou, R.M. Goldberg, D.K. Armstrong, K.M. Bever, A.N. Fader, J. Taube, F. Housseau, D. Spetzler, N. Xiao, D.M. Pardoll, N. Papadopoulos, K.W. Kinzler, J.R. Eshleman, B. Vogelstein, R.A. Anders, L.A. Diaz, Mismatch repair deficiency predicts response of solid tumors to PD-1 blockade, *Science* 357 (6349) (2017) 409–413.

173. A.O. Kamphorst, A. Wieland, T. Nasti, S. Yang, R. Zhang, D.L. Barber, B.T. Konieczny, C.Z. Daugherty, L. Koenig, K. Yu, G.L. Sica, A.H. Sharpe, G.J. Freeman, B.R. Blazar, L.A. Turka, T.K. Owonikoko, R.N. Pillai, S.S. Ramalingam, K. Araki, R. Ahmed, Rescue of exhausted CD8 T cells by PD-1-targeted therapies is CD28-dependent, *Science* 355 (6332) (2017) 1423–1427.

174. K.E. Pauken, M.A. Sammons, P.M. Odorizzi, S. Manne, J. Godec, O. Khan, A.M. Drake, Z. Chen, D.R. Sen, M. Kurachi, R.A. Barnitz, C. Bartman, B. Bengsch, A.C. Huang, J.M. Schenkel, G. Vahedi, W.N. Haining, S.L. Berger, E.J. Wherry, Epigenetic stability of exhausted T cells limits durability of reinvigoration by PD-1 blockade, *Science* 354 (6316) (2016) 1160–1165.

175. N.A. Rizvi, M.D. Hellmann, A. Snyder, P. Kvistborg, V. Makarov, J.J. Havel, W. Lee, J. Yuan, P. Wong, T.S. Ho, M.L. Miller, N. Rekhtman, A.L. Moreira, F. Ibrahim, C. Bruggeman, B. Gasmi, R. Zappasodi, Y. Maeda, C. Sander, E.B. Garon, T. Merghoub, J.D. Wolchok, T.N. Schumacher, T.A. Chan, Cancer immunology. Mutational landscape determines sensitivity to PD-1 blockade in non-small cell lung cancer, *Science* 348 (6230) (2015) 124–128.

176. H. Nishimura, T. Okazaki, Y. Tanaka, K. Nakatani, M. Hara, A. Matsumori, S. Sasayama, A. Mizoguchi, H. Hiai, N. Minato, T. Honjo, Autoimmune dilated cardiomyopathy in PD-1 receptor-deficient mice, *Science* 291 (5502) (2001) 319–322.

177. J.S. O'Donnell, G.V. Long, R.A. Scolyer, M.W.L. Teng, M.J. Smyth, Resistance to PD1/PDL1 checkpoint inhibition, *Cancer Treat. Rev.* 52 (2017) 71–81.

178. J. He, Y. Hu, M. Hu, B. Li, Development of PD-1/PD-L1 pathway in tumor immune microenvironment and treatment for non-small cell lung cancer, *Sci. Rep.* 5 (2015) 13110.

179. J.R. Brahmer, C.G. Drake, I. Wollner, J.D. Powderly, J. Picus, W.H. Sharfman, E. Stankevich, A. Pons, T.M. Salay, T.L. McMiller, M.M. Gilson, C. Wang, M. Selby, J.M. Taube, R. Anders, L. Chen, A.J. Korman, D.M. Pardoll, I. Lowy, S.L. Topalian, Phase I study of single-agent anti-programmed death-1 (MDX-1106) in refractory solid tumors: safety, clinical activity, pharmacodynamics, and immunologic correlates, *J. Clin. Oncol.* 28 (19) (2010) 3167–3175.

180. C. Robert, L. Thomas, I. Bondarenko, S. O'Day, J. Weber, C. Garbe, C. Lebbe, J.F. Baurain, A. Testori, J.J. Grob, N. Davidson, J. Richards, M. Maio, A. Hauschild, W.H. Miller, P. Gascon, M. Lotem, K. Harmankaya, R. Ibrahim, S. Francis, T.T. Chen, R. Humphrey, A. Hoos, J.D. Wolchok, Ipilimumab plus dacarbazine for previously untreated metastatic melanoma, *N. Engl. J. Med.* 364 (26) (2011) 2517–2526. doi:10.1056/NEJMoa1104621

181. P.T. Nghiem, S. Bhatia, E.J. Lipson, R.R. Kudchadkar, N.J. Miller, L. Annamalai, S. Berry, E.K. Chartash, A. Daud, S.P. Fling, P.A. Friedlander, H.M. Kluger, H.E. Kohrt, L. Lundgren, K. Margolin, A. Mitchell, T. Olencki, D.M. Pardoll, S.A. Reddy, E.M. Shantha, W.H. Sharfman, E. Sharon, L.R. Shemanski, M.M. Shinohara, J.C. Sunshine, J.M. Taube, J.A. Thompson, S.M. Townson, J.H. Yearley, S.L. Topalian, M.A. Cheever, PD-1 blockade with Pembrolizumab in advanced merkel-cell carcinoma, *N. Engl. J. Med.* 374 (26) (2016) 2542–2552.

182. J.R. Brahmer, S.S. Tykodi, L.Q. Chow, W.J. Hwu, S.L. Topalian, P. Hwu, C.G. Drake, L.H. Camacho, J. Kauh, K. Odunsi, H.C. Pitot, O. Hamid, S. Bhatia, R. Martins, K. Eaton, S. Chen, T.M. Salay, S. Alaparthy, J.F. Grosso, A.J. Korman, S.M. Parker, S. Agrawal, S.M. Goldberg, D.M. Pardoll, A. Gupta, J.M. Wigginton, Safety and activity of anti-PD-L1 antibody in patients with advanced cancer, *N. Engl. J. Med.* 366 (26) (2012) 2455–2465.

183. O. Hamid, C. Robert, A. Daud, F.S. Hodi, W.J. Hwu, R. Kefford, J.D. Wolchok, P. Hersey, R.W. Joseph, J.S. Weber, R. Dronca, T.C. Gangadhar, A. Patnaik, H. Zarour, A.M. Joshua, K. Gergich, J. Elassaiss-Schaap, A. Algazi, C. Mateus, P. Boasberg, P.C. Tumeh, B. Chmielowski, S.W. Ebbinghaus, X.N. Li, S.P. Kang, A. Ribas, Safety and tumor responses with lambrolizumab (anti-PD-1) in melanoma, *N. Engl. J. Med.* 369 (2) (2013) 134–144. doi:10.1056/NEJMoa1305133

184. R.S. Herbst, J.C. Soria, M. Kowanetz, G.D. Fine, O. Hamid, M.S. Gordon, J.A. Sosman, D.F. McDermott, J.D. Powderly, S.N. Gettinger, H.E. Kohrt, L. Horn, D.P. Lawrence, S. Rost, M. Leabman, Y. Xiao, A. Mokatrin, H. Koeppen, P.S. Hegde, I. Mellman, D.S. Chen, F.S. Hodi, Predictive correlates of response to the anti-PDL1 antibody MP-DL3280A in cancer patients, *Nature* 515 (7528) (2014) 563–567.

185. R.J. Motzer, B.I. Rini, D.F. McDermott, B.G. Redman, T.M. Kuzel, M.R. Harrison, U.N. Vaishampayan, H.A. Drabkin, S. George, T.F. Logan, K.A. Margolin, E.R. Plimack, A.M. Lambert, I.M. Waxman, H.J. Hammers, Nivolumab for metastatic renal cell carcinoma: results of a randomized phase II trail, *J. Clin. Oncol.* 33 (13) (2015) 1430–1437.

186. T. Powles, J.P. Eder, G.D. Fine, F.S. Braiteh, Y. Loriot, C. Cruz, J. Bellmunt, H.A. Burris, D.P. Petrylak, S.L. Teng, X. Shen, Z. Boyd, P.S. Hegde, D.S. Chen, N.J. Vogelzang, MPDL3280A (anti-PD-L1) treatment leads to clinical activity in metastatic bladder cancer, *Nature* 515 (7528) (2014) 558–562.

187. S.M. Ansell, A.M. Lesokhin, I. Borrello, A. Halwani, E.C. Scott, M. Gutierrez, S.J. Schuster, M.M. Millenson, D. Cattry, G.J. Freeman, S.J. Rodig, B. Chapuy, A.H. Ligon, L. Zhu, J.F. Grosso, S.Y. Kim, J.M. Timmerman, M.A. Shipp, P. Armand, PD-1 blockade with nivolumab in relapsed or refractory Hodgkin's lymphoma, *N. Engl. J. Med.* 372 (4) (2015) 311–319.

188. M.A. Postow, R. Sidlow, M.D. Hellmann, Immune-related adverse events associated with immune checkpoint blockade, *N. Engl. J. Med.* 378 (2) (2018) 158–168.

189. I. Sagiv-Barfi, H.E. Kohrt, D.K. Czerwinski, P.P. Ng, B.Y. Chang, R. Levy, Therapeutic antitumor immunity by checkpoint blockade is enhanced by ibrutinib, an inhibitor of both BTK and ITK, *Proc. Natl. Acad. Sci. U. S. A.* 112 (9) (2015) E966–E972.

190. S. Wang, J. Campos, M. Gallotta, M. Gong, C. Crain, E. Naik, R.L. Coffman, C. Guiducci, Intratumoral injection of a CpG oligonucleotide reverts resistance to PD-1 blockade by expanding multifunctional CD8+ T cells, *Proc. Natl. Acad. Sci. U. S. A.* 113 (46) (2016) E7240–E7249.

191. J. Folkman, K. Watson, D. Ingber, D. Hanahan, Induction of angiogenesis during the transition from hyperplasia to neoplasia, *Nature* 339 (6219) (1989) 58–61.

192. N. Ferrara, A.P. Adamis, Ten years of anti-vascular endothelial growth factor therapy, *Nat. Rev. Drug Discov.* 15 (6) (2016) 385–403.

193. M. Schmittnaegel, N. Rigamonti, E. Kadioglu, A. Cassará, C. Wyser Rmili, A. Kiialainen, Y. Kienast, H.J. Mueller, C.H. Ooi, D. Laoui, M. De Palma, Dual angiopoietin-2 and VEGFA inhibition elicits antitumor immunity that is enhanced by PD-1 checkpoint blockade, *Sci. Transl. Med.* 9 (385) (2017) eaak9670.

194. X. Duan, C. Chan, N. Guo, W. Han, R.R. Weichselbaum, W. Lin, Photodynamic therapy mediated by nontoxic core-shell nanoparticles synergizes with immune checkpoint blockade to elicit antitumor immunity and antimetastatic effect on brease cancer, *J. Am. Chem. Soc.* 138 (51) (2016) 16686–16695.

195. C. He, X. Duan, N. Guo, C. Chan, C. Poon, R.R. Weichselbaum, W. Lin, Core-shell nanoscale coordination polymers combine chemotherapy and photodynamic therapy to potentiate checkpoint blockade cancer immunotherapy, *Nat. Commun.* 7 (2016) 12499.

196. C. Wang, Y. Ye, G.M. Hochu, H. Sadeghifar, Z. Gu, Enhanced cancer immunotherapy by microneedle patch-assisted delivery of anti-PD1 antibody, *Nano Lett.* 16 (4) (2016) 2334–2340. doi:10.1021/acs.nanolett.5b05030.

197. Y. Ye, J. Wang, Q. Hu, G.M. Hochu, H. Xin, C. Wang, Z. Gu, Synergistic transcutaneous immunotherapy enhances antitumor immune responses through delivery of checkpoint inhibitors, *ACS Nano* 10 (9) (2016) 8956–8963.

198. C. Wang, W. Sun, G. Wright, A.Z. Wang, Z. Gu, Inflammation-triggered cancer immunotherapy by programmed delivery of CpG and anti-PD1 antibody, *Adv. Mater.* 28 (40) (2016) 8912–8920.

199. C. Wang, W. Sun, Y. Ye, Q. Hu, H.N. Bomba, Z. Gu, In situ activation of platelets with checkpoint inhibitors for post-surgical cancer immunotherapy, *Nat Biomed Eng.* 1 (2017) 0011.

200. C. Wang, J. Wang, X. Zhang, S. Yu, D. Wen, Q. Hu, Y. Ye, H. Bomba, X. Hu, Z. Liu, G. Dotti, Z. Gu, In situ formed reactive oxygen species-responsive scaffold with gemcitabine and checkpoint inhibitor for combination therapy, *Sci. Transl. Med.* 10 (429) (2018) eaan3682.

201. H. Yin, R.L. Kanasty, A.A. Eltoukhy, A.J. Vegas, J.R. Dorkin, D.G. Anderson, Nonviral vectors for gene-based therapy, *Nat Rev Genet.* 15 (8) (2014) 541–555.

202. E. Miele, G.P. Spinelli, E. Miele, E. Di Fabrizio, E. Ferretti, S. Tomao, A. Gulino, Nanoparticle-based delivery of small interfering RNA: challenges for cancer therapy, *Int. J. Nanomed.* 7 (2012) 3637–3657.

203. D. Wang, T. Wang, J. Liu, H. Yu, S. Jiao, B. Feng, F. Zhou, Y. Fu, Q. Yin, P. Zhang, Z. Zhang, Z. Zhou, Y. Li, Acid-activatable versatile micelleplexes for PD-L1 blockade-enhanced cancer photodynamic immunotherapy, *Nano Lett.* 16 (9) (2016) 5503–5513.

204. J.R. Moffett, M.A. Namboodiri, Tryptophan and the immune response, *Immunol. Cell Biol.* 81 (4) (2003) 247–265.

205. J.L. Adams, J. Smothers, R. Srinivasan, A. Hoos, Big opportunities for small molecules in immuno-oncology, *Nat. Rev. Drug Discov.* 14 (9) (2015) 603–622.

206. A.L. Mellor, D.H. Munn, IDO expression by dendritic cells: tolerance and tryptophan catabolism, *Nat. Rev. Immunol.* 4 (10) (2004) 762–774.

207. R. Metz, J.B. Duhadaway, U. Kamasani, L. Laury-Kleintop, A.J. Muller, G.C. Prendergast, Novel tryptophan catabolic enzyme IDO2 is the preferred biochemical target of the antitumor indoleamine 2,3-dioxygenase inhibitory compound D-1-methyl-tryptophan, *Cancer Res.* 67 (15) (2007) 7082–7087.

208. F. Fallarino, U. Grohmann, S. You, B.C. McGrath, D.R. Cavener, C. Vacca, C. Orabona, R. Bianchi, M.L. Belladonna, C. Volpi, P. Santamaria, M.C. Fioretti, P. Puccetti, The combined effects of tryptophan starvation and tryptophan catabolites down-regulate T cell receptor zeta-chain and induce a regulatory phenotype in naive T cells, *J. Immunol.* 176 (11) (2006) 6752–6761.

209. C. Uyttenhove, L. Pilotte, I. Théate, V. Stroobant, D. Colau, N. Parmentier, T. Boon, B.J. Van den Eynde, Evidence for a tumoral immune resistance mechanism based on tryptophan degradation by indoleamine 2, 3-dioxygenase, *Nat. Med.* 9 (10) (2003) 1269–1274.

210. X. Liu, R.C. Newton, S.M. Friedman, P.A. Scherie, Indoleamine 2, 3-dioxygenase, an emerging target for anticancer therapy, *Curr. Cancer Drug Targets* 9 (8) (2009) 938–952.

211. D.Y. Hou, A.J. Muller, M.D. Sharma, J. Duhadaway, T. Banerjee, M. Johnson, A.L. Mellor, G.C. Prendergast, D.H. Munn, Inhibition of indoleamine 2,3-dioxygenase in dendritic cells by stereoisomers of 1-methyl-tryptophan correlates with antitumor responses, *Cancer Res.* 67 (2) (2007) 792–801.

212. E. Vacchelli, F. Aranda, A. Eggermont, C. Sautès-Fridman, E. Tartour, E.P. Kennedy, M. Platten, L. Zitvogel, G. Kroemer, L. Galluzzi, Trial watch: IDO inhibitors in cancer therapy, *Oncoimmunology* 3 (10) (2014) e957994.

213. G.L. Beatty, P.J. O'Dwyer, J. Clark, J.G. Shi, R.C. Newton, R. Schaub, J. Maleski, L. Leopold, T. Gajewski. Phase I study of the safety, pharmacokinetics (PK), and pharmacodynamics (PD) of the oral inhibitor of indoleamine 2,3-dioxygenase (IDO1) INCB024360 in patients (pts) with advanced malignancies, *J. Clin. Oncol.* 31 (2013) 3025–3025.

214. G.T. Gibney, O. Hamid, T.C. Gangadhar, J. Lutzky, A.J. Olszanski, T. Gajewski, B. Chmielowski, P.D. Boasberg, Y. Zhao, R.C. Newton, P.A. Scherle, J. Bowman, J. Maleski, L. Leopold, J.S. Weber, Preliminary results from a phase 1/2 study of INCB024360 combined with ipilimumab (ipi) in patients (pts) with melanoma, *J. Clin. Oncol.* 32 (2014) 3010.

215. M. Li, A.R. Bolduc, M.N. Hoda, D.N. Gamble, S.B. Dolisca, A.K. Bolduc, K. Hoang, C. Ashley, D. McCall, A.M. Rojiani, B.L. Maria, O. Rixe, T.J. MacDonald, P.S. Heeger, A.L. Mellor, D.H. Munn, T.S. Johnson, The indoleamine 2,3-dioxygenase pathway controls complement-dependent enhancement of chemo-radiation therapy against murine glioblastoma, *J Immunother. Cancer.* 2 (2014) 21.

216. M. Figueiredo, Keytruda-Epacadostat combo fails primary goal in phase 3 trail for melanoma, companies announce, Accessed (April, 2018), https://immuno-oncologynews.com/2018/04/11/keytruda-epacadostat-fails-primary-goal-phase-3-trial-melanoma/

217. K. Lu, C. He, N. Guo, C. Chan, K. Ni, R.R. Weichselbaum, W. Lin, Chlorin-based nanoscale metal–organic framework systemically rejects colorectal cancers via synergistic photodynamic therapy and checkpoint blockade immunotherapy, *J. Am. Chem. Soc.* 138 (38) (2016) 12502–12510.

218. K. Lu, C. He, N. Guo, C. Chan, K. Ni, G. Lan, H. Tang, C. Pelizzari, Y.X. Fu, M.T. Spiotto, R.R. Weichselbaum, W. Lin, Low-dose X-ray radiotherapy-radiodynamic therapy via nanoscale metal-organic frameworks enhances checkpoint blockade immunotherapy, *Nat. Biomed. Eng.* (2018). doi:10.1038/s41551-018-0203-4.

219. J. Sun, Y. Chen, Y. Huang, W. Zhao, Y. Liu, R. Venkataramanan, B. Lu, S. Li, Programmable co-delivery of the immune checkpoint inhibitor NLG919 and chemotherapeutic doxorubicin via a redox-responsive immunostimulatory polymeric prodrug carrier, *Acta Pharmacol. Sin.* 38 (6) (2017) 823–834.

220. L. Zhang, D. Liu, S. Wang, X. Yu, M. Ji, X. Xie, S. Liu, R. Liu, MgAl-layered double hydroxide nanoparticles co-delivering siIDO and Trp2 peptide effectively reduce IDO expression and induce cytotoxic T-lymphocyte responses against melanoma tumor in mice, *J. Mater. Chem. B* 5 (2017) 6266.

221. E. Sick, A. Jeanne, C. Schneider, S. Dedieu, K. Takeda, L. Martiny, CD47 update: a multifaceted actor in the tumor microenvironment of potential therapeutic interest, *Br. J. Pharmacol.* 167 (7) (2012) 1415–1430.

222. M.P. Chao, I.L. Weissman, R. Majeti, The CD47-SIRP pathway in cancer immune evasion and potential therapeutic implications, *Curr. Opin. Immunol.* 24 (2) (2012) 225–232.

223. D. Tseng, J.P. Volkmer, S.B. Willingham, H. Contreras-Trujillo, J.W. Fathman, N.B. Fernhoff, J. Seita, M.A. Inlay, K. Weiskopf, M. Miyanishia, I.L. Weissmana, Anti-CD47 antibody-mediated phagocytosis of cancer by macrophages primes an effective antitumor T-cell response, *Proc. Natl. Acad. Sci. U. S. A.* 110 (27) (2013) 11103–11108.

224. N.G. Ring, D. Herndler-Brandstetter, K. Weiskopf, L. Shan, J.P. Volkmer, B.M. George, M. Lietzenmayer, K.M. McKenna, T.J. Naik, A. McCarty, Y. Zheng, A.M. Ring, R.A. Flavell, I.L. Weissman, Anti-SIRPα antibody immunotherapy enhances neutrophil and macrophage antitumor activity, *Proc. Natl. Acad. Sci. U. S. A.* 114 (49) (2017) E10578–E10585.

225. X. Liu, Y. Pu, K. Cron, L. Deng, J. Kline, W.A. Frazier, H. Xu, H. Peng, Y.X. Fu, M.M. Xu, CD47 blockade triggers T cell–mediated destruction of immunogenic tumors, *Nat. Med.* 21 (10) (2015) 1209–1215.

226. A. Chatzigeorgiou, M. Lyberi, G. Chatzilymperis, A. Nezos, E. Kamper, CD40/CD40L signaling and its implication in health and disease, *Biofactors* 35 (6) (2009)474–483.

227. M.F. Fransen, R.A. Cordfunke, M. Sluijter, M.J. van Steenbergen, J.W. Drijfhout, F. Ossendorp, W.E. Hennink, C.J. Melief, Effectiveness of slow-release systems in CD40 agonistic antibody immunotherapy of cancer, *Vaccine* 32 (15) (2014)1654–1660.

228. Y. Li, J. Yuan, Q. Yang, W. Cao, X. Zhou, Y. Xie, H. Tu, Y. Zhang, S. Wang, Immunoliposome co-delivery of bufalin and anti-CD40 antibody adjuvant induces synergetic therapeutic efficacy against melanoma, *Int. J. Nanomed.* 9 (2014) 5683–5700.

229. T. Bartkowiak, M.A. Curran, 4-1BB agonists: multi-potent potentiators of tumor immunity, *Front. Oncol.* 5 (2015) 117.

230. T. Bartkowiak, S. Singh, G. Yang, G. Galvan, D. Haria, M. Ai, J.P. Allison, K.J. Sastry, M.A. Curran, Unique potential of 4-1BB agonist antibody to promote durable regression of HPV+ tumors when combined with an E6/E7 peptide vaccine, *Proc Nati Acad Sci U. S. A.* 112 (38) (2015) E5290–E5299.

231. Q. Zhang, J. Bi, X. Zheng, Y. Chen, H. Wang, W. Wu, Z. Wang, Q. Wu, H. Peng, H. Wei, R. Sun, Z. Tian, Blockade of the checkpoint receptor TIGIT prevents NK cell exhaustion and elicits potent antitumor immunity, *Nat. Immunol.* 19 (2018) 723–732.

232. P. Sharma, J.P. Allison, The future of immune checkpoint therapy, *Science* 348 (6230) (2015) 56–61.

233. J. Larkin, F.S. Hodi, J.D. Wolchok, Combined nivolumab and ipilimumab or monotherapy in untreated melanoma, *N. Engl. J. Med.* 373 (13) (2015) 1270–1271.

234. C. Robert, J. Schachter, G.V. Long, A. Arance, J.J. Grob, L. Mortier, A. Daud, M.S. Carlino, C. McNeil, M. Lotem, J. Larkin, P. Lorigan, B. Neyns, C.U. Blank, O. Hamid, C. Mateus, R. Shapira-Frommer, M. Kosh, H. Zhou, N. Ibrahim, S. Ebbinghaus, A. Ribas, Pembrolizumab versus ipilimumab in advanced melanoma, *N. Engl. J. Med.* 372 (62) (2015) 2521–2532. doi:10.1056/NEJMoa1503093

235. J.E. Rosenberg, J. Hoffman-Censits, T. Powles, M.S. van der Heijden, A.V. Balar, A. Necchi, N. Dawson, P.H. O'Donnell, A. Balmanoukian, Y. Loriot, S. Srinivas, M.M. Retz, P. Grivas, R.W. Joseph, M.D. Galsky, M.T. Fleming, D.P. Petrylak, J.L. Perez-Gracia, H.A. Burris, D. Castellano, C. Canil, J. Bellmunt, D. Bajorin, D. Nickles, R. Bourgon, G.M. Frampton, N. Cui, S. Mariathasan, O. Abidoye, G.D. Fine, R. Dreicer, Atezolizumab in patients with locally advanced and metastatic urothelial carcinoma who have progressed following treatment with platinum-based chemotherapy: a single-arm, multicentre, phase 2 trial, *Lancet* 387 (10031) (2016) 1909–1920.

236. A.V. Kroll, R.H. Fang, Y. Jiang, J. Zhou, X. Wei, C.L. Yu, J. Gao, B.T. Luk, D. Dehaini, W. Gao, L. Zhang, Nanoparticulate delivery of cancer cell membrane elicits multiantigenic antitumor immunity, *Adv. Mater.* 29 (47) (2017) 1703969.

237. R. Kuai, L.J. Ochyl, K.S. Bahjat, A. Schwendeman, J.J. Moon, Designer vaccine nanodiscs for personalized cancer immunotherapy, *Nat. Mater.* 16 (4) (2017) 489–496.

238. S.N. Linch, M.J. Kasiewicz, M.J. McNamara, I.F. Hilgart-Martiszus, M. Farhad, W.L. Redmond, Combination OX40 agonism/CTLA-4 blockade with HER2 vaccination reverses T-cell anergy and promotes survival in tumor-bearing mice, *Proc. Natl. Acad. Sci. U. S. A.* 113 (3) (2016) E319–E327.

239. S.L. Uprichard, The therapeutic potential of RNA interference, *FEBS Lett.* 579 (26) (2005) 5996–6007.

240. R.T. Manguso, H.W. Pope, M.D. Zimmer, F.D. Brown, K.B. Yates, B.C. Miller, N.B. Collins, K. Bi, M.W. Lafleur, V.R. Juneja, S.A. Weiss, J. Lo, D.E. Fisher, D. Miao, E. Van Allen, D.E. Root, A.H. Sharpe, J.G. Doench, W.N. Haining, In vivo CRISPR screening identifies Ptpn2 as a cancer immunotherapy target, *Nature* 547 (7664) (2017) 413–418.

241. H. Zhu, F. Bengsch, N. Svoronos, M.R. Rutkowski, B.G. Bitler, M.J. Allegrezza, Y. Yokoyama, A.V. Kossenkov, J.E. Bradner, J.R. Conejo-Garcia, R. Zhang, BET bromodomain inhibition promotes anti-tumor immunity by suppressing PD-L1 expression, *Cell Rep.* 16 (11) (2016) 2829–2837.

242. T. Wang, D. Wang, H. Yu, B. Feng, F. Zhou, H. Zhang, L. Zhou, S. Jiao, Y. Li, A cancer vaccine-mediated postoperative immunotherapy for recurrent and metastatic tumors, *Nat. Commun.* 9 (2018) 1532.

243. T. Wu, D. Zhang, Q. Qiao, X. Qin, C. Yang, M. Kong, H. Deng, Z. Zhang, Biomimetic nanovesicles for enhanced antitumor activity of combinational photothermal and chemotherapy, *Mol. Pharm.* 15 (3) (2018) 1341–1352.

244. T. Wu, Y. Qi, D. Zhang, Q. Song, C. Yang, X. Hu, Y. Bao, Y. Zhao, Z. Zhang, Bone marrow dendritic cells derived microvesicles for combinational immunochemotherapy against tumor, *Adv. Funct. Mater.* 27 (2017) 1703191.

245. X. Zhang, C. Wang, J. Wang, Q. Hu, B. Langworthy, Y. Ye, W. Sun, J. Lin, T. Wang, J. Fine, H. Cheng, G. Dotti, P. Huang, Z. Gu, PD-1 blockade cellular vesicles for cancer therapy, *Adv. Mater.* 30 (22) (2018) e1707112.

246. X. Zhang, J. Wang, Z. Chen, Q. Hu, C. Wang, J. Yan, G. Dotti, P. Huang, Z. Gu, Engineering PD-1-presenting platelets for cancer immunotherapy, *Nano Lett.* 18 (9) (2018) 5716–5725.

247. A. Takahashi, K. Kono, F. Ichihara, H. Sugai, H. Amemiya, H. Iizuka, H. Fujii, Y. Matsumoto, Macrophages in tumor-draining lymph node with different characteristics induce T-cell apoptosis in patients with advanced stage-gastric cancer, *Int. J. Cancer* 104 (4) (2003) 393–399. doi:10.1002/ijc.10973

248. V. Carriere, R. Colisson, C. Jiguet-Jiglaire, E. Bellard, G. Bouche, T. Al Saati, F. Amalric, J.P. Girard, C. M'Rini, Cancer cells regulate lymphocyte recruitment and leukocyte-endothelium interactions in the tumor-draining lymph node, *Cancer Res.* 65 (24) (2005) 11639–11648. doi:10.1158/0008-5472.CAN-05-1190

249. D.H. Munn, A.L. Mellor, The tumor-draining lymph node as an immune-privileged site, *Immunol. Rev.* 213 (1) (2006) 146–158. doi:10.1111/j.1600-065X.2006.00431.x

250. K. Imai, Y. Minamiya, S. Koyota, M. Ito, H. Saito, Y. Sato, S. Motoyama, T. Sugiyama, J. Ogawa, Inhibition of dendritic cell migration by transforming growth factor-β1 increases tumor-draining lymph node metastasis, *J. Exp. Clin. Cancer Res.* 31 (1) (2012) 3. doi:10.1186/1756-9966-31-3

251. L.M. Habenicht, T.C. Albershardt, B.M. Iritani, A. Ruddell, Distinct mechanisms of B and T lymphocyte accumulation generate tumor-draining lymph node hypertrophy, *OncoImmunology* 5 (8) (2016) e1204505. doi:10.1080/2162402X.2016.1204505

252. L. Jeanbart, M. Ballester, A. de Titta, P. Corthesy, P. Romero, J.A. Hubbell, M.A. Swartz, Enhancing efficacy of anticancer vaccines by targeted delivery to tumor-draining lymph nodes, *Cancer Immunol. Res.* 2 (5) (2014) 436–447. doi:10.1158/2326-6066.CIR-14-0019-T

253. T. Kang, Y. Huang, Q. Zhu, H. Cheng, Y. Pei, J. Feng, M. Xu, G. Jiang, Q. Song, T. Jiang, H. Chen, X. Gao, J. Chen, Necroptotic cancer cells-mimicry nanovaccine boosts anti-tumor immunity with tailored immune-stimulatory modality, *Biomaterials* 164 (2018) 80–97. doi:10.1016/j.biomaterials.2018.02.033

254 F.W. Cao, Y.X. Guo, Y. Li, S.Y. Tang, Y.D. Yang, H. Yang, L.Q. Xiong, Fast and accurate imaging of lymph node metastasis with multifunctional near-infrared polymer dots, *Adv. Funct. Mater.* 28 (2018). doi:10.1002/adfm.201707174.

255. N.H. Cho, T.C. Cheong, J.H. Min, J.H. Wu, S.J. Lee, D. Kim, J.S. Yang, S. Kim, Y.K. Kim, S.Y. Seong, A multifunctional core-shell nanoparticle for dendritic cell-based cancer immunotherapy, *Nat. Nanotechnol.* 6 (10) (2011) 675–682. doi:10.1038/nnano.2011.149

256. K. Sehgal, R. Ragheb, T.M. Fahmy, M.V. Dhodapkar, K.M. Dhodapkar, Nanoparticle-mediated combinatorial targeting of multiple human dendritic cell (DC) subsets leads to enhanced T cell activation via IL-15–dependent DC crosstalk, *J. Immunol.* 193 (5) (2014) 2297–2305. doi:10.4049/jimmunol.1400489

257. T.Z. Chang, S.S. Stadmiller, E. Staskevicius, J.A. Champion, Effects of ovalbumin protein nanoparticle vaccine size and coating on dendritic cell processing, *Biomater. Sci.* 5 (2) (2017) 223–233. doi:10.1039/c6bm00500d

258. R. Liang, J. Xie, J. Li, K. Wang, L. Liu, Y. Gao, M. Hussain, G. Shen, J. Zhu, J. Tao, Liposomes-coated gold nanocages with antigens and adjuvants targeted delivery to dendritic cells for enhancing antitumor immune response, *Biomaterials* 149 (2017) 41–50. doi:10.1016/j.biomaterials.2017.09.029

259. C. Zhang, J. Zhang, G. Shi, H. Song, S. Shi, X. Zhang, P. Huang, Z. Wang, W. Wang, C. Wang, D. Kong, C. Li, A light responsive nanoparticle-based delivery system using pheophorbide a graft polyethylenimine for dendritic cell-based cancer immunotherapy, *Mol. Pharm.* 14 (5) (2017) 1760–1770. doi:10.1021/acs.molpharmaceut.7b00015

260. Y. Wang, L. Zhang, Z. Xu, L. Miao, L. Huang, mRNA vaccine with antigen-specific checkpoint blockade induces an enhanced immune response against established melanoma, *Mol. Ther.* 26 (2) (2018) 420–434. doi:10.1016/j.ymthe.2017.11.009

261. Q. Liu, H. Zhu, Y. Liu, S. Musetti, L. Huang, BRAF peptide vaccine facilitates therapy of murine BRAF-mutant melanoma, *Cancer Immunol. Immunother.* 67 (2018) 299–310. doi:10.1007/s00262-017-2079-7

262. X.Y. He, B.Y. Liu, J.L. Wu, S.L. Ai, R.X. Zhuo, S.X. Cheng, A dual macrophage targeting nanovector for delivery of oligodeoxynucleotides to overcome cancer-associated immunosuppression, *ACS Appl. Mater. Interfaces* 9 (49) (2017) 42566–42576. doi:10.1021/acsami.7b13594

263. V.V. Temchura, D. Kozlova, V. Sokolova, K. Uberla, M. Epple, Targeting and activation of antigen-specific B-cells by calcium phosphate nanoparticles loaded with protein antigen, *Biomaterials* 35 (23) (2014) 6098–6105. doi:10.1016/j.biomaterials.2014.04.010

264. O. Meurette, P. Mehlen, Notch signaling in the tumor microenvironment, *Cancer Cell* 34 (4) (2018) 536–548. doi:10.1016/j.ccell.2018.07.009

265. L.M. Zahn, Photosynthesis evolution in Cyanobacteria, *Science* 355 (6332) (2017) 1386–1388. doi:10.1126/science.355.6332.1386-o

266. W. Tomaszewski, L. Sanchez-Perez, T.F. Gajewski, J.H. Sampson, Brain tumor microenvironment and host state: implications for immunotherapy, *Clin. Cancer Res.* 25 (14) (2019) 4202–4210. doi:10.1158/1078-0432.CCR-18-1627

267. L. Meyaard, The inhibitory collagen receptor LAIR-1 (CD305), *J. Leukocyte Biol.* 83 (4) (2008) 799–803. doi:10.1189/jlb.0907609

268. H.C. Hope, R.J. Salmond, Targeting the tumor microenvironment and T cell metabolism for effective cancer immunotherapy, *Eur. J. Immunol.* 49 (8) (2019) 1147–1152. doi:10.1002/eji.201848058

269. G.M. Rodriguez, K.J.C. Galpin, C.W. McCloskey, B.C. Vanderhyden, The tumor microenvironment of epithelial ovarian cancer and its influence on response to immunotherapy, *Cancer* 10 (8) (2018). doi:10.3390/cancers10080242

270. J.S. Fang, R.D. Gillies, R.A. Gatenby, Adaptation to hypoxia and acidosis in carcinogenesis and tumor progression, *Semin. Cancer Biol.* 18 (5) (2008) 330–337. doi:10.1016/j.semcancer.2008.03.011

271. B. Keith, M.C. Simon, Hypoxia-inducible factors, stem cells, and cancer, *Cell* 129 (3) (2007) 465–472. doi:10.1016/j.cell.2007.04.019

272. G. Lin, S. Chen, P. Mi, Nanoparticles targeting and remodeling tumor microenvironment for cancer theranostics, *J. Biomed. Nanotechnol.* 14 (2018) 1189–1207. doi:10.1166/jbn.2018.2546

273. J.E. Park, B. Dutta, S.W. Tse, N. Gupta, C.F. Tan, J.K. Low, K.W. Yeoh, O.L. Kon, J.P. Tam, S.K. Sze, Hypoxia-induced tumor exosomes promote M2-like macrophage polarization of infiltrating myeloid cells and microRNA-mediated metabolic shift, *Oncogene* 38 (2019) 5158–5173. doi:10.1038/s41388-019-0782-x

274. Y. Li, S.P. Patel, J. Roszik, Y. Qin, Hypoxia-driven immunosuppressive metabolites in the tumor microenvironment: new approaches for combinational immunotherapy, *Front. Immunol.* 9 (2018) 1591. doi:10.3389/fimmu.2018.01591

275. S. Im, J. Lee, D. Park, A. Park, Y.M. Kim, W.J. Kim, Hypoxia-triggered transforming immunomodulator for cancer immunotherapy via photodynamically enhanced antigen presentation of dendritic cell, *ACS Nano* 13 (1) (2019) 476–488. doi:10.1021/acsnano.8b07045

276. G.B. Yang, L.G. Xu, Y. Chao, J. Xu, X.Q. Sun, Y.F. Wu, R. Peng, Z. Liu, Hollow MnO$_2$ as a tumor-microenvironment-responsive biodegradable nanoplatform for combination therapy favoring antitumor immune responses, *Nat. Commun.* 8 (1) (2017) 902. doi:10.1038/s41467-017-01050-0

277. G. Molema, B. Kroesen, W. Helfrich, D. Meijer, L. de Leij, The use of bispecific antibodies in tumor cell and tumor vasculature directed immunotherapy, *J. Controlled Release* 64 (1–3) (2000) 229–239. doi:10.1016/S0168-3659(99)00137-6

278. E. Lanitis, M. Irving, G. Coukos, Targeting the tumor vasculature to enhance T cell activity, *Curr. Opin. Immunol.* 33 (2015) 55–63.

279. Q. Chen, L. Xu, J. Chen, Z. Yang, C. Liang, Y. Yang, Z. Liu, Tumor vasculature normalization by orally fed erlotinib to modulate the tumor microenvironment for enhanced cancer nanomedicine and immunotherapy, *Biomaterials* 148 (2017) 69–80.

280. A. Gupte, R.J. Mumper, Elevated copper and oxidative stress in cancer cells as a target for cancer treatment, *Cancer Treat. Rev.* 35 (1) (2009) 32–46.

281. H. Xie, Y.J. Kang, Role of copper in angiogenesis and its medicinal implications, *Curr. Med. Chem.* 16 (10) (2009) 1304–1314.

282. P. Zhou, J. Qin, C. Zhou, G. Wan, Y. Liu, M. Zhang, X. Yang, N. Zhang, Y. Wang, Multifunctional nanoparticles based on a polymeric copper chelator for combination treatment of metastatic breast cancer, *Biomaterials* 195 (2019) 86–99.

283. J.E. Rundhaug, Matrix metalloproteinases and angiogenesis, *J. Cell. Mol. Med.* 9 (2) (2005) 267–285.

284. K. Kessenbrock, V. Plaks, Z. Werb, Matrix Metalloproteinases: Regulators of the Tumor Microenvironment, *Cell* 141 (1) (2010) 52–67.

285. C.M. Overall, C. Lopez-Otin, Strategies for MMP inhibition in cancer: innovations for the post-trial era, *Nat. Rev. Cancer* 2 (9) (2002) 657–672.

286. J.M. Shin, S.J. Oh, S. Kwon, V.G. Deepagan, M. Lee, S.H. Song, H.J. Lee, S. Kim, K.H. Song, T.W. Kim, J.H. Park, PEGylated hyaluronic acid conjugate for targeted cancer immunotherapy, *J. Controlled Release* 267 (2017) 181–190.

287. M.J. Heffernan, N. Murthy, Disulfide-crosslinked polyion micelles for delivery of protein therapeutics, *Ann. Biomed. Eng.* 37 (2009) 1993–2002. doi:10.1007/s10439-009-9734-x

288. D. Xiao, J.J. Hu, J.Y. Zhu, S.B. Wang, R.X. Zhuo, X.Z. Zhang, A redox-responsive mesoporous silica nanoparticle with a therapeutic peptide shell for tumor targeting synergistic therapy, *Nanoscale* 8 (2016) 16702–16709. doi:10.1039/C6NR04784J

289. K. Wang, Y. Yang, W. Xue, Z. Liu, Cell penetrating peptide-based redox-sensitive vaccine delivery system for subcutaneous vaccination, *Mol. Pharm.* 15 (3) (2018) 975–984. doi:10.1021/acs.molpharmaceut.7b00905

290. E. Verdegaal, Adoptive cell therapy: a highly successful individualized therapy for melanoma with great potential for other malignancies, *Curr. Opin. Immunol.* 39 (2016) 90–95. doi:10.1016/j.coi.2016.01.004

291. S. Rosenberg, M. Dudley, Adoptive cell therapy for the treatment of patients with metastatic melanoma, *Curr. Opin. Immunol.* 21 (2) (2009) 233–240. doi:10.1016/j.coi.2009.03.002

292. J. Cohen, S. Merims, S. Frank, R. Engelstein, T. Peretz, M. Lotem, Adoptive cell therapy: past, present and future, *Immunotherapy* 9 (2) (2017) 183–196. doi:10.2217/imt-2016-0112

293. S. Mardiana, B. Solomon, P. Darcy, P. Beavis, Supercharging adoptive T cell therapy to overcome solid tumor-induced immunosuppression, *Sci. Transl. Med.* 11 (495) (2019). doi:10.1126/scitranslmed.aaw2293

294. A. Wallace, V. Kapoor, J. Sun, P. Mrass, W. Weninger, D. Heitjan, C. June, L. Kaiser, L. Ling, S. Albelda, TGF-β receptor blockade augments the effectiveness of adoptive t-cell therapy of established solid cancers, *Clin. Cancer Res.* 14 (12) (2008) 3966–3974. doi:10.1158/1078-0432.CCR-08-0356

295. Y. Zheng, L. Tang, L. Mabardi, S. Kumari, D.J. Irvine, Enhancing adoptive cell therapy of cancer through targeted delivery of small-molecule immunomodulators to internalizing or noninternalizing receptors, *ACS Nano* 11 (3) (2017) 3089–3100.

296. S.B. Stephan, A.M. Taber, I. Jileaeva, E.P. Pegues, C.L. Sentman, M.T. Stephan, Biopolymer implants enhance the efficacy of adoptive T-cell therapy, *Nat. Biotechnol.* 33 (1) (2015) 97–101. doi:10.1038/nbt.3104

297. A. Grakoui, S.K. Bromley, C. Sumen, M.M. Davis, A.S. Shaw, P.M. Allen, M.L. Dustin, The immunological synapse: a molecular machine controlling T cell activation, *Science* 285 (5425) (1999) 221–227. doi:10.1126/science.285.5425.221

298. F.D. Brown, S.J. Turley, Fibroblastic reticular cells: Organization and regulation of the T lymphocyte life cycle, *J. Immunol.* 194 (4) (2015) 1389–1394.

299. E.H. Neto, A.L. Coelho, A.L. Sampaio, M. Henriques, C. Marcinkiewicz, M.S. De Freitas, C. Barja-Fidalgo, Activation of human T lymphocytes via integrin signaling induced by RGD-disintegrins, *Biochim. Biophys. Acta* 1773 (2) (2007) 176–184.

300. J. Guasch, C.A. Muth, J. Diemer, H. Riahinezhad, J.P. Spatz, Integrin-assisted T-cell activation on nanostructured hydrogels, *Nano Lett.* 17 (10) (2017) 6110–6116.

301. K. Perica, J.G. Bieler, C. Schutz, J.C. Varela, J. Douglass, A. Skora, Y.L. Chiu, M. Oelke, K. Kinzler, S. Zhou, B. Vogelstein, J.P. Schneck, Enrichment and expansion with nanoscale artificial antigen presenting cells for adoptive immunotherapy, *ACS Nano* 9 (7) (2015) 6861–6871.

302. A. Ghaemi, H. Soleimanjahi, T. Bamdad, S. Soudi, E. Arefeian, S.M. Hashemi, et al., Induction of humoral and cellular immunity against latent HSV-1 infections by

DNA immunization in BALB/c mice, *Comp. Immunol. Microbiol. Infect. Dis.* 30 (4) (2007) 197–210. doi:10.1016/j.cimid.2007.01.002

303. A. Ghaemi, H. Soleimanjahi, P. Gill, Z.M. Hassan, S. Razeghi, M. Fazeli, et al., Protection of mice by a λ-based therapeutic vaccine against cancer associated with human papillomavirus type 16, *Intervirology* 54 (3) (2011) 105–112. doi:10.1159/000320197

304. B. Zhang, CD73: a novel target for cancer immunotherapy, *Cancer Res.* 70 (16) (2010) 6407–6411. doi:10.1158/0008-5472.CAN-10-1544

305. F. Jadidi-Niaragh, F. Atyabi, A. Rastegari, N. Kheshtchin, S. Arab, H. Hassannia, et al., CD73 specific siRNA loaded chitosan lactate nanoparticles potentiate the antitumor effect of a dendritic cell vaccine in 4T1 breast cancer bearing mice, *J. Control. Release* 246 (2017) 46–59. doi:10.1016/j.jconrel.2016.12.012

306. H. Xiong, Z.-G. Zhang, X.-Q. Tian, D.-F. Sun, Q.-C. Liang, Y.-J. Zhang, et al., Inhibition of JAK1, 2/STAT3 signaling induces apoptosis, cell cycle arrest, and reduces tumor cell invasion in colorectal cancer cells, *Neoplasia* 10 (3) (2008) 287–297. doi:10.1593/neo.07971

307. C.H. Yang, M. Fan, A.T. Slominski, J. Yue, L.M. Pfeffer, The role of constitutively activated STAT3 in B16 melanoma cells, *Int. J. Interferon. Cytokine Mediat. Res.* 2010 (2) (2010) 1. doi:10.2147/IJICMR.S6657

308. D. Gabrilovich, A role for STAT3 in dendritic cell regulation by tumor-derived factors: dendritic cells in cancer. In *Dendritic Cells in Cancer* (eds. R. Salter, M. Shurin) 143–155 (Springer, New York, 2009).

309. Y. Nefedova, M. Huang, S. Kusmartsev, R. Bhattacharya, P. Cheng, R. Salup, et al., Hyperactivation of STAT3 is involved in abnormal differentiation of dendritic cells in cancer, *J. Immunol.* 172 (1) (2004) 464–474. doi:10.4049/jimmunol.172.1.464

310. Z. Luo, C. Wang, H. Yi, P. Li, H. Pan, L. Liu, et al., Nanovaccine loaded with poly I: C and STAT3 siRNA robustly elicits anti-tumor immune responses through modulating tumor-associated dendritic cells in vivo, *Biomaterials* 38 (2015) 50–60. doi:10.1016/j.biomaterials.2014.10.050

311. Z. Luo, P. Li, J. Deng, N. Gao, Y. Zhang, H. Pan, et al., Cationic polypeptide micelle-based antigen delivery system: a simple and robust adjuvant to improve vaccine efficacy, *J. Control. Release* 170 (2) (2013) 259–267. doi:10.1016/j.jconrel.2013.05.027

312. J.R. Cubillos-Ruiz, X. Engle, U.K. Scarlett, D. Martinez, A. Barber, R. Elgueta, et al., Polyethylenimine-based siRNA nanocomplexes reprogram tumor-associated dendritic cells via TLR5 to elicit therapeutic antitumor immunity, *J. Clin. Invest.* 119 (8)(2009) 2231–2244. doi:10.1172/JCI37716

313. M.B. Heo, M.Y. Cho, Y.T. Lim, Polymer nanoparticles for enhanced immune response: combined delivery of tumor antigen and small interference RNA for immunosuppressive gene to dendritic cells, *Acta Biomater.* 10 (5) (2014) 2169–2176. doi:10.1016/j.actbio.2013.12.050

314. S. Liang, J. Hu, Y. Xie, Q. Zhou, Y. Zhu, X. Yang, A polyethylenimine-modified carboxyl-poly (styrene/acrylamide) copolymer nanosphere for co-delivering of CpG and TGF-β receptor I inhibitor with remarkable additive tumor regression effect against liver cancer in mice, *Int. J. Nanomed.* 11 (2016) 6753. doi:10.2147/IJN.S122047

315. M.B. Heo, S.-Y. Kim, W.S. Yun, Y.T. Lim, Sequential delivery of an anticancer drug and combined immunomodulatory nanoparticles for efficient chemoimmunotherapy, *Int. J. Nanomed.* 10 (2015) 5981. doi:10.2147/IJN.S90104

316. J.M. Silva, E. Zupancic, G. Vandermeulen, V.G. Oliveira, A. Salgado, M. Videira, et al., In vivo delivery of peptides and Toll-like receptor ligands by mannosefunctionalized polymeric nanoparticles induces prophylactic and therapeutic antitumor immune responses in a melanoma model, *J. Control. Release* 198 (2015) 91–103. doi:10.1016/j.jconrel.2014.11.033

317. Z. Xu, S. Ramishetti, Y.-C. Tseng, S. Guo, Y. Wang, L. Huang, Multifunctional nanoparticles co-delivering Trp2 peptide and CpG adjuvant induce potent cytotoxic T-lymphocyte response against melanoma and its lung metastasis, *J. Control. Release* 172 (1) (2013) 259–265. doi:10.1016/j.jconrel.2013.08.021

318. L.J. Cruz, P.J. Tacken, R. Fokkink, C.G. Figdor, The influence of PEG chain length and targeting moiety on antibody-mediated delivery of nanoparticle vaccines to human dendritic cells, *Biomaterials* 32 (28) (2011) 6791–6803. doi:10.1016/j.biomaterials.2011.04.082

319. L. Bonifaz, D. Bonnyay, K. Mahnke, M. Rivera, M.C. Nussenzweig, R.M. Steinman, Efficient targeting of protein antigen to the dendritic cell receptor DEC-205 in the steady state leads to antigen presentation on major histocompatibility complex class I products and peripheral CD8+ T cell tolerance, *J. Exp. Med.* 196 (12) (2002) 1627–1638. doi:10.1084/jem.20021598

320. Y. Delneste, G. Magistrelli, J.-F. Gauchat, J.-F. Haeuw, J.-P. Aubry, K. Nakamura, et al., Involvement of LOX-1 in dendritic cell-mediated antigen cross-presentation, *Immunity* 17 (3) (2002) 353–362. doi:10.1016/S1074-7613(02)00388-6

321. R.W. Carter, C. Thompson, D.M. Reid, S.Y. Wong, D.F. Tough, Preferential induction of CD4+ T cell responses through in vivo targeting of antigen to dendritic cell-associated C-type lectin-1, *J. Immunol.* 177 (4) (2006) 2276–2284. doi:10.4049/jimmunol.177.4.2276

322. C. Fayolle, P. Sebo, D. Ladant, A. Ullmann, C. Leclerc, In vivo induction of CTL responses by recombinant adenylate cyclase of Bordetella pertussis carrying viral CD8+ T cell epitopes, *J. Immunol.* 156 (12) (1996) 4697–4706.

323. L. Zhang, Y. Tang, H. Akbulut, D. Zelterman, P.-J. Linton, A.B. Deisseroth, An adenoviral vector cancer vaccine that delivers a tumor-associated antigen/CD40-ligand fusion protein to dendritic cells, *Proc. Natl. Acad. Sci. U. S. A.* 100 (25) (2003) 15101–15106. doi:10.1073/pnas.2135379100

324. C.L. Van Broekhoven, C.R. Parish, C. Demangel, W.J. Britton, J.G. Altin, Targeting dendritic cells with antigen-containing liposomes: a highly effective procedure for induction of antitumor immunity and for tumor immunotherapy, *Cancer Res.* 64(12) (2004) 4357–4365. doi:10.1158/0008-5472.CAN-04-0138

325. T.T. Beaudette, E.M. Bachelder, J.A. Cohen, A.C. Obermeyer, K.E. Broaders, J.M. Frechet, et al., In vivo studies on the effect of co-encapsulation of CpG DNA and antigen in acid-degradable microparticle vaccines, *Mol. Pharm.* 6 (4) (2009) 1160–1169. doi:10.1021/mp900038e

326. C. Bourquin, D. Anz, K. Zwiorek, A.-L. Lanz, S. Fuchs, S. Weigel, et al., Targeting CpG oligonucleotides to the lymph node by nanoparticles elicits efficient antitumoral immunity, *J. Immunol.* 181 (5) (2008) 2990–2998. doi:10.4049/jimmunol.181.5.2990

327. C. Bourquin, C. Wurzenberger, S. Heidegger, S. Fuchs, D. Anz, S. Weigel, et al., Delivery of immunostimulatory RNA oligonucleotides by gelatin nanoparticles triggers an efficient antitumoral response, *J. Immunother.* 33 (9) (2010) 935–944. doi:10.1097/CJI.0b013e3181f5dfa7

328. R.A. Kokate, P. Chaudhary, X. Sun, S.I. Thamake, S. Maji, R. Chib, et al., Rationalizing the use of functionalized poly-lactic-co-glycolic acid nanoparticles for dendritic cell-based targeted anticancer therapy, *Nanomedicine* 11 (5) (2016) 479–494. doi:10.2217/nnm.15.213

329. S.M. Geary, Q. Hu, V.B. Joshi, N.B. Bowden, A.K. Salem, Diaminosulfide based polymer microparticles as cancer vaccine delivery systems, *J. Control. Release* 220 (2015) 682–690. doi:10.1016/j.jconrel.2015.09.002

330. V. Shukla, M. Dalela, M. Vij, R. Weichselbaum, S. Kharbanda, M. Ganguli, et al., Systemic delivery of the tumor necrosis factor gene to tumors by a novel dual DNA-nanocomplex in a nanoparticle system, *Nanomedicine* 13 (5) (2017) 1833–1839. doi:10.1016/j.nano.2017.03.004

331. X. Guan, M. Nishikawa, S. Takemoto, Y. Ohno, T. Yata, Y. Takakura, Injection sitedependent induction of immune response by DNA vaccine: comparison of skin and spleen as a target for vaccination, *J. Gene Med.* 12 (3) (2010) 301–309. doi:10.1002/jgm.1432

332. G. Von Maltzahn, J.-H. Park, A. Agrawal, N.K. Bandaru, S.K. Das, M.J. Sailor, et al., Computationally guided photothermal tumor therapy using long-circulating gold nanorod antennas, *Cancer Res.* 69 (9) (2009) 3892–3900. doi:10.1158/0008-5472.CAN-08-4242

333. H. Kang, H. Liu, X. Zhang, J. Yan, Z. Zhu, L. Peng, et al., Photoresponsive DNA cross-linked hydrogels for controllable release and cancer therapy, *Langmuir* 27(1) (2010) 399–408. doi:10.1021/la1037553.

334. A.A. Ali, C.M. McCrudden, J. McCaffrey, J.W. McBride, G. Cole, N.J. Dunne, et al., DNA vaccination for cervical cancer; a novel technology platform of RALA mediated gene delivery via polymeric microneedles, *Nanomedicine* 13 (3) (2017) 921–932. doi:10.1016/j.nano.2016.11.019

335. W. Yao, Y. Peng, M. Du, J. Luo, L. Zong, Preventative vaccine-loaded mannosylated chitosan nanoparticles intended for nasal mucosal delivery enhance immune responses and potent tumor immunity, *Mol. Pharm.* 10 (8) (2013) 2904–2914. doi:10.1021/mp4000053

336. M. Chieppa, G. Bianchi, A. Doni, A. Del Prete, M. Sironi, G. Laskarin, et al., Crosslinking of the mannose receptor on monocyte-derived dendritic cells activates an anti-inflammatory immunosuppressive program, *J. Immunol.* 171 (9) (2003) 4552–4560. doi:10.4049/jimmunol.171.9.4552

337. M.D. Bhavsar, M.M. Amiji, Polymeric nano-and microparticle technologies for oral gene delivery, *Expert Opin. Drug. Deliv.* 4 (3) (2007) 197–213. doi:10.1517/17425247.4.3.197

338. M. Terme, S. Pernot, E. Marcheteau, F. Sandoval, N. Benhamouda, O. Colussi, et al., VEGFA-VEGFR pathway blockade inhibits tumor-induced regulatory T-cell proliferation in colorectal cancer, *Cancer Res.* 73 (2) (2013) 539–549. doi:10.1158/0008-5472.CAN-12-2325

339. H. Suzuki, H. Onishi, J. Wada, A. Yamasaki, H. Tanaka, K. Nakano, et al., VEGFR2 is selectively expressed by FOXP3high CD4+ Treg, *Eur. J. Immunol.* 40 (1) (2010) 197–203. doi:10.1002/eji.200939887

340. Y. Huang, S. Goel, D.G. Duda, D. Fukumura, R.K. Jain, Vascular normalization as an emerging strategy to enhance cancer immunotherapy, *Cancer Res.* 73 (10) (2013) 2943–2948. doi:10.1158/0008-5472.CAN-12-4354

341. Q. Hu, M. Wu, C. Fang, C. Cheng, M. Zhao, W. Fang, et al., Engineering nanoparticle-coated bacteria as oral DNA vaccines for cancer immunotherapy, *Nano Lett.* 15 (4) (2015) 2732–2739. doi:10.1021/acs.nanolett.5b00570

342. T.H. Kim, J.W. Nah, M.-H. Cho, T.G. Park, C.S. Cho, Receptor-mediated gene delivery into antigen presenting cells using mannosylated chitosan/DNA nanoparticles, *J. Nanosci. Nanotechnol.* 6 (9–10) (2006) 2796–2803. doi:10.1166/jnn.2006.434

343. P. Daftarian, A.E. Kaifer, W. Li, B.B. Blomberg, D. Frasca, F. Roth, et al., Peptideconjugated PAMAM dendrimer as a universal DNA vaccine platform to target antigen-presenting cells, *Cancer Res.* 71 (24) (2011) 7452–7462. doi:10.1158/0008-5472.CAN-11-1766

344. C. Lai, X. Yu, H. Zhuo, N. Zhou, Y. Xie, J. He, et al., Anti-tumor immune response of folate-conjugated chitosan nanoparticles containing the IP-10 gene in mice with hepatocellular carcinoma, *J. Biomed. Nanotechnol.* 10 (12) (2014) 3576–3589. doi:10.1166/jbn.2014.2051

345. T. Yata, Y. Takahashi, M. Tan, H. Nakatsuji, S. Ohtsuki, T. Murakami, et al., DNA nanotechnology-based composite-type gold nanoparticle-immunostimulatory DNA hydrogel for tumor photothermal immunotherapy, *Biomaterials* 146 (2017) 136–145. doi:10.1016/j.biomaterials.2017.09.014

346. G. Zhu, L. Mei, H.D. Vishwasrao, O. Jacobson, Z. Wang, Y. Liu, et al., Intertwining DNA-RNA nanocapsules loaded with tumor neoantigens as synergistic nanovaccines for cancer immunotherapy, *Nat. Commun.* 8 (1) (2017) 1482. doi:10.1038/s41467-017-01386-7

347. R. Juliano, J. Bauman, H. Kang, X. Ming, Biological barriers to therapy with antisense and siRNA oligonucleotide, *Mol. Pharm.* 6 (2009) 686–695. doi:10.1021/mp900093r

348. J.P. Yang, L. Huang, Time-dependent maturation of cationic liposome-DNA complex for serum resistance, *Gene Ther.* 5 (1998) 380–387. doi:10.1038/sj.qt.3300596

349. S.C. Semple, S.K. Klimuk, Harasym TO, M.J. Hope, Lipid-based formulations of antisense oligonucleotides for systemic delivery applications, *Methods Enzymol.* 313 (2000) 322–341. doi:10.1016/S0076-6879(00)13020-4

350. M.B. Bally, P. Harvie, F.M. Wong, S. Kong, E.K. Wasan, D.L. Reimer, Biological barriers to cellular delivery of lipid-based DNA carriers, *Adv. Drug Deliv. Rev.* 38 (3) (1999) 291–315. doi:10.1016/S0169-409X(99)00034-4

351. N. Maurer, K.F. Wong, H. Stark, L. Louie, D. McIntosh, T. Wong, et al., Spontaneous entrapment of polynucleotides upon electrostatic interaction with ethanol-destabilized cationic liposomes, *Biophys. J.* 80 (5) (2001) 2310–2326. doi:10.1016/S0006-3495(01)76202-9.

352. Y. Qian, S. Qiao, Y. Dai, G. Xu, B. Dai, L. Lu, et al., Molecular-targeted immunotherapeutic strategy for melanoma via dual-targeting nanoparticles delivering small interfering rna to tumor-associated macrophages, *ACS Nano* 11 (9) (2017) 9536–9549. doi:10.1021/acsnano.7b05465

353. H.E. Daldrup-Link, D. Golovko, B. Ruffell, D.G. DeNardo, R. Castaneda, C. Ansari, et al., MRI of tumor-associated macrophages with clinically applicable iron oxide nanoparticles, *Clin. Cancer Res.* 17 (17) (2011) 5695–5704. doi:10.1158/1078-0432.CCR-10-3420

354. S. Zhu, M. Niu, H. O'Mary, Z. Cui, Targeting of tumor-associated macrophages made possible by PEG-sheddable, mannose-modified nanoparticles, *Mol. Pharm.* 10 (9) (2013) 3525–3530. doi:10.1021/mp400216r

355. D. Chen, J. Koropatnick, N. Jiang, X. Zheng, X. Zhang, H. Wang, et al., Targeted siRNA silencing of indoleamine 2, 3-dioxygenase in antigen-presenting cells using mannose-conjugated liposomes: a novel strategy for treatment of melanoma, *J. Immunother.* 37 (2) (2014) 123–134. doi:10.1097/CJI.0000000000000022

356. H. Akita, K. Kogure, R. Moriguchi, Y. Nakamura, T. Higashi, T. Nakamura, et al., Nanoparticles for ex vivo siRNA delivery to dendritic cells for cancer vaccines: programmed endosomal escape and dissociation, *J. Control. Release* 149 (1) (2011) 58–64. doi:10.1016/j.jconrel.2010.01.012

357. W. Hobo, T.I. Novobrantseva, H. Fredrix, J. Wong, S. Milstein, H. Epstein-Barash, et al., Improving dendritic cell vaccine immunogenicity by silencing PD-1 ligands using siRNA-lipid nanoparticles combined with antigen mRNA electroporation, *Cancer Immunol. Immunother.* 62 (2) (2013) 285–297. doi:10.1007/s00262-012-1334-1

358. T.O. Kabilova, A.V. Sen'kova, V.P. Nikolin, N.A. Popova, M.A. Zenkova, V.V. Vlassov, et al., Antitumor and antimetastatic effect of small immunostimulatory RNA against B16 melanoma in mice, *PLoS One* 11 (3) (2016) e0150751. doi:10.1371/journal.pone.0150751

359. M. Olejniczak, P. Galka-Marciniak, K. Polak, A. Fligier, W.J. Krzyzosiak, RNAimmuno: a database of the non-specific immunological effects of RNA interference and microRNA reagents, *RNA* 18 (5) (2012) 930–935. doi:10.1261/rna.025627.110

360. C.J. Desmet, K.J. Ishii, Nucleic acid sensing at the interface between innate and adaptive immunity in vaccination, *Nat. Rev. Immunol.* 12 (7) (2012) 479–491. doi:10.1038/nri3247

361. Y.-J. Liu, X.-Q. Dou, F. Wang, J. Zhang, X.-L. Wang, G.-L. Xu, et al., IL-4Rα aptamer-liposome-CpG oligodeoxynucleotides suppress tumour growth by targeting the tumour microenvironment, *J. Drug Target.* 25 (3) (2017) 275–283. doi:10.1080/1061186X.2016.1258569

362. H. Miyabe, M. Hyodo, T. Nakamura, Y. Sato, Y. Hayakawa, H. Harashima, A new adjuvant delivery system 'cyclic di-GMP/YSK05 liposome' for cancer immunotherapy, *J. Control. Release* 184 (2014) 20–27. doi:10.1016/j.jconrel.2014.04.004

363. W. Zhou, Y. Kaneda, S. Huang, R. Morishita, D. Hoon, Protective immunization against melanoma by gp100 DNA–HVJ-liposome vaccine, *Gene Ther.* 6 (10) (1999) 1768. doi:10.1038/sj.gt.3300998

364. G.J. Nabel, D. Gordon, D.K. Bishop, B.J. Nickoloff, Z.-Y. Yang, A. Aruga, et al., Immune response in human melanoma after transfer of an allogeneic class I major histocompatibility complex gene with DNA–liposome complexes, *Proc. Natl. Acad. Sci. U. S. A.* 93 (26) (1996) 15388–15393. doi:10.1073/pnas.93.26.15388

365. E. Yuba, Y. Kanda, Y. Yoshizaki, R. Teranishi, A. Harada, K. Sugiura, et al., pH sensitive polymer-liposome-based antigen delivery systems potentiated with interferon-γ gene lipoplex for efficient cancer immunotherapy, *Biomaterials* 67 (2015) 214–224. doi:10.1016/j.biomaterials.2015.07.031

366. A. Garu, G. Moku, S.K. Gulla, A. Chaudhuri, Genetic immunization with in vivo dendritic cell-targeting liposomal DNA vaccine carrier induces long-lasting antitumor immune response, *Mol. Ther.* 24 (2) (2016) 385–397. doi:10.1038/mt.2015.215

367. T. Yamano, Y. Kaneda, S. Hiramatsu, S. Huang, A. Tran, A. Giuliano, et al., Immunity against breast cancer by TERT DNA vaccine primed with chemokine CCL21, *Cancer Gene Ther.* 14 (5) (2007) 451. doi:10.1038/sj.cgt.7701035

368. S. Persano, M.L. Guevara, Z. Li, J. Mai, M. Ferrari, P.P. Pompa, et al., Lipopolyplex potentiates anti-tumor immunity of mRNA-based vaccination, *Biomaterials* 125 (2017) 81–89. doi:10.1016/j.biomaterials.2017.02.019

369. C. Voshavar, R.C. Meka, S. Samanta, S. Marepally, A. Chaudhuri, Enhanced spacer length between mannose mimicking shikimoyl and quinoyl headgroups and hydrophobic region of cationic amphiphile increases efficiency

370. of dendritic cell based dna vaccination: a structure–activity investigation, *J. Med. Chem.* 60 (4) (2017) 1605–1610. doi:10.1021/acs.jmedchem.6b01556

370. N. Pardi, M.J. Hogan, R.S. Pelc, H. Muramatsu, H. Andersen, C.R. DeMaso, et al., Zika virus protection by a single low-dose nucleoside-modified mRNA vaccination, *Nature* 543 (7644) (2017) 248. doi:10.1038/nature21428

371. M.A. McNamara, S.K. Nair, E.K. Holl, RNA-based vaccines in cancer immunotherapy, *J. Immunol. Res.* 2015 (2015). doi:10.1155/2015/794528

372. K.-J. Kallen, A. Thes, A development that may evolve into a revolution in medicine: mRNA as the basis for novel, nucleotide-based vaccines and drugs, *Ther. Adv. Vaccines* 2 (1) (2014) 10–31. doi:10.1177/2051013613508729

373. E.J. Sayour, G. De Leon, C. Pham, A. Grippin, H. Kemeny, J. Chua, et al., Systemic activation of antigen-presenting cells via RNA-loaded nanoparticles, *Oncoimmunology* 6 (1) (2017) e1256527. doi:10.1080/2162402X.2016.1256527

374. J.M. Richner, S. Himansu, K.A. Dowd, S.L. Butler, V. Salazar, J.M. Fox, et al., Modified mRNA vaccines protect against Zika virus infection, *Cell* 168 (6) (2017) 1114–1125.

375. L.M. Kranz, M. Diken, H. Haas, S. Kreiter, C. Loquai, K.C. Reuter, et al., Systemic RNA delivery to dendritic cells exploits antiviral defence for cancer immunotherapy, *Nature* 534 (7607) (2016) 396. doi:10.1038/nature18300

376. D.E. Speiser, K. Schwarz, P. Baumgaertner, V. Manolova, E. Devevre, W. Sterry, et al., Memory and effector CD8 T-cell responses after nanoparticle vaccination of melanoma patients, *J. Immunother.* 33 (8) (2010) 848–858. doi:10.1097/CJI.0b013e3181f1d614

377. S.M. Goldinger, R. Dummer, P. Baumgartnet, D. Mihic-Probst, K. Schwarz, A. Hammann-Haenni, et al., Nanoparticle vaccination combined with TLR-9 and -9 ligands triggers memory and effector CD8+ T-cell responses in melanoma patients, *Eur. J. Immunol.* 42 (2012) 3049–3061. doi:10.1002/eji.201142361

378. L.M. Weiner, M.V. Dhodapkar, S. Ferrone, Monoclonal antibodies for cancer immunotherapy, *Lancet* 373 (9668) (2009) 1033–1040. doi:10.1016/S0140-6736(09)60251-8

379. C. Kyi, M.A. Postow, Checkpoint blocking antibodies in cancer immunotherapy, *FEBS Lett.* 588 (2) (2014) 368–376. doi:10.1016/j.febslet.2013.10.015

380. A.A. Sarnaik, J.S. Weber, Recent advances using anti-CTLA-4 for the treatment of melanoma, *Cancer J.* 15 (3) (2009) 169–173. doi:10.1097/PPO.0b013e3181a7450f

381. S.L. Topalian, F.S. Hodi, J.R. Brahmer, S.N. Gettinger, D.C. Smith, D.F. McDermott, et al., Safety, activity, and immune correlates of anti-PD-1 antibody in cancer, *N. Engl. J. Med.* 366 (26) (2012) 2443–2454. doi:10.1056/NEJMoa1200690

382. A.J. Rech, R. Mick, S. Martin, A. Recio, N.A. Aqui, D.J. Powell, et al., CD25 blockade depletes and selectively reprograms regulatory T cells in concert with immunotherapy in cancer patients, *Sci. Transl. Med.* 4 (134) (2012) 134ra62.

383. C.S. Lee, M. Cragg, M. Glennie, P. Johnson, Novel antibodies targeting immune regulatory checkpoints for cancer therapy, *Br. J. Clin. Pharmacol.* 76 (2) (2013) 233–247. doi:10.1111/bcp.12164

384. Y.Y. Syed, Durvalumab: first global approval, *Drugs* 77 (12) (2017) 1369–1376. doi:10.1007/s40265-017-0782-5

385. E.S. Kim, Avelumab: first global approval, *Drugs* 77 (8) (2017) 929–937. doi:10.1007/s40265-017-0749-6

386. T. Sirkka, J. Skiba, S. Apell, Wound pH Depends on Actual Wound Size, (2016) arXiv preprint arXiv: 1601.06365.

387. K.S. Paudel, M. Milewski, C.L. Swadley, N.K. Brogden, P. Ghosh, A.L. Stinchcomb, Challenges and opportunities in dermal/transdermal delivery, *Ther. Deliv.* 1 (1) (2010) 109–131. doi:10.4155/tde.10.16

388. A. Gdowski, A. Ranjan, A. Mukerjee, J. Vishwanatha, Development of biodegradable nanocarriers loaded with a monoclonal antibody, *Int. J. Mol. Sci.* 16 (2) (2015) 3990–3995. doi:10.3390/ijms16023990

389. R. Kuai, X. Sun, W. Yuan, Y. Xu, A. Schwendeman, J.J. Moon, Subcutaneous nanodisc vaccination with neoantigens for combination cancer immunotherapy, *Bioconjug. Chem.* 29 (3) (2018) 771–775. doi:10.1021/acs.bioconjchem.7b00761

390. L. Liu, Y. Wang, L. Miao, Q. Liu, S. Musetti, J. Li, et al., Combination immunotherapy of MUC1 mRNA nano-vaccine and CTLA-4 blockade effectively inhibits growth of triple negative breast cancer, *Mol. Ther.* 26 (1) (2018) 45–55. doi:10.1016/j.ymthe.2017.10.020

391. J. Cano-Mejia, R.A. Burga, E.E. Sweeney, J.P. Fisher, C.M. Bollard, A.D. Sandler, et al., Prussian blue nanoparticle-based photothermal therapy combined with checkpoint inhibition for photothermal immunotherapy of neuroblastoma, *Nanomedicine* 13 (2) (2017) 771–781. doi:10.1016/j.nano.2016.10.015

392. Y. Shi, W. Zheng, K.L. Rock, Cell injury releases endogenous adjuvants that stimulate cytotoxic T cell responses, *Proc. Natl. Acad. Sci. U. S. A.* 97 (26) (2000) 14590–14595. doi:10.1073/pnas.260497597

393. B. Sauter, M.L. Albert, L. Francisco, M. Larsson, S. Somersan, N. Bhardwaj, Consequences of cell death: exposure to necrotic tumor cells, but not primary tissue cells or apoptotic cells, induces the maturation of immunostimulatory dendritic cells, *J. Exp. Med.* 191 (3) (2000) 423–434. doi:10.1084/jem.191.3.423

394. D.E. Dolmans, D. Fukumura, R.K. Jain, Photodynamic therapy for cancer, *Nat. Rev. Cancer* 3 (5) (2003) 380. doi:10.1038/nrc1071

395. X.F. Huang, W. Ren, L. Rollins, P. Pittman, M. Shah, L. Shen, et al., A broadly applicable, personalized heat shock protein-mediated oncolytic tumor vaccine, *Cancer Res.* 63 (21) (2003) 7321–7329.

396. R. Rai, C. Richardson, P. Flecknell, H. Robertson, A. Burt, D. Manas, Study of apoptosis and heat shock protein (HSP) expression in hepatocytes following radiofrequency ablation (RFA), *J. Surg. Res.* 129 (1) (2005) 147–151. doi:10.1016/j.jss.2005.03.020

397. W.R. Chen, A.K. Singhal, H. Liu, R.E. Nordquist, Antitumor immunity induced by laser immunotherapy and its adoptive transfer, *Cancer Res.* 61 (2) (2001) 459–461.

398. Q. Chen, L. Xu, C. Liang, C. Wang, R. Peng, Z. Liu, Photothermal therapy with immune-adjuvant nanoparticles together with checkpoint blockade for effective cancer immunotherapy, *Nat. Commun.* 7 (2016) 13193. doi:10.1038/ncomms13193

399. D. Schmid, C.G. Park, C.A. Hartl, N. Subedi, A.N. Cartwright, R.B. Puerto, et al., T cell-targeting nanoparticles focus delivery of immunotherapy to improve antitumor immunity, *Nat. Commun.* 8 (1) (2017) 1747. doi:10.1038/s41467-017-01830-8

400. M.A. Shetab Bousheri, M.M.A. Abel-Mootaaleb, A. Beduneau, Y. Pellequer, A. Lamprecht, A nanoparticle-based approach to improve the outcome of cancer active immunotherapy with lipopolysaccharides, *Drug Deliv.* 25 (1) (2018) 1414–1425. doi:10.1080/10717544.2018.1469684

401. R. Yang, J. Xu, L. Xu, X. Sun, Q. Chen, Y. Zhao, et al., Cancer cell membrane-coated adjuvant nanoparticles with mannose modification for effective anticancer vaccination, *ACS Nano* (2018). doi:10.1021/acsnano.7b09041

402. J. Widmer, C. Thauvin, I. Mottas, V.N. Nguyen, F. Delie, E. Allemann, et al., Polymer-based nanoparticles loaded with a TLR7 ligand to target the lymph node for immunostimulation, *Int. J. Pharm.* 535 (2018) 444–451. doi:10.1016/j.ijpharm.2017.11.031

403. A. Seth, H. Lee, M.Y. Cho, C. Park, S. Korm, J.Y. Lee, et al., Combining vasculture disrupting agent and toll-like receptor 7/8 agonist for cancer therapy, *Oncotarget* 8 (3) (2017) 5371–5381.

404. B. Cheng, W.E. Yuan, J. Su, Y. Liu, J. Chen, Recent advances in small molecule based cancer immunotherapy, *Eur. J. Med. Chem.* 157 (2018) 582–598. doi:10.1016/j.ejmech.2018.08.028

405. J. Ozao-Choy, G. Ma, J. Kao, G.X. Wang, M. Meseck, M. Sung, et al., The novel role of tyrosine kinase inhibitor in the reversal of immune suppression and modulation of tumor microenvironment for immune-based cancer therapies, *Cancer Res.* 69 (2009) 2514–2522. doi:10.1158/0008.5472.CAN-08-4709

406. H. Xin, C. Xhang, A. Herrmann, Y. Du, R. Figlin, H. Yu, Sunitinib inhibition of Stat3 induces renal cell carcinoma tumor cell apoptosis and reduces immunosuppressive cells, *Cancer Res.* 69 (2009) 2506–2513. doi:10.1158/0008.5472.CAN-08-4323

407. J.S. Ko, A.H. Zea, B.I. Rini, J.L. Ireland, P. Elson, P. Cohen, Sunitinib mediates reversal of myeloid-derived suppressor cell accumulation in renal cell carcinoma patients, *Clin. Cancer Res.* 15 (2009) 2148–2157. doi:10.1158/1078-0432.CCR-08-1332

408. M. Huo, Y. Zhao, A.B. Satterlee, Y. Wang, Y. Xu, L. Huang, Tumor-targeted delivery of sunitinib base enhances vaccine therapy for advanced melanoma by remodeling the tumor microenvironment, *J. Control. Release* 245 (2017) 81–94. doi:10.1016/j.jconrel.2016.11.013

409. W. Ou, R.K. Thapa, L. Jiang, Z.C. Soe, M. Gautam, J.H. Chang, et al., Regulatory T cell-targeted hybrid nanoparticles combined with immuno-checkpoint blockage for cancer immunotherapy, *J. Control. Rel.* 281 (2018) 84–96. doi:10.1016/j.jconrel.2018.05.018

410. L. Jeanbart, I.C. Kourtis, A.J. Van Der Vlies, M.A. Swartz, J.A. Hubbell, 6-Thioguanine-loaded polymeric micelles deplete myeloid-derived suppressor cells and enhance the efficacy of T cell immunotherapy in tumor-bearing mice, *Cancer Immunol. Immunother.* 64 (8) (2015) 1033–1046. doi:10.1007/s00262-015-1702-8

411. S.M. Garg, M.R. Vakili, O. Molavi, A. Lavasanifar, Self-associating poly (ethylene oxide)-block-poly (α-carboxyl-ε-caprolactone) drug conjugates for the delivery of STAT3 inhibitor JSI-124: potential application in cancer immunotherapy, *Mol. Pharm.* 14 (8) (2017) 2570–2584. doi:10.1021/acs.molpharmaceut.6b01119

412. A. Nel, T. Xia, L. Madler, N. Li, Toxic potential of materials at the nanolevel, *Science* 311 (5761) (2006) 622–627.

413. C. Medina, M.J. Santos-Martinez, A. Radomski, O.I. Corrigan, M.W. Radomski, Nanoparticles: pharmacological and toxicological significance, *Br. J. Pharmacol.* 150 (5) (2007) 552–558.

414. M.A. Dobrovolskaia, P. Aggarwal, J.B. Hall, S.E. McNeil, Preclinical studies to understand nanoparticle interaction with the immune system and its potential effects on nanoparticle biodistribution, *Mol. Pharm.* 5 (4) (2008) 487–495.

415. K. Greish, G. Thiagarajan, H. Herd, R. Price, H. Bauer, D. Hubbard, A. Burckle, S. Sadekar, T. Yu, A. Anwar, A. Ray, H. Ghandehari, Size and surface charge significantly influence the toxicity of silica and dendritic nanoparticles, *Nanotoxicology* 6 (2012) 713–723.

416. C.L. Slingluff, V.H. Engelhard, S. Ferrone, Peptide and dendritic cell vaccines, *Clin. Cancer Res.* 12 (2006) s2342–s2345. doi:10.1158/1078-0432.CCR-05-2541

417. S. Grabbe, H. Hass, M. Diken, L.M. Kranz, P. Langguth, U. Sahin, Translating nanoparticulate-personalized cancer vaccines into clinical applications: case study with RNA-lipoplex for the treatment of melanoma, *Nanomedicine* 11 (20) (2016) 2723–2734. doi:10.2217/nnm-2016-0275

418. J. Wolfram, M. Zhu, Y. Yang, J. Shen, E. Gentile, D. Paolino, et al., Safety of nanoparticles in medicine, *Curr. Drug. Targets* 16 (14) (2015) 1671–1681.

419. H.S. Sharma, A. Sharma, Nanoparticles aggravate heat stress induced congnitive deficits, blood-brain barrier disruption, edema formation, and brain pathology, *Prog. Brain Res.* 162 (2007) 245–273. doi:10.1016/S0079-6123(06)62013-X

420. J.V. Jokerst, T. Lobovkina, R.N. Zare, S.S. Gambhir, Nanoparticle PEGylation for imaging and therapy, *Nanomedicine* 6 (2011) 715–728. doi:10.2217/nnm.11.19

421. Y. Min, K.C. Roche, S. Tian, M. Eblan, K.P. McKinnon, J.M. Caster, et al., Antigencapturing nanoparticles improve the abscopal effect and cancer immunotherapy, *Nat. Nanotechnol.* 12 (9) (2017) 877–882. doi:10.1038/nnano.2017.113

422. M.J. Ernsting, M. Murakami, A. Roy, S.D. Li, Factors controlling the pharmacokinetics, biodistribution and intratumoral penetration of nanoparticles, *J. Control. Release* 172 (3) (2013) 782–794. doi:10.1016/j.jconrel.2013.09.013

423. W.-L. Tang, W.-H. Tang, A. Szeitz, J. Kulkarni, P. Cullis, S.-D. Li, Systemic study of solvent-assisted active loading of gambogic acid into liposomes and its formulation optimization for improved delivery, *Biomaterials* 166 (2018) 13–26. doi:10.1016/j.biomaterials.2018.03.004.

424. W.-L. Tang, W.C. Chen, A. Roy, E. Undzys, S.-D. Li, A simple and improved active loading method to efficiently encapsulate staurosporine into lipid-based nanoparticles for enhanced therapy of multidrug resistant cancer, *Pharm. Res.* 33 (5) (2016) 1104–1114. doi:10.1007/s11095-015-1854-4

425. W.L. Tang, W.H. Tang, W.C. Chen, C. Diako, C.F. Ross, S.D. Li, Development of a rapidly dissolvable oral pediatric formulation for mefloquine using lipsomes, *Mol. Pharm.* 14 (6) (2017) 1969–1979. doi:10.1021/acs.molpharmaceut.7b00077

426. T.G. Popova, A. Teunis, R. Magni, A. Luchini, V. Espina, L.A. Liotta, et al., Chemokine-releasing nanoparticles for manipulation of the lymph node microenvironment, *Nanomaterials* 5 (1) (2015) 298–320. doi:10.3390/nano5010298

427. S. Wilhelm, A.J. Tavares, Q. Dai, S. Ohta, J. Audet, H.F. Dvorak, W.C.W. Chan, Analysis of nanoparticle delivery to tumours, *Nat. Rev. Mat.* 1 (5) (2016) 16014.

428. S.K. Hobbs, W.L. Monsky, F. Yuan, et al., Regulation of transport pathways in tumor vessels: role of tumor type and microenvironment. *Proc. Natl. Acad. Sci. U. S. A.* 95 (1998) 4607–4612.

429. H.I. Hurwitz, L. Fehrenbacher, J.D. Hainsworth, et al., Bevacizumab in combination with fluorouracil and leucovorin: an active regimen for first-line metastatic colorectal cancer. *J. Clin. Oncol.* 23 (2005) 3502–3508.

430. B. Coiffier, E. Lepage, J. Brière, et al., CHOP chemotherapy plus rituximab compared with CHOP alone in elderly patients with diffuse large-B-cell lymphoma. *N. Engl. J. Med.* 346 (2002) 235–242.

431. V.P. Torchilin, Recent advances with liposomes as pharmaceutical carriers. *Nat. Rev. Drug Discov.* 4 (2005) 145–160.

432. B.J. Druker, M. Talpaz, D.J. Resta, et al., Efficacy and safety of a specific inhibitor of the BCR-ABL tyrosine kinase in chronic myeloid leukemia. *N. Engl. J .Med.* 2001 (2001) 1031–1037.

433. A.Z. Wang, F. Gu, L. Zhang, et al., Biofunctionalized targeted nanoparticles for therapeutic applications. *Expert Opin. Biol. Ther.* 8 (2008) 1063–1070.

434. M. Dehghan-Manshadi, A.R. Nikpoor, H. Hadinedoushan, F. Zare, M. Sankian, F. Fesahat, H. Rafatpanah, Protective immune response against P32 oncogenic peptide-pulsed PBMCs in mouse models of breast cancer. *Int. Immunopharmacol.* 93 (2021) 107414 doi:10.1016/j.intimp.2021.107414

List of Abbreviations

α GC:	Alpha-galactosylceramide
α GC/R8-NP:	αGC-loaded R8-NP
α HSP70p:	α-helix HSP70 functional peptide
α-TOS:	α-tocopheryl succinate
(β+):	beta plus
β-CD:	β-cyclodextrin
β-FeOOH:	akaganeite nanorods
(β-FeOOH):	NPs beta-iron oxyhydroxide nanoparticles
γ-Fe$_2$O$_3$:	maghemite
1D:	one-dimensional
1-MT:	1-methyl-DL-tryptophan
2-APB:	2-aminoethoxydiphenyl borate
2D:	two-dimensional
2IT:	2- iminothiolane
2OME:	2'-O-methyl
3D:	three-dimensional
5-FC:	5-fluorocytosine
5-FU:	5-fluorouracil
2"OCH$_3$:	methyl group
2'-OCH$_2$CH$_3$:	ethyl group
2'-O-Me:	2'-O-methyl-RNA units
3'-UTRs:	3'-untranslated regions
A2AR:	A2A adenosine receptors
A2V:	bispecific antibody
AAM:	acrylamide
AAS:	atomic absorption analysis
AAV:	adeno-associated virus
Ab:	antibody
ABC:	ATP-binding cassette family
(acan):	aggrecan
AC-NP:	antigen capturing nanoparticles
ACT:	Adoptive cell therapy
ADCC:	antigendependent cellular cytotoxicity
AD-PEG:	PEG modified with a terminal adamantane group
AD-PEG-Tf and AD-PEG:	conjugated to human transferrin
AET:	cysteamine
AFM:	Atomic force microscopy
AG:	aminoglycoside drug
Ag:	silver
Ag-NPs:	silver nanoparticles
AGO:	Argonaute
Ago$_2$:	Argonaute 2
Alg:	alginate
ALL:	acute B and T leukemias
ALN-RSV:	Alnylam Pharmaceuticals
ALT:	alanine aminotransferase
AMD:	age-related macular degeneration
AMF:	alternating magnetic field

AML:	acutemyelogenous leukemia
AMOs:	anti-miRNA oligonucleotides
AMPK:	5' adenosine monophosphate-activated protein kinase
AnxA2:	antibody against annexinA2
APC:	adenomatous polyposis coli
APCs:	antigen-presenting cells
aPD1:	anti-PD-1 antibody
ApoA1:	apolipoprotein A1
APOB:	Ap B
ASGPR:	asialoglycoprotein receptor
ASOs:	antisense oligonucleotides
ATA:	American Thyroid Association
ATP:	adenosine triphosphate
ATRA:	all-trans retinoic acid
ATRP:	atom transfer radical polymerization
ATTR:	amyloidosis transthyretin
Au:	gold
AUC:	area under curve
AuNPs:	Gold nanoparticle
Au@SiO$_2$:	mesoporous silica-coated gold nanorods
A2V:	bispecific antibody
BAC:	N, N'-bis(acryloyl) cystamine
Baf:	A1 bafilomycin A1
BBB:	blood–brain barrier
bCD:	bacterial cytosine deaminase
Bcl-2:	B-cell lymphoma 2
Bcl2L12:	Bcl2Like12
Bcl-XL:	B-cell lymphoma-extra large
BCR:	B-cell receptor
BD:	biodistribution
BDNF:	brain-derived neurotrophic factor
BDP-I2:	borondipyrromethene
BEAS-2B cells:	bronchial epithelial cell line
BLI:	bioluminescence imaging
BMDCs:	bone marrow-derived dendritic cells
BM(PEG)$_2$:	1,8-bis(maleimidodiethylene) glycol
bPEI:	Branched PEI
BSA:	bovine serum albumin
BTB:	blood–tumor barrier
BTZ:	Bortezomib
CA:	cis-aconitic anhydride
Ca^{2+}:	calcium ion
CAEC:	cholesteryl-2 aminoethylcarbamate
CAFs:	cancer-associated fibroblasts
Calu:	6 human lung carcinoma
CaP:	Calcium phosphate
CaPh:	calcium phosphate siRNA nanoparticles
CAR T:	cytotoxic T lymphocyte-associated antigen 4

CAs:	contrast agents	**CR:**	complete response
CAT:	catalase	**cRCT:**	complementary rolling circle transcription
CBP:	cysteine bridge peptide		
CC:	Cervical cancer	**cRGD:**	cyclic form of the RGD peptide
cccDNA:	covalently closed circular DNA	**CRGDKGPDC:**	conjugation of PTX with iRGD peptide NPs
CCD:	charge-coupled device		
CD:	Chron's disease	**cRGDyK:**	cyclic Arg- Gly-Asp
CD:	cyclodextrin	**CS:**	chitosan
CDC:	complement-dependent cytotoxicity	**CSCs:**	cancer stem cells
CDC6:	cell division cycle 6	**CSF-1R:**	colony stimulating factor-1 receptor
c-di-GMP:	Cyclic di-GMP	**cSLN:**	cationic solid lipid nanoparticles
C-dots:	Carbon nanodots	**C/S-SiNPs:**	core/shell silica nanoparticle
CDKs:	cyclin-dependent kinases	**CT:**	computed tomography
CDP:	cyclodextrin-based polymer	**CTAC:**	Community Training and Assistance Center
Cds:	cadmium sulfide		
CdS:	NPs cadmium sulphide nanoparticles	**CTL:**	cytotoxic T cell
		CTLA-4:	cytotoxic T lymphocyte antigen-4
Ce6:	Chlorin e6	**CTX:**	Cabazitax / chlorotoxin
CEA:	carcinoembryonic antigen	**CuO:**	copper oxide
CFA:	complete Freund's adjuvant	**CuO:**	NPs copper oxide nanoparticles
−(CH₂CH₂NH)ₙ:	aminoethylene unit	**CUR:**	curcumin
Chk-α:	choline kinase-α	**Cy5:**	5 cyanines dye
Chol-PVA-PEG:	PEGpoly(vinyl alcohol)	**CyA:**	cyclosporin A
Chol-siRNA:	cholesterol-modified siRNA	**Cys:**	cysteine
CHP:	cholesterol-bearing pullulan	**DAG:**	diacylglycerol
CHS:	chalcone synthase	**DAMPs:**	damage-associated molecular patterns
CI:	confidence interval		
CIN:	cervical intraepithelial neoplasia	**DAN:**	dopaminergic neuronal
CL:	cardiolipin	**DAPI:**	4′, 6-diamidino-2-phenylindole
Cl:	lower plasma clearance	**DAVID:**	Database for Annotation, Visualization, and Integration Discovery
CLIO:	crosslinked iron oxide nanoparticles		
CLL:	chronic lymphocytic leukemia		
CLRs:	C−type lectin receptors	**DCE-MRI:**	Dynamic contrast-enhanced MRI images
CLSM:	confocal laser scanning microscopy		
CMC:	critical micelle concentration	**DCF:**	dichlorofluorescein
CMC/GO:	carboxymethyl cellulose/ graphene oxide	**DCFH-DA:**	2′, 7-dichlorofluoresceindiacetate
		DCs:	Dendritic cells
CML:	chronic myelogenous leukemia	**DCF:**	dichlorofluorescein
CNL:	chronic neutrophilic leukemia	**DDSs:**	drug delivery systems
CNS:	central nervous system	**DEX:**	dextran
CNTs:	carbon nanotubes	**DEX-DOCA:**	dextran-deoxycholic acid
col2a1:	type II collagen	**DG:**	N′, N″-dioleylglutamide
Comb-Apt–siR:	comb-type aptamer–siRNA conjugates	**DGTmulti-siRNA:**	Dual gene targeted multimeric siRNA
COPA:	Cholesteryloxypropan-1-amine	**DIC:**	disseminated intravascular coagulation
COX-2:	cyclooxygenase		
CP:	cisplatin	**di-Pal-MTO:**	dipalmitoleys-MTO
CPE:	C-phycoerythrin	**DLinDMA:**	1,2- dilinoleyloxy-3-dimethylaminopropane
CpG:	deoxycytidine−deoxyguanosine dinucleotide		
		DLin-MC3-DMA:	dilinol eylmethyl-4-dimethylaminobutyrate
CPM:	crosslinked polymeric micelles		
CPN:	Calcium phosphate nanocrystals	**DLS:**	Dynamic light scattering
CPPs:	Cell-penetration peptides	**DMSO:**	dimethylsulfoxide
CPT:	Camptothecin	**DNA:**	deoxyribonucleic acid
CPT-FUDR:	camptothecin-fluorouridine	**DNA:**	NFs DNA nanoflowers
CPX-351:	cytarabine and daunorubicin approved for the treatment of adults with newly diagnosed	**DNAPAMAM:**	DNA-polyamides clustering DNA-poly (amidoamine)
		DNR:	DNA nanoribbon

DNR-T:	three DNA nanoribbons
DODAG:	N', N'-dioctadecyl-N-4,8-diaza-10-aminodecanoyl-glycylamide
DODAP:	1,2-dioleoyl-3- dimethylammonium propane
DODAP-MEND:	1,2-dioleoyl-3- dimethylammonium propane- multifunctional envelope-type nano device
DOPC:	1,2-dioleoyl-sn-glycero-3-phosphatidyl-choline
DOPE:	1,2-dioleoyl-sn-glycero-3-phosphoethanolamine
DOTA:	1,4,7,10-tetraazacyclododecane-1,4,7,10- tetraacetic acid
DOTAP:	1,2-dioleyloxy-3-trimethylammonium propane
DOX:	Doxorubicin
DOX:	HCl doxorubicin hydrochloride
DPA/Zn:	phosphate receptor Zn (II)-dipicolylamine
DPP:	1, 2-dioleoyl-3-trimethylammonium propane/methoxy poly(ethyleneglycol)
DSAA:	N, N-distearyl-N-methyl-N-2-(N-arginyl) aminoethyl ammonium chloride
DSC:	Differential Scanning Calorimetry
DSPC:	1,2-distearoyl-sn-glycero-3-phosphocholine
dsRNA:	double-stranded RNA
DTNB:	5,5'-dithio-bis(2-nitrobenzoic acid)
DTT:	dithiothreitol
DTX:	Docetaxel
EBOV:	Ebola virus
EC:	endometrial cancer
ECM:	extracellular matrix
ECs:	endothelial cells
ED50:	50% effective dose
EDAX:	energy dispersive spectroscopy
EDC:	1-ethyl-3-(3-dimethylaminopropyl) carbodiimide hydrochloride
EDOPC:	1,2-dioleoyl-snglycero-3-ethylphosphocholine
EDS:	energy dispersive spectroscopy
EGF:	epidermal growth factor
EGFP:	enhanced green fluorescent protein
EGFR:	Epidermal Growth Factor Receptor
EGFR-siRNA:	epidermal growth factor receptor (EGFR)-directed siRNA (EGFR-siRNA)
EGTA:	ethylene glycol tetraacetic acid
eIF5A:	eukaryotic translation initiation factor 5A
EMT:	epithelial-mesenchymal transition
ENaC:	Epithelial sodium channel
EPC:	egg phosphatidylcholine
EphA2:	Ephrin type-A receptor2

EEP:	ethyl ethylene phosphate
EPR:	Enhance Permeation and Retention
EPSs:	extracellular polysaccharides
ER:	endoplasmic reticulum
ERK:	extracellular-signal-regulated kinase
ESCs:	embryonic stem cells
ESF:	Expression Systems' F
EUS:	endoscopic ultrasound
EZH2:	Enhancer of Zeste Homolog 2
F7:	factor 7
FA:	folic acid
Fab:	antigen-binding fragment
FACS:	fluorescence-activated cell sorting
FAK:	focal adhesion kinase
Fc:	fragment crystallisable
FDA:	Food and Drug Administration
Fe_3O_4:	magnetite
$Fe_3O_4@mSiO_2$:	magnetic iron oxide nanoparticle in mesoporous silica nanoparticles
F-FMSNs:	folic acid modified fluorescent silica nanoparticles
FGF:	fibroblast growth factor
FIGO:	Federation of Gynecology and Obstetrics
FITC:	fluorescein isothiocyanate
fLuc:	firefly luciferase
(Fmoc)2KH7-TAT:	amphiphilic chimeric peptide
FMR:	ferromagnetic resonance
FMSNs:	fluorescent silica nanoparticle
FPBA:	3-fluoro-4-carboxyphenylboronic acid
FR:	folate receptor
FR-α:	folate receptor isoform α
FRET:	fluorescence resonance energy transfer
FRS2:	fibroblast growth factor substrate 2
(^{18}F-SFB):	^{18}F-fluorobenzoate
FTIR:	Fourier transform infrared spectroscopy
FUDR:	fluorouridine
G12D:	glycine at codon 12 with aspartate
GA:	glutaraldehyde
GalNAc:	N-acetyl-galactosamine
GalNAc:	tri-N-acetylgalactosamine
GBM:	glomerular basement membrane
GBM:	glioblastoma multiforme
GC:	glycol chitosan
GCs:	Gynecological cancers
GD2:	disialoganglioside
GdIO:	gadolinium-embedded iron oxide nanoclusters
GEM:	gemcitabine
GEO:	Gene Expression Omnibus
GFNs:	graphene family of nanomaterials
GFP:	green fluorescent protein
Glu:	thioglucose
Gly:	glycine

GM:	glioblastoma mutiforme/gentamicin	**HSPC:**	hydrogenated soy phosphatidylcholine
GNPs:	gold nanoparticles	**HSV2:**	herpes simplex virus 2
GO:	Graphene oxide	**HU:**	Hounsfield units
GOD:	glucose oxidase	**HUVECs:**	human umbilical vein ECs
GOx:	glucose oxidase	**HVJ:**	hemagglutinating virus of Japan
gp60:	glycoprotein receptor	**HYNIC:**	hydrazinonicotinamide
GPCR:	G protein-coupled receptor	**IC50:**	half maximal (50%) inhibitory concentration
GQDs:	graphene quantum dots		
GR:	glutathione reductase	**ICAM-1:**	Intercellular adhesion molecule-1
GSH:	oxidized form of glutathione	**ICB:**	immune checkpoint blockade
GSSG:	Glutathione disulfide	**ICD:**	immunogenic cell death
H2TPyP:	5, 10, 15, 20-tetro (4-pyridyl) porphyrin and perylene	**ICG:**	Indocyanine green
		ICP:	isocyanatopropyl
HA:	hyaluronic acid	**(ID/g):**	injected dose per gram
HAI-NGs:	hyaluronic acid-iodixanol nanogels	**IDM:**	Indomethacin
HAuCl₄:	auric chloride	**iDR-NC:**	intertwining hybrid DNA-RNA nanocapsule
HAuNS:	hollow gold nanospheres		
Hb:	hemoglobin	**IDO:**	indoleamine 2, 3-dioxygenase
HB:	hypocrellin	**IFA:**	incomplete Freund's adjuvant
HBeAg:	HBV e antigen	**IFN:**	interferon
HBsAg:	HBV surface protein	**IFN-α:**	interferon alpha
HBV:	hepatitis B virus	**IFN-β:**	interferon beta
HCC:	hepatocellular carcinoma	**IFN-γ:**	interferon gama
HCPT:	10-Hydroxycamptothecin	**IFNAR1:**	IFN-α receptor 1
HCR:	histidineand cysteine- modified polyarginine peptide	**IFNs:**	I interferons
		IGF1R:	Insulin like Growth Factor 1 Receptor
HCT116:	human colon cancer		
HCV:	hepatitis C virus	**IHC:**	immunohistochemistry
HDI:	Hexamethylene diisocyanate	**IKKβ:**	IκB kinase beta
HDL:	high density lipoprotein	**IL-10:**	interleukin 10
HE4:	human epididymis protein 4	**INPs:**	inorganic nanoparticles
H&E:	hematoxylin and eosin	**IP3:**	inositol 1,4,5-trisphosphate
HeLa:	cervical cancer cells	**IP3R:**	inositol 1,4,5-trisphosphate receptor
HeLa-Luc:	human cervical cancer cell line	**IRES:**	internal ribosome entering site
HER2:	Human Epidermal Growth Factor Receptor 2	**IRF3:**	interferon regulator factor 3
		IRR:	infusion-related reactions
HgS:	mercury sulfide	**(i.t.):**	intratumoral
HIF-1α:	transcription factor hypoxia-inducible factor-1α	**IVRT-CLSM:**	intravital confocal laser scanning microscopy
HII:	inverted hexagonal		
HIV-1:	human immunodeficiency virus type 1	**JCFC:**	Janus camptothecin-floxuridine conjugates
HMONs:	hollow manganese oxide nanoparticles	**JEV:**	Japanese encephalitis Virus
		JNK:	c-Jun N-terminal kinase
HO-1:	heme oxygenase 1	**KB:**	Cationic liposomes have the highest serum protein binding affinity
homo-FRET:	homo Förster resonance energy transfer		
		KD:	equilibrium dissociation constant
HPLC:	High-Performance Liquid Chromatography	**KDR:**	Kinase insert domain receptor
		KEGG:	Kyoto Encyclopedia of Genes and Genomes
HPMA:	poly (lactic-co-glycolic acid), N-(2 hydroxypropyl)-methacrylamide		
		KIF11:	kinesin family member **11**
HPPH:	hydrophobic photosensitizer, 2-devinyl-2-(1-hexyloxyethyl) pyropheophorbide	**KSP:**	kinesin spindle protein
		Kyn:	kynurenine
		LA:	lipoic acid
HPV:	human papilloma virus	**LAG3:**	Lymphocyte activation gene 3
HSA:	human serum albumin	**LAIR-1:**	Leukocyte-associated immunoglobulin-like receptor-1

LaP:	laponite silicate clay		**MGO:**	micrometer-sized GO
LbL:	layer-by-layer		**MHC:**	major histocompatibility complex
LC3:	protein 1A/1B-light chain 3		**MHC-I:**	major histocompatibility complex class I
LCP:	Lipid calcium phosphate			
LCST:	lower critical solution temperature		**MIAME:**	minimal information about a microarray experiment
LDHs:	layered double hydroxides			
LDL:	low-density lipoprotein		**MION:**	Monocrystalline iron oxide nanoparticles
LE:	loading efficiency			
LET:	linear energy transfer		**miRNAs:**	microRNAs
LF:	lipofectamine 2000		**MLP:**	melittin-like peptide
LF2000:	Lipofectamine 2000		**MLV:**	multilamellar vesicles
LMW-PEI:	low molecular weight polyethylenimine		**MM:**	multiple myeloma
			MMP:	matrix metalloproteinase
LNA:	Locked Nucleic Acid		**MMP2:**	matrix metalloproteinase 2
LNP:	lipid nanoparticles		**MMP3:**	matrix metalloproteinase 3
LNPs:	lipidoid nanoparticles		**M-MSN:**	magnetic mesoporous silicaNPs
LN-R:	nitrate based LDH		**MN:**	microneedles
LODER:	LOcal Drug EluteR		**MnMEIO:**	magnetismengineered iron oxide
LPA:	LPA		**MNPs:**	metal nanoparticles
LPD:	liposome–polycation–DNA		**MNPs:**	Magnetic nanoparticles
LPEI:	linear PEI		**mono-Pal-MTO:**	monopalmitoleys-MTO
lPEI-NH2:	linear PEI with primary amino terminals		**mPEG:**	methoxy-PEG
			mPEG-PCL:	methoxy PEG-PCL
LPH:	liposome–polycation–hyaluronic acid		**mPEG-PLA-Ch:**	Cholesterol-modified mPEG–PLA micelles
LP-R:	phosphate bound LDH-drug		**MPLA:**	monophosphoryl lipid A
LPS:	lipopolysacharide		**MPP:**	mitochondrial–penetrating peptides
LSECs:	liver sinusoidal endothelial cells		**MPPs:**	membrane permanent peptides
LTI:	lysine triisocyanate		**MPS:**	mononuclear phagocyte system
LUC:	luciferase reporter genes		**MPTS:**	3-mercaptopropyltrimethoxysilane
mAb:	monoclonal antibodies		**MR:**	magnetic resonance imaging
MALDI-MSI:	matrix-assisted laser desorption ionization mass spectrometry imaging		**MRI:**	magnetic resonance imaging
			mRNAs:	messenger RNAs
			MRP1:	multidrug resistance protein 1
MAN:	mannose		**MRP2:**	multidrug resistance protein 2
MAPK:	mitogen-activated protein kinase		**MRT:**	mean retention time
MB:	Methylene blue		**MRX34:**	cancer-targeting miRNA mimic of miR-34
MB-encapsulated PSiNPs:	methylene blue-encapsulated phosphonate-terminated silica nanoparticles			
			MSCs:	mesenchymal stem cells
			M-siRNA:	multimerized siRNA
MCF-7:	Michigan Cancer Foundation		**MSNPs:**	mesoporous mechanized silica nanoparticles
MCL:	mantle cell lymphoma cells			
Mcl-1:	myeloid cell leukemia sequence 1		**MSNs:**	Mesoporous silica nanoparticles
MCMC:	mannosylated carboxymethyl chitosan		**Mt:**	montmorillonite
			mtDOX:	amitochondrial targeted version of DOX
MDEF:	macroscopic dose enhancement factors			
			MTO:	mitoxantrone
MDNCs:	multidrug nanocrystals		**mTOR:**	mammalian target of rapamycin
MDR:	multiple-drug resistance		**MTX:**	methotrexate
MDR1:	multidrug resistance protein 1		**MTX-GEM:**	MTX and GEM conjugate
MDSCs:	myeloidderived suppressor cells		**MTX-CPT NPs:**	MTX-CPT conjugates nanoparticles
MEK:	mitogen-activated protein kinase		**MUC1:**	Amucin 1
MEND:	multifunctional envelope-type nano device		**multi-siRNA:**	Multimerized siRNA
			MWCNT:	multiwalled CNTs
MFI:	mean fluorescence intensity		**MWNTs:**	multi-walled nanotubes
MFs:	microflowers		**N2:**	atmospheric nitrogen
MGED:	Microarray Gene Expression Data		**NAG:**	N-acetylgalactosamine

NBD:	7-nitrobenz-2-oxa-1, 3-diazole	**PBAVE:**	polymer backbone, poly(vinyl ether)
NBSCs:	Nickel-Based Single Crystal Superalloy	**PBNP:**	Prussian blue nanoparticles
NCs:	Nanocarriers	**PBS:**	phosphate buffered saline
NFκB:	nuclear factor kappa B	**PC:**	phosphatidylcholine
NFs:	nanoflowers	**PC3:**	prostate cancer cell line
NGO:	nanometer-sized GO	**PC-3:**	human prostatic carcinoma
(−NH₂):	primary amines	**PCA:**	poly citric acid
NIPAM:	N-isopropylacrylamide	**PCL:**	poly(ε-caprolactone)
NIR:	near-infrared	**PCR:**	polymerase chain reaction
NIRF	near-infrared fluorescence	**PCSK9:**	proprotein convertase subtilisin/ kexin type 9
NIS:	National Institute Of Standards	**PD:**	progressive disease
NIST:	National Institute of Standards and Technology	**PD-1:**	programmed cell death protein 1 (programmed death signal-1)
NK:	Natural Killer	**PD-1/L1:**	programmed death/ligand 1
nLGs:	nano-lipogels	**PDA:**	pancreatic ductal adenocarcinoma
NLRs:	nucleotide-binding and oligomerization domain NOD-like receptors	**PDCD4:**	downstream target, programmed cell death 4
NLS:	nuclear localization signal-	**PDEAAm:**	poly(N, N-diethylacrylamide)
nMOF:	nanoscale metal-organic framework	**PDI:**	polydispersity
NMR:	nuclear magnetic resonance spectroscopy	**PD-L1:**	programmed cell death-ligand 1
N/P:	nitrogen/phosphate ratio	**PDMAAm:**	poly(N, N-dimethylacrylamide)
NP:	Nucleocapsid protein gene	**P(DMAEMA):**	poly (2-(N, N-dimethyl aminoethyl) methacrylate)
NPs:	Nanoparticles	**pDNA:**	plasmid DNA
NPV:	negative predictive value	**PDMAEMA:**	poly 2-dimethylamino ethyl methacrylate
Nrp1:	neurophilin-1		
NSCLC:	non-small-cell lung cancer	**Pd:**	NPs palladium nanoparticles
OC:	ovarian cancer	**PDPA:**	PEG-b-P(DPA-co-HEA)
ODN:	oligodeoxynucleotides	**PDT:**	photodynamic therapy
ODN-MS:	Oligonucleotide antisense microsponge particles	**PDTC:**	pyrrolidine dithiocarbamate
		PEG:	poly(ethylene glycol)
ODNs:	oligodeoxynucleotides	**PEGPAsp(DET):**	diethylenetriamine [−(CH₂CH₂NH)₂−, DET]
OEIeC14:	1,2-epoxytetradecane alkylated oligoethylenimine	**PEG-g-PEI:**	polyethylene glycol-graft-polyethylenimine
ONB:	o-nitrobenzyl		
ONPs:	oligonucleotide nanoparticles	**PEG-PAsp(TEP):**	tetraethylenepentamine [−(CH₂CH₂NH)₄−, TEP]
ORFs:	open reading frames		
OVA:	ovalbumin	**PEG-PLL:**	PEG-poly(L-lysine) block-co-polymer
(o/w):	oil in water ratio	**PEGylated:**	polyethylene glycol-conjugated
PA:	phosphatidic acid	**PEI:**	polyethyleneimine
Pa:	pheophorbide a	**PEM:**	pemetrexed
PAAc:	poly acrylic acid	**PET:**	positron emission tomography
PAC:	Paclitaxel	**PEO-PCL:**	poly(ethylene oxide)-poly(epsilon caprolactone)
PAMA:	poly(amidoamine)		
PAMAM:	poly-(amidoamine)	**PEOb-PCCL:**	poly (ethylene oxide)-*block*-poly (α-carboxylate-ε-caprolactone)
PAMAM-PEG-PAMAM:			
	polyamidoamine–polyethylene glycol–polyamidoamine	**PEOb-PCL:**	Poly(ethylene oxide)-block-poly(ε-caprolactone)
PAMP:	pathogen−associated molecular patterns	**PEO-PbAE:**	poly(ethylene oxide)-modified poly(beta aminoester)
PAR-1:	protease-activated receptor-1	**PET:**	Positron emission tomography
PAsp(DET):	(−CH₂CH₂NH−CH₂CH₂NH₃⁺)	**PEUR:**	Poly(ester urethane)
PATK	performance analysis tool kit	**PFBT:**	3-pseudotropyl-4-fluorobenzoate
PBA:	Phenylboronic acid	**PFS:**	progression-free survival
PBAEs:	poly(β-amino esters)	**PG:**	phosphatidylglycerol

PGA:	3-Phosphoglyceric acid
PGE2:	prostaglandin E2
P-gp:	P-glycoprotein
pGRP:	pDNA encoding gastrin releasing peptide
PhD:	hydrazone bond to form Pa-h- DOX conjugates
PHD2:	prolyl hydroxlase domain 2
PHPMA:	poly(N-(2-hydroxypropyl) methacrylamide)
PI:	phosphatidylinositol
(PI):	propidium iodide
PICs:	polyion complexes
PIK3:	phosphoinositide 3-kinase
PIP2:	phosphatidylinositol-4,5-bisphosphate
PIV:	parainfluenza virus
PK:	pharmacokinetics
PKN3:	protein kinase N3
PKR:	RNA activated protein kinase
PL:	phospholipid
PLA:	poly (lactic acid)
PLA2:	phosphatidylcholine 2-acetylhydrolase
PLD:	pegylated liposomal doxorubicin
PLGA:	poly (lactic-co-glycolic acid)
pLHMGA:	Poly(lactic-co-hydroxymethyl-glycolic acid)
PLK1:	polo-like kinase 1
PLL:	poly-L-lysine
PLLA:	poly(L-lactide)
PLLA-PEG-PLLA:	poly (L-lactide)-poly(ethyleneglycol)-poly(L-lactide)
PMAA:	poly (methacrylic acid)
P(MDS-co-CES):	Poly[(N-methyldietheneamine sebacate)-co-[(cholesteryl oxocarbonylamido ethyl) methyl bis(ethylene) ammonium bromide] sebacate]
PMNT:	poly[4-(2,2,6,6-tetramethylpiperidine-N-oxyl) aminomethylstyrene])
PMPs:	platelet microparticles
pNIPAAM:	poly(N-isopropylacrylamide)
P(NIPAM-ss-AA):	poly(N-isopropylacrylamide)-ss-acrylic acid
PNPs:	Polymeric nanoparticles
poly-siRNA:	polymerized siRNA
POPE:	phosphoethanolamine
PPa:	pyropheophorbide-a/pheophorbide A
PP2A:	protein phosphatase 2A
PPI:	poly(propylenimine)
PPT-g-PEG:	PEG-grafted polypeptide
PPV:	positive predictive value
PR:	partial response
prM-E:	pre-membrane and enveloped
pre-RISC:	precursor RNAi-induced silencing complex
pRNA:	packaging RNAs
PrS:	protamine sulfate
PRRs:	pattern recognition receptors
PS:	photosensitizer
PS:	phosphatidylserine
PS2	phosphorodithioate
PSMA:	prostate-specific membrane antigen
Pt:	platinum
PTEN:	phosphatase and tensin homolog
Pt:	NPs platinum nanoparticles
p-Trp2:	phosphorylated Trp2 peptide
PTT:	photothermal therapy
PTX:	paclitaxel
PV:	polycythemia Vera
PVAX:	personalized cancer vaccine
PVCL:	poly(vinylcaprolactam)
PVP:	poly (Nvinyl pyrrolidone)
QDs:	Quantum dots
qRT-PCR:	quantitative reverse transcription-polymerase chain reaction
QWBA:	quantitative whole-body autoradiography
R2:	ribonucleotide reductase
R8:	octaarginine
RA:	LC-MS-radioactivity
RAFT:	reversible addition-fragmentation chain transfer
RAI:	radioactive iodine
RARB:	retinoic acid receptor beta
RBC:	red blood cell
RCA:	rolling circle amplification
RCC:	renal cell carcinoma
RCR:	rolling circle replication
RCT:	rolling circle transcription
RES:	reticular endothelial system
RF:	radiofrequency
RFP:	red fluorescent protein
RGD:	arginine-glycine-aspartic acid
RGDS:	Arg-Gly-Asp-Ser
RH:	raloxifene hydrochloride
RHAMM:	Receptor for Hyaluronan Mediated Motility
rhApo:	apolipoprotein
R1G1:	retinoic acid inducible gene-1 like helicase
RISC:	RNA-induced silencing complex
rLuc:	Renilla luciferase
RNA:	ribonucleic acid
RNAi:	RNA interference
RNAiMAX:	maximum gene silencing efficiency of Lipofectamine RNAiMAX
RNase:	Ribonuclease
ROC:	receiver operating characteristic
ROI:	regions of interest
ROS:	reactive oxygen species

RRM2:	ribonucleotide reductase subunit M2
RSEM:	remote scanning electron microscopy
RSV:	respiratory syncytial virus
RT:	reverse transcriptase
(-S-):	thioether
(-2S-):	dithioether
SA:	sialic acid
SA:	stearic acid
SAHA:	suberoylanilide hydroxamic acid
SB:	silybin
SCC7:	squamous cell carcinoma
scFv:	single chain variable fragment
SCLC:	small cell lung carcinoma
SD:	standard deviations
SEM:	Scanning electron microscopy
semi-IPN:	semi-interpenetrating polymer network
SGO:	submicrometer-sized GO
sHDL:	synthetic high-density lipoprotein
SHP2 Src:	homology phosphotyrosyl phosphatase 2
shRNA:	short hairpin RNA
shRNAi:	short hairpin RNA interference
siBcl-2:	silence Bcl-2 genes
siIDO:	indoleamine 2,3-dioxygenase siRNA
siLuc:	silencing the luciferase-expressing gene
SiNPs:	silica based nanoparticles
siRNA:	small interfering RNA
SIRPα:	signal regulatory protein alpha
siTOX:	cytotoxic siRNA sequence
SKOV3:	ovarian cancer cells
SKOV-3TR:	paclitaxelresistant ovarian cancer cell line
SLNs:	solid lipid nanoparticles
SM:	sphingomyelin
SMCC:	succinimidyl-4-(N-maleimido methyl)cyclohexane-1-carboxylate
SNA:	spherical nucleic acid
SNALPs:	stabilized nucleic acid lipid particles
SncRNAs:	Small non-coding RNAs
snRNA:	small nuclear RNA
SOG:	singlet oxygen generation
SOCS1:	suppressor of cytokine signaling 1
SOX4:	SRY-related high mobility group box 4
SPECT:	single-photon emission computed tomography
(Sph):	succinoyl-pentaethylene hexamine
SPIO:	super paramagnetic iron oxide
SPIONs:	superparamagnetic iron oxide nanoparticles
SPIOs:	superparamagnetic iron oxide nanoparticles

SQUID:	superconducting quantum interference device
SR-B1:	scavenger receptor B type 1
SRF:	Sorafenib
SRY:	sex-determining region Y protein
(-S-S-):	disulfide
(ss):	single-stranded
ssiRNA:	carrier of siRNA with sticky overhangs
STAT3:	signal transducer and activator of transcription 3
STING:	stimulate an interferon gene protein
STIs:	sexually transmitted infections
STMN1:	stathmin 1
(Stp):	succinoyl-tetraethylene pentamine
stPEI:	polyethylenimine
STR-R8:	DOPE/sphingomyelin (SM)/ stearylated R8
sulfo-SMCC:	sulfosuccinimidyl-4-(N-maleimido methyl)cyclohexane-1-carboxylate
SWCNTs:	single-walled CNTs
SWNTs:	single-walled CNTs
$(t_{1/2})$:	half-life
TAAs:	tumor-associated antigens
TBA:	thrombin binding aptamer
TBK1:	tank binding kinase 1
TCGA:	The Cancer Genome Atlas
TCL-SPIONs:	thermally crosslinked superparamagnetic iron oxide nanoparticles
TCPP:	4-tetracarboxyphenyl porphyrin
TCR:	T-cell receptor
TCPs:	targeted combinatorial polyplexes
TCV:	tumour cell vaccines
TDLNs:	tumor-draining lymph nodes
TDPA:	tumor-derived protein antigens
TDS:	thyroid differentiation score
TEM:	transmission electron microscopy
TEOS:	tetraethyl orthosilicate
TERT:	telomerase reverse transcriptase
TF:	Transferrin
TFR:	transferrin receptors
TGA:	thermogravimetric analysis
TGC:	thiolated glycol chitosan
TGF-β:	transforming growth factor beta
tHSA:	thiolated human serum albumin
TIGIT:	T cell Ig and ITIM domain
TILs:	tumor infiltrating lymphocytes
TIM-3:	T cell immunoglobulin and mucin-domain containing-3
TK:	thioketal linker
TKIs:	tyrosine kinase inhibitors
tLNPs:	targeted lipid nanoparticles
TLRs:	Toll-like receptors
TME:	Total mesorectal excision
TMEA:	tri-[2-maleimidoethyl]-amine
TNBC:	triple negative breast cancer

(TNF)-α:	tumor necrosis factor alpha	**USPIO:**	Ultra-small superparamagnetic iron oxide nanoparticles
TNFR:	tumor necrosis factor receptor	**UTP:**	uridine triphosphate
TPGS:	tocopheryl polyethylene glycol 1000 succinate mono-ester	**UV:**	ultraviolet
TPP:	triphenylphosphine	**VEGF:**	Vascular endothelial growth factors
TPP-LP:	TPP-modified liposome	**VEGFA:**	vascular endothelial growth factor A
Tregs:	regulatory T cells	**VLP:**	virus-like nanoparticle
Trk:	NGF tyrosine kinase nerve growth factor	**VSM:**	vibrating sample magnetometer
Trp:	tryptophan	**WebGestalt:**	Web-based Gene Set Analysis Toolkit
Trp2:	tyrosine-related protein 2	**WHO:**	World Health Organization
tTF:	thiolated TF	**(W/O):**	water-in-oil
TTR:	transthyretin	**(WT):**	wild-type
T-UCRs:	UCRs are transcribed	**WT1:**	Wilms' tumour protein
TumourP:	tumour lysate protein	**Xgene:**	X-treme GENE
TUNEL:	transferase-mediated deoxy uridine triphosphate (UTP) nick end labeling	**XPA3:**	Audiophile Home Theater Power Amplifier
U87:	human primary glioblastoma cell line that is commonly used in brain cancer research	**XPS:**	X-ray photo-electron spectroscopy
		X-ray:	CT X-ray computed tomography
		XRD:	X-ray diffraction
		(Z):	atomic number
UCNPs:	upconversion nanoparticles	**ZEB1:**	Zinc finger E-box-binding homeobox 1
UNA:	Unlocked Nucleic Acid	**ZEB2:**	Zinc finger E-box-binding homeobox 2
uPA:	urokinase-type plasminogen activator	**ZEBOV:**	Zaire Ebola virus
uPIC:	unimer polyion complex	**ZnO:**	zinc oxide
uPIC-AuNP:	unimer polyion complex-assembled gold nanoparticle	**ZnO:**	NPs zinc oxide nanoparticle
		ZnP:	Zn-pyrophosphate
US:	United States	**ZnPc:**	zinc phthalocyanine

Index

Note: **Bold** page numbers refer to tables and *italic* page numbers refer to figures.

For Product Safety Concerns and Information please contact our EU
representative GPSR@taylorandfrancis.com
Taylor & Francis Verlag GmbH, Kaufingerstraße 24, 80331 München, Germany

www.ingramcontent.com/pod-product-compliance
Lightning Source LLC
Chambersburg PA
CBHW060949210326
41598CB00031B/4768